CLINICAL PEDIATRIC NEPHROLOGY

NOTICE

CLINICAL PEDIATRIC NEPHROLOGY

EDITORS

Kanwal K. Kher, M.D.

Assistant Professor of Pediatrics
George Washington University School of Medicine
Director of Dialysis and Attending Nephrologist
Children's National Medical Center
Washington, D.C.

Sudesh P. Makker, M.D.

Professor of Pediatrics
Director of Pediatric Nephrology
University of California Davis School of Medicine
Davis, California

McGRAW-HILL, INC.
HEALTH PROFESSIONS DIVISION

New York St. Louis San Francisco Auckland Bogotá
Caracas Lisbon London Madrid Mexico Milan Montreal
New Delhi Paris San Juan Singapore Sydney Tokyo Toronto

CLINICAL PEDIATRIC NEPHROLOGY
International Editions 1992

1 2 3 4 5 6 7 8 9 0 KKP UPE 9 6 5 4 3 2

ISBN 0-07-034543-0

This book was set in Meridien by University Graphics, Inc.
The editors were Edward M. Bolger and Muza Navrozov;
the production supervisor was Richard Ruzycka;
the cover was designed by N.S.G. Design;
the index was prepared by Alexandra Nickerson.

Library of Congress Cataloging-in-Publication Data

Clinical pediatric nephrology / editors, Kanwal K. Kher, Sudesh P.
Makker.
p. cm.
Includes index.
ISBN 0-07-034543-0
1. Pediatric nephrology. I. Kher, Kanwal K. II. Makker, Sudesh
P.
[DNLM: 1. Kidney Diseases-diagnosis. 2. Kidney Diseases-in infancy & childhood. 3. Kidney Diseases-therapy. WS 320 C641]
RJ476.K5C56 199
618.92'61-dc20
DNLM/DLC
for Library of Congress 91-37495
CIP

When ordering this title, use ISBN 0-07-112678-3

Printed in Singapore

Dedicated to my parents and my teachers.

Kanwal K. Kher

Dedicated to my parents and my mentors,
the late Walter Heymann, M.D., Warren
Grupe, M.D., and Malcolm Holliday, M.D.

Sudesh P. Makker

CONTENTS

PART V NEONATAL NEPHROLOGY

CONTRIBUTORS*

Lamya Alarif, M.D. [19]
Director
Medlantic Immunogenetic Laboratory
Washington Hospital Center
Washington, D.C.

Mary P. Andrich, M.D. [3]
Senior Staff Physician
Nuclear Medicine Department
Clinical Center
National Institutes of Health
Bethesda, Maryland

Billy S. Arant, Jr., M.D. [*9*]
Professor and Director
Pediatric Nephrology
The University of Texas Southwestern Medical Center at Dallas
Dallas, Texas

A. Barry Belman, M.D. [*9*]
Professor and Chairman
Department of Pediatric Urology
George Washington University School of Medicine
Children's National Medical Center
Washington, D.C.

Glen H. Bock, M.D. [15]
Associate Professor of Pediatrics
George Washington University School of Medicine
Vice Chairman, Nephrology
Children's National Medical Center
Washington, D.C.

James C. M. Chan, M.D. [21]
Professor of Pediatrics
Chairman, Division of Pediatric Nephrology
Medical College of Virginia
Virginia Commonwealth University
Richmond, Virginia

Russell W. Chesney, M.D. [*16, 17*]
LeBonheur Professor and Chairman
Department of Pediatrics
The University of Tennessee
LeBonheur Children's Medical Center
Memphis, Tennessee

Richard N. Fine, M.D. [*18*]
Professor and Chairman
Department of Pediatrics
State University of New York at Stony Brook
Stony Brook, New York

Philip G. Guzzetta, M.D. [19]
Associate Professor of Surgery
George Washington University School of Medicine
Attending Renal Transplant Surgeon
Children's National Medical Center
Washington, D.C.

James D. Hanna, M.D. [21]
Fellow, Pediatric Nephrology
Children's Medical Center
Division of Pediatric Nephrology
Medical College of Virginia
Virginia Commonwealth University
Richmond, Virginia

*The numbers in brackets following the contributor name refer to chapter(s) authored or coauthored by the contributor. Italic numbers in brackets refer to commentaries contributed to the chapter.

Gary L. Hedlund, D.O. [3]
Clinical Assistant Professor of Radiology
University of Alabama at Birmingham
Attending Radiologist
The Children's Hospital of Alabama
Birmingham, Alabama

Julie R. Ingelfinger, M.D. [*10*]
Co-Director, Pediatric Nephrology Unit
The Children's Service
Massachusetts General Hospital
Harvard Medical School
Boston, Massachusetts

Kanwal K. Kher, M.D. [1, 2, 4, 7, 9, 10, 11, 13, 14, 16, 17, 18, 19, 22, 23, 24]
Assistant Professor of Pediatrics
George Washington University School of Medicine
Director of Dialysis and Attending Nephrologist
Children's National Medical Center
Washington, D.C.

Heinz E. Leichter, M.D. [9, 18]
Assistant Professor of Pediatrics
Medical College of Wisconsin
Medical Director, ESRD Program
Children's Hospital of Wisconsin
Milwaukee, Wisconsin

Massoud Majd, M.D. [3]
Professor of Radiology and Pediatrics
George Washington University School of Medicine
Director, Section of Nuclear Medicine
Children's National Medical Center
Washington, D.C.

Sudesh P. Makker, M.D. [5, 6, 8]
Professor of Pediatrics
Director of Pediatric Nephrology
University of California Davis School of Medicine
Davis, California

Cynthia G. Pan, M.D. [20]
Assistant Professor of Pediatrics
Medical College of Wisconsin
Attending Nephrologist
Children's Hospital of Wisconsin
Milwaukee, Wisconsin

H. Gil Rushton, M.D. [12]
Associate Professor of Urology and Pediatrics
George Washington University School of Medicine
Vice Chairman, Department of Urology
Children's National Medical Center
Washington, D.C.

Fernando Santos, M.D. [21]
Visiting Scientist
Children's Medical Center
Division of Pediatric Nephrology
Virginia Commonwealth University
Richmond, Virginia
Professor of Pediatrics
Division of Pediatric Nephrology
University of Oviedo
Oviedo, Spain

H. William Schnaper, M.D. [7]
Associate Professor of Pediatrics
George Washington University School of Medicine
Washington, D.C.

Eglal Shalaby-Rana, M.D. [3]
Attending Radiologist
George Washington University School of Medicine
Attending Radiologist
Children's National Medical Center
Washington, D.C.

F. Bruder Stapleton, M.D. [*22*]
Professor and Chairman
Department of Pediatrics
State University of New York at Buffalo
Pediatrician-in-Chief
Children's Hospital of Buffalo
Buffalo, New York

PREFACE

This book was conceived as a primer of pediatric nephrology devoted to the clinical discussion of commonly encountered renal disorders in children. The focus of the book is on the day-to-day clinical care of children with such disorders, and a conscious effort has been made by the authors and the editors to maintain this objective and to sustain the clinical flavor of the text throughout the book. Extensive use of tables, flow diagrams, and actual case histories in the book is intended to provide the reader with a helpful and a quick resource of the clinically relevant information.

The book has been arbitrarily divided into five parts. Part I deals with the diagnostic evaluation of patients with renal diseases. Renal function, urinalysis, radiology of the urinary tract, and renal biopsy are discussed. Part II consists of chapters dealing with specific renal diseases. Glomerular diseases, nephrotic syndrome, urinary tract infection, and hypertension are discussed in detail. Two of the common clinical urologic problems—obstructive uropathy and enuresis—are also dealt with to familiarize the reader with the clinically relevant pathophysiologic events in these two conditions. Acute and chronic renal failure and renal transplantation have been discussed in detail in Part III. Common renal metabolic disorders encountered by the nephrologists are discussed in Part IV. Neonatal nephrology is a growing field of pediatric nephrology, and Part V has been devoted to the evaluation of renal function in the newborn and common neonatal renal problems. Although this book is not intended to be an exhaustive reference source, every effort has been made to include pertinent up-to-date references for the subjects under discussion.

One of the unique features of this book is the inclusion of commentaries by leading authorities in the fields of pediatric nephrology and urology, at the end of selected chapters. The purpose of these commentaries is to share the clinical experience of these experts with the readers of the book. We have allowed the authors of these commentaries a free hand in their approach to the content and writing style, and these comments have been published without any editorial alterations. Consequently, the format in which these commentaries have been written varies throughout the book. At times, the reader may even find the expert's comments at variance with the author's view in the main body of the chapter. We have not attempted to soften such differences of opinion, since they provide an alternative point of view, as is commonly experienced during academic discussions in clinical medicine.

Although primarily meant to fulfill the needs of pediatric and adult nephrology fellows, we hope that this book will also be helpful to the medical students, house officers, and the practicing physicians in the diagnosis and management of their patients with renal disorders.

Many individuals have contributed materials to this book. Our special thanks go to Dr. Sudesh Kapur, Dr. Kathleen Patterson, Dr. Fermin Tio, Dr. Edward J. Ruley, and Dr. Howard Austin—all of whom provided photomicrographs for several chapters. Dr. Steven Wasner provided the table of growth standards for children. The entire staff of the medical library at the Children's National Medical Center, Washington, D.C., especially Shirley S. Knobloch, provided excellent library support. Almost always did we seem to need the Med-Line literature search done and journal articles obtained "yesterday", and not even once have we been let down. We also wish to thank Patty Hill and Gail Higgins for their excellent typing of parts of the manuscript for the book. Karen Seddon, Toni Smith, Alexis Barthlett, and Maria Chatman helped with their secretarial assistance during the preparation of the book.

We wish to express our profound gratitude to Dr. Julie R. Ingelfinger, Dr. Russell W. Chesney, Dr. H. William Schnaper, Dr. Billy S. Arant, Dr. A. Barry Belman, Dr. F. Bruder Stapleton, Dr. Richard N. Fine, and Dr. James C. M. Chan for reviewing manuscripts and their willingness to share their personal views in the form of commentaries.

The editorial staff of McGraw-Hill has provided exceptional help in the completion of this book. Their constant encouragement throughout the project has gone a long way in making us feel, often at times when finishing the book appeared as a distant dream, that "there is light at the end of the tunnel". Our special thanks, among this excellent crew, go to Muza Navrozov, area editing supervisor, for going over each line, figure, and table of the text and arranging even the last-minute corrections to be accommodated; and to Edward Bolger, for keeping faith in our project and providing whatever help we needed.

Finally, we want to thank our family members: Shashi, Sidarth, Tapasya, Kadambari, Donna Vishal, and Kirin, who stood by us throughout and encouraged us to meet this challenge.

CLINICAL PEDIATRIC NEPHROLOGY

I

DIAGNOSTIC NEPHROLOGY

1

EVALUATION OF RENAL FUNCTIONS

Kanwal K. Kher

The kidneys are highly vascular organs that receive approximately 25 percent of the cardiac output at any given time. Each kidney has about 1 million nephrons, which develop in the fetus by the 35th week of gestation. Each nephron consists of a filtering unit, or glomerulus, and a tubule which conducts and alters the constitution of the glomerular ultrafiltrate. Although ultrafiltration of plasma in the glomerulus is the primary and an essential event in the formation of urine, intact tubular functions are equally important in modulating the final constitution of urine and preserving the body's internal milieu. Normal renal function is characterized by three essential attributes: (1) glomerular ultrafiltration, (2) tubular reabsorption of the filtered solutes and water, and (3) tubular secretion of organic and nonorganic ions. This chapter discusses the principles and techniques of laboratory tests used for the evaluation of renal functions in children.

GLOMERULAR STRUCTURE

The glomerulus consists of a network of capillaries that function as a complex sieve and filter water and solutes from the capillary lumen into the urinary space (Bowman's space). The glomerular capillary filtration barrier is composed of three distinct anatomic structures: (1) the endothelial cell, (2) the glomerular basement membrane (GBM), and (3) the epithelial cell (Fig. 1–1). Endothelial cells comprise the innermost layer of the glomerular capillaries. These cells rest directly on the GBM and are in contact with the blood flowing through the capillary lumen. The cytoplasm of the endothelial cell has numerous openings known as *endothelial fenestrations,* which range from 500 to 1000 Å in diameter.

The GBM makes up the middle layer of the glomerular capillary barrier and consists of a central dense core known as the *lamina densa,* which is surrounded on the inner and the outer sides by less compact portions referred to as the *lamina rara interna* and *lamina rara externa,* respectively. The GBM functions as a selectively permeable membrane with functional pores, but no anatomically distinct pores have been identified in it by electron microscopy. The outermost

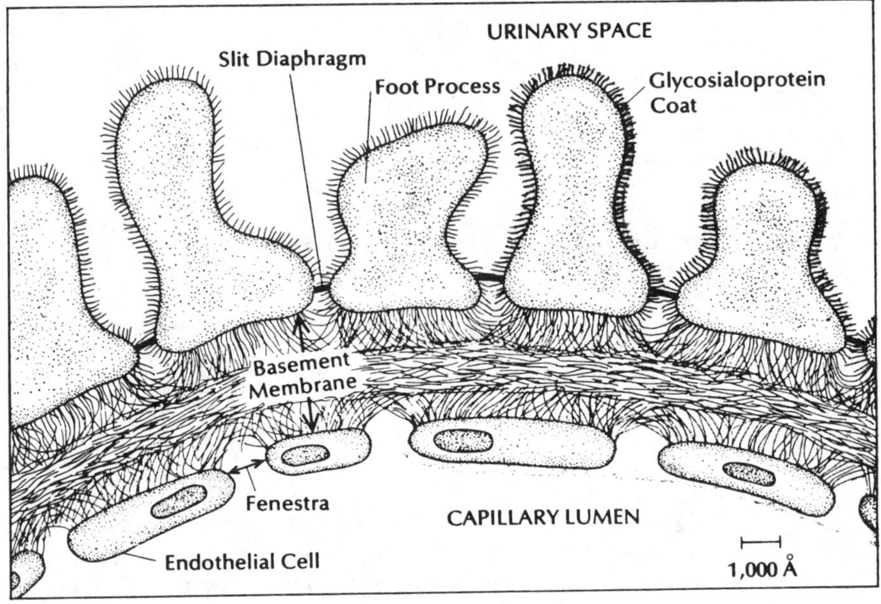

A

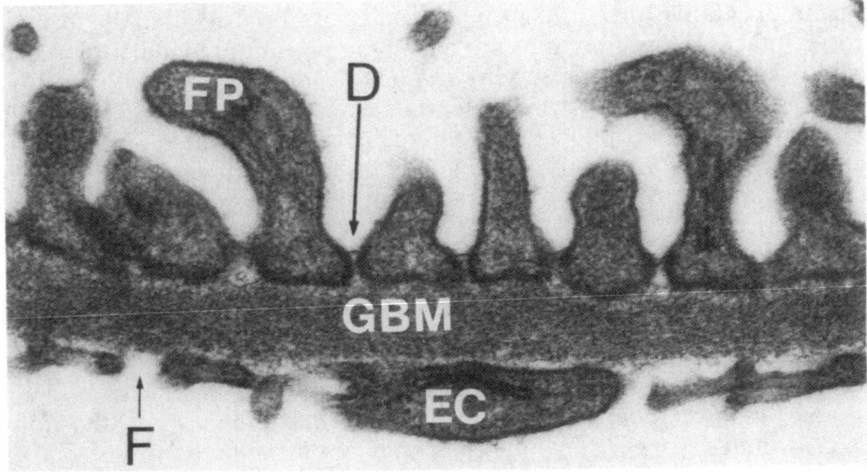

B

FIG. 1–1. *A:* A diagrammatic representation of the glomerular capillary wall in cross section. The endothelial cells lining the capillary lumen have fenestrations. The epithelial cells and their foot processes are present on the urinary side of the glomerular basement membrane. Epithelial cell foot processes are separated by slit diaphragms. (From Brenner BM, Beeuwkes III, R: The renal circulation. *Hosp Pract* 13:35, 1978. Illustrator: NL Gahan Markris. Reproduced by permission.) *B:* Electron microscopic section of a normal human glomerular capillary wall. GBM = glomerular basement membrane; FP = foot process; EC = endothelial cell; F = endothelial cell fenestration; D = epithelial cell slit diaphragm. (Photograph kindly provided by Dr. Fermin Tio, University of Texas Health Science Center, San Antonio, Texas.)

layer of the glomerular filtration barrier consists of the epithelial cell, which is anchored to the GBM by numerous cytoplasmic extensions known as the *podocytes* or foot processes. Individual podocytes appear on electron microscopy as distinct structures, and the spaces between the adjoining podocytes are referred to as *epithelial slit pores.* These pores are covered by a membrane known as the *slit diaphragm.* The GBM is negatively charged due to the presence of various glycosaminoglycans, such as heparan sulfate.[1–3]

GLOMERULAR ULTRAFILTRATION

Filtration of plasma across the glomerular filtration barrier of the glomerular capillary is governed by Starling forces (Fig. 1–2).[4] Of these, glomerular capillary hydrostatic pressure is the main factor that permits ultrafiltration of plasma from the capillary lumen into the urinary space. Plasma oncotic pressure within the glomerular capillary lumen and hydrostatic pressure within the Bowman's capsule oppose glomerular ultrafiltration. In addition to net positive Starling forces, the filtration function of the glomerular capillaries is further ensured by a high coefficient of ultrafiltration (K_f), which is the product of the capillary surface area (S) and hydraulic capillary permeability (k).

$$\text{SNGFR} = K_f\{(P_{GC} - P_t) - (\pi_{GC} - \pi_t)\} \quad (1\text{–}1)$$

$$\text{SNGFR} = k \times S\{(P_{GC} - P_t) - (\pi_{GC} - \pi_t)\} \quad (1\text{–}2)$$

where SNGFR = single nephron glomerular filtration rate; P_{GC} = hydrostatic pressure within glomerular capillary lumen; P_t = hydrostatic pressure within Bowman's capsule; π_{GC} = plasma oncotic pressure in glomerular capillary lumen; and π_t = oncotic pressure within Bowman's space.

CLINICAL EVALUATION OF RENAL FUNCTIONS

Renal functions can be evaluated by several easily available laboratory tests (Table 1–1). The first step in such an evaluation consists of a complete urinalysis, including examination of the spun urinary sediment. A wealth of useful information regarding the functional state of the kidneys can be obtained from a well-performed urinalysis (Chap. 2). Determination of blood urea nitrogen

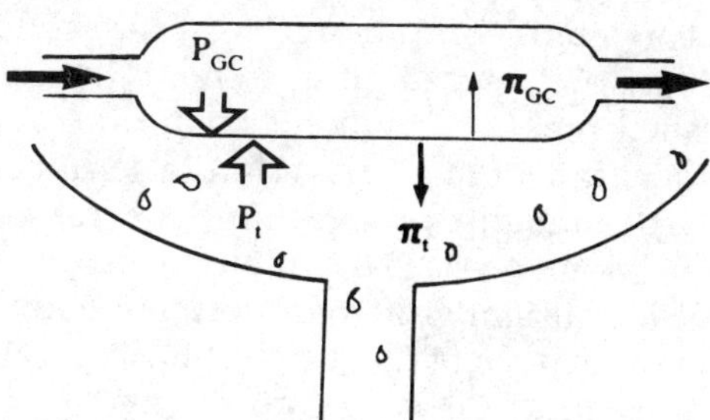

FIG. 1–2. Starling forces governing filtration of plasma in the glomerular capillary. See text for details.

TABLE 1–1. Laboratory Tests Used to Evaluate Renal Functions in Children

Glomerular Functions	Tubular Functions	Hormonal Functions
BUN Serum creatinine Creatinine clearance Inulin clearance	Water metabolism Urine specific gravity Urine osmolality Maximal urine concentrating capacity Acid-base metabolism Urine pH Urine titrable acid excretion Urine ammonium excretion Urine-blood P_{CO_2} Fractional excretion of bicarbonate at normal serum bicarbonate level	Erythropoietin Hematocrit Reticulocyte count Vitamin D Serum 1,25-$(OH)_2D_3$ concentration Serum calcium concentration

(BUN) and serum creatinine are commonly used laboratory tests for the overall assessment of renal functions. Even with their inherent limitations, these two tests provide a reasonably accurate estimation of glomerular filtration rate (GFR). For a more precise determination of GFR, clearance of endogenous creatinine or exogenously administered inulin and radionuclide GFR methods are necessary. Detailed evaluation of tubular functions may be indicated in some children. These tests include assessment of renal handling of water, mineral metabolism, and acid-base balance.

SERUM CREATININE

Creatinine, a product of creatine and phosphocreatine metabolism, is synthesized predominantly in the skeletal muscles; minor contributions to the total creatinine pool are also made by its synthesis in the liver, pancreas, and kidneys.[5] Creatinine is exclusively excreted through the kidneys, predominantly by the process of glomerular filtration and to a lesser extent by tubular secretion. Urinary creatinine contributed by tubular secretion in normal individuals does not exceed 10 to 15 percent,[6] but it is significantly higher in patients with chronic renal failure.[7] In most clinical conditions, the rate of creatinine synthesis remains constant and its serum concentration reflects the rate of renal elimination. Elevated serum creatinine concentration, therefore, denotes diminished renal clearance of creatinine and a decline in GFR. Even with normal renal function, an elevation in serum creatinine may sometimes be seen where large amounts of creatinine are released from muscles, as in crush injury or rhabdomyolysis. The intake of large quantities of well-cooked (red) meat can also transiently increase serum creatinine concentration by providing an exogenous source of creatinine.[8] Each gram of ingested meat provides 3.5 to 5.0 mg of creatine. Cooking converts about 65 percent of this to creatinine, which can then be absorbed from the gastrointestinal tract.[9] Conversely, serum creatinine

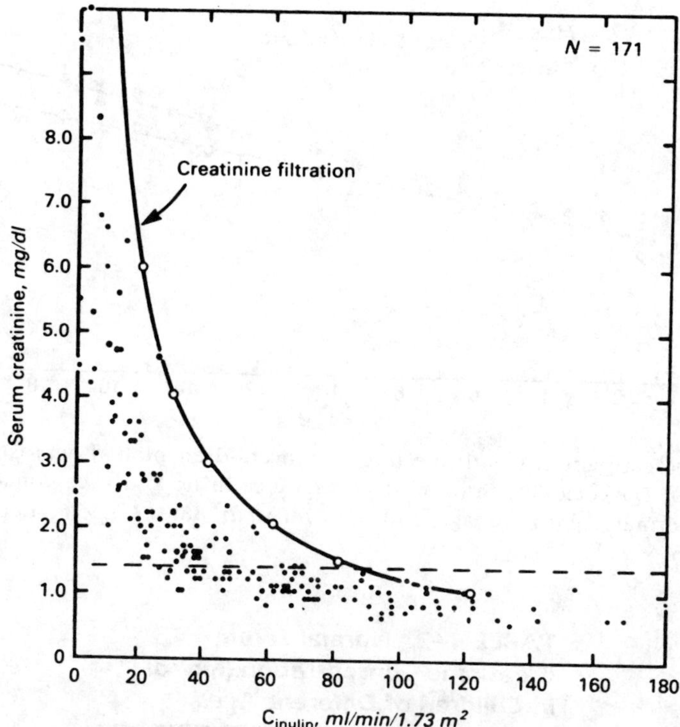

FIG. 1–3. Relationship of serum creatinine to GFR. (From Shemesh O, Golbetz H, Kriss JP, et al: Limitation of creatinine as a filtration marker in glomerulopathic patients. *Kidney Int* 28:830, 1985. Reproduced by permission.)

concentration may be inappropriately low in patients with reduced muscle mass resulting from malnutrition or advanced muscle diseases. Certain drugs—such as cimetidine, trimethoprim, and probenecid—can falsely increase serum creatinine by competing for renal tubular transport of creatinine.

During steady state, a 50 percent reduction of GFR results in a doubling of serum creatinine. As is apparent from Fig. 1–3, the relationship between serum creatinine and GFR is not linear. A doubling of serum creatinine from its baseline value in the initial portion of this curve signifies a greater reduction of GFR than for a similar rise in the absolute serum creatinine concentration when GFR is diminished to a moderate or severe degree. For example, a rise (or doubling) of serum creatinine from 1.0 mg/dL to 2.0 mg/dL reflects a 50-percent reduction of GFR, while an increment of serum creatinine by a similar amount (i.e., 1.0 mg/dL), from 5.0 mg/dL to 6.0 mg/dL, only indicates a further decrease of GFR by only about 5 percent.

NORMAL SERUM CREATININE

Serum creatinine concentration is low at birth and increases as a child's muscle mass increases from the neonatal period through infancy (Fig. 1–4).[10] Failure to appreciate this fact can be a potential source of error in calculating GFR on

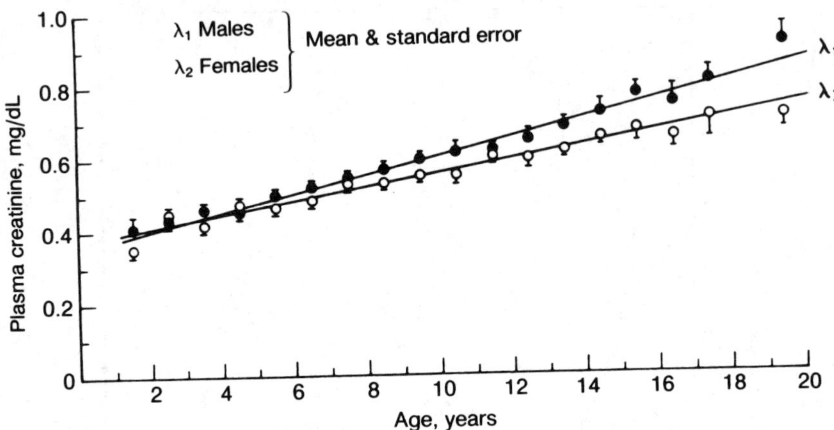

FIG. 1–4. Mean serum creatinine (mg/dL) in children plotted against age. (From Schwartz GJ, Haycock GB, Spitzer A: Plasma creatinine and urea concentration in children: Normal values for age and sex. *J Pediatr* 88:828, 1976. Reproduced by permission.)

TABLE 1–2. Normal Serum Creatinine Concentration (mg/dL) in Children of Different Ages

Age, Years	Girls	Boys
1	0.35 ± 0.05	0.41 ± 0.10
2	0.45 ± 0.07	0.43 ± 0.12
3	0.42 ± 0.08	0.46 ± 0.11
4	0.47 ± 0.12	0.45 ± 0.11
5	0.46 ± 0.11	0.50 ± 0.11
6	0.48 ± 0.11	0.52 ± 0.12
7	0.53 ± 0.12	0.54 ± 0.14
8	0.53 ± 0.11	0.57 ± 0.16
9	0.55 ± 0.11	0.59 ± 0.16
10	0.55 ± 0.13	0.61 ± 0.22
11	0.60 ± 0.13	0.62 ± 0.14
12	0.59 ± 0.13	0.65 ± 0.16
13	0.62 ± 0.14	0.68 ± 0.21
14	0.65 ± 0.13	0.72 ± 0.24
15	0.67 ± 0.22	0.76 ± 0.22
16	0.65 ± 0.15	0.74 ± 0.23
17	0.70 ± 0.20	0.80 ± 0.18
18–20	0.72 ± 0.19	0.91 ± 0.17

Source: From Schwartz GJ, Haycock GB, Spitzer A: Plasma creatinine and urea concentration in children: Normal values for age and sex. *J Pediatr* 88:828, 1976. Reproduced by permission.

the basis of serum creatinine concentration. For example, a concentration of 0.8 mg/dL, considered normal in a child 4 to 5 years age, would indicate about a 50-percent decrement of renal function in a newborn infant, in whom normal serum creatinine is only 0.4 mg/dL. Normal serum creatinine concentrations for both sexes from 1 through 20 years of age are given in Table 1–2. Norms for neonates of various gestational ages are discussed in Chap. 23.

PREDICTING GFR FROM SERUM CREATININE

While serum creatinine provides an approximate estimate of GFR, a better projection can be obtained by using one of the several available mathematical formulas and nomograms. Most such formulas are based on the following relationship of GFR (expressed as mL/min/1.73 m^2) to serum creatinine concentration:

$$GFR = \frac{k \times L}{P_{cr}} \quad (1\text{–}3)$$

where L = length in centimeters; k = constant of proportionality, which is related to creatinine excretion per unit body size; and P_{cr} = plasma creatinine.

In their early studies, Schwartz et al.[11] found the value of k to be 0.55, but later studies reported by the same investigators suggest that the value of k should be age-dependent in order to accurately reflect the changes in true muscle mass that occur during childhood (Table 1–3).[12–14] Nomograms derived from Eq. (1–3) are also available for clinical use (Fig. 1–5).

USING THE RECIPROCAL OF SERUM CREATININE

Several workers have shown that by plotting the reciprocal of serum creatinine ($1/S_{cr}$) against time (in months or years), the rate of deterioration or improvement in GFR can be predicted.[15,16] In patients with stable renal function, the $1/S_{cr}$ plot demonstrates a flat slope, while progressive deterioration or improvement of GFR is represented, respectively, by a downward or upward slant of the

TABLE 1–3. Formulas Used in Assessing Creatinine Clearance

Age Group	Formula	References
Full-term newborn through first year:	$\frac{0.45 \times \text{length (cm)}}{\text{Plasma creatinine (mg/dL)}}$	12
Children (up to 13 years):	$\frac{0.55 \times \text{length (cm)}}{\text{Plasma creatinine (mg/dL)}}$	11
Adolescents (13 to 21 years)		13
Males:	$\frac{0.7 \times \text{height (cm)}}{\text{Plasma creatinine (mg/dL)}}$	
Females:	$\frac{0.57 \times \text{height (cm)}}{\text{Plasma creatinine (mg/dL)}}$	

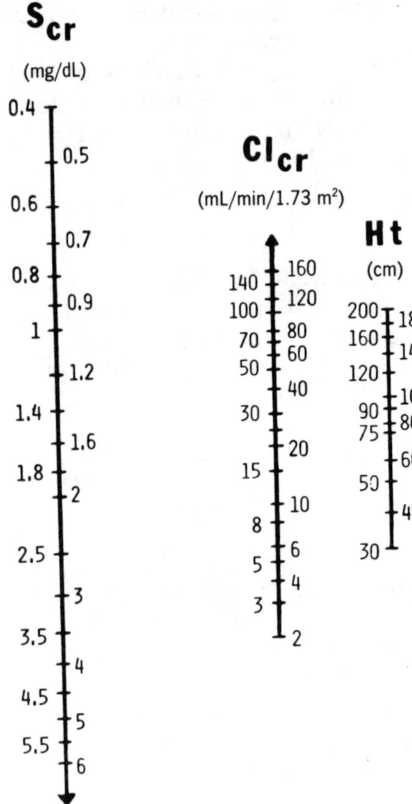

FIG. 1–5. Nomogram for rapid evaluation of endogenous creatinine clearance in children (1 to 18 years of age). To predict creatinine clearance, connect the child's serum creatinine concentration and height with a ruler and read the creatinine clearance where the ruler intersects the central line. (From Traub SC, Johnson CE: Comparison of methods of estimating creatinine clearance in children. *Am J Hosp Pharm* 37:195, 1980. Reproduced by permission.)

$1/S_{cr}$ slope (Fig. 1–6). Apart from monitoring the rate of decline of GFR, the $1/S_{cr}$ plot can also be used to predict the time of onset of end-stage renal disease in patients whose illness is chronic and progressive. For this purpose, however, one presumes that the rate of decline of renal function is steady and follows a linear course. Yet many patients may not have such a course and experience an accelerated decline. Accelerated deterioration of GFR is common in patients with uncontrolled hypertension, urinary tract obstruction, urinary tract infection, or underlying systemic diseases such as lupus erythematosus or vasculitides.

BLOOD UREA NITROGEN AS AN INDICATOR OF GFR

Normal BUN in a well-nourished and well-hydrated healthy child can be regarded as a reflection of a normal GFR. Compared to serum creatinine, BUN should be considered a less reliable index of GFR primarily because several extrarenal factors affect its serum concentration. This may lead to erroneously high or low laboratory values even in patients with normal renal function (Table 1–4). Additionally, renal excretion of urea and its concentration in the blood are significantly altered by the state of hydration and urine flow.

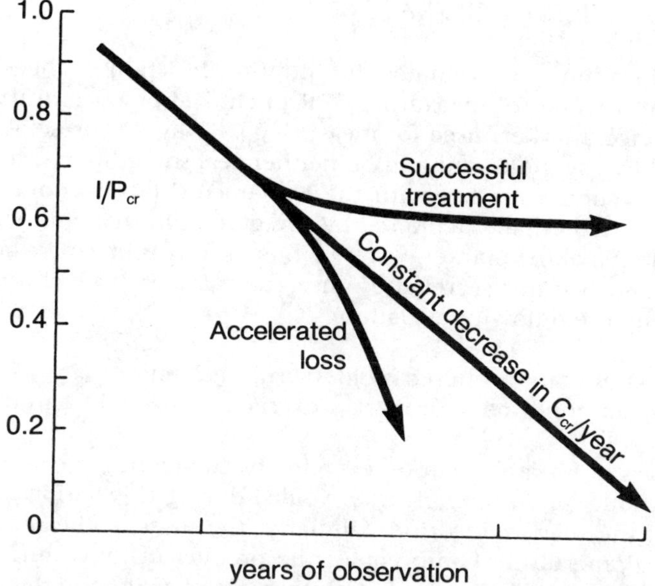

FIG. 1–6. Use of the reciprocal of serum creatinine concentration ($1/P_{cr}$) to follow progression of renal disease. (From Sullivan LP, Grantham JJ: *Physiology of the Kidney*. Philadelphia, Lea & Febiger, 1982, p 53. Reproduced by permission.)

Although freely filtered in the glomeruli, urea undergoes significant reabsorption in the renal tubules. A variable amount of the filtered urea is reabsorbed in the proximal tubule, the loop of Henle, and the medullary collecting duct. While urea reabsorption along the proximal tubule and the loop of Henle is passive, reabsorption in the collecting duct is highly dependent on the presence of vasopressin. During antidiuresis or when there is a low urine flow rate, urea absorption in the distal nephron increases; it decreases during diuresis. Complex tubular handling of urea by the kidney further reduces the usefulness of BUN as an indicator of GFR.

TABLE 1–4. Factors Affecting Serum BUN Concentration That May Lead to Falsely Increased or Decreased Values

Increased	Decreased
Gastrointestinal hemorrhage	Decreased protein intake
Dehydration	Advanced starvation
Increased protein intake	Liver disease
Increased protein catabolism	
Systemic infection	
Burns	
Glucocorticoid therapy	
Early phase of starvation	

GLOMERULAR FILTRATION RATE

Glomerular filtration rate evaluates the filtration function of the kidney. The most common methods of measuring GFR in clinical practice utilize the principle of clearance. Markers used for measuring GFR by this principle should be freely filtered by the glomeruli and be neither reabsorbed nor secreted by the renal tubules. When a marker with these characteristics is administered, the amount (mass) of the marker filtered by the glomeruli in 1 min should equal the amount (mass) of the marker excreted in urine in 1 min, since the substance is neither reabsorbed nor secreted by the renal tubules. This relationship can be expressed by the following equation:

Amount (mass) of marker filtered by glomeruli in 1 min
= amount (mass) of marker excreted in urine in 1 min (1–4)

The net mass of filtration marker excreted by the kidneys in 1 min (Eq. 1–4) equals the product of volume of urine voided during this period and the concentration of the marker in urine. Similarly, the mass of the marker filtered through the glomeruli in 1 min equals the product of the volume of plasma filtered by the glomeruli per minute (in other words, GFR) and the plasma concentration of the marker. Therefore, Eq. (1–4) can be rewritten as

$$\mathrm{GFR} \times \mathrm{P} = \mathrm{U} \times \mathrm{V} \tag{1–5}$$

where GFR = glomerular filtration rate; P = plasma concentration of marker agent; U = urinary concentration of marker agent; and V = volume of urine voided during test period.

Equation (1–5) can be further rearranged as follows:

$$\mathrm{GFR} = \frac{\mathrm{U} \times \mathrm{V}}{\mathrm{P}} \tag{1–6}$$

Thus, if the volume of urine (V) elaborated during the test and the concentrations of marker substance in plasma (P) and urine (U) are known, GFR can easily be estimated by using Eq. (1–6).

MARKERS FOR ESTIMATING GFR

The characteristics of an ideal marker for measuring GFR are listed in Table 1–5. Inulin, a fructose polymer obtained from Jerusalem artichokes and dahlia roots, meets all the requirements of such a marker. Inulin clearance is regarded as the reference standard for determining GFR in both adults and children. However, a major drawback of using inulin clearance is that the procedure requires extensive preparation of the patient and attention to detail. The inulin must be injected intravenously until a steady blood level is achieved; multiple blood samples must then be drawn from the patient; and corresponding urine samples must be collected at regular intervals after catheterizing and air-wash-

TABLE 1–5. Characteristics of an Ideal Marker Agent for Studying GFR

Should be nontoxic when given exogenously
Should achieve a stable plasma concentration in a steady state
Should not be bound to plasma proteins
Should be freely filtered by glomeruli
Should not be secreted by renal tubules
Should not be reabsorbed by renal tubules

ing the bladder. Additionally, special arrangements must be made to measure the inulin concentration in plasma and urine, since this assay is not routinely available in most clinical laboratories. For these reasons, despite its exceptional accuracy, inulin clearance is seldom used routinely in clinical practice.

Endogenous creatinine is extensively used as a marker for determining GFR by the clearance method. Although creatinine is freely filtered by the glomeruli, its tubular secretion can potentially lead to an overestimation of GFR by 10 to 15 percent. However, this overestimation is minimized, though not completely eliminated in normal individuals, by the fact that serum creatinine concentration measured by the Auto Analyser method in most clinical laboratories is also overestimated by 10 to 15 percent due to the presence of noncreatinine chromogens in the serum. This reduces the error in computing the true GFR by creatinine clearance method.*

Although several studies have shown a good correlation between GFR measured by creatinine clearance and by inulin clearance,[17] a high degree of variability in the results of creatinine clearance tests, even under ideal circumstances, is well known. In a study of 5 normal adults, Chantler et al.[18] reported that the mean coefficient of variation of creatinine clearance was 11.6 percent. In patients with chronic renal failure, who undergo increased tubular secretion of creatinine, GFR can be significantly overestimated by the creatinine clearance method.[9,19] However, despite these shortcomings, creatinine clearance remains a reasonably accurate and a readily available test for determining GFR for most clinical purposes.

Urea, like creatinine, is synthesized endogenously and is also filtered freely by the glomeruli. However, urea does not meet the criteria of an ideal marker for measuring GFR, since it undergoes significant reabsorption in the renal tubules. Urea clearance usually underestimates GFR by 30 to 50 percent.[20] On the other hand, in patients with chronic renal failure, osmotic diuresis in the surviving nephrons leads to a decreased urea reabsorption in the renal tubules; therefore urea clearance in these patients approximates true GFR.[7] Since creatinine clearance overestimates and urea clearance underestimates GFR, an average of the two clearances approximates inulin clearance or true GFR in normal individuals.

* $\frac{U_{cr} \text{ (overestimated by 15\%)} \times V}{P_{cr} \text{ (overestimated by 15\%)}}$.

PROCEDURE FOR PERFORMING THE CREATININE CLEARANCE TEST

The creatinine clearance method of determining GFR demands an accurate, timed collection of urine. Although 24-h urine collection is used as a standard method of measuring creatinine clearance, a short urine collection time (1 to 2 h) has also been reported to produce acceptable and reproducible results.[21] On the day of the test the child is asked to void and empty the bladder in the morning (7 A.M.), the urine discarded, and the time noted to denote the start of urine collection. All urine voided in the next 24 h is collected in a container and is either stored in a refrigerator or placed on ice. At the end of 24 h (7 A.M. on the next day), the bladder is emptied and the last void is deposited in the container as part of the collection. The volume of urine collected is noted accurately, and the urine is sent to the laboratory for estimation of creatinine concentration. Blood for creatinine estimation is preferably drawn at the midpoint of urine collection (around 12 h); in case this is not possible, blood may be collected at the end of urine collection. Creatinine clearance is calculated by using Eq. (1–5).

In order to adhere to a uniform standard for the purpose of comparison, creatinine clearance as well as other representations of GFR (such as inulin clearance) are expressed in relation to body surface area (mL/min/1.73 m²). Therefore, the final representation of Eq. (1–6) for calculating creatinine clearance is as follows:

$$C_{cr}\ (\text{mL/min}/1.73\ \text{m}^2) = \frac{U_{cr}\ (\text{mg/dL}) \times V\ (\text{mL}) \times 1.73}{P_{cr}\ (\text{mg/dL}) \times 1440 \times SA\ (\text{m}^2)} \qquad (1\text{–}7)$$

where C_{cr} = creatinine clearance; U_{cr} = urine creatinine concentration; V = urine volume obtained in 24 h; P_{cr} = plasma creatinine; SA = patient's surface area; and 1440 = time in minutes during which urine was collected (24 h × 60 min = 1440 min).

JUDGING THE COMPLETENESS OF URINE COLLECTION: CREATININE INDEX

The accuracy of endogenous creatinine clearance measurements depends on the completeness of urine collection, and it is essential to ascertain whether the collected urine represents an adequate sample for the test. The relative constancy of creatinine production and its urinary excretion in a steady state is utilized for evaluating completeness of the collected sample. Urinary creatinine excretion in healthy children varies with age, ranging from 8 to 10 mg/kg/day in premature infants to more than 20 mg/kg/day in adolescent males (Table 1–6).[12,22–24] Twenty-four-hour urine collections containing less than 15 mg/kg/day of creatinine in children over 3 years of age suggest that the urine has been either collected for less than 24 h or all of the urine voided during this interval has not been included in the specimen. Estimation of creatinine clearance in such a sample will lead to a falsely low value. On the other hand, daily urine creatinine excretion of more than 23 mg/kg probably indicates that the urine may have been collected for more than 24 h. This may result in a falsely elevated creatinine clearance value.

TABLE 1–6. Daily Urine Creatinine Excretion in Children

Age Group		Urine Creatinine, mg/kg/24 h
Neonates[a]		8–12
1 month to 1 year[a]		12–14
3–4.9 years[b]	Boys	20.9 ± 5.7
	Girls	18.9 ± 4.4
5–6.9 years	Boys	23.3 ± 7.3
	Girls	21.9 ± 4.3
7–8.9 years	Boys	23.3 ± 7.9
	Girls	24.4 ± 5.7
9–10.9 years	Boys	23.9 ± 5.1
	Girls	25.5 ± 7.1
11–12.9 years	Boys	23.4 ± 4.5
	Girls	24.2 ± 5.6
13–14.9 years	Boys	25.6 ± 5.2
	Girls	23.6 ± 3.7
15 years and up	Boys	27.0 ± 3.4
	Girls	21.9 ± 4.2

[a]Values derived from Refs. 12 and 23.

[b]Data on children 3 years and beyond reproduced with permission from Reynolds EL, Clark LC: Creatinine excretion, growth progress and body structure in normal children. *Child Dev* 18:155, 1947. Copyright by the Society for Research in Child Development, Inc.

DETERMINING GFR BY RADIONUCLIDE SCANS

Determination of GFR by the use of radioactive isotopes is becoming an increasingly attractive option in children. This method of estimating GFR is particularly useful in newborn infants and young children, from whom it is usually difficult to obtain an accurate timed collection of urine. Several radioisotopes meeting the criteria of clearance markers—such as ^{99m}Tc-diethylenetriaminepentacetic acid (^{99m}Tc-DTPA), ^{125}I-iothalamate, and ^{51}Cr-ethylenediaminetetraacetic acid (^{51}Cr-EDTA)—are available for GFR estimation in clinical practice. Two separate techniques of obtaining GFR by radioisotopes are available. In the first method, GFR is calculated from the uptake of labeled tracer in each kidney.[25] By this method, split renal function of each kidney can be assessed separately. The second technique utilizes the disappearance of the labeled GFR marker from plasma as an index.[26] The radioisotope method of estimating GFR is discussed in Chap. 3.

NORMAL VALUES OF GFR IN CHILDREN

The GFR is considerably lower in neonates than it is in adults; most studies have reported values ranging from 20 to 25 mL/min/1.73 m^2 (20 percent of adult

TABLE 1–7. Normal Values for GFR in Children

Age	GFR, mL/min/1.73 m^2	References[a]
Birth	20.8 ± 1.9	28
1 week	46.6 ± 5.2	28
3–5 weeks	60.1 ± 4.6	28
6–9 weeks	67.5 ± 6.5	29,30
3–6 months	73.8 ± 7.2	30
6 months–1 year	93.7 ± 14.0	30
1–2 years	99.1 ± 18.7	29,30
2–5 years	126.5 ± 24.0	29,30
5–15 years	116.7 ± 20.2	30

[a]GRF derived from data given in the references.

GFR).[27,28] Premature infants have an even lower GFR at birth than do full-term infants.[28] A rapid improvement in GFR occurs in the first 2 weeks of life; it usually doubles during this time (Table 1–7). A GFR comparable to that of adults is reached by the end of the second year of life (Fig. 1–7).[29,30] Neonatal and developmental aspects of GFR are discussed in detail in Chap. 23.

TESTS EVALUATING TUBULAR FUNCTIONS

The renal tubules perform several important functions that are essential to maintaining a normal fluid, electrolyte, and acid-base balance. These functions

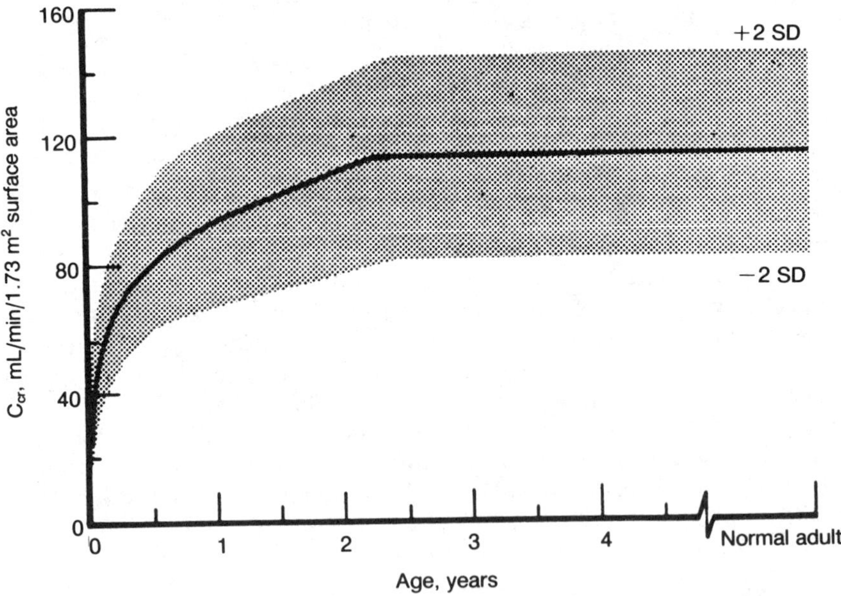

FIG. 1–7. Changes in normal value for GFR from birth to later childhood. The GFR was derived by endogenous creatinine clearance. (Reprinted by permission of the publishers from *Developmental Nephrology* by Wallace W. McCrory, Cambridge, Massachusetts: Harvard University Press, 1972, p 98. Copyright ©1972 by the President and Fellows of Harvard College.)

include reabsorption of water and solutes from the glomerular ultrafiltrate, secretion of various toxic organic ions, and excretion of hydrogen ions generated by normal metabolic activity. Evaluation of urine specific gravity and pH are the commonest tests used for studying tubular functions. These tests provide useful information regarding tubular concentrating ability and the urinary acidification mechanism. Detailed evaluation of renal tubular functions is not routinely performed but may be necessary if specific tubular transport defects such as renal bicabonate wasting, acidification defects, defective concentrating ability, etc. are suspected.

URINARY CONCENTRATING ABILITY

Renal concentrating ability is tested by determining urinary specific gravity or osmolality. Urinary osmolality is a more precise method of determining the renal concentrating ability than is specific gravity. Although mild proteinuria (less than 2+ by dipstick) does not alter urine specific gravity significantly,[31] the presence of large amounts of protein in the urine induces a serious error in the estimation of urinary concentrating ability as determined by specific gravity. Other causes of falsely elevated urine specific gravity include the presence of glucose, various pharmaceutical agents, and contrast media in the urine sample. Methodologic details of testing urine specific gravity and osmolality are discussed in Chap. 2.

DEVELOPMENTAL ASPECTS

Newborn infants are not able to concentrate urine well during the first month of life, especially in the first 7 days. Fisher et al.[32] noted that the mean urinary osmolality in normal healthy newborn infants was only 291 mosmol/L and 309 mosmol/L at 12 and 24 h, respectively.[32] Maximal urine osmolality after 72 h of fluid deprivation in normal neonates has been found to reach only to about 600 mosmol/L—half the value that adults are able to generate.[33] A gradual improvement in urinary concentrating capacity is seen during the first 2 years of life, and maximal renal concentrating capacity—comparable to that of adults (>1362 mosmol/L)—is reached by puberty (14 to 18 years).[34]

The inability of neonates to concentrate urine is best explained by the developmental immaturity of their kidneys. Newborn infants respond poorly to exogenously administered pitressin as well as to DDAVP. Svenningsen and Aronson[35] noted that the urine osmolality following pitressin (0.5 units/kg) and DDAVP (10 μg) challenge rose only to a mean value of 369 mosmol/L and 430 mosmol/L, respectively, in healthy full-term 1- to 3-week-old newborn infants. Maximal urine concentrating capacity in this study improved markedly when the test was repeated at 4 to 6 weeks of age. These findings suggest that the renal tubules of the neonate are relatively insensitive to vasopressin. Another factor considered important in the pathogenesis of impaired urinary concentrating ability in the first month of life is a lack of adequate medullary hyperosmolality. Urea, a product of protein metabolism, contributes almost half of the osmolality for the hypertonic medullary environment and forms an essential element in the optimal functioning of the countercurrent multiplier mechanism for urinary concentration. Although newborn infants take adequate amounts of dietary protein, low medullary urea concentration is believed to result from their highly anabolic state. Increased protein intake in the neonatal period has been demonstrated to enhance renal concentrating ability, possibly by providing the additional urea necessary for establishing a hypertonic medullary environment.[36]

TEST FOR MAXIMAL URINE CONCENTRATING ABILITY

A test of maximal urine concentrating ability is indicated in patients who are unable to concentrate their urine and have polyuria. Routine evaluation of urine samples in these patients demonstrates low specific gravity ($\leq$1.010) or osmolality. Because of excessive renal water loss, many such patients may have evidence of hypernatremia. This test is designed to differentiate patients whose polyuria is due to a lack or insufficiency of vasopressin (central diabetes insipidus) from those who have an inadequate renal tubular response to vasopressin (nephrogenic diabetes insipidus). The test is conducted as follows:[31]

- After a light dry supper (without fluids), the patient is asked to empty the bladder (start time). Baseline urine (U_1) and blood (S_1) samples are assessed for osmolality. Fluids and food are withheld for the next 12 h. The first voided sample of urine (U_2) is collected at the end of 12 h and a corresponding blood sample (S_2) is also obtained for assessing osmolality. Plasma arginine vasopressin (AVP) may also be obtained at the end of the fluid deprivation period to provide data about the status of the patient's antidiuretic hormone.
- A test of the response to exogenously administered pitressin or the synthetic analogue of arginine vasopressin (DDAVP)[37] can be performed at the end of the test described above or may be conducted as a separate procedure at another time. DDAVP (10 to 20 μg) is given intranasally at the end of the fluid deprivation period and the patient is monitored for further 3 to 4 h. Fluid intake to match urine output is allowed during this phase of the test. Urine and plasma samples are obtained at the end of the test (labeled U_3 and S_3, respectively) for determining osmolality. Careful attention is paid to fluid intake during the next 12 h to prevent water intoxication and hyponatremia.

It is important to note that children with a known defect in urinary concentrating ability should not be subjected to prolonged water restriction, since severe dehydration, shock, and compromise of renal perfusion may result in a further deterioration of their renal function. In such patients, a less intense water deprivation test lasting only 7 h, as proposed by Frasier et al.,[38] may be advised. As an added safeguard, the test should be performed during the day and may be abandoned if the patient loses more than 3 percent of body weight at any time during the test.

INTERPRETATION OF THE TEST

Edelmann et al.[31] noted that mean urinary osmolality following a 12-h fluid deprivation test was 1089 mosmol/L (range: 873 to 1305 mosmol/L) in children

TABLE 1–8. Diagnostic Findings Differentiating Nephrogenic from Idiopathic Diabetes Insipidus in Children

	Initial Values				Values after Water Deprivation				Values after Vasopressin				
	U_1	S_1	$\frac{U_1}{S_1}$	Urine SG	U_2	S_2	$\frac{U_2}{S_2}$	Urine SG	U_3	S_3	$\frac{U_3}{S_3}$	Urine SG	Vasopressin Preparation Used
Idiopathic diabetes insipidus	95	293	0.32	1.002	219	308	0.69	1.005	552	300	1.84	1.019	DDAVP
Nephrogenic diabetes insipidus	68	297	0.23	1.005	107	329	0.33		68	330	0.21	1.004	DDAVP
									110	320	0.34	1.007	Pitressin-in-oil

SG = specific gravity.

[a]Not obtained.

Note: Urine and serum osmolality (U_1, U_2, U_3, S_1, S_2, S_3) expressed as mosmol/L at various times during the test as described in the text.

Source: From Hendricks SA, Lippe B, Kaplan SA, Lee W-N P: Differential diagnosis of diabetes insipidus: Use of DDAVP to terminate the seven-hour water deprivation test. *J Pediatr* 98:244, 1981. Modified and reproduced by permission.

TABLE 1–9. Nephrogenic Causes of Diabetes Insipidus in Children

Primary
Secondary
- Prematurity
- Chronic renal failure
- Acute tubular necrosis (ATN): nonoliguric variety and during diuretic phase of oliguric ATN
- Posturinary tract obstruction diuresis
- Developmental renal malformations: renal dysplasia, cystic renal diseases
- Sickle cell disease and trait
- Hypokalemic nephropathy, hypercalcemia
- Drugs: demeclocycline, amphotericin B, lithium

aged 2 to 16 years. Children with normal renal concentrating ability should be able to achieve a U_1/S_1 ratio above 1.5 following a fluid deprivation test. Determining the response to pitressin or DDAVP and pitressin is essential in differentiating various types of polyuria. Patients with central diabetes insipidus demonstrate a decrease in urine output, they also show an increase in urine osmolality and a U_3/S_3 ratio that exceeds 1.5. Lack of such a response to DDAVP and/or pitressin suggests the diagnosis of nephrogenic diabetes insipidus (Table 1–8). Nephrogenic causes of diabetes insipidus are given in Table 1–9.

RENAL TUBULAR ACIDIFICATION FUNCTION

Maintaining acid-base status is an important aspect of renal tubular function. Renal regulation of acid-base balance involves (1) reclaiming bicarbonate filtered by the glomeruli and (2) excreting the hydrogen ions and generating new bicarbonate to replenish the bicarbonate pool of the body. Detailed evaluation of the functions maintaining renal acid-base status is required in patients who are suspected of having renal tubular acidosis. These patients have a characteristic hyperchloremic metabolic acidosis that is associated with a normal anion gap. Urine pH in such patients is inappropriately high (>5.5) in face of metabolic acidosis. Tests available to diagnose various types of renal tubular acidosis are discussed in detail in Chap. 21.

SUMMARY

The kidney is a complex organ that is responsible for maintaining fluid and electrolyte balance, fine tuning acid-base status, and excreting nitrogenous waste products. Evaluation of all these functional aspects of the kidney requires an understanding of its workings. In order to obtain an accurate assessment of renal function, both glomerular and tubular functions need to be evaluated. Measuring BUN and serum creatinine provides a reasonably accurate estimate of glomerular filtration rate. This can be further supplemented by estimation of creatinine clearance based on one of the several (Schwartz's) formulas. This method of estimating creatinine clearance is especially helpful in young children, in whom obtaining an accurate timed urine collection is always difficult. Urinalysis and measurement of serum electrolytes constitute essential components of evaluating renal functions; these tests provide information regarding renal concentrating function and urinary acidification. Further evaluation of tubular functions such as maximal renal concentrating ability and excretion of ammonium and titratable acids, of course, requires detailed testing.

REFERENCES

1. Kanwar YS, Liu ZZ, Kashihara N, et al: Current status of the structural and functional basis of glomerular filtration and proteinuria. *Semin Nephrol* 11:390, 1991.
2. Rennke HG, Patel Y, Venkatachalam MA: Effect of molecular change on glomerular permeability to proteins in the rat: Clearance studies using neutral, anionic and cationic horseradish peroxidase. *Kidney Int* 13:278, 1978.
3. Kanwar YS: Biophysiology of glomerular filtration and proteinuria. *Lab Invest* 51:7, 1984.
4. Starling EH: On the absorption of fluids from the connective tissue spaces. *J Physiol* 19:312, 1896.
5. Hoberman HD, Sims EAH, Peters JH: Creatine and creatinine metabolism in the normal adult studied with the aid of isotope nitrogen. *J Biol Chem* 172:45, 1948.
6. Doolan PD, Alpen EL, Theil GB, et al: A clinical appraisal of the plasma concentration and endogenous clearance of creatinine. *Am J Med* 32:65, 1962.
7. Lubowitz H, Slatopolsky E, Shankel S, et al: Glomerular ultrafiltration: Determination in patients with chronic renal disease. *JAMA* 199:252, 1967.
8. Jacobsen FK, Christensen CK, Morgensen CE, et al: Pronounced increase in serum creatinine concentration after eating cooked meat. *Br Med J* 1:1049, 1979.
9. Levey AS: Measurement of renal function in chronic renal disease. *Kidney Int* 38:167, 1990.
10. Schwartz GJ, Haycock GB, Spitzer A: Plasma creatinine and urea in children: Normal values for age and sex. *J Pediatr* 88:828, 1976.
11. Schwartz GJ, Haycock GB, Edelmann CM, et al: A simple estimate of glomerular filtration rate in children derived from body length and plasma creatinine. *Pediatrics* 58:259, 1976.
12. Schwartz GJ, Feld LG, Langford DJ: A simple estimate of glomerular filtration rate in full-term infants during the first year of life. *J Pediatr* 104:849, 1984.
13. Schwartz GJ, Gauthier B: A simple estimate of glomerular filtration rate in adolescent boys. *J Pediatr* 106:522, 1985.
14. Brion LP, Fleischman AR, McCarton C, et al: A simple estimate of glomerular filtration rate in low birth weight infants during the first year of life: Noninvasive assessment of body composition and growth. *J Pediatr* 109:698, 1986.
15. Mitch WE, Walser M, Buffington GA, et al: A simple method for estimating progression of chronic renal failure. *Lancet* 2:1326, 1976.
16. Reimold EW: Chronic progressive renal failure: Rate of progression monitored by change of serum creatinine. *Am J Dis Child* 135:1039, 1981.
17. Arant BS, Edelmann CM, Spitzer A: The congruence of creatinine and insulin clearances in children: Use of Technicon Auto Analyser. *J Pediatr* 81:559, 1972.

18 Chantler C, Barret TM: Estimation of GFR from plasma clearance of 51 chromium eidetic acid. *Arch Dis Child* 47:613, 1972.

19 Shemesh O, Golbetz H, Kriss JP, et al: Limitations of creatinine clearance as a filtration marker in glomerulopathic patients. *Kidney Int* 28:830, 1985.

20 Smith HW, Goldring W, Chasis H: The measurement of the tubular excretory mass, effective blood flow and filtration rate in the normal human kidney. *J Clin Invest* 17:263, 1938.

21. Richardson JA, Philbin PE: The one hour creatinine clearance rate in healthy men. *JAMA* 216:987, 1971.

22. Stuphen JL: Anthropometric determinants of creatinine excretion in preterm infants. *Pediatrics* 69:719, 1982.

23. Al-Dahhan J, Stimmler L, Haycock GB: Urinary creatinine excretion in the newborn. *Arch Dis Child* 63:398, 1988.

24. Reynolds EL, Clark LC: Creatinine excretion, growth progress and body structure in normal children. *Child Dev* 18:155, 1947.

25. Piepsz A, Denis R, Ham RH, et al: A simple method of measuring separate glomerular filtration rate using a single injection of ^{99m}Tc-DTPA and scintillation camera. *J Pediatr* 93:769, 1978.

26. Chantler C, Barratt TM: Estimation of glomerular filtration rate from plasma clearance of 51-chromium eidetic acid. *Arch Dis Child* 47:613, 1972.

27. Oh W, Oh MA, Lind J: Renal function and the blood volume in the newborn infants related to placental transfusion. *Acta Paediatr Scand* 56:197, 1966.

28. Aperia A, Broberger O, Elinder G, et al: Postnatal development of renal function in pre-term and full-term infants. *Acta Paediatr Scand* 70:183, 1981.

29. Rubin M, Brick E, Rapoport M, et al: Maturation of renal function in childhood: Clearance studies. *J Clin Invest* 28:1144, 1949.

30. Winberg J: The 24-hour true endogenous creatinine clearance in infants and children without renal disease. *Acta Paediatr* 48:433, 1959.

31. Edelmann CM Jr, Barnett HL, Stark H, et al: A standardized test of renal concentrating capacity in children. *Am J Dis Child* 114:693, 1967.

32. Fisher DA, Pyle HR, Porter JC, et al: Control of water balance in the newborn. *Am J Dis Child* 106:51, 1963.

33. Hansen JDL, Smith CA: Effect of withholding fluid in the immediate postnatal period. *Pediatrics* 12:99, 1953.

34. Polacek E, Vocel J, Neugebauerova L, et al: The osmotic concentrating ability in healthy infants and children. *Arch Dis Child* 40:291, 1965.

35. Svenningsen NW, Aronson AS: Postnatal development of renal concentrating capacity as estimated by DDAVP-test in normal and asphyxiated neonates. *Biol Neonate* 25:230, 1974.

36. Edelmann CM Jr, Barnett HL, Troupkou V: Renal concentrating mechanism in newborn infants: Effect of dietary protein and water content, role of urea, and responsiveness to antidiuretic hormone. *J Clin Invest* 39:1062, 1960.

37. Hendricks SA, Lippe B, Kaplan SA, et al: Differential diagnosis of diabetes insipidus: Use of DDAVP to terminate the seven-hour water deprivation test. *J Pediatr* 98:244, 1981.

38. Frasier SD, Kutnik LA, Schmidt RT, et al: A water deprivation test for the diagnosis of diabetes insipidus in children. *Am J Dis Child* 114:157, 1967.

2

URINALYSIS

Kanwal K. Kher

Urinalysis (UA) is a valuable diagnostic aid for the evaluation of patients with renal disease. This use of UA dates back to the Middle Ages.[1,2] The practice of diagnosing diseases by examining the urine was known as *uroscopy* and was highly regarded as a science during that era. It is clear from a review of the literature that many authorities on the subject made exaggerated claims about their ability to diagnose diseases by the color and smell of the urine alone.[2] By present standards, some of these claims may be considered quackery. The development of the modern microscope refined the technique of examining urinary sediment, enhanced the usefulness of UA, and legitimized UA as a diagnostic tool. More recently, phase contrast microscopy for cellular morphology and determination of red cell volume have been included as additional components of UA for the investigation of renal disorders. The commercial availability of reagent test strips for the chemical analysis of urine has rendered UA more practical and accessible in a busy office practice.

COLLECTING URINE

Asepsis and midstream urine collection, as required for urine culture, are unnecessary for samples that are to be evaluated by UA alone. However, urine should be collected and stored in a clean container. Urine can be obtained on voluntary voiding in older children but obtaining urine samples in infants usually necessitates the use of some type of collection device. The most common such device consists of a plastic bag that is applied to the infant's perineum (U-Bag, Hollister, Illinois) so that the urine is collected when the child voids spontaneously. Sometimes, the Perez reflex may be used to obtain urine from infants. This involves holding the infant face-down in one hand and firmly stroking its back in the paraspinal area with the other hand in order to stimulate voiding (Fig. 2–1). An assistant then collects the urine in a container.

In order to preserve cell structure in the sediment, UA is best performed on a freshly voided urine. In case delay in examining the urine is anticipated, the sample may be refrigerated. Acidification of the urine to a pH of 6.0 also helps

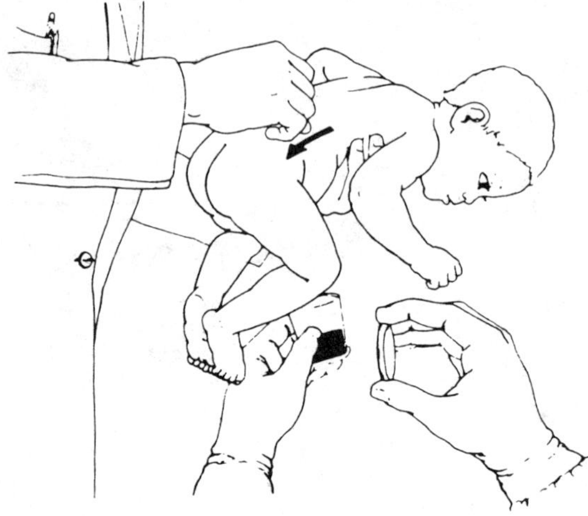

FIG. 2–1. Perez reflex to induce urination in infants. [From Kory M, Waife SO (eds): *Kidney and Urinary Tract Infections*. Eli Lilly and Company, 1971. Reproduced by permission.]

in preserving the architecture of cellular casts. A first morning void is preferred for determining urinary concentrating ability following overnight water deprivation.

TECHNIQUE OF URINALYSIS

Complete UA involves three essential steps: (1) observing the color and physical characteristics of the urine, (2) determining its specific gravity and chemical composition; and (3) performing a microscopic examination of the spun urinary sediment. In order to perform UA, the office laboratory should be equipped with a tabletop centrifuge, a refractometer, glass slides, cover slips, pipettes, centrifuge tubes, reagent test strips, and a light microscope. A polarizing filter is often helpful to differentiate the various crystals in urine, while a phase contrast microscope may be required for special circumstances (see below).

URINE COLOR

Normal urine is of amber color but may appear lighter following intake of a large volume of fluid. The urine's color may provide clues to several underlying renal and nonrenal disorders (Table 2–1). Red discoloration, a common clinical issue for practicing nephrologists, may be caused by the presence of blood (hematuria), hemoglobin (hemoglobinuria), or myoglobin (myoglobinuria). Urine tests positive for blood with reagent test strips (dipsticks) in all these conditions, but red blood cells (RBCs) are seen in the urinary sediment only of patients with hematuria; they are absent in those with hemoglobinuria and myoglobinuria. Features differentiating these three conditions are listed in Table 2–2. Urinary bleeding originating in the bladder and other parts of the collecting system renders the urine pink or red in color; on the other hand,

TABLE 2–1. Conditions Associated with Abnormal Urine Color

Appearance	Cause	Remarks
Colorless	Very dilute urine	Polyuria, diabetes insipidus
Cloudy	Phosphates, carbonates	Soluble in dilute acetic acid
	Urates, uric acid	Dissolve at 60°C and in alkali
	Leukocytes	Insoluble in dilute acetic acid
	Red cells ("smoky")	Lyse in dilute acetic acid
	Bacteria, yeasts	Insoluble in dilute acetic acid
	Spermatozoa	Insoluble in dilute acetic acid
	Prostatic fluid	
	Mucin, mucous threads	May be flocculent
	Calculi, "gravel"	Phosphates, oxalates
	Clumps, pus, tissue	
	Fecal contamination	Rectovesical fistula
	Radiographic dye	In acid urine
Milky	Many neutrophils (pyuria)	Insoluble in dilute acetic acid
	Fat	
	Lipiduria, opalescent	Nephrosis, crush injury—soluble in ether
	Chyluria, milky	Lymphatic obstruction—soluble in ether
	Emulsified paraffin	Vaginal creams
Yellow	Acriflavine	Green fluorescence
Yellow-orange	Concentrated urine	Dehydration, fever
	Urobilin in excess	No yellow foam
	Bilirubin	Yellow foam if sufficient bilirubin
Yellow-green	Bilirubin-biliverdin	Yellow foam
Yellow-brown	Bilirubin-biliverdin	"Beer" brown, yellow foam
Red	Hemoglobin	Positive } reagent strip for blood
	Red blood cells	Positive } reagent strip for blood
	Myoglobin	Positive } reagent strip for blood
	Porphyrin	May be colorless
	Fuscin, aniline dye	Foods, candy
	Beets	Yellow alkaline, genetic
	Menstrual contamination	Clots, mucus
Red-purple	Porphyrins	May be colorless
Red-brown	Red blood cells	
	Hemoglobin on standing	
	Methemoglobin	Acid pH
	Myoglobin	Muscle injury
	Bilifuscin (dipyrrole)	Result of unstable hemoglobin
Brown-black	Methemoglobin	Blood, acid pH
	Homogentisic acid	On standing, alkaline; alkaptonuria
	Melanin	On standing, rare
Blue-green	Indicans	Small intestine infections
	Pseudomonas infections	
	Chlorophyrll	Mouth deodorants

Source: From Bradley M, Schumann GB: Examination of Urine, in Henry JB (ed): *Clinical Diagnosis and Management by Laboratory Methods*. Philadelphia, Saunders, 1984, p. 380. Reproduced by permission.

TABLE 2–2. Clinical and Laboratory Tests Differentiating Hematuria, Hemoglobinuria, and Myoglobinuria

		Urine Dipstick					
	Urine Color	Blood	Protein	Urinary Sediment	Serum Color	Supportive/Confirmatory Test	Remarks
Hematuria	Smoky or tea-colored in glomerular hematuria, pink in nonglomerular hematuria	Positive	May be elevated	RBCs, granular or RBC casts may be seen	Clear	Document RBCs in urinary sediment	Hypotonic urine may cause RBC lysis. Urine sediment in such cases may not show RBC.
Hemoglobinuria	Pink or brown	Positive	Minimal proteinuria	Generally unremarkable. Hemosiderin within epithelial cells or as casts may be seen.	Pink	Low serum haptoglobin, normal serum CPK, negative ammonium sulfate precipitation. Spectroscopic analysis of urine and plasma for myoglobin is negative.	Disorder predisposing to intravascular hemolysis is usually present.
Myoglobinuria	Red, turns brown on standing	Positive	Moderate proteinuria	Generally unremarkable.		Normal serum haptoglobin. Elevated serum CPK. Positive urine and plasma ammonium sulfate precipitation and spectroscopic analysis for myoglobin.	Crush injury, polymyositis, or inherited muscular disorders are present.

hematuria due to glomerular diseases is rusty brown (it may also be described as "coke-" or tea-colored). Red urine may also be seen in patients with porphyrias as well as those who have ingested beets, certain food additives, or some drugs.

Leukocytes in the urine of patients with urinary tract infection usually render it cloudy. Cloudy urine may also be observed normally when excessive amounts of phosphates are present in an alkaline urine. Acidification of such a urine by the addition of a few drops of acetic acid should clear turbidity of this type. Sometimes, urates present in the urine may also make it look cloudy. Such cloudiness clears upon warming the sample to 60°C. Prostatic secretions and spermatozoa in the urine of a healthy adolescent male may render the urine somewhat turbid, and this does not clear on warming or acidification. Mucous threads may someimtes be observed in patients with urinary tract infection or those with urinary diversion (such as ileal conduits).

URINARY CONCENTRATION

One of the key functions of the kidney is to modulate fluid balance by regulating the renal excretion of water. This is achieved by concentrating or diluting the urine in the states of water deprivation and water overload, respectively. In addition to the structural and functional integrity of the nephrons, renal concentrating ability is also dependent on the presence of an appropriate amount of circulating antidiuretic hormone (ADH), or vasopressin. Urinary concentrating ability may be one of the first kidney functions to be affected by renal parenchymal diseases, especially those involving the tubulointerstitium. Urinary concentration can be assessed by determining either specific gravity or osmolality.

SPECIFIC GRAVITY

Specific gravity is defined as a ratio between the weight of a defined volume of urine and that of the same volume of distilled water. Since the weight of urine is determined by the number of dissolved solute particles, specific gravity indirectly reflects the concentration of these solutes in urine. In general, a higher specific gravity indicates a more concentrated urine. However, the presence of heavier solutes such as proteins, glucose, and radiocontrast materials will increase the specific gravity of the urine significantly and out of proportion to the number of dissolved solutes in the sample. This represents a limitation of the use of specific gravity as a method for measuring urinary concentration. Corrected specific gravity in the presence of glucose and protein can be calculated by subtracting 0.004 and 0.003 from the measured specific gravity for each gram per deciliter of glucose and protein present in the urine sample, respectively. The term *isothenuria* is used to denote a fixed low urine specific gravity of 1.010, while *hyposthenuria* indicates specific gravity of 1.007 or less.

Urinary specific gravity is determined by the Total Solids Refractometer (American Optical Company), an instrument based on the principle that the refractive index of any solution is determined by the number of particles dissolved in it. Thus, urine with a greater number of dissolved particles—in other words, a more concentrated urine—will have a higher refractive index and, accordingly, a higher specific gravity. A refractometer uses only one or two drops of urine to analyze specific gravity, which is read directly from the scale within the instrument. Recently, several types of reagent test strips have incorporated an indirect method of determining specific gravity (e.g., Ames N-Multistix SG). The polyelectrolyte reagents in the test strip for specific gravity respond to changes in the ionic concentration of the urine samples being tested. Urinary solute ions react with the polyelectrolyte in the test strip, releasing free acid radicals which trigger a change in the test strip's pH. This change is detected by a pH indicator present in the test strip; the degree of the change determines the specific gravity. By this method, urinary specific gravity can be measured in the range of 1.000 through 1.030 in increments of 0.005.

It may be mentioned that specific gravity can also be determined by another, older instrument known as the *urinometer*. Because this instrument requires a large volume of urine (15 to 20 mL) and is cumbersome to use, it has been abandoned for the more convenient technology now available.

OSMOLALITY

In contrast to specific gravity, *urine osmolality* refers to the number of osmotically active molecules of solute dissolved in a unit of solution and is represented as mosmol/L of water. Determination of osmolality is, therefore, a more accurate method of evaluating urinary concentration than is specific gravity. In the absence of protein, glucose, or radiocontrast materials, however, urinary specific gravity bears a close relationship to urinary osmolality (Fig.2–2).

Osmolality is determined by freezing-point depression using an instrument called an *osmometer*. The test is based on the principle that the freezing point of any solution is determined by the number of solute particles dissolved in it. The presence of 1 osmol (or 1000 mosmol) of solute in one 1 kg of water depresses the freezing point of the solution by 1.86°C. Thus, a lower freezing point denotes a higher osmolality. Another way of measuring osmolality is by the vapor pressure method.

Urine osmolality is generally not determined in the office setting, since it calls for sophisticated equipment. An approximate estimation of osmolality based on the results of specific gravity can be made by the following formula[3,4]:

$$\text{Urine osmolality} = (\text{specific gravity} - 1.000) \times 40{,}000$$

The concentration of a random sample of urine, in terms of either specific gravity or osmolality, provides little information about the concentrating ability of the kidney. A water deprivation test is required to assess renal concentrating ability. (This test is discussed in detail in Chap. 1.) Maximal urine concentrating ability is age-dependent in infancy and early childhood and almost reaches adult capacity by age 2 (Fig. 2–3). Renal concentrating ability is impaired in patients with chronic renal failure and renal diseases that primarily affect the renal tubules and interstitium. These include chronic pyelonephritis, sickle cell

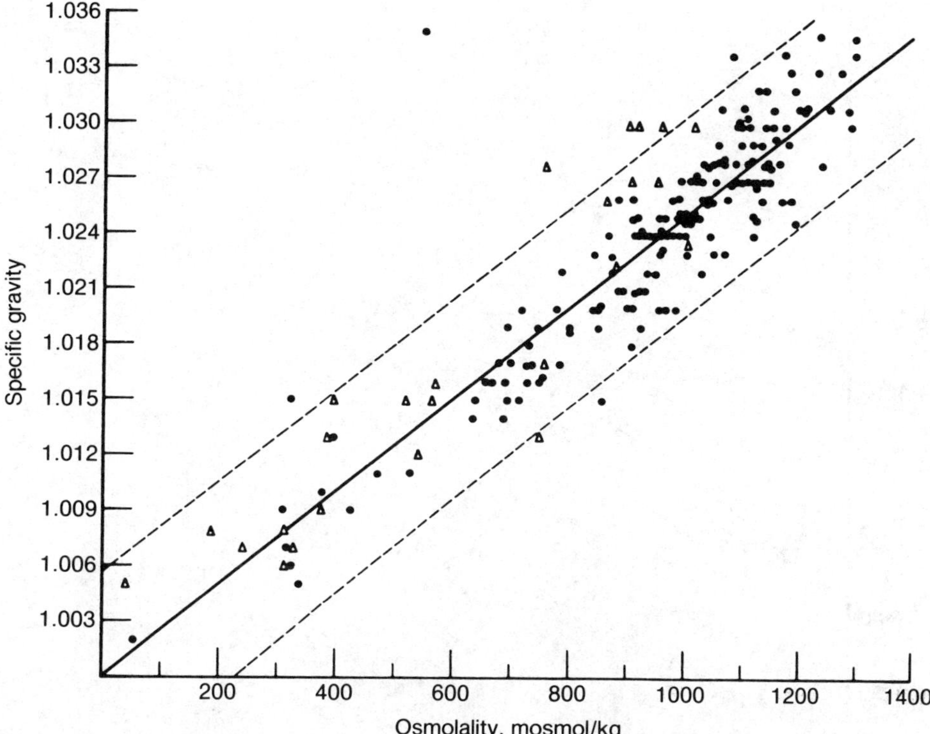

FIG. 2–2. Relationship of urinary osmolality and specific gravity. (From Edelmann CM Jr, Barnett HL, Stark H, et al: A standard test of renal concentrating capacity in children. *Am J Dis Child* 114:639, 1967. Copyright © 1967 American Medical Association. Reproduced by permission.)

anemia, interstitial nephritis, acute tubular necrosis, hypokalemic nephropathy, and hypercalcemia. Failure of the posterior pituitary to secrete vasopressin (central diabetes insipidus) or renal tubular unresponsiveness to the hormone (nephrogenic diabetes insipidus) is also characterized by inability to concentrate urine.

CHEMICAL ANALYSIS

The chemical analysis of urine has been made convenient and practical by the development of reagent test strips that provide an instant report about the chemical constitution of the test sample. Several types of reagent test strips are commercially available for office use. Most consist of plastic strips with individual absorbent pads that are impregnated with chemical reagents. Each area of the test strip is designed to detect and quantitate a single chemical constituent in urine. The test strip is dipped in the urine sample and allowed to stand for

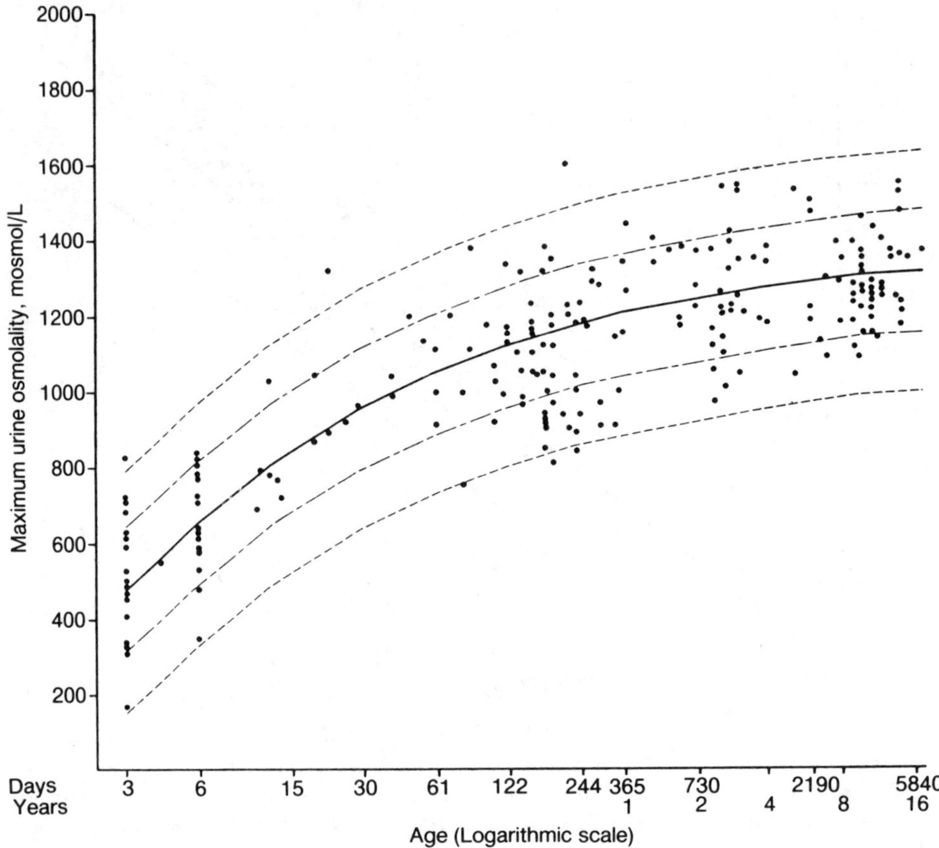

FIG. 2–3. Maximum urine osmolality in children aged 3 days through 16 years. (From Polacek E, Vocel J, Neugebauerova M, et al: The osmotic concentrating ability in healthy infants and children. *Arch Dis Child* 40:291, 1965. Reproduced by permission.)

the time interval recommended by the manufacturer. A change in the color of any component of the test strip is compared with the standard provided with the kit (usually on the container label), and the results are noted in terms of either a semiquantitative scale (e.g., trace to 4+) or mg/dL values.

URINE pH

Renal excretion of endogenously produced acid is an important aspect of maintaining a normal acid-base equilibrium. The degree of acidification of urine is assessed in clinical laboratories by determining the pH using either reagent test strips or Nitrazine Paper. For a more accurate assessment, urine pH may be measured by a pH meter. Urine pH should always be measured in a freshly voided sample, since standing permits the bacterial breakdown of urea to ammonia as well as loss of carbon dioxide by evaporation, both of which falsely raise the sample's pH. The normal pH of urine varies from 5.0 to 8.0. A high urine pH in face of systemic metabolic acidosis is indicative of a defect in renal acidification (renal tubular acidosis). A persistently alkaline urine with normal acid-base status may be encountered in individuals consuming a vegetarian diet.

PROTEIN

Except when it is of postural nature, proteinuria is considered an important indicator of renal parenchymal diseases. Samples of urine can be checked with any of the commercially available reagent test strips for a semiquantitative estimation of proteinuria. The test strip for the detection of protein consists of an absorbent area impregnated with tetrabromophenol, which changes its color from yellow in the unaltered state to green or blue with increasing concentrations of protein in the urine. A highly alkaline or a concentrated urine may lead to falsely higher semiquantitative results by this method. The reagent strip is more sensitive to albumin than globulin in the urine.

Sulfosalicylic acid precipitation can also be used as a semiquantitative method of estimating urine protein. The test is performed by placing 3 mL of urine in a test tube and adding an equal volume of 3 percent sulfosalicylic acid solution. The test tube is then shaken to mix the two solutions and allowed to stand. Modifications of the procedure include using 2 drops of 20 percent sulfosalicylic acid per milliliter of urine. The degree of turbidity is noted and semiquantitative estimation of proteinuria is made, as shown in Table 2–3.

For the quantitation of urinary protein, a timed collection of urine, preferably over 24 h, is necessary. Normal children and adults excrete a small amount of protein in urine. The range of daily urinary protein excretion varies with age but does not exceed 250 mg in older children.[5] Ratio of the urinary protein (U_p) to the urinary creatinine (U_{cr}) obtained in a spot urine sample has been shown to correlate well with proteinuria assessed in a timed urine collection.[6] A U_p/U_{cr} ratio of 0.2 is considered normal in children more than 2 years of age.[7] U_p/U_{cr} ratio exceeding 3.5 corresponds to nephrotic-range proteinuria in adults;[6] the same value is applicable for children with proteinuria.[7] U_p/U_{cr} is especially useful in following proteinuria in patients in whom a timed urine collection is difficult to obtain.

TABLE 2–3. Semiquantitative Estimation of Urinary Protein by the Sulfosalicylic Acid Precipitation Test

Degree of Turbidity	Interpretation
No turbidity	Negative results
Slight turbidity	Trace (20 mg/dL)
Turbidity without granule formation	1+ (50 mg/dL)
Turbidity with granule formation	2+ (200 mg/dL)
Turbidity with flocculation and granule formation	3+ (500 mg/dL)
Precipitated protein	4+ (1000 mg/dL or more)

ful in following proteinuria in patients in whom a timed urine collection is difficult to obtain.

Proteinuria may be postural or fixed. *Postural proteinuria* (also known as *orthostatic proteinuria*) is demonstrable only when the individual has assumed an upright posture for some time and disappears when he or she lies down. Postural proteinuria is usually encountered in older children who are otherwise well, is of moderate degree, and does not usually reach nephrotic proportions.[8] In contrast, proteinuria that is demonstrated persistently and is not postural in character is known as *fixed proteinuria.* By implication, fixed proteinuria indicates an underlying renal disorder.

Testing for postural proteinuria can usually be done at home by the patient. The patient is directed to empty his or her bladder prior to going to bed at night. On the following morning, the patient is asked to obtain a sample of the first void immediately upon waking up—even before brushing the teeth. Multiple urine samples are collected during the day at various levels of physical activity; at least one is obtained following some form of exercise. The patient can test the urine for protein by using reagent test strips (dipsticks). The results are then recorded, along with the type of activity undertaken by the patient at the corresponding time. Alternatively, the urine samples may be tested in the physician's office. Absence of proteinuria in the first morning void with increasing amount of protein noted during the day and with activity suggests the diagnosis of postural proteinuria. The subject of proteinuria is discussed in detail in Chap. 6.

BLOOD

Blood in the urine, or hematuria, is a common manisfestation of a variety of renal diseases. The test for hematuria is based on the detection of hemoglobin that is liberated in the urine or on the test strip upon lysis of the red blood cells (RBCs). The hemoglobin-detecting reagent strip contains orthotoluidine and buffered organic peroxide. In the presence of hematuria, the color of the test strip changes to blue. Since the test strips detect heme moiety, both hemoglobin and myoglobin produce a positive reaction. When such a positive result is obtained *without* concomitant evidence of RBCs in the urine, intravascular hemolysis resulting in hemoglobinemia and hemoglobinuria or myoglobinuria should be suspected. Further differentiation of the three disorders is outlined in Table 2–2. Significance of hematuria in the diagnosis of renal disease is discussed in detail in Chap. 5.

GLUCOSE

Most of the presently available multiple-reagent urine testing strips can detect glucose qualitatively. These test strips specifically react to the presence of glucose. In case the urinary excretion of other sugars requires evaluation, testing with Clinitest or Benedict's reagent may be indicated. Excretion of glucose in urine (also known as *glucosuria* or *glycosuria*) may be due to either diabetes mellitus or a defect in the absorption of glucose in the proximal renal tubules, as in Fanconi syndrome, heavy metal poisoning, and interstitial nephritis.

NITRITE

Detection of urinary nitrites is considered to be diagnostic of urinary tract infection. This test is based on the fact that dietary nitrate excreted in the urine is transformed into nitrite by the nitrate-splitting bacteria that may invade the urinary tract and cause infection. For this reaction to take place, bacteria require incubation with urinary nitrate within urinary bladder. Under circumstances where urine cannot incubate with the infecting organisms, as in patients with increased frequency of micturition or those in whom urine bypasses anatomic urinary bladder (e.g., in the presence of a ureterostomy, nephrostomy, or ileal loop), the nitrite test may yield false-negative results. The test may also be false-negative if the urinary tract infection is caused by bacteria that do not split nitrate.

MICROSCOPIC EXAMINATION

GENERAL PRINCIPLES

Examination of urinary sediment provides important clues about the nature of renal disease. For an optimal evaluation of urinary sediment, about 10 to 12 mL of freshly voided urine is poured into a conical test tube and spun in a centrifuge at 3000 rpm for 3 min. The supernatant is then drained from the tube and the sediment resuspended in about 0.5 mL of urine in the test tube. A drop of the resultant suspension is withdrawn by pipette and placed on a slide, which is covered with a cover slip. The slide is examined under the low power (10 × 10) of a light microscope. It is helpful to decrease the intensity of the microscope's light source by lowering the condenser while examining urinary sediment, since identification of cells and casts, particularly hyaline casts, is difficult under bright light. The slide is scanned systematically from edge to edge, and any areas that need further scrutiny are examined under high power (40 × 10). The cells (Table 2–4) and casts (Table 2–5) in the slide preferentially localize toward the edges of the cover slip, and these areas should be searched carefully. Experience is necessary to identify the various cellular and formed elements accurately.

For better identification of urinary cells and casts, the urinary sediment may be stained with various commercially available stains. We have found staining of the urinary sediment with Sedi Stain (Clay Adams) to be helpful, quick, and easy under office conditions. One drop of the urinary sediment is mixed in the test tube with a drop of the stain, and the mixture can be examined immediately. Phase contrast microscopy is superior to conventional light microscopy in delineating the outlines of cells and casts. This technique is of particular interest to the nephrologist who wishes to differentiate glomerular from nonglomerular hematuria using RBC morphology. A conventional light microscope

TABLE 2–4. Diagnostic Significance of Cells in the Urinary Sediment

Formed Element Category	Detected in Normal Urine	Clinical Significance
Red blood cells	<5/HPF	Dysmorphic RBCs seen in glomerular bleeding. Nondysmorphic RBCs in hypercalciuria, hyperuricemia, sickle cell trait, and nonglomerular bleeding.
Leukocytes	<5/HPF	Urinary tract infection, acute interstitial nephritis, acute glomerulonephritis.
Renal tubular epithelial cells	Occasional	Large numbers are seen in tubular disorders, acute tubular necrosis, tubulointerstitial nephritis, and (sometimes) renal cystic diseases.
Oval fat bodies	No	Nephrotic syndrome of any etiology—especially in minimal change nephrotic syndrome. These appear as "Maltese crosses" under polarized light.

TABLE 2–5. Diagnostic Significance of Casts in the Urinary Sediment

Formed Element Category	Detected in Normal Urine	Clinical Significance
Hyaline casts	Occasional	Dehydration, following exercise, fever, diuretic use, congestive cardiac failure, and nephrotic syndrome
Granular casts	Occasional	Dehydration, glomerulonephritis, tubulointerstitial diseases, and acute transplant rejection
Red cell casts	None	Glomerulonephritis
Leukocytes casts	None	Acute pyelonephritis, acute interstitial nephritis, acute glomerulonephritis
Broad waxy casts	None	Chronic renal disease possibly associated with tubular hypertrophy
Fatty casts	None	Severe proteinuria, nephrotic syndrome
Tubular cell casts	None	Acute tubular necrosis, acute allograft rejection, cytomegalovirus infection, heavy metal poisoning

can be fitted with a polarizing filter which helps in identifying crystals and other noncellular sediments in the urine. Polarized light is particularly helpful in identifying fat-laden epithelial cells or oval fat bodies. Fat within these cells appears in a characteristic Maltese-cross pattern under polarizing light.

RED BLOOD CELLS

Red blood cells are normal constituents of urine; excretion of 500,000 RBCs/24h (assessed by Addis count) is considered normal.[9] This generally amounts to less than 1 to 2 cells per high power field (HPF) in the spun urinary sediment of normal healthy children. Hematuria is defined as an erythrocyte count exceeding 5 cells per HPF in centrifuged urine sediment. Red blood cells in urine appear as light-refractive biconcave disks under high-power magnification. They may become deformed and hemolyze easily in a dilute or alkaline urine. It has been shown that dysmorphic urinary RBCs are of glomerular origin.[10] Although it is possible to identify such dysmorphic urinary RBCs by routine light microscopy, they are best visualized with the help of a phase contrast microscope (Fig. 2–4). Pollock et al.[11] recently contested the view that urinary RBC dysmorphism represents glomerular hematuria. They demonstrated that RBC dysmorphism could also be seen in patients with hematuria following renal biopsy. In their view, dysmorphic RBCs indicate hematuria of renal rather than glomerular origin. It has also been suggested that RBC volume may be of

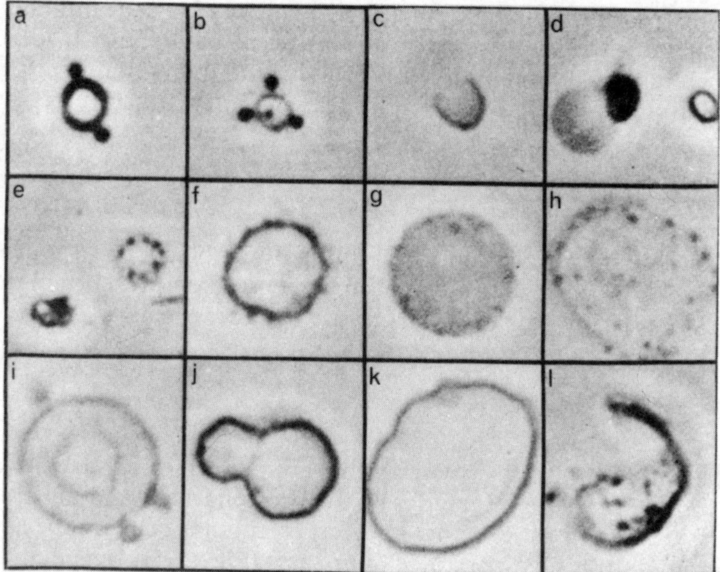

FIG. 2–4. Dysmorphic red cells in hematuria of glomerular origin. Shown is the variety of RBC shapes that can be considered dysmorphic. (From Fairly KF, Birch DF: Hematuria: A simple method for identifying glomerular bleeding. *Kidney Int* 71:105, 1982. Reproduced by permission.)

diagnostic help in differentiating glomerular hematuria from nonglomerular hematuria.[12] Urinary RBCs associated with glomerular diseases are smaller in size than those stemming from nonglomerular hematuria. Further work, however, must be done in this field before the test can be utilized in clinical practice. Hematuria may be encountered in renal parenchymal diseases such as glomerulonephritis or interstitial nephritis, disorders associated with hypercalciuria, urinary tract infection, and trauma.

LEUKOCYTES

Normal urinary sediment may contain leukocytes as well as erythrocytes. The presence of 1 to 2 leukocytes per HPF in a spun sediment is regarded as normal. Leukocytes appear as multinucleated cells that are approximately 1.5 times the size of erythrocytes. Leukocyturia is a prominent feature of urinary tract infection. It may also be seen in conditions other than urinary tract infection such as dehydration, meatal irritation, vaginitis, renal stones, interstitial nephritis, and glomerulonephritis. Lymphocytes may be present in the urine in acute renal transplant rejection, and eosinophils are seen in acute interstitial nephritis.

RENAL TUBULAR EPITHELIAL CELLS

Renal tubular cells are nucleated cells resembling leukocytes, but they are larger in size and have a single nucleus. Renal tubular cells are derived from the renal tubules; they are found in the urine of patients with renal tubular damage such as in acute tubular necrosis and acute interstitial nephritis. Sometimes, renal tubular cells may also be seen in patients with cystic renal diseases.

SQUAMOUS CELLS

These cells originate from the mucosal lining of the bladder and appear as large square cells with a single centrally placed nucleus. Their presence in the urinary sediment is not of any particular diagnostic significance.

URINARY CASTS

Urinary casts are cylindrical structures that are present in the urinary sediment. They are formed in the renal tubules by the precipitation of Tamm-Horsfall tubuloprotein. Cells such as RBCs, leukocytes, or tubular cells trapped within the tubuloprotein matrix give rise to cellular casts (Fig. 2–5). Degeneration of the cells incorporated in the protein matrix probably occurs and leads to the formation of granular casts. Urinary casts carry different diagnostic and prognostic connotations depending on the structure and type of cell present in the cast.

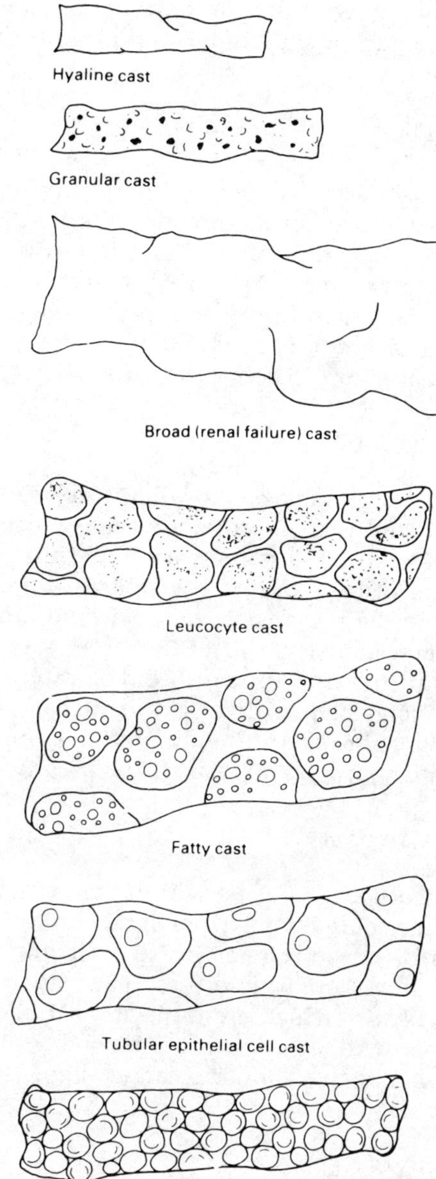

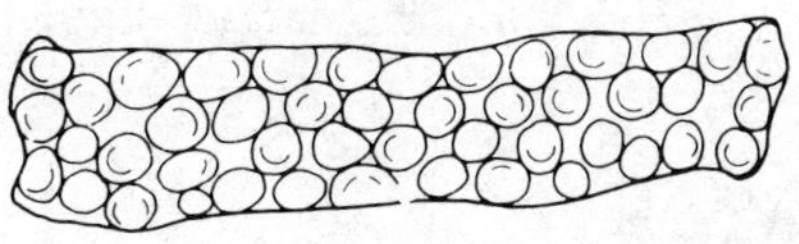

FIG. 2–5. Urinary casts. [From Sweny P, Farrington K, Moorhead JF (eds): *The Kidney and Its Disorders*. London, Blackwell Scientific Publications, 1989. Reproduced by permission.]

HYALINE CASTS

These casts are made of Tamm-Horsfall protein and look like translucent, cylindrical structures with tapering ends. Hyaline casts may be missed if the light source of the microscope is too bright. A few hyaline casts (0 to 2 per HPF) may normally be seen in urine, but greater numbers are seen in fever, following exercise, with dehydration, upon diuretic use, in congestive heart failure, and in nephrotic syndrome. Hyaline casts can be easily dissolved by alkalinizing the urine.

WAXY CASTS

Waxy casts are similar to hyaline casts in their translucent and refractile appearance but are broader in size. Unlike hyaline casts, waxy casts are resistant to alkalinization. Their origin is unclear; they may derive from degenerating granular casts. Waxy casts are seen in many chronic renal diseases and are not diagnostic of any specific renal pathology. Large waxy casts, also known as *broad casts* (or renal failure casts), are characteristically seen in patients with renal failure. These casts usually have blunt ends.

RED CELL CASTS

These casts appear as cylindrical structures of the urinary glycoprotein matrix (Tamm-Horsfall protein) within which the round, discoid RBCs are embedded. The red cell casts can vary from short segments to elongated structures. Disruption of casts during the centrifugation and resuspension of urine may sometimes be responsible for a variation in the size of the RBC casts that are seen. In the course of time, RBCs in these casts undergo degeneration, leaving a granular cast with brownish discoloration. The presence of RBC casts in the urine denotes hematuria of glomerular origin and supports the diagnosis of glomerulonephritis. Another important component of glomerulonephritis, in addition to hematuria and casts, is the presence of proteinuria.

FATTY CASTS

Incorporation of fat within the Tamm-Horsfall protein gives rise to fatty casts. Viewed under polarized light, cholesterol within these casts appears as Maltese-cross structures. Fatty casts are commonly seen in patients with nephrotic syndrome. The urine of such patients may also contain structures known as *oval fat bodies,* which are fat-laden, denuded renal tubular epithelial cells. As is the case with fatty casts, oval fat bodies also demonstrate Maltese-cross appearance when viewed under polarized light.

CRYSTALS

Normal urine contains several types of crystals. The presence of these structures in the urinary sediment is of limited diagnostic value except in patients who are likely to have urolithiasis. Hypercalciuria[13] and hyperuricosuria[14] have both been implicated in the etiology of hematuria, and urinary sediment in these clinical conditions may demonstrate calcium oxalate and uric acid crystals (Fig. 2–6). Hexagonal (benzene ring structure) cystine crystals in cystinuria (cystine stone formers) and fine, needlelike crystals in tyrosinosis are of diagnostic

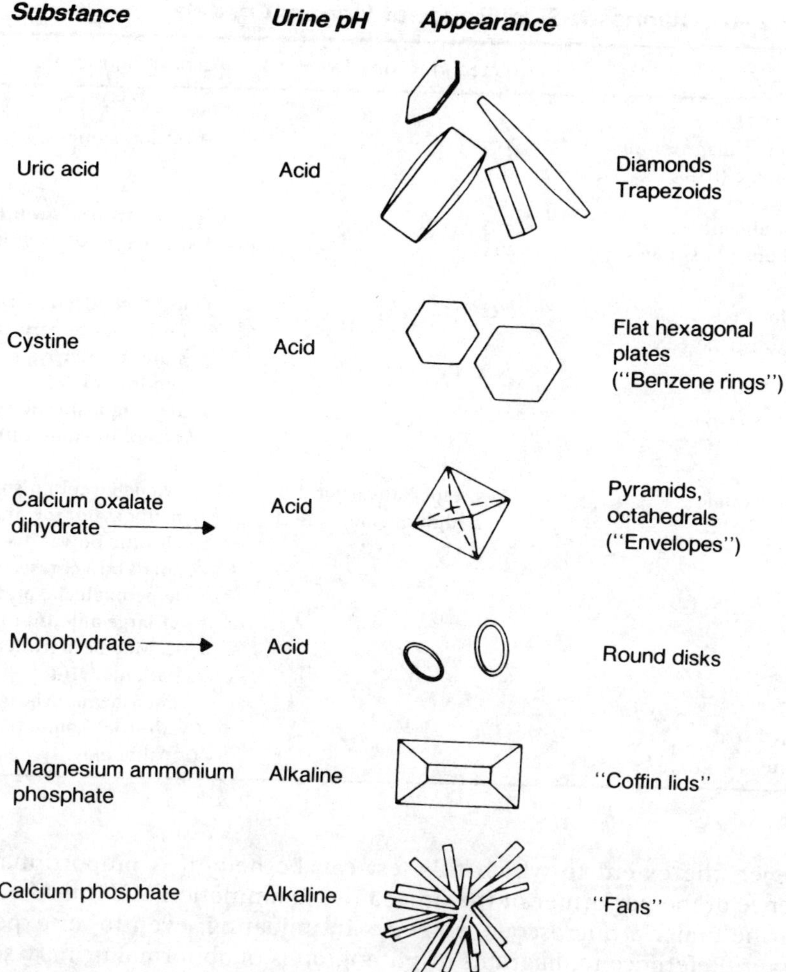

FIG. 2–6. Urinary crystals. [From Sweny P, Farrington K, Moorhead JF (eds): *The Kidney and Its Disorders.* London, Blackwell Scientific Publications, 1989. Reproduced by permission.]

value. The significance of commonly encountered urinary crystals is discussed in Table 2–6.

SUMMARY

Urinalysis is an inexpensive and easy to perform test that reveals a wealth of information about renal disease. Some have likened it to a "fluid renal biopsy."

TABLE 2–6. Diagnostic Significance of Urinary Crystals

Type of Crystals	Detected in Normal Urine	Clinical Significance
PHOSPHATES		
Ammonium magnesium phosphate (triple phosphate)	Yes	Infection stones
Calcium phosphate	Yes	Hypercalciuria, urolithiasis
Amorphous phosphate	Yes	Little diagnostic significance
URATES		
Uric acid	Yes	Gout, Lesch-Nyhan syndrome, and other hyperuricemic states (tumor lysis syndrome)
Amorphous urates	Yes	Little diagnostic significance except in stone formers
OTHERS		
Calcium oxalate	Yes, especially after a high-oxalate diet	Ethylene glycol poisoning, methoxyflurane anesthetic, chronic bowel disease, small bowel resection, hyperoxaluria, and intake of large amount of vitamin C. May be significant in patients with microhematuria.
Cystine	No	Cystinuria, homocystinuria
Tyrosine	No	Tyrosinemia

However, the extent to which this test can be helpful is proportional to the diligence of the performer of the procedure. Examination and interpretation of the urine under a microscope is always intimidating, even to an experienced observer. Reference to diagrams or photographs of abnormal urinary sediment lessens this "fear of the unknown."

REFERENCES

1. Haber MH: Pisse prophecy: A brief history of urinalysis. *Clin Lab Med* 8:415, 1988.
2. White WI: A new look at the role of urinalysis in the history of diagnostic medicine. *Clin Chem* 37:119, 1991.
3. Edelmann CM Jr, Barnett HL, Stark H, et al: A standardized test of renal concentrating capacity in children. *Am J Dis Child* 114:639, 1967.
4. Goldsmith DI: Clinical and laboratory evaluation of renal function, in Edelmann CM Jr (ed): *Pediatric Renal Disease,* Boston, Little Brown, 1978, p. 213.
5. Miltenyi M: Urinary protein excretion in healthy children. *Clin Nephrol* 12:216, 1979.

6. Ginsberg JM, Chang BS, Materese AR, et al: Use of single voided urine samples to estimate quantitative proteinuria. *N Engl J Med* 309:1543, 1983.
7. Houser M: Assessment of proteinuria using random urine samples. *J Pediatr* 104:845, 1984.
8. Rytand DA, Spreiter S: Prognosis in postural proteinuria: Forty to fifty year follow-up of six patients after diagnosis by Thomas Addis. *N Engl J Med* 305:618, 1981.
9. Addis T: The number of formed elements in the urinary sediment of normal individuals. *J Clin Invest* 2:409, 1926.
10. Fairly KF, Birch DF: Hematuria: A simple method for identifying glomerular bleeding. *Kidney Int* 21:105, 1982.
11. Pollock C, Pei-Ling L, Gyory AZ, et al: Dysmorphism of urinary red blood cells—Value in diagnosis. *Kidney Int* 36:1049, 1989.
12. Oner A, Ahmad TM, Besbas N, et al: Identification of the source of hematuria by automated measurement of mean corpuscular volume of urinary red cells. *Pediatr Nephrol* 5:54, 1991.
13. Stapelton FB, Roy S III, Noe HN, et al: Hypercalciuria in children with hematuria. *N Engl J Med* 310:1345, 1984.
14. Andres A, Parga M, Bello I, et al: Hematuria due to hypercalciuria and hyperuricosuria in adult patients. *Kidney Int* 36:96, 1989.

3

RADIOLOGY OF THE URINARY TRACT

Radiographic investigations, especially renal ultrasound and radionuclide imaging, are frequently utilized in the workup of children with renal diseases. These two imaging modalities are taking over the role that was previously reserved for the plain radiographic view of the kidney, ureter, and bladder (KUB) and intravenous pyelography (IVP). Ultrasound offers the advantage of being a noninvasive procedure that does not involve the risk of exposure to ionizing radiation and provides excellent visualization of the anatomy of the kidney and the urinary tract. Although radionuclide imaging is used primarily for studying filtration and excretory functions of the kidney, this investigative modality can also be helpful in detecting obstructive lesions of the urinary tract. This chapter discusses the practical aspects of conventional imaging techniques, including ultrasonography, and radionuclide tests employed in the diagnosis of renal diseases.

CONVENTIONAL IMAGING TECHNIQUES

Gary L. Hedlund

Until recently, it was possible to study the anatomy of the urinary tract using radiocontrast agents only. With technical improvements in ultrasound equipment, last decade has seen a progressive increase in the clinical use of ultrasound. Consequently IVP, which has been the standard imaging test for investigating the kidneys and urinary tract, is now utilized less often. Effective and safe use of radiocontrast-based conventional imaging modalities demands an understanding of the nuances of each of these diagnostic procedures.

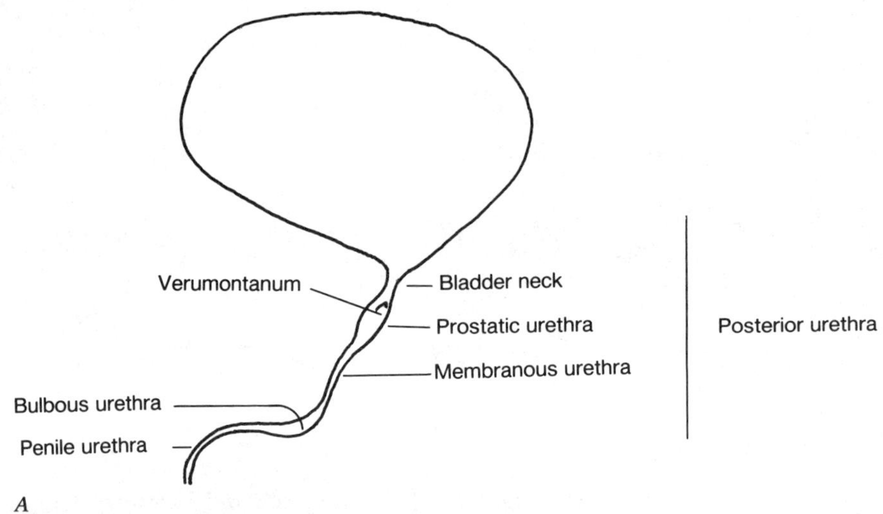

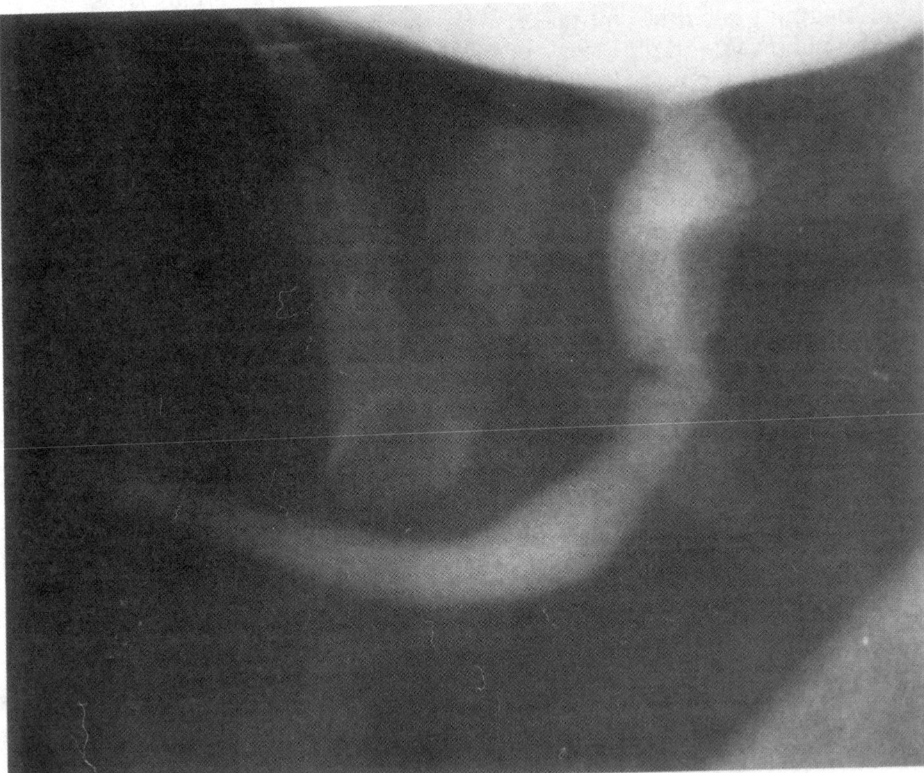

B

FIG. 3–1. Cystourethrogram. *A*. Normal anatomy of the urinary bladder and urethra in a male child. *B*. Normal cystourethrogram in a male child. *C*. Male infant with posterior urethral valves showing area of dilatation of the posterior urethra above the site of obstruction.

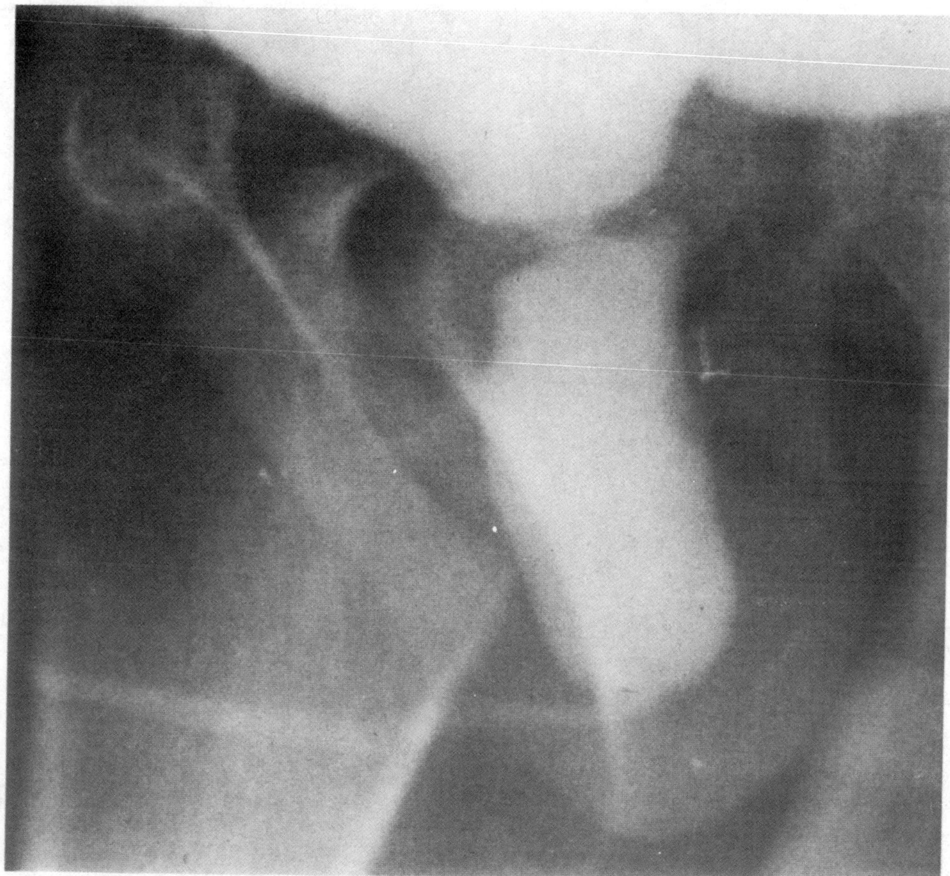

C

FIG. 3–1 (*Continued*).

VOIDING CYSTOURETHROGRAM

The voiding cystourethrogram (VCUG) using *radiocontrast* agents is the preferred method for evaluating bladder contour, vesicoureteral reflux, and urethral anatomy. Other than direct visualization by cystoscopy, the VCUG is the only method available for diagnosing posterior urethral valves in boys. The VCUG using *radionuclide* agents is usually reserved for the evaluation of vesicoureteral reflux in children who are not likely to have other anatomic abnormalities of the lower urinary tract. Radionuclide VCUG is discussed in the detail in the second half of this chapter.

PROCEDURE

Performing a VCUG necessitates aseptic catheterization of the urinary bladder. Taking the time to explain the procedure to the patient and the parent goes a long way toward ensuring a successful study. For the infant and young child, immobilization (swaddling, octagon board) is usually necessary. The parents' presence in the room is helpful, as they may comfort the child during the procedure. Catheterization of the preteen and teenager is best accomplished by a nurse or physician of the same sex. In boys over 2 years of age, the placement of a water-soluble anesthetic gel into the urethral meatus makes the process of catheterization more tolerable. Straight catheters or feeding tubes are preferred over Foley catheters. Iodinated contrast material is instilled by gravity flow into the urinary bladder through the urethral catheter. The approximate volume of contrast material to be used for a VCUG can be determined by the following formula:

$$\text{Bladder volume (ounces)} = \text{age (years)} + 2$$

Intermittent fluoroscopy is used to view the filling of the bladder and ureters, and radiographs are obtained for permanent records. The urethral catheter is then removed and radiographs are obtained during the act of voiding in order to assess the patency and structure of the urethral passage.

Standard VCUG involves a radiation exposure of 68 to 199 mrads in males and 252 to 327 mrads in females.[1] Potential complications of VCUG include infection, perforation of the bladder, vagal response, and chemical cystitis.[2] Because of the risk of retrograde spread of infection from the lower urinary tract into the kidneys, VCUG should not be attempted in patients suffering from acute lower urinary tract infection. A negative urine culture following appropriate therapy should always be sought in such patients prior to this procedure.

INTERPRETATION

The normal bladder is seen in the VCUG as a centrally placed round structure with smooth walls, and the urethra demonstrates unobstructed flow of the contrast agent (Fig. 3–1). In patients with severe bladder outlet obstruction, the muscular wall of the bladder hypertrophies, leading to a distended bladder with irregular and trabeculated walls. Posterior urethral valves are identified by the characteristic dilatation of the posterior urethra above the area of obstruction in the VCUG (Fig. 3–1*C*).

Vesicoureteral reflux can be identified on VCUG by passage of the contrast agent into the ureters. Vesicoureteral reflux is classified according to severity as follows: grade I, reflux into the ureter; grade II, reflux into the ureter and kidney without distortion of the calyces (Fig. 3–2); grade III, reflux into mildly dilated ureters and renal collecting structures without or with only slight blunting of the calyces; and grade IV, reflux into a moderately dilated ureter with ballooning of the pelvis and collecting system and with calyceal blunting; and grade V, reflux into a grossly dilated and tortuous ureter, with papillary impressions no longer visible in the majority of calyces.[3]

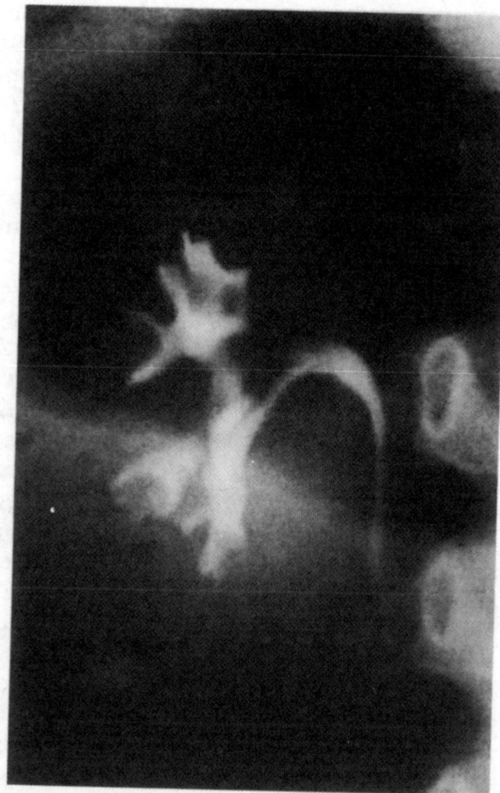

FIG. 3–2. Vesicoureteral reflux showing flow of the contrast material into the renal pelvis with no distension of the intrarenal collecting system.

INTRAVENOUS PYELOGRAPHY

Intravenous pyelography (IVP) is used for evaluating the anatomy of the kidneys and collecting system (i.e., pelvicalyceal structures, ureters, and bladder). This test also provides information regarding the perfusion and filtration functions of the kidneys. Since the kidneys of neonates cannot concentrate the injected contrast material adequately, their IVP images are sometimes of poor quality. IVP is of limited diagnostic help in patients with poor renal function, such as acute or chronic renal failure.

PROCEDURE

Intravenous pyelography is performed by injecting iodinated contrast agents intravenously, and radiographs are obtained at periodic intervals to visualize renal contour and the contrast-filled urinary collecting system. The usual dose of contrast agent used is 2 to 3 mL/kg. A scout radiograph is usually obtained prior to injecting the contrast material and may be helpful in detecting nephrolithiasis, nephrocalcinosis, or ureterolithiasis. The nephrogram or early film taken at 1 min following injection of the contrast reflects its filtration by the glomeruli and flow through the proximal renal tubules. The central renal collecting structures (calyces, infundibuli, and renal pelvis) are first visualized by the contrast at about 2 to 3 min and are well seen on the 5-min supine film. Films obtained between 5 to 15 min are used to evaluate the ureters and urinary bladder.

The contrast agents used for IVP fall into two broad categories: ionic, or hyperosmolar, and nonionic, or low osmolar (Table 3–1). Adverse reactions that occur with iodinated contrast agents are related in large part to hyperosmolality of the solutions used. The overall incidence of adverse reactions reported with the use of hyperosmolar agents is 5 to 8 percent, whereas the rate with the low osmolar agents is only about 2 percent.[4] In adults, the risk of mortality associated with the use of high osmolar contrast agents is estimated to be 1:40,000 to 1:66,500; with low osmolar contrast agents, the figure is 1:250,000 to 1:300,000.[4] Patients with a history of "allergy" and those with prior adverse reactions to iodinated contrast have an increased risk of experiencing a severe reaction. Neonates and pediatric cardiac patients receiving high osmolar contrast agents may experience pulmonary edema secondary to expansion of the intravascular volume.[5] High osmolar contrast agents are also well known to precipitate acute renal failure, especially in patients with diabetes mellitus or intravascular volume depletion such as that caused by nephrotic syndrome and dehydration.

Steps that can be taken to minimize contrast-related adverse effects include adequate hydration of the patient prior to the examination, limiting contrast volume to a maximum of 3 mL/kg of body weight, and using low osmolar contrast agents or steroid pretreatment of the patient. Low osmolar contrast agents are preferable in imaging procedures in neonates or cardiac patients and in patients with sickle cell disease, renal failure, or known prior contrast reactions.

TABLE 3–1. Contrast Agents Commonly Used in Imaging of the Urinary Tract

Category	Compound	Trade Name	Osmolality, mosmol/L
High osmolar	Diatrizoate meglumine sodium	Renografin 60[a]	1402
Ionic	Diatrizoate meglumine	Hypaque Meglumine 60[b]	1115
	Iothalamate meglumine	Conray 60[c]	1400
Low osmolar			
Nonionic	Iopamidol	Isovue 300[a]	616
	Iohexol	Omnipaque[b]	709
Ionic	Ioxaglate sodium meglumine	Hexabrix[c]	600

[a]Squibb Pharmaceuticals.

[b]Winthrop Pharmaceuticals.

[c]Mallincrodt Pharmaceuticals.

Source: From Slovis TL, Sty JR, Haller JO (eds): *Imaging of the Pediatric Urinary Tract.* Philadelphia, Saunders, 1989, p 16. Modified and reproduced by permission.

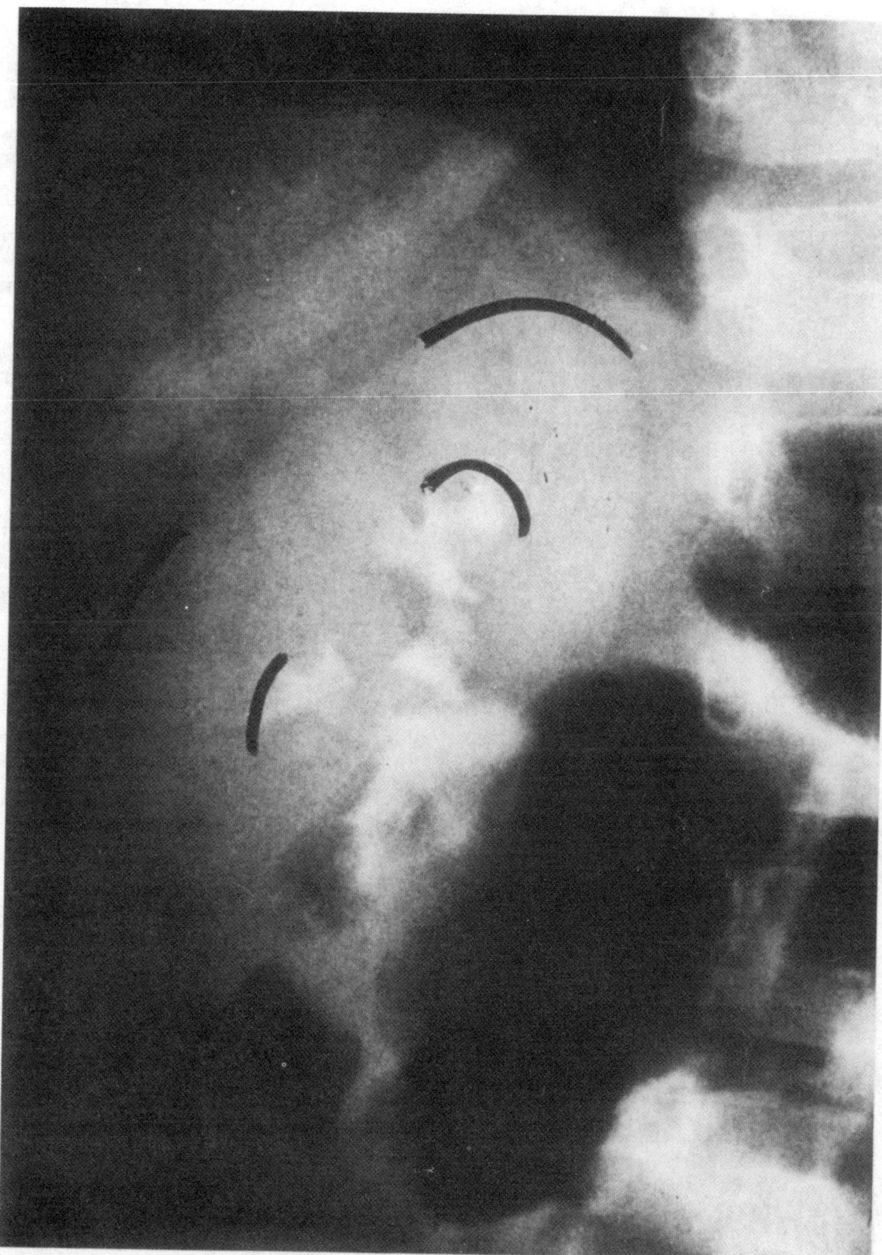

FIG. 3–3. Method of determining cortical thickness using IVP.

INTERPRETATION

The nephrogram phase of the IVP is useful in assessing the size, shape, and orientation of the kidneys. A delay of 1 min or more in the appearance of the nephrogram phase on one side is highly suggestive of a perfusion abnormality, such as renal artery stenosis. The thickness of the cortical tissue is evaluated by judging the distance between the calyces and the cortical margin (Fig. 3–3).[6] This assessment helps to distinguish normal variations in renal contour such as those due to splenic impression and fetal lobulation from renal scarring, where cortical thickness is expected to be decreased. Various diagnostic nephrographic patterns have been described in several disease states. Faint persistence of the nephrogram is seen in patients with severe impairment of filtration, as in chronic glomerular disease. Immediate but persistently dense nephrograms without effective visualization of the collecting system are seen in acute tubular necrosis (ATN) and rarely in acute pyelonephritis. Slowly appearing dense nephrograms may be seen in acute urinary tract obstruction, hypotension, renal ischemia, or acute renal failure (Fig. 3–4).[7]

Hydronephrosis caused by obstruction of the urinary tract is evident in the IVP as ballooning of the renal pelvis and blunting of the calyces. A large extra-

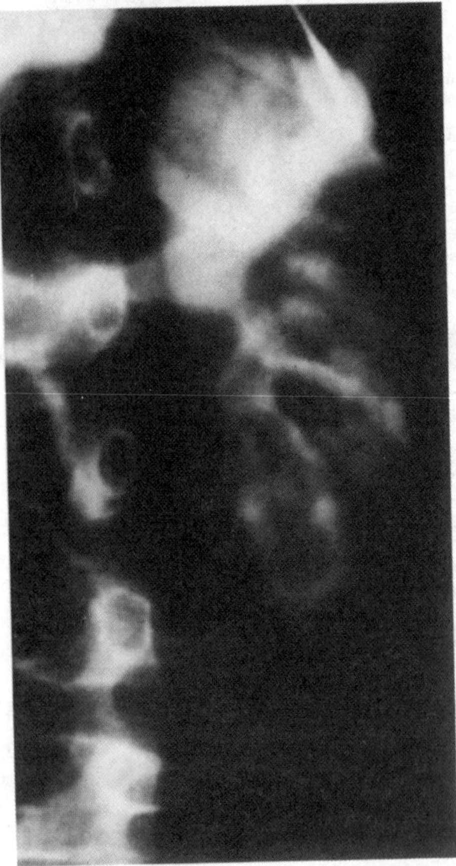

FIG. 3–4. IVP. Dense nephrogram seen in a child with acute oliguric renal failure.

renal pelvis may mimic hydronephrosis, especially if the bladder is distended.[8] Under these circumstances, obtaining radiograms after voiding or catheterization will be of help in differentiating factitious hydronephrosis due to an extrarenal pelvis from true hydronephrosis. Ureters are commonly seen segmentally in their abdominal and pelvic course in the IVP. Use of supplemental films (prone, upright) often enhances visualization of the ureters. The normal ureter as seen on the frontal projection courses over the transverse processes of the vertebrae (Fig. 3–5). Intrarenal masses (cystic or solid) may distort the renal contour, displace collecting elements, or appear as a hypodense or hyperdense region on the nephrogram.

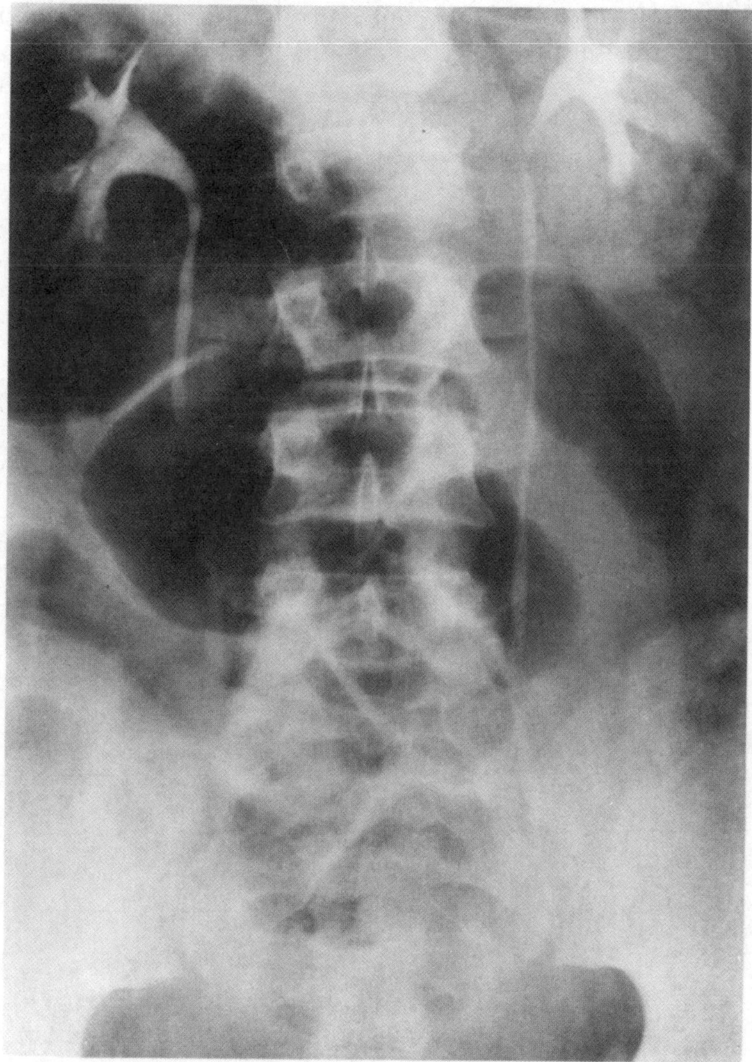

FIG. 3–5. Course of normally placed abdominal and pelvic portions of ureters seen in IVP.

RENAL ULTRASONOGRAPHY

Real-time ultrasonography requires little or no patient preparation, is a non-contrast examination, involves no ionizing radiation, and has multiplanar capabilities. Renal ultrasonography can be used to evaluate renal size and position, renal architecture, cortical thickness, and to investigate pelvicalyceal and ureteral anatomy. Ultrasound also has the advantage of providing information about other intraabdominal viscera, regional vascular structures, and portions of the peritoneal cavity, in addition to renal anatomy. Renal ultrasonography is also used for guiding percutaneous renal procedures such as drainage of an obstructed kidney or kidney biopsy. Ultrasound examination of kidneys may be hindered by bowel gas. For most clinical applications, ultrasonography has replaced IVP as the imaging test of choice for studying renal anatomy in children and adults.

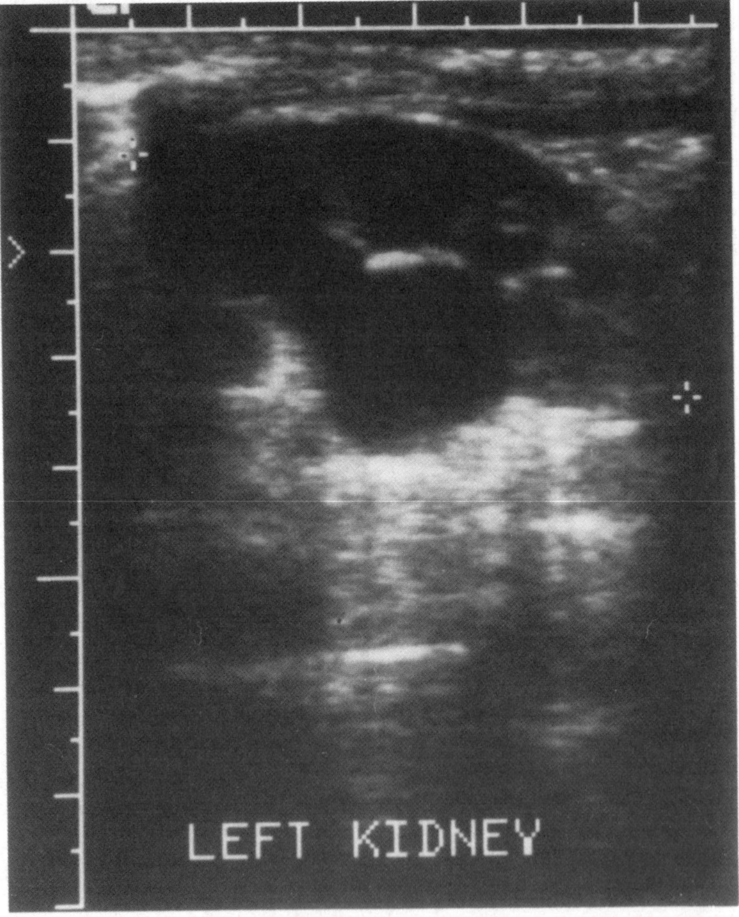

FIG. 3–6. Ureteropelvic junction obstruction seen by renal sonography. Marked pelvocalyceal dilatation with rapid tapering of the pelvis at ureteropelvic junction is seen.

Currently available ultrasound equipment provides outstanding resolution of the images obtained; not only does it allow delineation of normal renal parenchyma but it also can accurately characterize renal mass lesions (cystic, solid, complex). The ability to characterize the renal parenchyma and subtle variations in tissue echotexture makes ultrasound an excellent modality for investigating both congenital disorders such as cystic renal diseases, renal dysplasia, developmental obstructive lesions of the urinary tract (Fig. 3–6) and acquired lesions such as renal ischemia, renal artery thrombosis, and cortical necrosis. Patients with nephrocalcinosis and nephrolithiasis can also be diagnosed and followed by serial real-time ultrasound examination. The architecture of the kidney as characterized by ultrasound changes with age. In the normal neonate, the renal cortex is echogenic compared to that of the older infant or child. The renal medulla appears prominent and hypoechoic. There is also a paucity of renal sinus fat in the neonate (Fig. 3–7).[9]

Renal ultrasound with duplex Doppler scanning can characterize renal vascular flow. The major renal vessels (main renal artery and vein) and smaller intrarenal vessels (arcuate arteries) can be surveyed with this imaging technique. Conditions where duplex Doppler evaluation is helpful include renovascular hypertension (renal artery stenosis), venous and arterial vascular thrombosis, and renal transplant rejection.[10]

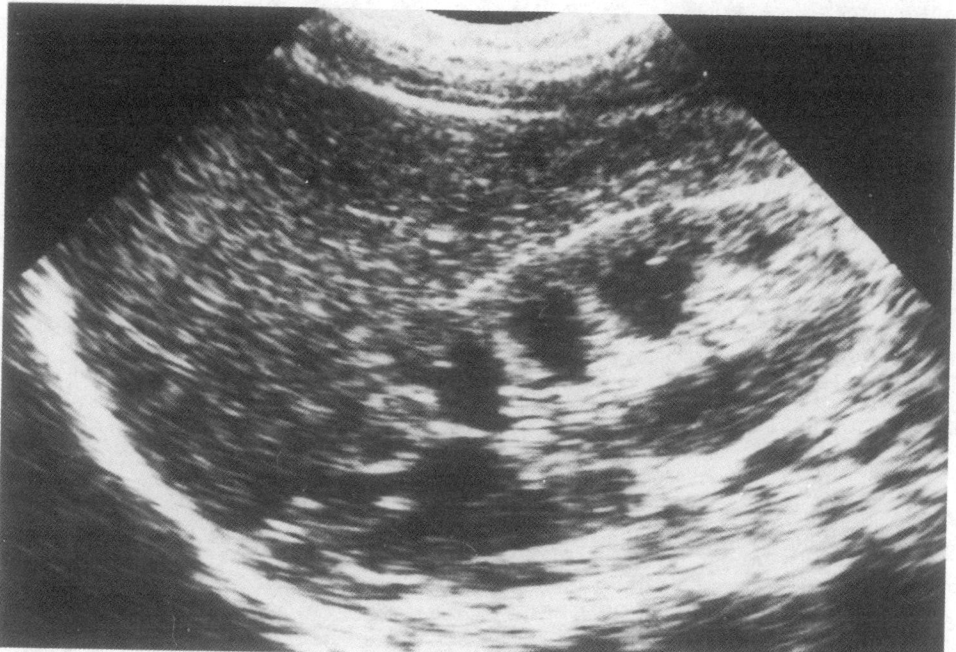

FIG. 3–7. Sonographic features of a normal neonatal kidney. The cortex is isoechoic in comparison to liver; prominent hypoechoic pyramids and paucity of renal sinus fat are seen.

URINARY TRACT INFECTION

In many institutions, ultrasound examination of the kidneys and collecting system has become the imaging study of choice in evaluating patients presenting with their first urinary tract infection. Clinically useful information related to renal size, shape, and presence or absence of urinary tract obstruction in association with urinary tract infection can be determined by ultrasonography. In acute pyelonephritis, the kidney shows enlargement with preservation of normal renal architecture. Complications of acute renal infection such as acute focal pyelonephritis (lobar nephronia) or perirenal abscess can also be identified by renal ultrasonography.[11] In the setting of focal renal infection, one must consider other causes of a renal parenchymal mass lesion, including lymphoma, nephroblastomatosis, or a prominent normal column of Bertin. A renal parenchymal scintigram adds further data to the evaluation of a focal renal lesion.[12] A renal sonogram done soon after the detection of acute pyelonephritis also provides a baseline measurement of kidney size, which can then be used to study future renal growth.

TABLE 3–2. Renal Size in Children as Determined by Sonography

Age[a]	Mean Renal Length, cm	SD	Inches
0–1 week	4.48	0.31	10
1 week–4 months	5.28	0.66	54
4–8 months	6.15	0.67	20
8 months–1 year	6.23	0.63	8
1–2	6.65	0.54	28
2–3	7.36	0.54	12
3–4	7.36	0.64	30
4–5	7.87	0.50	26
5–6	8.09	0.54	30
6–7	7.83	0.72	14
7–8	8.33	0.51	18
8–9	8.90	0.88	18
9–10	9.20	0.90	14
10–11	9.17	0.82	28
11–12	9.60	0.64	22
12–13	10.42	0.87	18
13–14	9.79	0.75	14
14–15	10.05	0.62	14
15–16	10.93	0.76	6
16–17	10.04	0.86	10
17–18	10.53	0.29	4
18–19	10.81	1.13	8

[a]Years unless specified otherwise.

Source: From Rosenbaum DM, Korngold E, Teele RL: Sonographic assessment of renal length in normal children. *AJR* 142:467, 1984. © 1984 by American Roentgen Ray Society. Reproduced by permission.

RENAL SIZE

Ultrasound examination is an excellent noninvasive modality for determining renal size.[13] Such information may be useful for following renal growth in patients with established renal scars. Normal values of renal size determined by sonography are given in Table 3–2 and also illustrated in Fig. 3–8. Conditions associated with alteration in renal size are listed in Table 3–3.

RENAL COMPUTED TOMOGRAPHY

Transaxial display of information with computed tomography (CT) provides descriptive anatomic information about renal abnormalities and characterizes adjacent organs and vascular structures. The true extent of a renal lesion is well seen. The most common indication for performing dedicated renal CT in the pediatric population is to examine the origin, internal character, and extent of the renal mass lesion. These lesions may be of infectious, inflammatory, developmental, or neoplastic etiologies. CT plays an important role in defining the extent of renal trauma.[14] Based on the severity of renal injury (minor, major, catastrophic), medical and surgical management can be optimized.

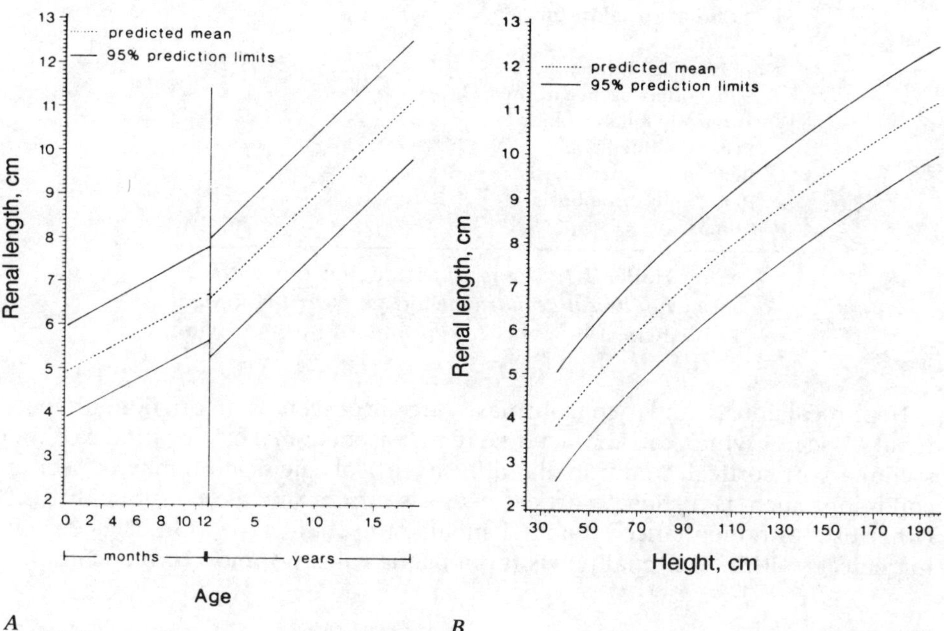

FIG. 3–8. Nomogram for renal size in children determined by ultrasonography. (From Han BK, Babcock DS: Sonographic measurements and appearance of the normal kidneys in children. *AJR* 145:611, 1985. © 1985 by American Roentgen Ray Society. Reproduced by permission.)

TABLE 3–3. Differential Diagnosis of Enlarged, Small, and Nonvisualized Kidneys in Children

Large kidneys
- Single large kidney
  - Tumor
  - Renal vein thrombosis
  - Pyelonephritis
  - Abscess
  - Hematoma
  - Obstruction
- Two large kidneys
  - Polycystic disease
  - Hydronephrosis due to neurogenic bladder, posterior urethral valves, or other obstruction
  - Glycogen storage disease
  - Amyloid
  - Bilateral Wilms tumor
  - Acute glomerulonephritis

Small kidneys
- Single small kidney
  - Chronic renal disease
  - Congenital hypoplastic kidney (renal artery stenosis)
  - Reflux
- Two small kidneys
  - Chronic renal insufficiency
  - Reflux

Nonvisualized kidney
- Congenital absence of the kidney
- Surgically removed kidney
- Ectopic kidney
- Renal artery thrombosis
- Renal vein thrombosis
- Tumor

Source: Haller JO, Slovis TL, Reed JO: *Introduction to Radiology in Clinical Pediatrics.* Chicago, Year Book Medical Publishers, 1984, p 122. Reproduced by permission.

Nephrocalcinosis and nephrolithiasis are also seen well on nonenhanced renal CT scans, which can characterize renal parenchymal calcification as either medullary or cortical. Additionally, diffuse cortical calcification may be seen in conditions such as oxalosis, cortical necrosis, or chronic glomerulonephritis.[14] Other uses of nonenhanced renal CT include the characterization of lucent filling defects within the renal pelvis (nonopaque calculi, tumor, or blood clot).

MAGNETIC RESONANCE IMAGING OF THE KIDNEY

Although ultrasound can generally characterize the presence, position, and orientation of the kidneys, there are times when their localization is difficult. In this setting, magnetic resonance imaging (MRI) provides an overall view of the abdomen that allows easy differentiation between renal agenesis and renal ectopia.[15,16] In the evaluation of an intrarenal mass, characterization of the origin and extent of disease is key in planning appropriate therapy. The multiplanar capability of MRI provides useful information as to the origin of intraabdominal tumors (hepatic, renal, adrenal) as well as the extent of disease. The superior depiction of vascular structures as they relate to an intrarenal or intraabdominal tumor aids in the planning of surgery.

The dialysis patient with chronic renal disease is an ideal candidate for MRI, given its ability to evaluate, without iodinated contrast, the diseased native kidneys for renal cysts or tumors.[15] MRI has also proven useful in evaluating complications of renal biopsy after renal transplant. Intuitively, renal MRI will be more sensitive than ultrasound and CT in detecting diseases that cause little or no change in the size, contour, or architecture of the kidney such as leukemia, lymphoma, and glycogen storage diseases.

REFERENCES

1. Aspin N: The gonadal x-ray dose to children from diagnostic radiographic technics. *Radiology* 85:944, 1969.
2. McAlister WH, Cacciarelli A, Schackelford GD: Complications associated with cystography in children. *Radiology* 111:167, 1974.
3. Report of the International Reflux Study Committee: Medical versus surgical treatment of primary vesicoureteral reflux. *Pediatrics* 67:392, 1981.
4. McClennan BL: Low-osmolality contrast media: Premises and promises. *Radiology* 162:1, 1987.
5. Wolf GL: Safer, more expensive iodinated contrast agents: How do we decide? *Radiology* 159:557, 1986.
6. Hodson CJ, Davies Z, Prescod A: Renal parenchymal radiographic measurement in infants and children. *Pediatr Radiol* 3:16, 1975.
7. Fry IK, Cattell WR: The nephropathic pattern during excretory urology. *Br Med Bull* 28:227, 1972.
8. Berdon WE, Baker DH: The significance of a distended bladder in the interpretation of intravenous pyelograms obtained on patients with "hydronephrosis." *Am J Radiol* 120:402, 1974.
9. Haller JO, Berdon WE, Friedman AP: Increased renal cortical echogenicity: A normal finding in neonates and infants. *Radiology* 142:173, 1982.
10. Taylor KW, Morse SS, Rigsby CM, et al: Vascular complications in renal allografts: Comparison in normal and rejected transplants with pathologic correlation. *Radiology* 162:31, 1987.
11. Schneider M, Becker JA, Staiano S, et al: Sonographic-radiographic correlation of renal and perirenal infections. *Am J Roentgenol* 127:1007, 1976.
12. Davis ER, Roberts M, Roylance J: The renal scintigram in pyelonephritis. *Clin Radiol* 23:370, 1972.
13. Han BK, Babcock DS: Sonographic measurements and appearance of normal kidneys in children. *Am J Roentgenol* 145:611, 1985.
14. Kaufman RA, Towbin R, Babcock DS, et al: Upper abdominal trauma in children: Imaging evaluation. *Am J Roentgenol* 142:449, 1984.

15. Dietrick RB, Kangerloo H: Kidneys in infants and children: Evaluation with MR. *Radiology* 159:215, 1986.
16. Hricak H, Crooks L, Sheldon P, et al: Nuclear magnetic resonance imaging of the kidney. *Radiology* 146:425, 1986.

RADIONUCLIDE IMAGING

Mary P. Andrich
Eglal Shalaby-Rana
Massoud Majd

The evaluation of the urinary tract by radionuclide imaging techniques can provide information about both function and morphology. The ability to obtain quantitative functional data distinguishes these studies from other imaging modalities. Pharmacologic interventions, such as the administration of furosemide (Lasix) or captopril in association with renal imaging, may be utilized to improve diagnostic accuracy. Radionuclide imaging procedures are relatively noninvasive, do not require patient preparation such as fasting or enemas, can be performed without sedation, and do not require hospitalization. Allergic reactions and toxic side effects are extremely rare. Visualization of structures is not impaired by overlying gas, stool, or plastic tubing. In some cases, the radiation exposure for the patient is significantly less than that resulting from the comparable radiographic procedure. For these reasons, radionuclide imaging techniques are being utilized more frequently to study diseases of the urinary tract in children (Table 3–4). In many institutions, renal scintigraphy, in conjunction with renal sonography, has become the primary imaging technique for the evaluation and management of urinary tract disorders.

TABLE 3–4. Common Applications of Radionuclide Studies in the Evaluation of the Pediatric Urinary Tract

Evaluation of renal function
Evaluation and management of
Urinary tract infection
Hypertension
Hydronephrosis
Renal transplant
Detection of vesicoureteral reflux

RADIOPHARMACEUTICALS

Several different radiopharmaceuticals are currently available for imaging of the urinary tract. Each compound is labeled with a radionuclide, and the one most commonly used is technetium 99m (^{99m}Tc). This radionuclide has a half-life of 6 h and emits 140 keV photons. It is inexpensive, readily available, and provides good-quality images. A less commonly used radionuclide is iodine 131 (^{131}I), which emits 364 keV photons, making collimation more difficult. ^{131}I has a half-life of 8 days and emits beta particles. Therefore, the radiation absorbed dose with ^{131}I, particularly in the presence of obstruction or poor renal function, is high, necessitating the use of the smallest possible dose for adequate visualization. An alternative is iodine 123 (^{123}I), which has a half-life of 13 h and emits 159 keV photons. This radionuclide is more expensive, requires a cyclotron for synthesis, and is not readily available.

The properties of each radiopharmaceutical determine the specific diagnostic uses. ^{99m}Tc-DTPA (diethylenetriamine pentaacetic acid) is primarily filtered at the glomerulus. Its initial transit through the kidney is related to renal perfusion, and early images give information regarding renal blood flow. Between 1 and 3 min after injection, the tracer accumulation in each kidney reflects its glomerular filtration. Subsequent excretion is rapid, resulting in a high concentration of tracer in the urine. This provides excellent visualization of the pelvicalyceal systems, ureters, and bladder. DTPA is used to determine the glomerular filtration rate (GFR), evaluate renovascular etiologies of hypertension, perform diuretic renography in patients with hydronephrosis, and assess renal transplant function. An example of a normal DTPA scan is shown in Fig. 3–9.

^{99m}Tc-DMSA (dimercaptosuccinic acid) is bound to the cortical tubular cells, with only a small percentage excreted in the urine. This makes it an excellent imaging agent for the evaluation of renal parenchyma without interference from pelvicalyceal activity. Delayed images can define small cortical lesions such as those seen with acute pyelonephritis, cortical scarring, masses, or infarcts.

^{99m}Tc-GHA (glucoheptonate) combines characteristics of both DTPA and DMSA. GHA is cleared by a combination of glomerular filtration and tubular secretion, giving moderately good images of the collecting systems, ureters, and bladder. In addition, approximately 20 percent of the administered dose remains in the renal cortex, bound to the tubular cells, thus allowing for delayed cortical imaging.

^{131}I-orthoiodohippurate (OIH) is primarily a tubular agent. Eighty percent is secreted by the renal tubular cells, while only 20 percent is filtered at the glomerulus. This agent is commonly used for adult studies, but it has little place in the practice of pediatric nuclear medicine because of the imaging characteristics of ^{131}I as described above. ^{123}I-OIH is a good alternative radiopharmaceutical but is not readily available.

^{99m}Tc MAG3 (mercaptoacetyltriglycine) is a new radiopharmaceutical which is cleared by tubular secretion. It combines the physical properties of ^{99m}Tc with the biologic properties of OIH.[1,2] MAG3 is rapidly gaining favor for pediatric studies as a substitute for OIH. It is particularly useful for diuretic renography

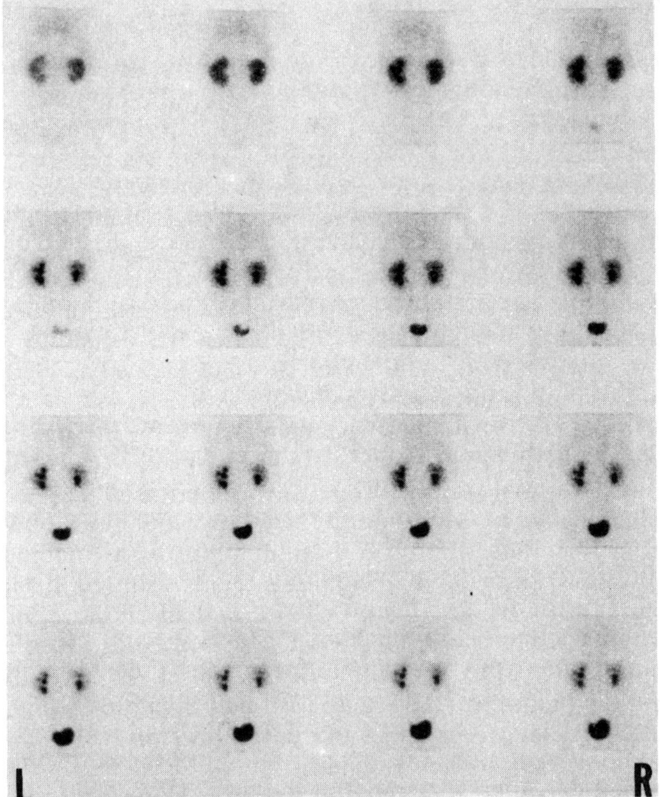

FIG. 3–9. Normal DTPA renal scan. Posterior 1-min images: symmetric cortical uptake, prompt excretion at 3 min, good drainage of tracer, and clearance of the cortex by the end of the sequence.

in place of DTPA. MAG3 may also prove to be a better agent for the evaluation of renal transplant function and for studying patients with hypertension.

DIFFERENTIAL RENAL FUNCTION

Differential renal function can be calculated during renal scanning with either DTPA, MAG3, GHA, or DMSA. Differential and segmental renal function may be obtained based on the amount of radiopharmaceutical extracted by the kidneys. Regions of interest are drawn around the kidneys or the specific renal segments. The total number of counts in each region are added, then the relative percentages are determined. The renal differential can be calculated with DTPA during the period of glomerular filtration just prior to the appearance of tracer in the renal collecting systems. Similarly, when imaging with MAG3, quantitation of the renal differential may be done prior to its passage from the tubules into the collecting systems. During delayed imaging with either GHA or DMSA, a differential can be obtained which reflects tracer bound to the tubular cells in the renal cortex. The renal differential reflects glomerular and/or tubular function, depending on the radiopharmaceutical used for the study.

GLOMERULAR FILTRATION RATE

The agent for the measurement of GFR should meet several criteria. It should be freely filtered at the glomerulus without secretion or reabsorption by the renal tubules, and it should not interfere with renal function. The agent should not bind to plasma proteins and should have no extrarenal modes of excretion. Although inulin is an ideal agent for GFR measurement, its clinical use is cumbersome. The creatinine clearance can be used as an alternative method of determining GFR, but the collection of a 24-h urine specimen is often difficult in children. Furthermore, creatinine is partly secreted by the renal tubules, particularly in pathologic states. Therefore, creatinine clearance often overestimates the GFR in patients with decreased renal function. The use of radionuclide techniques eliminates the need for urine collection and is the method of choice for determining an accurate GFR in infants and children.

The radioactive tracers used for the determination of GFR include carbon-14 (^{14}C) inulin, iodine-125 (^{125}I) iothalamate, chromium-51 (^{51}Cr) ethylenediaminetetraacetic acid (EDTA), and ^{99m}Tc-DTPA. ^{51}Cr EDTA is commonly used in Europe, but ^{99m}Tc-DTPA is the most widely used tracer in the United States. DTPA meets the criteria for an ideal GFR agent except for the fact that 5 to 10 percent of the injected dose becomes protein-bound.[3] Even so, there is a good correlation between inulin clearance and GFR calculated with DTPA.[4]

There are three major methods for determining GFR using DTPA: (1) plasma sampling, (2) imaging (camera-based), and (3) imaging coupled with plasma sampling.

PLASMA SAMPLING METHODS

Calculation of GFR is based on plasma clearance of the tracer. The mathematical formulas used are based on either the compartmental model or the volume distribution method. The compartmental model probably yields the most accurate GFR measurement. After the intravenous injection of DTPA, the tracer clears from the plasma in two phases. In the first phase, there is rapid decrease in the plasma activity due to a combination of glomerular filtration and redistribution of the tracer between the intravascular and extravascular spaces. Once the exchange of the tracer between these compartments reaches equilibrium, the second phase begins. During this time, there is a gradual decrease in plasma concentration of DTPA, which is directly related to glomerular filtration (Fig. 3–10).

The number and timing of the blood samples depends upon which compartmental model is used: (1) the multicompartment (multiexponential), (2) the two-compartment (biexponential), or (3) the one-compartment (monoexponential).[5] The multiexponential method analyzes the plasma clearance curve in its

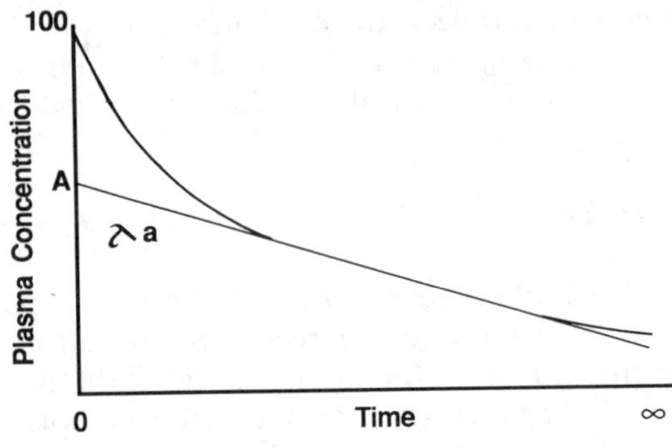

FIG. 3–10. Time-activity curve of plasma clearance of DTPA.

entirety. Although it is the most accurate, its use is limited primarily to research because of the need for numerous blood samples. The two-compartment technique, outlined by Sapirstein et al.[6] in 1955, also requires several blood samples in both phases. The most practical technique for clinical use is based on the monoexponential model, which analyzes only the second part of the curve when equilibrium between the intra- and extravascular spaces has been reached. This usually occurs at about 2 h after injection, when the first blood sample is drawn. One or two additional samples are drawn, with 30 min intervening between each sample. Using the following formula, a computer-generated calculation of the GFR may be obtained:

$$\text{GFR} = \frac{Q\lambda_a}{A}$$

where Q is the administered dose, λ_a the slope of the second phase of the curve, and A the intercept at $t = 0$.

The formula is a simplification of the multiexponential analysis and may be derived as follows:

$$\text{GFR} = \frac{\text{Rate of excretion}}{[P]} = \frac{dU/dt}{[P]}$$

where [P] is the mean plasma level, U the total quantity excreted, and dU/dt the differential of that quantity excreted over time.

Integrating the numerator and the denominator, we obtain

$$\text{GFR} = \frac{U}{\int_0^\infty [P]dt}$$

where $\int_0^\infty$ [P]dt represents the total area under the plasma curve from $t = 0$ to $t =$ infinity. When $t =$ infinity, the total dose injected (Q) equals the total amount excreted; the equation can be rewritten:

$$\text{GFR} = \frac{Q}{\int_0^\infty [P]dt}$$

In a single-compartment system, at t = infinity:

$$\int_0^\infty [P]dt = \frac{A}{\lambda_a}$$

where A is the intercept derived from extrapolating the slope λ_a of the plasma curve back to t = 0.

So by substitution we obtain:

$$GFR = \frac{Q}{A/\lambda_a} = \frac{Q \times \lambda_a}{A}$$

Although GFR is calculated from the plasma samples only, concomitant renal imaging may also be performed. This provides information as to morphology and function of the kidneys as well as drainage of the tracer. In addition, as the calculated GFR represents the total value, the individual GFR for each kidney can be computed by multiplying the total GFR by the percentages obtained from the differential renal function.

Another plasma sampling technique is the volume distribution method, which requires only one blood sample. This principle, using a theoretical volume of distribution obtained from the injected dose, was initially introduced by Tauxe et al.[7] to measure the effective renal plasma flow using ^{131}I-OIH. Later, it was extended for the calculation of GFR.[8] More recently, Ham and Piepsz,[9] using this same method, have developed a formula for the determination of GFR in children requiring only one blood sample. This new technique is attractive because of the need for only one blood drawing; however it has yet to be validated.

IMAGING-BASED METHODS

Imaging or camera-based techniques for the determination of GFR rely on the assumption that accumulation of the tracer in each kidney during the 2 to 3 min after injection represents glomerular filtration. A time-activity curve for each kidney is generated. Uptake by each kidney, expressed as a percentage of the administered dose, is quantitated. Using a regression formula, GFR is calculated.[10–12] Although these methods are acceptable in adults, their reliability in the pediatric age group has yet to be established.

COMBINED IMAGING AND PLASMA SAMPLING METHOD

Imaging together with plasma sampling can be used to determine GFR.[13,14] Time-activity curves over the kidneys and heart are generated for 20 min after injection. At that point, a blood sample is obtained and the activity in this blood sample is used to convert the heart (plasma) time-activity curve to the plasma concentration of isotope. Calculation of GFR is based on the plasma concentration of isotope and the accumulated activity in the kidneys between 60 and

180 s postinjection. Because many factors interfere with the determination of the plasma concentration, this is not considered a very accurate method.

RADIONUCLIDE IMAGING AND URINARY TRACT INFECTION

While the majority of children with urinary tract infection (UTI) do not have any anatomic or functional abnormalities of the urinary tract, a significant number have underlying congenital anomalies which may be associated with infection. After a first infection has been diagnosed in infants and young children, those with anomalies should be identified. General diagnostic evaluation of the child with a urinary tract infection is discussed in Chap. 9. Vesicoureteral reflux is the most common problem and can be identified by cystography. Other anomalies associated with UTI include obstructive uropathies (posterior urethral valves, ureteropelvic junction obstruction, or ureterovesical junction obstruction), duplication, and ectopic ureterocele. Nonobstructive hydronephrosis or neuropathic functional disorders may also be present. These can be diagnosed by first performing sonography, and then, if indicated, diuretic renography with either DTPA or MAG3.

Urinary tract infection may affect the bladder (cystitis) or upper collecting system (ureteritis, pyelitis) or may involve the renal parenchyma (pyelonephritis). Of particular concern is the case of the young infant or child with a febrile UTI where the failure to treat pyelonephritis aggressively may result in significant renal damage. Studies have shown that the potential for renal cortical scarring and consequent sequelae of hypertension and chronic renal failure can be decreased by early diagnosis and appropriate treatment of acute pyelonephritis.[15–19]

Recently a prospective study has demonstrated that the diagnosis of renal parenchymal infection in children cannot be reliably made on the basis of standard clinical criteria alone.[20] In this group of children hospitalized with febrile urinary tract infections, neither clinical parameters nor laboratory results accurately determined which patients had renal parenchymal involvement. The current "gold standard" for the diagnosis of pyelonephritis in children is renal cortical scintigraphy using DMSA. DMSA scans have been shown to accurately identify experimental acute pyelonephritis in animals models. In one study, there was 94 percent agreement between changes seen on scans and histopathologic findings.[21] Other investigators have shown similar results.[22,23]

Cortical uptake of DMSA is related to intrarenal blood flow and proximal renal tubular cell membrane transport function. Acute pyelonephritis and other pathologic processes which alter these parameters are manifest as areas of decreased uptake. The scintigraphic picture of acute pyelonephritis is one of decreased uptake without loss of cortical volume. There may be three different patterns: focal, multifocal, or diffuse (Fig. 3–11). Although not specific for pyelonephritis, within the clinical context it is a very reliable sign of acute renal parenchymal infection. Occasionally renal sonography is required to further characterize the photopenic lesions seen on DMSA scans. Areas of decreased uptake (photopenia) associated with volume loss are usually due to scars and

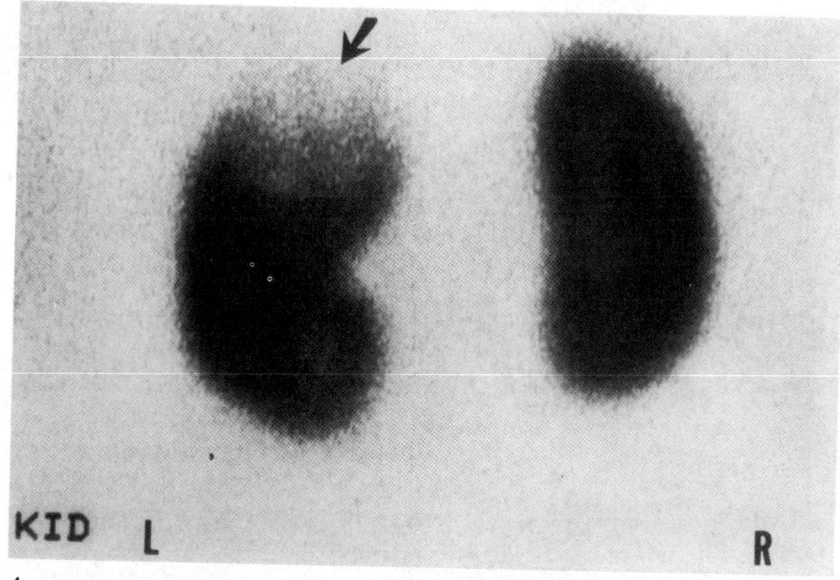

A

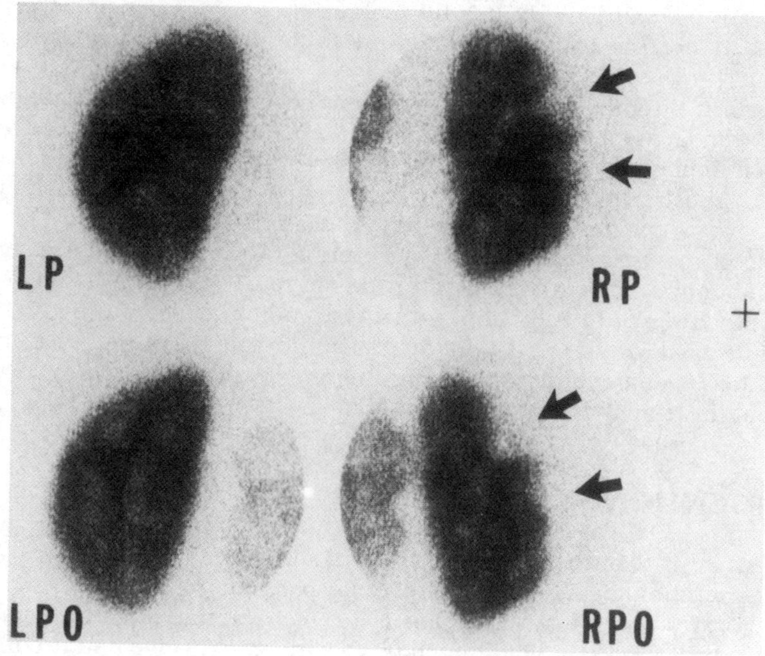

B

FIG. 3–11. Acute pyelonephritis. Delayed DMSA, posterior, and posterior oblique images. *A*. Focal: localized photopenic defect at upper pole of left kidney with preservation of cortical volume and contour (*arrow*). *B*. Multifocal: several photopenic defects in the right kidney without volume loss (*arrows*). RP = right posterior; RPO = right posterior oblique; LP = left posterior; LPO = left posterior oblique.

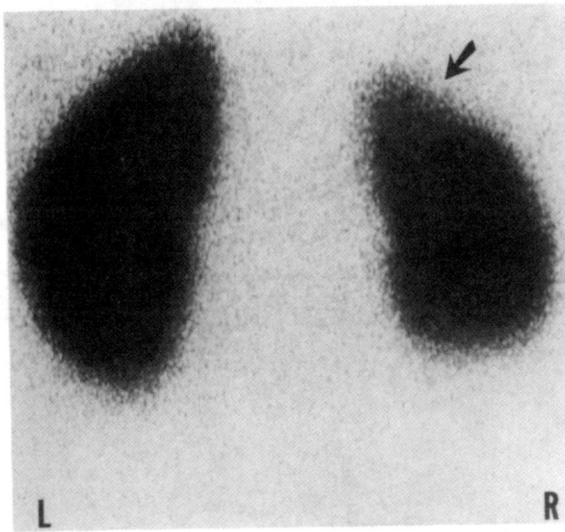

FIG. 3–12. Renal scarring. Delayed DMSA, posterior images—overall decreased size of right kidney with focal scar in the upper pole (*arrow*); normal left kidney.

suggest that previous episodes of pyelonephritis have occurred (Fig. 3–12). DMSA scans are particularly helpful in the follow-up of patients with pyelonephritis to document either resolution of lesions or progression to scar formation.

Renal cortical scintigraphy with DMSA has been demonstrated to be superior to other standard imaging techniques for the detection of pyelonephritis.[24–31] Computed tomography (CT) may be sensitive, but it is not practical for routine use in diagnosing pyelonephritis in children. Other nuclear imaging techniques, such as gallium-67 scintigraphy or scanning with indium-111-labeled white blood cells, are probably very accurate for localizing renal parenchymal infection but are not routinely used for this purpose for the following reasons. The absorbed doses of radiation with these radionuclides are high; imaging must be delayed for 24 to 48 h following administration of the tracer in order to allow for adequate target-to-background ratios; and these studies do not provide renal functional or morphologic data.

HYPERTENSION

Hypertension is seen in 1 to 2 percent of children and in the majority of these patients the etiology is secondary to renal parenchymal or renovascular diseases.[32] A rare cause of hypertension is a catecholamine-secreting tumor such as a pheochromocytoma. Radionuclide imaging is a reliable and useful tool in the evaluation of children with hypertension. Infarction, postpyelonephritic cortical scarring, and posttraumatic injuries are easily diagnosed with conventional renal scanning, while the diagnosis of renal vascular causes may be more difficult. An accurate determination of renal vascular causes of hypertension requires renal arteriography and renal vein renin measurements. The morbidity associated with arteriography obviates its use as a screening procedure. While less invasive, the use of digital subtraction angiography for this purpose has yet to be defined for pediatric studies. The hypertensive excretory urogram is not sensitive enough to be reliable for screening. Currently, a modified renal scanning method using angiotensin converting enzyme (ACE) inhibitor appears to be the most reliable screening technique for renovascular hypertension (RVH).[33–36]

CAPTOPRIL-ENHANCED RENAL SCINTIGRAPHY

When hemodynamically significant renal arterial stenosis is present, there is a reduction in renal perfusion. The affected kidney attempts to maintain adequate intrarenal perfusion through constriction of efferent arterioles. Because of this autoregulatory mechanism, the GFR is maintained and renal scans may be normal. In these patients, blockade of the renin-angiotensin system results in dilation of the efferent arterioles, causing a decrease in the transcapillary pressure gradient. This leads to a measurable but reversible deterioration of renal function, which is easily detectable on renal scanning (Fig. 3–13).

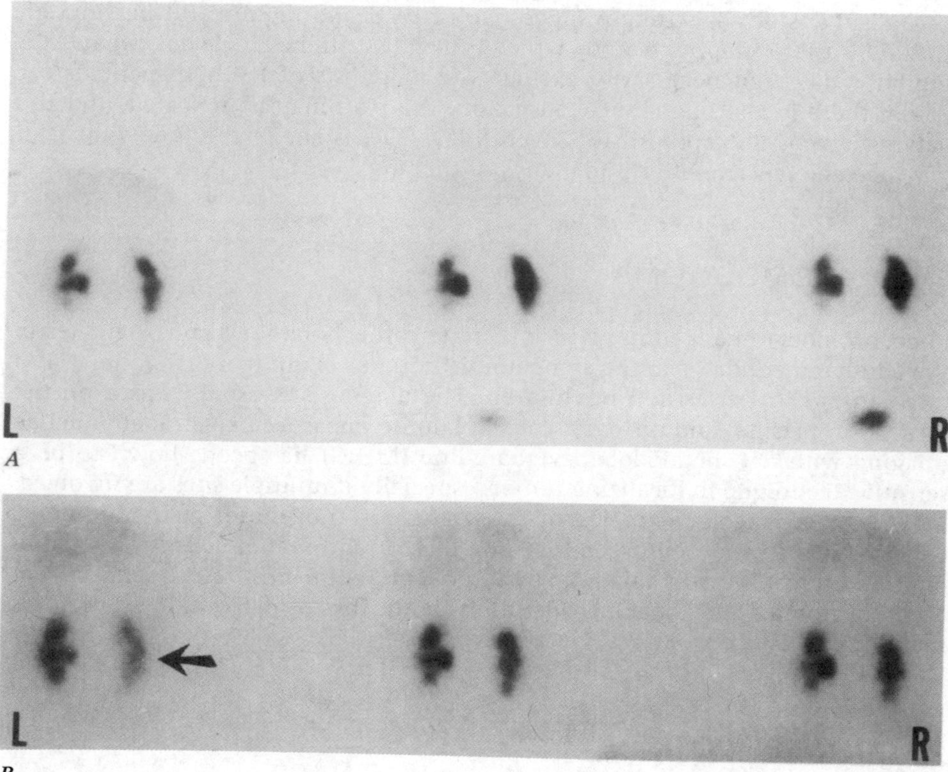

FIG. 3–13. Right renal artery stenosis. DTPA, posterior 2-min images. *A*. Normal baseline scan. *B*. Decreased function of right kidney after single dose of captopril (*arrow*).

The choice of radiopharmaceutical, ACE inhibitor, and technique of examination varies among institutions.[34–36] Renal scanning can be performed with ^{99m}Tc-DTPA, ^{99m}Tc-MAG3, ^{99m}Tc-DMSA, or ^{131}I-OIH. The original work in pediatric patients was done with DTPA and captopril.[33] Subsequent experience has shown this to be a reliable method. At the present time MAG3, which has replaced OIH for clinical use, is being evaluated and appears to be very promising, especially in cases of segmental renal artery stenosis. For blockade of the renin-angiotensin system, either captopril or enalaprilat can be used. Their mechanism of action is similar, but the advantage of enalaprilat is that it is given intravenously, allowing better control of the dose without having to rely on variable rates of GI absorption. We routinely obtain a baseline renal scan, followed by a second study 1 h after oral administration of captopril (0.5 to 1 mg/kg, maximum 50 mg) or 10 min after intravenous injection of enalaprilat (0.03 to 0.05 mg/kg).

The scintigraphic manifestation of decreased renal function after administration of ACE inhibitor depends on the choice of radiopharmaceutical. With DTPA there is decreased extraction and delayed appearance of tracer in the collecting system. MAG3, a tubular agent, demonstrates a prolonged parenchymal retention of activity.

A positive study is strongly suggestive of RVH and requires further investigation by arteriography. A study which is negative after a single dose of an ACE inhibitor does not necessarily exclude the diagnosis of RVH. In patients for whom there is a strong clinical suspicion, the scan may be repeated after the patient is kept on captopril for several days. Occasionally the follow-up scan may become positive after 3 to 4 days of therapy.

PHEOCHROMOCYTOMA

Pheochromocytoma, a tumor which secretes cathecholamines and originates in the adrenal medulla or in the sympathetic nervous chain (paraganglioma), is a rare cause of hypertension in children. The diagnosis is usually based on the results of plasma and urinary catecholamine measurements. Radionuclide imaging with ^{131}I metaiodobenzylguanidine (MIBG) has been shown to be a sensitive technique in localizing tumor, especially if multiple sites are involved. MIBG, a pharmacologic analog of the false neurotransmitter guanethidine, is concentrated in the neurosecretory granules of chromaffin cells.[37] This radiopharmaceutical is avidly taken up by tumors of neural crest cells, such as pheochromocytoma, and imaging identifies both the primary site as well as metastases.[38]

HYDRONEPHROSIS

Hydroureteronephrosis is most often initially detected by ultrasound. However, the distinction between obstructive and nonobstructive dilatation cannot be made on sonography. With the furosemide-augmented renal scan (diuretic renography), the presence and level of obstruction can be determined.[39,40] In addition, the function of the affected system can be assessed. Obstruction can be at the level of the ureteropelvic junction, in the ureter, or at the ureterovesical junction. Dilatation of the collecting system is often detected during workup for urinary tract infection, hematuria, search for urinary tract anomalies in patients with known syndromes, and during routine prenatal ultrasound exams.

DIURETIC RENOGRAPHY

Diuretic renography is indicated when hydronephrosis or hydroureteronephrosis is present. This examination has become of paramount importance in the evaluation of neonates with dilatation of the urinary tract discovered on prenatal sonography.[41] Techniques for this examination may differ slightly from one institution to another. The parents are instructed to maintain the child's normal hydration status (i.e., feedings are not withheld). An indwelling bladder catheter is inserted, intravenous hydration is begun followed by the injection of DTPA or MAG3, and a standard renal scan is then obtained. When the dilated system is completely filled with tracer, furosemide 1 mg/kg (maximum 40 mg) is injected intravenously. Urine output is recorded during this 30-min diuretic renogram to assess adequate response of the kidneys to the diuretic. In addition to monitoring urinary output, placement of the catheter is necessary for bladder decompression to eliminate interference with drainage of the upper tracts, reduce patient discomfort and thus movement, decrease the likelihood of vesicoureteral reflux, and reduce gonadal radiation exposure from radioactive urine.

After completion of imaging, time-activity curves are generated and clearance half-times calculated by computer. The half-time represents the time needed for half of the activity to clear from the collecting system after administration of diuretic. Interpretation is made by examining the images in conjunction with the quantitative data and the shape of the curve. The majority of nonobstructed systems will drain with a half-time of less than 15 min, while most obstructed systems will drain with a half-time of 20 min or more. Half-times between 15 and 20 min are in the indeterminate range.[39]

Diuretic renography is valuable in directing patient management and has been shown to be almost as sensitive in the detection of obstruction when compared to pressure perfusion studies, such as the Whitaker test.[42] The diuretic-augmented renal scan is frequently used in the postoperative evaluation of surgically corrected obstruction to evaluate drainage and kidney function (Fig. 3–14). It is important to note however, that the diagnosis of obstruction may not always be clear-cut on each examination. Factors affecting the shape of the renogram curve and the rate of washout of tracer from the kidney include the degree of obstruction, renal function, capacity and compliance of the dilated system, state of hydration, bladder fullness, dose and timing of diuretic injection, patient position, and radiopharmaceutical used.

Radionuclide renography is a practical and reliable tool in the evaluation and management of hydronephrosis in children. Its usefulness depends on the technique of examination, careful analysis of the drainage pattern on the images and on the curve, and recognition of its limitations.

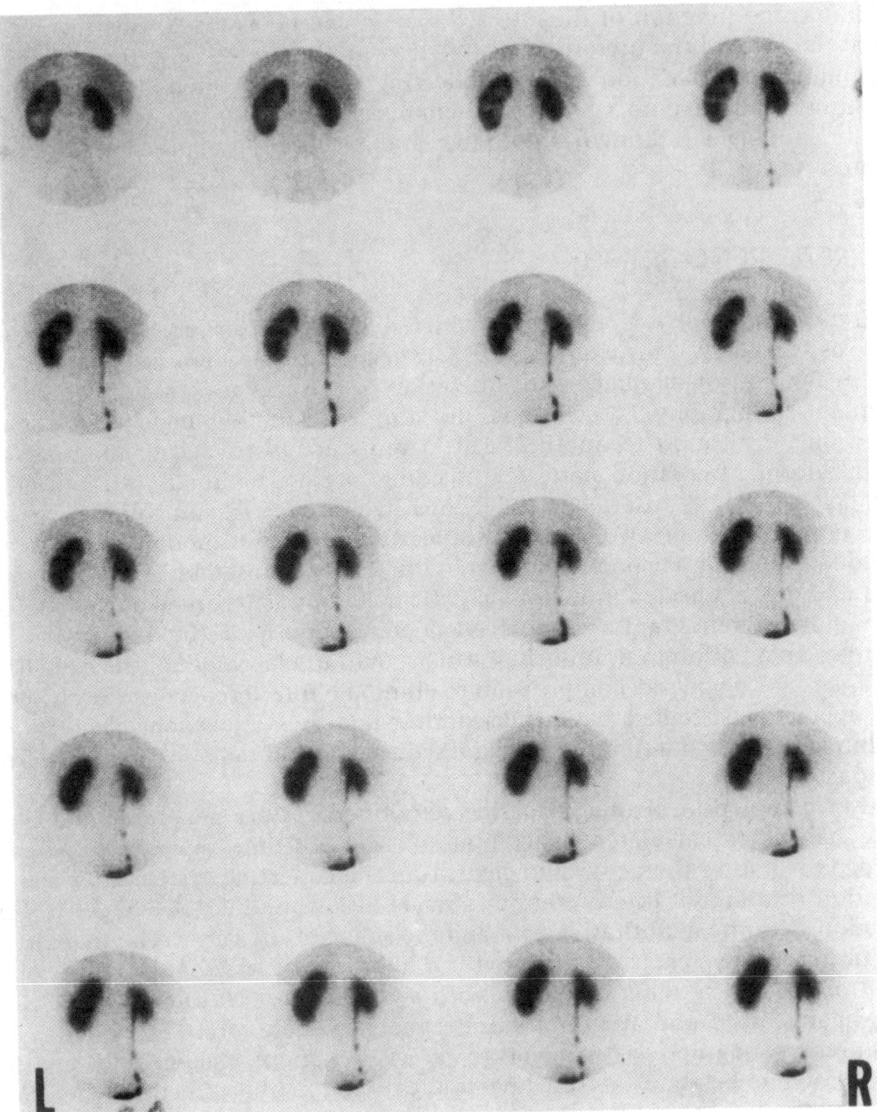

A

FIG. 3–14. Ureteropelvic junction obstruction: preoperative (*A, B, C*) and postoperative (*D, E, F*) MAG-3, posterior 1-min images. *A*. Left hydronephrosis with preserved renal function.

(Fig. 3–14 continues on pages 71–73.)

RENAL TRANSPLANT EVALUATION

Renal scintigraphy plays an important role in the evaluation of both the donor (living-related) and the recipient. It is an accurate and noninvasive method of evaluating flow and function of the transplanted kidney both in the immediate postoperative period and for long-term follow-up (Fig. 3–15). The complica-

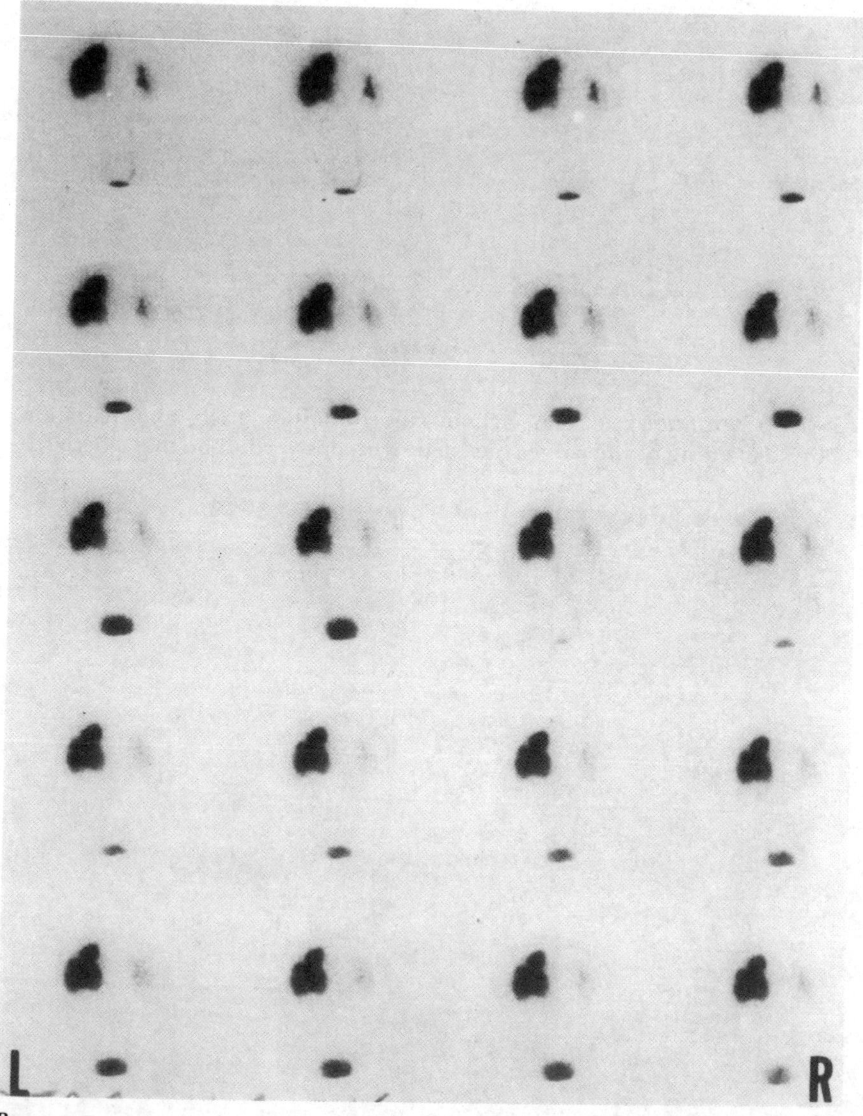

B

FIG. 3–14 (*Continued*). *B*. Obstructed left collecting system after administration of Lasix; right kidney drains well.

tions which can follow renal transplantation may be grouped into two categories: (1) renal parenchymal problems, which include acute tubular necrosis (ATN), acute rejection (AR) and chronic rejection (CR), infection, and cyclosporine toxicity, and (2) mechanical problems, which include obstruction of the blood vessels, obstruction of the ureter, urine leak, hematoma, and lymphocele.[43] These complications occur at various times during the postoperative course, and the time of onset may aid in the differential diagnosis.[44]

Absence of flow on the initial posttransplant scan indicates either vascular

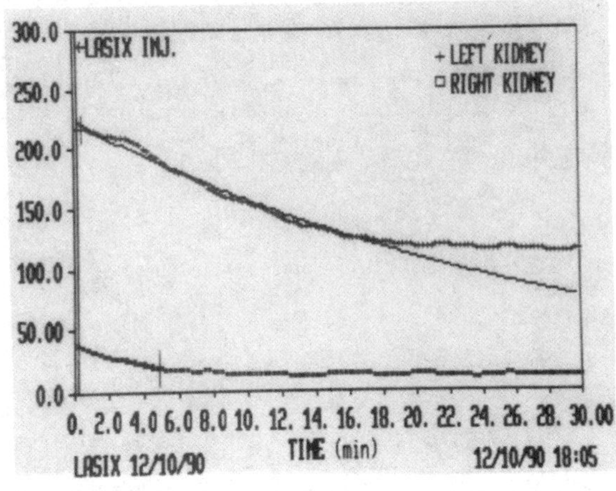

C

FIG. 3–14 (*Continued*). *C*. Time-activity curve following Lasix administration. Left side shows flattening of the curve consistent with obstruction on that side.

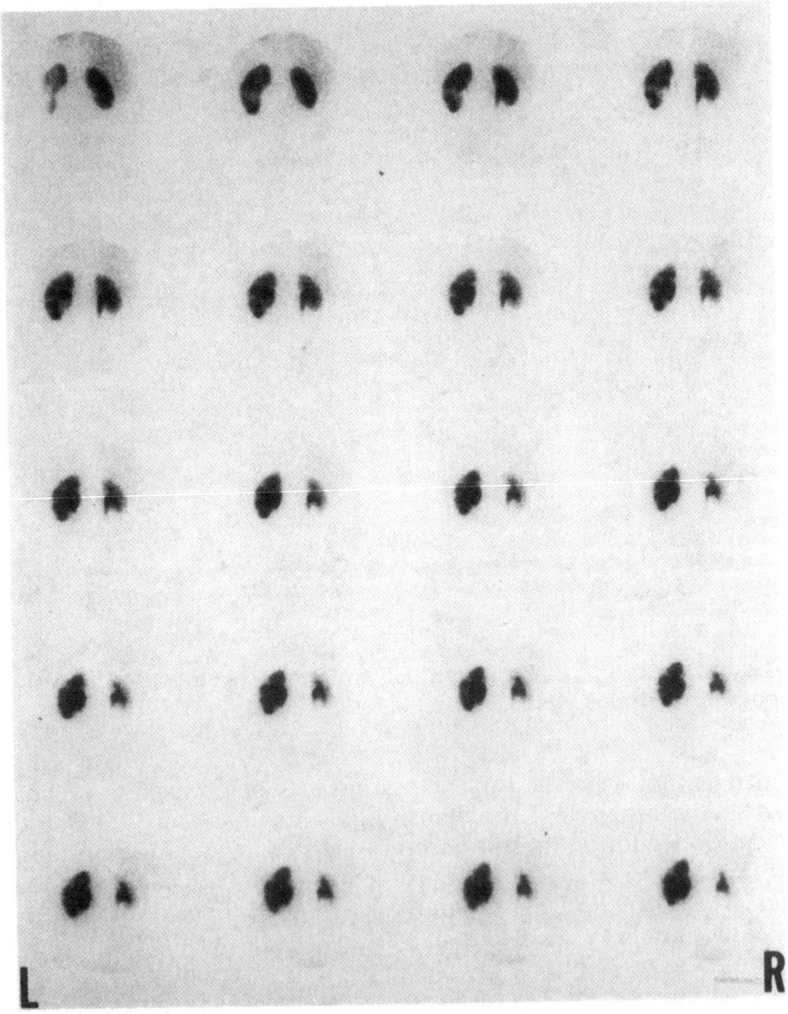

D

FIG. 3–14 (*Continued*). *D*. Hydronephrosis on left.

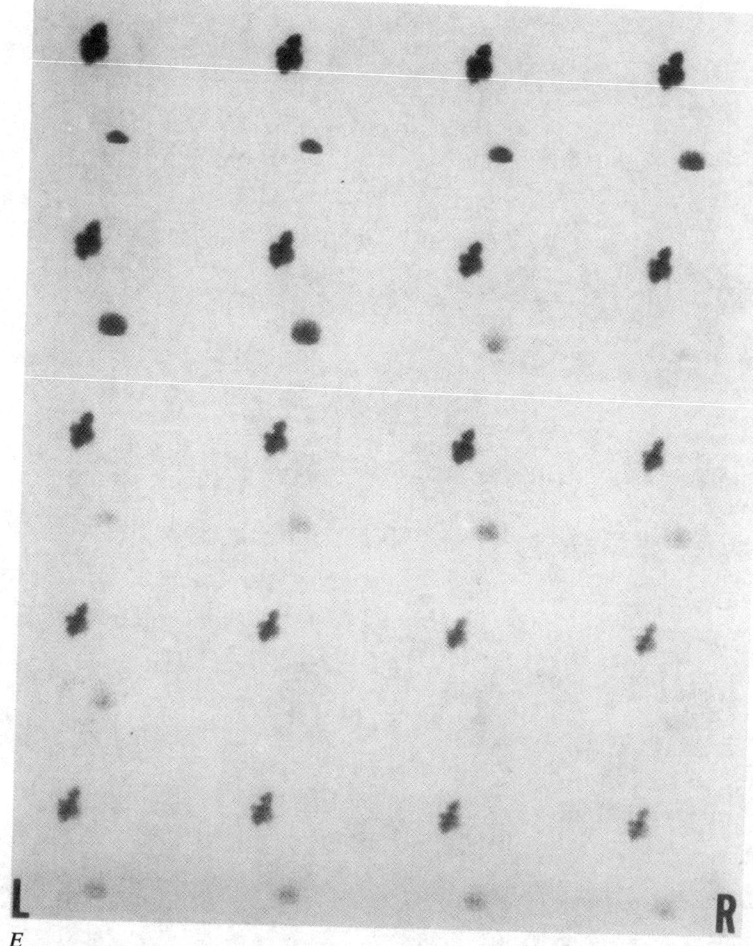

E

FIG. 3–14 *(Continued)*. *E.* Good drainage on the left after administration of Lasix.

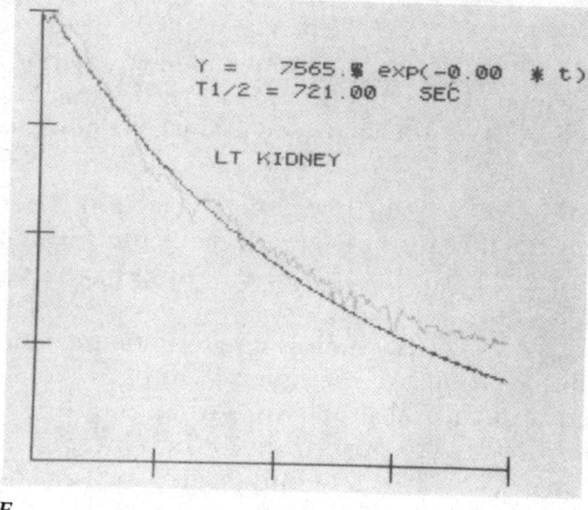

F

FIG. 3–14 *(Continued)*. *F.* Normal-appearing time-activity curve of left kidney with half-time of 12 min.

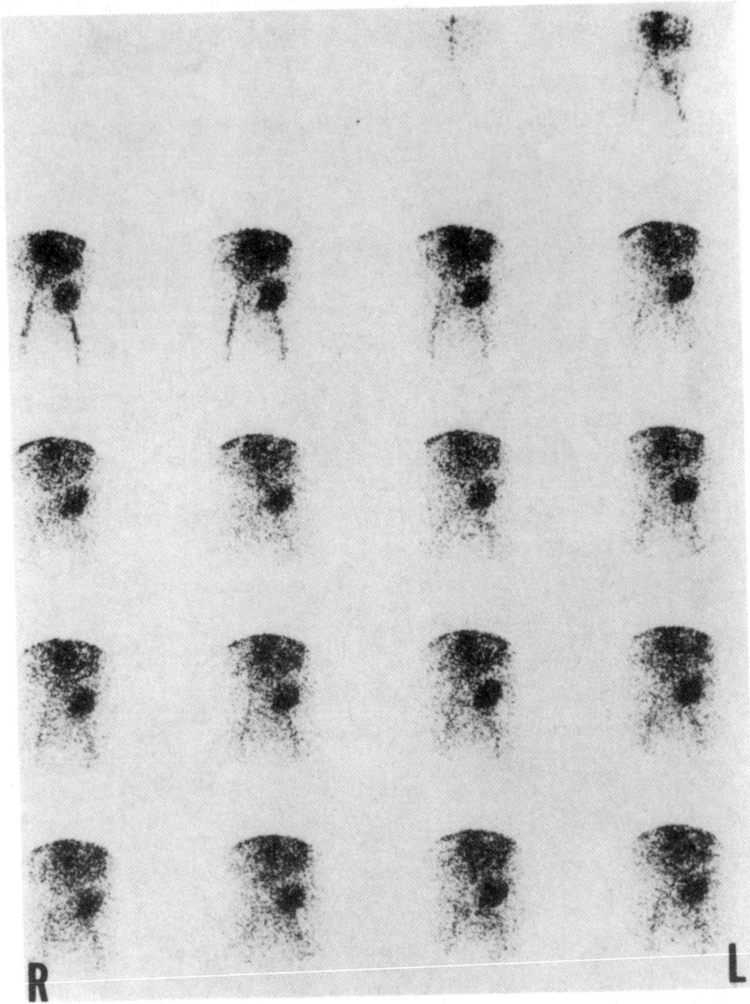

A

FIG. 3–15. Normal DTPA scan of transplanted kidney, anterior images. *A*. Prompt blood flow to the transplant in the left iliac fossa (3-s images). *B*. Homogeneous cortical uptake, excretion at 2 to 3 min, and good drainage (1-min images).

obstruction (arterial or venous) or hyperacute rejection. These entities cannot be distinguished on renal scan; however, hyperacute rejection is almost nonexistent now due to extensive preoperative testing of the recipient. In either case, emergency surgery is indicated.

Acute tubular necrosis (ATN), which is due to ischemic damage, is present in most cadaveric kidneys. It occurs infrequently in living-related donor kidneys and may be related to technical problems during grafting, a hypotensive episode, or toxicity from x-ray contrast media. When present, ATN is evident on the first postoperative scan. It is generally at its worst in the first 24 to 48 h posttransplant and tends to improve over time. Scintigraphically the flow is nor-

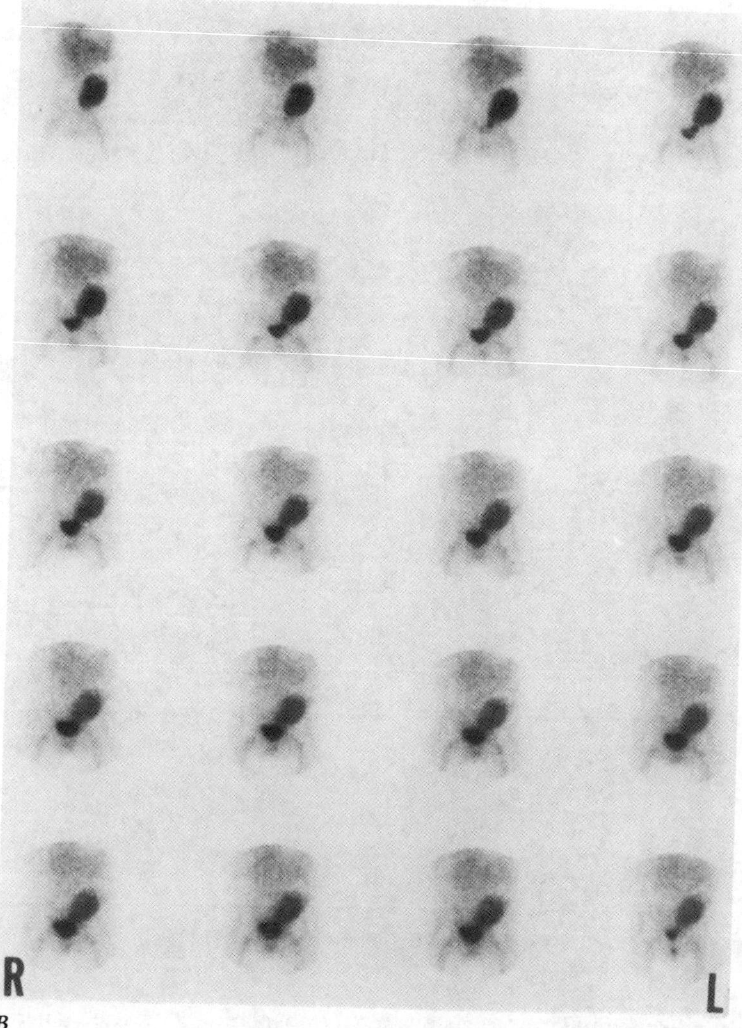

B

FIG. 3–15 (*Continued*).

mal but the function is decreased, which may be manifest by decreased cortical uptake, delay in excretion, or nonexcretion over the 20-min imaging sequence (Fig. 3–16).

Cyclosporine is an immunosuppressive drug commonly used in renal transplant patients. It is also nephrotoxic and may cause scintigraphic changes similar to those of ATN. Distinction between these two entities may be difficult; however, the time of onset may be helpful in that cyclosporine toxicity does not usually occur until 2 to 3 weeks postoperatively.

Acute rejection (AR) usually occurs 5 to 7 days after transplantation. Findings on renal scan are decreased perfusion and decreased function (Fig. 3–17). In contrast to ATN, renal perfusion and function will deteriorate over time if left

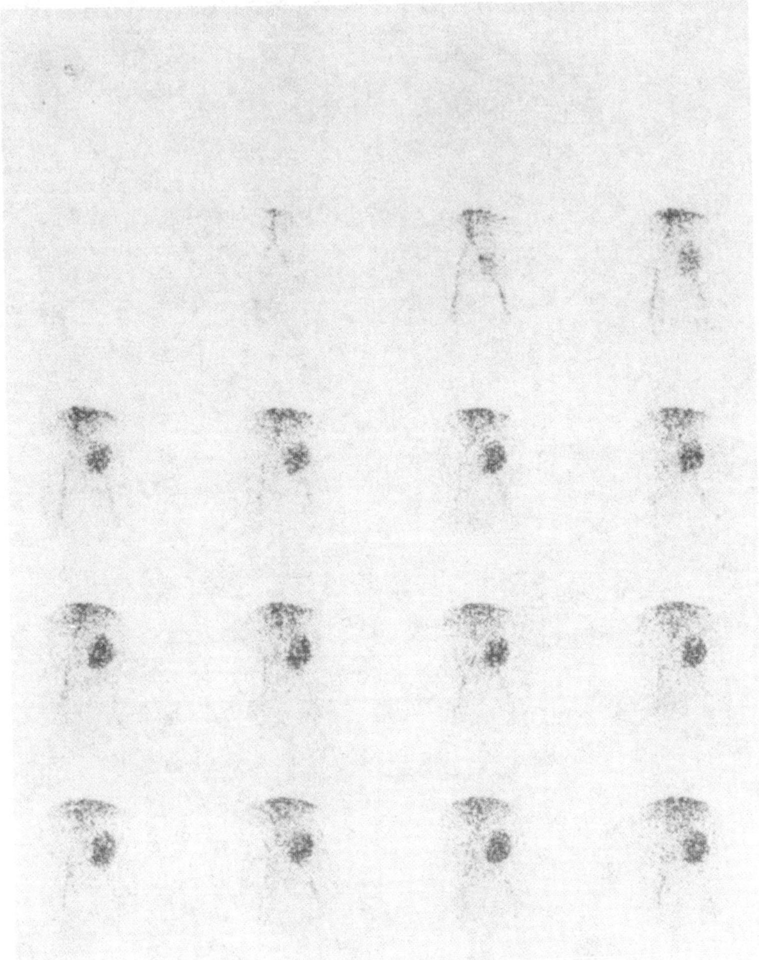

A

FIG. 3–16. Acute tubular necrosis in a renal transplant. DTPA scan, anterior images. *A*. Prompt blood flow to the transplant in the left iliac fossa (3-s images). *B*. Good cortical uptake with marked delay in excretion of tracer (1-min images).

untreated. Most cases of AR are treated successfully. The time of onset and course of the disease on serial scans help to differentiate ATN from AR. However, they may sometimes coexist and differentiation may be difficult. Chronic rejection occurs a few months to years after renal transplantation and evolves slowly. There is a gradual decrease in perfusion and function as seen on serial scans.

In addition to flow and function of the transplant, drainage of the upper tracts and ureter is also assessed. A full bladder may interfere with drainage. If, despite an empty bladder, the collecting system and/or ureter are dilated, furosemide may be administered intravenously to evaluate for obstruction.

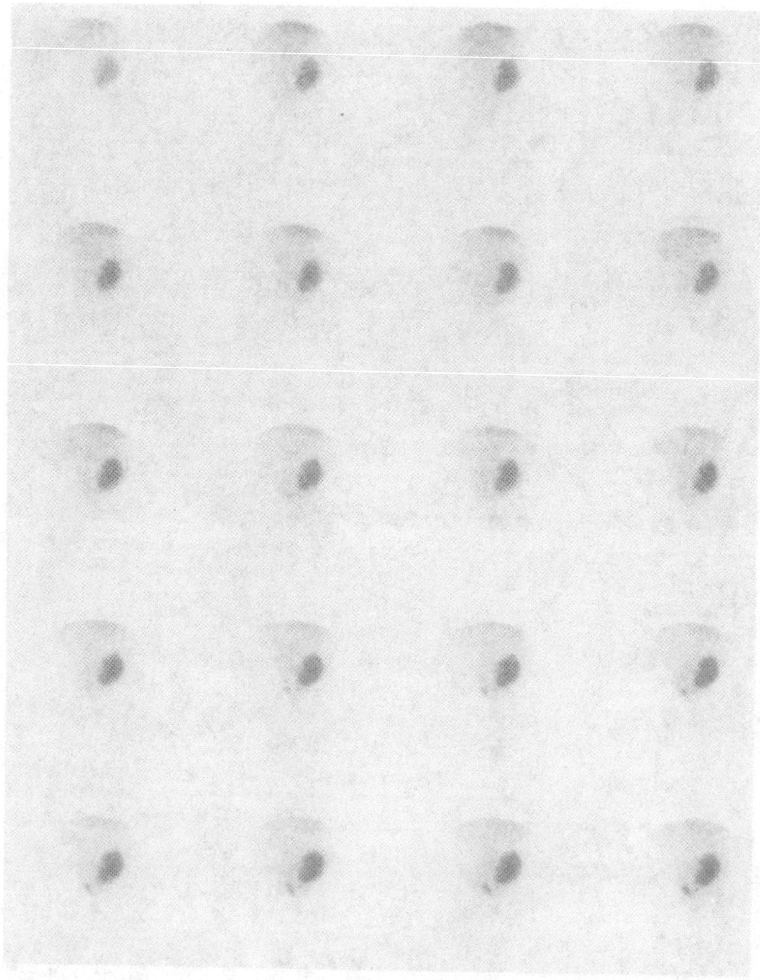

B

FIG. 3–16 *(Continued)*.

Leakage of blood, urine, or lymph can occur, leading to the formation of a hematoma, urinoma, or lymphocele, respectively. Hematoma usually occurs just days after transplant, urinoma days to weeks after grafting, and lymphocele even later. Renal scans show a photopenic area in the early phase of the scan with all three types of collections. Delayed imaging will show accumulation of tracer in this area with urinoma but will remain photon-deficient with hematoma or lymphocele. Ultrasound is useful as a complementary imaging modality in the evaluation of these fluid collections.

The use of OIH in children is limited due to the high radiation burden. At the present time, the radionuclide of choice for evaluation of renal transplants is DTPA. However, in the future, MAG3 may prove to be useful and may possibly even replace DTPA.

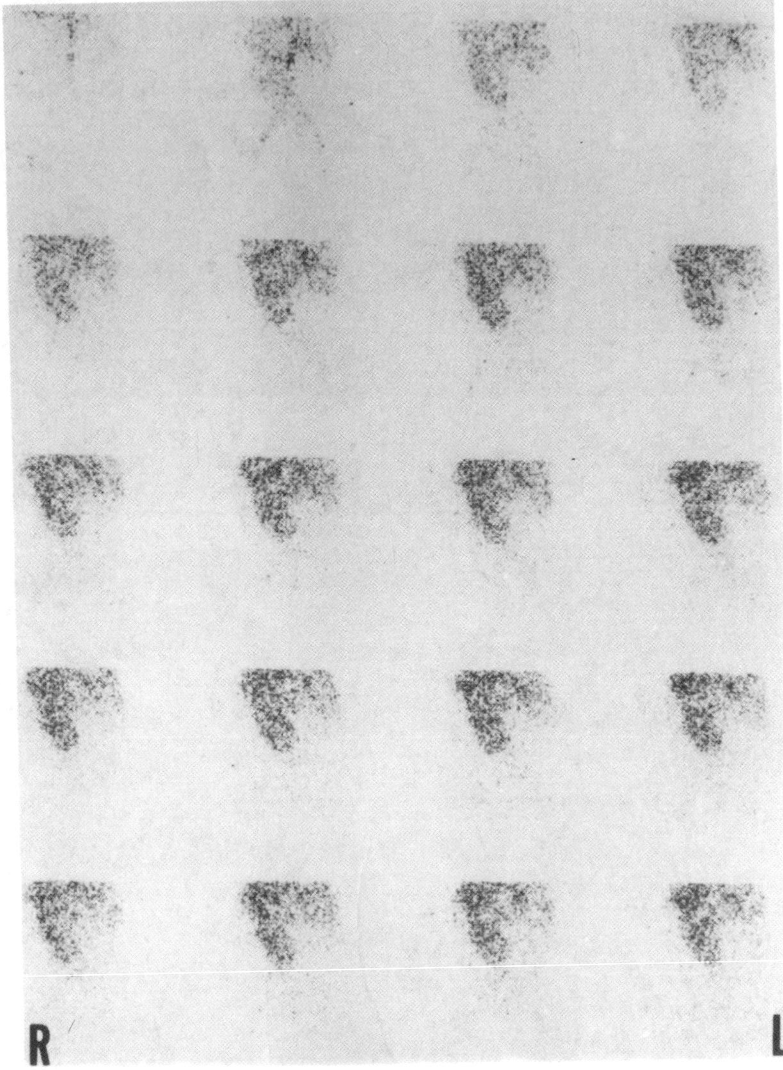

A

FIG. 3–17. Acute renal transplant rejection. DTPA scan, anterior images. *A*. Prompt but markedly decreased blood flow to the transplant in the right iliac fossa (3-s images). *B*. Good cortical uptake with significant delay in appearance of tracer in the collecting system at 17 to 18 min (1-min images).

RADIONUCLIDE CYSTOGRAPHY

The conventional method for diagnosing vesicoureteral reflux is the radiographic VCUG. In addition to grading the reflux, this type of study provides excellent delineation of bladder and urethral anatomy. An alternative method for the detection of reflux is radionuclide cystography (RNC), of which there

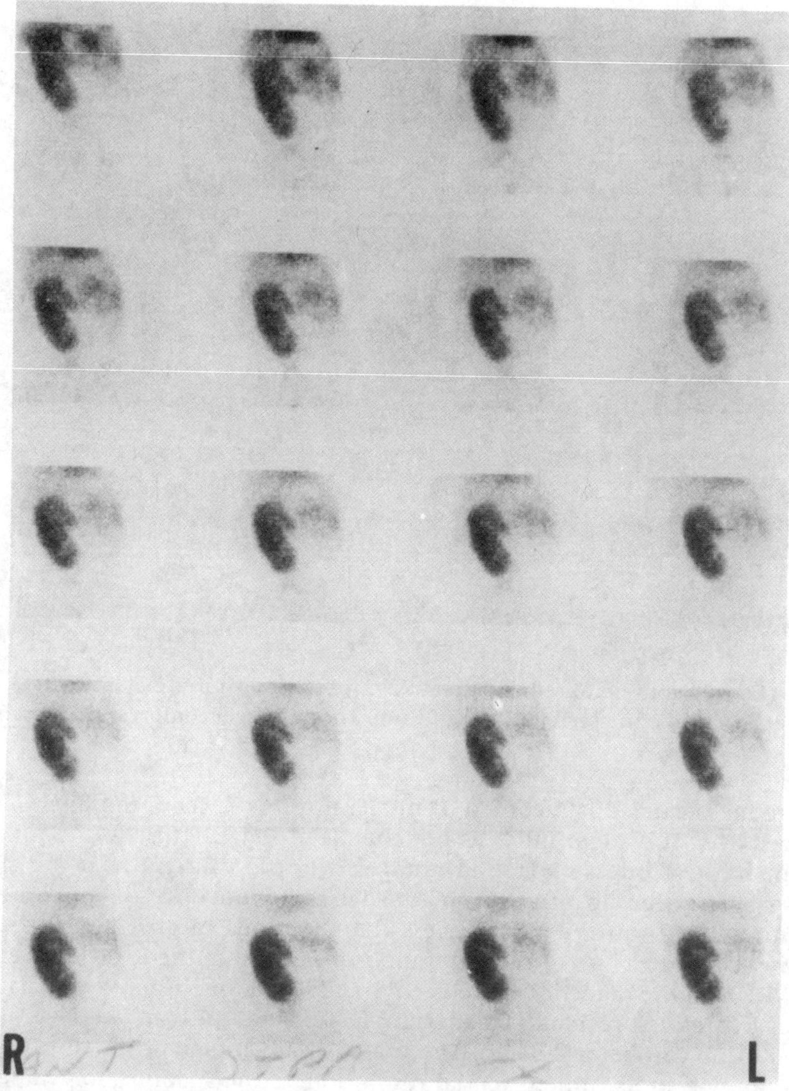

B

FIG. 3–17 (*Continued*).

are two types: the more commonly used direct (retrograde) RNC and the indirect (intravenous) RNC.

DIRECT (RETROGRADE) RADIONUCLIDE CYSTOGRAPHY

The direct RNC is performed easily without sedation. The technique is similar to that of the VCUG except that radioisotope and saline instead of radioopaque contrast media are instilled into the bladder. If reflux is seen, the volume at

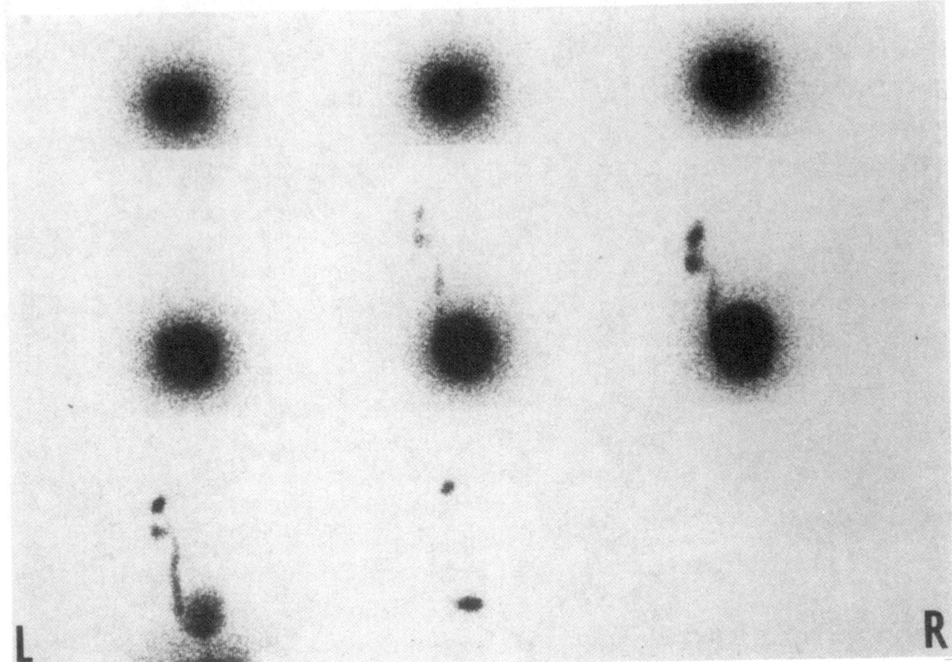

FIG. 3–18. Vesicoureteral reflux. Direct RNC, posterior 1-min images: reflux into the left ureter and collecting system during filling. The system decompresses after voiding.

which reflux occurred is recorded. If bilateral reflux is seen, the flow of saline is stopped even if bladder filling is not complete (Fig. 3–18).

The direct RNC offers several advantages over the VCUG. By far the greatest of these is the significantly lower gonadal radiation dose—about one hundredth the dose from the VCUG—less than 5 mrads in girls and less than 2 mrads in boys.[45] Because of the continuous monitoring, the RNC is as sensitive as the VCUG in the detection of reflux.[46] In addition, quantitative estimation of volumes of reflux, residual bladder capacity, and the rate of clearance of refluxed urine can be calculated. The major disadvantage of the direct isotope cystogram, due to its limited spatial resolution, is the inability to evaluate the urethra and grade reflux accurately. Minor bladder wall abnormalities such as small diverticula may also remain undetected.

The applications for RNC relate to its relatively low radiation burden.[47] Direct RNC is the method of choice in the follow-up in patients with known reflux. The radiation dose is of particular importance in this group of children, who undergo serial examinations. The isotope cystogram is also ideal as a screening tool in the evaluation of asymptomatic siblings of patients with known reflux. The prevalence of sibling reflux may be as high as 32 percent.[48] Direct RNC is also used in the assessment for reflux after ureteral reimplantation. Finally, the direct radionuclide cystogram is quite suitable in the initial workup of vesicoureteral reflux in girls, in whom the incidence of urethral anomalies is rare. Because the urethra is not evaluated on this study, the direct RNC is not recommended for the initial evaluation in boys.

INDIRECT (INTRAVENOUS) RADIONUCLIDE CYSTOGRAPHY

Indirect RNC is another method for the detection of vesicoureteral reflux—however, without the need for urethral catheterization. This technique utilizes an intravenously injected radionuclide (usually DTPA) for bladder filling. The patient is monitored for the length of the renal scan and instructed not to void. Once the renal collecting systems have emptied and most of the tracer is in the bladder, the patient is instructed to void and images are taken during voiding. Although this technique obviates the need for catheterization and provides renal functional information, there are several disadvantages. Only reflux which occurs during voiding is detected. Also, the radiation dose is higher than that from the direct RNC. In addition, the success of the indirect RNC depends upon adequate renal function, rapid clearance of tracer from the upper tracts, urinary continence, and the ability of the patient to void upon request. Thus this method is not suitable for children with decreased renal function or those who are not toilet-trained.

Comparative studies using DTPA have shown that the indirect RNC is not as sensitive as the direct RNC in detecting vesicoureteral reflux.[49] This is especially the case with the lower grades of reflux. With the advent of MAG3, the ability of the indirect RNC to detect reflux may improve because of better renal tracer clearance of this new agent.

REFERENCES

1. Russell CD, Thorstad B, Yester MV, et al: Comparison of technetium-99m MAG3 with iodine-131 hippuran by a simultaneous dual channel technique. *J Nucl Med* 29:1189, 1988.
2. Taylor A, Ziffer JA, Steves A, et al: Clinical comparison of I-131 orthoiodohippurate and the kit formulation of Tc-99m mercaptoacetyltriglycine. *Radiology* 170:721, 1989.
3. Klopper JF, Hauser W, Atkins HL, et al: Evaluation of 99mTc-DTPA for the measurement of glomerular filtration rate. *J Nucl Med* 13:107, 1971.
4. Huttunen K, Huttunen NP, Koivula A, et al: 99mTc-DTPA—A useful clinical tool for the measurement of glomerular filtration rate. *Scand J Urol Nephrol* 16:237, 1982.
5. Cohen ML: Radionuclide clearance techniques. *Semin Nucl Med* 4:23, 1974.
6. Sapirstein LA, Vidt DG, Mandeel MJ, Hanusek G: Volumes of distribution and clearance of intravenously injected creatinine in the dog. *Am J Physiol* 181:330, 1955.
7. Tauxe WN, Maher FT, Taylor WF: Effective renal plasma flow: Estimation from theoretical volumes of distribution of intravenously injected ^{131}I-orthoiodohippurate. *Mayo Clin Proc* 46:524, 1971.
8. Fisher M, Veall N: Glomerular filtration rate estimation based on a single blood sample. *Br Med J* 2:542, 1975.
9. Ham H, Piepsz A: Estimation of glomerular filtration rate in infants and children using a single plasma sample method. *J Nucl Med* 32:1294, 1991.
10. Gates GF: Glomerular filtration rate: Estimation from fractional renal accumulation of 99m Tc-DTPA. *AJR* 138:565, 1982.
11. Shore RM, Koff SA, Mentser M, et al: Glomerular filtration rate in children—Determination from the Tc-99m-DTPA renogram. *Radiology* 151:627, 1984.

12. Piepsz A, Froideville JL, Kinthaert J, Ham HR: Reproducibility of three methods of renal clearance estimation without blood samples by measurement of 99mTc-DTPA. *Contrib Nephrol* 56:77, 1987.
13. Piepsz A, Dobbleir A, Erbsmann F: Measurement of separate kidney clearance by means of 99mTc-DTPA complex and a scintillation camera. *Eur J Nucl Med* 2:173, 1977.
14. Piepsz A, Denis R, Ham HR, et al: A simple method for measuring separate glomerular filtration rate using a single injection of 99mTc-DTPA and the scintillation camera. *J Pediatr* 93:769, 1978.
15. Winberg J, Bollgren I, Kallenius G, et al: Clinical pyelonephritis and focal renal scarring: A selected review of pathogenesis, prevention, and prognosis. *Pediatr Clin North Am* 29:801, 1982.
16. Winter AL, Hardy BE, Alton DJ, et al: Acquired renal scars in children. *J Urol* 129:1190, 1983.
17. Ransley PG, Risdon RA: Reflux nephropathy: Effects of antimicrobial therapy on the evolution of the early pyelonephritic scar. *Kidney Int* 20:733, 1981.
18. Glauser MP, Lyons JM, Braude AI: Prevention of chronic experimental pyelonephritis by suppression of acute suppuration. *J Clin Invest* 61:403, 1978.
19. Miller T, Phillips S: Pyelonephritis: The relationship between infection, renal scarring and antimicrobial therapy. *Kidney Int* 19:654, 1981.
20. Majd M, Rushton HG, Jantausch B, Wiedermann BL: Relationship among vesicoureteral reflux, p-fimbriated *E. coli* and acute pyelonephritis in children with febrile urinary tract infection. J *Pediatr* 119:578, 1991.
21. Rushton HG, Majd M, Chandra R, Yim D: Evaluation of 99m-technetium-dimercaptosuccinic acid renal scans in experimental acute pyelonephritis in piglets. *J Urol* 140:1169, 1988.
22. Parkhouse HF, Godley ML, Cooper J, et al: Renal imaging with 99Tc-labelled DMSA in the detection of acute pyelonephritis: An experimental study in the pig. *Nucl Med Commun* 10:63, 1989.
23. Arnold AJ, Brownless SM, Carty HM, et al: Detection of renal scarring by DMSA scanning—An experimental study. *J Pediatr Surg* 25:391, 1990.
24. Bjorgvinsson E, Majd M, Eggli KD: Diagnosis of acute pyelonephritis in children: Comparison of sonography and 99mTc-DMSA scintigraphy. *AJR* 157:539, 1991.
25. Conway JJ: The role of scintigraphy in urinary tract infection. *Semin Nucl Med* 18:308, 1988.
26. Kogan BA, Kay R, Wasnick RJ, et al: 99Tc-DMSA scanning to diagnose pyelonephritic scarring in children. *Urology* 21:641, 1983.
27. Merrick MV, Uttley WS, Wild SR: The detection of pyelonephritic scarring in children by radioisotope imaging. *Br J Radiol* 53:544, 1980.
28. Traisman ES, Conway JJ, Traisman HS, et al: The localization of urinary tract infection with 99mTc glucoheptonate scintigraphy. *Pediatr Radiol* 16:403, 1986.
29. Monsour M, Azmy AF, MacKenzie JR: Renal scarring secondary to vesicoureteric reflux: Critical assessment and new grading. *Br J Urol* 60:320, 1987.
30. Sty JR, Wells RG, Starshak RJ, Schroeder BA: Imaging in acute renal infection in children. *AJR* 148:471, 1987.
31. Verber IG, Strudley MR, Meller ST: 99mTc dimercaptosuccinic acid (DMSA) scan as first investigation of urinary tract infection. *Arch Dis Child* 63:1320, 1988.
32. Dillon MJ: Investigation and management of hypertension in children. *Pediatr Nephrol* 1:59, 1987.
33. Majd M, Potter BM, Guzzetta PC, et al: Effect of captopril on the efficacy of renal scintigraphy in the detection of renal artery stenosis. *J Nucl Med* 24:23, 1983.

34. Sfakianakis GN, Bourgoignie, JJ, Jaffe D, et al: Single-dose captopril scintigraphy in the diagnosis of renovascular hypertension. *J Nucl Med* 28:1383, 1987.
35. Hovinga TKK, de Jong PE, Piers DA, et al: Diagnostic use of angiotensin converting enzyme inhibitors in radioisotope evaluation of unilateral renal artery stenosis. *J Nucl Med* 30:605, 1989.
36. Dondi, M, Franchi R, Levorato M, et al: Evaluation of hypertensive patients by means of captopril enhanced renal scintigraphy with technetium-99m DTPA. *J Nucl Med* 30:615, 1989.
37. Wieland DM, Wu JL, Brown LE, et al: Radiolabeled adrenergic neuron-blocking agents: Adrenomedullary imaging with 131I-iodobenzylguanidine. *J Nucl Med* 21:349, 1980.
38. Shapiro B, Copp JE, Sisson JC, et al: Iodine-131 metaiodobenzylguanidine for the location of suspected pheochromocytoma: Experience in 400 cases. *J Nucl Med* 26:576, 1985.
39. Kass E, Majd M: Evaluation and management of upper urinary tract obstruction in infancy and childhood. *Urol Clin North Am* 12:133, 1985.
40. Ireton RC, Parker RM, Hayden P: Diuretic renography in evaluating dilated upper urinary tract in children. *Urology* 29:178, 1987.
41. Heyman S: An update of radionuclide renal studies in pediatrics. *Nucl Med Ann* 179, 1989.
42. Kass EJ, Majd M, Belman AB: Comparison of the diuretic renogram and the pressure perfusion study in children. *J Urol* 134:92, 1985.
43. Majd M: Nuclear medicine in pediatric urology, in Kelalis PP, King LR, Belman AB (eds): *Clinical Pediatric Urology.* Philadelphia, Saunders, 1985, p 163.
44. Dubovsky E, Russell C: Radionuclide evalution of renal transplants. *Semin Nucl Med* 18:181, 1988.
45. Majd M, Belman AB: Nuclear cystography in infants and children. *Urol Clin North Am* 6:395, 1979.
46. Conway JJ, King LR, Belman AB, Thorson T: Detection of vesicoureteral reflux with radionuclide cystography—A comparison study with roentgenographic cystography. *Am J Roentgenol Rad Ther Nucl Med* 115:720, 1972.
47. Majd M: Radionuclide imaging in clinical pediatrics. *Pediatr Ann* 15:396, 1986.
48. Jerkins GR, Noe HN: Familial vesicoureteral reflux—A prospective study. *J Urol* 128:774, 1982.
49. Majd M, Kass EJ, Belman AB: Radionuclide cystography in children: Comparison of direct (retrograde) and indirect (intravenous) techniques. *Ann Radiol* 28:322, 1984.

4

RENAL BIOPSY

Kanwal K. Kher

Renal biopsy is frequently performed to establish diagnosis and prognosis in patients with renal disease. Most renal biopsies performed by nephrologists are done by the percutaneous technique, open surgical biopsy being reserved for special circumstances. The technique of percutaneous renal biopsy has undergone several important modifications since its first widespread clinical introduction in the 1950s.[1,2] The introduction of ultrasound for guiding the biopsy needle as well as the development of newer biopsy instruments have significantly contributed toward making the procedure safer and more efficient. This chapter discusses indications, technique, complications, and other practical aspects of renal biopsy in children.

INDICATIONS FOR RENAL BIOPSY

The purpose of renal biopsy as an investigative tool is threefold: (1) to confirm the histologic diagnosis, (2) to characterize prognosis for the patient, and (3) to assist in developing treatment strategies. The most frequent indication for renal biopsy in children is nephrotic syndrome that is either steroid-resistant (unresponsive) or steroid-dependent. Perhaps the second most common use of renal biopsy in children is to evaluate "hematuria syndrome." The disease categories included in this diagnostic subgroup are IgA nephropathy, Alport syndrome, and the benign hematuria syndromes. Since the diagnosis of rapidly progressive glomerulonephritis rests solely on demonstrating crescentic glomerular lesions, renal biopsy is essential in the evaluation of patients who may have this condition. Renal biopsy is not generally undertaken in patients with acute renal failure unless acute or chronic glomerulonephritis (membranoproliferative glomerulonephritis, systemic lupus erythematosus nephritis, rapidly progressive glomerulonephritis, etc.) or acute tubulointerstitial nephritis is suspected to be the underlying etiology. In patients presenting for the first time with advanced chronic renal failure or end-stage renal failure (small, scarred kidneys on ultrasound), renal biopsy usually provides little or no diagnostic information. Advanced glomerulosclerosis with tubular atrophy (end-stage kidney) forbids

TABLE 4–1. Indications for Renal Biopsy in Children

Well-established indications
- Steroid-resistant or -dependent nephrotic syndrome
- Rapidly progressive glomerulonephritis
- Atypical or nonresolving acute glomerulonephritis
- Suspected acute tubulointerstitial nephritis
- Recurrent hematuria syndromes
- Nonorthostatic persistent proteinuria
- Diagnosis of renal allograft rejection
- Renal involvement in systemic diseases such as SLE,
  Henoch-Schönlein purpura, vasculitis syndromes, Fabrey disease, etc.

"Fuzzy" indications
- Chronic renal failure of unknown etiology
- Acute renal failure not due to a glomerular or tubulointerstitial disease
- Evaluation of renal response to therapy

the establishment of any firm morphologic diagnosis. At times, renal biopsy may be used as a measure of success (or failure) of therapy. Table 4–1 lists the indications for renal biopsy in children.

PREPARING THE PATIENT

Adequate preparations and arrangements must be made to ensure the safe performance of a renal biopsy. In most institutions patients are admitted to the hospital and the procedure is usually conducted in the radiology suite, where facilities for real-time ultrasound examination of the kidney are available. Therefore, the procedure must usually be scheduled ahead of time. The pathology department must also be informed so that the biopsy specimen can be processed without delay. The patient should be instructed to take nothing by mouth for 6 h prior to the biopsy procedure. Laboratory evaluation of hemoglobin or hematocrit, coagulation status, and urinalysis should be ordered and reviewed prior to the procedure. One unit of packed red blood cells should be available for use in case of a postbiopsy hemorrhagic event. An intravenous access should be established before the biopsy is undertaken; this intravenous line can be used to infuse maintenance fluids, since these patients usually cannot take anything by mouth for 8 to 10 h in the pre- and postbiopsy periods. Other steps involved in the preparation of patients are listed in Table 4–2.

The patient should receive premedication about 30 min prior to the procedure. Most institutions use the conventional *DPT premedication protocol* of Demerol (meperidine), Phenergan (promethazine), and Thorazine (chlorpromazine) in the doses listed in Table 4–3. The injection is given intramuscularly in leg. This premedication protocol can be modified on the basis of personal and insti-

TABLE 4–2. Prebiopsy Order Sheet

- Obtain consent for the procedure
- Obtain and check the following laboratory tests:
  - Urinalysis
  - Complete blood count, including platelet count
  - Coagulation panel, prothrombin time, partial thromboplastin time, and (in selected cases) bleeding time
- Type and hold one unit of packed red blood cells
- Arrange pathology and radiology services for the biopsy
- Patient should be instructed to take nothing by mouth for 6 h prior to the procedure
- Start an intravenous access through which the patient may be given required maintenance fluids
- Premedicate the patient 30 min before the procedure
- Transport the patient, accompanied by a nurse, to the radiology suite on a stretcher

tutional preferences. In young children (3 years of age of less) or those who are expected to be uncooperative during biopsy, general anesthesia may be required. Premedication under these conditions should accord with the recommendations of the anesthesia service.

Accompanied by a nurse, the patient should be wheeled to the ultrasound suite on a stretcher. Some institutions require that a pulse oximeter or cardiac rate monitor be available during patient transportation as well as during the biopsy procedure.

BIOPSY INSTRUMENTS

VIM-SILVERMAN NEEDLE

Traditionally, the Franklin modification of the Vim-Silverman biopsy needle has been used in performing renal biopsies (Fig. 4–1). This device consists of a

TABLE 4–3. Premedication for Percutaneous Renal Biopsy

Meperidine (Demerol)	2 mg/kg (max., 50 mg)
Promethazine (Phenergan)	1 mg/kg (max., 25 mg)
Chlorpromazine (Thorazine)	1 mg/kg (max., 25 mg)

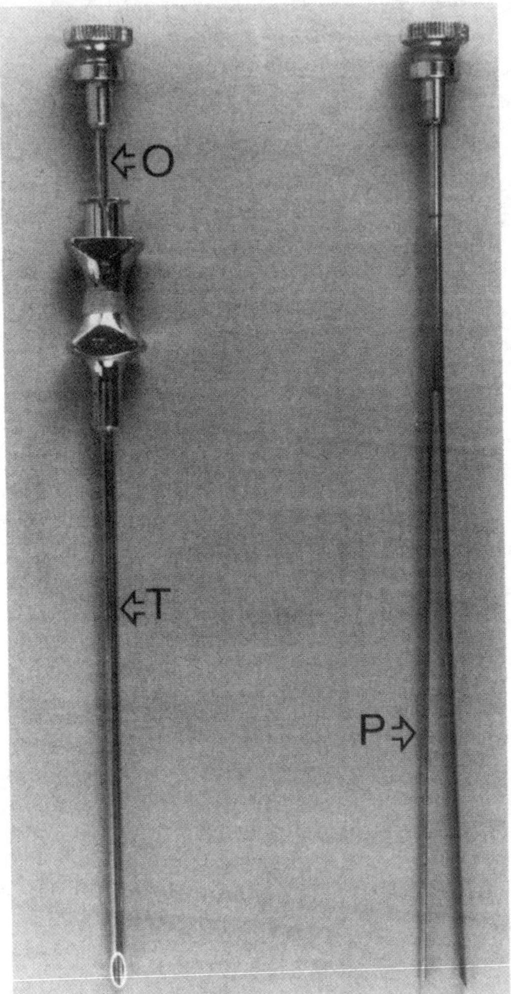

FIG. 4–1. Franklin modification of the Vim-Silverman needle. The trocar (T) is fitted with the obturator (O); the cutting prongs (P) are shown on the side.

trocar and a fitting obturator, which are introduced together into the renal cortex. The obturator is then removed and the cutting needle with prongs is introduced through the trocar. The cutting needle is advanced rapidly into the renal cortex, quickly followed by the trocar. Finally, the biopsy needle (both the trocar and the cutting needle) is quickly removed from the patient without disturbing the relative position of any of its components. Renal tissue core is gathered between the two prongs of the cutting needle.

The Vim-Silverman needle is not disposable and must be cleaned and sterilized like any other surgical instrument. With time, however, the needle loses its sharpness; it must therefore be resharpening periodically.

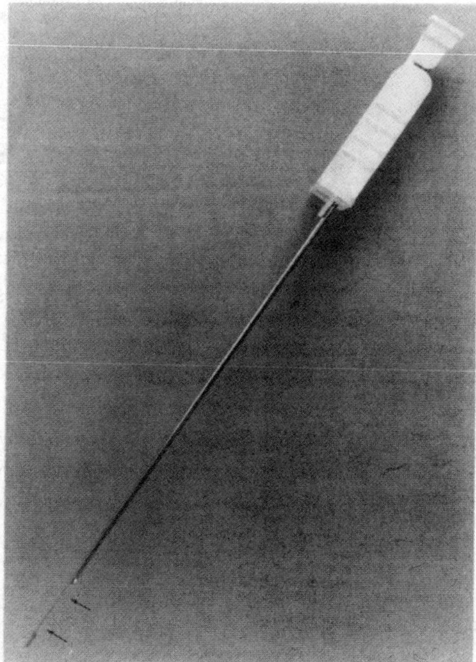

FIG. 4–2. Disposable True-Cut biopsy needle (Baxter Healthcare Corporation, Valencia, California). Arrows point to the specimen notch.

TRUE-CUT NEEDLE

In the last 10 years, a disposable renal biopsy needle (the True-Cut biopsy needle from Baxter Healthcare Corporation, Valencia, California) has been available for use in children and adults (Fig. 4–2). Because of its advantage of being disposable, assured sharpness, and simplicity, the True-Cut needle has become the preferred instrument for renal biopsy in many institutions. True-cut needle consists of a trocar encasing the cutting needle, which slides within the trocar to a predetermined fixed depth. In order to obtain a tissue core, the trocar and the cutting needle are advanced together to the level of renal cortex. At this point the cutting needle is advanced into the renal cortex, followed by the trocar. The needle and the torcar are removed from the patient and the tissue lifted from the cutting needle (Fig. 4–3).

BARD MONOPTY NEEDLE

A third type of renal biopsy needle (Bard Monopty Biopsy Instrument, Bard Urologic Division, Covington, Georgia) has recently been introduced (Fig. 4–4).[3] The Bard Monopty needle is particularly useful for the biopsy of renal allografts. This instrument consists of a cutting needle encased in a trocar, both of which are mounted on a spring-loaded handle. The tissue core is obtained by pressing a button on the handle of the biopsy needle. The manual dexterity

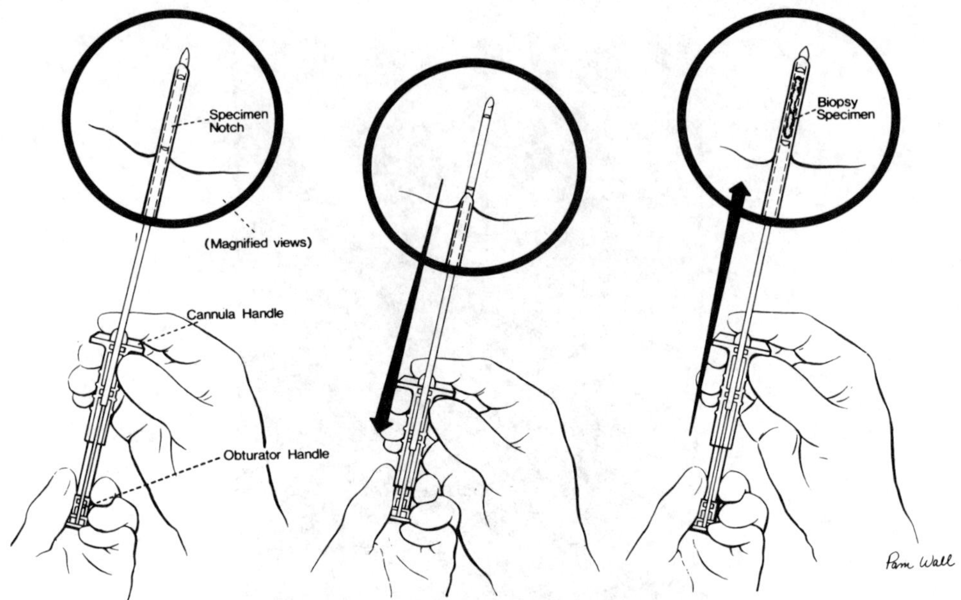

FIG. 4–3. Technique of obtaining the tissue core by the True-Cut biopsy needle. (Reproduced by permission of Baxter Healthcare Corporation, Valencia, California, from package insert.)

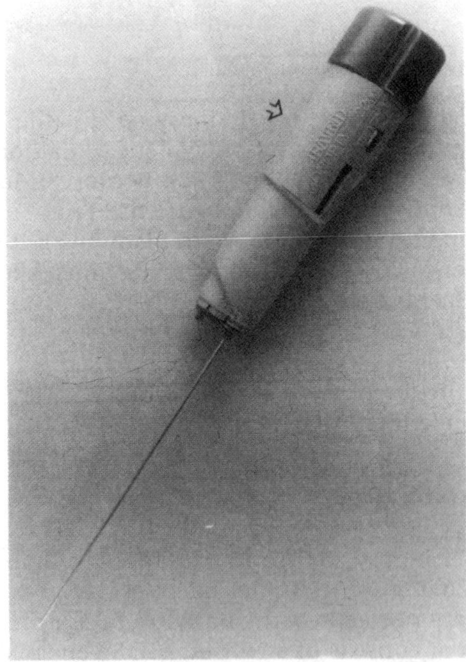

FIG. 4–4. Bard Monopty Biopsy Instrument (Bard Urological Division, Covington, Georgia). Arrow points to the handle, which contains the spring-loaded mechanism for automatic cutting and removal of the tissue core.

required for obtaining tissue by the Vim-Silverman needle and the True-Cut biopsy needle is not necessary for this device. A significant drawback of this needle, however, is that the tissue cores available are thin (22-gauge). In order to collect enough tissue for processing, more than one core is almost always necessary.

BIOPSY PROCEDURE[4]

In the ultrasound suite, the patient is placed prone on the biopsy table. A roll of towels is placed under his or her abdomen in order to stabilize the kidney and push it up toward the operator. An ultrasound examination of kidneys is undertaken to ensure that both kidneys are present and to evaluate their structural normality. The lower pole of the left kidney is localized and its outline marked on the patient's back. Next, the depth of the kidney from the skin is measured by the ultrasound probe. The biopsy needle's optimal point and angle of entry is determined by ultrasound probe. The area is next prepared with povidone-iodine and covered with sterile drapes.

The skin around the planned point of entry is anesthetized by injecting 1% lidocaine intradermally and then subcutaneously. With the help of a long, 22-gauge spinal tap needle, the entire path to be taken by the biopsy needle to the renal surface (as determined earlier by ultrasound probe) is anesthetized. The spinal tap needle is then used to confirm the location and depth of the kidney and to judge the angle at which the biopsy needle must be directed. The spinal tap needle is then withdrawn and the depth to which it was advanced noted on the biopsy needle. The skin over the biopsy site is next nicked with a surgical blade longitudinally (3 to 4 mm) so as to permit the entry of the biopsy needle. The biopsy needle is then advanced toward the underlying kidney at the same angle and to the same depth as determined by the spinal tap needle. The patient is instructed not to breathe as the needle is advanced into the kidney. Its position is then assessed by the pattern of its movement during respiration or by real-time ultrasound examination. An appropriately placed needle (i.e., anchored in the kidney's cortex) swings with each respiratory excursion. Absence of such a movement indicates that the biopsy needle is not within the kidney and must be removed and repositioned. If the biopsy needle is properly positioned, the patient is again instructed not to breathe and a core of tissue is punched from the kidney by whatever maneuver is called for by the instrument in use. Both the needle and tissue core are removed from the patient in one quick motion.

Renal tissue thus obtained is placed in normal saline and examined under a dissection microscope for the number of glomeruli present. The glomeruli, which appear as pink dots under such microscopic examination, should be counted. Six to ten glomeruli should be present in a tissue core for it to be designated as adequate. If enough glomeruli are not present in the tissue, another core of biopsy material may have to be obtained. Usually the pathology technician is handed the tissue specimen for division into three parts to be processed for light, immunofluorescence, and electron microscopy.

BIOPSY IN A RENAL TRANSPLANT

The procedure for biopsying the renal transplant is essentially similar to that for the native kidney except that the kidney is present anteriorly and usually palpable. Accordingly, the patient is placed supine (rather than prone) on the biopsy table, the kidney is palpated, and an ultrasound examination is undertaken. Based on the position of the kidney in the pelvic fossa, the upper pole or lateral aspect of the kidney is selected for biopsy. The remaining steps of the biopsy procedure are similar to those outlined above. It may be difficult to biopsy a kidney that has been placed intraperitoneally, especially if loops of bowel surround the transplanted organ. An open biopsy is preferable under those circumstances. Contraindications to a percutaneous renal biopsy of a transplanted kidney are similar to those cited for the native kidney.

POSTRENAL BIOPSY CARE

After the biopsy procedure has been completed, the kidney should be examined by ultrasound so as to determine whether any subcapsular hematoma has developed. The patient's biopsy site is cleaned with povidone-iodine and an adhesive strip is placed over the site. Vital signs, including blood pressure, are noted, and the patient is taken either to the recovery room or the nephrology floor. Nursing orders, as listed in Table 4–4, should be placed in the patient's chart and adhered to immediately. These orders are designed to ensure that any clinically

TABLE 4–4. Postbiopsy Orders

Place patient flat on back for 12 h
Monitor vital signs, including blood pressure:
- q 15 min X 4
- q 30 min X 4
- q 1 h X 4
- If stable, then monitor q 4 h
- Inform house officer about changes beyond set parameters

Obtain hematocrit 4 h and 24 h after biopsy
Report any abdominal or back pain to the house officer
Observe biopsy site for pain and swelling
Stack samples of voided urine and observe for macroscopic/microscopic hematuria and clots
Report occurrence of gross hematuria to the house officer
Resume diet as tolerated after patient is fully awake; encourage fluid intake
Inform house officer if patient has not voided by 6 h
Discharge patient after 24 h if stable
Clinic follow-up in 1 week

significant hemorrhagic event resulting from the biopsy will be detected at the earliest possible moment and dealt with in a timely fashion. The patient should remain prone for at least 12 h (preferably 24 h) following renal biopsy; even bathroom privileges are restricted during this time. If there is no evidence of clinically significant renal bleeding and the patient is stable, plans for discharge from the hospital can be made after 24 h.

COMPLICATIONS FOLLOWING RENAL BIOPSY

The overall incidence of complications related to renal biopsy has been reported to be about 10 percent, most of these being due to hemorrhage associated with the procedure.[5–7] Death resulting directly from percutaneous renal biopsy has been reported rarely (0.1 percent).[8,9] Improving operator skills and application of modern technologic advances such as continuous real-time ultrasound guidance in directing the biopsy needle can reduce the risk of complications associated with renal biopsy but may not entirely eliminate it.[10] Table 4–5 lists the complications that are associated with renal biopsy.

GROSS HEMATURIA

The incidence of macroscopic hematuria following renal biopsy in children has been reported to range from 5 to 16 percent.[7,11–13] Microscopic hematuria, on the other hand, occurs in almost all patients undergoing renal biopsy and may not be considered a complication of the procedure.[11,14,15] Macroscopic hematuria following renal biopsy usually resolves spontaneously within 24 to 48 h; in some cases, however, patients may require blood transfusion to correct a decreasing hematocrit. Profuse macroscopic hematuria may be indicative of a vascular bleed into the calyceal system and requires urgent surgical exploration.

TABLE 4–5. Incidence of Common Complications of Percutaneous Renal Biopsy

Complication Category	Incidence, Percent	References
Gross hematuria	5–16	5,11–13
Microscopic hematuria	100	11,14
Perirenal hematoma		
Clinical studies	1.5	9
Ultrasound	13–64	20,21
CT scan	60–90	22,23
Renal A-V fistula	6–18	19,25,26
Clinically significant decrease of hematocrit (requiring blood transfusion)	1–3	11,15
Death directly related to biopsy	0.1	8,9

Angiographic obliteration of the bleeding lesions has also been used successfully in managing hematuria following percutaneous renal biopsy.[16] In some patients, severe macroscopic hematuria may lead to the formation of blood clots within the collecting system and cause obstruction of the urinary tract.[17,18]

PERINEPHRIC HEMATOMA

Prior to the availability of ultrasound and computerized tomography (CT), Diaz-Buxo and Donadio reported the incidence of clinically apparent hematoma formation following renal biopsy to be 1.4 percent.[9] Obviously, patients detected to have subcapsular hematomas by clinical examination represent the most severe cases; a vast majority of smaller hematomas probably remain asymptomatic and are therefore not included in such an estimation. The formation of perinephric hematomas in the subcapsular area around the biopsy site has recently been reported to be more common than had previously been thought. Using angiography as a method of study, Jorstad et al. demonstrated subcapsular hematomas developed in 23 percent of patients following renal biopsy.[19] The incidence of subcapsular hematomas detected by ultrasound examination following renal biopsy has ranged from 13 to 64 percent.[20,21] Examination of the kidney by CT scan, on the other hand, has revealed a strikingly high incidence of perirenal hematomas following percutaneous renal biopsy, ranging from 60 percent to more than 90 percent.[22,23] Most perinephric hematomas are, however, small, self-limiting, and resolve with time. In renal transplants, compression by large subcapsular hematomas may compromise renal function.[24]

FORMATION OF ARTERIOVENOUS FISTULAS

It is well known that renal biopsy can result in the development of intrarenal arteriovenous fistulas. This complication, as visualized by renal angiography, has been reported to occur in 6 to 18 percent of patients undergoing renal biopsy.[19,25,26] Presence of an abdominal bruit following renal biopsy should suggest the development of an intrarenal arteriovenous fistula, other manifestations include hypertension and hematuria.[27] Recently, color-coded Doppler sonography has been found to be useful as a noninvasive diagnostic test in the diagnosis of renal arteriovenous fistulas.[28] Although many patients remain asymptomatic, surgical ligation of the arterial end of the fistula may be necessary in those with significant symptomatology. Embolization of the affected arterial branch has also been used in treating intrarenal arteriovenous fistulas.[29]

MISCELLANEOUS COMPLICATIONS

Perforation of the gastrointestinal tract, pancreatic pseudocyst formation,[30] injury to the liver if biopsy is performed on the right side, injury to lumbar arteries with serious hemorrhage,[31] and infection at the biopsy site[18] have all

TABLE 4–6. Contraindications to Renal Biopsy

Absolute contraindications
Solitary kidney (except renal transplant)
Coagulation abnormalities
Severe uncontrolled hypertension
Uncooperative or inadequately sedated patient
Presence of acute pyelonephritis
Relative contraindications
End-stage renal failure
Anatomic anomalies of renal size, shape, and/or position
Chronic pyelonephritis
Hydronephrosis
Conditions where renal biopsy is of limited diagnostic value
Renal cystic disease
Renal tubular disorders
Postural proteinuria

been reported. The performance of the biopsy with radiologic guidance (ultrasound or CT scan) may reduce the occurrence of such complications.

CONTRAINDICATIONS TO RENAL BIOPSY[32,33]

Several clinical conditions are associated with an extraordinarily high risk of complications following renal biopsy, and in some instances the yield from the procedure does not justify risk (Table 4–6). Since renal biopsy is generally an elective surgical procedure, each patient should be evaluated for possible contraindications.

If it is essential to obtain a diagnostic renal biopsy in patients with known contraindications to the percutaneous procedure, an open surgical biopsy may be planned.

SUMMARY

Several technical advances in the last decade have made performance of renal biopsy a safer and less technically complicated procedure. Use of ultrasound guidance in renal biopsy ensures proper placement of the needle in the renal parenchyma and reduces the risk of accidental injury to other abdominal organs.

Prudence, however, dictates that in order to ensure patient safety, each case be evaluated well in advance for both indications and contraindications. An adequately trained and experienced operator is essential for an optimal outcome.

REFERENCES

1. Perez A: La biopsia puntural del rinon no megalico consideraciones generales y aportacion de un nuevo metod. *Boln Liga Cancer* 25:121, 1950.
2. Iversen P, Brun C: Aspiration biopsy of the kidney. *Am J Med* 11:324, 1951.
3. Komaiko MS, Jordan SC, Querfeld U, et al: A new percutaneous renal biopsy device for pediatric patients. *Pediatr Nephrol* 3:191, 1989.
4. Kark RM, Muehrcke RC: Biopsy of the kidney in prone position. *Lancet* 1:1047, 1954.
5. Altebarmakian VK, Guthinger WP, Yakub YN, et al: Percutaneous kidney biopsies: Complications and their management. *Urology* 18:118, 1981.
6. Abdurrahman MB: Percutaneous renal biopsy in a developing country: Experience with 300 cases. *Ann Trop Paediatr* 4:25, 1984.
7. Sweet M, Brouhard BH, Ramirez-Seijas F, et al: Percutaneous renal biopsy in infants and young children. *Clin Nephrol* 26:192, 1986.
8. Slotkin EA, Madsen PO: Complications of renal biopsy: Incidence in 5000 reported cases. *J Urol* 87:13, 1962.
9. Diaz-Buxo JA, Donadio JV: Complications of percutaneous renal biopsy: an analysis of 1000 consecutive biopsies. *Clin Nephrol* 4:223, 1975.
10. Bachmann H, Heckemann R, Olbing H: Percutaneous renal biopsy in children under guidance of ultrasonic real-time technique. *Int J Pediatr Nephrol* 5:175, 1984.
11. Dodge WF, Daeschner CW Jr, Brennan JC, et al: Percutaneous renal biopsy in children. I. General considerations. *Pediatrics* 30:287, 1962.
12. White RHR: Observations on percutaneous renal biopsy in children. *Arch Dis Child* 38:260, 1963.
13. Karafin L, Kendall AR, Fliesher DS: Urologic complications in percutaneous renal biopsy in children. *J Urol* 103:332, 1970.
14. Muth RG: The safety of percutaneous renal biopsy: an analysis of 500 consecutive cases. *J Urol* 94:1, 1965.
15. Bolton WK, Vaughan ED: A comparative study of open surgical and percutaneous renal biopsies. *J Urol* 117:696, 1977.
16. Makita Y, Hori K, Osato S, et al: Successful treatment of massive hemorrhage after percutaneous renal biopsy with transcatheter arterial embolization. *Am J Neprhol* 9:513, 1989.
17. Fruhwald F, Harmuth P, Kovarik J, et al: Bladder obstruction—a rare complication after percutaneous renal biopsy. *Eur J Radiol* 4:225, 1984.
18. Rao KV: Urologic complications associated with a kidney transplant biopsy: Report of 3 cases and review of the literature. *J Urol* 135:768, 1986.
19. Jorstad S, Borander U, Berg KJ, et al: Evaluation of complications due to percutaneous renal biopsy: A clinical and angiographic study. *Am J Kid Dis* 4:162, 1984.
20. Helenius H, Lasonen L, Forslund T, et al: Ultrasonic scanning after percutaneous renal biopsy. *Scand J Urol Nephrol* 17:213, 1983.
21. Nybonde T, Mortensson W: Ultrasonography of the kidney following renal biopsy in children. *Acta Radiol* 29:151, 1988.

22. Ginsburg JC, Fransman SL, Singer MA, et al: Use of computed tomography to evaluate bleeding after renal biopsy. *Nephron* 26:240, 1980.
23. Ralls PW, Barakos JA, Kaptein EM, et al: Renal biopsy-related hemorrhage: Frequency and comparison of CT and sonography. *J Comput Assist Tomogr* 11:1031, 1987.
24. Figueroa TE, Frentz GE: Anuria secondary to percutaneous needle biopsy of a transplant kidney: A case report. *J Urol* 140:355, 1988.
25. Bennett AR, Weiner SN: Intrarenal fistula and aneurysm: a complication of percutaneous renal biopsy. *Am J Roentgenol* 95:372, 1965.
26. Ekelund L, Lindholm T: Arteriovenous fistulae following percutaneous renal biopsy. *Acta Radiol* 11:38, 1971.
27. De Beukelaer MM, Schreiber MH, Dodge WF, et al: Intrarenal arteriovenous fistulas following needle biopsy of the kidney. *J Pediatr* 78:266, 1971.
28. Hubsch PJ, Mostbeck G, Barton PP, et al: Evaluation of arteriovenous fistulas and pseudoaneurysms in renal allografts following percutaneous needle biopsy: Color-coded Doppler sonography versus duplex Dopper sonography. *J Ultrasound Med* 9:95, 1990.
29. Brookstein JJ, Goldstein HM: Successful management of postbiopsy arteriovenous fistula with selective arterial embolization. *Radiology* 109:535, 1973.
30. Ibarguen E, Sharp HL: Gastrointestinal complications following percutaneous kidney biopsy. *J Pediatr Surg* 24:286, 1989.
31. Wall B, Keller FS, Spalding DM, et al: Massive hemorrhage from lumbar artery bleeding following percutaneous renal biopsy. *Am J Kid Dis* 7:250, 1986.
32. Gault MH, Muehrcke RC: Renal biopsy: Current views and controversies. *Nephron* 34:1, 1983.
33. Wickre CG, Golper TA: Complications of percutaneous needle biopsy of the kidney. *Am J Nephrol* 2:173, 1982.

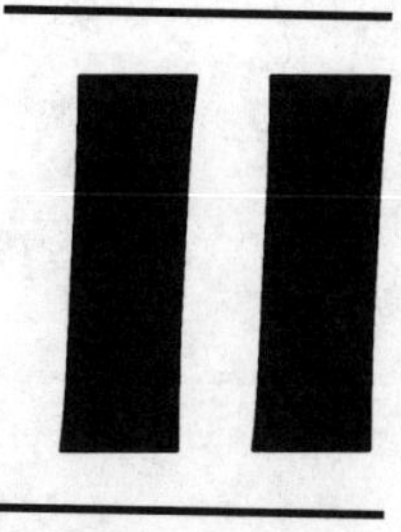

SPECIFIC RENAL DISORDERS

5

HEMATURIA SYNDROMES

Sudesh P. Makker

Hematuria may be defined as the excretion in urine of abnormal amounts of red blood cells (RBCs) or their hemoglobin. It is important to stress that RBCs can be present in normal urine. The presence of six or more RBCs per 0.9 mm^3 counted in a counting chamber in fresh uncentrifuged midstream urine was considered abnormal in a large study in children.[1] In another study in children, the presence of five or more RBCs per high power field in the centrifuged urine sediment was defined as hematuria.[2] In general, three RBCs per high power field are commonly accepted as the upper limit of normal.[3] These definitions are not applicable to females who are menstruating or to catheterized urine samples. In both these situations, excessive excretion of RBCs would be expected. Red blood cells and their hemoglobin are included in the definition because the cells may be lysed during excretion (hypotonic urine) or storage of urine (alkaline pH). This situation is to be differentiated from hemoglobinuria, where free hemoglobin is filtered at the glomerulus and then excreted in the urine as such.

CLINICAL TERMS

Hematuria is a common presentation of the disorders of the urinary tract in children. It is termed *gross* or *macroscopic* when a sufficient amount of blood is present in the urine to discolor it red or brown. If the urine is of normal yellowish color and the blood in it can be detected only by a chemical test or by visualization of RBCs following microscopic examination, it is termed *micro* or *microscopic.* It should be pointed out that only a small amount of blood is needed to discolor urine and thus to fulfill the definition of gross hematuria. For example, the addition of only 1 mL of whole blood to 1000 mL (normal daily volume of urine for most children) of a normal saline solution will produce a red color.

Hematuria detected in each and every urine in a patient is termed *persistent;* if interspersed between normal urines, it is termed *intermittent* or *recurrent.* It is termed *asymptomatic* when it is painless and *symptomatic* when accompanied by symptoms such as pain. These terms are useful because certain renal disorders are more likely than others to follow particular patterns and because these terms are often used in medical papers.

DETECTION

The detection of hematuria has been simplified by the availability of Hemastix (Ames) paper test strips. This strip is impregnated with orthotoluidine and buffered organic peroxide. Orthotoluidine forms a blue-colored compound when hemoglobin is present in urine—either in its free form or within red blood cells—and catalyzes the oxidation reaction of orthotoluidine with peroxide. The color of the strip is compared with a color chart 30 s after the strip is dipped in the urine. The color blocks indicate negative, small, moderate, or large amounts of hemoglobin and range in color through different shades of blue. This test is very sensitive and will give a positive result in a urine where as few as three to five RBCs per high power field would be detected in the urine sediment if the urine were examined microscopically.[3–5] Therefore, a positive (small to large) Hemastix test should be considered significant. The test is much more specific for the presence of free hemoglobin than intact RBCs and will also be positive in myoglobinuria. In hemoglobinuria and myoglobinuria, the paper strip generally shows a diffuse positive reaction, while a speckled appearance is seen if the RBCs are intact. False-negative results may be obtained when large amounts of ascorbic acid are present in urine or when formalin is used to preserve the urine.[6] False-positives may be produced by residues of strongly oxidizing cleaning agents in the urine container or by povidone-iodine.[7]

Microscopic examination of the urine is an essential accompaniment of the paper strip test and should be performed on all patients. Preferably, fresh urine is centrifuged in a conical tube for 3 to 5 min at 2000 to 3000 rpm. The supernatant is then decanted and the sediment redissolved in a small volume of residual urine and layered on a glass slide for microscopic examination. Red blood cells can be identified from their reddish-yellow color and their shape, which may vary depending upon the tonicity of urine. In hypotonic urine, the cells look like swollen spheres or are lysed; in isotonic urine, they may appear as spheres or biconcave disks; and in hypertonic urine, they may look like small, crenated spheres. Sometimes *Candida* spores, spherical calcium oxalate crystals, and air bubbles may be mistaken for RBCs; however, the Hemastix test will be negative for all these situations. If the Hemastix test is negative and no RBCs are found in the urine sediment but the urine is discolored red, other causes such as the ingestion of anthrocyanins (beets and berries), phenindione, pyridium, phenolphthalein, food colorings, porphyrin, etc. should be considered. Heavy urate concentration in urine can give it a pinkish hue ("pink diaper" in infants).

QUANTITATION

Quantitation of microhematuria (Addis count) is rarely indicated and generally not very helpful in clinical decision making. Addis's studies showed that normal individuals excrete between 500,000 and 2 million RBCs per day (1500/min).[8]

Quantitation of gross hematuria may be obtained by performing a hematocrit on urine (urocrit) in a manner similar to that used for a hematocrit on whole blood.

GLOMERULAR VERSUS NONGLOMERULAR HEMATURIA

A careful look at the morphology of the red cells with the knowledge of the tonicity (specific gravity) of the urine can be helpful in differentiating glomerular from nonglomerular microhematuria. Red blood cells originating from a glomerular leak show great variation in size, shape, and hemoglobin content, often appearing fragmented and crenated (Fig. 5–1), whereas those coming from lesions such as tumors, calculi, infections, and other nonglomerular sources are uniform in size and shape and usually retain a high hemoglobin content except when the urine is strongly acidic.[9] These findings are best observed under phase contrast microscopy. In addition to the glomerular morphology of RBCs, the presence of RBC casts and heavy proteinuria also suggests that the hematuria is of glomerular origin.

ETIOLOGY OF HEMATURIA

Hematuria may originate from any site in the urinary tract, from the glomerular capillaries to the anterior urethra, and it can be due to a variety of causes, from trauma to disorders of coagulation. It may be due to inherited defects or acquired disorders. Common causes of hematuria in children are listed in Table 5–1, and Table 5–2. In each category the disease entities are listed in approximate order of prevalence.

EVALUATION OF CHILDREN WITH HEMATURIA

A careful history, physical examination, and urinalysis (including microscopic examination of sediment) will in most cases give the necessary clues for further diagnostic studies (Fig. 5–2).

HISTORY

Symptoms of frequency, urgency, dysuria, hesitancy, enuresis, suprapubic heaviness, flank pain, fever, etc., suggest urinary tract infection. Renal colic-like pain in the loin region or radiating to the groin region suggests calculi or blood clots in the kidney or ureter. Dysuria with hematuria in the beginning of micturition suggests anterior urethritis, and dysuria with terminal hematuria usually indicates posterior urethritis or a bladder calculus. Painless gross hematuria with brown tea- or coke-colored urine usually indicates glomerulonephritis, and painless red- or pink-colored urine is usually associated with nonglomerular causes such as trauma, tumors, coagulation disorders, renal tuberculosis, etc.

Gross hematuria following upper respiratory infection is frequently seen in

TABLE 5–1. Etiology of Hematuria

- Parenchymal Renal Disorders
  - Glomerular
    - Inherited
      - Alport syndrome
      - Familial benign hematuria
      - Nail-patella syndrome
      - Fabry disease
    - Acquired
      - Primary glomerular diseases
      - IgA nephropathy
      - Mesangial proliferative glomerulonephritis
      - Membranoproliferative glomerulonephritis
      - Crescentic glomerulonephritis
      - Membranous glomerulonephritis
      - Focal glumerulosclerosis
      - Minimal change disease
    - Glomerular disease as part of a systemic disease
      - Systemic lupus erythematosus
      - Henoch-Schönlein purpura
      - Vasculitis, including polyarteritis nodosa, Wagner granulomatosis and other collagen vascular diseases
      - Hemolytic uremic syndrome
      - Goodpasture syndrome
      - Diabetes mellitus
      - Amyloidosis
    - Infectious
      - Poststreptococcal glomerulonephritis
      - Subacute bacterial endocarditis
      - "Shunt" nephritis
      - Hepatitis B–associated glomerulonephritis
      - Congenital syphilis–associated glomerulonephritis
      - Malaria
      - Schistosomiasis
      - Filariasis
      - Toxoplasmosis
  - Tubulointerstitial
    - Congenital or inherited
      - Polycystic kidney disease (infantile or adult type)
      - Medullary cystic disease (juvenile nephronophthisis)
      - Congenital nephrotic syndrome (microcystic disease)
      - Ask-Upmark kidney
      - Cystinosis
      - Oxalosis
      - Renal dysplasia
      - Nephrocalcinosis associated with renal tubular acidosis
      - Tuberous sclerosis
    - Acquired
      - Renal transplant rejection
      - Nephrolithiasis
      - Exogenous toxins
      - Aminoglycoside toxicity
      - Cyclosporine toxicity
      - Cytotoxic drugs used for cancer therapy (cisplatin, etc.)

TABLE 5–1 (*Continued*). Etiology of Hematuria

Tubulointerstitial *(cont'd)*
- Acquired *(cont'd)*
  - Heavy metal toxicity (lead, mercury)
  - Radiation injury
  - Radiocontrast medium injury
  - Analgesic abuse
  - Infectious (bacterial, viral, fungal, rickettsial, protozoal)
  - Obstructive uropathy
  - Reflux nephropathy
  - Hypersensitivity to drugs (penicillin, sulfa drugs, nonsteroidal anti-inflammatory drugs, diuretics, and others)
  - Metabolic disorders
  - Hypercalcemia, hypercalciuria
  - Hyperuricemia
  - Tumors
  - Wilms tumor and other neoplasias
  - Leukemic or lymphomatous infiltrates
  - Multisystem disorders
  - Systemic lupus erythematosus
  - Sarcoidosis
  - Sjögren syndrome
  - Idiopathic interstitial nephritis
  - Renal papillary necrosis (sickle cell disease, diabetes, analgesic abuse)

Vascular
- Sickle cell disease
- Renal vein thrombosis
- Renal arterial thrombosis or embolism
- Loin pain hematuria
- Arteriovenous malformations
- Malignant hypertension

Urinary Tract Disorders
- Urinary tract infections (bacterial, fungal, viral, protozoal, rickettsial)
- Calculi
- Trauma
- Hydronephrosis
- Periureteritis (appendicitis, etc.)
- Ureterocele
- Cyclophosphamide cystitis
- Prostatitis
- Foreign body
- Urethritis

Associated Bleeding and Coagulation Defects
- Hemophilia
- Thrombocytopenic purpura
- Anticoagulants
- Other congenital or acquired defects of coagulation

Factitious Hematuria

---

various forms of glomerulonephritis. In poststreptococcal glomerulonephritis, the sore throat precedes the onset of gross hematuria by 7 to 14 days, and the symptoms of sore throat have usually resolved by the time the hematuria appears. In IgA nephropathy, the gross hematuria develops along with the

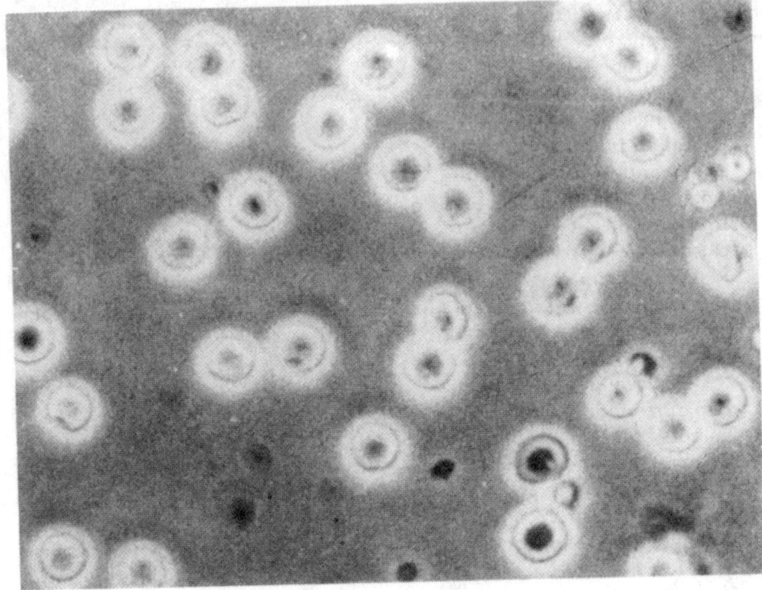

A

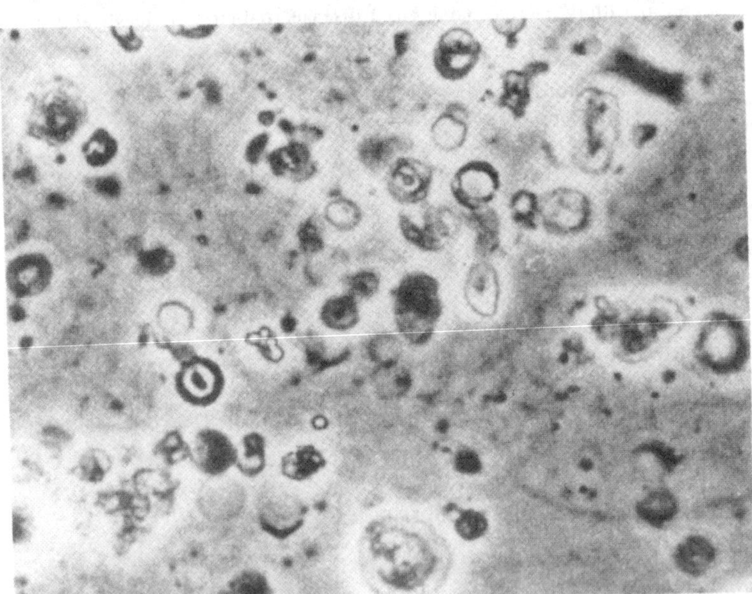

B

FIG. 5–1. *A*. Nonglomerular hematuria, characterized by well-demarcated red cell boundaries. *B*. Glomerular hematuria, characterized by irregular, dysmorphic red cells. (Reproduced with permission from Fairley KF, Birch DF: Hematuria: A simple method for identifying glomerular bleeding. *Kidney Int* 21:105, 1982.)

TABLE 5–2. Causes of Asymptomatic Hematuria with No or Minimal Proteinuria

Glomerular
IgA nephropathy
Poststreptococcal glomerulonephritis
Henoch-Schönlein purpura
Benign familial hematuria
Mesangioproliferative glomerulonephritis
Systemic lupus erythematosus
Alport syndrome
Membranoproliferative glomerulonephritis
Exercise-induced hematuria
Nonglomerular renal
Sickle cell disease
Polycystic kidney disease
Renovascular hypertension
Hypercalciuria
Renal vein thrombosis
Nephrocalcinosis
Renal tumors
Leukemic or lymphomatous infiltrates in kidney
Hydronephrosis
Renal tuberculosis
Renal hemangioma
Nonrenal
Calculi[a]
Urinary tract infection[a]
Foreign body (urethra or bladder)[a]
Bladder tumors and arteriovenous malformations

[a]Hematuria may be painful.

upper respiratory infection and usually clears as the infection subsides. This is a very useful differentiating clue to the diagnosis of IgA nephropathy versus poststreptococcal glomerulonephritis.

It should be kept in mind that poststreptococcal glomerulonephritis and IgA nephropathy are not the only glomerulonephritides where gross hematuria is associated with upper respiratory infection. Respiratory infections may lead to flare-ups of any underlying chronic glomerulonephritis, resulting in gross hematuria.

A history of purpuric skin rash, joint pain, abdominal pain, fever, etc., would suggest Henoch-Schönlein purpura or systemic lupus erythematosus. Weight loss and poor appetite may be seen in tuberculosis, systemic lupus erythematosus, or with tumors. Weight gain may indicate fluid retention, as a result of either associated renal failure or nephrotic syndrome. A recent throat or skin infection may indicate poststreptococcal glomerulonephritis, and a history of previous heart murmurs or atrioventricular shunts for hydrocephalus with fever would suggest, respectively, subacute bacterial endocarditis and shunt nephritis. A careful history should be taken, including previous renal calculi or bleeding or clotting disorders (hemophilia), drug ingestion (e.g., anticoagulants, antibiotics, particularly aminoglycosides), administration of cyclophosphamide

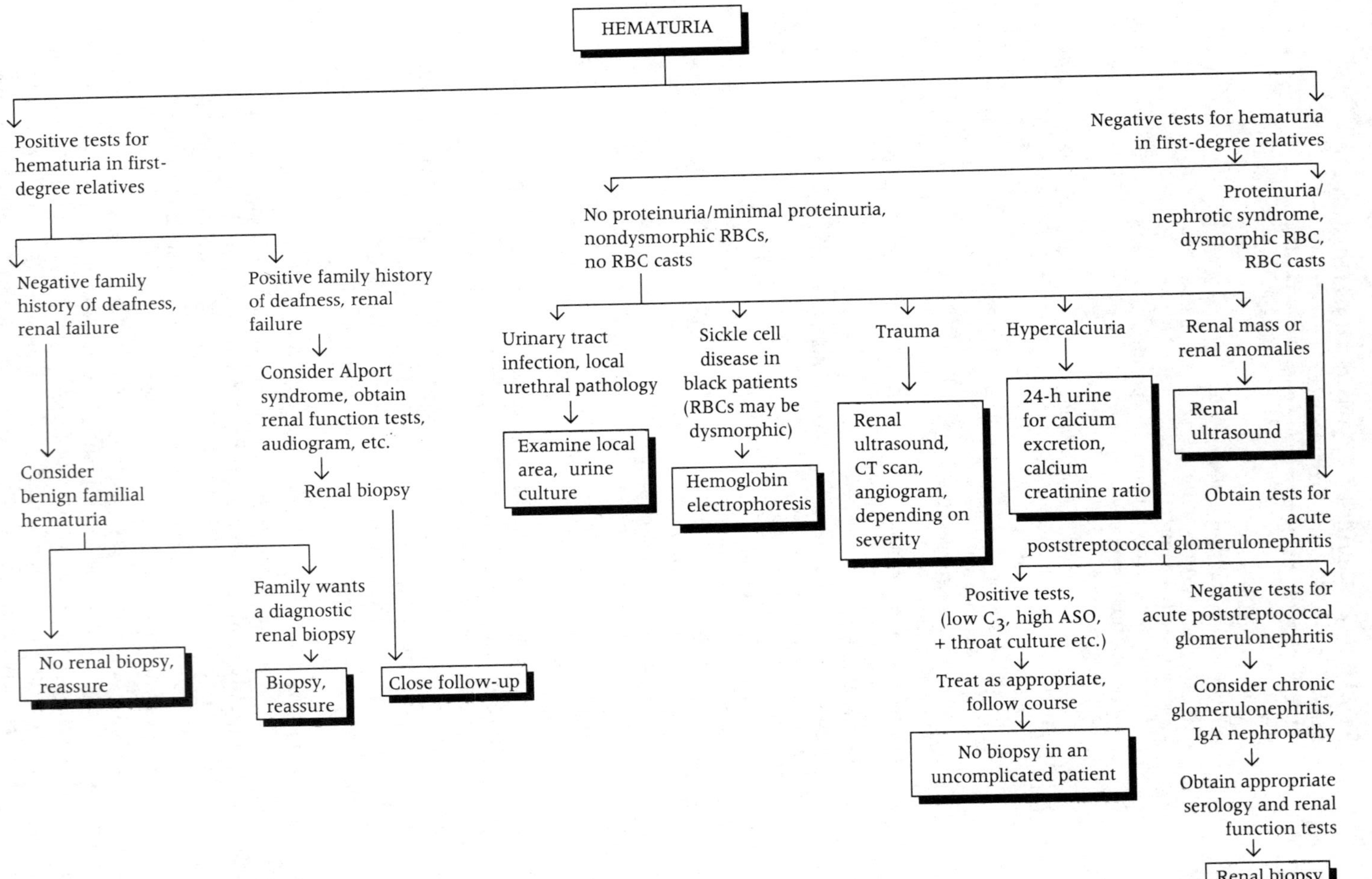

FIG. 5–2. Algorithm for the evaluation of hematuria in children.

or nitrogen mustard (chemical cystitis), analgesic abuse (papillary cystitis), necrosis, etc.

A family history of chronic glomerulonephritis and renal failure with or without deafness is suggestive of Alport syndrome. In familial benign hematuria, several members of the family may have the condition, but the course is benign and renal failure is not seen. A family history of polycystic kidney disease, sickle cell disease, and/or bleeding/clotting disorders (hemophilia) will be helpful in diagnosing these conditions.

PHYSICAL EXAMINATION

Physical examination is frequently normal; however, certain findings can be very helpful in diagnosis and must be recorded. High blood pressure usually indicates either an underlying parenchymal renal disease or renal failure. Occasionally severe hypertension (malignant hypertension) itself may produce microscopic hematuria. Eye grounds should be examined for hypertensive retinopathy and papilledema whenever blood pressure is elevated. Corneal and lens abnormalities may indicate Alport syndrome. Additionally, sensorineural deafness may be detected in the latter condition. Pallor (anemia) is usually the result of associated renal failure but may also be seen in systemic lupus erythematosus or hemolytic uremic syndrome due to hemolytic anemia. Poststreptococcal glomerulonephritis frequently produces some anemia, and anemia may also be seen in other forms of chronic glomerulonephritis. Anemia generally does not develop as a result of the minimal blood loss associated with gross hematuria. A purpuric skin rash is always present in Henoch-Schönlein purpura and may also be seen in systemic lupus erythematosus and other forms of vasculitis. Generalized edema indicates fluid retention associated with renal failure or the nephrotic syndrome. Heart murmurs may indicate subacute bacterial endocarditis, and abnormal heart rhythm may be associated with emboli. Kidneys may be enlarged and palpable in polycystic kidney disease, hydronephrosis, renal vein thrombosis, or renal tumors. Tenderness in the costovertebral areas may indicate urinary tract infection or loin pain hematuria. The anterior urethral meatus should be examined for evidence of urethritis, and rectal examination should be performed in teenage boys when prostatitis is suspected.

URINALYSIS

The importance of a careful urinalysis, including examination of the urine sediment, cannot be overemphasized. This procedure should be performed by the *physician.* Brown tea- or coke-colored urine generally suggests a diagnosis of glomerulonephritis. The presence of RBC casts is essentially pathognomic of glomerulonephritis. White blood cell casts, granular casts, epithelial cell casts, and waxy casts may be present in glomerulonephritis or tubulointerstitial nephritis. Detection of dysmorphic RBCs will also suggest a glomerular disease. Heavy proteinuria (3 to 4+) almost always indicates glomerular parenchymal disorders. This is particularly true if it is detected in a yellow urine in the absence of gross hematuria. With gross hematuria of nonglomerular origin, some protein in urine (part of the blood protein) would be expected; however, this rarely exceeds 1 to 2+ on dipstick tests for proteinuria. This is because it only takes a few milliliters of blood to discolor the urine. For example, if 10 mL of whole blood (6 mL of plasma) were to be added to the urine from a bladder bleed and the normal volume of urine is 1000 mL, it will amount to the addition of only 420 mg of blood protein (7 g/100 mL of plasma), providing a concentration of 42 mg/100 mL. This would only give a 2+ result on dipsticks, yet the urine would be grossly bloody. As pointed out earlier, even 1 milliliter of whole blood can produce the appearance of gross hematuria. Any of the conditions listed in Table 5–1 can produce hematuria with no or minimal proteinuria.

> **Comments (Kanwal Kher).** Tapp and Copley[10] evaluated the effect of varying degrees of hematuria on urinary protein concentration. They added blood from healthy volunteers to urine of varying osmolalities to produce a urocrit ranging from 0.01 to 3.0 percent. A urocrit of 0.05 percent or less (the equivalent of microscopic hematuria) was never associated with proteinuria. On the other hand, the urinary protein concentration in a grossly bloody urine (urocrit, 3.0 percent) in an isotonic or hypertonic urine resulted in a moderate degree of proteinuria (69 to 97 mg/dL), while the same urocrit in a hypotonic urine resulted in a urinary protein concentration of 1302 mg/dL. The authors suspected hemolysis of RBCs, leading to the release of hemoglobin (and the cause for increased urinary protein) in a hypotonic urinary environment. Protein electrophoresis, indeed, revealed hemoglobin to be the protein responsible for a positive test. Therefore, in a patient with macroscopic hematuria, falsely elevated urinary protein excretion can be observed due to hemoglobin derived from red blood cells as a result of hemolysis.

Based on urinalysis, most children with hematuria can be placed in one of the two following categories: (1) hematuria with minimal or no proteinuria and (2) hematuria associated with proteinuria.

Hematuria with Minimal or No Proteinuria. This is a common problem in children. This diagnosis is made if no proteinuria is detected in *yellow* urine. If the hematuria is gross, some protein (part of blood proteins) would be expected. Hematuria may be painful or asymptomatic. Painful hematuria is less common and often due to urinary tract infection or urinary calculi, hypercalciuria sometimes due to IgA nephropathy and less commonly due to the syndrome of "loin pain hematuria." This last condition was first described by Little et al.[11] in 1967 as one that is usually seen in teenage girls and young women who present with recurrent episodes of severe and at times incapacitating pain in the loin area associated with gross hematuria. The urine may be normal between episodes, and there is no detectable abnormality on intravenous pyelography or cystoscopy. Renal biopsy specimens show only minor changes in the glomeruli (increased mesangial matrix).[12] Granular staining for C3 complement may be present in the walls of small arteries and arterioles on immunofluorescence,[13] and abnormal intrarenal vasculature may be seen on angiography.[9] There is no satisfactory treatment for this condition; analgesics, antiplatelet agents, anticoagulants, and fibrinolytic agents are unhelpful. Renal denervation and autotransplantation have been shown to result in relief of pain.[14] This procedure, however, does not stop the hematuria.

Asymptomatic hematuria with minimal or no proteinuria is more common than painful hematuria in children. Common causes of this condition are listed in Table 5–2. It must be remembered, however, that although the glomerular diseases listed in Table 5–2 may present with isolated hematuria, they can also present with hematuria and greater amounts of proteinuria.

Hematuria Associated with Proteinuria. Hematuria associated with heavy proteinuria (3 to 4+), particularly if detected in a yellow urine, invariably indicates glomerular disease. Although mild to moderate proteinuria (1 to 2+) is not uncommon in glomerular diseases, it may also be seen in tubulointeristitital diseases. In the latter conditions, it is usually less than 1 g/day; in glomerular diseases, it is frequently but not always greater than 1 g/day. Glomerular diseases are discussed in Chaps. 7 and 8. It should be remembered that gross hematuria from nonglomerular causes, as pointed out earlier, can be associated with mild proteinuria (1 to 2+) on dipsticks. Also, glomerular diseases may present with microscopic hematuria only and no abnormal proteinuria (e.g., IgA nephropathy).

OTHER LABORATORY TESTS

1. A complete blood count (CBC), including erythrocyte sedimentation rate (ESR), can provide leads toward some of the causes of hematuria. Anemia with sickle cells would suggest sickle cell disease. Microangiopathic anemia with distorted RBCs and thrombocytopenia should suggest the possibility of hemolytic uremic syndrome. Normocytic normochromic anemia with a high reticulocyte count (indicating a hemolytic process) may be seen in systemic lupus erythematosus. Normocytic normochromic anemia with normal or low reticulocyte count would indicate bone marrow suppression, which can be seen with chronic renal failure (suggesting parenchymal disease) or with chronic conditions such as glomerulonephritis or systemic disorders such as tuberculosis, systemic lupus erythematosus, etc. The ESR may be elevated in a multitude of conditions listed under parenchymal renal disorders and is not diagnostic of any specific one. However, ESR can be a useful parameter for monitoring the activity of a given condition and will generally decrease or increase in parallel with its severity.

2. A urine culture should be obtained if hematuria is symptomatic. Generally, if a urinary tract infection is severe enough to produce hematuria, it is likely to be associated with symptoms like dysuria, frequency, urgency, enuresis, suprapubic tenderness, costovertebral angle tenderness, fever, etc. If there are no other symptoms, it is unlikely that the urine culture would show significant bacterial growth. However, the urine should probably be cultured in all cases. It is also well to remember that the hematuria caused by renal tuberculosis is asymptomatic.

3. Basic blood chemistries should be obtained for every patient early in evaluation and should include at least blood urea nitrogen (BUN) and serum creat-

inine to rule out renal failure, which may be seen in many conditions, particularly those affecting the renal parenchyma. Other serum chemistries such as serum electrolytes, calcium, phosphorus, uric acid, total serum protein, serum albumin, and serum cholesterol should be performed if evaluation to this point (history, physical examination, urinalysis, CBC, BUN, and serum creatinine) has led to the suspicion of parenchymal renal disease. Some causes of hematuria such as renal tubular acidosis with nephrocalcinosis and hyperuricemia, etc. would be uncovered by these tests. Low total serum proteins, low serum albumin, and high serum cholesterol would indicate the presence of a nephrotic syndrome, which invariably would indicate a parenchymal glomerular disease.

4. An ultrasound examination of the abdomen can be performed to uncover conditions such as polycystic kidney disease, hydronephrosis, renal tumors, renal calculi, and even renal vein thrombosis. This noninvasive test can be very helpful in the initial assessment of the conditions mentioned above. For more definitive information, other tests can then be performed, such as an intravenous urogram (hydronephrosis, renal stones, polycystic kidneys, tumors), angiogram (tumors, renal arterial obstruction), CT scan (tumors), and inferior venacavogram (renal vein thrombosis).

5. If parenchymal glomerular disease is suspected (brown- or tea-colored urine, heavy proteinuria, red blood cell casts and dysmorphic RBCs in urine sediment), additional blood and urine studies should be obtained and should include the following: throat culture and culture of skin impetigo lesions (poststreptococcal glomerulonephritis), a 24-h urine for total protein to assess the presence of heavy proteinuria and calcium/creatinine ratio for hypercalciuria (>0.2), serum total hemolytic complement, C3 and C4 complement, antinuclear antibody test, hepatitis-associated antigen (HAA) test, antistreptolysin O (ASO) and serologic test for syphilis, etc. If poststreptococcal disease is suspected and the ASO titer is not high, other tests for antibodies to streptococcal antigens may be necessary (antihyaluronidase, anti-DNase B). If the antinuclear antibody test is positive, then the anti-DNA antibody test should be performed to further assist in the diagnosis of systemic lupus erythematosus. Blood cultures may be useful if subacute bacterial endocarditis or shunt nephritis is suspected; eosinophils in urine may be detected in hypersensitivity interstitial nephritis. Goodpasture syndrome is rare in children, but if it is suspected, serum should be tested for antiglomerular basement membrane antibodies.

6. If Alport syndrome or familial hematuria is suspected, other members of the family should be screened for hematuria. This can easily be done by giving Hemastix to the family and asking them to check the first morning urine specimen. An audiogram may be obtained if Alport syndrome is suspected.

7. A skin test for tuberculosis may be performed to rule out renal tuberculosis (painless hematuria, absence of features of glomerular disease, negative urine cultures for bacteria, absence of renal masses, high erythrocyte sedimentation rate, and evidence of primary tuberculosis elsewhere). For culturing the tubercle bacillus, three 24-h urine or three full first morning urines should be obtained.

8. Cystoscopy is rarely needed for the diagnosis of hematuria in children. It should be considered if it is necessary to localize the side (right versus left ureter) or if it is suspected that the site of bleeding is in the bladder. The latter

TABLE 5–3. Evaluation of Hematuria

History
Physical examination
Urinalysis, including microscopic examination
Urinalysis on family members (Alport syndrome, familial benign hematuria)
Urine culture
Skin test for TB
Complete blood counts, including reticulocyte count, examination of peripheral smear, and erythrocyte sedimentation rate (ESR)
Serum chemistries, including BUN, creatinine, electrolytes, calcium, phosphorus, total proteins, albumin, and cholesterol, etc.
24-h urine for total protein, calcium, creatinine, and creatinine clearance
Throat culture, skin impetigo culture (poststreptococcal glomerulonephritis)
Serum C3, C4, antinuclear antibody (ANA), hepatitis-associated antigen (HAA), antistreptolysin O (ASO) titer, serologic test for syphilis (VDRL), antineutrophil antibodies, etc.
Audiogram (Alport syndrome)
Ultrasound examination of abdomen
Intravenous urogram and cystourethrogram
Angiography
Renal biopsy
Cystoscopy

would be indicated by nonrenal hematuria (pink urine; absence of proteinuria in a yellow urine or minimal proteinuria when hematuria is gross; no RBCs, WBCs, epithelial cells, or granular casts in the urine sediment; normal morphology of RBCs), a negative urine culture, a normal ultrasound examination of the urinary tract and abdomen, and a negative workup for parenchymal renal disease and a systemic bleeding or clotting disorder.

9. A percutaneous renal biopsy may be necessary for a definitive diagnosis of glomerular and or tubulointerstitial disease.

The above plan will uncover the cause of hematuria in most patients (Table 5–3). However, it should be kept in mind that all of these diagnostic tests are not necessary in every case and an algorithm presented in Fig. 5–2 may be followed as a guide.

EXERCISE-RELATED HEMATURIA

Micro- or macrohematuria has been documented following prolonged running in otherwise healthy persons. Earlier it was thought that it resulted from impaction of the flaccid posterior wall of the bladder against the base of the bladder during running, because ecchymoses and congestion of the posterior bladder were seen on cystoscopy in these subjects.[15] In a recent study an appreciable increase in the number of RBCs in urine was seen in 44 of 48 runners, with the numbers clearly exceeding normal limits in 33.[16] Further, the red cell morphology indicated hematuria of glomerular origin and 46 subjects showed increases in hyaline casts as well as granular casts, while 10 showed RBC casts. If the urinalysis is normal otherwise and hematuria is detected only following exercise, further work is usually not necessary.

TABLE 5–4. Differentiating Features of Benign Hematuria, Alport Syndrome, and IgA Nephropathy

	Benign Familial Hematuria	Alport Syndrome	IgA Nephropathy
Sex	F<M	M>F	M>F
Family history of hematuria	+	+	−
Family history of ESRD	−	+	−
Deafness	−	+	−
Blood pressure	Normal	Hypertension in many	Usually normal
Proteinuria	Minimal	Can be severe	Moderate
Serum creatinine	Normal	May be abnormal	Usually normal
Outcome	Benign	Declining renal function	Usually benign

BENIGN FAMILIAL HEMATURIA

This disorder is characterized by hematuria in the patients and some of their first-degree family members; however, a family history of sensorineural deafness and end-stage renal failure is lacking.[17,18] In most patients, the hematuria is microscopic in nature and is detected on routine physical examination. Some, however, may develop macroscopic hematuria at onset or during follow-up.[18,19] Proteinuria is generally absent or minimal, and blood pressure and renal function are normal in all. The mode of inheritance of benign hematuria has been suggested to be autosomal dominant, with a strong predominance of the disease in females.[18,19] Age at the time of detection of benign familial hematuria in children has been reported to be about 5 years.[18,21]

Renal biopsy of these patients usually shows normal or minimal glomerular abnormalities on light and immunofluorescence microscopy.[18,21,23] Electron microscopy, on the other hand, may show a thinned lamina densa of the glomerular basement membrane in some patients.[18–22] Splitting or lamination of the glomerular basement membrane seen in Alport syndrome is absent in patients with benign familial hematuria.[18,20–22]

The clinical course of patients with benign familial hematuria is generally favorable. Several studies have documented well-preserved renal function in children during prolonged follow-up.[18,20] A similarly benign outcome has been reported in adults by Blumenthal et al.[19] Clinical features differentiating benign familial hematuria from Alport syndrome and IgA nephropathy are listed in Table 5–4.

HEMATURIA IN SICKLE CELL DISEASE

Hematuria is a common manifestation of sickle cell hemoglobinopathy.[23] It is reported to be more common in patients with sickle cell trait (SA) than in those with sickle cell anemia (SS)[24–26]; however, this may be due to the fact that there are more patients with SA than with SS in the general population. Hematuria due to sickle cell hemoglobinopathy is more common in males, and may be microscopic or macroscopic hematuria. In patients with macroscopic hematuria, the left kidney is affected more often than the right one.[27]

The etiopathogenesis of hematuria in sickle cell disease is unclear, but the condition is believed to result from obstruction and rupture of the vasa recta in the renal medullary circulation.[28] The process of sickling and microvascular thrombosis in the vasa recta is facilitated by medullary hypertonicity, low oxygen tension, and acidosis. Resulting vascular stasis and obstruction leads to rupture of these vessels into the urinary collecting system. Papillary necrosis has also been reported in sickle cell disease.[29]

REFERENCES

1. Vehaskari VM, Rapola J, Koskimies O, et al: Microscopic hematuria in schoolchildren: Epidemiology and clinicopathologic evaluation. *J Pediatr* 95:676, 1979.
2. Dodge WF, West EF, Smith EK, et al: Proteinuria and hematuria in schoolchildren: Epidemiology and early natural history. *J Pediatr* 88:327, 1976.
3. Glassock RJ: Hematuria and pigmenturia, in: Massry SG, Glassock RJ (eds): *Textbook of Nephrology.* Baltimore, Williams & Wilkins, 1983, pp 4, 12.
4. Shaw ST, Poon SY, Wong T: Routine urinalysis. *JAMA* 253:1596, 1985.
5. Look S, Scottolini AG, Luangphinith S, et al: Urine screening strategy employing dipstick analysis and selective culture: An evaluation. *Am J Clin Pathol* 81:634, 1984.
6. White-Stevens RH: Interference by ascorbic acid in test systems involving peroxidase: I. Reverse indicators and the effects of copper, iron and mercury. *Clin Chem* 28:578, 1982.
7. Litwin MS, Graham SD: False positive hematuria. *JAMA* 254:1724, 1985.
8. Addis T: The number of formed elements in the urinary sediment of normal individuals. *J Clin Invest* 2:409, 1926.
9. Fairley KF, Birch DF: Hematuria: A simple method for identifying glomerular bleeding. *Kidney Int* 21:105, 1982.
10. Tapp DC, Copley JB: Effect of red blood cell lysis on protein quantification in hematuric states. *Am J Nephrol* 8:190, 1988.
11. Little PJ, Sloper JS, de Wardner HE: A syndrome of loin pain and hematuria associated with disease of peripheral renal arteries. *Q J Med* 36:253, 1967.
12. Burden RP, Dathan JR, Etherington MD, et al: The loin-pain/haematuria syndrome. *Lancet* 1:897, 1979.
13. Naish PF, Aber GM, Boyd WN: C3 deposition in renal arterioles in the loin pain hematuria syndrome. *Br Med J* 3:746, 1975.
14. Bloom PB, Viner ED, Mazala M, et al: Treatment of loin pain hematuria syndrome by renal autotransplantation. *Am J Med* 87:228, 1989.
15. Siegel AJ, Hennekens CH, Solomon HS, et al: Exercise-related hematuria: Findings in a group of marathon runners. *JAMA* 241:391, 1979.
16. Fassett RG, Owen JE, Fairley J, et al: Urinary red-cell morphology during exercise. *Br Med J* 285:1455, 1982.
17. McConville J, West C, McAdams A: Familial and non-familial benign hematuria. *J Pediatr* 69:207, 1966.

18. Yoshikawa N, Matsuyama S, Iijima K, et al: Benign familial hematuria. *Arch Pathol Lab Med* 112:794, 1988.
19. Blumenthal SS, Fritsche C, Lemann J: Establishing the diagnosis of benign familial hematuria: The importance of examining urine sediment of family members. *JAMA* 259:2263, 1988.
20. Tina L, Jenis E, Jose P, et al: The glomerular basement membrane in benign familial hematuria. *Clin Nephrol* 17:1, 1982.
21. Piel CF, Biava CG, Goodman JR: Glomerular basement membrane attenuation in familial nephritis and "benign" hematuria. *J Pediatr* 101:358, 1982.
22. Tiebosch ATMG, Frederik PM, van Breda Vriesman PJC, et al: Thin-basement-membrane nephropathy in adults with persistent hematuria. *N Engl J Med* 320:14, 1989.
23. Sears DA: The morbidity of sickle cell trait: A review of the literature. *Am J Med* 64:1021, 1978.
24. Lucas WM, Bullock WH: Hematuria in sickle cell disease. *J Urol* 83:733, 1960.
25. Alleyne GAO, Statius van Eps LW, Addae CK, et al: The kidney in sickle cell anemia. *Kidney Int* 5:371, 1975.
26. Allen TD: Sickle cell disease and hematuria: A report of 29 cases. *J Urol* 91:177, 1964.
27. Mostofi FK, Vorder Bruegge CF, Diggs LW: Lesions in kidneys removed for unilateral hematuria in sickle cell disease. *Arch Pathol Lab Med* 63:336, 1957.
28. de Jong PE, Statius van Eps LW: Sickle cell nephropathy: New insights into its pathophysiology. *Kidney Int* 27:711, 1985.
29. Harrow BR, Sloane JA, Liebman NC: Roentgenologic demonstration of renal papillary necrosis in sickle cell disease. *N Engl J Med* 268:969, 1963.

6

PROTEINURIA

Sudesh P. Makker

Proteinuria has been known to be associated with renal disease since the days of Richard Bright, over 150 years ago.[1] Like hematuria, it is one of the most common urine abnormalities seen in children with parenchymal renal disease; when present with hematuria in the absence of gross hematuria, it almost always indicates an underlying renal disease. On the other hand, isolated proteinuria, albeit transient, may also accompany several nonrenal diseases and such varied conditions as febrile illness, seizures, pneumonia, chronic obstructive lung disease, congestive heart failure, changes in posture, after strenuous exercise, during emotional stress, after administration of epinephrine, etc.[2,3] Heavy proteinuria or low-grade persistent proteinuria generally indicate a renal disease and should be investigated. It is also important to remember that proteinuria with other symptoms (such as dysuria, frequency of urination, abdominal pain, and hematuria) may be seen in urinary tract infections.

PROTEIN IN NORMAL URINE

Normal urine contains protein. Nearly 60 percent of the proteins are plasma proteins; the remaining 40 percent originate from the secretions of the urinary tract.[4] The major plasma protein is albumin, but 32 plasma proteins have been detected in normal urine, including small amounts of immunoglobulins G, A, and D, immunoglobulin fragments (Fc fragment, light chains, heavy chains), transferrin, beta$_2$ microglobulin, haptoglobin, ceruloplasmin, and several enzymes like amylase, lysozyme, and kallikrein, etc.[5,6] Tissue proteins originating from the urinary tract are Tamm-Horsfall mucoproteins, urokinase, secretory IgA, and small amounts of glomerular basement membrane-like and tubular epithelial cell proteins.[6] The bulk of the tissue protein is made up of Tamm-Horsfall protein, a large mucoglycoprotein secreted by the distal tubule and involved in cast formation.[6,7] Briefly, normal urine contains 40 percent albumin, 40 percent Tamm-Horsfall protein, 15 percent immunoglobulins, and 5 percent other plasma proteins and enzymes.[6] The total amount of protein in a

TABLE 6–1. Normal 24-h Urine Protein

	Total, mg	mg/m^{2a}
Premature babies (5–30 days)	14–60	88–377
Full-term babies (7–30 days)	15–68	68–309
Infants (2–12 months)	17–85	48–244
Children 2–4 years	20–121	37–223
4–10 years	26–194	31–234
10–16 years	29–238	22–181

[a]mg/m^2 = milligrams per square meter of body surface area.

Source: Adapted from Miltényi M: Urinary protein excretion in healthy children. *Clin Nephrol* 12:216, 1979. Reproduced by permission from Dustri-Verlag, Deisenhofen, Germany.

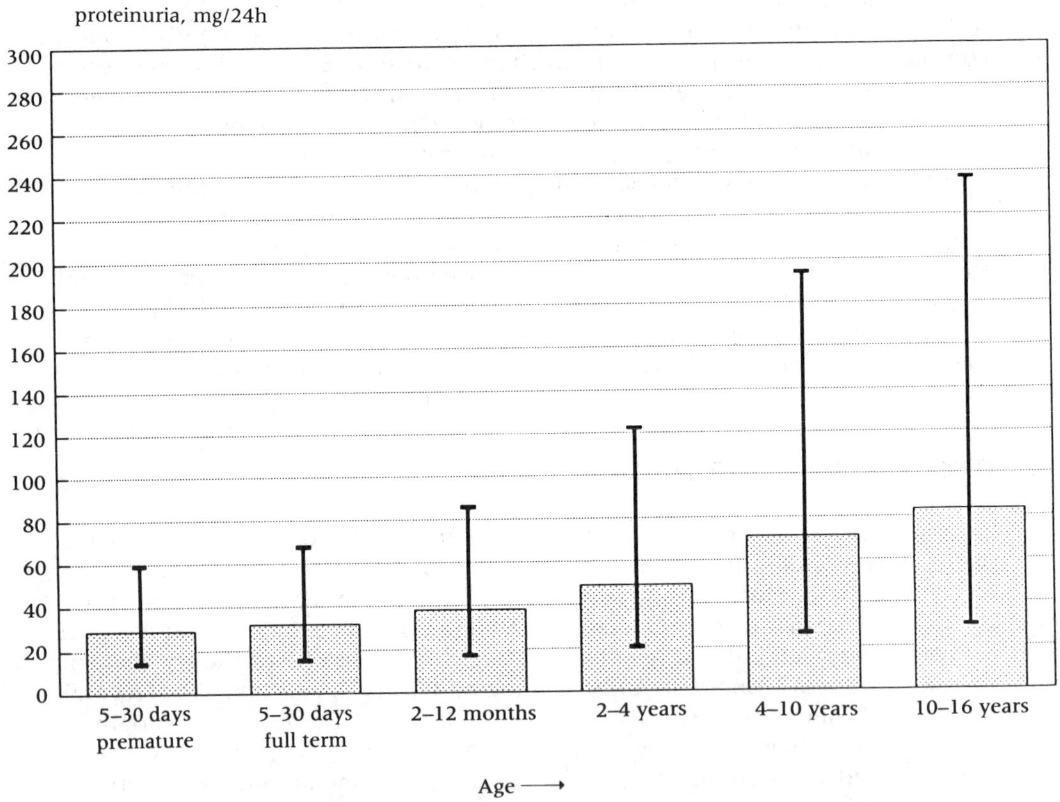

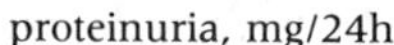

FIG. 6–1. A graphic representation of urinary protein excretion in normal children of various ages. (Data source from Miltényi M: Urinary protein excretion in healthy children. *Clin Nephrol* 12:216, 1979. Reproduced by permission from Dustri-Verlag, Deisenhofen, Germany.)

24-h sample from an adult is less than 150 mg.[5,6] In children, the amount varies with age (Table 6–1 and Fig. 6–1).[8]

DETECTION

Protein in urine can easily be detected by two simple methods. The first, a colorimetric method, involves a protein-induced change in the color of a dye (tetrabromophenol blue) impregnated on a dipstick (Albustix, Combistix); the second, a turbidimetric method, involves precipitation of protein by an acid (sulfosalicylic acid) or by heat and acid. On dipsticks, the intensity of color change from yellow to blue is correlated to the amount of protein in urine and expressed from the color chart with various shades of blue as trace = 10 mg/dL, 1+ = 30 mg/dL, 2+ = 100 mg/dL, 3+ = 300 mg/dL, and 4+ = 1000 mg/dL. In the absence of protein, the dipstick will remain yellow. This method is more sensitive for detecting albumin than other proteins.

Among the turbidimetric methods, the sulfosalicylic acid method is the most popular. First, 5 mL of urine is placed in a test tube; then three drops of 20% sulfosalicylic acid added and mixed with the urine. If protein is present, various grades of turbidity from minimal (trace) to heavy flocculation (4+) are noted. The grades of turbidity from trace to 4+ are obviously somewhat subjective. This test is quite sensitive and can detect 3 to 5 mg/dL of protein. In addition, it is equally sensitive for all proteins.[6]

Although both the dipstick and sulfosalicylic acid tests are simple and easily performed, errors in their interpretation can occur, as can false-positive or false-negative results (Table 6–2). Therefore, it is advised that both tests be performed

TABLE 6–2. False-Positive and False-Negative Results of Tests for Proteinuria

	False-Positive	False-Negative
Dipstick	Highly concentrated urine Highly alkaline buffered urine (pH>8) Gross hematuria Pyuria Skin cleanser chlorhexidine Quarternary ammonium compounds Phenazopyridine	Dilute urine Light chains of immunoglobulin
Sulfosalicylic acid	Highly concentrated urine Gross hematuria Pyuria Radiologic contrast media High levels of penicillins, cephalosporins Metabolites of sulfonamide Tolbutamide Tolmetin	Dilute urine

on urine whenever possible and the results interpreted in light of the urine's specific gravity. For example, a child excreting 100 mg/day of protein (normal amount) in 400 mL of highly concentrated urine will have 25 mg/dL of protein and will probably test 1+ on a dipstick and sulfosalicylic acid. However, the same protein in 2000 mL of dilute urine will have 5 mg/dL of protein and will test negative on a dispstick and probably trace on sulfosalicylic acid. Clearly, then, it is possible for normal children to test positive for protein on a random concentrated urine and patients with low-grade proteinuria to test trace or negative on a very dilute urine. Gross hematuria without parenchymal renal disease (urolithiasis, trauma, etc.), discussed in Chap. 5, will produce a positive test for proteinuria because of the presence of plasma proteins. Similarly, an inflammatory exudate from a urinary tract infection may also test positive for proteinuria because of the tissue proteins. Highly alkaline urine (pH > 8) may overcome the buffer of the dye on dipstick and thus produce a blue color, giving a false-positive result. Such highly alkaline urine is generally seen in patients with urinary tract infections due to urea-splitting organisms (e.g., *Proteus*).

QUANTITATION

Traditionally, quantitation of proteinuria has been done on 24-h urine samples. However, it is usually difficult to collect accurate 24-h urines on infants and children. Recent studies suggest that the ratio of protein (mg/dL)/creatinine (mg/dL) on a single urine correlates well with the total 24-h urine protein (Fig. 6–2).[9] The normal ratio for adults (mg/dL protein/mg/dL creatinine) is reported to be less than 0.2.[9] In children under 2 years of age, the ratio is 0.5; in those over 2 years of age, it is less than 0.2 (Table 6–3).[10] A ratio of 3.5 represents heavy proteinuria, in the range of nephrotic syndrome.[9] On the basis of these studies, it would appear that the practice of 24-h urine collection can be substituted by the simple measurements described above. However, if a 24-h urine is collected, it is important to make sure that the collection is complete. This is easily done by simultaneously measuring creatinine clearance and calculating the amount of creatinine excreted per kilogram of body weight. Since the daily production of creatinine is related to the muscle mass (body weight) and creatinine is almost entirely eliminated in urine, the total daily excretion of creatinine and thus the amount of creatinine excreted per kilogram of body weight in a steady state is essentially the same from day to day. The daily steady-state creatinine excretion varies with age and sex. The reported values for both sexes in infants are approximately 14 mg/kg/day and beyond 1 year approximately 20 mg/kg/day. After 12 years of age, the creatinine excretion is a little higher in boys (25 mg/kg/day) than in girls (22 mg/kg/day).[11–14]

MECHANISM

In order to understand the mechanism of proteinuria, it is essential to know how the normal kidney handles proteins presented to it from the circulation.

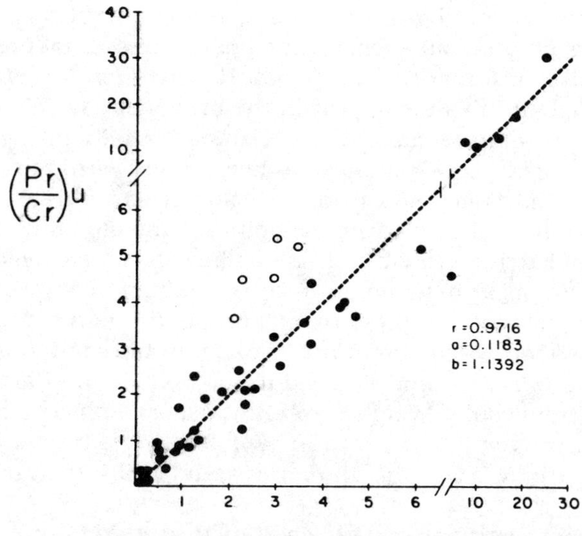

FIG. 6–2. Ratio of urinary protein to creatinine concentration [(Pr/Cr)u] of random single voided urine samples expressed as a function of protein excretion per 24 h/1.73 m^2. The concentrations of protein and creatinine were measured in milligrams per deciliter. The five open circles denote values for patients who had a protein/creatinine ratio of more than 3.5 and a protein excretion rate of less than 3.5 g/24 h/1.73 m^2. (From Ginsberg JM, Chang B, Matarese RA, Garella S: Use of single voided urine samples to estimate quantitative proteinuria. Reprinted by permission of *The New England Journal of Medicine* 309:1543, 1983.)

PROTEIN HANDLING BY THE NORMAL KIDNEY

Fluid from the early proximal convoluted tubule (presumably glomerular filtrate) in the rat, obtained by micropuncture techniques, contains 1 to 10 mg/L of albumin.[15,16] If similar concentration exists in humans, then—assuming that 180 liters of glomerular filtrate is formed per day (125 mL/min) in an adult

TABLE 6–3. Urine Protein/Creatinine in Random Urine in Children

Subject	Protein (mg/dL)/Creatinine (mg/dL)
Normal children	
<2 years	<0.5
>2 years	<0.2
Children with proteinuria[a]	>1.5

[a] >1 g/m^2/day.

Source: Adapted from Houser M: Assessment of proteinuria using random urine samples. *J Pediatr* 104:845, 1984. Reproduced by permission from Mosby-Year Book, Inc.

human—the amount of albumin filtered at the glomerulus would be 180 to 1800 mg/day. As pointed out earlier, the upper limit of total protein excretion in a normal adult is 150 mg/day, and about 40 percent of this is albumin. Thus about 60 mg of albumin would appear in the urine per day. We also know that the normal concentration of albumin in plasma is 35,000 mg/L (3.5 g/dL). This line of reasoning leads to two important conclusions: *First,* miniscule amounts of albumin from plasma appear in the glomerular filtrate (1 to 10 mg/ 35,000 mg); therefore, under normal conditions, the glomerular capillary acts as a very efficient barrier to the filtration of albumin. *Second,* most of the filtered albumin does not appear in urine. It must therefore be reabsorbed and, in fact, is known to be reabsorbed by the proximal tubule through the process of endocytosis.[17,18] The endocytosed albumin is broken up into amino acids inside the cell by lysosomal enzymes and returned to the body pool of amino acids. Several other small molecular weight proteins such as light chains of immunoglobulins, $beta_2$ microglobulin, insulin, amylase, parathyroid hormone, and glucagon are also filtered at the glomerulus and reabsorbed by the proximal tubule.[19]

How does the glomerular capillary wall function as an effective filtration barrier to the plasma proteins? There is considerable evidence that it selectively limits the filtration of macromolecules on the basis of size and charge. To grasp the basis of this selectivity, it is important to understand the ultrastructure and biochemical composition of the glomerular capillary wall. Ultrastructurally, this wall has three distinct components: the endothelium, with fenestrations 1000 Å wide; the 3000 Å-thick glomerular basement membrane; and the epithelial cells, with their interdigitating foot processes abutting against the basement membrane and bridged by slit diaphragms. The gaps between the foot processes, called *slit pores,* are approximately 250 Å wide.

Biochemically, the entire glomerular capillary wall is anionic (negatively charged). The endothelium and the epithelial cell layer are covered with anionic sialoglycoproteins,[20–23] and the glomerular basement membrane contains highly anionic heparan sulfate proteoglycans.[23–25] The latter contribute significantly to the anionic charge of the glomerular basement membrane.[23–25]

Much of the evidence for the size and charge basis of the glomerular capillary wall's selective permeability to macromolecules has been obtained by studies utilizing fractional clearance of dextran.[26–30] Dextran is a polymer of glucose which can be made into macromolecules of various sizes and charges. The principle of fractional clearance utilizes the clearance of an unknown macromolecule relative to inulin. Inulin, a 5200-Da molecule which is completely filtered at the glomerular capillary wall, is neither reabsorbed nor secreted by the tubule and appears intact in the urine. Dextran has similar characteristics. The fractional clearance of dextran can be calculated by the formula $(u/p)\mathrm{D}/(u/p)\mathrm{I}$, where u is urine concentration and p the plasma concentration of dextran (D) and inulin (I). Two facts emerge from these studies. *One:* There is an inverse relationship between the fractional clearance of dextran and its size (effective molecular radius expressed in angstrom units), with 18-Å size molecules having the same clearance as inulin and molecules greater than 44 Å having no clearance (not filtered). *Two:* For any given size of dextran macromolecules, the fractional clearance is as follows—cationic (positively charged) $>$ neutral $>$

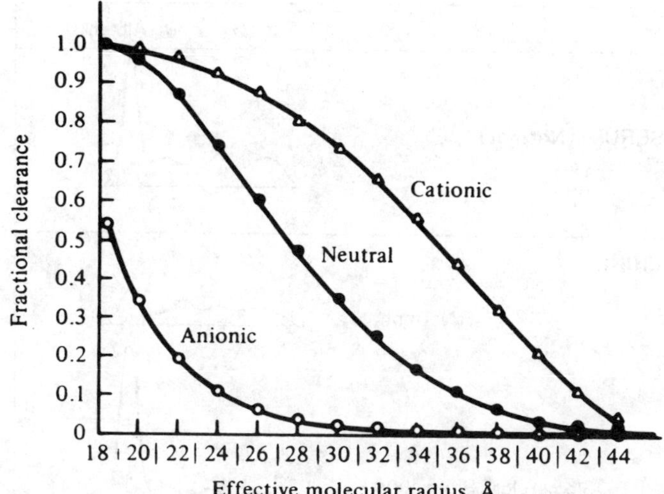

FIG. 6–3. Fractional clearance (clearance of dextran/clearance of inulin) of anionic, neutral, and cationic dextrans as a function of molecular radius (size). Both molecular size and charge influence clearance. (From Bohrer MP, Baylis C, Humes HD, Glassock RJ, Robertson CR, Brenner BM: *J Clin Invest* 61:72, 1978, by copyright permission of the American Society for Clinical Investigation.)

anionic (negatively charged). In other words, the filtration of anionic macromolecules is retarded while that of cationic macromolecules facilitated (Fig. 6–3).

The physiologic implications of these size- and charge-selective mechanisms are that normally only very small amounts of plasma protein are filtered by the glomerular capillary. This is because most of the plasma proteins at physiologic pH are anionic and greater than or equal to 36 Å in size (molecular size of albumin). Macromolecules below the molecular weight of albumin (60,000) are filtered in progressively greater amounts (listed above). Evidence for the size and charge basis of selective permeability has also been obtained by electron microscopy, using electron-dense tracers of various sizes and charges. These are injected intravenously into experimental animals and their site of localization visualized in the glomerular capillary wall. Tracers varying in size from 61 Å (ferritin, with molecular weight 480,000) to 30 Å (horseradish peroxidase, with molecular weight 40,000) and a same-size tracer with varying charge (ferritin, with isoelectric points from 4.5 to 11.5) have been used in various studies.[31–34] The results of tracer studies in general corroborate the results of fractional clearance studies with dextran.

ABNORMAL PROTEINURIA

Based on the preceding discussion of normal kidney function, abnormal proteinuria may be categorized as follows (Fig. 6–4):

1. Glomerular proteinuria
2. Tubular proteinuria
3. Overload proteinuria
4. Proteinuria due to hemodynamic alterations

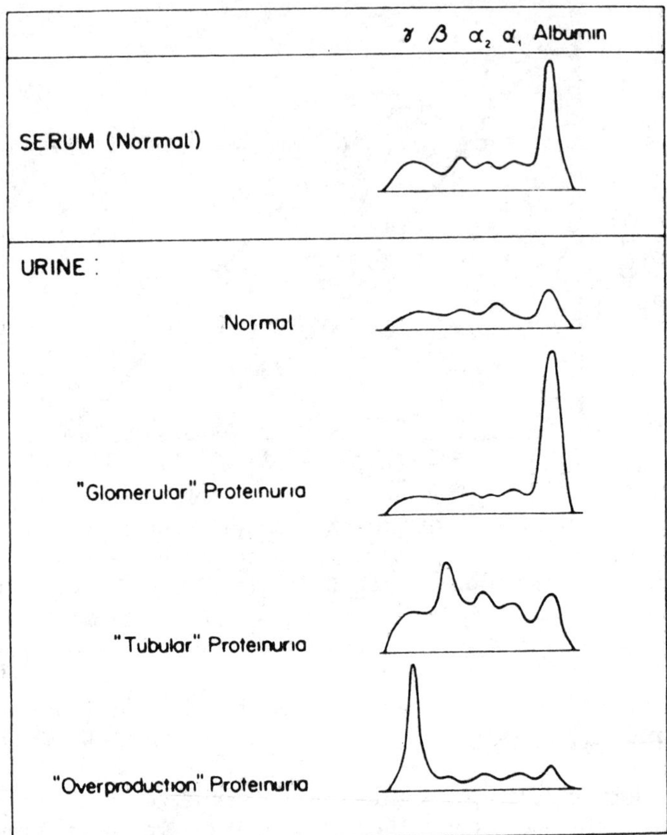

FIG. 6–4. Serum protein electropheresis *(top)* compared with urinary protein electropheresis pattern in normal individuals *(middle)* and patients with glomerular, tubular, and overproduction proteinuria *(bottom)*. [From Kassiyev JP, Harrington JT: Laboratory evaluation of renal function, in Schrier RW, Gottschalk CW (eds): *Diseases of the Kidney*, 4th ed., Boston, Little, Brown and Company, 1988, p. 393. Reproduced by permission.]

GLOMERULAR PROTEINURIA

Since the glomerular capillary wall acts as a charge- and size-selective barrier to circulatory proteins, any alteration in the characteristics of this barrier will lead to increased permeability and glomerular leakage of plasma proteins. Indeed, this occurs in several experimental models of glomerular disease in animals.[28,35–37] In human glomerular diseases, it appears that the proteinuria in minimal change disease is associated with disruption of the charge barrier (Fig. 6–5).[38,39] In addition, histochemical staining for the assessment of negative charge on the glomerular capillary wall shows reduction of charge in several of the glomerular diseases in humans, suggesting defects in the charge barrier.[40] Reduction of heparan sulfate proteoglycan has been reported in congenital

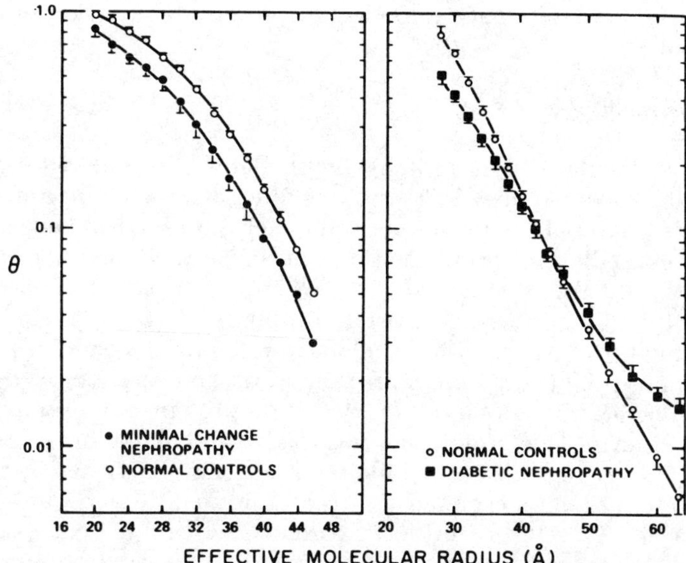

FIG. 6–5. Mean fractional clearance of dextran (θ) as a function of effective molecular radius (size) in 10 patients with minimal change disease nephrotic syndrome (•), *left panel,* and 16 patients with diabetic nephropathy (■), *right panel,* compared with normal controls (○). In minimal change disease, the clearance of dextran is less than controls over the entire range of size from 22 to 44 Å. In diabetic nephropathy, clearance of small-size dextran is less but of larger size than in controls. [From Deen WM, Myers BD, Brenner BM: The glomerular barrier to macromolecules: theoretical and experimental considerations, in Brenner BM, Stein JH (eds): *Contemporary Issues in Nephrology.* New York, Churchill Livingstone, vol. 9, 1982, p. 22. Reproduced by permission.]

nephrotic syndrome.[41] Alteration of the size-selective barrier has been observed in patients with diabetic nephropathy[42] and idiopathic membranous glomerulopathy.[43] Patients with diabetic nephropathy also have some alteration in the charge barrier (Fig. 6–5).[42] It is likely that a combination of charge and size alteration of varying magnitude is present in most of the human glomerulonephritides. How these alterations in charge and size occur in various immunologically and nonimmunologically mediated glomerular diseases remains to be elucidated.

Glomerular proteinuria may be selective or nonselective. Proteinuria is considered selective when the glomerular capillary wall selectively allows leakage of predominantly small molecular weight proteins such as albumin and nonselective when there is leakage of small and large molecular weight proteins. The selectivity of proteinuria index (SPI) can be measured by determining the clearance of a small molecular weight protein (transferrin) and a large molecular weight protein (IgG). An SPI of <0.1 denotes highly selective proteinuria and a ratio of >0.3 as nonselective proteinuria. This measurement has clinical utility. Patients with minimal change disease generally have highly selective proteinuria and respond to corticosteroids, while patients with other glomerular proteinurias generally have nonselective proteinuria and do not respond to corticosteroids.[44,45]

TUBULAR PROTEINURIA

If the small molecular weight proteins (light chains of immunoglobulins, $beta_2$ microglobulin and lysozyme, etc.) normally filtered at the glomerulus and reabsorbed by the proximal tubule are not completely absorbed and appear in urine in amounts exceeding albumin, the proteinuria is called *tubular proteinuria.*[6] It should be obvious that this would occur when the proximal tubules are damaged. Indeed, it can be seen in a variety of tubular disorders (Table 6–4). The amount of total protein in urine in tubular proteinuria is generally much less than the amount seen in glomerular proteinuria and rarely exceeds 2 g/day.[6] Excretion of $beta_2$ microglobulin, an 11,600-Da protein, is a useful marker for tubular proteinuria. This protein normally exists in circulation at a concentration of 1 to 2.5 μg/mL. Most of the filtered protein is reabsorbed by the tubules and only 30 to 370 μg is excreted in urine in normal humans; amounts up to 100 mg may be excreted in urine in patients with tubular diseases.[46] Other markers known to assist with the diagnosis of tubular proteinuria include excretion of high amounts of lysozyme,[47] retinol-binding protein,[48] and $alpha_1$ microglobulin.[49] Because $beta_2$ microglobulin deteriorates in acid urine and its concentration in serum can vary independently of glomerular function (lymphoid malignancies), the last two tests may be preferred.[50]

OVERLOAD PROTEINURIA

If low molecular weight proteins that are normally filtered by the glomerulus and reabsorbed by the tubule are present in excessive amounts and overwhelm the reabsorptive capacity of the tubule, proteinuria will result. This form of proteinuria is called *overload proteinuria.* It may result from the excessive delivery of light chains (multiple myeloma), lysozyme (myelocytic leukemia),[51] myoglobulin (rhabdomyolysis), or hemoglobulin (hemolysis (Table 6–4). The molecular weights of light chains of immunoglobulin, lysozyme, and myoglobin are 23,000, 14,000, and 19,000, respectively. As pointed out earlier, lysozyme can also be seen in tubular diseases due to defective reabsorption in the absence of overproduction. Excessive amounts of light chains in urine are detected as Bence Jones protein.

PROTEINURIA DUE TO HEMODYNAMIC ALTERATIONS

Alterations of intrarenal hemodynamic factors may affect glomerular permselectivity and produce proteinuria. Much of the evidence for this comes from studies of the remnant kidney adaptation model seen in uninephrectomy rats.[30,52–54] Uninephrectomy in normal rats is followed by a 40 to 50 percent increase in glomerular filtration rate (GFR) and a threefold increase in proteinuria in the remnant kidney.[53,55] There is an increase in single-nephron GFR, dilatation of afferent and to a lesser degree efferent arterioles, and an increase in glomerular plasma flow and hydrostatic pressure.[53] These alterations produce

TABLE 6–4. Classification of Proteinuria

I. Orthostatic
II. Transient: Fever, exercise-induced, congestive heart failure, exposure to cold, epinephrine infusion, seizures, emotional stress, etc.
III. Persistent
 A. Glomerular
  1. Congenital or hereditary: Congenital nephrotic syndrome, Alport syndrome
  2. Acquired
   a. Primary or idiopathic: Minimal change disease, focal segmental glomerulosclerosis, membranoproliferative glomerulonephritis, membranous nephropathy, some cases of IgA nephropathy, proliferative glomerulonephritis, unclassified chronic glomerulonephritis
   b. Secondary
    (1) Infection: Poststreptococcal glomerulonephritis, other postinfectious glomerulonephritis, shunt nephritis, subacute bacterial endocarditis, hepatitis B, secondary syphilis, malaria, schistosomiasis, AIDS, etc.
    (2) Multisystem disorders: Systemic lupus erythematosus, Henoch-Schönlein purpura, hemolytic uremic syndrome, diabetes mellitus, other collagen vascular diseases (i.e., polyarteritis nodosa, Wagner's granulomatosis, vasculitis, rheumatoid arthritis, etc.), Goodpasture syndrome, amyloidosis, etc.
    (3) Drugs: Penicillamine, nonsteroidal anti-inflammatory drugs, captopril, gold salts, "street" heroin, trimethadione, lithium, mercury, etc.
    (4) Neoplasia: leukemia, lymphoma, carcinoma
    (5) Miscellaneous: Chronic renal transplant rejection, reflux nephropathy, renal vein thrombosis, sickle cell anemia, renal artery stenosis, hypertension, etc.
 B. Tubular
  1. Congenital or hereditary: Fanconi syndrome, oculocerebral-renal syndrome (Lowe syndrome), Lawrence-Moon-Biedl syndrome, Bartter syndrome, renal tubular acidosis, cystinosis, oxalosis, medullary cystic disease, polycystic kidney disease, renal dysplasia, Wilson disease, hereditary fructose intolerance, glycogen storage disease, galactosemia, etc.
  2. Acquired: Interstitial nephritis, pyelonephritis, renal transplant rejection, acute tubular necrosis, sarcoidosis, nephrocalcinosis, hypercalcemia, gout, hypokalemia, drugs (aminoglycosides, methicillin, cyclosporine, analgesics, lithium, cisplatin), metal toxicity (lead, aluminum, mercury, etc.), obstructive uropathy, reflux nephropathy, Balkan nephropathy, etc.
 C. Overland
  Light chains: Plasma cell dyscrasias
  Lysozyme: Monocytic and myelocytic leukemias
  Myoglobin: Rhabdomyolysis
  Hemoglobin: Hemolysis

a state of intraglomerular "hyperfiltration and hypertension" which apparently leads to glomerular capillary damage and proteinuria.[30,54] It may be that the glomerular proteinuria seen with reflux nephropathy[56] and possibly in other nonglomerular progressive tubulointerstitial diseases results from these alterations. Other instances where hemodynamic alterations may be involved in the genesis of proteinuria include congestive heart failure,[57] some forms of hypertension (salt-sensitive in rats),[58] exercise-induced proteinuria,[59] and orthostatic proteinuria.[60]

CLINICAL TERMS

Several of the most common clinical terms used to describe patients with proteinuria are defined as follows:

1. *Transient proteinuria* exists when proteinuria is not present in each and every urine.
2. *Persistent,* or *fixed, proteinuria* exists when all urine specimens from a patient test positive for protein.
3. *Orthostatic proteinuria* is considered to be present when urine produced in the recumbent position tests negative but that produced in the erect position tests positive for protein.

CLASSIFICATION

On the basis of the mechanisms of proteinuria discussed earlier and the clinical terms defined above, proteinuria may be classified as outlined in Table 6–4.

EVALUATION

HEALTHY PATIENT WITH A POSITIVE TEST FOR PROTEIN

Detection of proteinuria on a routine physical examination is a common clinical occurrence in pediatric practice. School surveys in children have shown the prevalence of proteinuria to range from 0.53 percent in Canadian schoolgirls to 6 percent in Texan boys (Table 6–5).[61–65] In the evaluation of such patients, the following plan may be adopted. If the history and physical examination do not reveal any abnormality and both the blood pressure and growth percentiles are normal, a urinalysis should be performed by the *physician.* Both the dipstick and the sulfosalicylic acid tests for proteinuria should be performed and the results interpreted in light of the specific gravity of the urine and the false-positive and false-negative conditions of these tests. If proteinuria is definitely

TABLE 6–5. Prevalence of Proteinuria in Schoolchildren

Study Group	Number with Proteinuria/ Number Screened	Prevalence, %
Canadian schoolgirls[61] age 5–14 years	125/23,427	0.53
Finnish schoolboys and schoolgirls[62] age 8–15 years	223/8,954	2.5
Virginian schoolgirls[63] age 6–8 years	24/804	2.98
Texan schoolboys and schoolgirls[64] age 6–12 years	736/12,252	6
Texas Primary Care Center, boys and girls[65] age 1–17 years	125/2,288	5.46

present and no other urine abnormalities are detected on urinalysis (including a careful examination of the urine sediment), tests for quantitative proteinuria and orthostatic proteinuria should be performed next.

Since most children attend school during weekdays, timed collection of urine for these tests is best obtained on a Sunday. If a special container is not available, a clean gallon milk jug can be used. On Sunday morning, upon awakening (7 A.M.), the child empties his or her bladder and this urine is not saved. From that time onward, all urine is saved in the container, including the urine voided before going to bed (10 P.M.). The child must empty his or her bladder completely, and this urine is saved in the collection from 7 A.M. to 10 P.M. Throughout the collection period, the urine is saved in the refrigerator. Upon awakening on Monday morning (7 A.M.) the child empties his or her bladder, and this urine is saved in a separate container. Both urine containers are labeled appropriately and delivered to the laboratory for analysis. Protein is assayed in both urine collections, either by dipstick or analytically. The two urine samples are mixed together; total volume of urine is noted and protein as well as creatinine are measured in the timed urine collection. From these values, the following can be determined: (1) Whether the urine is a complete 24-h collection. This is determined as discussed earlier (under quantitation) by calculating the creatinine excretion per kilogram of body weight. If the creatinine per kilogram is not normal, the urine collection is not complete. (2) A quantitative assessment of proteinuria by the total protein content and the protein/creatinine ratio. (3) If the urine collected in recumbent position (10 P.M. to 7 A.M.) is negative while the urine collected during day two from 7 A.M. to 10 P.M. is positive for protein, then the proteinuria is orthostatic. (4) If protein is present in both samples, the proteinuria is considered persistent, or fixed, and should be evaluated further. If proteinuria is orthostatic, the patient should be evaluated for renal function (BUN, serum creatinine) and followed yearly to make sure that the proteinuria remains orthostatic and renal function remains normal. Orthostatic proteinuria is a benign condition and may be seen in 2 to 5 percent of adolescents.[66] Generally the total 24-h protein excretion is less than 1 g, but values up to 3 g have been reported.[67] It is believed that hemodynamic alterations induced by the upright posture produce proteinuria in this condition.[60,68] Although mild histologic abnormalities in glomeruli may be present in 50 percent of these patients, the long-term prognosis is excellent and renal failure does not develop.[66,69] In some patients, orthostatic proteinuria disappears over time.[68]

PERSISTENT PROTEINURIA

Patients with persistent, or fixed, proteinuria should be investigated further for evidence of renal disease.

HISTORY AND PHYSICAL EXAMINATION

The clinical presentation of these patients can have a wide spectrum. They may be completely asymptomatic or may have a variety of clinical symptoms, ranging from manifestations of nephrotic syndrome to acute or chronic renal failure, with or without symptomatology of systemic disorders such as lupus erythematosus. Any of the conditions listed under *persistent proteinuria* in Table 6–4 may be responsible in any patient. History and physical examination should be performed in order to find clues to any of these conditions. If renal disease is present in the family or the condition is detected early in life, hereditary and congenital conditions should first be considered. A family history of deafness may suggest Alport syndrome. Polyuria may suggest tubular disease or chronic renal failure. Gross hematuria with tea- or coke-colored urine usually means the presence of an underlying glomerular disease. Duration of proteinuria may also assist in assessing the seriousness of the condition. If the proteinuria has been present in a healthy patient for several years, it may indicate a slow, progressive disease. A history of a recent sore throat or impetigo may suggest a poststreptococcal glomerulonephritis. If there is edema, nephrotic syndrome or renal failure is likely. Hypertension in children generally suggests intrinsic renal disease. Physical growth retardation or failure to thrive suggests a chronic renal disease.

URINALYSIS

After a careful history has been taken and a physical examination performed, a complete urinalysis is the first test to be done. This should include both the dipstick test and sulfosalicylic acid test for proteinuria as well as examination of the urine sediment. The latter must be done by the physician and requires patience and careful scrutiny. Results of tests for proteinuria, as discussed earlier, must be interpreted in light of the specific gravity of the urine and the false-positive and -negative conditions associated with these tests. Heavy proteinuria (4+) is generally seen in glomerular rather than tubular diseases. If, in addition, edema is present, it is likely to be due to nephrotic syndrome. Proteinuria with hematuria, particularly when it ranges from 3 to 4+, is almost always due to a glomerular lesion. The presence of glucose may indicate diabetes mellitus or disorders associated with damage to the proximal tubules. Red blood cell casts with proteinuria and hematuria are almost always due to a glomerulonephritis. White blood cells, white blood cell casts, and renal epithelial cell casts suggest tubulointerstitial disease, including pyelonephritis.

QUANTITATION OF PROTEINURIA

Quantitation of proteinuria is helpful in differentiating glomerular from tubular proteinuria. In adults, it is rare for tubular proteinuria to exceed 2 g/day. In children, this figure is probably lower, but the exact data, to my knowledge, are not available. Therefore, if proteinuria is >2 g/day, it is most likely glomerular in origin; however, if it is <2 g/day, it may be glomerular or tubular. Heavy glomerular proteinuria is seen in nephrotic syndrome and may range from 2 to 10 g or even higher in children with nephrotic syndrome. For purposes of standardization, proteinuria exceeding 40 mg/h/m^2 of body surface may be considered heavy.[70] If a 24-h urine is not collected, as discussed earlier, an estimate of quantity may be obtained by urine protein/urine creatinine (mg/dL) on a random sample.

OTHER TESTS

From the history, physical examination, urinalysis, quantitation of proteinuria, and test for orthostatic proteinuria, it should be possible to diagnose orthostatic proteinuria and have a reasonable impression of the condition's severity and also whether the patient has (1) a glomerular disease, (2) a nephrotic syndrome secondary to the glomerular disease, (3) a tubular disorder, (4) an acute versus chronic disease, (5) a hereditary versus an acquired form of the disease, or (6) a multisystemic or an isolated disease. However, additional laboratory tests will be required for a definitive diagnosis. Baseline complete blood counts and serum chemistries should be obtained in all patients. The latter should include serum sodium, potassium, chloride, CO_2, glucose, BUN, creatinine, uric acid, calcium, phosphorus, alkaline phosphatase, total proteins, albumin, cholesterol, etc. These baseline studies can uncover information about several conditions associated with glomerular proteinuria (i.e., nephrotic syndrome, hemolytic uremic syndrome, diabetes mellitus, etc.) or tubular proteinuria (i.e., renal tubular acidosis, hypercalcemia, etc.). In addition, the studies will show the presence or absence of renal failure. Anemia may indicate chronic renal failure, chronic multisystem disease or hemolytic uremic syndrome, etc.

The results of these tests may determine what tests should be done next. If nephrotic syndrome is uncovered, then tests to find its cause should be performed (see Chap. 7). These generally will include C3, C4, and total hemolytic complement, antinuclear antibody test (ANA), serological test for syphilis, hepatitis screen, test for selectivity of proteinuria and antistreptolysin O (ASO) titer. The test for the selectivity of proteinuria can be done on a spot urine sample along with a serum obtained at the same time. Since the test measures a *ratio* of the clearance of IgG to transferrin, a 24-h urine is not necessary. If tubular proteinuria is suspected, 24-h urine may be quantitated for beta$_2$ microglobulin, alpha$_1$ microglobulin, retinol-binding protein, and lysozyme. It is important to remember that increased urinary lysozyme excretion can result from excessive production in myelocytic leukemia. If excessive loss of light chains due to plasma cell dyscrasias is suspected, the urine should be tested for these by immunoelectrophoresis.

Ultrasound examination of the abdomen is noninvasive and can provide valuable information about a number of conditions, such as polycystic kidneys, renal dysplasia, nephrocalcinosis, and oxalosis. It should be performed in proteinuria that has not been explained by the above tests. A voiding cystogram will be necessary to diagnose vesicoureteral reflux.

The plan for the evaluation of patients with persistent proteinuria is summarized in Table 6–6. A flow diagram for the assessment of proteinuria is presented in Fig. 6–6.

RENAL BIOPSY

If, from the above tests, the diagnosis is not clear, a renal biopsy may be necessary. A renal biopsy is recommended in the following situations:

Steroid-resistant nephrotic syndrome
Nephrotic syndrome associated with low serum complement

TABLE 6–6. Evaluation of Persistent Proteinuria

History and physical examination
Urinalysis, including examination of sediment
Quantitation of proteinuria
Complete blood counts
Serum chemistries, including sodium, potassium, chloride, CO_2, glucose, BUN, creatinine, uric acid, calcium, phosphorus, total proteins, albumin, cholesterol, etc.
Serum total hemolytic complement, C3, C4
Antinuclear antibody test, serologic test for syphilis, hepatitis screen, antistreptococcal antibodies (antistreptolysin O, streptozyme, anti-DNase B)
Test for selectivity of proteinuria
Urine $beta_2$ microglobulin, $alpha_1$ microglobulin, retinal binding protein, lysozyme, etc.
Urine immunoelectrophoresis
Abdominal ultrasound
Renal biopsy

Nephrotic syndrome associated with persistent hematuria, hypertension, or renal failure
Persistent proteinuria with hematuria
Persistent proteinuria with renal failure

Children with isolated mild to moderate proteinuria who are otherwise healthy and have no other evidence of renal disease may be watched and followed reg-

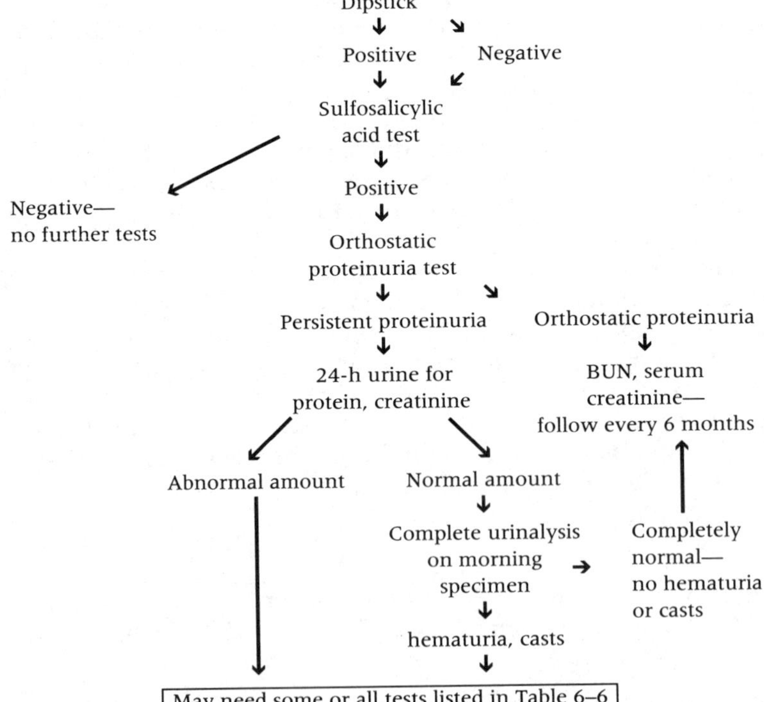

FIG. 6–6. A suggested flow diagram for the evaluation of patients with proteinuria.

ularly at 3- to 6-month intervals. If any other abnormalities suggestive of renal involvement, such as those listed above, develop, a renal biopsy should be considered.

REFERENCES

1. Bright R: *Reports of Medical Cases Selected with a View of Illustrating the Symptoms and Cures of Diseases by Reference to Morbid Anatomy.* London, Longman, Rees, Orme, Brown & Green, 1827.
2. Ruen DB, Wachtel TJ, Brown PC, et al: Transient proteinuria in emergency medical admissions. *N Engl J Med* 306:1031, 1982.
3. Poortmans JR: Postexercise proteinuria in humans. *JAMA* 253:236, 1985.
4. Hemmingsen L, Skarrup P: The 24-hr excretion of plasma proteins in the urine of apparently healthy subjects. *Scand J Clin Lab Invest* 35:347, 1975.
5. Berggard I: Plasma proteins in normal human urine, in Manuel Y, Betrel H, Revilland JP (eds): *Proteins in Normal and Pathological Urine.* Baltimore, University Park Press, 1970, pp 7–19.
6. Pesce AJ, First MR: *Proteinuria: An Integrated Review.* New York, Marcel Dekker, 1979.
7. Tamm I, Horsfall FL: A mucoprotein derived from human urine which reacts with influenza, mumps, and Newcastle disease viruses. *J Exp Med* 95:71, 1952.
8. Miltenyi M: Urinary protein excretion in healthy children. *Clin Nephrol* 12:216, 1979.
9. Ginsberg JM, Chang BS, Materese RA, et al: Use of single voided urine samples to estimate quantitative proteinuria. *N Engl J Med* 309:1543, 1983.
10. Houser M: Assessment of proteinuria using random urine samples. *J Pediatr* 104:845, 1984.
11. Hunter A: *Creatine and Creatinine.* New York, Longmans-Green, 1928.
12. Clark LC, Thompson HL, Beck EI, et al: Excretion of creatine and creatinine excretion in children. *Am J Dis Child* 81:774, 1951.
13. Novak LP: Age and sex differences in body density and creatinine excretion of high school children. *Ann NY Acad Sci* 110:545, 1963.
14. Schwartz GJ, Feld LG, Langford DJ: A simple estimate of glomerular filtration rate in full-term infants during the first year of life. *J Pediatr* 104:849, 1984.
15. Oken DE, Kirschbaum BB, Landwehr DM: Micropuncture studies of the mechanisms of normal and pathologic albuminuria: Experimental and clinical aspects of proteinuria. *Contr Nephrol* 24:1, 1981.
16. Oken DE, Flamenbaum W: Micropuncture studies of proximal tubule albumin concentrations in normal and nephrotic rats. *J Clin Invest* 50:1498, 1971.
17. Maunsbach AB: Absorption of ^{125}I-homologous albumin by rat kidney proximal tubular cells. *J Ultrastruct Res* 15:197, 1966.
18. Maack T, Kinter WB: Transport of protein by flounder kidney tubules during long-term incubation. *Am J Physiol* 216:1034, 1969.
19. Carone FA, Peterson DR, Fluret G: Renal tubular handling of small peptide hormones. *J Lab Clin Med* 100:1, 1982.
20. Latta H, Johnson WH, Stanley TM: Sialoglycoproteins and filtration barriers in the glomerular capillary wall. *J Ultrastruct Res* 51:354, 1975.
21. Jones DB: Mucosubstances of the glomerulus. *Lab Invest* 21:119, 1969.

22. Mohos SC, Skoza L: Histochemical demonstration and localization of sialoglycoproteins in the glomerulus. *Exp Mol Pathol* 12:316, 1970.
23. Kanwar YS: Biology of disease: Biophysiology of glomerular filtration and proteinuria. *Lab Invest* 51:7, 1984.
24. Kanwar S, Farquhar MG: Presence of heparin sulfate proteoglycan in the glomerulus basement membrane. *Proc Nat Acad Sci USA* 76:1303, 1979.
25. Kanwar YS, Veis A, Kimura JH, et al: Characterization of heparin sulfate proteoglycan of glomerulus basement membrane. *Proc Nat Acad Sci USA* 81:762, 1984.
26. Pappenheimer JR: Passage of molecules through capillary walls. *Physiol Rev* 33:387, 1953.
27. Wallenius G: Renal clearance of dextran as a measure of glomerular permeability. *Acta Soc Med Uppsala* 59:1, 1954.
28. Bennett CM, Glassock RJ, Chang RLS, et al: Permselectivity of the glomerular capillary wall: Studies of experimental glomerulonephritis in the rat using dextran sulfate. *J Clin Invest* 57:1287, 1976.
29. Bohrer MP, Baylis C, Humes MD, et al: Permselectivity of the glomerular capillary walls. *J Clin Invest* 61:72, 1978.
30. Brenner BM, Hostettler TH, Humes MD: Molecular basis of proteinuria of glomerular origin. *N Engl J Med* 298:826, 1978.
31. Farquhar MG, Wissig SL, Palade GE: Glomerular permeability: I. Ferritin transfer across the normal capillary wall. *J Exp Med* 113:47, 1961.
32. Graham RC, Karnovsky MJ: Glomerular permeability: Ultrastructural cytochemical studies using peroxidase as protein tracers. *J Exp Med* 124:1123, 1966.
33. Venkatachalam MA, Karnovsky JJ, Fahimi HD, et al: An ultrastructural study of glomerular permeability using catalase and peroxidase as tracer proteins. *J Exp Med* 132:1153, 1970.
34. Rennke HG, Cotran RS, Ventatachalam MA: Role of molecular charge in glomerular permeability: Tracer studies with cationized ferritin. *J Cell Biol* 67:638, 1975.
35. Bohrer MP, Baylis C, Robertson CR, et al: Mechanism of puramycin-induced defects in the transglomerular passage of water and macromolecules. *J Clin Invest* 60:152, 1977.
36. Kanwar YS, Linker AM, Farquhar MG: Increased permeability of the glomerular basement membrane to ferritin after removal of glycosaminoglycans by enzyme digestion. *J Cell Biol* 86:688, 1980.
37. Michael AF, Blau EB, Vernier RL: Glomerular polyanion: Alterations in aminonucleoside nephrosis. *Lab Invest* 23:649, 1970.
38. Winetz JA, Robertson CR, Colbetz HV, et al: The nature of the glomerular injury in minimal change and focal sclerosing glomerulopathies. *Am J Kid Dis* 1:91, 1981.
39. Carrie BJ, Salyer WR, Myers BD: Minimal change nephropathy: An electrochemical disorder of the glomerular membrane. *Am J Med* 70:262, 1981.
40. Blau EB, Haas DE: Glomerular sialic acid and proteinuria in human renal disease. *Lab Invest* 28:477, 1973.
41. Vernier RL, Klein DJ, Sisson SP, et al: Heparin sulfate-rich anionic sites in the human glomerular basement membrane: Decreased concentration in congenital nephrotic syndrome. *N Engl J Med* 309:1001, 1983.
42. Myers BD, Winetz JA, Chin F, et al: Mechanisms of proteinuria in diabetic nephropathy. *Kidney Int* 21:633, 1982.
43. Shemesh O, Rose JC, Deen WM, et al: Nature of glomerular capillary injury in human membranous glomerulonephropathy. *J Clin Invest* 77:868, 1986.
44. Makker SP, Heymann W: The idiopathic nephrotic syndrome of childhood: A clinical evaluation of 148 cases. *Am J Dis Child* 127:830, 1974.

45. Cameron JS, Blandford G: The simple assessment of selectivity in heavy proteinuria. *Lancet* 2:242, 1966.
46. Peterson PA, Evin PE, Berggard I: Differentiation of glomerular, tubular, and normal proteinuria: Determinations of urinary excretion of β-2 microglobulin, albumin, and total protein. *J Clin Invest* 48:1189, 1969.
47. Harrison JF, Lunt GS, Scott P, et al: Urinary excretion of lysozyme, ribonuclease, and low molecular weight protein in renal disease. *Lancet* 1:371, 1968.
48. Bernard AM, Moreau D, Lanweys R: Comparison of retinal binding protein and β_2 microglobulin in urine in the early detection of ambular proteinuria. *Clin Chim Acta* 126:1, 1982.
49. Yu H, Yanagisawa Y, Forbes MA, et al: Alpha-1 microglobulin: An indicator protein for renal tubular function. *J Clin Pathol* 36:253, 1983.
50. Hardwicke J: Proteinuria—The future. *Clin Nephrol* 21:50, 1984.
51. Osserman EF, Lawlor DP: Serum and urinary lysozyme in monomyelocytic leukemia. *J Exp Med* 124:921, 1966.
52. Chanulin A, Ferris EB: Experimental renal insufficiency produced by partial nephrectomy: I. Control diet. *Arch Intern Med* 49:767, 1932.
53. Deen WM, Maddox DA, Robertson CR, et al: Dynamics of glomerular ultrafiltration in the rat: VII. Response to reduced renal mass. *Am J Physiol* 227:556, 1974.
54. Brenner BM: Nephron adaptation to renal injury or ablation. *Am J Physiol* 249:F324, 1985.
55. Robson AM, Mor J, Root ER, et al: Mechanism of proteinuria in non-glomerular renal disease. *Kidney Int* 16:426, 1979.
56. Bhathena DB, Weiss JH, Holland NH, et al: Focal and segmental glomerular sclerosis in reflux nephropathy. *Am J Med* 68:886, 1980.
57. Albright R, Brensilver J, Cortell S: Proteinuria in congestive heart failure. *Am J Nephrol* 3:272, 1983.
58. Azar S, Johnson MA, Iwai J, et al: Single nephron dynamics in post salt rats with chronic hypertension. *J Lab Clin Med* 91:156, 1978.
59. Castenford J, Massfeldt F, Piscator M: Effect of prolonged heavy exercise on kidney function and urinary protein excretion. *Acta Physiol Scand* 70:194, 1967.
60. Grenier T, Henry JP: Mechanism of postural proteinuria. *JAMA* 157:1373, 1955.
61. Silverberg DS, Allard MJ, Ulan RA, et al: City-wide screening for urinary abnormalities in school girls. *Can Med Assoc J* 109:981, 1973.
62. Vehaskari VM, Rapola J: Isolated proteinuria: Analysis of a school-age population. *J Pediatr* 101:661, 1982.
63. Kunin CM: Emergence of bacteriuria, proteinuria, and symptomatic urinary tract infections among a population of school girls followed for 7 years. *Pediatrics* 41:968, 1968.
64. Dodge WF, West EF, Smith EH, et al: Proteinuria and hematuria in school children: epidemiology and early natural history. *J Pediatr* 88:327, 1976.
65. Gutgesell M: Practicality of screening urinalyses in asymptomatic children in a primary care setting. *Pediatrics* 62:103, 1978.
66. Robinson RR: Isolated proteinuria in asymptomatic patients. *Kidney Int* 18:395, 1980.
67. Rytand DA, Spreiter S: Prognosis in postural proteinuria: Forty to fifty year follow-up of six patients after diagnosis by Thomas Addis. *N Engl J Med* 305:618, 1981.
68. Epstein FH, Goddyer An, Lauroson FD, et al: Studies of the antidiuresis of quiet standing: The importance of changes in plasma volume and glomerular filtration rate. *J Clin Invest* 30:62, 1951.

69. Springberg PD, Garrett LE, Thom AL, et al: Fixed and reproducible orthostatic proteinuria: Results of a 20-yr follow-up. *Ann Intern Med* 97:516, 1982.
70. International Study of Kidney Disease in Children: The nephrotic syndrome in children: Prediction of histopathology from clinical and laboratory characteristics at the time of diagnosis. *Kidney Int* 13:43, 1978.

7

NEPHROTIC SYNDROME

Kanwal K. Kher

Nephrotic syndrome, one of the commonest renal diseases in childhood, is characterized by proteinuria, hypoalbuminemia, hypercholesterolemia, and edema. An increased glomerular permeability resulting in proteinuria is the primary renal abnormality in nephrotic syndrome, while hypoalbuminemia, edema, and hypercholesterolemia are believed to be secondary pathophysiologic events. Studies of Rothenberg and Heymann[1] and Schlesinger et al.[2] suggest that the incidence of nephrotic syndrome is 2.0 new patients per 100,000 children per year in the United States. A similar incidence has also been reported from the United Kingdom.[3] Nephrotic syndrome appears to be slightly more common in black children than in white children.[1,2]

CLASSIFICATION OF NEPHROTIC SYNDROME

Nephrotic syndrome can result from a variety of morphologically distinct renal diseases that give rise to significant proteinuria. *Minimal change,* or *nil disease,* is the most frequent cause of childhood nephrotic syndrome, accounting for 80 to 85 percent of all cases. Various types of chronic glomerulonephritides and inherited renal diseases account for the remaining 15 to 20 percent of cases of nephrotic syndrome in children.[4,5] The terms *minimal change, minimal change nephrotic syndrome* (MCNS), and *nil disease* only reflect a lack of specific and definable pathologic abnormalities such as cellular proliferation, inflammatory cells, or other evidence of glomerular injury in the renal biopsy of such patients. To a large extent, clinical course, prognosis, and response of nephrotic patients to therapy is determined by the underlying glomerular pathology and the etiology of nephrotic syndrome. To be useful, any classification of nephrotic syndrome must take into account both the renal histopathology and the etiology. Traditionally, nephrotic syndrome is classified into primary and secondary subtypes. Primary refers to the patients in whom the etiology of nephrotic syndrome is not known, while secondary nephrotic syndrome is seen in the course of systemic diseases such as connective tissue disorders, neoplasms, infections and use of drugs. Classification of nephrotic syndrome is given in Table 7–1, and the relative frequency of various causes of nephrotic syndrome in children is listed in Table 7–2.

PATHOPHYSIOLOGY

Increased glomerular permeability leading to proteinuria is the pathophysiologic hallmark of nephrotic syndrome. Albumin is the predominant plasma pro-

TABLE 7–1. Classification of Nephrotic Syndrome

Primary nephrotic syndrome
- Minimal change nephrotic syndrome (MCNS)
- Chronic glomerulonephritis
  - Focal glomerulosclerosis
  - Membranous glomerulonephritis
  - Membranoproliferative glomerulonephritis
  - Mesangial proliferative glomerulonephritis
    - with IgM deposition
    - with IgA-IgG deposition (Berger's disease)
- Congenital nephrotic syndrome (Finnish type)

Nephrotic syndrome secondary to renal involvement in systemic disorders
- Henoch-Schönlein purpura
- Systemic lupus erythematosus
- Systemic infections
  - Hepatitis B
  - Congenital and secondary syphilis
  - Ventriculoatrial shunt infections
  - Subacute bacterial endocarditis
  - Malaria
  - Varicella
  - Acquired immune deficiency syndrome (AIDS)
- Sickle cell disease
- Diabetes mellitus
- Drugs
  - Gold
  - D-penicillamine
  - Mercury
  - Tridione
  - Captopril
  - Heroin
  - Nonsteroidal anti-inflammatory drugs
- Neoplasms: Hodgkin's disease and other lymphomas
- Chronic inflammatory diseases
  - Familial mediterranean fever
  - Amyloidosis
- Hereditary disorders
  - Alport's syndrome

Source: From Kher KK, Sweet M, Makker SP: Nephrotic syndrome in children. *Curr Probl Pediatr* 18:199, 1988. Reproduced with permission of Year Book Medical Publishers Inc., Chicago.

TABLE 7–2. Histopathologic Distribution of Nephrotic Syndrome in Children

	White et al.[5] (146 Patients), Percent 1970	Habib and Kleinknecht[47] (406 Patients), Percent 1971	ISKDC[4] (521 Patients), Percent 1978
Minimal change	76.5	51.5	76.4
Focal glomerulosclerosis	8.2	11.5	6.9
Membranous glomerulonephritis	1.3	9	1.5
Membranoproliferative glomerulonephritis	6.2	13	7.5
Microcystic disease	—	1.5	—
Others	7.8	13.5	7.7

Source: From Kher KK, Sweet M, Makker SP: Nephrotic syndrome in children. *Curr Probl Pediatr* 18:199, 1988. Reproduced with permission of Year Book Medical Publishers Inc., Chicago.

tein lost in urine in nephrotic patients, but other plasma proteins such as immunoglobulins, various coagulation factors, vitamin D-binding protein, and metalloproteins are also excreted in significant amounts in urine. Consequences of urinary loss of various plasma proteins in nephrotic syndrome are outlined in Table 7–3. Clinical and laboratory features of nephrotic syndrome such as edema, hypoproteinemia, and hypercholesterolemia develop as a consequence of albuminuria. These pathophysiologic alterations are observed in all nephrotic patients, irrespective of their underlying renal morphology or etiology.

PROTEINURIA

The urine of healthy children contains only a small amount of protein, usually not exceeding 100 mg/day.[6] Passage of plasma proteins from the glomerular capillary lumen is prevented by the complex anatomic and electrostatic properties of the glomerular filtration barrier. Glomerular proteinuria develops as a consequence of the qualitative alterations in the glomerular capillary filtration barrier. The glomerular filtration barrier consists of endothelial cell, glomerular basement membrane (GBM), and epithelial cell (Fig. 7–1*A* and *B*). Although pathways for filtration through the glomerular capillary wall have not been well characterized, functional "pores" have been proposed to be present in the GBM. The glomerular capillary is not a freely permeable membrane; it restricts molecular traffic from the capillary lumen into the urinary space by acting as a size as well as an electrical charge selective barrier. While being freely permeable to molecules less than 20 Å in radius, the glomerular capillary increasingly restricts the passage of molecules whose radius is between 20 and 40 Å and is impermeable to molecules greater than 42 Å in radius.[7] Additionally, anionic charge on the glomerular filtration surface is also believed to play an important role in preventing escape of plasma proteins and other molecules from the glo-

TABLE 7–3. Effects of Protein Losses in Nephrotic Syndrome

Protein	Consequences
Albumin	Hypoalbuminemia and edema
Lecithin-cholesterol acyltransferase High-density lipoproteins	Altered cholesterol and triglyceride metabolism, with resultant hyperlipidemia
Antithrombin III Plasminogen Antiplasmin	Abnormal fibrinolysis and increased risk of thrombosis
IgG Factor B	Hypogammaglobulinemia and altered opsonization, with increased risk of infection
Transferrin	Iron-resistant hypochromic microcytic anemia
Loss of other metal-binding proteins (Zn, Cu)	Dysgeusia, poor wound healing
Loss of vitamin D-binding protein	Altered vitamin D metabolism, with risk of metabolic bone disease
Transcortin	Altered cortisol metabolism
Thyroxin-binding globulin	Altered thyroid function tests with increased total T3, T4

Source: From Kher KK, Sweet M, Makker SP: Nephrotic syndrome in children. *Curr Probl Pediatr* 18:199, 1988. Reproduced with permission of Year Book Medical Publishers Inc., Chicago.

merular capillary lumen into urine. It is now well established that the filtration barrier, particularly the GBM and the epithelial cell, possesses anionic electrostatic surface charge due to the presence of sialoglycoproteins and proteoglycans. Negative electrostatic charge on the filtration barrier hinders passage of anionically charged molecules such as plasma proteins by electrostatic repulsion. On the other hand, filtration of molecules with cationic or neutral charge through the filtration barrier is favored.[8] Abolition of glomerular capillary anionic surface charge in rats by infusion of cationic molecules has been shown to result in a loss of charge-dependent permselectivity and in heavy proteinuria.[9] Based on these observations, a diminution or elimination of the anionic charge on the glomerular filtration barrier is believed to be the primary factor giving rise to increased glomerular permeability and proteinuria in nephrotic syndrome.[7,10] However, the mechanism by which these changes are initiated, particularly in MCNS, remains a subject of intense discussion and speculation. The possible role played by an increased glomerullar capillary pore size and loss of anionic surface charge in the pathogenesis of proteinuria in nephrotic syndrome is being actively debated. Bridges et al.[10] have suggested that glomerular capillary pore size remains unchanged in MCNS and that proteinuria in this disease can be entirely explained by loss of surface anionic charge of the glomerular capillary filtration barrier. On the other hand, proteinuria and nephrotic syndrome associated with chronic glomerulonephritis may result from a combination of an increased pore size, reduction in the anionic charge

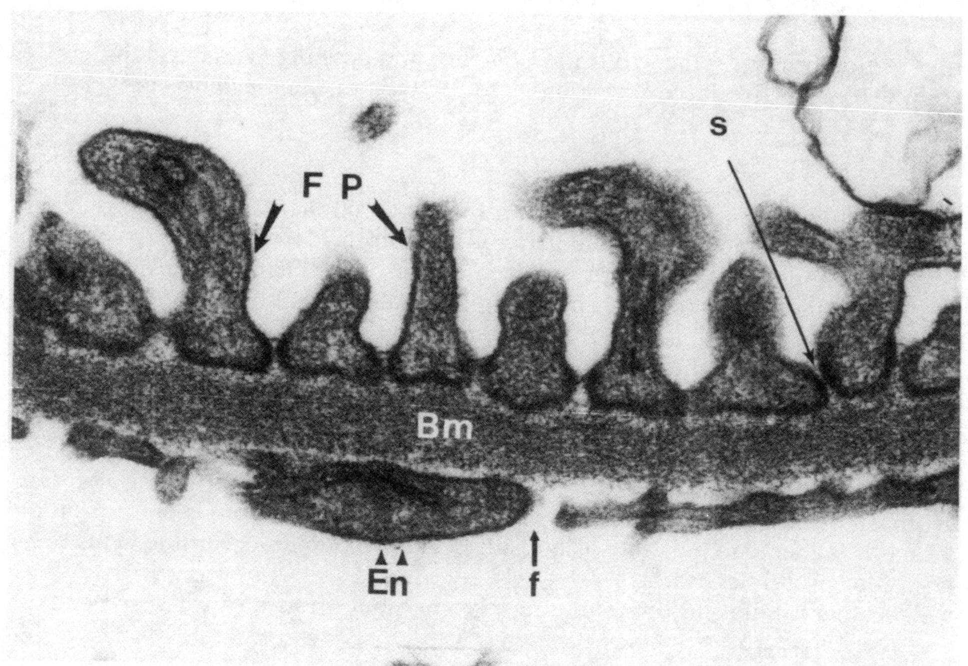

A

B

FIG. 7–1. *A*. Electron micrograph of a normal glomerular capillary wall showing endothelial cell (En) with fenestrae (f), basement membrane (Bm), foot processes of the epithelial cells (FP), and slit pores (S). (Photograph courtesy of Dr. Firmin Tio.) *B*. A cross-sectional representation of the glomerular capillary wall, detailing the structures shown in Fig. 7–1*A*. (From Brenner BM, Beeuwkes R: The renal circulation. *Hosp Pract* 13:35, 1978. Reproduced with permission of Hospital Practice Publishing Company, New York.)

on the glomerular capillary filtration barrier, and possibly even development of charge-nonselective large-sized pores (70 to 90 Å) or *shunt pathway*.[11,12]

HYPOALBUMINEMIA

Hypoalbuminemia is an integral feature of the clinico-laboratory profile of nephrotic syndrome.[13] Excessive urinary albumin loss is the primary cause of hypoalbuminemia in nephrotic syndrome, but other factors such as the rate of hepatic albumin synthesis and albumin catabolism also determine the net balance of plasma albumin. Experimental and clinical studies suggest that hepatic albumin synthesis is accelerated rather than decreased in nephrotic patients.[14] In fact, hepatic synthesis of albumin closely follows the rate of urinary albumin excretion in nephrotic syndrome (Fig. 7–2). Available evidence indicates that enhanced hepatic albumin synthesis is stimulated by a decrease in plasma oncotic pressure resulting from hypoalbuminemia.[15] Hepatic albumin synthesis is adversely affected in nephrotic patients in whom dietary protein intake is inadequate, possibly as a result of nonavailability of amino acids necessary for protein synthesis.[15]

Excessive catabolism of circulating plasma albumin as a cause of hypoalbu-

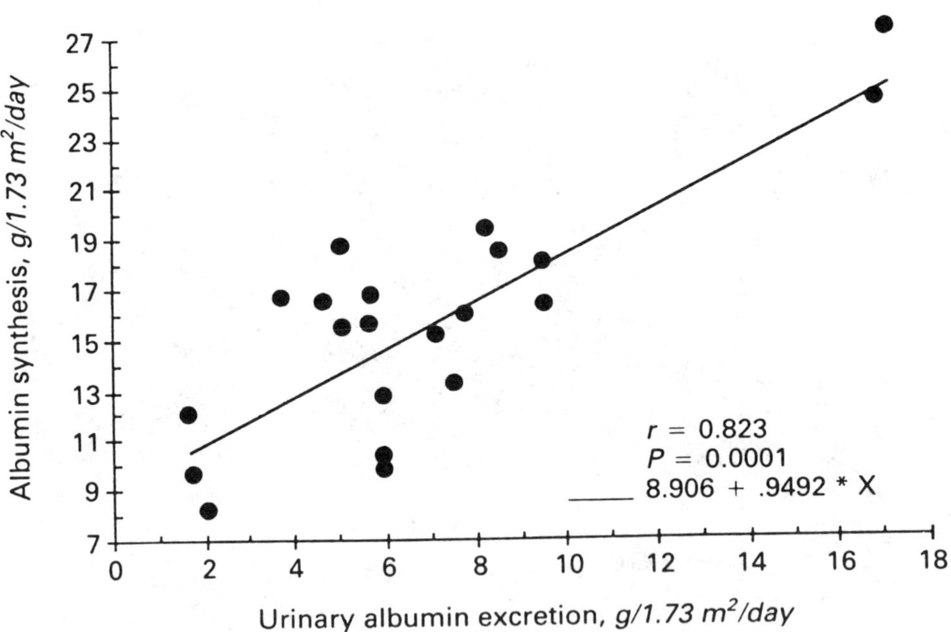

FIG. 7–2. Correlation between the rate of albumin synthesis and average albumin excretion. Hepatic albumin synthesis enhances with increasing proteinuria. (From Kaysen GA, Gambertoglio T, Felts J, et al: Albumin synthesis, albuminuria and hyperlipidemia in nephrotic patients. *Kidney Int* 31:1368, 1987. Reproduced with permission.)

minemia in nephrotic syndrome has also received considerable attention in the past. Normally, about 10 percent of circulating albumin undergoes catabolism daily, mostly in non-renal tissues.[15,15a] Although the absolute rate of albumin catabolism is reduced in nephrotic syndrome, fractional albumin catabolic rate (or the fraction of circulating albumin pool undergoing catabolism over given time) is elevated.[15] It has long been held that kidneys are responsible for excessive catabolism of albumin in the nephrotic state: the suggested mechanism is that a large portion of the filtered albumin undergoes tubular reabsorption and is catabolized into aminoacids within the tubular cells.[15b] Work by Kayson and colleagues, however, suggests that renal catabolism of albumin contributes little towards development of hypoalbuminemia in nephrotic syndrome.[15,15c] Gastrointestinal loss of albumin in nephrotic syndrome has been a subject of controversy, but probably does not contribute significantly to the development of hypoalbuminemia in these patients.[16]

The severity of hypoalbuminemia in nephrotic syndrome varies from patient to patient, and serum albumin can range from 0.5 g/dL to 2.5 g/dL during a relapse. In general, serum albumin bears an inverse relationship to the severity of proteinuria.[13] Since several factors other than urinary protein excretion influence the net albumin metabolism, patients with a similar degree of proteinuria often have variable serum albumin concentration.[16]

EDEMA

Edema is the principal clinical manifestation of nephrotic syndrome in both children and adults. Edema in nephrotic syndrome develops from decreased intravascular colloid oncotic pressure secondary to hypoalbuminemia and resultant transcapillary passage of water and solutes into the subcutaneous tissues. As a consequence of these hemodynamic events, contraction of intravascular volume occurs and the renin-angiotensin-aldosterone system is activated, leading to renal sodium and water retention and perpetuation of the edematous state in nephrotic patients (Fig. 7–3).[17] While this conventional view of edema formation may be operative in many nephrotic patients, particularly those with MCNS, several recent observations have questioned the application of this hypothesis to all cases of nephrotic syndrome. In fact, plasma volume determinations in nephrotic patients have revealed conflicting results (in part due to the problem of measuring plasma volume accurately) and the intravascular volume has been found to be diminished, normal, or even elevated in these patients.[18] Also, plasma renin activity (PRA) is not elevated universally in nephrotic syndrome. Of the 123 nephrotic patients reviewed by Dorhout Mees et al.,[19] 64 had either normal or low PRA. Intravascular volume expansion by albumin infusion and suppression of the renin-angiotensin-aldosterone system by oral captopril administration has not been shown to ameliorate the sodium retaining state in nephrotic patients.[20] Similar findings have been reported in experimental animals by others.[21] This has led some to conclude that sodium retention in nephrotic syndrome is caused by an intrarenal defect in sodium handling.[21] The precise location and nature of this abnormality in renal sodium handling in nephrotic syndrome has not yet been fully characterized.

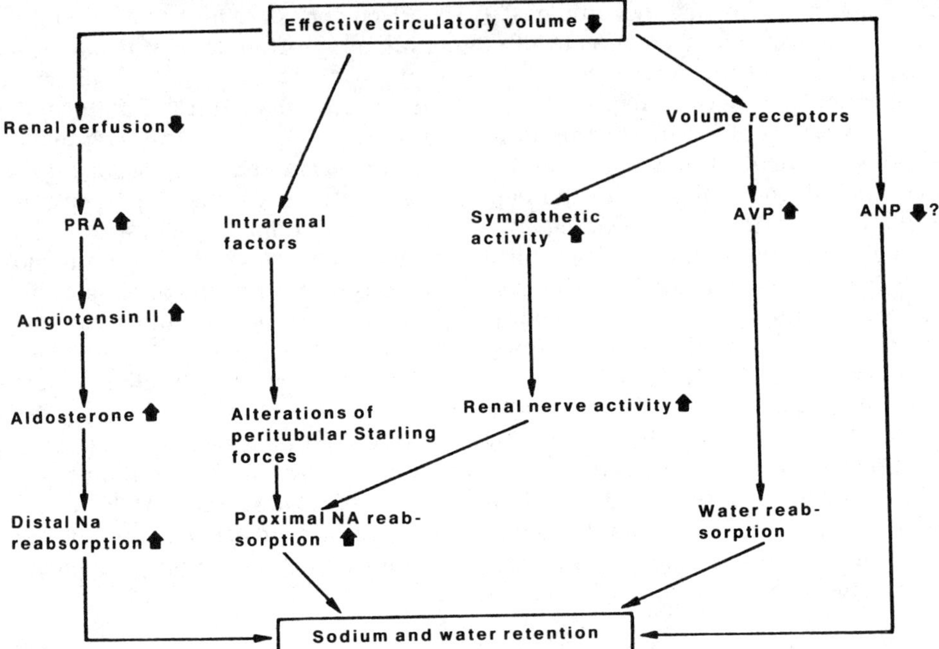

FIG. 7–3. Proposed mechanisms involved in the pathogenesis of edema in nephrotic syndrome. PRA = plasma renin activity, AVP = arginine vasopressin, ANP = atrial natriuretic peptide, and Na = sodium. (From Tulassay T, Rascher W, Scharer K: Intra- and extrarenal factors of oedema formation in the nephrotic syndrome. *Pediatr Nephrol* 3:92, 1989. Reproduced with permission.)

While plasma concentration of antidiuretic hormone (ADH) has been shown to be elevated in nephrotic patients, the role of this water-retaining hormone in the pathogenesis of edema of nephrotic syndrome remains controversial.[22] Atrial natriuretic peptide (ANP) has been shown to be involved in diuresis and natriuresis associated with albumin infusion in nephrotic patients, but it is unclear if ANP is necessary in the pathogenesis of edema.[23]

HYPERLIPIDEMIA AND HYPERLIPOPROTEINEMIA

Hyperlipidemia is a well-described laboratory feature of nephrotic syndrome, and an elevated plasma concentration of cholesterol, triglycerides, phospholipids, and fatty acids is usually observed in these patients. While serum cholesterol concentration is consistently elevated, serum triglyceride and phospholipids may not be elevated in all patients. Abnormalities in the lipoprotein metabolism have also been described in nephrotic patients. Serum high-density lipoprotein (HDL) concentration is usually normal, but low-density lipoprotein (LDL) and very low density lipoprotein (VLDL) concentration is generally elevated during relapse of nephrotic syndrome.[13,24–26]

An inverse relationship between serum cholesterol concentration and serum albumin is well known; a similar relationship between serum albumin and serum triglycerides is observed frequently.[13,14] The severity of hypercholesterolemia and hypertriglyceridemia correlates well with the severity of hypoalbuminemia and albuminuria (Fig. 7–4).[14] Other factors that determine the degree of hyperlipidemia in nephrotic syndrome are patient's age, diet, presence of renal failure, and use of corticosteroids. For unknown reasons, hyperlipidemia is less commonly associated with nephrotic syndrome resulting from glomerulonephritis of systemic lupus erythematosus and amyloidosis.

Plasma lipid and lipoprotein abnormalities in nephrotic syndrome primarily result from an enhanced hepatic synthesis of lipids and lipoproteins, particularly VLDL.[24,26] Additionally, decreased catabolism of lipids may also significantly contribute to hyperlipidemia of nephrotic syndrome.[24,25] Available evidence suggests that a decrease in plasma oncotic pressure due to hypoalbuminemia triggers increased hepatic lipid and lipoprotein synthesis in nephrotic patients.[13,14,26] Resolution of lipid abnormalities is usually noted with onset of remission of nephrotic syndrome.[25,26] The significance of serum lipid and lipoprotein abnormalities in relation to long-term cardiovascular morbidity and mortality in nephrotic children is not entirely settled. While patients with MCNS are probably at a minimal risk for such complications, hyperlipidemia may be a significant determinant of long-term outcome in patients with nonremitting nephrotic syndrome.

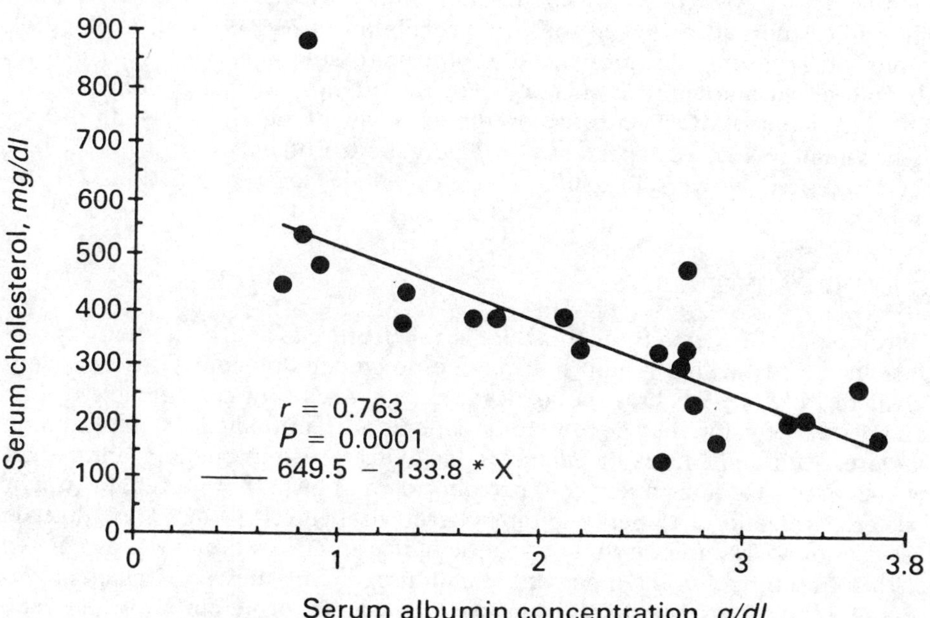

FIG. 7–4. Correlation between serum cholesterol and serum albumin in nephrotic syndrome. (From Kaysen GA, Gambertoglio T, Felts J, et al: Albumin synthesis, albuminuria and hyperlipidemia in nephrotic patients. *Kidney Int* 31:1368, 1987. Reproduced with permission.)

PRIMARY NEPHROTIC SYNDROME

MINIMAL CHANGE NEPHROTIC SYNDROME

Albuminuria without any demonstrable renal inflammatory lesion has been well known since the beginning of this century. Several descriptions such as *lipoid nephrosis, foot process disease,* and *childhood nephrosis* have been used in the past to define this clinicopathologic entity. The term *minimal change* was coined by Hamburger (1961)[27] to denote an obvious lack of pathologic changes in the renal tissues of these patients. The term *minimal change nephrotic syndrome* (MCNS) is currently preferred to include patients with nephrotic syndrome previously described under several of the above definitions.

EPIDEMIOLOGY

Approximately 80 percent of all forms of nephrotic syndrome in children result from MCNS; the remaining 20 percent are due to chronic glomerulonephritis and inherited renal diseases. In the International Study of Kidney Disease in Children (ISKDC), MCNS constituted the etiology of nephrotic syndrome in 76.45 percent of all patients. In another study by White et al.,[5] the incidence of MCNS in unselected patients with nephrotic syndrome was reported to be 88 percent. Although MCNS may occur in patients of any age, including adults, onset of this disorder in children usually occurs between 1 and 6 years of age. Median age at onset of MCNS in children studied by the ISKDC was 3 years.[4] The same study also showed that the probability of MCNS as an etiology of nephrotic syndrome declines steadily with increasing age, while that due to chronic glomerulonephritis increases correspondingly during childhood (Fig. 7–5). In adults, MCNS constitutes the etiology of nephrotic syndrome in approximately 15 to 25 percent. A preponderance of males with MCNS has been reported universally, and male to female ratio approaches 2:1 in childhood.[4]

CLINICAL MANIFESTATIONS

Development of edema is the most noticeable feature of MCNS. It often appears first in the periorbital region but may be noted simultaneously in dependent areas of the body, such as the ankles and legs. Ascites of considerable degree and pleural effusion may be present in patients with untreated or long-standing disease. Although onset of edema is insidious and without any antecedent events in most, some patients (30 percent) report a history of preceding viral or bacterial infection.[3] Upper respiratory tract viral infection may also precede relapses of MCNS. In one study,[28] relapse of nephrotic syndrome was associated with a viral infection in 70 percent of children; among these, a viral agent was identified in 51.6 percent. With the onset of edema, urine output is generally reduced and the urine appears concentrated in color. Gross hematuria is not seen in uncomplicated MCNS. When it is present, it should alert the physician to the diagnostic possibilities of an associated renal vein thrombosis or chronic glomerulonephritis as an etiology of nephrotic syndrome. On the other hand,

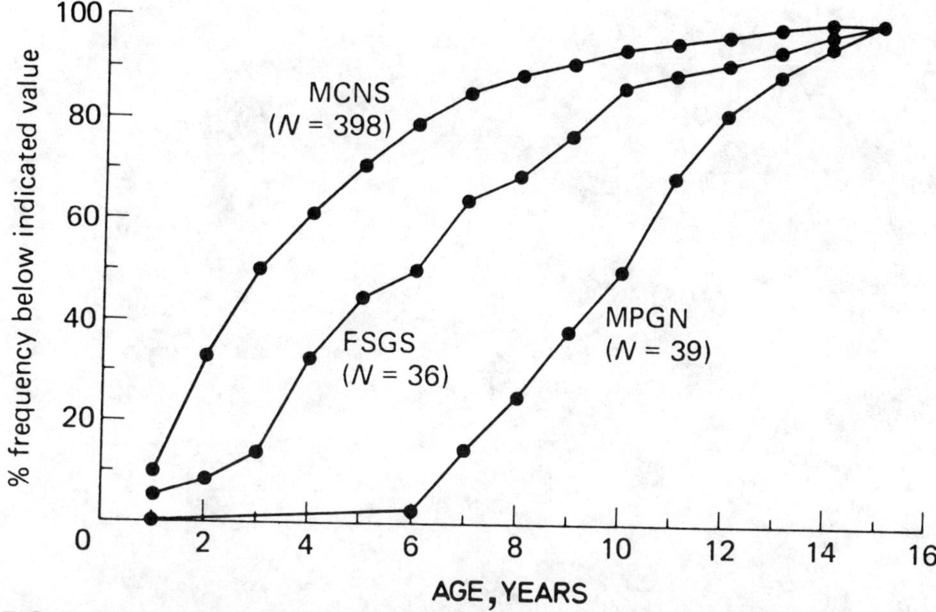

FIG. 7–5. Age at the time of diagnosis of patients with minimal change nephrotic syndrome (MCNS), focal segmental glomerulonephritis (FSGS), and membranoproliferative glomerulonephritis (MPGN). (From International Study of Kidney Disease in Children: Prediction of histopathology from clinical and laboratory characteristics at the time of diagnosis. *Kidney Int* 13:159, 1978. Reproduced with permission.)

transient microscopic hematuria at onset occurs in about 15 percent of children with MCNS.[4] Blood pressure is normal in most children at the onset of MCNS, but mild hypertension may be noted in about 15 percent.[4] Severe hypertension should generally be regarded as evidence against the diagnosis of MCNS. Renal function tests are normal in patients with MCNS, but transiently diminished creatinine clearance due to a decrease in the intravascular volume may occur in up to 30 percent of children with MCNS.[4] Acute renal failure has been reported only rarely in such children.[29]

PATHOLOGY

The pathologic hallmark of MCNS on light microscopic examination of renal tissue is absence of any significant glomerular or interstitial inflammation (Fig. 7–6). Electron microscopy shows fusion of the foot processes of the epithelial cells (Fig. 7–7). Electron-dense deposits are not seen and immunofluorescence examination does not reveal any immune deposits. Renal biopsy in some nephrotic patients may demonstrate a varying degree of proliferation of mesangial matrix, with deposits of IgM and C3 in the mesangial location. There is an ongoing debate whether this pathologic description should be regarded as a separate entity (IgM nephropathy) or be considered a variant of MCNS. The generally held view is that nephrotic syndrome associated with mesangial IgM deposits and mesangial cell or matrix proliferation represents a variant of

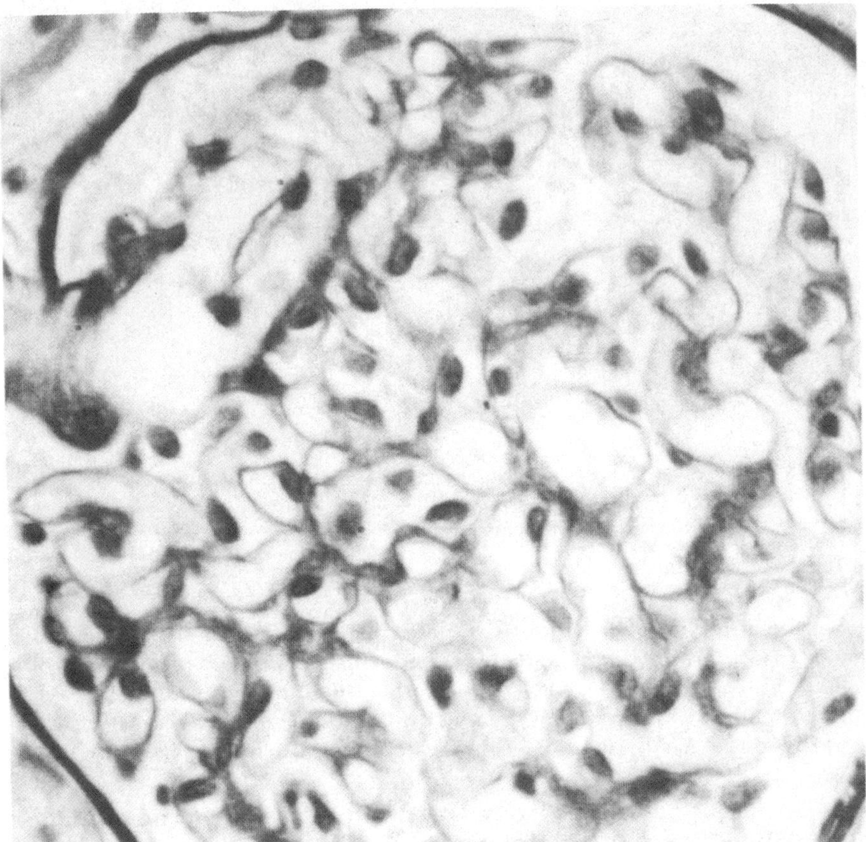

FIG. 7–6. Minimal change nephrotic syndrome. Light microscopy showing normal-looking glomerulus. Lack of cellular proliferation in the glomerulus, open capillary lumens, and thin basement membrane are characteristic features. (From Kher KK, Sweet M, Makker SP: Nephrotic syndrome in children. *Curr Probl Pediatr* 18:199, 1988. Reproduced with permission of Year Book Medical Publishers Inc., Chicago.)

MCNS.[30,31] Some have also argued that nephrotic syndrome with minimal change glomerular morphology and mesangial IgM deposition represents an early stage of focal segmental glomerulosclerosis.[32]

ETIOLOGY

The etiology and pathogenesis of MCNS is not entirely clear. The prevailing view suggests that MCNS is an immunologic disorder characterized by circulating lymphokines that are toxic to the renal filtration barrier. Factors pertinent in the etiopathogenesis of MCNS are discussed below.

Genetics. MCNS is not a genetically determined disorder but has been reported in more than one member of the same family.[33] An increased frequency of

DRw8 and DRw3 has been reported in Japanese adults with MCNS and may represent a genetic predisposition to this disorder.[34] A strong relationship between steroid sensitive nephrotic syndrome and HLA-DQw2 haplotype has been reported in children.[34a] However, McEnery and Welch[35] were unable to find any association between steroid-responsive nephrotic syndrome (presumed MCNS) and the major histocompatibility complex in children.

Immunology. Despite absence of any immune deposits in the renal biopsy specimens of patients with MCNS, the immune system is thought to play a central role in the etiopathogenesis of this disorder. Shalhoub [36] proposed in 1974 that (a) MCNS is a T-cell disorder that results from persistence and proliferation of an abnormal T-cell clone or subclass and (b) proteinuria results from a lymphocyte-derived circulating lymphokine. Evidence favoring such a hypothesis is derived from the following observations: (a) T-lymphocyte disorders such as Hodgkin's lymphoma can lead to MCNS,[37] (b) remission of MCNS is seen following natural measles infection—a condition known to cause depression of cell-mediated immunity,[38] and (c) induction of prolonged remission with cytotoxic drugs such as cyclophosphamide, which cause impairment of suppressor T-cell function. Conclusive evidence of T-lymphocyte dysfunction as an etiology of MCNS has, however, yet to be presented. Cultured lymphocytes of patients

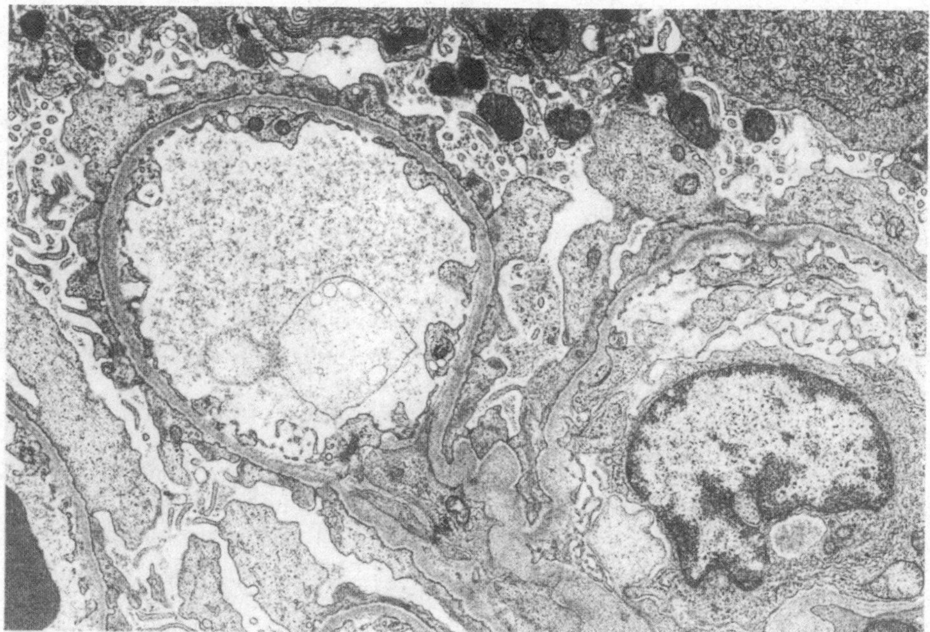

FIG. 7–7. Low-power electron micrograph of a glomerular capillary loop in a patient with MCNS. Fusion of the epithelial foot processes is seen all along the urinary side of the basement membrane. (Photograph provided by Sudesh Kapur, M.D. Children's National Medical Center, Washington D.C.)

with MCNS have been reported to produce lymphokine(s),[39,40] and these lymphokine(s) have been shown to increase permeability of guinea pig skin capillaries as well as to induce proteinuria in rats.[40–42] Circulating immune complexes have been reported in some studies in children and adults with MCNS,[43,44] but the significance of these observations in view of absence of immune-complex deposition in the glomeruli remains undetermined.

Allergy. Some studies have reported an increased incidence of atopic symptoms, positive skin tests, and higher mean serum concentration of IgE in patients with MCNS. In one report,[45] such allergic manifestations were present in about 40 percent of children with MCNS, in contrast to only 22 percent of controls. Others have not found any evidence of increased incidence of allergic manifestations in these patients.[46]

CHRONIC GLOMERULONEPHRITIS AS A CAUSE OF NEPHROTIC SYNDROME

Most subtypes of chronic glomerulonephritis result in severe proteinuria and represent an important cause of nephrotic syndrome in children (20 percent of all pediatric nephrotic patients). Of these subtypes, focal glomerulosclerosis is the most frequent morphologic variety encountered in children, followed by membranoproliferative glomerulonephritis and membranous glomerulonephritis.[4,5,47] Occasionally chronic glomerulonephritis secondary to systemic disorders also leads to nephrotic syndrome in children.

FOCAL GLOMERULOSCLEROSIS

Focal glomerulosclerosis leads to nephrotic syndrome that may be clinically indistinguishable from MCNS at onset. Focal glomerulosclerosis constitutes 6 to 12 percent of all cases of nephrotic syndrome in childhood.[4,5,47] Children with focal glomerulosclerosis are slightly older at onset (median age, 6 years) than are those with MCNS (median age, 3 years).[4] A predominance of males, as in MCNS, is also observed in focal glomerulosclerosis.

Nephrotic syndrome is the presenting manifestation of focal glomerulosclerosis in a majority of cases (80 percent), but asymptomatic proteinuria may be the presenting feature at onset in some (20 percent).[48] The incidence of asymptomatic proteinuria at presentation has been reported to be higher among Japanese children.[49] Those presenting with asymptomatic proteinuria often develop nephrotic syndrome during the course of the disease. Although gross hematuria is uncommon, microscopic hematuria is detected at onset in 50 to 60 percent of cases. Hypertension is also present in approximately 40 percent of patients, and impaired renal function may be observed in 30 to 40 percent of cases at onset.[48] Multiple defects of tubular functions—such as glycosuria, hyperaminoaciduria, phosphaturia, and renal tubular acidosis—are often seen in patients with focal glomerulosclerosis.[50]

The characteristic pathologic feature of focal glomerulosclerosis is the patchy distribution of glomerular disease, with many glomeruli appearing entirely normal in the renal biopsy. Affected glomeruli may exhibit either segmental areas of sclerosis (focal segmental glomerulosclerosis—FSGS), where only certain segments of the glomerulus are involved by the sclerotic process, or as sclerosis of the entire glomerulus (focal global sclerosis—FGS). The former (FSGS) is the more common clinicopathologic form of glomerulosclerosis (Fig. 7–8).[51] Intraglomerular intracapillary foam cells are present in 40 to 60 percent of cases.[48] Tubular atrophy is seen in patients with advanced glomerular disease. Diffuse mesangial cell prominence is seen in some patients. Immunofluorescence microscopy shows IgM and complement C3 deposits in the sclerotic areas, but other immunoglobulins can also be seen in similar locations. Fusion of foot processes of the epithelial cell and mesangial electron-dense deposits are seen by electron microscopy.[48] Glomerulosclerosis is usually first seen in the juxta-

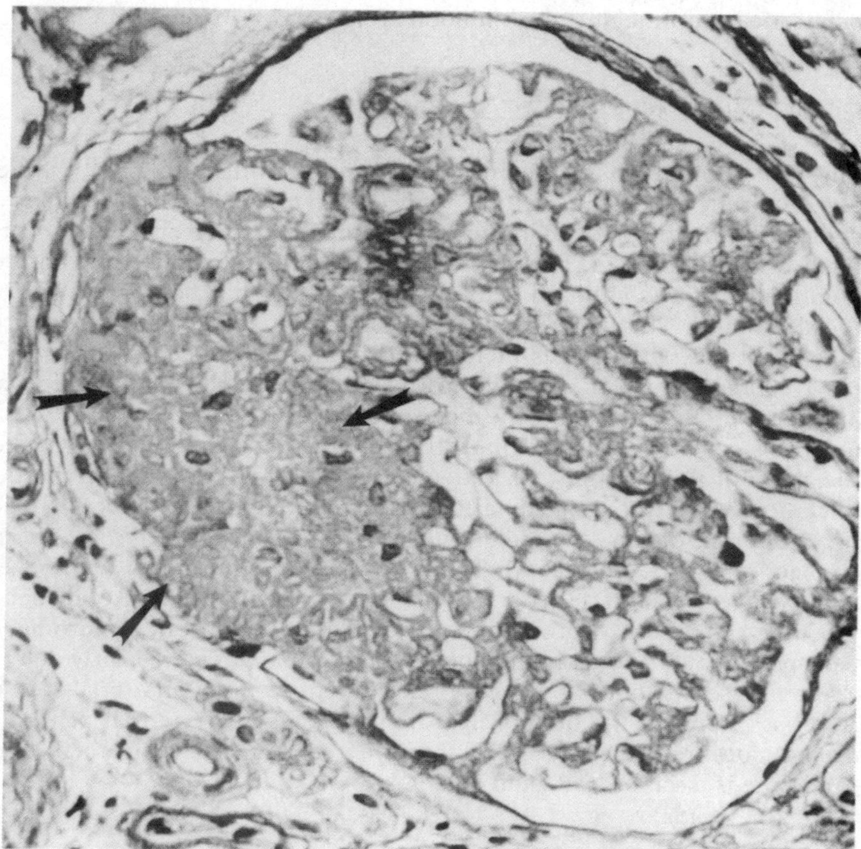

FIG. 7–8. Focal segmental glomerulosclerosis. Light microscopy showing an area of the glomerulus affected by sclerosis *(arrows)*. (From Kher KK, Sweet M, Makker SP: Nephrotic syndrome in children. *Curr Probl Pediatr* 18:199, 1988. Reproduced with permission of Year Book Medical Publishers Inc., Chicago.)

medullary glomeruli. Therefore, diagnosis of early focal glomerulosclerosis may be missed if the renal biopsy specimen does not include the juxtamedullary area for evaluation.

The pathogenesis of focal glomerulosclerosis is unknown. Since it has been reported to occur in a variety of disease states such as vesicoureteral reflux, intravenous drug abuse, and acquired immunodeficiency syndrome (AIDS), glomerular sclerosis may merely represent the end result of diverse renal injuries. An increased frequency of HLA-DR4 in patients with idiopathic FSGS has been reported recently and may represent a genetic predisposition for this disease.[52] Among patients who undergo renal transplantation for end-stage renal disease, FSGS recurs in the renal allografts of 30 to 40 percent.[53,54] At times, the recurrence of proteinuria in such patients begins within days of transplantation. The serum of patients who develop recurrent FSGS in the renal transplants has been shown to induce proteinuria when infused in rats.[55] These observations suggest that a humoral factor may be involved in the pathogenesis of FSGS.

Other subtypes of primary chronic glomerulonephritis that result in nephrotic syndrome during childhood are discussed in detail in Chap. 8.

CONGENITAL NEPHROTIC SYNDROME

This rare disorder usually begins in the first 3 months of life, with proteinuria and nephrotic syndrome. In their study, Habib and Kleinknecht[47] reported that congenital nephrotic syndrome represented 1.5 percent of all forms of nephrotic syndrome in children. Although congenital nephrotic syndrome predominantly affects children of Finnish descent, it has been reported in other racial groups.[56] The mode of inheritance of congenital nephrotic syndrome is autosomal recessive and its incidence in Finland has been reported to be 1.2 per 10,000 population.[57] Children with congenital nephrotic syndrome are usually born prematurely and the placenta is characteristically large. Antenatal diagnosis can be made by demonstration of a high alpha fetoprotein level in the amniotic fluid of high-risk patients. Renal biopsy shows characteristic cystic dilatation of the proximal renal tubules, also known as microcysts, and foot-process fusion of the glomerular epithelial cells is usually present. These renal changes may be seen in aborted fetuses also. Proteinuria is usually severe and microscopic hematuria generally present. Corticosteroids are ineffective in inducing remission of proteinuria in congenital nephrotic syndrome. In the past, patients with congenital nephrotic syndrome often died early due to overwhelming sepsis, but the success of early nephrectomy and renal transplantation has improved the outlook for these patients.[58] Congenital nephrotic syndrome does not recur in the transplanted kidney. Congenital nephrotic syndrome is discussed in detail in Chap. 8.

SECONDARY NEPHROTIC SYNDROME

Renal involvement due to systemic disorders may result in proteinuria and secondary nephrotic syndrome. Henoch-Schönlein purpura and systemic lupus erythematosus are the most frequent causes of secondary nephrotic syndrome in children. Bacterial infections such as subacute bacterial endocarditis and ventriculoatrial shunt infections also result in chronic glomerulonephritis and nephrotic syndrome. Malaria is the most common etiology of nephrotic syndrome in black children in Africa, and sickle cell nephropathy may cause nephrotic syndrome in black children in this country. Systemic viral infections such as hepatitis B, varicella, and AIDS may lead to chronic glomerulonephritis and nephrotic syndrome. Since the secondary causes of nephrotic syndrome are diverse, the morphologic features of each of these are also variable. Secondary forms of chronic glomerulonephritides are discussed in Chap. 8.

LABORATORY EVALUATION OF NEPHROTIC SYNDROME

Laboratory investigations of nephrotic patients are performed in order to (1) establish the diagnosis and severity of nephrotic syndrome, (2) attempt to elucidate its etiology, and (3) determine the morphologic diagnosis by renal biopsy. While tests in the first two categories should be performed in all nephrotic patients, renal biopsy is necessary for diagnostic or prognostic purposes in only a small number of patients.

URINALYSIS

Semiquantitative estimations of urinary protein excretion and microscopic hematuria by commercially available test strips (dipsticks) must be made as the first step in the evaluation of nephrotic patients. Confirmation of hematuria is done by microscopic examination of the spun urinary sediment. While transient microscopic hematuria may be seen in about 15 percent of patients with MCNS, the presence of macroscopic hematuria in a nephrotic child should arouse suspicion of chronic glomerulonephritis. Hematuria may also result from renal vein thrombosis in nephrotic patients. Hyaline casts and oval fat bodies are seen in the urine of most nephrotic patients, including those with MCNS. Red blood cell casts, granular casts, as well as waxy and broad casts in the urinary sediment support the diagnosis of chronic glomerulonephritis as the underlying etiology for nephrotic syndrome.

QUANTIFYING PROTEINURIA

A timed collection of urine for protein excretion, preferably over 24 h, should be obtained in all children to establish the severity of proteinuria. The upper limit of urinary protein excretion in normal children, defined by the ISKDC, is 4 $mg/h/m^2$ in an overnight timed urine collection. Nephrotic range proteinuria is defined as urinary protein excretion in excess of 40 $mg/h/m^2$.[59] Several authors have recently advocated the use of a urinary protein (Up)/urinary creatinine (Ucr) ratio, obtained in a spot-voided sample of urine, as a reasonably accurate method of quantifying urinary protein excretion. Because of diurnal fluctuations, an early-morning void is preferred for determining proteinuria by Up/Ucr ratio. The upper limit for Up/Ucr (mg/mg) in normal children is 0.2,[60] while nephrotic-range proteinuria corresponds to Up/Ucr (mg/mg) of 3.5.[60a]

SERUM PROTEIN, CHOLESTEROL, AND RENAL FUNCTION TESTS

In order to evaluate the severity of nephrotic syndrome, serum total protein, albumin, and cholesterol concentration should be evaluated in all patients. Serum albumin concentration should be 2.5 g/dL or less in order to qualify for the diagnosis of hypoalbuminemia and nephrotic syndrome. Serum concentration of $alpha_2$ globulin and beta globulin may be elevated because of enhanced hepatic synthesis. On the other hand, serum IgG is reduced, while serum IgM and IgE concentration is increased. Serum cholesterol and triglycerides should also be obtained in order to assess the severity of nephrotic syndrome. Blood urea nitrogen (BUN) and serum creatinine concentration should be included in the initial screening of these patients to evaluate renal function. While transient, mild deficits of renal function due to hypovolemia may be seen in MCNS, persistent and severe renal failure is usually indicative of nephrotic syndrome due to chronic glomerulonephritis.

SERUM COMPLEMENT

Serum complement (CH50 or C3) should be obtained in the initial evaluation of nephrotic patients. This is particularly important if hypertension, macroscopic hematuria, or decreased renal function is also present. Serum complement level is normal in MCNS, but it may be decreased in patients in whom nephrotic syndrome is caused by membranoproliferative glomerulonephritis, glomerulonephritis associated with systemic lupus erythematosus, poststreptococcal glomerulonephritis, shunt nephritis, or partial lipodystrophy.

SEROLOGIC EVIDENCE OF INFECTION

Serologic tests for hepatitis B infection should be included in the initial workup of all newly diagnosed nephrotic patients. Since AIDS is being increasingly recognized in children and can also lead to nephrotic syndrome, it may be necessary to obtain diagnostic tests for AIDS in high-risk patients. Serologic tests for syphilis may be obtained in selected patients.

SEROLOGIC EVIDENCE FOR COLLAGEN VASCULAR DISORDERS

Systemic lupus erythematosus is a common cause of secondary nephrotic syndrome. Serologic tests for this disorder (ANA, anti-DNA) should be obtained in all newly diagnosed nephrotic patients. This is particularly important in

TABLE 7–4. Investigative Studies in Nephrotic Syndrome

Recommended in all patients
Urinalysis
Estimation of proteinuria by a timed urine collection
Blood urea nitrogen (BUN) and serum creatinine
Serum electrolytes, serum total protein, and albumin
Serum cholesterol and triglycerides
Recommended in patients suspected to have glomerulonephritis
Antinuclear antibody
Serum complements C3, C4 (or CH 50)
Antistreptolysin O
Throat culture
Serologic tests for syphilis
Hepatitis B surface antigen
Renal biopsy

Source: Modified from Kher KK, Sweet M, Makker SP: Nephrotic syndrome in children. *Curr Probl Pediatr* 18:199, 1988. Reproduced with permission of Year Book Medical Publishers Inc., Chicago.

patients with clinical manifestations compatible with this diagnosis, evidence of hematuria, or diminished serum complement concentration (Table 7–4).

WHEN TO PERFORM RENAL BIOPSY IN NEPHROTIC SYNDROME

Diagnostic renal biopsy is not necessary in most children with nephrotic syndrome. This thinking has been reinforced by several clinicopathologic studies of children with nephrotic syndrome.[4,61,62] Whether or not a child with nephrotic syndrome has MCNS can be predicted reasonably accurately by clinical features and response to corticosteroid therapy. In one study,[61] the ISKDC showed that remission of proteinuria by corticosteroids in the initial episode of nephrotic syndrome was predictive of MCNS in 91.8 percent of cases. However, a lack of response to corticosteroids cannot always rule out MCNS; in the above study, 25 percent of patients not responding to an 8-week course of corticosteroid therapy had MCNS by renal biopsy. Therefore, based on these observations, all children presenting with their first episode of nephrotic syndrome should receive a trial of corticosteroids unless chronic glomerulonephritis is strongly suspected to be the underlying cause. Patients responding to such a therapy can be presumed to have MCNS and need not undergo a renal biopsy, since a histologic diagnosis does not provide additional information needed for therapeutic or prognostic purposes. On the other hand, failure to respond to corticosteroid treatment (steroid nonresponsive) is highly indicative of FSGS or other forms of glomerulonephritis as a cause of nephrotic syndrome.[61,62] These patients should undergo a diagnostic renal biopsy. Nephrotic patients with clinical or laboratory evidence of chronic glomerulonephritis should be considered for a renal biopsy early in the course of their disease. Many physicians consider renal biopsy to be essential prior to starting cytotoxic therapy in frequently relapsing nephrotic patients.

TREATMENT OF NEPHROTIC SYNDROME

Corticosteroids remain the drugs of choice for inducing remission of nephrotic syndrome in children, while cytotoxic agents are reserved for patients who respond poorly to corticosteroid therapy. Both these groups of drugs have dramatically improved the outlook for children with nephrotic syndrome in the last 40 years. Adjuncts such as intravenous albumin administration, salt restriction, and diuretics have an important but limited role in the management of these patients. Families of nephrotic children should be trained to check the patients' urine with dipsticks and to maintain a log of proteinuria during treatment, particularly in the initial few relapses of the disease. A pattern of response to corticosteroid therapy developed from these data is often helpful in directing the treatment of future nephrotic relapses in MCNS.

CORTICOSTEROIDS

Patients presenting for the first time with nephrotic syndrome can be presumed to have MCNS and should be considered for corticosteroid therapy unless clinical, laboratory, or biopsy evidence contrary to this diagnosis is present. Each patient must be carefully evaluated for any contraindications to corticosteroid use, and an intradermal purified protein derivative (PPD) test or tine test for tuberculosis should be done on all patients considered for such therapy. Several protocols for use of corticosteroids in childhood nephrotic syndrome have been published in the literature; some of the frequently used protocols are given in Table 7–5. In treating an initial episode of nephrotic syndrome, prednisone or prednisolone (Table 7–6) is administered daily until remission of proteinuria is achieved.* This is followed by a maintenance phase during which corticosteroids are prescribed on an alternate-day basis and discontinued either after a slow tapering schedule or abruptly. The ISKDC[61] recommends use of prednisone on 3 consecutive days out of the 7 days of the week during the maintenance phase of the treatment. Other studies have, however, documented superiority of the alternate-day treatment in reducing the frequency of relapses, and this is the recommended method of maintenance corticosteroid therapy.[63] Relapses of nephrotic syndrome can be treated in a similar manner. Spontaneous remission, without any therapy, may be observed in some patients with MCNS; the occurrence of such remissions is, however, unpredictable.[64,65] In one study,[65] at least one spontaneous remission of nephrotic syndrome was noted in 23 percent of frequently relapsing patients and in 10 percent of corticosteroid-dependent patients. The authors of this study have suggested that initiation of corticosteroids may be delayed for 7 to 10 days in order to observe whether or not remission can be induced spontaneously, without treatment. However, an

*Remission is defined as urine being negative for protein by dipstick for 3 to 4 days consecutively.

TABLE 7–5. Treatment Regimens

Makker and Heymann[67] 1974	ISKDC[62] 1981	Arbeitsgemeinschaft für Pädiatrische Nephrologie[63] 1981
First Episode	*First Episode*	*First Episode*
Prednisone 2 mg/kg/day (max. up to 60 mg/day) in three or four divided doses until urine is protein-free for 3 days. Prednisone is continued for 2 weeks beyond this point and then tapered over 2 to 4 weeks.	Prednisone 60 mg/24 h/m^2 (max. dosage 80 mg/24 h) in divided doses for 4 weeks, followed by prednisone 40 mg/m^2/24 h given on 3 consecutive days out of the 7 days per week for 4 weeks.	Prednisone 60 mg/m^2/24 h (max. 80 mg/day) in divided doses for 4 weeks. Followed by prednisone 40 mg/m^2/48 h for 4 weeks, given on alternate days.
Subsequent Episodes	*Subsequent Relapses*	*Subsequent Episodes*
Prednisone started at the same dose as for initial episode and continued until urine is negative for protein for 3 consecutive days, followed by twice the daily dose (up to a maximum of 80 mg) given as a single morning dose on alternate days for 8 weeks. Prednisone is then tapered over 5 to 6 weeks.	Prednisone is started in the dose of 60 mg/m^2/24 h (max. dosage 80 mg/24 h) for 4 weeks and intermittent maintenance treatment given for another 4 weeks as outlined above for initial episode.	Prednisone is started in the dose of 60 mg/m^2/24 h until the urine is protein-free for 3 days. Prednisone is then continued in the dose of 40 mg/m^2/48 h for 4 weeks on an alternate-day basis.

Source: From Kher KK, Sweet M, Makker SP: Nephrotic syndrome in children. *Curr Probl Pediatr* 18:199, 1988. Reproduced with permission of Year Book Medical Publishers Inc., Chicago.

undue delay in initiating corticosteroid treatment should be avoided, since such a delay has been shown to increase the morbidity and mortality rates in nephrotic children.[66]

The response of nephrotic children to treatment with corticosteroids is determined largely by the underlying renal histology. In an unselected population of nephrotic children (MCNS as well as those with chronic glomerulonephritis), Makker and Heymann[67] observed that approximately 75 percent of the patients responded to treatment with corticosteroids. In biopsy-proven MCNS, remission of proteinuria is observed in over 95 percent cases during an 8 week course of corticosteroids.[5,61] In the steroid-responsive patients, proteinuria disappears between 1–2 weeks in 75 percent of cases, an additional 20 percent patients respond between 2 and 4 weeks, and the remainder require more than 4 weeks to achieve remission.[61,67,68] Frequently relapsing course of nephrotic syndrome is observed in many patients despite adequate corticosteroid therapy, renal biopsy studies reported by ISKDC demonstrated that most such patients have MCNS.[61] Whether or not a great majority of children with frequently relapsing nephrotic syndrome can be presumed to have MCNS has, however, been contested by Trachtman et al.[69] These authors found that only 25 percent of

TABLE 7–6. Available Oral Corticosteroid Preparations

	Generic Corticosteroid	Available Size/Preparation
Tablets		
Deltasone (Upjohn)	Prednisone	2.5, 5, 10, 20, and 50 mg
Medrol (Upjohn)	Prednisolone	2, 4, 8, 16, 24, and 32 mg
Liquid		
Prelone Syrup (Fisons Corp)	Prednisolone	5 mg/5 mL and 15 mg/5 mL
Pediapred (Muro Pharmaceutical)	Prednisolone	5 mg/5 mL

patients demonstrating frequently relapsing course within the first six months following onset of nephrotic syndrome had MCNS, others had either FSGS or mesangial proliferative lesions with or without IgM deposition. Similarly, corticosteroid dependence and late resistance to corticosteroids in nephrotic patients have also been reported to be indicative of an underlying morphologic lesion other than MCNS.[70,71]

CYTOTOXIC THERAPY

Indications for use of cytotoxic drugs in the treatment of nephrotic syndrome are less clearly defined than those for corticosteroids. In general, cytotoxic drugs are employed in the treatment of nephrotic syndrome under the following clinical circumstances: (a) in the treatment of those who develop corticosteroid toxicity due to prolonged use of these drugs, (b) to induce prolonged remission in patients who have frequent lapses of nephrotic syndrome, and (c) to induce remission of proteinuria in patients who are unresponsive to corticosteroid treatment. Because of a potential for serious side effects, close medical supervision is necessary for patients receiving cytotoxic drug therapy. The patient and his or her family must have full comprehension of the risks involved with cytotoxic drug therapy. A renal biopsy for morphologic diagnosis of nephrotic syndrome is generally recommended prior to initiating cytotoxic drug therapy.

Cyclophosphamide and chlorambucil are the two commonly used cytotoxic drugs in the treatment of nephrotic syndrome in children. Azathioprine has not been shown to be any more effective than prednisone alone in the treatment of nephrotic syndrome.[72] Cyclophosphamide is generally prescribed in a dose of 2.0 to 2.5 mg/kg/day, aiming for a cumulative dose of about 150 mg/kg given over 8 to 12 weeks. Total dose and duration of cyclophosphamide therapy may be an important determinant of the length of remission induced by such treatment. In the German cooperative study,[73] 12 weeks of cyclophosphamide therapy (total dose: 168 mg/kg) was found to be superior to 8 weeks of treatment (total dose: 112 mg/kg) in inducing longer-lasting remissions. The daily recommended dose of chlorambucil is 0.1 to 0.2 mg/kg/day and is prescribed for 8 to 10 weeks.[74] The total cumulative dose of chlorambucil should not exceed 7 to 10 mg/kg. Prednisone is usually continued on an alternate-day basis during cytotoxic therapy and is tapered gradually toward the completion of treatment. Continued use of prednisone during chlorambucil therapy has been shown to reduce the risk of azoospermia in boys.[75] Since bone marrow suppression is a frequently observed side effect of cytotoxic drugs, white blood cell count and other hematologic parameters should be monitored weekly during such therapy. Cytotoxic drug treatment should be discontinued temporarily if the total white blood cell count drops below $4000/mL^3$. It is not uncommon for the white blood cell count to continue to decline even after discontinuation of these drugs. On recovery of the white blood cell count to normal, cytotoxic drugs can be resumed at a reduced dose. Cyclophosphamide should be administered in the morning to reduce the risk of hemorrhagic cystitis.

The response of patients with nephrotic syndrome to cytotoxic therapy is determined by the underlying renal pathology. A long-lasting or permanent remission is induced in 80 to 90 percent of children with MCNS.[76,77] The remaining patients often show an improvement in the course of the disease. In contrast, remission of nephrotic syndrome is observed in only 25 percent of patients with FSGS in whom cytotoxic drugs are used. Remission of proteinuria induced by cytotoxic drugs in FSGS is often shorter-lasting than that seen in patients with MCNS.[62]

Gonadal toxicity and an increased risk of carcinogenesis is a significant concern in children treated with cytotoxic drugs.[75,78,79] Azoospermia and oligospermia occur in 40 to 50 percent of prepubertal boys treated with such drugs. The risk of gonadal toxicity due to cytotoxic drugs is considerably less in females. Menstrual cycle, gonadal function, and subsequent childbearing ability have been reported to be normal in prepubertal girls treated with cytotoxic drugs.[75,78–80]

RESPONSE OF FSGS AND FGS TO CORTICOSTEROID AND CYTOTOXIC THERAPY

Approximately 30 percent of children with FSGS and 75 percent with FGS will undergo remission of the initial episode of nephrotic syndrome with standard corticosteroid therapy alone.[51,62] The remaining patients usually fail to respond to such a therapy, although a partial response may be noted in a minority of patients. The failure of FSGS patients to respond to initial corticosteroid therapy or development of resistance to such treatment during the course of the disease often indicates (a) poor response to subsequent cytotoxic therapy[62,81] and (b) greater risk for decline of renal function to end-stage renal failure (Fig. 7–9).[71,81,82] End-stage renal failure requiring dialysis or transplantation can be expected to occur in 20 to 25 percent of children with FSGS within 5 years of disease onset.[48,82] Published studies do not suggest that the long-term outcome of FSGS is influenced by cytotoxic drug therapy. The remission induced by such therapy in these patients is often shorter than that seen in patients with MCNS.[62,71]

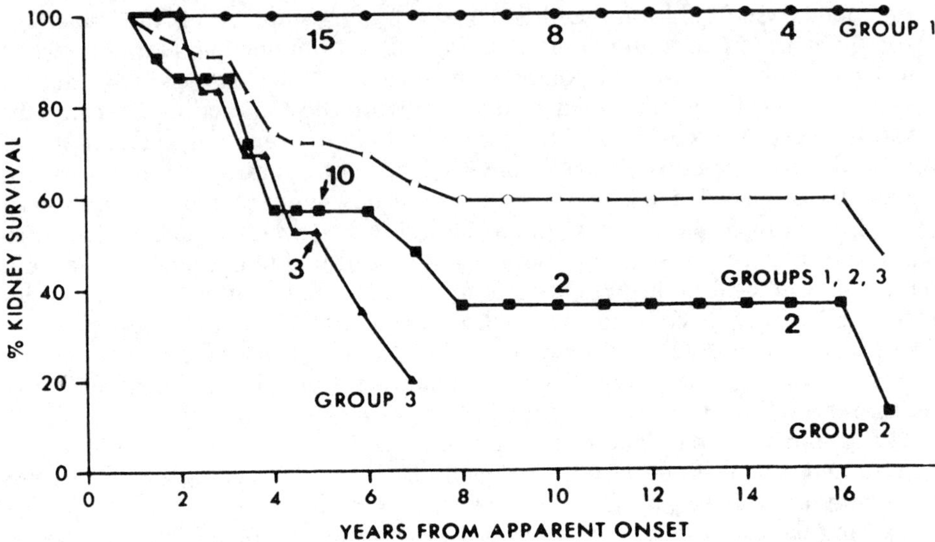

FIG. 7–9. Cumulative renal survival results of children with FSGS. Group 1 responded consistently to treatment with corticosteroids and/or cyclophosphamide and none developed end-stage renal disease. Group 2 patients did not demonstrate remission of nephrotic syndrome with treatment. Group 3 patients were corticosteroid-responsive initially but developed corticosteroid resistance subsequently in the course of their disease. Numbers within the figure represent the number of patients with surviving kidneys at 5, 10, and 15 years from the time of apparent onset of the disease. (From Arbus GS, Poucell S, Bacheyie GS, et al: Focal segmental glomerulosclerosis with idiopathic nephrotic syndrome: Three types of clinical response. *J Pediatr* 101:40, 1982. Reproduced with permission.)

NEWER IMMUNOREGULATORY DRUGS

Other forms of therapy aimed at altering the immune response in MCNS are currently under study. Levamisole, an antihelminthic drug with T-cell stimulating properties, has been employed in a few clinical trials in children with nephrotic syndrome. From the available data, it appears that levamisole may induce remission in both steroid-responsive and steroid-resistant MCNS.[83] Clear indications, dose, and duration of therapy with this drug have yet to be well defined. Cyclosporine, a novel immunosuppressive agent with T-cell suppressive properties, has also been used to treat nephrotic syndrome due to MCNS and FSGS.[84,85] Despite early enthusiasm, the role of cyclosporine in the treatment of nephrotic syndrome remains controversial and is being debated. When used in a conventional dose of 5 mg/kg/day, cyclosporine was not found to be beneficial in treatment of patients with corticosteroid-resistant nephrotic syndrome (FSGS and MCNS).[86] Because of its cost, potential for long-term side effects, and lack of clear superiority over conventional therapy, cyclosporine has not yet been accepted as an alternative form of therapy for nephrotic syndrome.

The use of "pulse" methylprednisolone therapy to significantly decrease proteinuria and improve the outlook for patients with FSGS has recently been suggested.[87] Data on long-term follow-up of patients treated with this form of therapy are still awaited. According to the authors of the study, methylprednisolone is administered intravenously on alternate days at a dose of 30 mg/kg for a total of six treatments. Intravenous methylprednisolone is continued once weekly for 2 months. Alternate-day administration of oral prednisone therapy (2 mg/kg/dose) is initiated after the first course of intravenous methyl prednisolone and is continued for six months.

ADJUNCTS IN THE TREATMENT OF NEPHROTIC SYNDROME

Diet and Activity. The dietary management of nephrotic syndrome is important but need not be complex. A "no added salt" diet is recommended in order to avoid further renal salt and water retention and aggravation of edema formation. Precooked, preserved, and packaged salty foods such as soups, pickles, and potato chips should be avoided. Fluid restriction may be prescribed, but is usually unnecessary in most children if salt intake is curtailed. In order to prevent protein malnutrition, an adequate intake of high-biologic-value protein (recommended daily allowance) should be provided. Patients' physical activity should not be restricted and mild edema should not serve as an excuse to stay home from school.

Albumin Infusion. Use of salt-poor albumin (25 percent solution contains 130 to 160 meq sodium ions per liter), usually combined with furosemide, is indicated in severely edematous patients, especially those with scrotal or labial swelling and ascites or pleural effusion. The usual dose of albumin is 1 g/kg/day infused over 2 to 4 h and followed immediately by 1 to 2 mg/kg of intravenous furosemide. Risks of albumin infusion therapy include hypertension, circulatory overload, and pulmonary edema due to the movement of the subcutaneous edema fluid into the intravascular compartment. Since most of the albumin administered intravenously is eliminated in urine in the subsequent 24 to 48 h, results of this therapy are usually transient.

Diuretics. Diuretic therapy is usually unnecessary in the treatment of MCNS. The only well-defined indication for diuretic use is in corticosteroid-nonresponsive nephrotic patients who are feeling significant discomfort due to severe fluid retention and edema. Edema in nephrotic syndrome tends to be resistant to mild diuretics in the usual doses, furosemide (1 to 2 mg/kg/dose) given once or twice daily is the diuretic of choice. The combination of hydrochlorothiazide and furosemide has been found to be more effective in nephrotic patients than furosemide alone.[88] Nonpharmacologic methods of diuresis may appeal to some patients. Standing in a water bath with the head out produces an effect similar to that produced by wearing a pressurized suit and helps to move fluid from the subcutaneous space into the intravascular compartment, thus inducing diuresis.[89] In order to decrease the risk of shock, thrombotic complications, and acute renal failure, overly vigorous diuresis should be avoided in nephrotic patients.

COMPLICATIONS OF NEPHROTIC SYNDROME

INFECTIONS

High morbidity and mortality of nephrotic patients in the pre-antibiotic era was primarily due to infection related complications. Serious infections were noted to occur in 56 percent of nephrotic children followed by Metcoff[90] between 1943 and 1956. Of these, cellulitis was the most common form of infection, followed closely by peritonitis and bacteremia. Despite a significant decrease in the incidence of infection in nephrotic children in the last forty years, infection continues to remain the primary cause of mortality in these patients.[91] In a recent study, peritonitis was reported to affect almost 17 percent of nephrotic children.[92] Multiple episodes of infection in the same patient are not unusual.

Infections in nephrotic patients are usually caused by *Streptococcus pneumoniae* but may also be due to gram-negative bacteria. Studies done at the Children's Medical Center in Boston between 1970 and 1980 documented the emergence of *Escherichia coli* as an important etiology of peritonitis (25 percent of cases) in nephrotic children.[93] Other studies have, however, failed to demonstrate any increasing incidence of gram negative infections in nephrotic patients.[92] In order to protect nephrotic children from pneumococcal infection, immunization with a vaccine containing pneumococcal polysaccharide antigen (Pneumovax) has been advocated and practiced for several years. However, serum titer of protective IgG antibody against *S. pneumoniae* has been shown to be low in immunized nephrotic patients.[94] The protective role of immunization with pneumococcal polysaccharide antigen has been questioned by these observations. Infections due to *S. pneumoniae* have been reported despite adequate immunization.[95]

Several factors are responsible for nephrotic patients' increased susceptibility to infection. Serum immunoglobulin concentration is abnormal in nephrotic syndrome. While serum IgM and IgE concentration is elevated, serum IgG concentration is decreased. Deficiency of IgG may lead to defective opsonization of bacteria in nephrotic patients.[95,96] Defective lytic activity of the monocyte-macrophage function has been noted in nephrotic syndrome and may contribute toward enhanced susceptibility to infection in these patients. On the other hand, polymorphonuclear functions have been shown to be normal in nephrotic patients.[97] Some components of the complement cascade are low (C1q, C2, B, I, C8, and C9), but others are normal or elevated.[98] The role played by the subnormal serum concentration of some complement components in increasing susceptibility to infection in nephrotic patients has not been well characterized.

THROMBOEMBOLIC COMPLICATIONS

Nephrotic syndrome is well known to be associated with an increased risk of vascular thrombosis. Renal vein thrombosis is especially common in these patients. The incidence of renal vein thrombosis in adult nephrotic patients has been variously reported to range from 5 to 54 percent, often occurring in patients with membranous glomerulonephritis.[98–101] It has been argued that

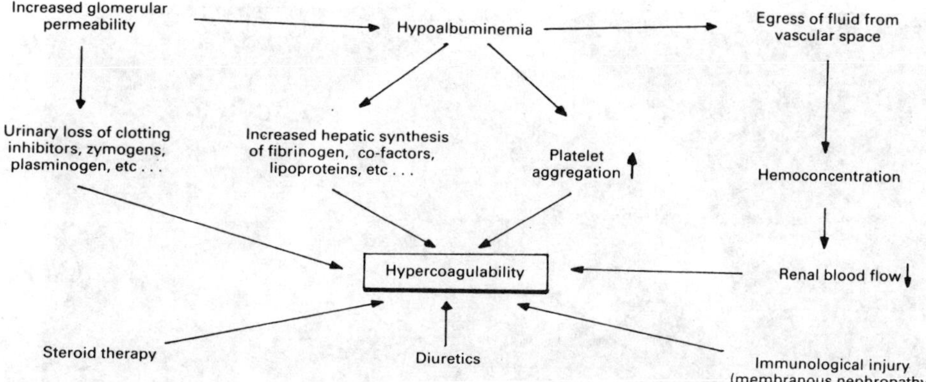

FIG. 7–10. **Schematic representation of pathogenetic factors leading to hypercoagulability and thromboembolic phenomenon in nephrotic syndrome. (From Llach F: Hypercoagulability, renal vein thrombosis and other thrombotic complications of nephrotic syndrome. *Kidney Int* 28:429, 1985. Reproduced with permission.)**

renal vein thrombosis may be the cause rather than the effect of nephrotic syndrome in these patients. Currently available evidence, however, suggests that—rather than being the etiology of membranous glomerulonephritis—renal vein thrombosis be considered a complication of the hypercoagulable state in this disease.[101] A precise incidence of thromboembolic complications in nephrotic syndrome in children is not known, but thrombosis in a variety of sites has been reported.[102,103]

Increased risk of thrombosis in nephrotic syndrome is multifactorial in origin (Fig. 7–10). Hyperfibrinogenemia resulting from enhanced hepatic synthesis of this clotting factor contributes significantly to the state of hypercoagulability in nephrotic patients. Abnormalities of several zymogens and cofactors involved in the process of clotting have also been described in nephrotic syndrome. While plasma concentration of factors II, V, VII, VIII, and X is elevated, concentration of factors IX, XI, and XII is generally low.[101,104] Decreased plasma concentration of naturally occurring inhibitors of coagulation, particularly antithrombin III, results from enhanced urinary losses in nephrotic syndrome and adds to the risk of spontaneous thrombosis in these patients.[105] Thrombocytosis is common in MCNS, but the role of platelets in enhancing the risk of thrombosis in these patients remains unresolved. Finally, hyperviscosity of the plasma resulting from hyperfibrinogenemia and volume depletion further increases the risk of thrombosis in nephrotic syndrome (Fig 7–11).[101]

GROWTH IN NEPHROTIC SYNDROME

Growth retardation has been recognized as a significant problem in nephrotic children, particularly in those who manifest a frequently relapsing course and have received prolonged corticosteroid therapy.[106] Although the exact mechanism of growth failure in children treated with corticosteroids is not fully known, interference with chondrocyte function has been proposed.[107] Recent

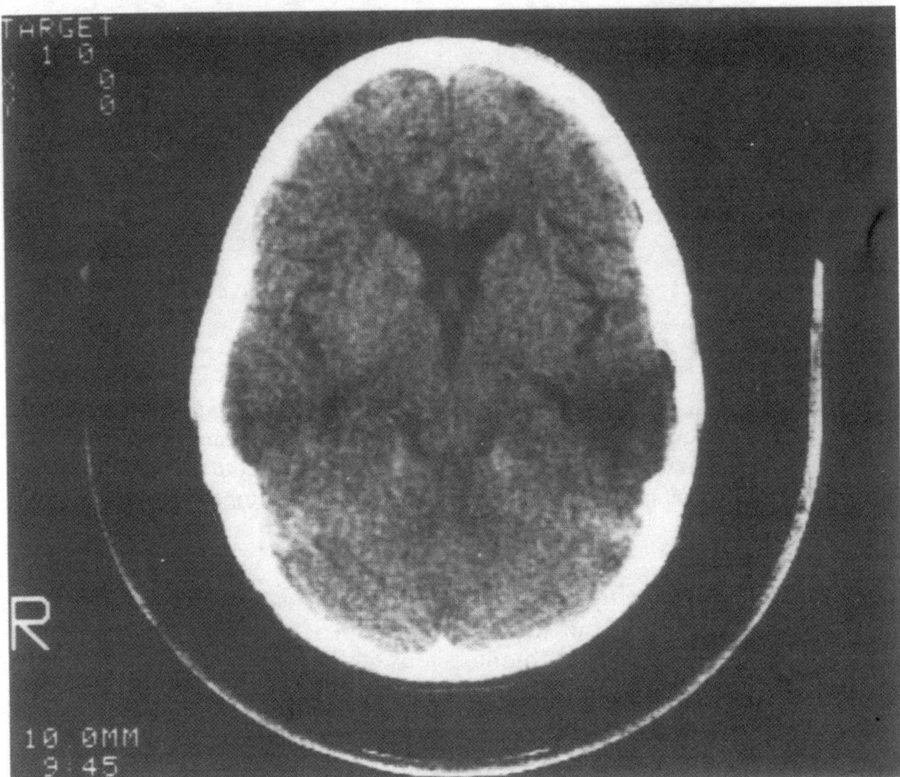

FIG. 7–11. An unenhanced computerized axial tomogram (CAT) of a child with nephrotic syndrome who developed intracerebral thrombosis and hemiplegia. A triangular area of increased density on the left parietal region reflects an area of infarction. (From Kher KK, Sweet M, Makker SP: Nephrotic syndrome in children. *Curr Probl Pediatr* 18:199, 1988. Reproduced with permission of Year Book Medical Publishers Inc., Chicago.)

studies have shown that corticosteroids may adversely affect somatomedin activity and produce an inhibitory effect on collagen metabolism, and thereby affect bone growth.[107a] Serum concentration of insulin like growth factors 1 and 2 (IGF 1 and 2) has also been reported to be low in children with active nephrotic syndrome, but the significance of these observations in relation to growth failure is not clear yet.[107b] Some studies have suggested that the ultimate height attained by nephrotic children treated with corticosteroids is not seriously affected, especially when they are treated with alternate-day corticosteroid therapy.[108,109] The effects of nephrotic syndrome and corticosteroid therapy on puberty are not well characterized. Growth failure and delayed onset of puberty has been reported in adolescent nephrotic boys in one study, despite use of low-dose alternate-day corticosteroid therapy.[110] The authors of this study have noted that the amplitude of growth hormone and gonadotrophin secretion was reduced in these patients and that these hormonal aberrations returned to normal after discontinuation of corticosteroids. These observation may implicate hypothalamic-pituitary dysfunction in growth retardation associated with the use of corticosteroids. Others have reported less growth suppression by using alternate day corticosteroid therapy.[111]

MANAGEMENT ISSUES

Q. How does nephrotic syndrome alter the pharmacokinetics of prednisone?

Prednisone requires hepatic conversion to prednisolone in order to be metabolically active. In plasma, glucocorticoids are transported bound with transcortin, albumin, and to lesser extent with α-1-acidglycoprotein; the pharmacologic actions of glucocorticoids are, however, determined by the plasma concentration of the free or unbound fraction. Abnormalities reported in the pharmacokinetics of prednisolone in nephrotic patients are as follows: (1) plasma-free prednisolone concentration bears an inverse relationship to plasma albumin concentration during relapse of nephrotic syndrome, and (2) clearance of both bound and unbound prednisolone is decreased.[112,113] The implications of these observations for the treatment of nephrotic patients, however, remain unclear. One interpretation can be that the dose of corticosteroids required by severely nephrotic patients may need to be lower (due to a greater availability of unbound prednisolone) than it would be for those with only mild disease.

Q. How should prednisone be administered to nephrotic patients?

ISKDC and other studies have recommended that prednisone be administered in several divided doses in the initial phase of nephrotic syndrome until remission of proteinuria is achieved. Warshaw and Hymes[114] have, however, recently reported that a single daily dose is as effective as multiple divided doses in inducing remission of nephrotic relapses. These authors have also questioned the need for using prednisone in the dose of 2 mg/kg/day in nephrotic syndrome, since they were able to achieve remission in 55 of 63 relapses by using a significantly lower dose (0.2 to 1.5 mg/kg/day).

Q. Is there any relationship between adrenal suppression caused by corticosteroids and the frequency of relapses?

Leisti et al.[115] have written several papers on this issue. These authors believe that adrenal suppression resulting from standard corticosteroid therapy in nephrotic children predisposes them to an increased frequency of early relapses (within 6 months of corticosteroid treatment). Increased risk of early relapse was, however, present only in patients in whom severe adrenocortical suppression was documented by a 2-h ACTH test; those with only moderate adrenocortical dysfunction were not shown to be at a greater risk of developing early relapses. Of interest is the fact that when replacement cortisol was provided to nephrotic children with documented severe adrenocortical dysfunction, the authors were unable to find any beneficial effect on the frequency of relapses. Therefore, despite the evidence that an 8-week treatment with prednisone suppresses normal adrenal response, the argument for its link to increased frequency of relapse in these patients is less than compelling.

Q. Does hyperlipidemia of nephrotic syndrome need to be treated?

A clear link between the lipid abnormalities in nephrotic syndrome and enhanced cardiovascular mortality has been difficult to establish, and the results of various studies in the published literature have been conflicting. As an example, while the incidence of ischemic heart disease was found to be high in the nephrotic patients reported by Berlyne and Mallick,[116] others were unable to find such an increased risk in adult nephrotic patients.[117] In one study, nephrotic patients (15 to 35 years of age) were shown to have a higher incidence of coronary atherosclerosis on necropsy than age-matched controls.[118] Cases of premature atherosclerosis have also been reported among children with nephrotic syndrome.[119]

Until recently, treatment of hyperlipidemia in nephrotic syndrome has received scant attention. Several papers reporting the effect of cholesterol-lowering agents in patients with nephrotic syndrome have been published in the last few years. The administration of lovastatin, an inhibitor of cholesterol synthesis, results in a decrease of total cholesterol, LDL cholesterol, VLDL cholesterol, and triglyceride concentration in nephrotic syndrome. On the other hand, HDL concentration has been reported to remain unchanged.[120,121] Apart from its effect of improving the lipid profile in nephrotic syndrome and possibly improving cardiovascular morbidity and mortality, treatment of hypercholesterolemia may also be beneficial in retarding the progression of renal disease in patients in whom nephrotic syndrome results from chronic glomerular diseases such as FSGS and other glomerulonephritides.[122] Lovastatin has not yet been approved for use in children.

Q. Should steroid-dependent or steroid-resistant patients with MCNS receive a second course of cytotoxic agents?

A minority of patients (10 to 15 percent) with MCNS will not experience prolonged remission of nephrotic syndrome after treatment with one course of chlorambucil or cyclophosphamide.[76,77] Although some physicians recommend a second course of cytotoxic agents for such patients, little information about the effects of such therapy in children is available in the published literature. Jones et al.[123] have recently reviewed their experience in treating 9 children with MCNS who received two courses of cytotoxic drugs. These children represented 15 percent of MCNS patients who had previously received cytotoxic therapy and 6 percent of the investigators' total MCNS population. Although no unusual side effects of a second course were apparent, gonadal toxicity was not evaluated. One female patient, however, later gave birth to a normal infant. Longer remissions of nephrotic syndrome were observed in children treated with a second course of cytotoxic agents. Of note is the finding that patients who were previously corticosteroid-resistant became responsive to it following such a therapy.

Q. What is the expected prognosis of nephrotic syndrome in a child who has frequent relapses?

Various studies of ISKDC have reported that 40 percent of steroid-responsive MCNS patients develop a frequently relapsing clinical course.[124]* On the basis

*Frequent relapses: A patient is considered to have frequent relapses if he or she has either two relapses in 6 months or four relapses in any 12-month period (ISKDC).

of single renal biopsy data, these investigators also concluded that 95 percent of the frequently relapsing patients had MCNS and were expected to have a favorable outcome.[69] Some studies have, however, reported a less benign outcome for frequently relapsing nephrotic patients. Tejani[125] performed repeat biopsies in 33 children with early frequently relapsing nephrotic syndrome in whom first biopsies had shown MCNS. Of these, 45 percent had developed FSGS, while 27 percent each had minimal change and mesangial IgM deposition. Transition of MCNS to FSGS has also been reported by other workers.[69,70,71] One of the renal biopsy features of children with apparent MCNS who evolve into FSGS/FGS has been reported to be glomerular hypertrophy.[126]

What We Do Not Know about Nephrotic Syndrome: A Commentary

H. William Schnaper

Many questions remain in our understanding of childhood nephrotic syndrome. These relate to etiology, pathogenesis, and treatment of nephrotic syndrome and are of clinical significance, since they affect our approach to the diagnosis and treatment of children with this disorder.

What is the cause of MCNS, the most common form of nephrotic syndrome in childhood? MCNS is believed to be an immunologically mediated disorder. The effectiveness of corticosteroids and alkylating agents in inducing remission of the nephrotic state—as well as altered immune responsiveness during relapse—support an immune etiology. Although numerous abnormalities have been described in MCNS, the primary immune defect remains unknown. The relationship of the immune abnormalities to the pathogenesis of proteinuria in MCNS is also not fully understood. The fact that proteinuria in MCNS occurs without any definable glomerular inflammation is both critical and baffling. Alterations in both the size selectivity and electrostatic charge of the glomerular filtration barrier have been implicated in the pathogenesis of proteinuria. In MCNS, the absence of disruption of the glomerular filter has suggested that loss of charge selectivity is the primary pathogenetic event. However, recent observations have seriously questioned the hypothesis. Obviously, more work needs to be done in this area.

Do corticosteroids play a role in the development of some histopathologic variants of MCNS? Corticosteroids are known to retard clearance of large immune complexes from the mesangium. Since most pediatric patients are biopsied after a trial of corticosteroids, it is unclear whether mesangial IgM deposition represents the end result of prior treatment with this drug or a different process from that involved in uncomplicated MCNS.

Little has changed in the therapy of MCNS in the past 15 to 20 years. Cyclosporine has been advocated as a new, effective treatment, but its toxicity and cost, as well as the fact that it is most effective in patients who respond to corticosteroids, have limited its use. Treatment of steroid-dependent and steroid-resistant nephrotic patients has received relatively little coverage in the published literature. Extended corticosteroid and diuretic therapy in such patients requires constant observation to avoid potential toxic effects of therapy. Every pediatric nephrologist has encountered one or two such patients who have continued problems—with severe edema, recurrent peritonitis, and potential for thrombosis. This remains a major challenge for the physician. The management of these cases involves balancing the need to keep intravascular fluid volume within safe limits against the desire to minimize edema. Aggressive diuresis in severely nephrotic patients may be unwise.

Finally, much recent attention has been centered on the hyperlipidemia of nephrosis. Although the primary cause of this phenomenon is not known, pharmacologic intervention has become possible for this problem. It is both expensive and complicated, so that its use is not warranted in steroid-responsive patients. However, the potential for long-range cardiovascular complications and recent evidence that hyperlipidemia may accelerate the development of glomerulosclerosis indicate that treatment of lipid abnormalities in the steroid-resistant patient, especially one with FSGS, should be seriously considered.

REFERENCES

1. Rothenberg MB, Heymann W: The incidence of nephrotic syndrome in children. *Pediatrics* 19:446, 1957.
2. Schlesinger ER, Sultz MA, Mosher WE, et al: The nephrotic syndrome: Its incidence and implications for the community. *Am J Dis Child* 116:623, 1968.
3. Arneil GC: 164 children with nephrotic syndrome. *Lancet* 2:1103, 1961.
4. International Study of Kidney Disease in Children. Nephrotic syndrome in children: Prediction of histopathology from clinical and laboratory characteristics at time of diagnosis. *Kidney Int* 13:159, 1978.
5. White RHR, Glasgow EF, Mills RJ: Clinicopathologic study of nephrotic syndrome in children. *Lancet* 1:353, 1970.
6. Miltenyi M: Urinary protein excretion in healthy children. *Clin Nephrol* 12:216, 1979.
7. Brenner BM, Hostetter TH, Humes HD: Molecular basis of proteinuria of glomerular origin. *N Engl J Med* 298:826, 1978.
8. Rennke HG, Patel Y, Venkatachalam MA: Glomerular filtration of proteins, clearance of anionic, neutral and cationic horseradish peroxide in the rat. *Kidney Int* 13:278, 1978.
9. Hunsicker LG, Shearer TP, Shaffer SJ: Acute reversible proteinuria induced by infusion of polycationic hexadimethrine. *Kidney Int* 20:7, 1981.
10. Bridges CR, Myers BD, Brenner BM, et al: Glomerular charge alterations in human minimal change nephropathy. *Kidney Int* 22:677, 1982.
11. Myers BD, Okarma TB, Friedman S, et al: Mechanisms of proteinuria in human glomerulonephritis. *J Clin Invest* 70:732, 1982.

12. Bertolatus JA, Abuyousef M, Hunsiker LG: Glomerular seiving of high molecular weight proteins in proteinuric rats. *Kidney Int* 31:1257, 1987.
13. Kaysen GA, Gambertoglio J, Felts J, et al: Albumin synthesis, albuminuria and hyperlipidemia in nephrotic patients. *Kidney Int* 31:1368, 1987.
14. Appel GB, Blum CB, Chien S, et al: The hyperlipidemia of nephrotic syndrome: Relation to plasma albumin concentration, oncotic pressure and viscosity. *N Engl J Med* 312:1544, 1985.
15. Kaysen GA: Albumin metabolism in nephrotic syndrome: The effect of dietary protein intake. *Am J Kid Dis* 12:461, 1988.
15a. Sellers AL, Katz J, Bonorris G, et al: Determination of extravascular albumin in the rat. J Lab Clin Med 68:177, 1966.
15b. Spector WG: The reabsorption of labelled protein by the normal and nephrotic rat kidney. *J Pathol Bacteriol* 68:187, 1954.
15c. Kaysen GA, Kirkpatrick WG, Couser WG: Albumin homeostasis in the nephrotic rats: Nutritional considerations. *Am J Physiol* 247:F192, 1984.
16. Kaysen GA, Gambertoglio J, Jiminez J, et al: Effect of dietary protein intake on albumin synthesis in nephrotic patients. *Kidney Int* 29:572, 1986.
17. Schrier RW: Pathogenesis of sodium and water retention in high-output and low-output cardiac failure, nephrotic syndrome, cirrhosis and pregnancy. Part 1. *N Engl J Med* 319:1065, 1988.
18. Dorhout Mees EJ, Roos JC, et al: Observations on edema formation in nephrotic syndrome in the adults with minimal change lesion. *Am J Med* 67:378, 1979.
19. Dorhout Mees EJ, Geers AB, et al: Blood volume and sodium retention in the nephrotic syndrome: A controversial pathophysiologic concept. *Nephron* 36:201, 1984.
20. Brown EA, Sagnella GA, Jones BE: Evidence that some mechanism other than the renin system causes sodium retention in nephrotic syndrome. *Lancet* 2:1237, 1982.
21. Ichikawa I, Rennke HG, Hoyer JR, et al: Role for intra renal mechanism in the impaired salt excretion of experimental nephrotic syndrome. *J Clin Invest* 71:91, 1983.
22. Usberti M, Federico S, Meccareiello S, et al: Role of plasma vasopressin in impairment of water excretion in nephrotic syndrome. *Kidney Int* 25:422, 1984.
23. Tulassay T, Rascher W, Lang RE, et al: Atrial natriuretic peptide and other vasoactive hormones in nephrotic syndrome. *Kidney Int* 31:1391, 1987.
24. Kaysen GA, Myers BD, Couser WG, et al: Biology of disease: Mechanisms and consequences of proteinuria. *Lab Invest* 54:479, 1986.
25. Querfeld U, Gnasso A, Haberbosch W, et al: Lipoprotein profiles at different stages of nephrotic syndrome. *Eur J Pediatr* 147:233, 1988.
26. Joven J, Villabona C, Vilella E, et al: Abnormalities of lipoprotein metabolism in patients with nephrotic syndrome. *N Engl J Med* 323:579, 1990.
27. Hamburger J: Discussion on glomerular structure in Bright's disease, in Wolstenholme GEN, Cameron MP (eds): *Ciba Foundation Symposium on Renal Biopsy.* London, Churchill Livingstone, 1961, p 139.
28. Macdonald NE, Wolfish N, McLaine P, et al: Role of respiratory viruses in exacerbation of primary nephrotic syndrome. *J Pediatr* 108:378, 1986.
29. Springate JE, Coyne JF, Karp MP, et al: Acute renal failure in minimal change nephrotic syndrome. *Pediatrics* 80:946, 1987.
30. Pardo V, Riesgo I, Zilleruello G, et al: The clinical significance of mesangial IgM deposits and mesangial hypercellularity in minimal change nephrotic syndrome. *Am J Kid Dis* 3:264, 1984.
31. Habib R, Girardin E, Gagnadou MF, et al: Immunopathologic findings in idiopathic

nephrosis: Clinical significance of glomerular "immune deposits." *Pediatr Nephrol* 2:402, 1988.

32. Hirszel P, Yamase HT, Carney R, et al: Mesangial proliferative glomerulonephritis with IgM deposits: Clinicopathologic analysis and evidence for morphologic transition. *Nephron* 38:100, 1984.
33. Norio R: The nephrotic syndrome and heredity. *Hum Hered* 19:11, 1970.
34. Kobayashi Y, Meichen X, Hiki Y, et al: Association of HLA-DRw8 and DQw3 with minimal change nephrotic syndrome in Japanese adults. *Kidney Int.* 28:193, 1985.

34a. Lagueruela CC, Buettner TL, Cole BR, et al: HLA extended haplotypes in steroid-responsive nephrotic syndrome of childhood. *Kidney Int* 38:145, 1990.

35. McEnery PT, Welch TR: Major histocompatibility complex antigens in steroid-responsive nephrotic syndrome. *Pediatr Nephrol* 3:33, 1989.
36. Shalhoub RJ: Pathogenesis of lipoid nephrosis: A disorder of T cell function. *Lancet* 2:556, 1974.
37. Moorthy AV, Zimmerman SW, Burkholdre PM: Nephrotic syndrome in Hodgkin's disease: Evidence for pathogenesis alternative to immune complex deposition. *Am J Med* 61:471, 1976.
38. Janeway CA, Mokk GH, Armstrong SH, et al: Diuresis in children with nephrosis: Comparison of response to normal human serum albumin and to infection, particularly measles. *Trans Assoc Am Physicians* 61:108, 1948.
39. Maruyama K, Tomizawa S, Shimabukuru N, et al: Effect of supernatants derived from T lymphocyte culture in minimal change nephrotic syndrome on rat kidney capillaries. Nephron 51:73, 1989.
40. Yoshizawa N, Kusumi Y, Matsumoto K, et al: Studies of a glomerular permeability factor in patients with minimal-change nephrotic syndrome. *Nephron* 51:370, 1989.
41. Lagrue G, Xheneumont S, Branellec A, et al: Vascular permeability factor elaborated from lymphocytes: Demonstration in patients with nephrotic syndrome. *Biomedicine* 23:37, 1975.
42. Boulton-Jones JM, Tulloch I, Dore B, et al: Changes in glomerular capillary wall induced by lymphocyte products and serum of nephrotic patients. *Clin Nephrol* 20:72, 1983.
43. Levinsky RJ, Malleson PN, Barrat JM: Circulating immune complexes in steroid responsive nephrotic syndrome. *N Engl J Med* 298:126, 1978.
44. Abress CK, Hall CL, Border WA, et al: Circulating immune complexes in adults with nephrotic syndrome. *Kidney Int* 17:545, 1980.
45. Groshong T, Mendelson L, Mendoza S, et al: Serum IgE in patients with minimal change nephrotic syndrome. *J Pediatr* 83:767, 1973.
46. Meadow SR, Sarsfield JK, Scott DG, et al: Steroid responsive nephrotic syndrome and allergy. *Arch Dis Child* 56:517, 1981.
47. Habib R, Kleinknecht C: The primary nephrotic syndrome of children: Classification and clinicopathologic study of 406 children, in Sommers SC (ed): *Pathology Annual.* New York, New York, Appleton-Century-Crofts, 1971, p 17.
48. South West Pediatric Nephrology Study Group: Focal segmental glomerulosclerosis in children with idiopathic nephrotic syndrome. *Kidney Int* 27:442, 1985.
49. Yoshikawa N, Ito H, Akamatsu R, et al: Focal segmental glomerulosclerosis with and without nephrotic syndrome in children. *J Pediatr* 109:65, 1986.
50. McVicar M, Exeni R, Susin M: Nephrotic syndrome and multiple tubular defects in children: An early sign of focal segmental glomerulosclerosis. *J Pediatr* 97:918, 1980.

51. Mongeau JG, Corneille L, Robitaille P, et al: Primary nephrosis in children associated with focal glomerulosclerosis: Is long-term prognosis that severe? *Kindey Int* 20:743, 1981.
52. Glicklich D, Hastell L, Senitzer D, et al: Possible genetic predisposition to focal segmental glomerulosclerosis. *Am J Kid Dis* 12:26, 1988.
53. Sigel JE, Sibley RK, Fryd DS, et al: Recurrence of focal segmental glomerulosclerosis in children following renal transplantation. *Kidney Int* 30:S-44, 1986.
54. Cameron JS, Senguttvan P, Hartley B, et al: Focal segmental glomerulosclerosis in fifty-nine renal allografts from a single center: Analysis of risk factors for recurrence. *Transplant Proc* 21:2117, 1989.
55. Zimmerman SW, Mann S: Increased urinary protein excretion in the rat produced by serum from a patient with recurrent focal glomerulosclerosis. *Clin Nephrol* 22:32, 1984.
56. Kendall-Smith IM, Pullon DHH, Tomlinson BE: Congenital nephrotic syndrome in Maori siblings. *New Zealand Med J* 68:156, 1968.
57. Huttunen N: Congenital nephrotic syndrome of Finnish type. *Arch Dis Child* 51:344, 1976.
58. Holmberg C, Jalanko H, Koskimies O, et al: Renal transplantation in children with congenital nephrotic syndrome of Finnish type. *Transplant Proc* 22:158, 1990.
59. International Study of Kidney Disease in Children: Prospective controlled trial of cyclophosphamide therapy in children with nephrotic syndrome. *Lancet* 2:423, 1974.
60. Houser MT, Jahn MF, Kobayashi A, et al: Assessment of urinary protein in adolescent: Effect of body position and exercise. *J Pediatr* 109:556, 1986.
60a. Houser MT: Unpublished data. Personal communication. 1991.
61. International Study of Kidney Disease for Children: The primary nephrotic syndrome in children: Identification of patients with minimal change nephrotic syndrome from initial response to prednisone. *J Pediatr* 98:561, 1981.
62. Schulman SL, Kaiser BA, Polinsky MS, et al: Predicting the response to cytotoxic therapy for childhood nephrotic syndrome: Superiority of response to corticosteroid therapy over histopathologic patterns. *J Pediatr* 113:996, 1988.
63. Arbeitsgemeinschaft für Pädiatrische Nephrologie: Alternate-day prednisone is more effective than intermittent prednisone in frequenty relapsing nephrotic syndrome. *Eur J Pediatr* 135:229, 1981.
64. Barness LA, Moll GH, Janeway CA: Nephrotic syndrome: I. Natural history of the disease. *Pediatrics* 5:486, 1950.
65. Wingen AM, Muller-Wifel DE, Scharer K: Spontaneous remissions in frequently relapsing and steroid dependent idiopathic nephrotic syndrome. *Clin Nephrol* 23:35, 1985.
66. Heymann W, Hunter JLP: Importance of early treatment of nephrotic syndrome. *J Am Med Assoc* 175:563, 1961.
67. Makker SP, Heymann W: The idiopathic nephrotic syndrome: A clinical reevaluation of 148 cases. *Am J Dis Child* 127:830, 1981.
68. Koskimies O, Vilski J, Rapola J, et al: Long-term outcome of primary nephrotic syndrome. *Arch Dis Child* 57:544, 1982.
69. Trachtman M, Carrol F, Phadke, et al: Paucity of minimal-change lesion in children with early frequently relapsing steroid-responsive nephrotic syndrome. *Am J Nephrol* 7:13, 1987.
70. Srivastava RN, Agarwal RK, Moudgil A, et al: Late resistance to corticosteroids in nephrotic syndrome. *J Pediatr* 107:66, 1985.

71. Siegel NJ, Gaudio KM, Krassner LS, et al: Steroid-dependent nephrotic syndrome: Histopathology and relapses after cyclophosphamide treatment. *Kidney Int* 19:454, 1981.
72. International Study of Kidney Disease in Children: Controlled trial of azathioprine in children with nephrotic syndrome. *Lancet* 2:959, 1976.
73. Arbeitsgemeinscharft für Pädiatrische Nephrologie: Cyclophosphamide treatment of steroid dependent nephrotic syndrome: Comparison of eight week course with 12 week course. *Arch Dis Child* 62:1102, 1987.
74. Guesry P, Lenoir G, Broyer M: Gonadal effect of chlorambucil given to prepubertal and pubertal boys for nephrotic syndrome. *J Pediatr* 92:299, 1978.
75. Kashtan C, Melvin T, Kim Y: Long-term follow-up of patients with steroid-dependent, minimal change nephrotic syndrome. *Clin Nephrol* 29:79, 1988.
76. Williams SA, Makker SP, Ingelfinfer JR, et al: Long-term evaluation of chlorambucil plus prednisone in the idiopathic nephrotic syndrome of childhood. *N Engl J Med* 302:929, 1980.
77. Berns JS, Gaudio KM, Krassner LS, et al: Steroid-responsive nephrotic syndrome of childhood: A long-term study of clinical course, histopathology, efficacy of cyclophosphamide therapy, and effect on growth. *Am J Kid Dis* 9:108, 1987.
78. Lentz RD, Berstein J, Steffes MW, et al: Postpubertal evaluation of gonadal function following cyclophosphamide therapy before and during puberty. *J Pediatr* 91:385, 1977.
79. Callis L, Nieto J, Vila A, et al: Chlorambucil treatment in minimal lesion nephrotic syndrome: A reappraisal of its gonadal toxicity. *J Pediatr* 97:653, 1980.
80. Pennisi AJ, Grushkin AM, Lieberman E: Gonadal function in children with nephrosis treated with cyclophosphamide. *Am J Dis Child* 129:315, 1975.
81. Arbus, GS, Poucell S, Bachyie GS, et al: Focal segmental glomerulosclerosis with idiopathic nephrotic syndrome: Three types of clinical responses. *J Pediatr* 101:40, 1982.
82. Tejani A, Nicastri AD, Sen D, et al: Long-term evaluation of children with nephrotic syndrome and focal segmental glomerulosclerosis. *Nephron* 35:225, 1983.
83. Mongeau JG, Robitaille PO, Roy F: Clinical efficacy of levamisol in the treatment of primary nephrosis in children. *Pediatr Nephrol* 2:398, 1988.
84. Tejani A, Butt KM, Trachtman H, et al: Cyclosporine induced remission of relapsing nephrotic syndrome in children. *Kidney Int* 33:729, 1988.
85. Brodehl J, Hoyer PF, Oemar BS, et al: Cyclosporine treatment of nephrotic syndrome in children. *Transplant Proc* 20:269, 1988.
86. Garin EH, Orak JK, Hiott KL, et al: Cyclosporine therapy for steroid resistant nephrotic syndrome: A controlled study. *Am J Dis Child* 142:985, 1988.
87. Griswold WR, Tune BM, Reznik VM, et al: Treatment of prednisone-resistant nephrotic syndrome and focal glomerulosclerosis with intravenous methylprednisolone and oral alkylating agents. *Nephron* 46:73, 1987.
88. Nakahama H, Otita Y, Yamazaki M, et al: Pharmacokinetics and pharmacodynamic interactions between furosemide and hydrochlorothiazide in nephrotic patients. *Nephron* 49:223, 1988.
89. Rascher W, Tulassy T, Seyberth HW, et al: Diuretic and hormonal responses to head-out immersion in nephrotic syndrome. *J Pediatr* 104:69, 1986.
90. Metcoff J (ed): *Proceedings of the Eighth Annual Conference on the Nephrotic Syndrome.* New York, National Nephrosis Foundation Inc, 1957, p 152.
91. International Study of Kidney Disease in Children: Minimal change nephrotic

syndrome in children: Deaths during the first 5–15 years' observations. *Pediatrics* 73:497, 1984.

92. Gorensek MJ, Lebel MH, Nelson JD: Peritonitis with nephrotic syndrome. *Pediatrics* 81:849, 1988.
93. Kernsky AM, Ingelfinger JR, Grupe WE: Peritonitis in nephrotic syndrome. *Am J Dis Child* 136:732, 1987.
94. Garin EH, Barrett DJ: Pneumococcal polysaccharide immunization in patients with active nephrotic syndrome. *Nephron* 50:383, 1988.
95. Moore DH, Shackelford PG, Robson AM, et al: Recurrent pneumococcal sepsis and defective opsonization after pneumococcal capsular polysaccharide vaccination in a child with nephrotic syndrome. *J Pediatr* 96:882, 1980.
96. Chan MK, Chan KW, Jones B: Immunoglobulins (IgG, IgA, IgM, IgE) and complement components (C_3,C_4) in nephrotic syndrome due to minimal change and other forms of glomerulonephritis, a clue for steroid therapy? *Nephron* 47:125, 1987.
97. Estevez ME, Voyern LE, Craviotto RJ, et al: Dysfunction of monocyte-macrophage system in the idiopathic minimal change nephrotic syndrome. *Acta Paediatr Scand* 78:87, 1989.
98. Strife FC, Jackson EC, Forristal J, et al: Effect of nephrotic syndrome on the concentration of serum complement components. *Am J Kid Dis* 8:37, 1986.
99. Bennet WM: Renal vein thrombosis and nephrotic syndrome. *Ann Intern Med* 83:577, 1975.
100. Wagoner RD, Stanson AW, Holly KE, et al: Renal vein thrombosis in idiopathic membranous glomerulopathy and nephrotic syndrome. *Kidney Int* 23:368, 1983.
101. Llach F: Hypercoagulability, renal vein thrombosis and other thrombotic complications of nephrotic syndrome. *Kidney Int* 28:429, 1985.
102. Alkjaersig N, Fletcher AP, Narayan M, et al: Course and resolution of coagulopathy in nephrotic children. *Kidney Int* 31:772, 1987.
103. Cameron JS, Ogg CS, Ellis FG, et al: Femoral artery thrombosis in nephrotic syndrome. *Arch Dis Child* 46:216, 1971.
104. Thomson C, Forbes CD, Prentice CRM, et al: Changes in blood coagulation and fibrinolysis in nephrotic syndrome. *Q J Med* 43:399, 1974.
105. Viziri ND, Paule P, Toohey J, et al: Acquired deficiency and urinary excretion of antithrombin III in nephrotic syndrome. *Arch Intern Med* 144:1802, 1984.
106. Lam CN, Arneil GC: Long-term dwarfing effect of corticosteroid treatment for childhood nephrosis. *Arch Dis Child* 43:589, 1968.
107. Preece MA: The effect of administered corticosteroids on growth of children. *Postgrad Med J* 52:625, 1967.

107a. Hyams JS, Carey DE: Corticosteroids and growth. *J Pediatr* 113:249, 1988.

107b. Garin EH, Grant MD, Silverstein JH: Insulinlike growth factors in patients with active nephrotic syndrome. *Am J Dis Child* 143:865, 1989.

108. Foote KD, Brocklebank JT, Meadow SR: Height attainment in children with steroid responsive nephrotic syndrome. *Lancet* 2:917, 1985.
109. Trompeter RS, Lloyd BW, Hicks J, et al: Long-term outcome for children with minimal change nephrotic syndrome. *Lancet* 1:368, 1985.
110. Reese L, Greene SA, Adlard P, et al: Growth and endocrine function in steroid sensitive nephrotic syndrome. *Arch Dis Child* 63:484, 1988.
111. Polito C, Oporoto R, Totino SF, et al: Normal growth of nephrotic children during long-term alternate-day prednisone therapy. *Acta Paediatr Scand* 75:245, 1986.
112. Gatti G, Perucca E, Frigo GM: Pharmacokinetics of prednisone and its metabolite

prednisolone in children with nephrotic syndrome during active phase and in remission. *Br J Clin Pharmacol* 17:423, 1984.

113. Miller PFW, Bowmer CJ, Wheeldon J, et al: Pharmacokinetics of prednisolone in children with nephrosis. *Arch Dis Child* 65:196, 1990.
114. Warshaw BL, Hymes LC: Daily single-dose and daily reduced-dose prednisone therapy for children with nephrotic syndrome. *Pediatrics* 83:694, 1989.
115. Leisti S, Koskimies O: Risk of relapse in steroid sensitive nephrotic syndrome: Effect of stage of post-prednisone adrenocortical suppression. *J Pediatr* 103:553, 1983.
116. Berlyne MG, Mallick NP: Ischemic heart-disease as a complication of nephrotic syndrome. *Lancet* 2:399, 1969.
117. Wass VJ, Jarret RJ, Chilvers C, et al: Does nephrotic syndrome increase the risk of cardiovascular disease? *Lancet* 2:664, 1979.
118. Curry RC, Robers WC: Status of the coronary arteries in the nephrotic syndrome: Analysis of 20 necropsy patients aged 15–35 years to determine if coronary atherosclerosis is accelerated. *Am J Med* 63:183, 1977.
119. Kallen RJ, Brynes RK, Aronson AJ, et al: Premature coronary atherosclerosis in a 5-year-old with corticosteroid-refractory nephrotic syndrome. *Am J Dis Child* 131:976, 1977.
120. Kasiske BL, Velosa JA, Halstenson CE, et al: The effect of lovastatin in hyperlipidemic patients with nephrotic syndrome. *Am J Kid Dis* 15:8, 1990.
121. Harris KPG, Purkerson ML, Yates J, et al: Lovastatin ameliorates the development of glomerulosclerosis in experimental nephrotic syndrome. *Am J Kid Dis* 15:16, 1990.
122. Diamond JR, Karnovsky MJ: Exacerbation of chronic aminonucleoside nephrosis by dietary cholesterol supplementation. *Kidney Int* 32:671, 1987.
123. Jones DP, Stapleton B, Roy S, et al: Beneficial effect of second courses of cytotoxic therapy in children with minimal change nephrotic syndrome. *Pediatr Nephrol* 2:291, 1988.
124. Barnett HL: The natural and treatment history of glomerular disease in children: What can we learn from international cooperative studies? *A report of the International Study of Kidney Disease in Children, in Proceedings of the 6th International Congress of Nephrology.* S Karger, Basel, 1976, p 470.
125. Tejani A: Morphologic transition in minimal change nephrotic syndrome. *Nephron* 39:157, 1985.
126. Fogo A, Hawkins EP, Berry PL, et al: Glomerular hypertrophy in minimal change disease predicts subsequent progression to focal glomerulosclerosis. *Kidney Int* 38:115, 1990.

8

GLOMERULAR DISEASES

Sudesh P. Makker

Glomerular diseases are the most common cause of end-stage renal failure in humans and are responsible for significant rates of morbidity in both children and adults. Most glomerular diseases are chronic in nature and of unknown etiology; however, a majority of these appear to be immunologically mediated. In addition to etiology, the classification of glomerular diseases involves consideration of histologic, immunohistologic, and electron microscopy findings observed in the renal biopsy. In order to grasp the morphologic classification of glomerulonephritis, it is essential to have an understanding of the normal structure of the glomerulus and the terms used to describe the morphology of the diseased glomerulus.

GLOMERULAR STRUCTURE

LIGHT MICROSCOPY

The normal glomerulus is a network of branching capillary vessels interfaced between the afferent and the efferent arterioles (Fig. 8–1). The capillaries are hung around a supporting tissue called *mesangium,* which consists of extracellular tissue (mesangial matrix) and mesangial cells. When sections of renal tissue 4 to 8 μm thick are studied by routine light microscopy, the open capillary loops, mesangial matrix, and mesangial cells can easily be identified (Fig. 8–2). Four types of cells making up the glomerular complex are *mesangial, endothelial, visceral epithelial,* and *parietal epithelial* cells. The parietal epithelial cells lining the Bowman's capsule can easily be identified and the visceral epithelial cells outlining the capillary loops are also not difficult to find, but differentiating between the mesangial and endothelial cells is not always easy. The mesangium (matrix and cells) is located in the central part of the tuft.

IMMUNOFLUORESCENCE MICROSCOPY

When frozen sections (4 to 8 μm) of renal biopsy tissue are stained with fluorescein-labeled antibodies that are specifically directed against immunoglobu-

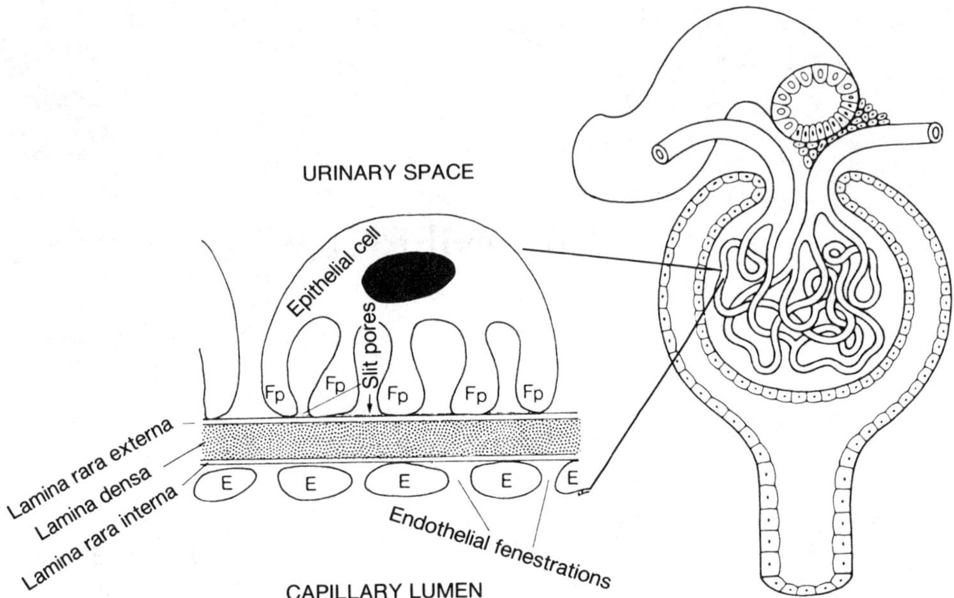

FIG. 8–1. A diagrammatic representation of the glomerulus and a cut section of the glomerular capillary loop.

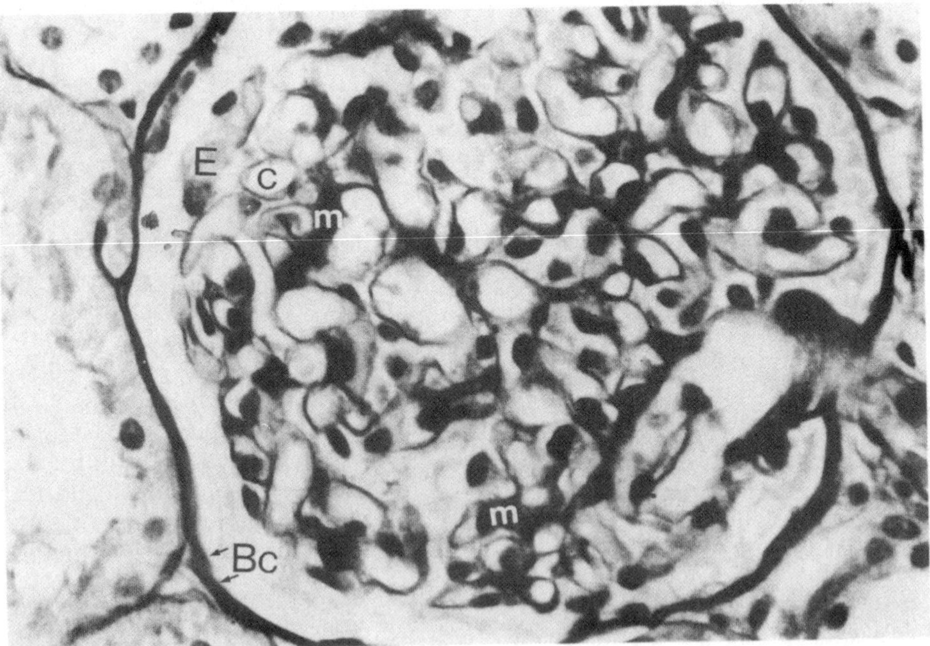

FIG. 8–2. Light microscopic picture of a normal glomerulus showing capillary loops (C), mesangial cells (m), visceral epithelial cells (E), and Bowman capsule (Bc).

lins (anti-IgG, IgA, IgM) and complement components (anti-C1q, C3, C4, C5b-9, etc.) and the sections are then examined under the ultraviolet light of a fluorescence microscope, the existence and location (mesangial versus capillary loop) of the endogenously deposited antibodies and complement in the diseased glomerulus can be determined. Normal glomerulus is devoid of any immune deposits. In disease states, the fluorescent reactants in the glomerulus may appear granular in nature in various locations such as mesangium (as in IgA nephropathy) (Fig. 8–3) or along the capillary loop (as in membranous glomerulonephropathy, Fig. 8–4) or they may appear as smooth linear staining (Fig. 8–5) outlining the glomerular capillary wall, as in Goodpasture syndrome.

Immunofluorescence technique demonstrates the existence of antibodies and/or complement in the diseased glomerulus, and these findings are accepted as an evidence for immune mediation of the glomerular disease. Linear immunofluorescence along the glomerular capillary wall indicates that the immune reactants (IgG, complement, etc.) have bound to endogenous structural antigens of the glomerulus, as in Goodpasture syndrome. On the other hand, granular immunofluorescence in the glomeruli denotes deposition of immune complexes. These immune complexes can result either from entrapment of circulating immune complexes in the glomeruli or from the binding of an anti-

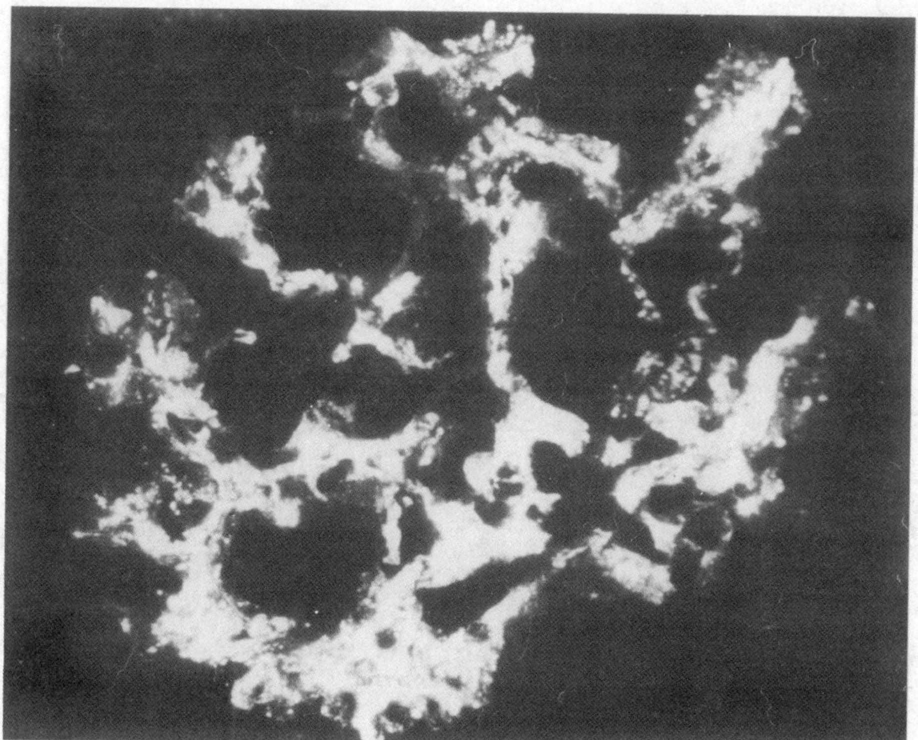

FIG. 8–3. Granular immune deposits in the mesangial region in a patient with IgA nephropathy.

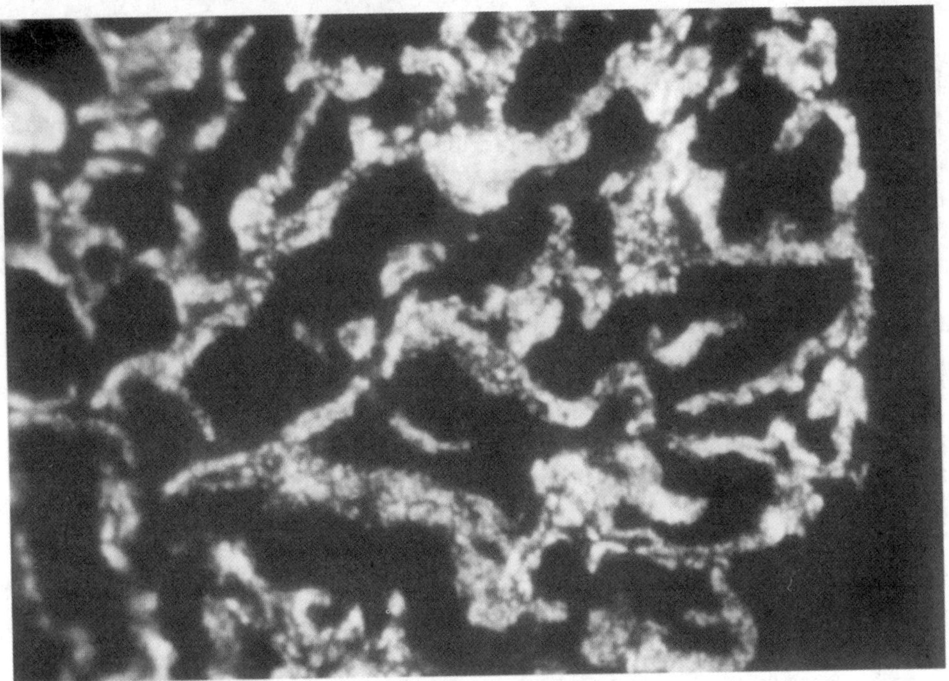

FIG. 8–4. Granular immune deposits along the capillary loop in membranous glomerulonephropathy (IgG).

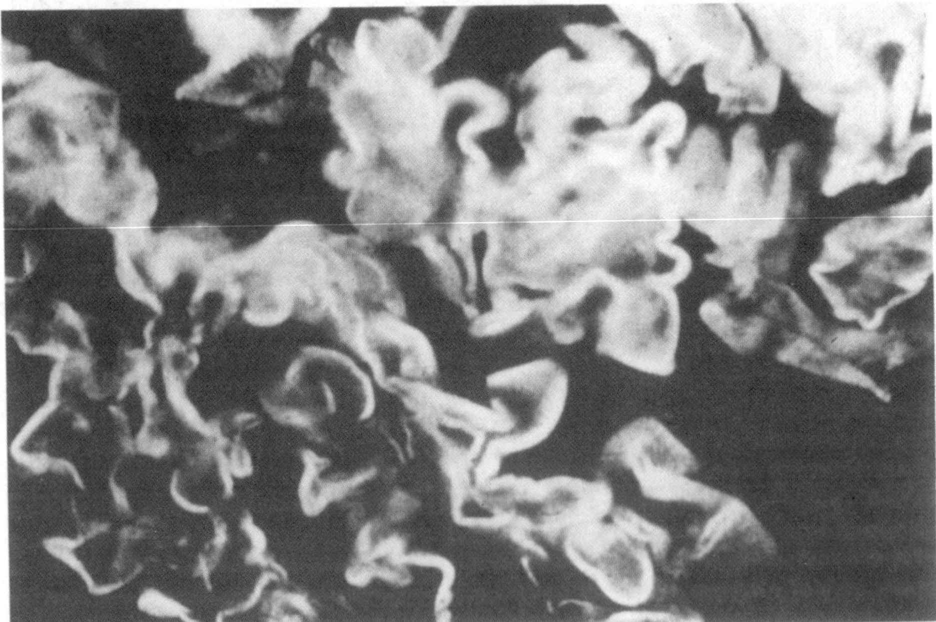

FIG. 8–5. Goodpasture syndrome, immunofluorescence microscopy demonstrating linear immune deposits along the capillary loop (IgG). (Courtesy of Dr. E. J. Ruley, Children's Hospital National Medical Center, Washington, D.C.)

body to the endogenous structural or planted antigens in the glomerulus (in situ immune complex formation).

ELECTRON MICROSCOPY

When a glomerular capillary is studied by electron microscopy, it is seen to consist of three distinct layers. The *innermost layer* (toward the lumen) is formed by the fenestrated endothelial cells, the *middle layer* is formed by the basement membrane, and the *outermost layer* (toward Bowman's space) is composed of the visceral epithelial cells, with their interdigitating cytoplasmic extensions (foot processes) resting against the basement membrane. The spaces between adjoining foot processes are called *slit pores;* these are closed by a very thin membrane known as *slit diaphragm* (Fig. 8–6). Electron microscopy aids in revealing abnormalities of the glomerular basement membrane (e.g., lamination, as in Alport syndrome), abnormalities of glomerular cells (e.g., fusion of foot process of visceral epithelial cells, as in proteinuric state), and the location of electron-dense deposits. The latter correspond to the antigen-antibody complexes detected on immunofluorescence and may be present in four locations. Identification of the location of deposits can be very helpful in the diagnosis of a glomerular disease. For example, in membranous glomerulonephropathy, the electron-dense deposits are located exclusively in the subepithelial region.

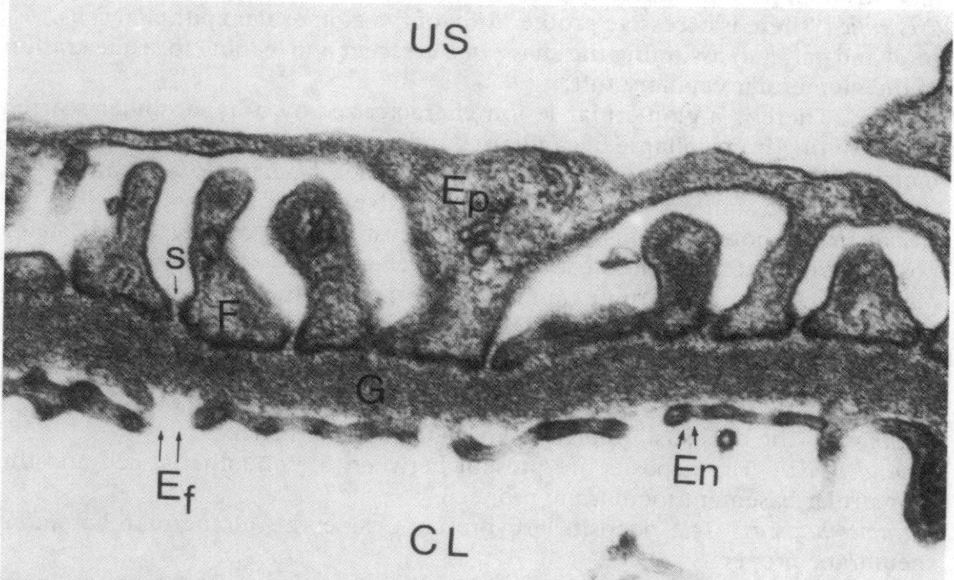

FIG. 8–6. Electron micrograph of a normal glomerular capillary loop showing epithelial cells (Ep), foot processes (F), slit pore with slit diaphragm (S), endothelial cell cytoplasm (En), endothelial fenestrations (Ef), urinary space (US), capillary lumen (CL), and glomerular basement membrane (G). (Courtesy of Dr. Fermin Tio, University of Texas Health Science Center, San Antonio.)

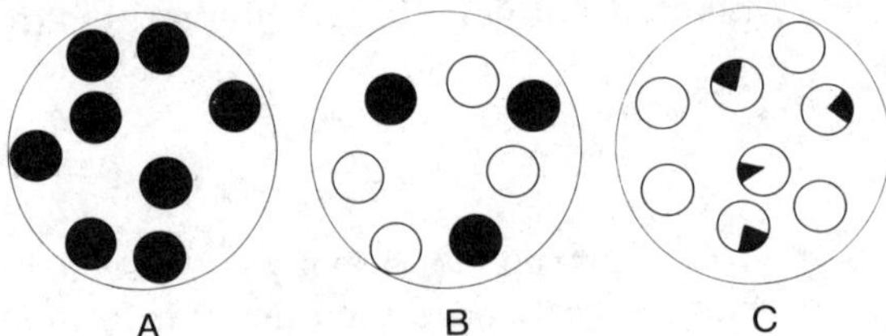

FIG. 8–7. A diagrammatic representation of renal biopsy sections showing glomerular involvement in diffuse (*A*), focal (*B*), and segmental (*C*) glomerulonephritis.

MORPHOLOGIC TERMS

The following terms are used to describe structural abnormalities in the diseased glomeruli.

LIGHT MICROSCOPY

Diffuse Refers to the involvement of every visible glomerulus (Fig. 8–7*A*).
Focal Only some glomeruli are involved, while others are normal (Fig. 8–7*B*).
Segmental Only a segment of a glomerulus is involved; other parts of the same glomerulus are normal (Fig. 8–7*C*).
Global All capillaries of a glomerulus are involved. This term is generally used in describing sclerosis.
Proliferative There is an increase in the number of intrinsic cells of the glomerulus (i.e., mesangial, endothelial, or epithelial).
Crescentic There is excessive proliferation of the glomerular epithelial cells (visceral and parietal) assuming the shape of a crescent and leading to sequestration of the glomerular capillary tuft.
Sclerosis There is a glomerular lesion characterized by a hypocellular scarred area resulting from collapse of capillaries and an excessive amount of mesangial matrix. The material is eosinophilic when stained by hematoxylin and eosin (H&E) and also stains positive with PAS and silver stains.
Hyalinosis A homogeneous, hypocellular, eosinophilic change which stains positive with PAS stain but *negative* with silver stain.
Membranous The glomerular capillary wall appears thickened due to the existence of antigen-antibody complexes.

ELECTRON MICROSCOPY

Mesangial The deposits are present in the mesangial matrix.
Subendothelial The deposits are present between the endothelial cell and the glomerular basement membrane proper.
Intramembranous The deposits are present inside the glomerular basement membrane proper.
Subepithelial The deposits are present between the glomerular basement membrane proper and the visceral epithelial cell.

CLASSIFICATION

Based on the morphologic terminology and known or unknown etiology and whether the disease is congenital-inherited or acquired, the glomerular diseases

TABLE 8–1. Classification of Glomerulonephritis

Congenital or inherited
- Alport syndrome
- Congenital nephrotic syndrome (Finnish type)
- Familial hematuria
- Nail patella syndrome

Acquired
- *Primary or idiopathic*
  - Minimal change disease
  - Mesangial proliferative glomerulonephritis
  - Focal segmental glomerulosclerosis
  - Membranoproliferative glomerulonephritis types I, II, III
  - Membranous glomerulonephropathy
  - IgA nephropathy
  - Rapidly progressive glomerulonephritis
  - Focal proliferative glomerulonephritis
  - Diffuse proliferative glomerulonephritis
  - Unclassified chronic glomerulonephritis
- *Secondary*
  - Infection-related
    - Poststreptococcal glomerulonephritis
    - Hepatitis B
    - Subacute bacterial endocarditis
    - Shunt nephritis
    - Postpneumococcal glomerulonephritis
    - Congenital syphilis
    - Malaria
    - Leprosy
    - Schistosomiasis
    - Filariasis
    - AIDS, etc.
  - Associated with a multisystem disease
    - Henoch-Schönlein purpura
    - Systemic lupus erythematosus
    - Hemolytic uremic syndrome
    - Diabetes mellitus
    - Other collagen vascular diseases: polyarteritis nodosa, mixed connective tissue disease, Wagner's granulomatosis, vasculitis, rheumatoid arthritis
    - Goodpasture syndrome
    - Amyloidosis, etc.
  - Drugs
    - Penicillamine
    - Nonsteroidal anti-inflammatory drugs
    - Captopril
    - Gold salts
    - "Street" heroin
    - Trimethadione
    - Lithium
    - Mercury, etc.
  - Neoplasia
    - Leukemia
    - Lymphoma
    - Carcinoma
  - Miscellaneous
    - Chronic renal transplant rejection
    - Reflux nephropathy
    - Sickle cell disease, etc.

may be classified as shown in Table 8–1. Some of the glomerular diseases are rare and are mentioned only briefly. The more common glomerular diseases are discussed below.

CONGENITAL OR INHERITED GLOMERULAR DISEASES

ALPORT SYNDROME

Alport syndrome is an inherited disorder characterized by progressive familial glomerulonephropathy with or without accompanying nerve deafness and ocular abnormalities such as anterior lenticonus.[1] It has been described among many ethnic groups from various geographic locations. Although both males and females are affected, the disease is more severe in males. All affected males eventually develop chronic renal failure, but the progression to end-stage renal failure is variable. Alport syndrome accounts for approximately 3 percent of the children with chronic renal failure[2] and for 1 to 2 percent of adults receiving renal transplants.[3] In one series of children who underwent diagnostic renal biopsies for isolated hematuria, 11 percent were found to have Alport syndrome.[4]

PATHOLOGY[5–11]

Light microscopy findings of Alport syndrome are not specific and vary with age. Biopsies performed before 5 years of age may appear normal except for a few fetal glomeruli. With advancing age, glomerular changes consisting of mesangial cell and matrix proliferation, capillary wall thickening, and tubulointerstitial changes become evident. The latter consist of interstitial fibrosis, tubular atrophy and dilatation, thickened tubular basement membrane, and foam cells. With progression of the disease, glomerulosclerosis and severe tubulointerstitial lesions become prominent and the renal lesion looks like any other end-stage glomerular or tubulointerstitial disease.

Immunofluorescence studies in the early stage are negative. With advancing disease, granular deposits of C3 and IgM are frequently seen in the areas of glomerulosclerosis. This finding is not specific and is seen frequently in other nonimmunologically mediated progressive glomerular disorders.

The diagnostic morphologic changes in Alport syndrome are detected by electron microscopy in the glomerular basement membrane (GBM). The GBM shows splitting and lamination in the longitudinal axis and is typically described as having a laminated and "basket-weaving" appearance (Fig. 8–8). Also, the basement membrane is thinned at places and may contain microparticles. Similar changes may be present in the tubular basement membrane. The severity and diffuseness of these changes vary with the age and sex of the patient. These ultrastructural changes are more diffuse among males than females and increase with age. Young children and females often show only attenuation or thinning of the GBM, while older patients show thickening and the basket-weaving pattern.

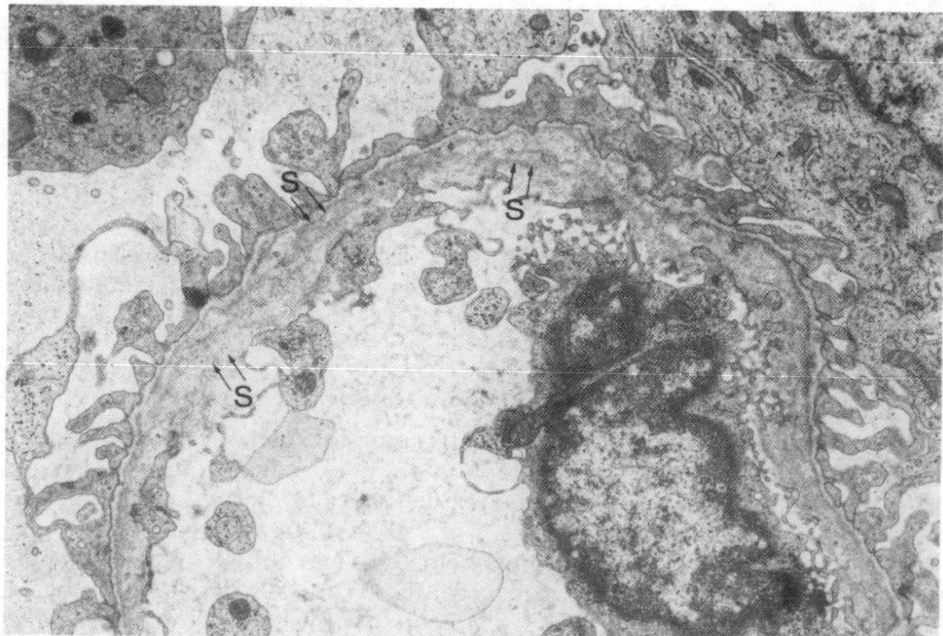

FIG. 8–8. **Alport syndrome, electron micrograph showing characteristic splitting (S) of glomerular basement membrane. (Courtesy of Dr. Sudesh Kapur, Children's Hospital National Medical Center, Washington, D.C.)**

MODE OF INHERITANCE

A satisfactory consensus-building statement regarding the mode of inheritance is yet to be developed. However, three modes of inheritance have been observed and include X-linked dominant, autosomal dominant preferentially segregating with X chromosome, and autosomal recessive.[12,13] In the X-linked type, the gene for Alport syndrome appears to be located in the middle of the long arm of the X chromosome.[14–16]

PATHOGENESIS

Although the exact pathogenesis of the Alport syndrome is not known, four observations suggest that this disorder is caused by a defective biosynthesis of basement membrane in the involved organs. These observations are (1) the specific ultrastructural abnormalities of thinning, lamination, splitting, and basket-weave appearance of the GBM and (2) the lack of Goodpasture antigen in the GBM. The latter hypothesis is based on the following clinical and laboratory findings: Goodpasture autoantibody, which—when tested by indirect immunofluorescence—shows a linear fluorescence on normal GBM but fails to react with the GBM of patients with Alport syndrome.[17] Some Alport syndrome patients who receive renal transplants from normal donors develop autoantibodies to GBM because of a lack of this antigen in their native basement membranes.[18] Fortunately, this, for yet unexplained reasons, occurs in only about 10 percent of cases.[19] Goodpasture epitopes (antigen) is localized on a 28-kDa polypeptide monomer and its dimers in the noncollagenous (NC1) domain of the type IV collagen molecule.[20] (3) The 28-kDa Goodpasture epitopes may be absent in the GBM isolated from patients with Alport syndrome.[21] Autoantibodies developing in some Alport syndrome patients who receive renal transplants from normal donors are directed against Goodpasture epitopes.[18,21]

Absence of Goodpasture antigen and ultrastructual abnormalities of basket-weaving of the GBM strongly suggest that the biosynthesis of GBM is disturbed in Alport syndrome. How these abnormalities result in progressive renal damage remains unknown.

CLINICAL MANIFESTATIONS

Patients with Alport syndrome usually present because of persistent microscopic hematuria or come to the attention of a physician as a result of an episode of gross hematuria. Others may be detected during testing of urines on family members during the evaluation of a child or an adult with Alport syndrome or hematuria. Episodes of gross hematuria may be precipitated by upper respiratory infections and can easily be confused clinically with other causes of hematuria, such as IgA nephropathy or acute postinfectious glomerulonephritis. The disease is considerably more severe in males than in females. Hematuria in the affected males may be detected as early as the first year of life[10] and has been reported to be present even at birth.[22] Although microscopic hematuria is present in most females it may be absent in 10 to 15 percent of females.[23] With progression of the disease, proteinuria appears in almost all males in late childhood or the early teen years and may be of sufficient degree to lead to a nephrotic syndrome in some. Hypertension and renal failure eventually develop in all affected males, although the rate of progression to end-stage renal failure is variable. In some families the end-stage renal failure may not develop until the third and fourth decade of life, while in others it may develop in the teen years.[24] Affected females generally do not develop end-stage renal failure, but exceptions are seen.[25]

The hearing deficit is bilateral and of sensorineural type. In the early stages it is in the 2000 to 8000 Hz frequency range and can be detected only by audiometry. With time it progresses to other frequencies and involves the conversational speech zone and can be quite severe. The hearing deficit is generally not detectable at birth but frequently develops in the early teen years.[10,26] Like the renal disease, hearing deficit is more severe in males than in females and does not improve upon renal transplantation.[27]

Among ocular abnormalities, anterior lenticonus is the most common lesion seen in these patients. It is absent at birth and usually appears in the second to third decade of life. Occular abnormalities are also more common in males and have been reported to occur in about 15 to 30 percent of patients.[10,26] Anterior lenticonus is usually associated with deterioration of vision and the development of axial myopia. When present, anterior lenticonus is highly suggestive of Alport syndrome. Perimacular and macular changes consisting of white or yellowish dotlike lesions may be seen in some cases and are usually bilateral.[10,26] In some children, disappearance of the foveal reflex may be an early abnormality.[11]

DIAGNOSIS AND TREATMENT

The diagnosis of Alport syndrome can be made from the family history, presence of sensorineural deafness, lenticonus, and the characteristic ultrastructural abnormalities seen in the GBM on renal biopsy. There is no therapy available for treatment of Alport syndrome at this time; therefore the disease generally progresses, ultimately, to end-stage renal failure in males, requiring dialysis and renal transplantation. Some patients, as pointed out earlier, will develop autoantibodies to the GBM when they receive a renal transplant from a normal donor. Fortunately, this is not common and should not be considered a contraindication to renal transplantation.

Case History 8–1. A 7-year-old white boy was seen by his pediatrician for acute painless gross hematuria (tea-colored) following an upper respiratory infection (URI) and referred for evaluation. Gross hematuria occurred when the child had symptoms of URI and a fever of 100°F. A throat culture obtained at the time of URI was reported to be negative for group A beta-hemolytic strep. Family history was significant for renal disease and deafness. A maternal uncle, who also had deafness, died at age 20 from kidney failure. On physical examination, the pertinent findings were as follows: BP, 100/60 mmHg; height and weight on 50th percentile; no edema, rash, arthritis, or other abnormal findings. Urinalysis showed yellow color; specific gravity, 1.019; 1+ protein; moderate blood; 7 to 15 red blood cells (RBCs); 1 to 3 white blood cells (WBCs); and occasional granular and RBC casts per high-power field (HPF) in the sediment. The 24-h urine protein estimation was 158 mg; BUN, 18 mg/dL; serum creatinine, 0.4 mg/dL; creatinine clearance, 138 mL/1.73 m^2 surface area; hematocrit, 37 percent; antinuclear antibody test, negative; an antistreptolysin O (ASO) titer of 250 Todd units; and the C3 serum complement, 225 mg/dL. Urinalyses were performed on all family members. The urinalyses were normal on the father and a 10-year-old sister, while the urinalysis on the mother and a 5-year-old brother showed hematuria and proteinuria. Audiograms on the patient and his brother were abnormal and showed bilateral sensorineural hearing loss. Retrospectively, the mother realized that the patient's hearing had probably been impaired since the age of 3 or 4 years. A renal biopsy was performed and was compatible with the diagnosis of Alport's syndrome. The patient's renal function and hearing gradually deteriorated, and he needed to wear hearing aids on both ears at the age of 11 years. At 16 years of age, his renal failure had reached end stage and he was started on hemodialysis. Three months later, he received a cadaver renal transplant. The renal transplant functioned for about 4 months, when it was lost to acute rejection. A month later the transplanted kidney and his own kidneys were removed. At that time his serum tested negative for antiglomerular basement antibodies and no linear fluorescence for IgG was seen along the glomerular basement membrane of the rejected kidney. Three months later, the patient received a second cadaver renal transplant, which remains functional at the patient's present age of 30. However, he continues to wear hearing aids and there has been no improvement in his hearing loss. The patient's brother developed end-stage renal failure at 19 years of age and also received a renal transplant. At age 32, his sister's urinalysis, blood pressure, and renal function are normal. His mother (age 55) has had proteinuria and hematuria for over 25 years and has not developed renal failure.

Comment. This patient presented at age 7 years with acute painless gross hematuria following an upper respiratory infection (URI) and his condition could easily have been confused with acute poststreptococcal, IgA, or membranoproliferative glomerulonephritis. Lack of renal failure, hypertension, and edema; normal ASO titer and C3 concentration; and negative throat culture for group A beta-hemolytic streptococcal infection do not favor the diagnosis of poststreptococcal glomerulonephritis. A combination of gross hematuria, normal C3, normal blood pressure, normal renal function, and an absence of edema would be unusual in membranoproliferative glomerulonephritis. However, this diagnostic possibility could not be entirely ruled out when the patient was first seen, since many such patients can develop these laboratory abnormalities subsequently, on follow-up. Without the family history, it also is difficult to rule out the diagnosis of IgA nephropathy. In the latter disorder, as in the case of this patient, hematuria occurs at the time of an upper respiratory infection (synpharyngitic hematuria) and usually improves upon resolution of the URI. A typical family history of hearing loss and renal failure were the two important clues to the diagnosis of Alport syndrome in this patient. This patient's clinical course, both before and after renal transplantation, was characteristic for patients with Alport syndrome.

CONGENITAL NEPHROTIC SYNDROME OF THE FINNISH TYPE

Congenital nephrotic syndrome of the Finnish type is an inherited disorder with autosomal recessive transmission which was first described from Finland by Hallman and associates.[28–30] The disorder, however, is not limited to Finland, and several cases have been described from other parts of the world.[31,32]

CLINICAL MANIFESTATIONS

In Finland the incidence of this form of congenital nephrotic syndrome is 1 per 8200 live births, with an estimated gene frequency of 1:200.[33] The course of pregnancy is usually unremarkable, but premature birth (33 to 37 weeks gestation) is common.[28–33] Other significant perinatal events include an increased incidence of breech presentation and asphyxia, with lower Apgar scores. The placenta is usually large and generally weighs more than 25 percent of the weight of the infant, but placental weights as large as 65 percent of the infant's weight have been recorded.[33] Other abnormal physical findings include low-bridged nose, wide-set eyes, low-set ears, widely separated cranial sutures, and large open anterior and posterior fontanelles. Postural deformities of flexion of hips, knees, and elbows are common.[34] Some of the babies are edematous at birth, with distended abdomens secondary to ascites, and nearly 50 percent become edematous in the first week of life.[29,33] Almost all newborn infants with the disease are edematous by the second month of life.[33]

Proteinuria is present in nearly all babies at birth, but exceptions to this generalization occur.[28,33] Microscopic hematuria is also common.[28] Blood urea nitrogen and serum creatinine are normal at birth in most but may be slightly elevated in some (10 percent).[33] Other laboratory findings of nephrotic syndrome (hypoproteinemia, hyperlipemia) are present concomitant with edema and are no different than the nephrotic syndrome from other causes. Serum albumin is generally very low; values of less than 1 g/dL are common. Serum IgG levels are low,[35] and these, along with urinary losses of complement factors B and D, may be responsible for an increased incidence of infections in such patients.[36] Urinary losses of several other proteins such as transferrin, vitamin D-binding proteins, and 25 hydroxycholicalciferol as well as thyroid-binding proteins may produce iron deficiency anemia, poor growth, delayed ossification, and hypothyroidism,[37] respectively, in some patients.

PATHOLOGY[38–43]

Histologic changes in the renal biopsy of patients with congenital nephrotic snydrome vary with age, and no single feature is pathognomonic. Kidneys from infants dying early in life show prominent microcysts, which appear to be due to dilatation of the proximal tubules (Fig. 8–9). Microcysts may not, however, be seen in all patients. Mesangial proliferation is common, but some cases may have minor glomerular abnormalities similar to those seen in the minimal change disease. Segmental and focal glomerulosclerosis, global hyalinosis, and interstitial inflammation have also been described. In later stages, the renal morphology looks like any other type of end-stage kidney disease. Immunofluorescence studies are generally negative, but focal staining for IgM and C3 may be seen, particularly in areas of glomerulosclerosis. Electron microscopy shows effacement of the foot processes of glomerular epithelial cells, but the basement membrane is generally normal.

PATHOGENESIS AND PRENATAL DIAGNOSIS

The pathogenesis of the Finnish type of congenital nephrotic syndrome is unknown. It is clear, however, that the abnormal pathology and proteinuria are present in fetal life.[28–30,43] It has been shown that the number of anionic sites in the GBM is decreased in infants with this disease, which may be due to a failure of the heparan sulfate-rich anionic sites to develop in the GBM.[44]

The Finnish type of congenital nephrotic syndrome can be diagnosed prenatally by showing increased levels of alpha fetoprotein in amniotic fluid and maternal serum.[45,46]

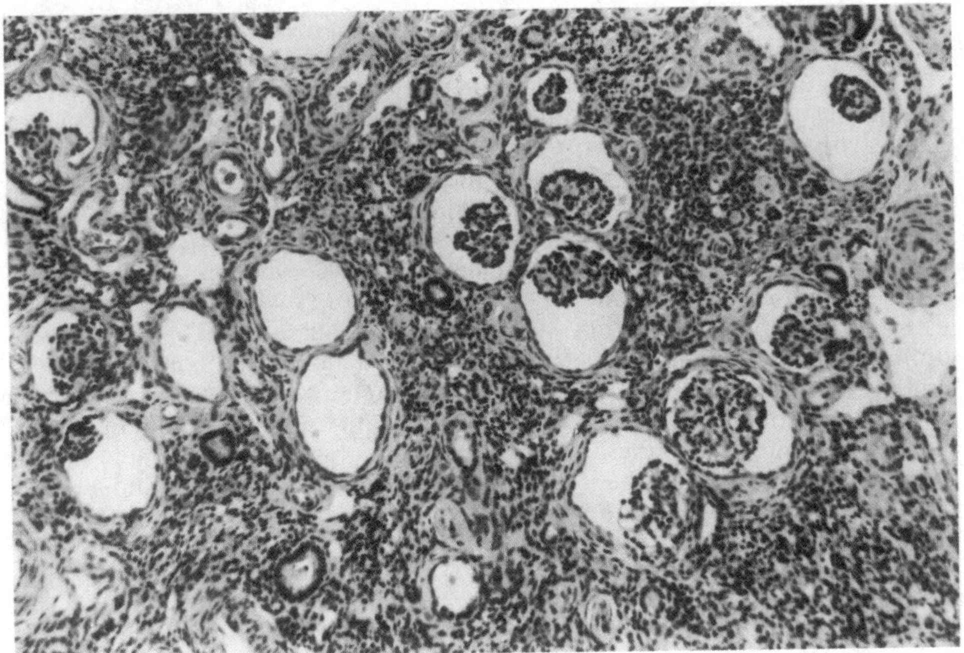

FIG. 8–9. Congenital nephrotic syndrome. Microcysts caused by dilated renal tubules are evident.

CLINICAL COURSE AND MANAGEMENT

The clinical course of patients with congenital nephrotic syndrome is marked by continued proteinuria, anasarca, poor growth, and recurrent infection. They frequently vomit their feeds and have a higher incidence of pyloric stenosis and gastroesophageal reflux.[47] Specific therapy for this disorder is not available, and corticosteroids and cytotoxic drugs are not helpful. Management should be aimed at providing adequate nutrition, control of edema, and prevention and prompt treatment of infections and thrombotic episodes. All of these are challenging problems and require a team approach as well as considerable cooperation from parents.

Adequate nutritional intake can be assured by providing formulas containing additional calories and protein. This may require continuous nocturnal nasogastric feeding. At times parenteral nutrition may be needed, but this should be avoided, if possible, because of the added risk of infection. Edema is difficult to control adequately in most cases, but judicious use of diuretics (hydrochlorothiazide, furosemide, etc.) and infusions of salt-poor albumins are quite helpful (see Chap. 7.).

Because of the increased risk of pneumococcal infections, prophylaxis with penicillin should be used in all infants. Once the patient has achieved a size where a renal transplantation can be performed, this mode of therapy offers the best chance of survival for the infant. Removal of the native kidneys, in order to eliminate proteinuria and nephrotic syndrome, can be done prior to or during transplantation. Results of renal transplantation in these patients are comparable to those seen in infants with other congenital or acquired diseases.[47]

Case History 8–2. This full-term baby weighed 6 lb, 1 oz at birth. No complications were noted during pregnancy. Both parents were white, and they were not sure about any Finnish background in their families. According to the mother, the baby was noted to be puffy within 2 h of birth and had some breathing difficulties. When she was 2 days old, her physical examination showed pitting edema of the limbs and ascites, but no other abnormalities were noted. Urinalysis showed 4+ protein, moderate blood, and 40 to 50 RBCs and 0 to 2 granular casts per HPF in the sediment. Total serum protein was 2.1 g/dL; albumin, 0.9 g/dL; cholesterol, 484 mg/dL; BUN, 6 mg/dL; serum creatinine, 0.3 mg/dL; sodium, 135 meq/L; potassium, 4.1 meq/L; chloride, 100 meq/L; CO_2, 25 meq/L; calcium, 7.5 mg/dL; and phosphorus, 5.3 mg/dL. TORCH titers (toxoplasmosis, rubella, cytomegalovirus inclusion disease, herpes) were negative, the serologic test for syphilis was negative, serum complement levels were normal, and the test for antinuclear antibody was negative. When a percutaneous renal biopsy was performed, 31 glomeruli were present in the sample. Nearly half the glomeruli showed dilatation of Bowman's space. The glomeruli were hypercellular, with an increased number of mesangial cells. There was dilatation of the proximal tubules but no cellular interstitial infiltrate or edema. Only an occasional lymphocyte was present in the interstitial tissue. On electron microscopy, the GBM was normal and there was a diffuse fusion of the foot processes of the glomerular epithelial cells. The immunofluorescence studies were negative. A diagnosis of congenital nephrotic syndrome was made. The patient was discharged on diuretics (furosemide 5 mg twice a day and spironolactone 5 mg twice a day) and penicillin prophylaxis (125 mg twice a day). Over the next several months, she had multiple hospital admissions for febrile episodes, some of which were documented gram-negative urinary tract infections and others which were thought to be viral. A variety of antimicrobial agents were used. On several occasions she received infusions of albumin and furosemide to reduce edema. She received pneumococcal vaccination in addition to routine immunizations for childhood diseases. Her urine continued to show 4+ proteinuria and trace to moderate blood, and she remained edematous. Her serum albumin remained low (0.9 to 1.7 g/dL) and cholesterol high (297 to 484 mg/dL). Despite nutritional supplementation with polycose and medium-chain triglycerides, her growth remained suboptimal and her weight remained below the fifth percentile. At 20 months of age, she was admitted with fever and shock, having been reported to be well 2 to 3 h prior to admission. She was in respiratory distress and quickly became hypotensive and developed ventricular tachycardia. Cardiopulmonary resuscitation was unsuccessful. Autopsy showed fibrin-platelet thrombi in lungs, kidney, liver, spleen, and adrenals, indicating disseminated intravascular coagulation. Evidence for severe acute and chronic pancreatitis, with abundant peripancreatic fat necrosis, as well as calcification and diffuse fibrosis of the pancreas was present. The kidneys showed dilatation of

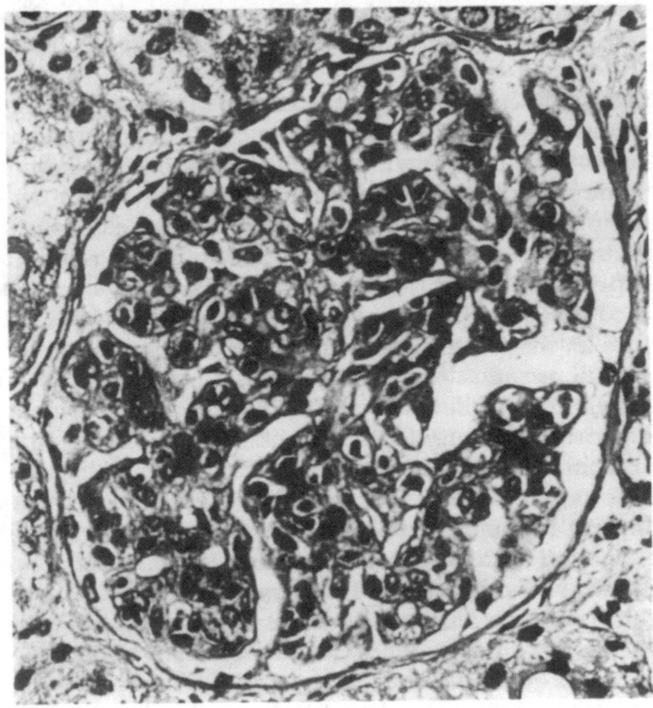

FIG. 8–10. *A*: Membranoproliferative glomerulonephritis showing obliteration of glomerular capillaries and cellular proliferation resulting in a lobular appearance of the glomerulus. The arrow points to the "double contour" appearance of capillary wall. (From Kher KK, Sweet M, Makker SP: Nephrotic syndrome. *Curr Prob Pediatr* 18:199, 1988. Reproduced with permission.) *B*: Electron micrograph of type II membranoproliferative glomerulonephritis demonstrating dense ribbonlike deposits within the lamina densa of the glomerular basement membrane. (Courtesy of Dr. Sudesh Kapur, Children's Hospital National Medical Center, Washington, D.C.)

the proximal tubules and microcyst formation. The glomeruli showed mild mesangial expansion and minimal focal sclerosis. The interstitium showed fibrosis and chronic inflammatory infiltrate. Immunofluorescence studies were negative. No organisms were identified in any organ either on fungal or Gram stain. All postmortem cultures were negative and no source of infection was identified.

Comment. This patient developed generalized edema on the first day of life, had heavy proteinuria and microscopic hematuria on the first urine tested, and developed hypoproteinemia and hypercholesteremia. With this picture the diagnosis of congenital nephrotic syndrome was apparent, and this was confirmed by a renal biopsy. The course of this patient highlights the problems of poor growth, serious infections, and lack of relief of nephrotic syndrome encountered in these patients. Other causes of congenital nephrotic syndrome, such as congenital syphilis or any other

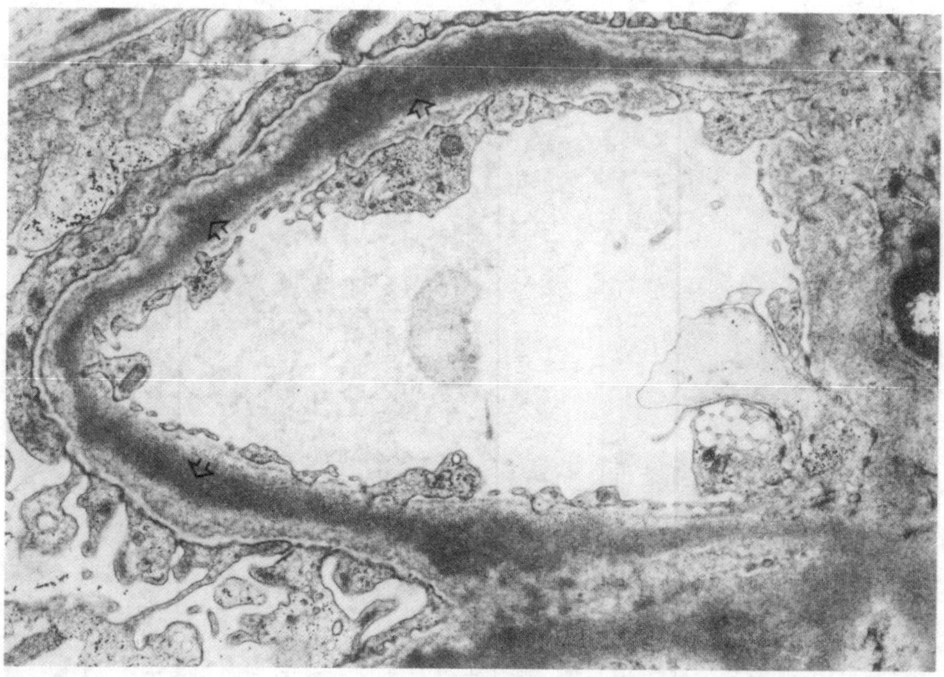

B

Figure 8–10 (*Continued*).

chronic intrauterine infections (e.g., toxoplasmosis, rubella, etc.), must be excluded in absence of a positive history of Finnish ancestry.

ACQUIRED PRIMARY GLOMERULAR DISEASES

MEMBRANOPROLIFERATIVE GLOMERULONEPHRITIS

Membranoproliferative glomerulonephritis (MPGN) is a chronic glomerulonephritis of unknown etiology which was first described as a distinct clinicopathologic entity in 1965.[48,49] It primarily affects older children and accounts for 6 to 13 percent of children presenting with idiopathic nephrotic syndrome.[50–52] MPGN, however, may remain asymptomatic for long periods of time and may come to light only after detection of chance microscopic hematuria or proteinuria on urinalysis. The probability of developing renal failure is high and MPGN can recur in the renal transplant. Other terms used to describe MPGN are *mesangiocapillary* and *lobular glomerulonephritis.*

PATHOLOGY[48,53,54]

Based on electron microscopy findings, three types of MPGN have been recognized. However, on light microscopy, all three forms may appear similar. By light microscopy, the predominant change in all types of MPGN is the severe proliferation of mesangial matrix and cells. Because of this, glomerular tufts

TABLE 8–2. Membranoproliferative Glomerulonephritis: Clinical, Laboratory and Pathologic Features Differentiating the Three Subtypes

	Electron Microscopy		Immunofluorescence Microscopy		Serum Complement				
MPGN Type	Location of Electron-Dense Deposits	Basement Membrane	C3	IgG	C3	C4	C3NeF	Activation of Complement	Recurrence in Renal Transplant
Type I	Mesangium Prominent Subendothelial	Intact	+	+ Fringe pattern	↓N	↓N	May be present	Classic	30% chance
Type II	Mesangium Subepithelial	Lamina densa replaced by continuous electron-dense material	+ Interrupted linear double contour	–	↓	N	Usually present	Alternate	90% chance
Type III	Mesangium Subepithelial Subendothelial Intramembranous	Disrupted	+	? Granular capillary loops	↓N	N	Usually absent	Alternate	?

Note: + = positive; – = negative; ? = insufficient data; N = normal; ↓ = decreased.

appear lobulated and the capillary lumens are occluded or compressed. Another typical feature of this severe mesangial proliferation is the interposition of the mesangial cytoplasm between the capillary endothelium and basement membrane. Newly synthesized basement membrane is laid between the endothelium and the interposed mesangium. When studied by the silver methenamine stain of Jones, the basement membranes show the characteristic double contour ("tram-track") appearance of the capillary wall, since the newly synthesized basement membrane and the basement membrane (lamina densa) both stain black but the interposed mesangium does not (Fig. 8–10*A*). The proliferative lesion of MPGN is usually diffuse, but focal and segmentally proliferative lesions have also been described in 5 to 10 percent of cases.[55] Although mesangial cells are the primary cells that proliferate in MPGN, some endothelial proliferation is also present. In cases with epithelial crescent formation, epithelial cell proliferation is obvious. Neutrophilic infiltration in the glomerulus may also be present.

MPGN is classified into three subtypes, based on the electron microscopic findings (Table 8–2). All three types have electron-dense deposits in the mesangium. In type I MPGN, large subendothelial deposits are prominent (Fig. 8–11). In type II MPGN (also known as *dense deposit disease*), a continuous, dense, ribbonlike material is present in the basement membrane, essentially replacing the lamina densa (Fig. 8–10*B*). Similar material may also be seen in the Bowman's capsule and the tubular basement membrane. In type III MPGN, the electron-dense deposits are present both in the subendothelial and subepithelial sites. In type I MPGN, the basement membrane is intact; in type II, it contains the continuous dense material; and in type III MPGN, it is disrupted and fenestrated at some places.

Immunofluorescence studies show positive staining for C3 in all three subtypes, but some distinction among them can be made based on the pattern of staining. In type I MPGN, the C3 staining is usually confined to the periphery of capillary loops (fringe pattern). In type II MPGN, the staining appears continuous with interruptions (pseudolinear) along the periphery of the capillary loops. In type III MPGN, the staining is granular and is present both along the capillary loops and in the mesangium. Staining for IgG is variable in the three types. In type I MPGN, staining for IgG is detected in 70 to 80 percent of cases, being located in the mesangium and along the periphery of capillary loops in the same location as C3. Staining for IgG is very faint in type II MPGN, and the dense intramembranous material does not stain for IgG. Insufficient data are available regarding IgG deposition in type III MPGN. Minimal staining for IgM and IgA may be present in all three types. Staining for early components of complement C1q and C4 is frequently present in type I MPGN but not in type II MPGN; it is occasionally seen in type III MPGN. These findings suggest that complement activation in type I occurs through the classical pathway and in type II and perhaps type III through the alternate pathway.[56]

CLINICAL MANIFESTATIONS

The exact incidence and prevalence of MPGN are not known. Most patients present after the age of 6 years, but the exact time of onset in many cases is

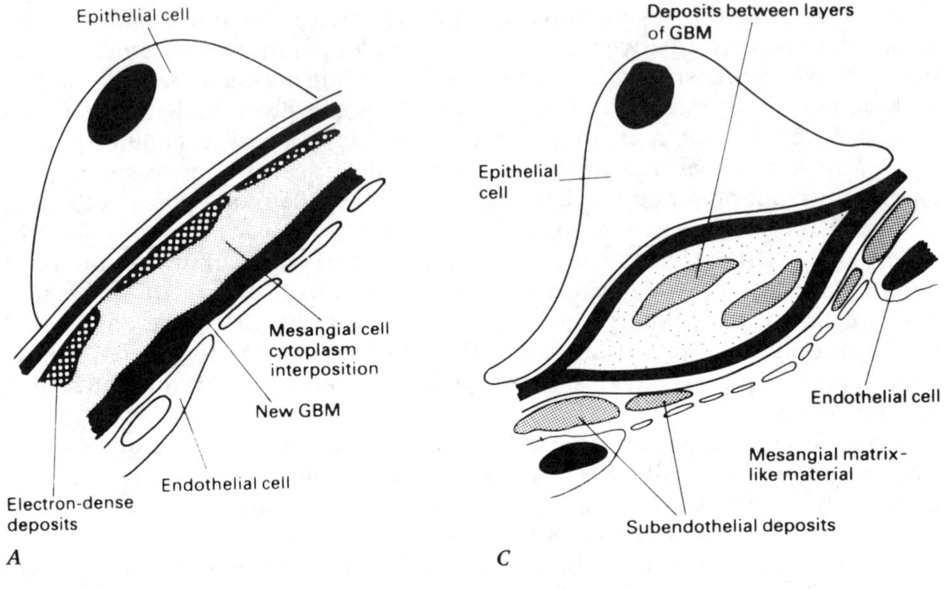

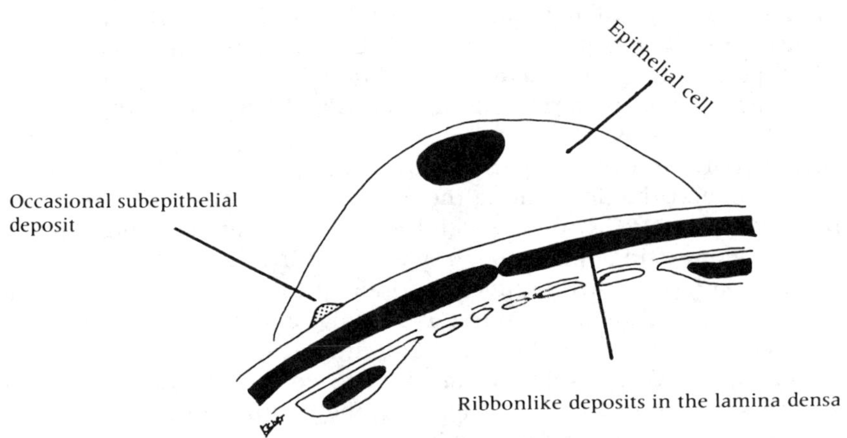

FIG. 8–11. A diagrammatic representation of the electron microscopic features of various types of membranoproliferative glomerulonephritis. Type I MPGN (*A*) shows interposition of the mesangial cell cytoplasm between the endothelial cell and the true basement membrane; electron dense deposits are present in the subendothelial location. Type II MPGN (*B*) is characterized by ribbonlike deposits that replace lamina densa. Type III MPGN (*C*) shows features of mesangial cell interposition in the subendothelial region, subendothelial electron dense deposits, and intramembranous electron dense deposits. (From Sweny P, Farrington K, Moorhead JF: *The Kidney*. Blackwell Scientific Publications, London, 1989. Reproduced with permission.)

difficult to ascertain.[50,53] There is no sex predominance and the disease appears to be uncommon in blacks[57] and perhaps also in orientals.[54]

At onset, MPGN may present with a broad spectrum of manifestations, varying from asymptomatic hematuria to rapidly progressive glomerulonephritis.[48,53,54,58–60] Roughly, a third (25 to 30 percent) of patients present with asymptomatic microhematuria and proteinuria, a third (30 percent) have an acute onset of glomerulonephritis with gross hematuria and edema (nephritic), and over a third (40 to 45 percent) have nephrotic syndrome. However, overlapping of the acute nephritic type and nephrotic syndrome presentation is not uncommon. It is also not uncommon (25 to 45 percent) to have a history of preceding upper respiratory infection, and the disease may be confused with acute poststreptococcal glomerulonephritis or IgA nephropathy. Hypertension, which can be severe, is common in MPGN, especially in patients who present with an acute nephritic onset.

LABORATORY DIAGNOSIS

Urinalysis in patients with MPGN shows the typical findings of a glomerular disease (hematuria, proteinuria, and abnormal casts). Depending upon the mode of presentation, laboratory evidence of nephrotic syndrome may be present and renal function may be normal, or there may be various grades of renal failure. Patients presenting with acute nephritic onset frequently have renal failure. In some patients, this may be very severe, resembling a rapidly progressive glomerulonephritis. The ASO titer may be elevated in some cases, but the frequency of this observation is similar to that seen in age-matched normal children.[48,53,54,58–60]

Serum concentration of C3 is low in approximately 60 percent of cases at the time of diagnosis.[54,61] Therefore, a normal C3 level does not rule out MPGN in a child with idiopathic nephrotic syndrome. The reasons for low C3 in MPGN are not completely understood and several factors may be involved. These include activation of complement and thus consumption of C3, reduced synthesis, and increased catabolism of C3.[62,63] Among the possible agents considered as activators of complement are circulating immune complexes[64] and C3NeF, an autoantibody against a determinant on factor B of the alternate pathway. Immune complexes activate and consume C3 through the classical pathway, whereas C3NeF disrupts the normal inactivation of C3bBb convertase, and this allows unchecked activation of C3 through the alternate pathway.[65] C3NeF is usually absent in type III MPGN, may be present in type I MPGN, but is frequently seen in patients with type II MPGN.[54] Low levels of early complement components C1q and C4 may be seen in type I but not in types II or III MPGN (Table 8–2).[54]

PATHOGENESIS

The exact pathogenesis of MPGN is not known and may possibly be different in different types. Type I appears to be an immune complex-mediated disease, possibly resulting from glomerular trapping of circulating immune complexes.

This is suggested by (1) the granular staining for IgG and C3 in the glomerulus both in the mesangium and along the capillary loops, (2) low levels of the early components of complement C1q and C4, and (3) the presence of circulating immune complexes in serum.[64] The immune complex hypothesis for type I MPGN is enhanced by the observation that certain glomerulonephritides (due to chronic infections such as shunt nephritis[66,67] and hepatitis B[68]) are often of the type I MPGN variety. However, the nature of the antigen(s) involved in the formation of these immune complexes in idiopathic MPGN remains unknown.

The pathogenesis of type II MPGN is also not well established. The nature of the dense material in the GBM is not known, and this material frequently recurs in the renal allografts, sometimes within 3 months of transplantation.[69] Despite morphologic recurrence of the electron-dense material in the GBM of the renal transplants, clinical evidence of glomerulonephritis may not be seen in all patients. The role of C3NeF in the pathogenesis of type II MPGN is also not clear. Clinically, there is no correlation between the presence of C3NeF and the course of MPGN.[61] The pathogenesis of type III MPGN is also not known, but the immunofluorescence findings in glomeruli suggest that it is an immune complex-mediated disease.

A high incidence of types I and III MPGN has been reported in families with inherited deficiency of complement, particularly those with deficiency of C2.[54,70,71] The pathogenesis of MPGN associated with complement deficiency states is not clear.

TREATMENT

A number of drugs—including oral corticosteroids,[54,72,73] large intravenous boluses of methylprednisolone,[74] combination therapy of cyclophosphamide, warfarin plus dipyridamole,[75,76] and aspirin plus dipyridamole[77]—have been tried in the treatment of MPGN, but a consensus regarding an optimal therapy has not emerged. This is not surprising, because of the chronic nature of the disease, the multiple variables that influence its course, and the fact that temporary remissions can occur in some patients without treatment.[53,78,79]

In an uncontrolled trial in Cincinnati, alternate-day prednisone was considered to be beneficial.[54,80,81] Prednisone was given in a dosage of 2 mg/kg/day (80 mg/day maximum) every other day for 1 year, followed by slow tapering to a maintenance dose of 20 mg every other day, which was continued for 2 to 15 years. Of the 37 patients followed for a total of 310 patient-years, only 3 (8 percent) developed end-stage renal failure, compared with over 50 percent from historic controls obtained from other published studies in the literature.[82] Improvement was noted in renal function, proteinuria, nephrotic syndrome, urinary abnormalities, and renal histology. Patients who relapsed (development of nephrotic syndrome, increased proteinuria) while receiving low-dose maintenance prednisone were treated with an increase in the dose of prednisone, and a symptomatic improvement was noted in these patients upon such retreatment. The most significant improvement was noted in type I MPGN, but other subtypes also demonstrated evidence of clinical improvement. Also, it was felt that institution of treatment earlier in the course of disease led to better results. The main side effect of prednisone was growth retardation, which was seen primarily in patients who had to receive higher dosages for extended periods.

A controlled trial with alternate-day prednisone in type I MPGN in 37 children was also conducted by the International Study of Kidney Disease in Children.[73] Prednisone was given to 23 children on alternate days in a single morning dose at dosage of 40 mg/m^2 (maximum 60 mg) and 14 children received placebo. Using a 50 percent reduction in glomerular filtration rate (GFR) as the end point, a 5-year success rate (end point not reached) was seen in 95 percent of treated and 57 percent of the placebo group. However, treatment with prednisone was associated with severe side effects, including hypertension and seizures.

In a controlled trial, treatment with dipyridamole (225 mg/day) and aspirin (975 mg/day) for 1 year in 45 patients significantly slowed the deterioration of renal function and progression to end-stage renal failure (ESRD). In the treated group, the average decrease in GFR at 12 months was 1.3 mL/min/1.73 m^2, while in the placebo group it was 19.6 mL/min/1.73 m^2. ESRD was noted in 14 percent of treated group at 62 months and in 47 percent of the placebo group at 33 months.[77]

The results of controlled trials of treatment with warfarin, dipyridamole, and cyclophosphamide are conflicting. In one study, treatment with warfarin and dipyridamole was considered to be beneficial,[83] while in another study, the addition of cyclophosphamide to the anticoagulant therapy given for 18 months was found to be of no benefit.[76] In both studies the incidence of side effects of anticoagulants and cyclophosphamide was substantial. Regression of dense deposits has been reported in type II MPGN following treatment with anticoagulants, prednisone, and cytotoxic drugs.[84]

Patients presenting with cresescentic or rapidly progressive glomerulonephritis (RPGN) associated with MPGN pose a challenge, and various modes of therapy (including the use of daily oral prednisone, immunosuppressive drugs, and anticoagulants[82,83,85] as well as intravenous boluses of methyl prednisolone[74] and plasmapheresis[86]) have been used, and improvements have been reported in individual cases. Whether these measures are effective in changing the long-term outcome of these patients remains unclear.

Membranoproliferative glomerulonephritis frequently recurs in the transplanted kidney.[69,87] The rate of recurrence of MPGN in renal transplants for type I is 30 percent and for type II 90 percent. However, this should not be considered a contraindication to renal transplantation, since loss of transplant due to recurrent disease is seen in only about 10 percent, and most cases remain asymptomatic.[87]

MPGN ASSOCIATED WITH OTHER CONDITIONS

In addition to the idiopathic type, MPGN can also be seen in a variety of conditions listed in Table 8–3. In most cases the morphology is of type I, but type II is seen in patients with lipodystrophy. The diagnosis and management of these cases is dependent upon the underlying condition.

Case History 8–3. A 9-year-old white girl presented with generalized swelling and was referred to the nephrology service for evaluation. The swelling developed gradually over 2 weeks and was accompanied by low-grade fever but no gross hematuria, rash, joint pain or swelling, abdominal

TABLE 8–3. Clinical Conditions Associated with Membranoproliferative Glomerulonephritis

Partial lipodystrophy[88]
Shunt nephritis[66,67]
Hepatitis B[68]
Visceral abscesses[89]
alpha$_1$-antitrypsin deficiency[90]
Chronic renal transplant rejection[91]
Schistosomiasis[92]
Leukemia[93]

pain, upper respiratory tract symptoms, or any other complaints. Past and family history were noncontributory. On physical examination her blood pressure was 120/80 mmHg; her height was on the 50th percentile for her age. There was generalized swelling, including ascites but no other abnormal findings. Laboratory tests: urinalysis—specific gravity, 1.032; pH,6; protein, 4+; blood, 1+; 8 to 10 RBCs; 10 to 12 WBCs; and several WBC casts in the sediment. Serum electrolytes were normal; BUN, 34 mg/dL; serum creatinine, 1.2 mg/dL; total proteins, 3.9 g/dL; albumin, 1.7 g/dL; cholesterol, 385 mg/dL; Hct, 42 percent; WBCs, 13,000/mm^3; normal differential and platelet counts; negative antinuclear antibody test; negative cryoglobulins; and an ASO titer of 250 Todd units. Throat culture was negative for group A beta-hemolytic streptococci; urine culture, negative; C3 complement, 95 mg/dL (normal); C4 complement, 20 mg/dL (normal). During this period her blood pressure on several occasions was 120 to 140/80 to 90 mmHg (see Table 8–4). A diagnostic percutaneous renal biopsy was performed, yielding 10 glomeruli for study under light microscopy. All showed moderate to marked generalized mesangial cell and matrix proliferation as well as lobular accentuation. Capillary loops were occluded in most glomeruli. Silver stain showed duplication, splitting, and fraying of the glomerular basement membrane. No necrosis or crescent formation was seen. Tubules showed cytoplasmic swelling, the interstitium was edematous, and the blood vessels were normal. Immunofluorescence studies showed fine granular staining along the capillary loops (fringe pattern) for IgG and C3. The intensity of staining for IgG was 1 to 2+ and for C3, 2 to 3+. Minimal staining of similar pattern was seen for IgA, IgM, and C1q; however, no staining was seen for C4 or properdin. Electron microscopy revealed a marked increase in mesangial cells and matrix, with interposition of mesangial matrix in the capillary walls. Most of the capillary lumens were occluded due to severe mesangial interposition. There were several large subendothelial electron-dense deposits. The foot processes of the glomerular epithelial cells were fused diffusely. A diagnosis of membranoproliferative glomerulonephritis type I was made. She was started on oral prednisone 10 mg four times a day (1.5 mg/kg/day). During therapy with prednisone, her hypertension worsened and required treatment with propranolol, hydrochlorothiazide, and spironolactone. Her edema also increased and she required periodic infusions of albumin and furosemide.

TABLE 8–4. Clinical Course of a Patient with Membranoproliferative Glomerulonephritis (Case History 8–3).

Time	BP	Urine		24-h Urine	Serum Chemistries							Therapy				Comment
		Protein	Blood	Protein, g	BUN, mg/dL	Cr, mg/dL	TP, g/dL	Alb, g/dL	Cholesterol, mg/dL	C3, mg/dL	C4, mg/dL	P, mg/day	PRO, mg/day	HCTZ, mg/day	SP, mg/day	
Onset	120/80	4+	1+	7.8	34	1.2	3.9	1.7	385	95	20					
2 weeks	140/90	4+	1+							55		40	40	25		
5 weeks	120/80	4+	2+	2.0	27	0.6	4.2	1.8	495	76		40	40	50	100	
8 weeks	110/86	4+	1+	9.37	25	0.5	4.4	1.5	403	132	26	80/0[a]	60	50	100	
11 weeks	105/85	4+	2+	3.78	23	0.7	5.0	2.1	341	132	30	80/0	80	50	100	
16 weeks	90/60	4+	3+	3.93	18	0.5	5.0	2.6	354			60/0	40	50	100	
5 months	90/60	4+	2+	1.93	19	0.5	5.3	2.9	298	151		50/0	40	50	100	
6 months	100/60	4+	2+	0.67	20	0.8	5.5	3.1				40/0	40	50	50	
8 months	90/60	2+	2+		16	0.8	5.6	3.3	222			30/0	40	50	50	
12 months	110/70	tr	3+		14	0.7	6.5	4.1	176	148	23.8	20/0	40	50	50	
1½ years	120/70	tr	tr	0.01	13	0.7	6.5	4.5	146	140	24.6	20/0	40	50	0	
2 years	110/80	—	—	0.01	14	0.8	6.0	4.1	137	105	15.3	20/0	0	0	0	
2½ years	110/70	—	—		12	0.8	6.2	4.3		111	22.1	20/0	0	0	0	
3 years	100/80	—	—	0.01	11	0.5	6.3	4.2	143	136	22.3	20/0	0	0	0	
4 years	100/80	—	—	0.01	12	0.6	6.5	4.3	143	126	18.1	20/0	0	0	0	Renal biopsy

Note: BP = blood pressure, mmHg; BUN = blood urea nitrogen; Cr = creatinine; TP = total protein; Alb = albumin; C3 = C3 complement; C4 = C4 complement; + = positive; – = negative; P = prednisone; PRO = propranolol; HCTZ = hydrochlorothiazide; SP = spironolactone.

[a] every-other-day prednisone.

With this regimen she became normotensive and her edema subsided. She remained in the hospital for approximately 5 weeks. Her clinical course is summarized in Table 8–4. A renal biopsy was performed after 4 years of therapy with prednisone. Fourteen glomeruli were available for study on light microscopy. There was minimal mesangial proliferation of matrix and cells, but the capillary loops were open and the GBM appeared normal and there was no lobular accentuation. One to two glomeruli showed partial sclerosis. No inflammatory cells were seen, and the tubules, vessels, and interstitium appeared normal. The immunofluorescence studies showed minimal fine granular staining for IgG only in an occasional capillary loop in a few glomeruli. Some glomeruli showed no staining. Staining for C3, C1q, C4, IgM, and IgA was negative. Electron microscopy of two glomeruli showed increased mesangial matrix and cells. A few electron-dense deposits were seen in the mesangium and paramesangial areas. A rare small intramembranous deposit was also seen, associated with cellular interposition, but the capillary loops were open and generally appeared normal.

Comment. This 9-year-old girl presented with acute onset of nephrotic syndrome without gross hematuria or a preceding sore throat. She had microscopic hematuria, WBC casts in the urine sediment, mild hypertension, and mild renal failure. Although her serum complement was initially normal, hypocomplementemia was noted within the first few weeks. Based on these findings, it was unlikely that the patient had minimal change disease as the underlying etiology for nephrotic syndrome. Accordingly, a renal biopsy was advocated, which demonstrated type I MPGN. Upon prolonged treatment with prednisone, the patient showed a gradual improvement in urinary protein losses, serum albumin, and cholesterol, and she normalized her serum complement. Her clinical improvement was sustained, and 4 years after onset she had a normal urinalysis and an improved renal histology even though the disease had not been cured. Although the role of corticosteroids in the treatment of MPGN is controversial, this patient demonstrated a considerable long-term benefit from such a therapy.

MEMBRANOUS GLOMERULONEPHROPATHY

The term *membranous glomerulonephritis* or *glomerulonephropathy* (MGN) was used first by Bell in 1938 to describe glomerular histology in patients dying of nephrotic syndrome, and this condition is characterized by two prominent features under light microscopy.[94] The first one is a thickened glomerular basement membrane and the second a lack of glomerular inflammation. Thickening of the basement membrane in MGN results from immune deposits, which are located in the subepithelial position. Membranous glomerulonephropathy is the most common cause of nephrotic syndrome in adults.[95,96] In children, it represents roughly 2 to 6 percent of cases of idiopathic nephrotic syndrome.[50–52]

PATHOLOGY

Membranous glomerulonephropathy is one of the best-characterized histologic lesions among various glomerulonephritides. Under light microscopy, using H&E stain, the glomeruli in early stages may appear essentially normal except for varying grades of thickening of the GBM. Thickened GBM appears as an eosinophilic homogeneous band outlining the capillary loops in H&E stain. The MGN lesion is best evaluated by Jones stain, which outlines the basement membrane black but does not stain the subepithelial immune deposits. Because the subepithelial deposits are surrounded on the sides by projections of GBM, this gives the appearance of spikes lining the peripheral capillary loops when biopsy sections are stained by Jones stain (Fig. 8–12). Membranous glomerulonephropathy is characterized by a lack of proliferation of mesangial and endothelial cells and by mesangial matrix or infiltration with inflammatory cells. Rarely, epithelial cells may proliferate and lead to the formation of crescents.

Immunofluorescence studies show typical granular staining of IgG and C3 along the capillary loops (Fig. 8–4). The staining for IgG is considerably more intense than C3. Weak but similar staining may also be seen for IgA and IgM in some of patients. Immune staining is absent in the mesangium or in other

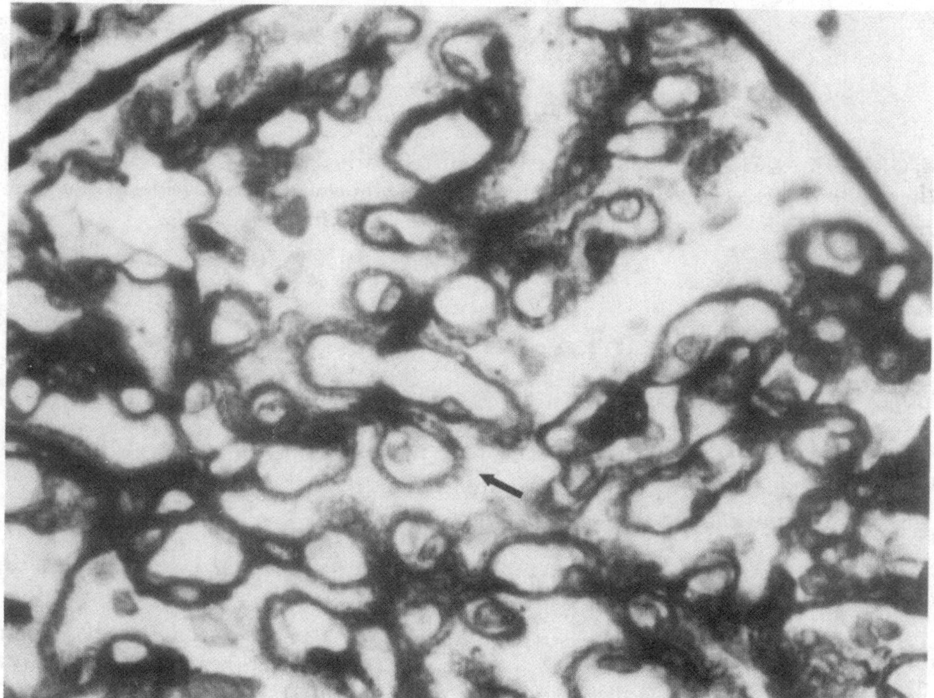

FIG. 8–12. Membranous glomerulonephritis. The capillary loops show the characteristic "spikes" (Jones silver stain). (From Kher KK, Sweet M, Makker SP: Nephrotic syndrome. *Curr Probl Pediatr* 18:199, 1988. Reproduced with permission.)

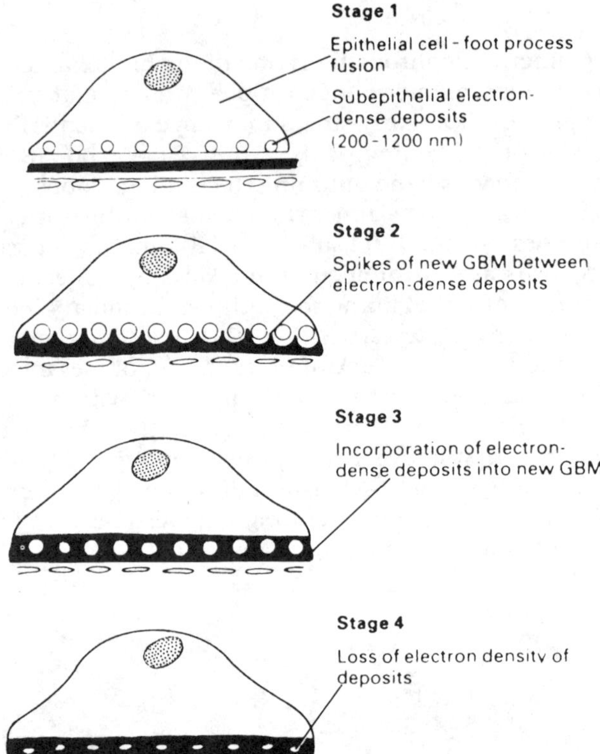

FIG. 8–13. A diagrammatic representation of various stages of membranous glomerulonephritis. (From Sweny P, Farrington K, Moorhead JF: *The Kidney.* Blackwell Scientific Publications, London, 1989. Reproduced with permission.)

parts of the the kidney. Using monoclonal antibodies, the IgG staining along the capillary loops appears to be primarily IgG4.[97]

The electron microscopy findings show the characteristic electron-dense deposits corresponding to the granular IgG staining seen on immunofluorescence. Depending upon the severity of disease, four stages of MGN can be recognized by electron microscopy (Fig. 8–13). In stage I, the electron-dense subepithelial deposits are discrete and small. The overlying foot processes of the visceral glomerular epithelial cell are usually fused at the site of the deposits and the deposits are frequently located opposite the slit diaphragms. In stage II, the deposits are larger and separated by projections of basement membrane corresponding to the spikes seen with Jones stain under light microscopy. In stage III, the deposits begin to be surrounded by the projections of the basement membrane noted in stage II and are in the process of being incorporated into the basement membrane. In stage IV, there is further incorporation of the deposits in the basement membrane and the deposits appear more lucent. Both stages III and IV are considered to be reparative in nature. It has been reported that various stages can exist at the same time and affect different capillary loops.[98] The clinical significance of these four stages is not clear.

PATHOGENESIS

The pathogenesis of MGN is not known. It is believed that the subepithelial granular deposits represent immune complexes. The antigen involved in these deposits and the process by which they are formed are not entirely clear. Whether the antigen is endogenous or exogenous is also not well established. Based on the studies of Heymann nephritis in the rat, it is possible that the immune complexes are formed in situ with an endogenous glomerular epithelial cell antigen.[99–101] Preliminary data are supportive of this view, but definitive evidence is lacking so far.[102–105] Also, based on studies of Heymann nephritis, it appears that following subepithelial deposition of immune complexes, complement activation ensues, leading to the formation of terminal membrane attack components (C5b-9), which may be an important mediator for induction of proteinuria.[106,107]

Membranous glomerulonephropathy can occur in association with other conditions or following treatment with certain drugs or toxic agents. A list of common conditions and drugs associated with MGN is given in Table 8–5. The most common of these are hepatitis B and systemic lupus erythematosus. Membranous glomerulonephropathy associated with drugs is not common (with pencillamine, 7 percent [108]; with captopril, <1 percent [109,110]; with gold, 1 to 3 percent[111]) but responds promptly to the discontinuation of drugs.[108–111] MGN associated with congenital syphilis should be treated with penicillin and is reversible. Membranous glomerulonephropathy can also occur in the course of malignancies.[93,112] Most of such cases have been reported in adults,[93,112] but isolated cases have also been seen in children.[113] MGN has also been reported in renal allografts in patients whose primary disease was not MGN.[114] The pathogenesis of de novo MGN occurring in allografts is not known.

CLINICAL FEATURES

Membranous glomerulonephropathy is not a common glomerular disease in children, and—as alluded to earlier—represents only 2 to 6 percent of the children presenting with nephrotic syndrome. Although mean age of presentation in most studies in children is 10 to 12 years,[126–129] children with onset of the

TABLE 8–5. Clinical Conditions Associated with Membranous Glomerulonephritis

Hepatitis B[115–122]
Systemic lupus erythematosus[123]
Congenital syphilis[124]
Malaria[125]
Drugs
Penicillamine[108]
Captopril[109,110]
Gold salts[111]
Malignancy[93,112,113]
Renal transplants[114]

TABLE 8–6. Clinical Features of 54 Children with Membranous Glomerulonephritis[a]

Number of patients	54
Age, years	10.6 ± 4.5 (53)[b]
Race, % white	48%
Sex, % female	48%
Hypertension	31% (52)
Nephrotic syndrome	85%
GFR, mL/min/1.73 m^2	97.5 ± 43.4 (32)
Serum albumin, g/dL	2.2 ± 0.8 (49)
Total serum protein, g/dL	5.1 ± 1.0 (50)
Serum ANA/% positive	0% (47)
Low serum C3	4% (47)
Hematuria	56%
Proteinuria	98%

[a]Results are expressed as mean ±1 standard deviation.

[b]Values in parentheses refer to number of patients in whom data were available (other than total in that group).

Source: Modified from Southwest Pediatric Nephrology Study Group: Comparison of idiopathic and systemic lupus erythematosus associated membranous glomerulonephritis in children. *Am J Kid Dis* 7:115, 1986. Reproduced with permission.

disease at less than 1 year of age have been reported.[129] There is no predilection for sex (Table 8–6). Proteinuria is present in almost all patients, and nephrotic syndrome has been reported in 80 percent to over 95 percent of children at onset. Hematuria is seen in 50 to 60 percent of these children, and hypertension is present in 30 percent. Renal function is well preseved in most patients when they are first seen.[126–129] Serum complement is normal in most children, but one study reported low C3 in 4 percent children with idiopathic MGN.[126]

COURSE AND TREATMENT

Reports of MGN in children have described a variable clinical course, ranging from complete remission (normal urinalysis) to persistent nephrotic syndrome and renal failure with or without treatment with corticosteroids.[98,126–129] Some have reported that early age of onset in children was a favorable factor for remission of proteinuria and nephrotic syndrome,[127] but others have not been able to confirm this.[128] In general, however, it appears that the course of MGN is more favorable in children than it is in adults.[113] Although corticosteroids have been used in uncontrolled studies in children with MGN,[98,126–129] there has not been sufficient experience in children to recommend a definitive treatment, and the experience in adults, even from controlled trials, remains controversial.[130–133] Recent studies from Italy suggest that alternating courses of corticosteroids and chlorambucil are beneficial[132] but a consensus for drug therapy for MGN has not emerged to date.

Case History 8–4. A 2-year-old white boy was admitted to the hospital for evaluation of nephrotic syndrome. Approximately 6 weeks prior to admission he developed swelling over his eyes, abdomen, and scrotum and was hospitalized by his physician at a local community hospital. His workup in the hospital at that time revealed normal blood pressure; urinalysis—4+ protein, moderate blood, greater than 50 RBCs/HPF in the sediment; 24-h urinary protein excretion of 3.1 g/day; total serum protein, 3.5g/dL; serum albumin, 1.6 g/dL; BUN, 8 mg/dL; serum creatinine, 0.4 mg/dL; normal serum electrolytes; serum complement C3, 95 mg/dL; ASO titer, less than 100 Todd units; and a negative antinuclear antibody test. He was started on prednisone 2 mg/kg/day and discharged. Follow-up in his physician's office continued to show 4+ protein and 4+ blood on dipsticks in his urine, and occasional RBC casts were reported in the sediment. Since his urine did not become negative for protein after 6 weeks of daily prednisone at 2 mg/kg/day, he was referred to the pediatric nephrology service for further evaluation. On physical examination, he was moderately cushingoid and had mild generalized edema; the blood pressure was 90/60 mmHg. Laboratory workup showed the following: urinalysis—4+ protein, moderate blood, 25 to 50 RBCs/HPF, and an occasional granular cast in the sediment. Total serum protein was 5.1 g/dL; albumin, 2.6 g/dL; cholesterol, 203 mg/dL; BUN, 11 mg/dL; creatinine, 0.2 mg/dL; serum complement C3, 87 mg/dL (normal); and C4, 17 mg/dL (normal); screen for hepatitis B surface antigen, B core IgM antibody, antihepatitis A IgM, and antihepatitis B surface antigen IgG was negative. A percutaneous renal biopsy was performed. More than 20 glomeruli were available for review on light microscopy. The GMB was diffusely thickened and the silver stain showed numerous spikes. The cellularity of the glomerulus was normal and the mesangium was not expanded. Occasional casts were noted in the tubules and focal, minimal interstitial fibrosis was present. An organizing thrombus was noted in two venous blood vessels. On immunofluorescence, 3+ granular staining for IgG was seen all along the capillary loops, and the staining for C3 was trace; C1q, trace; IgM, trace; and IgA, trace. Electron microscopy showed extensive fusion of foot processes and typical numerous electron-dense subepithelial deposits. No such deposits were seen in the mesangium. A diagnosis of idiopathic membranous glomerulonephropathy was made and the patient was discharged on the following medications: prednisone 12.5 mg twice a day (2 mg/kg/day), hydrochlorothiazide 25 mg, and spironolactone 12.5 mg once a day. Alternate-day prednisone therapy was initiated 3 months later, and this was slowly tapered over the following 3 years. A gradual improvement in proteinuria was noted after 3 months of starting treatment with prednisone; at 17 months of follow-up, the patient had only 79 mg protein in an adequate 24-h urine collection. Although he continues to have trace hematuria on urinalysis, he is free of proteinuria at 3 years. His blood pressure and renal function are normal.

Comment. This patient manifested features that are commonly seen in children with MGN. Persistent microscopic hematuria should have alerted the treating physician to the existence of a renal lesion other than minimal change as the cause of nephrotic syndrome in this child. Failure to respond to a 6-week course of corticosteroids further suggested this possibility. Renal biopsy was a necessary diagnostic test in this patient and confirmed the diagnosis of MGN. Although treatment of MGN with prednisone is controversial, long-term alternate-day prednisone therapy appears to have helped in the resolution of proteinuria and nephrotic syndrome in this child. It needs to be re-emphasized that the rate of spontaneous remission of nephrotic syndrome is also high in this disorder.

IgA NEPHROPATHY

IgA nephropathy (IgA-N), first described by Berger[134] as a distinct chronic glomerulonephritis with predominant IgA mesangial deposits, is probably one of the most common glomerulonephritides in the industrialized world.[135] Although much progress has been made since its description in 1968, it remains a disease of undetermined etiology with poorly understood pathogenesis. First thought to be a benign renal disease which rarely led to end-stage renal failure, it is now clear that IgA-N can lead to terminal renal failure, with an incidence as high as 20 to 30 percent in adults and 2.5 to 9 percent in children.[135–139] Although many large series have been reported in western Europe[136] and Japan,[138,139] few have appeared from the United States.[137,140] Because of the limited published data, the precise incidence and prevalence of IgA-N in children in the United States is not known. In one study of the 220 consecutive renal biopsies performed in children with glomerular disease in a single center, IgA-N was diagnosed in 9.5 percent of biopsied cases.[140]

CLINICAL MANIFESTATIONS

IgA-N is more common in males than in females, with the male-to-female ratio generally greater than 2:1.[136–140] It appears to be less common in blacks. In two reports from the United States in which racial distribution of the disease is discussed, only 7.5 percent were found to be black.[140,141]

Salient clinical features of IgA-N in children reported in studies from the United States, Europe, and Japan are shown in Table 8–7. Hematuria is the most common manifestation of IgA-N. Macroscopic hematuria at onset is frequent and has been reported in 70 to 90 percent of children from the United States and Europe[136,137,140,142] and in approximately 20 to 25 percent from Japan.[138,139] About 15 to 20 percent of children in the United States and Europe[136,140,142] and about 70 percent in Japan are asymptomatic and are diagnosed because of chance detection of microscopic hematuria.[138,139]

Episodes of macroscopic hematuria are usually precipitated by upper respiratory infections, but they can also occur with infections at other sites or by noninfectious events such as exercise and immunizations.[136,137,140] Most episodes of macroscopic hematuria are asymptomatic, but loin pain may occur in an

TABLE 8–7. Clinical Features at Onset in Children with IgA Nephropathy[a]

	Levy et al.[152] (1972) $n = 36$	Michalk et al.[142] (1980) $n = 19$	Kher et al.[140] (1983) $n = 21$	Levy et al.[136] (1985) $n = 91$	Yoshikawa et al.[138] (1987) $n = 200$
Microscopic hematuria with or without proteinuria	2 (5.5)	2 (10.5)	6 (28.5)	20 (22.0)	126 (63.0)
Macroscopic hematuria	29 (80.5)	17 (89.5)	15 (71.5)	62 (68.1)	40 (20.0)
Acute nephritic or nephrotic syndrome	1 (2.8)	0	0	7 (7.7)	22 (11.0)
Asymptomatic proteinuria	4 (11.2)	0	0	2 (2.2)	12 (6.0)

[a]Figures in parentheses represent percentages.

Source: Makker SP, Kher KK: IgA nephropathy in children. *Seminars in Nephrol* 9:112, 1989. Reproduced with permission.

occasional patient. Macroscopic hematuria typically starts within 72 h of the onset of infection (synpharyngetic hematuria) and generally lasts 3 to 7 days, with gradual clearing of the urine. Microscopic hematuria may persist for a variable time. In some patients the urine may be completely normal between episodes of gross hematuria, while others may continue to have persistent microhematuria.[140] Mild proteinuria (1 to 2+ on dipstick) is usually seen during episodes of macroscopic hematuria. Recurrent macroscopic hematuria is common and has been reported in about 80 percent of children in studies from the United States and France.[136,137,140]

Although proteinuria may accompany microscopic hematuria, isolated proteinuria as a manifestation at onset has been observed in only 1 to 6 percent of children.[136,138] Proteinuria is often of mild degree (<1 g/day), but it can be severe. Nephrotic-range proteinuria at onset has been reported in <5 percent of cases from the United States[137,140] and Europe,[136] but has been described more commonly (5 to 20 percent) in Japanese studies.[138,143,144] Hypertension has been noted at onset in 4 to 7 percent of cases and acute renal failure in 11 to 19 percent.[136,137] Acute renal failure is transient in most cases, but rapidly progressive renal failure leading to end-stage renal disease with epithelial cell crescents on renal biopsy may be seen occasionally (<1 percent).[144,145]

PATHOLOGY[136,137,140,144]

On light microscopy, 25 to 30 percent of children show either normal glomeruli or minimal increase in mesangial matrix. A majority of patients show varying grades of mesangial matrix and cellular proliferation, which (in 40 to 50 percent) is segmental and focal in nature (Fig. 8–14). Diffuse mesangial proliferation with or without epithelial crescents and glomerulosclerosis has been reported in 20 to 30 percent of the cases. Varying grades of tubulointerstitial changes—such as mononuclear cell infiltrate, fibrosis, and tubular atrophy—may be present in patients with morphologically severe disease, especially those with epithelial cell crescents.

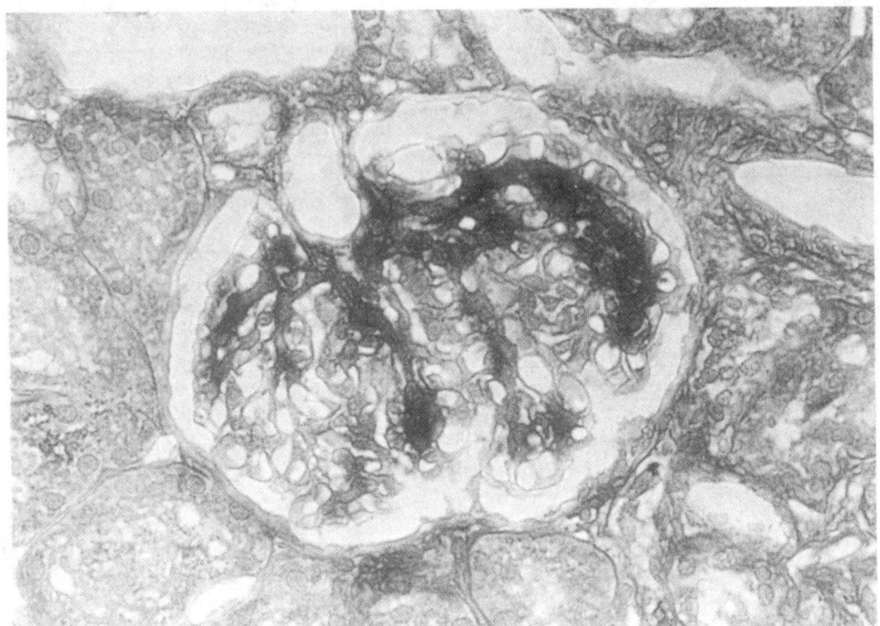

FIG. 8–14. IgA nephropathy. Light microscopy showing mesangial proliferation.

On immunofluorescence examination, a prominent fine to coarse granular staining of the mesangium for IgA is present in all cases (Fig. 8–3). IgA_1 is the predominant isotype of IgA found in the glomeruli, and, according to some reports, it is the only isotype.[146–148] The secretory component (SC) is absent in the glomerular deposits, but exogenous SC can be shown to bind in vitro, suggesting that at least some of the IgA_1 is polymeric.[146,148,149] IgA may be the only immunoglobulin deposited within the glomeruli in some cases (20 to 30 percent), but IgG (50 to 60 percent) and IgM (30 to 40 percent) are also present. Upon staining, C3 can be detected in 95 percent of cases, but staining for C1q and C4 is usually negative.[150] Also frequently detected are C9 and properdin.[151] These findings suggest that complement activation occurs through the alternate pathway.

Electron microscopy shows electron-dense deposits in the mesangium, corresponding to the areas of IgA deposition by immunofluorescence in all cases. However, subendothelial and subepithelial deposits have been reported in 10 to 50 percent of children.[137,142,143,152]

DIAGNOSIS

Although the diagnosis of IgA-N can be suspected in a patient with recurrent macroscopic hematuria or microscopic hematuria, it can only be established by a renal biopsy. Serum IgA levels are elevated in 10 to 20 percent of children,[136,140] but this finding is not specifically diagnostic of IgA-N. Serum complement levels (C3, C4) are normal or elevated. Increased levels of macromolecular (polymeric) IgA[146,153] and IgA-containing immune complexes have been

TABLE 8–8. Clinical Conditions Associated with Prominent Mesangial IgA Deposition and Glomerulonephritis

Henoch-Schönlein purpura[156]
Systemic lupus erythematosus[157]
Cirrhotic liver disease[158,159]
Celiac disease[160]
Ankylosing spondyloarthritis[161]
Rheumatoid arthritis[162]
Cytomegalovirus infection[163]
Hepatitis B virus infection[164]
Mycosis fungoides[165]
Dermatitis herpetiformis[166]

detected by various tests in many patients.[154,155] However, these specialized tests are available to only a few investigators at this time and need further evaluation of their diagnostic potential. In addition to the idiopathic variety of IgA-N, prominent staining for IgA in the glomerular mesangium (secondary IgA-N) may be observed in several unrelated types of glomerulonephritis. A list of these conditions is given in Table 8–8.

THERAPY

A specific and satisfactory treatment for IgA-N is unavailable at the present time. Asymptomatic patients with microscopic hematuria/proteinuria or those with recurrent macroscopic hematuria without nephrotic syndrome or renal failure are generally not considered for any therapeutic intervention. Patients with severe renal disease, such as renal failure and nephrotic syndrome, have been treated with corticosteroids, immunosuppressive agents (including azathioprine, chlorambucil, cyclophosphamide, and cyclosporine), anticoagulants, and plasma exchange.[136,138,167] Although improvements in individual patients have been observed, a consensus about the use of these agents in IgA-N is lacking. Phenytoin, a drug that reduces serum IgA levels, has been shown to be ineffective.[168] Corticosteroid-responsive nephrotic syndrome has been reported in some patients with IgA-N.[169] Renal histology in such cases generally shows minimal mesangial abnormalities. Whether the nephrotic syndrome in these children is due to IgA-N or represents concomitant minimal change disease remains uncertain. On the other hand, nephrotic syndrome in IgA-N that is associated with severe glomerular changes is usually an indicator of poor prognosis and does not respond to corticosteroids.[136]

COURSE AND PROGNOSTIC INDICATORS

The relatively short-term studies reported so far suggest that the clinical course of most children with IgA-N is benign and that they do not develop progressive renal failure. However, urinary abnormalities, including recurrent episodes of macroscopic hematuria, usually persist.[136,139,140]

In three large studies from the United States,[137] Europe,[136] and Japan[138] comprising 83, 91, and 200 patients, respectively, the incidence of chronic renal failure ranged from 5 to 9 percent during a follow-up of 1 month to 15 years. Longer follow-up studies in children are clearly needed. The severity of renal histologic changes, especially the presence of epithelial cell crescents, appears to be the most accurate predictor of development of chronic renal failure.[136,137,145] An inconsistent correlation between the long-term outcome and the age at onset, type of hematuria, severity of proteinuria, presence of nephrotic syndrome, and evidence of transient renal failure at onset has been reported in the published literature.[136,139]

PATHOGENESIS

Based on the immunofluorescence findings in the glomeruli, it can be assumed that IgA-N is an immune complex-mediated disease. Because of the similarities between the circulating macromolecular IgA material and the mesangial IgA (IgA isotype composition, presence of J chain, and the ability to bind SC), it is tempting to postulate that the material in the mesangium represents immune complexes entrapped from the circulation.[146–149] However, this does not rule out the possibility that the complexes are formed in situ in the mesangium by the reaction of polymeric IgA_1 with mesangial, endogenous, or planted antigens. The nature of the antigen in the circulating IgA complex is not known. Whether these antigens are derived from various viral or bacterial agents causing upper respiratory infection which could possibly leak from mucosal surfaces into the circulation and are responsible for the subsequent events (formation of immune complexes in serum or in situ in the glomerulus) remains unknown. The effector molecules that produce renal symptoms and damage remain to be determined. Complement may play a role in this process, since C3, properdin, C9, and membrane attack complex (MAC) are detected in the glomeruli by indirect immunofluorescence.[151,170] Frequent and quick occurrence of gross hematuria following upper respiratory infections suggests a role for antigenic stimulation at the mucosal level.

Relationship Between IgA Nephropathy and Henoch-Schönlein Purpura. Henoch-Schönlein purpura is a systemic disorder characterized by nonthrombocytopenic purpura and a variable involvement of the gastrointestinal tract, large joints, and the kidneys. Renal involvement of Henoch-Schönlein purpura can range from mild mesangial proliferation to severe proliferative glomerulonephritis with extra capillary crescent formation and a rapidly progressive clinical course. Both IgA-N and Henoch-Schönlein purpura nephritis are characterized by a predominant deposition of IgA in the glomerular mesangium. The light microscopic and ultrastructural findings of the two diseases are also strikingly similar.[171] Because of such morphologic similarities, it has been suggested that IgA-N and Henoch-Schönlein purpura represent two ends of the spectrum of a similar disease process. Further support for this notion has been derived from the clinical similarities of the two disorders.[172,173] The report by Meadow and Scott[172] is particularly striking and involved two identical twin brothers.

Both developed upper respiratory infection caused by the same adenovirus, but one of the brothers developed IgA-N while the other developed Henoch-Schönlein purpura.[172] Additional evidence cited to point to similarities between IgA-N and Henoch-Schönlein purpura includes (1) an elevated serum IgA level in some patients with both disorders,[152,174] (2) presence of circulating IgA containing immune complexes,[175] (3) IgA deposits in the skin capillaries of normal skin with both disorders,[176,177] (4) increased IgA-bearing lymphocytes in the peripheral blood,[178,179] and (5) an abnormally high number of IgA-secreting plasma cells in the tonsils with both these disorders.[180]

Further, in addition to the immunologic similarities outlined above, a review of the literature reveals that IgA-N is not a monosymptomatic disease affecting kidneys only. A variety of systemic symptoms similar to those encountered in Henoch-Schönlein purpura such as joint pain, abdominal pain, and loin pain have also been reported in patients with IgA-N.[181] Although the issue is far from settled, the currently held view is that IgA-N and Henoch-Schönlein purpura share a common etiopathogenesis, some having gone as far to characterize IgA-N as "Henoch-Schönlein purpura without rash."[172]

Case History 8–5. A 15-year-old white male was referred for evaluation of recurrent gross hematuria of 6 years duration. Episodes of gross hematuria were on all occasions precipitated by upper respiratory infections and were diagnosed at various times as acute nephritis, urinary tract infection, or prostatitis and were frequently treated with antibiotics. In between these episodes of gross hematuria, urinalyses were reported to be normal. An intravenous urogram and cystogram were reported to be normal. There was no history of trauma and the family history was noncontributory. On physical examination, the patient's blood pressure was 120/80 mmHg; height and weight were normal for his age. There were no clinically detectable abnormal findings. The laboratory data were as follows: urinalysis—specific gravity, 1.024; protein trace; blood, +; 5 to 10 RBCs; and an occasional granular cast in the sediment. Serum electrolytes were normal; calcium, 10.6 mg/dL; phosphorus, 3.3 mg/dL; BUN, 12 mg/dL; serum creatinine, 1.0 mg/dL; creatinine clearance, 131 mL/min/1.73 m^2; antinuclear antibody test, negative; serum C3, 111 mg/dL; serum C4, 36.6 mg/dL; ASO titer, 125 Todd units; 24-h urine protein, 130 mg; urine culture, negative; total serum proteins, 8.2 g/dL; serum albumin, 5.5 g/dL; and serum cholesterol, 140 mg/dL. A percutaneous renal biopsy was performed; 11 glomeruli were available for study. All glomeruli showed segmental mesangial cell proliferation and mesangial matrix expansion. No exudative changes or areas of necrosis were seen. There were areas of focal tubular atrophy, interstitial inflammation, and fibrosis. The vessels were normal. Immuofluorescence microscopy showed 3+ granular staining for IgA in the mesangium of all glomeruli. The staining for C3 was 2+ and IgG, 1+. There was minimal staining for IgM and properdin, but no staining was seen for C1q and C4. Electron microscopy showed electron-dense mesangial deposits. A diagnosis of IgA nephropathy was made, no treatment was prescribed, and follow-up every 6 months was suggested.

SECONDARY GLOMERULAR DISORDERS

POSTSTREPTOCOCCAL GLOMERULONEPHRITIS

It has been known for a long time that some children, after suffering from scarlet fever, can develop edema and gross hematuria; this disorder has been known as poststreptococcal glomerulonephritis (PSGN).[182,183] Since the advent of antibiotics and better public health, the incidence of this disease has decreased dramatically in the United States. In developing countries, however, PSGN remains a common form of glomerulonephritis in children. Fortunately, the disease is self-limiting in most children and the recovery is complete, but in an occasional child it may lead to acute renal failure.

PATHOLOGY

Poststreptococcal glomerulonephritis is a proliferative glomerulonephritis. On light microscopy, the severity and intensity of pathologic changes varies with the severity of disease. In mild cases, particularly in patients with subclinical disease, the abnormalities may be minimal, usually consisting of mild to moderate mesangial cell and matrix proliferation.[184,185] In severe cases, diffuse mesangial cell and matrix and endothelial cell proliferation as well as infiltration with polymorphonuclear cells and monocytes are seen and the capillary lumens may be occluded. The term *diffuse endocapillary exudative proliferative glomerulonephritis* is sometimes used to describe such a morphology. The glomerular basement membrane generally appears normal, and varying degrees of mild to moderate interstitial edema and infiltration with polymorphonuclear cells, monocytes, and occasional eosinophils are not uncommon.[186,187] In a minority of severe cases, extracapillary crescents are present, and the histologic and clinical picture resembles rapidly progressive crescentic glomerulonephritis. Necrotizing vasculitis in renal blood vessels may occur rarely.[188]

Electron microscopy shows electron-dense deposits in the mesangium and large, well defined deposits, known as *humps,* in the subepithelial location are characteristic (Fig. 8–15). Immunofluorescence microscopy typically shows irregular fine to coarse granular staining in the mesangium and along the capillary loops for IgG and C3. Although the predominant glomerular capillary immunoglobulin deposition consists of IgG, minimal staining for IgM or IgA may also be seen. Generally, staining for C1q and C4 is absent or is seen inconsistently and is minimal. Staining for fibrin is frequently present in the mesangium and in the crescents if the latter are present.

These abnormal histologic lesions resolve in almost all children with time, but the time taken for such a resolution can be variable. The electron-dense and immunofluorescence deposits usually disappear within a year.[189,190] Polymorphonuclear infiltration and mesangial and endothelial cell proliferation begin to resolve within 2 to 3 months but some mesangial proliferation and particularly mesangial matrix expansion can persist for several years.[186,191]

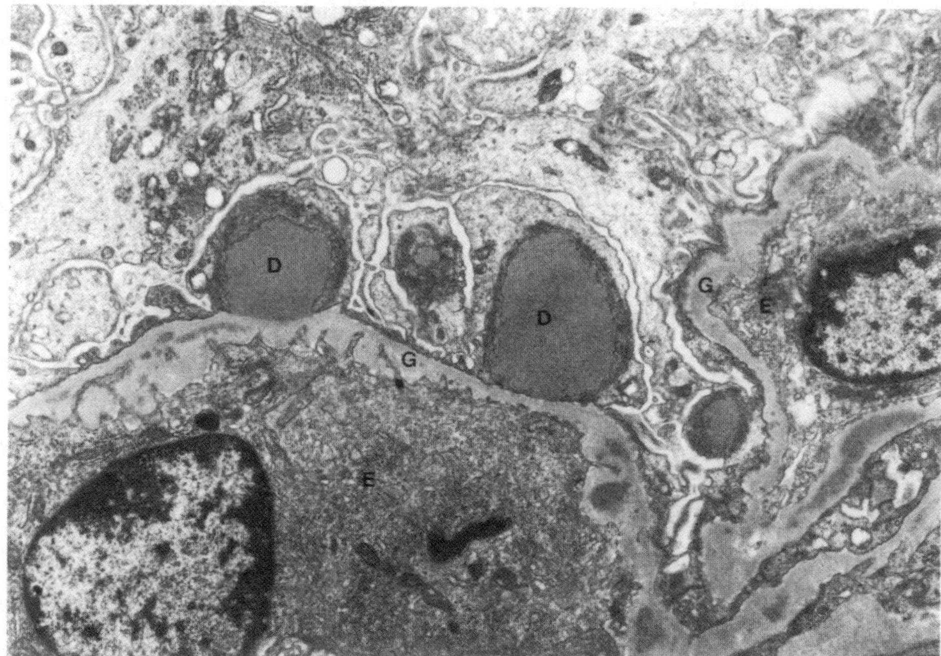

FIG. 8–15. Acute poststreptococcal glomerulonephritis. Electron micrograph showing large subepithelial electron dense deposits, or humps (D). (Courtesy of Dr. Fermin Tio, University of Texas Health Science Center, San Antonio.)

ETIOPATHOGENESIS

Poststreptococcal glomerulonephritis follows an infection with group A beta-hemolytic streptococci; rarely, however, other types of streptococci may also be involved.[192] Only a few nephritogenic strains of group A beta-hemolytic streptococci are capable of leading to PSGN (Table 8–9). The site of infection is usually in the upper respiratory tract, including the middle ear, or the skin. PSGN can occur after scarlet fever and has rarely been reported to occur in conjunction with acute rheumatic fever in the same patient.[193] Based on the relationship to streptococcal infection, clinical findings, and the immunofluorescence

TABLE 8–9. Nephritogenic Strains of Streptococci

Group A
Beta-hemolytic
Respiratory tract—M 1, 2, 4, 12, 18, 25
Skin—M 49, 55, 57, 60
Group C
Streptococci
Streptococcus zooepidermicus

findings in kidney, there are sufficient reasons to believe that PSGN is an immunologically mediated glomerulonephritis. However, despite considerable progress in the understanding of PSGN and the accumulation of a wealth of knowledge about the pathogenesis of glomerular diseases in general, the precise mechanisms of the development of the glomerular lesion and the ensuing proteinuria and hematuria in PSGN are not clear. Both "circulating immune complex formation"[194] and "in situ immune complex formation"[195] have been proposed as the mechanisms for pathogenesis of PSGN. Another hypothesis proposes that neuraminidase produced by streptococci alters endogenous IgG and makes it "autoantigenic." Autoantibodies are formed to the altered IgG, leading to the formation of circulating complexes, which are then deposited in the kidney.[196]

CLINICAL MANIFESTATIONS

PSGN may follow an infection of the upper respiratory tract or skin with nephritogenic strains of streptococci. The latent period for pharyngitis associated PSGN is usually 10 days; 21 days for the impetigo-associated disease.[197] Many children do not volunteer a history of pharyngitis or impetigo, and parents may not be aware of these infections or have considered them important. Therefore, it is essential to look for healed or healing skin lesions on physical examination.

Typically, children with PSGN present with sudden onset of painless gross hematuria ("coke- or tea-colored urine"), and some edema is usually present. The latter is often first noticed as puffy eyes but can also appear as generalized edema. Patients may also present with features of congestive heart failure or pulmonary edema. Hypertension is a common feature of PSGN and may lead to hypertensive encephalopathy characterized by headache, vomiting, lethargy, confusion, and seizures. Oliguria is often present, and anuria may be encountered in a rare patient with severe disease. Some patients may appear anemic.

LABORATORY FEATURES

Urinalysis in most cases shows proteinuria (1–4+), hematuria, and abnormal sediment, which may include dysmorphic RBCs, WBCs, and cellular and granular casts, including the RBC casts. Blood urea nitrogen and serum creatinine are generally elevated, but the degree of elevation is quite variable. While some patients have essentially normal renal function, others may have elevated BUN and serum creatinine. Other laboratory evidence of renal failure such as hyperkalemia, acidosis, hyperphosphatemia, and hypocalcemia may be present. Rarely, some patients may have heavy proteinuria and biochemical characteristics of nephrotic syndrome. Serum total hemolytic complement and C3 are low in almost all patients in the first week of disease, but C4 is generally normal or may be depressed only slightly.[198–201] Properdin levels have been reported to be decreased in over half the patients.[202] These findings suggest activation of the alternate pathway of complement. Depression of C3 is quite striking in patients with PSGN, and values of 20 to 40 mg/dL are common (normal range, 80 to 170 mg/dL). However, the degree of depression of C3 does not correlate with either the severity of disease or eventual recovery. The complement levels

TABLE 8–10. Clinical Conditions Associated with Glomerulonephritis and Low Serum Complement C3 Level

	Serum Complement		
	CH50, Units	C3, Units	C4, mg/dL
Acute poststreptococcal GN	↓	↓	N
Membranoproliferative GN			
Type I	↓	↓ N	↓
Type II	↓	↓	N
Type III	↓	↓ N	N
Lupus nephritis	↓	↓	↓
Shunt nephritis	↓	↓	↓
Subacute bacterial endocarditis	↓	↓	↓

Note: ↓ = decreased; N = normal.

become normal in 8 to 10 weeks.[200] This observation is of considerable diagnostic value, since in other glomerulonephritides (membranoproliferative glomerulonephritis, lupus nephritis) that are associated with low C3 levels on presentation (Table 8–10), hypocomplementemia may persist for a longer period or never normalize.

Laboratory evidence for a recent streptococcal infection should be searched for in all patients. Throat and skin cultures should be obtained but may be negative for group A beta-hemolytic streptococci, particularly if antimicrobial agents have been administered. Several serologic tests for streptococcal antigens are available and can be used to obtain corroborative evidence of a recent streptococcal infection. Among these are antistreptozyme, ASO, antihyaluronidase, and anti-DNase B. Antistreptozyme screening is quite useful because it measures antibodies against multiple streptococcal antigens.[203] Antistreptolysin O titer is raised in 75 to 80 percent of patients with pharyngitis-associated PSGN,[204] but some strains of streptococci do not produce streptolysin O[205] and it is preferred that sera be tested for antibodies against more than one streptococcal antigen. When all serologic tests are used, the evidence for streptococcal infection can be found in over 90 percent of cases. Antistreptolysin O titers are raised in only 50 percent of PSGN patients following impetigo, but antihyaluronidase or other antibodies to streptococcal antigens are usually positive.[204] It is important to remember that early in the course of the disease, titers of streptococcal antibodies may not be raised; serial titers must be performed in such cases. Serial titers showing two- to threefold increase indicate a recent infection. However, laboratory evidence of recent streptococcal infection does not imply that glomerulonephritis is of poststreptococcal etiology. Clinical features and the course of the patient are equally important in deciding the need for a renal biopsy and further investigations. Table 8–11 lists the clinical and laboratory tests that are helpful in the evaluation of patients with acute glomerulonephritis.

Cryoglobulins may be present in serum in PSGN and have been shown to contain IgG, IgM, and C3.[206] Circulating immune complexes may also be present in patients with PSGN.[207] However, these tests do not have any specific diag-

TABLE 8–11. Clinical and Laboratory Evaluation of Patients with Acute Glomerulonephritis

History (sore throat, impetigo)
Physical examination (blood pressure, fluid overload)
Urinalysis, 24-h urine for protein and creatinine
Throat culture, skin culture
Blood chemistries (serum electrolytes, BUN, creatinine, calcium, phosphorus, total proteins, albumin, and cholesterol)
Serum complement (CH50, C3, C4)
Serum for antistreptococcal antibodies (streptozyme, ASO, anti-DNase B, antihyaluronidase)
Antinuclear antibody test
Antiglomerular basement membrane antibodies and antineutrophil cytoplasmic antibodies in patients presenting with rapidly progressive glomerulonephritis
Renal biopsy (if unresolved)

nostic value and need not be performed routinely during the workup of patients with PSGN.

Epidemiologic studies done in microepidemics suggest that not all patients infected with nephritogenic strains develop glomerulonephritis. Only about 5 to 10 percent following pharyngitis and about 25 percent following impetigo developed glomerulonephritis in epidemics.[208,209]

DIAGNOSIS

The diagnosis of PSGN can be suspected in a patient with the clinical presentation of sudden onset of gross hematuria, edema, and acute renal failure following a recent streptococcal infection. Urinalysis findings characteristic of glomerulonephritis, laboratory evidence of recent streptococcal infection, and a low serum complement C3 concentration are supportive evidences for the diagnosis. However, other conditions can also mimic PSGN at onset. These include IgA nephritis and other chronic glomerulonephritides as well as inherited glomerulopathies. Children with IgA nephropathy often present with sudden onset of gross hematuria following an upper respiratory infection; this may be confused with PSGN. However, macroscopic hematuria in IgA nephropathy occurs at the time of pharyngitis (synpharyngetic hematuria), while in PSGN hematuria follows pharyngitis by about 10 days. Also, presence of hypertension and edema are less common as presenting features of IgA nephropathy in children, while both these features are common in PSGN.[210]

Other chronic glomerulonephritides can also manifest clinical features of acute onset of macroscopic hematuria, edema, hypertension, and renal failure. The most notable of these are the membranoproliferative glomerulonephritis (MPGN), lupus nephritis, and rapidly progressive glomerulonephritis (or crescentic glomerulonephritis). Differentiation of these diseases from PSGN may be difficult at onset. While the course of a patient with PSGN is one of progressive improvement in all parameters (i.e., hypertension, edema, and renal failure), this is rare with chronic glomerulonephritides. Also, nephrotic syndrome and heavy proteinuria are less commonly observed in patients with PSGN than in chronic glomerulonephritides. The pattern of serum complement C3 concentration during follow-up is an important marker of distinction between PSGN and other chronic glomerulonephritides associated with a low serum C3 concentration. The serum C3 concentration returns to normal in 6 to 8 weeks in PSGN, while a prolonged depression of C3 is usually seen in other disorders. Exacerbation of macroscopic hematuria may be seen in chronic glomerulonephritides as a result of infection by any of the several nonnephritogenic strains of streptococci. This has been particularly noted in patients with MPGN.[211] Most patients with PSGN do not have to undergo a renal biopsy for diagnosis, but if improvement in renal function is not noticed and nephrotic syndrome persists or worsens, a diagnostic renal biopsy is indicated.

MANAGEMENT

The management of PSGN is essentially supportive. Hypertension can be managed effectively by using peripheral vasodilators (hydralazine or nifedipine). Diuretics are also helpful in relieving fluid overload and hypertension in these patients. Most patients require a short course (days to weeks) of antihypertensive therapy. Patients who have symptoms of hypertensive encephalopathy require aggressive antihypertensive treatment. Fluids, sodium, and potassium should be restricted in the diet until the threat of hypertension, fluid overload, and hyperkalemia is resolved. There is no convincing evidence that treatment with antimicrobials alters the course of PSGN in a patient with established glomerulonephritis or prevents PSGN in a patient infected with nephritogenic strains of streptococci except when treatment is begun within 36 h of infection.[209] Throat and skin culture (if lesions are present) should be obtained from the patient and family members. Those with positive cultures for group A beta-hemolytic streptococci should be treated with appropriate antimicrobials, penicillin, or erythromycin (in allergic patients) in order to prevent the spread of infection to others. Asymptomatic PSGN, as evidenced by microhematuria/proteinuria and depression of C3, has been reported to occur in about 20 percent of family contacts of index cases with PSGN.[212] Bed rest is generally not necessary unless the patient is extremely sick (hypertensive encephalopathy), and most patients should have full ambulation.

Patients with acute renal failure from PSGN require appropriate management. This includes paying attention to fluid balance and serum electrolytes, particularly hyperkalemia. Most patients can be managed without dialysis, but it may be necessary in an occasional patient. Corticosteroids or other immunosuppressive agents have no proven role in the treatment of PSGN and should not be given to these patients. Treatment of RPGN resulting from PSGN is controversial; some authors have advocated the use of corticosteroids, cytotoxic agents, anticoagulants, and plasmapheresis.[212a] However, it is difficult to evaluate the efficacy of such treatment modalities since well-controlled studies are lacking.

COURSE AND PROGNOSIS

Almost all children with PSGN recover, but a rapidly progressive clinical course with glomerular epithelial crescent formation is seen in about 5 percent of cases.[186,191] Diuresis generally begins within 7 to 10 days of onset of the disease, with loss of edema and a gradual return of blood pressure towards normal. Renal function (BUN and creatinine) shows progressive improvement within a week but may not return to normal for 3 to 4 weeks.[186,213] Serum complement normalizes in 6 to 8 weeks. After loss of edema, abnormalities in the urinalysis persist for several months to years in most patients.[79–81]

It does not appear that PSGN leads to significant long-term sequelae such as renal parenchymal damage or hypertension in most children. In a study of 36 children with biopsy-confirmed PSGN followed for a mean period of 9.5 years, prognosis for complete recovery was determined to be excellent.[214] Hypertension was noted in 1 patient and 2 patients had persistent mild proteinuria. On the other hand, the prognosis of PSGN in adults has been a subject of considerable discussion. Potter et al.[215] found persistent urinary abnormalities (proteinuria and hematuria) in only 3.5 percent of the 534 patients they followed for 12 to 17 years in Trinidad. The prevalence of hypertension was not significantly different from that in the control population for this study. The authors of this study concluded that the long-term prognosis of PSGN was good. Other studies have, however, pointed to histologic progression of the renal disease in adult patients.[216,217] It is prudent to follow patients with PSGN until the serum complement C3 normalizes and microhematuria has disappeared in the urinalysis. Progression of PSGN patients with extracapillary crescentic formation to glomerulosclerosis and chronic renal insufficiency has been previously reported.[212a,217a]

Case History 8–6. An 11-year-old white boy was admitted with a 1-day history of passing "coke-colored" urine with pain. Eight days prior to admission he had had a sore throat, which resolved spontaneously in 2 to 3 days. No throat culture was taken and no treatment given. According to his mother, there was puffiness in his face 2 days prior to admission. On the day of admission he had an episode of epistaxis. There was no history of skin rash, abdominal pain, arthralgias, joint swelling, or vomiting. Past and family history were noncontributory. There was no history of renal disease or deafness in the family. On physical examination, the pertinent findings were blood pressure, 142/98 mmHg; temperature, 100.2°F; facial and pedal edema; normal pharynx and tonsils; normal chest, cardiovascular, and abdominal examination. Eye grounds were normal without papilledema. Laboratory workup revealed the following: urinalysis—4+ protein, 4+ blood, RBCs too numerous to count, 0 to 2 granular and 0 to 3 RBC casts in the sediment; 24-h urine protein, 2 g; Hct, 26; WBCs, 9400; neutrophils, 72 percent; lymphocytes, 24 percent; monocytes, 2 percent; eosinophils, 2 percent; platelets, 410,000; normocytic, normochromic RBCs with normal morphology; erythrocyte sedimentation rate (ESR) 40 mm first hour by Wintrobe method; serum chemistries: sodium, 140 meq/L, potassium, 4.9 meq/L; chloride, 112 meq/L; CO_2, 18 meq/L; BUN, 53 mg/dL; creatinine, 1.2 mg/dL; calcium, 7.1 mg/dL; phosphorus, 5.9 mg/dL; total protein, 5.5 g/dL; albumin, 3.2 g/dL; and cholesterol, 114 mg/dL; serum complement C3, 40 mg/dL; complement C4, 15 mg/dL; ASO titer, 200 Todd units; anti-DNase B titer, 640; negative antinuclear antibody test, throat-culture positive for group A beta-hemolytic streptococci. A chest radiograph showed small bilateral plural effusions.

The patient's blood pressure was initially controlled with intravenous hydralazine (0.2 to 0.3 mg/kg) and later with oral hydralazine 25 mg, given every 6 hours with intermittent use of 20 mg of oral furosemide. He continued to require treatment for hypertension for 9 days. On day 11 he was normotensive, off antihypertensive medications for 2 days, and had a BUN of 29 mg/dL, serum creatinine of 0.9 mg/dL, and Hct, 26. Renal biopsy was not performed and he was discharged from the hospital. A month later (6 weeks after onset), his serum complement C3 was 102 mg/dL (normal), blood pressure 113/73 mmHg, and he had no edema. Six months later his urine was normal without blood.

Case History 8–7. A 13-year-old white boy was referred because of worsening renal failure, which had recently been diagnosed. A month prior to admission, the patient presented to his physician with acute onset of facial edema, gross hematuria, and evidence of renal failure. A throat culture did not reveal group A streptococci, but the ASO titer was 333 Todd units and the streptozyme test was positive. Total serum complement was 21 mg/dL (normal, 61 to 232) and the antinuclear antibody test and Coombs' test were negative. The BUN was 75 mg/dL; serum creatinine, 1.9 mg/dL; total serum proteins, 5.8 g/dL; albumin, 2.5 g/dL; and cholesterol, 137 mg/dL. The 24-h urine protein was 2.1 g and erythrocyte sedimentation rate 42 mm by the Wintrobe method. Based on these findings, a diagnosis of poststreptococcal glomerulonephritis was made and he was discharged from the hospital by his physician with a serum creatinine of 1.5 mg/dL. During follow-up, his serum creatinine started to increase and he was hospitalized with a serum creatinine of 3.3 mg/dL. On physical examination, he appeared pale, his blood pressure was 140/100 mmHg, there was minimal facial and pedal edema, but the rest of his physical examination was normal. His urinalysis showed 4+ protein, 4+ blood, many RBCs, and RBC casts and granular casts in the sediment. The 24-h urine protein was 6 g. The ASO titer was 500 Todd units; C3 complement, 89 mg/dL (normal); C4 complement, 12.5 mg/dL (normal); antinuclear antibody test, negative; direct and indirect Coombs' test, negative; Hct, 17 percent; normal WBC, differential, and platelet count; normal peripheral smear; and low reticulocyte count.

A percutaneous renal biopsy was performed, providing 17 glomeruli for study under light microscopy. All glomeruli were hypercellular and had epithelial cellular and fibrocellular crescents. The increased glomerular cellularity was due to mesangial and endothelial cell proliferation and infiltration with polymorphonuclear cells and eosinophils. The mesangial matrix was increased and there was minimal glomerulosclerosis. The interstitium was slightly edematous and there was infiltration with lymphocytes, plasma cells, and eosinophils. Disruption of Bowman's capsule was noted in some areas. The blood vessels were normal. Immunofluorescence studies showed 2+ granular staining for C3 and 1+ staining for IgG along the capillary loops and mesangium. Minimal staining was seen for IgM, but staining for IgA, C1q, and C4 was negative. Crescents stained 2+ for fibrin. Electron microscopy showed increased cellularity of mesangial and endothelial cells. The visceral and parietal cells were also hyperplastic. The capillary lumens were obliterated by the proliferating swollen endothelial cells. Subepithelial humplike deposits were seen and a few intramembranous and mesangial deposits were also present. A diagnosis of poststreptococcal rapidly progressive glomerulonephritis was made.

The patient was managed with supportive care. The blood pressure was controlled with oral hydralazine 50 mg four times a day, propranolol 40 mg twice a day, and furosemide 20 mg once a day. Although he had heavy proteinuria and hypoalbuminemia, his serum cholesterol remained normal. His edema resolved and his serum creatinine decreased from 3.8 mg/dL to 1.0 mg/dL and the BUN dropped to 10 mg/dL 2 weeks later. The clinical course is summarized in Table 8–12.

Comment. Case History 8–7 represents a more severe variety of PSGN than Case History 8–6. Hypertension and renal failure in this patient were severe and prolonged, and proteinuria was in the nephrotic range. His renal biopsy showed a diffuse proliferative glomerulonephritis, with 100 percent of the glomeruli affected by crescents. Despite a severe clinical course and morphology, he made a complete recovery with only supportive therapy.

GLOMERULONEPHRITIS ASSOCIATED WITH OTHER INFECTIONS

Besides group A beta-hemolytic streptococci, a number of other infectious agents including bacteria, viruses, fungi, and parasites have been implicated in the genesis of glomerulonephritis. Although the literature abounds with individual case reports, the exact role of these agents in the causation and pathogenesis of the glomerular lesions in most cases is not completely understood. Generally, acute infections produce proliferative glomerulonephritis, which usually resolves following eradication of the organism, while more chronic infections lead to a membranous or membranoproliferative glomerular lesion. A list of the common organisms and their associated glomerulonephritides is given in Table 8–13, and the most common entities are discussed below.

HEPATITIS-ASSOCIATED GLOMERULONEPHRITIS

Since the original description of hepatitis B virus (HBV) infection associated membranous glomerulonephropathy (MGN) by Coombs et al in 1971,[115] several individual cases and series of cases have been reported by many investigators.[116–122] Most of these reports have come from Japan and southeast Asia. In the great majority of children with hepatitis B-associated glomerulonephritis, the renal lesion is MGN, but membranoproliferative (MPGN)[121,250] and mesangial proliferative lesions have also been described.[251] Hepatitis B-associated glomerulonephritis is believed to be an immune complex-mediated disease. Hepatitis B surface (HBs), hepatitis core (HBc), and hepatitis Be (HBe) antigens, along with immunoglobulins and complement (IgG and C3), have been demonstrated in the glomeruli of patients with HBV-associated glomerulonephritis.[230,252] Whether this represents trapping of circulating immune complex in the

TABLE 8–12. Clinical Course of a Patient with Acute Poststreptococcal Glomerulonephritis with Rapidly Progressive Course (Case History 8–7)

			Urine		24-h	Blood Counts			Serum Chemistries						Therapy		
Time	Edema	BP	Protein	Blood	Urine Protein, g	Hct, %	Retic, %	ESR, meq/h	BUN, mg/dL	Cr, mg/dL	Total, g/dL	Albumin, g/dL	Cholesterol, mg/dL	C3, mg/dL	HZ, mg/day	PRO, mg/day	FU, mg/day
Onset	+	140/90	4+	coke-colored	2.1				75	1.9	5.8	2.5	137	↓			
4 weeks	+	140/100	4+	coke-colored	6.0	17	<1.0			3.5		2.6		89	100	80	20
6 weeks	–	120/80	4+	coke-colored		24	9.0		10	1.0		3.0		93	100	80	20
8 weeks	–	110/70	4+	coke-colored	2.2	29.7		58	19	1.2				115	50	40	10
10 weeks	–	120/80	3+	4+	0.81	32.1		35	18	1.0	7.0	4.0			—	—	—
14 weeks	–	100/70	2+	4+	0.45	32.8		38	18	0.9							
20 weeks	–	100/70	2+	2+	0.256	38.4		18	13	0.8				111			
8 months	–	120/80	+	+	0.326	39.5		15	15	0.8							
11 months	–	120/80	+	+		39		8	16	0.5				110			
1¼ years	–	120/70	+	tr	0.183	40			15	1.0							
1¾ years	–	120/80	+	tr	0.123				14	0.8				113			
2 years	–	110/70	+	–	0.194				13	0.8							
2½ years	–	110/70	tr	–	0.102				9	0.4							
3 years	–	110/80	tr	–	0.213				8	0.8							
3¾ years	–	120/80	tr	–	0.199				19	0.6							
5¾ years	–	120/70	–	–	0.199				15	0.9							

[a]Creatinine clearance: 160 mL/min.

Note: BP = blood pressure, mmHg; Hct = hematocrit; ESR = erythrocyte sedimentation rate (Wintrobe method); BUN = blood urea nitrogen; Cr = serum creatinine; C3 = C3 complement; Hz = hydralazine; PRO = propranolol; FU = furosemide.

TABLE 8–13. Infections Associated with Immune Complex Glomerulonephritis

Bacterial
Group A beta-hemolytic streptococci
Group C streptococci *(Streptococcus zooepidermicus)*[192]
Pneumococcus (pneumonia)[218]
Streptococcus viridans (subacute bacterial endocarditis)[219]
Staphylococcus aureus (acute bacterial endocarditis,[219] pneumonia[220])
Staphylococcus albus (infected ventriculoatrial shunt)[66]
Diphtheroids (infected ventriculoatrial shunt)[67]
Meningococcus (sepsis)[221]
Klebsiella pneumoniae (pneumonia)[222]
Gram-negative organisms (sepsis)[89,223]
Gonococcus (endocarditis)[224]
Brucella[225]
Salmonella typhi (typhoid fever)[226]
Mycoplasma pneumoniae (pneumonia)[227]
Leptospira[228]
Treponema pallidum (congenital syphilis)[124]
Mycobacterium leprae[229]
Viral
Hepatitis B[230]
Varicella[231]
Measles[232]
Mumps[233,234]
Epstein-Barr (infectious mononucleosis)[235]
Cytomegalovirus[236]
Coxsackievirus B[237]
Echovirus[238]
Influenza virus[239]
Human immunodeficiency virus (HIV)[240]
Rickettsia
Rickettsia rickettsii (Rocky mountain spotted fever)[241]
Fungi
Histoplasma capsulatum (histoplasmosis)[242]
Protozoa
Plasmodium falciparum (malaria)[125,243,244]
Plasmodium malariae[125]
Toxoplasma gondii (congenital toxoplasmosis)[245]
Helminths
Schistosomiasis[92]
Leishmaniasis[246]
Trypanosomiasis[247]
Filariasis[248]
Trichinosis[249]

kidney or in situ formation of glomerular immune complexes is not entirely clear.

CLINICAL MANIFESTATIONS

Males predominate in most reported cases of HBV-associated MGN. A majority of children present at between 5 and 10 years of age, but the disease has been detected in children as young as 2 years of age.[116–122] The mean age of onset of HBV-associated MGN in the United States has been reported to be below that of idiopathic MGN (5.3 years versus 10.6 years), and the disease has been reported to be more common in black children.[117] Presenting features of HBV-associated glomerulonephritis are variable and can range from asymptomatic microscopic hematuria or proteinuria to fully developed nephrotic syndrome. Gross hematuria has also been described as a manifestation. Hypertension is usually not severe but has been reported at onset in 20 to 30 percent of children, and renal function is usually normal at onset.[116–122,253]

Clinical evidence of liver disease is generally absent at the time patients develop features of renal disease.[116–122] However, in one series, nearly 40 percent of patients had mild jaundice and hepatic enlargement.[116] On the other hand, laboratory evidence of hepatic involvement is more common, and elevated levels of serum transaminases (SGOT, SGPT) are either present at onset or develop subsequently during follow-up.[116–122,253,254] Low serum complement C3 level has been reported to be a feature of MGN associated with HBV. Hypocomplementemia was reported to be present during the disease course in 100 percent of such patients in one study, compared to only 4 percent of patients noted to have hypocomplementemia in idiopathic MGN.[117] Decreased serum C4 and C1q concentration has also been reported in some studies.[116]

DIAGNOSIS

A high index of suspicion of HBV-induced glomerulonephritis is necessary in patients presenting with nephrotic syndrome and a history of infection by the virus. A positive serology for HBV infection and evidence for hepatocellular dysfunction in a child with nephrotic syndrome associated with hematuria should suggest the diagnosis of HBV-associated glomerulonephritis. However, the diagnosis can be established only by a renal biopsy. Additional studies to document HBV antigens in the glomerular deposits by immunofluorescence, using specific antibodies to these antigens, may be necessary to establish a causal relationship between the infection and the renal lesion. All the HBV antigens may not be detected in the renal biopsy of these patients. In one study of children from Taiwan, hepatitis Be antigen was demonstrated in 95 percent of renal biopsies; in contrast, the HBV surface and core antigens were consistently absent in the renal tissues.[254]

MPGN is not common in HBV-infected children; when present, it is usually of the type 1 variety.[122,250,255,256] Serum complement (C3, C4) levels are usually low in these patients.[250,256]

MANAGEMENT AND COURSE

The number of patients and the duration of follow-up in the reported series in children are limited.[116–122,253,255,256] It is therefore difficult to draw firm conclusions regarding the long-term prognosis. Spontaneous remission of nephrotic syndrome has been reported to occur in most children (83 percent at 5 years), but proteinuria may persist in others.[254] The course can be prolonged, lasting several years, and an occasional patient develops end-stage renal failures.[117,254]

There is no evidence available to suggest that corticosteroids alter the course of the disease.[254]

GLOMERULONEPHRITIS ASSOCIATED WITH ENDOCARDITIS

The association of glomerulonephritis and endocarditis has been known for a long time.[257] Although the incidence has decreased considerably since the availability of antimicrobial drugs, sporadic cases in children are still seen. A variety of organisms may be responsible, but the most common ones are *Staphylococcus aureus* for acute and *Streptococcus viridans* for subacute bacterial endocarditis.[219] Most patients present with signs and symptoms of endocarditis, such as fever, heart murmurs, hepatosplenomegaly, rash, etc. The clinical manifestations of renal disease are variable. Some patients may present with gross hematuria; in others, however, microscopic hematuria, proteinuria and nephritic urinary sediment (RBCs, WBCs, and casts) may be detected incidentally during the workup of endocarditis. Nephrotic syndrome and hypertension are not common, but there is frequently some degree of renal failure and an occasional patient may present with a picture resembling "rapidly progressive crescentic glomerulonephritis."[258] Serum complement (C3, C4) is usually low and rheumatoid factor,[259] immune complexes,[260] and cryoglobulins[261] may be present in the serum.

Renal pathology in typical cases shows a focal proliferative glomerular lesion, predominantly involving mesangial and endothelial cells.[219,258] In some cases fibrinoid necrosis and capillary thrombi may also be present, and an occasional patient may show a diffuse proliferative glomerular lesion with crescents.[259] Immunofluorescence studies show granular capillary and mesangial staining for IgG, C3, IgM. In some patients, the offending bacterial antigens can be localized to the site of the glomerular lesions.[219] Electron microscopy usually shows subendothelial and mesangial deposits with or without subepithelial humps.[219,258–260,262,263] At one time it was thought that the glomerular lesion in subacute bacterial endocarditis resulted from bacterial embolization of the kidney, but this condition is now considered to be an immune complex-mediated disease.[263]

The diagnosis in most cases is quite straightforward and is easily made from history, physical examination, and positive blood cultures for the infectious organism. However, it may be difficult to differentiate this disease from systemic lupus erythematosus, which may present with the same findings (i.e., fever, heart murmurs, rash, evidence of glomerular disease and low C3 and C4). The treatment is aimed at eradication of the offending organism with appropriate antibiotics. Most patients recover with the above therapy, but chronic renal failure may develop in some, particularly those in whom the treatment is delayed.[219]

SHUNT NEPHRITIS

Since its first description by Black et al,[264] several cases of glomerulonephritis have been reported in children in association with infected ventriculoatrial shunts used for hydrocephalus.[66] The most common infectious organism implicated has been *Staphylococcus epidermidis,*[66] but diphtheroids[67] have also been isolated. Patients may present with evidence of increased intracranial pressure such as headache, vomiting, and visual disturbances or they may present with hematuria, proteinuria, renal failure, and hypertension. Nearly 30 percent of cases present with nephrotic syndrome.[66] Serum complement levels (C3, C4) are usually low[66,67,265,266] and as in the glomerular disease associated with endocarditis, rheumatoid factor and cryoglobulins may also present in blood.[265] The most common glomerular lesion detected upon renal biopsy is type 1 membranoproliferative glomerulonephritis.[66,67] Immunofluorescence studies usually show granular staining for C3, IgG, and IgM in the mesangium and along the capillary loops, and electron microscopy shows subendothelial and mesangial deposits.[66,67] Offending bacterial antigens have been detected in the glomerular lesions in some cases.[67,263–269] Based on these findings, the disease is considered to be an immune complex glomerulonephritis. Treatment consists of appropriate antimicrobial drugs and the removal of the infected shunt. In some cases the disease may not resolve despite appropriate therapeutic measures.[270]

HENOCH-SCHÖNLEIN PURPURA NEPHRITIS

Henoch-Schönlein purpura (HSP) is an immunologically mediated systemic vasculitis of small blood vessels that primarily involves skin, gastrointestinal tract, joints, and the kidneys. It has been recognized as a clinical syndrome in children since 1837[271] and is also known as anaphylactoid purpura.[272]

CLINICAL MANIFESTATIONS

Henoch-Schönlein purpura usually affects children between the ages of 5 and 15 years; males are affected more often than females (male:female ratio, 1.5:1). In colder climates, most cases occur in late winter and early summer, and a history of upper respiratory infection is present in over two-thirds of cases. Several other factors or events that may precipitate HSP or may be associated with it are listed in Table 8–14, but it is unclear whether they have any specific etiological significance. Family history is generally negative for HSP in other family members, but cases have been described where one member of the family had HSP and another developed IgA nephropathy.[172]

HSP in children manifests with skin rash, arthralgias, or arthritis and abdominal pain. Symptomatic renal involvement is not common, but patients may present with gross hematuria and acute renal failure. Skin rash is most often present on the lower extremities, particularly on buttocks, shins, and ankles, but it may also be present on other parts of the body (Fig. 8–16). It usually starts as a symmetrical erythematous macular rash that soon changes to a maculopapular and purpuric form. The purpura may coalesce into large ecchymoses and the rash may appear in crops in some patients. Edema of the scalp may be seen in some patients.[273] Arthralgias and arthritis commonly involve feet, ankles and knees, but hands may also be involved. Although the involved areas generally appear puffy, they are usually not hot or red and do not have joint

TABLE 8–14. Clinical Events That Can Precipitate Henoch-Schönlein Purpura

Infections
Upper respiratory infections
Streptococcal pharyngitis
Mycoplasma
Chickenpox
Measles
Rubella
Yersinia
Shigellosis
Food and drug allergy
Insect bites
Vaccination
Familial Mediterranean fever

effusions. Gastrointestinal symptoms usually consist of abdominal pain, vomiting, bloody diarrhea, or melena. Gastrointestinal involvement can be quite severe, and patients may present with ileus, severe melena, or acute abdomen from intussusception.

Renal involvement of HSP is variable both in incidence and severity. The reported incidence of renal involvement varies from 20 to 80 percent. In an unselected childhood population with HSP, Stewart et al. have reported that renal involvement occurred in 20 percent of patients.[275] The spectrum of symptoms related to the renal involvement also is wide, varying from isolated microscopic hematuria to gross hematuria, nephrotic syndrome, and acute renal failure with a picture resembling rapidly progressive crescentic glomerulonephritis. Henoch-Schönlein purpura-associated nephritis may coincide or follow skin, joint, and gastrointestinal involvement; in some cases, this may occur months after the initial episode of purpura. Ureteritis has been reported as a complication in some patients with HSP and can lead to gross hematuria and ureteric stenosis.[276]

Lesions affecting other organs can be seen in patients with HSP; lesions in the testis, pancreas, parotids, muscles, central nervous system and lungs have been reported.[274,276,277] The latter may present with hemoptysis, which may lead to a mistaken diagnosis of Goodpasture syndrome.

LABORATORY FINDINGS

Urinalysis may show only microscopic hematuria or may demonstrate a nephritic picture with hematuria, proteinuria, and granular and cellular casts, including RBC casts. Blood urea nitrogen and serum creatinine may be normal or elevated, depending upon the degree of renal involvement, and serum proteins and cholesterol may be normal or show values consistent with nephrotic syndrome. The ASO titers do not usually differ from those in normal children, and serum complement levels of C3 and C4 are usually normal. Tests for antinuclear antibodies are negative. Serum IgA is raised in nearly 50 percent of children, serum IgM may also be increased in some, but IgG levels have been

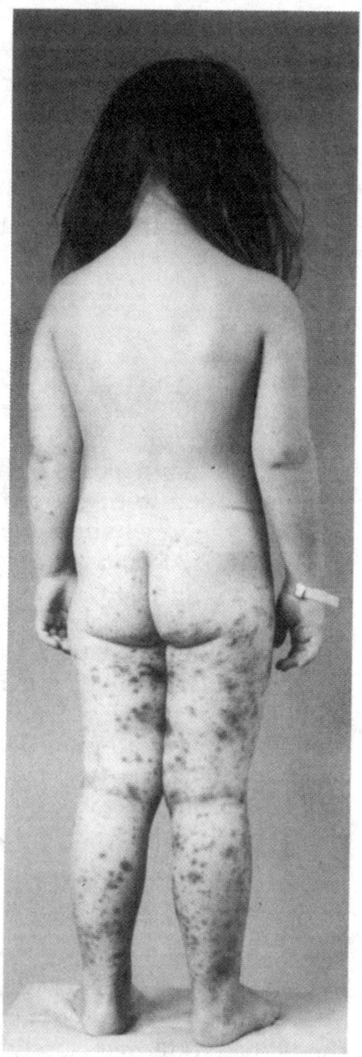

FIG. 8–16. Henoch-Schönlein purpura; distribution of rash.

reported to be normal.[278] Cryoglobulins containing IgA, IgA rheumatoid factor, and circulating immune complexes containing IgA have been reported in serum in some patients.[279–281] Platelet counts, prothrombin time (PT), and partial thromboplastin time (PTT) are normal.

PATHOLOGY

Henoch-Schönlein purpura is a proliferative glomerulonephritis, and the glomerular lesions are similar in many respects to those of IgA nephropathy. The most common lesion is a mild, focal, and segmental mesangial proliferative lesion. In severe cases, a diffuse proliferative glomerulonephritis with crescents—resembling rapidly progressive crescentic glomerulonephritis (RPGN)—

may be seen. Immunofluorescence examination of the renal biopsy shows granular staining for IgA and C3 in the mesangium, but in some cases the staining may also be seen along the capillary loops. IgG and IgM staining is seen less commonly, and staining for early components of complement (C1q, C4) is usually absent.[282] However, staining for fibrinogen is present in most cases.[277] Deposits of IgA have also been observed in the wall of the dermal vessels both in the purpuric lesion site and in the uninvolved normal skin.[274,277,282] Electron microscopy usually shows mesangial electron-dense deposits, but subendothelial and subepithelial deposit humps have also been observed.[283]

PATHOGENESIS

The exact pathogenesis of HSP is not known. Recently, a microepidemic and clustering of HSP has been described; this suggests the possible role of a transmissible agent (probably a virus) in the pathogenesis of this disease.[284] The presence of granular deposits of IgA and C3 in the glomerular lesion suggests that the renal lesion in HSP is immune complex-mediated. These granular deposits most likely represent immune complexes with IgA as the antibody. The antigen involved in the formation of immune complexes is not known. Increased serum IgA levels,[278] IgA containing serum cryoglobulins[279] and immune complexes[281] in serum in HSP suggest that the immune complexes detected in glomeruli come from the circulation. However, this does not rule out the possibility that the glomerular complexes may be formed in situ in glomeruli. Absence of C1Q and C4 and presence of C3 and properdin in the glomerular lesion suggest that complement activation in HSP occurs through the alternate pathway.[285] In susceptible individuals, host factors predisposing to the disease may be important; they include an increased incidence of histocompatibility antigen HLA-BW35[286] and inherited deficiency of C2 complement.[287]

MANAGEMENT

The management for a vast majority of patients with HSP is supportive and the prognosis good. Patients with joint involvement may be given analgesics for arthralgias. Those with abdominal pain and gastrointestinal hemorrhage should be monitored closely for intussusception. Although short-term corticosteroid therapy has been used empirically for relief of abdominal pain in severe cases, it is not established that such a treatment alters the course of the disease. Also, there is no evidence that corticosteroids are beneficial for skin involvement.

Most patients with renal involvement exhibit mild urinary abnormalities; renal failure, nephrotic syndrome, and hypertension are not seen. However, these patients need to be monitored for development of hematuria, renal dysfunction, and hypertension during the acute phase of the disease. Renal biopsy is not necessary, since most such patients show complete recovery over the next few months. Supportive care is all that is necessary. Some patients may have recurrences of HSP, and the degree of involvement may vary from one episode to the other.

Patients with severe renal disease (nephrotic syndrome, acute renal failure, and hypertension) need closer supervision. Their management is more complex and their prognosis guarded, because some of them develop end-stage renal failure. Management of hypertension and acute renal failure in HSP will require strict adherence to fluid balance, judicious use of various antihypertensive drugs and diuretics, management of hyperkalemia, and dialysis if indicated. A renal biopsy for diagnostic and prognostic purposes should be considered for patients with heavy proteinuria, nephrotic syndrome, and deteriorating renal function.

Pharmacologic agents used to treat severe HSP nephritis include oral corticosteroids, intravenous boluses of methyl prednisolone, cytotoxic drugs (azathioprine, cyclophosphamide), anticoagulatnts, antiplatelet drugs, and plasmapheresis.[288] The role of these measures in favorably influencing the course of renal disease has, however, not been fully established. In HSP-associated rapidly progressive glomerulonephritis, recovery of renal function has been reported after use of a combination of the above therapies.[277,282,288,289] These drugs may produce serious side effects, and the risks associated with such treatments should be weighed carefully prior to their use.

All patients with renal involvement in HSP should be followed until their urinalyses become normal. The author has seen children who had only mild urinary abnormalities (no renal failure, nephrotic syndrome, or hypertension) at onset who were lost to follow-up and eventually developed end-stage renal failure.

COURSE AND PROGNOSIS

The prognosis of HSP depends upon the extent and severity of renal involvement at onset. A majority of children with hematuria or hematuria with mild proteinuria undergo resolution of the urinary abnormalities over 2 to 4 months of follow-up.[275] In some studies, however, 5 to 10 percent of such patients have been reported to develop chronic renal failure over prolonged follow-up.[290,290a] On the other hand, patients with nephritic and/or nephrotic features at onset frequently continue to have abnormalities of urinalysis or develop chronic renal failure.[282,290,290a] Nearly 15 to 20 percent of all patients with HSP nephritis have been reported to develop end-stage renal failure (ESRD).[290,290a,290b] About half of these develop ESRD within the first few months of onset, especially patients with evidence of severe glomerulonephritis. In the remaining half, ESRD develops over a period of 5 to 15 years of follow-up.[282,290] The incidence of chronic renal failure, ESRD, hypertension, and persistent urinary abnormalities seems to be higher in adults than in children.[290c] Indicators of a poor prognosis include nephrotic syndrome, hypertension, renal failure at onset, and the presence of glomerular crescents on renal biopsy (Table 8–15).[282,289,290] However, some patients, despite having one or more of these poor prognostic features, do recover completely. Those developing ESRD can be considered for renal transplantation, but recurrence of the disease has been reported in the transplanted graft.[291]

Case History 8–8. A 7-year-old boy was referred for evaluation of HSP nephritis. Five months earlier, he presented to his physician with pain and

TABLE 8–15. Henoch-Schönlein Purpura: Correlation of Long-Term Outcome and the Severity of Epithelial Crescents

	No. of Patients				
Glomeruli Affected by Crescents	Total	Recovery	Minimal Renal Abnormality	Persisting Nephropathy	Terminal Renal Failure
>80%	19	2	4	1	12(60%)
50–80%	20	4	5	5	6(30%)
>50%	42	22	11	7	2(5%)

Source: From Cameron JS[314]: Henoch-Schönlein purpura nephritis: Renal involvement in multisystem and heredofamilial disease. In Massry SG, Glassock RJ (eds): *Textbook of Nephrology*, 2nd ed. Baltimore, Williams & Wilkins, 1989, vol 1, pp 714–719. Reproduced with permission. © 1989 Williams & Wilkins Co., Baltimore.

swelling of both ankles and was hospitalized elsewhere. While in that hospital, he developed purpuric rash on his back, buttocks, legs, and arms. He was discharged from the hospital with a diagnosis of HSP. Two days later, he started to have abdominal pain, was noted to be swollen, and was rehospitalized. He gave a history of sore throat 2 weeks prior to this illness, but no throat culture was obtained. Past and family history was unremarkable. On physical examination, he was well developed, well nourished, and in no acute distress. His blood pressure was 110/80 mmHg and temperature 98 °F. His face was puffy and he had 1+ pedal edema. He had purpuric lesions over his buttocks and lower extremities and some purplish spots on his upper extremities. There was no joint swelling or pain in any of the joints. He had slight epigastric tenderness on deep palpation, but there was no guarding or rebound. Normal bowel sounds were heard in all quadrants. The rest of the physical examination was normal. His urinalysis showed a specific gravity of 1.025, 4+ protein, moderate blood, and the sediment showed 12 to 15 RBCs, 5 to 6 WBCs, 0 to 2 WBC count, and 5 to 6 coarse and fine granular casts in the urine sediment. His Hct was 31.5 percent, WBC count, 11,000/mm^3; differential count, normal; platelet count, 457,000; prothrombin time, 12.8 s; and partial thromboplastin time, 24.2 s. All these were within the normal range. His BUN was 20 mg/dL; serum creatinine, 0.7 mg/dL; and serum albumin, 3.5 g/dL. Other tests included a positive throat culture for beta-hemolytic strep group A, ASO titer of 833 Todd units, negative antinuclear antibody test, C3 complement of 97 mg/dL (normal), C4 of 15 mg/dL (normal), negative cryoglobulins, negative Coombs' test, erythrocyte sedimentation rate of 50 mm by the Wintrobe method, and a 24-h urine protein of 3.1 g. His hospital course was unremarkable, and he was discharged 3 days later. In the 5 months between onset and his referral, he had had several episodes of gross hematuria, usually precipitated by upper respiratory infections and subsiding on their own. At no time did he have edema or recurrence of rash.

Case History 8–9. A 13-year-old white boy was referred for evaluation of HSP nephritis. Four weeks prior to admission, he developed sore throat, fever, and muscle aches. Four days after the onset of these symptoms, he developed a red, papular, nonpruritic rash over his lower extremities. A day later, he had swelling and pain on both ankles and also complained of abdominal pain. At this time he was seen by his physician and hospitalized. The following laboratory data were obtained: a positive throat culture for beta-hemolytic strep group A, an ASO titer of 625 Todd units, proteinuria, and hematuria. Red blood cell casts were seen in the urinalysis. Twenty-hour urinary collection on several occasions showed proteinuria of 3 to 4 g, BUN ranged from 30 to 40 mg/dL, and a serum creatinine was 1.0 mg/dL. He was treated with penicillin, a diagnosis of HSP nephritis was made, and he was referred to the nephrology service for further evaluation. Past and family histories were noncontributory. At this point his physical examination was as follows: blood pressure, 140/78 mmHg; purpuric rash present over lower extremities, including ankles, feet, and the buttocks; rash also present on the hands bilaterally. There was 1+ facial and ankle edema. The rest of the physical examination was normal. The laboratory data were as follows: urinalysis—pH, 5; specific gravity, 1.013; albumin, 3+; blood, 2+; many RBCs, RBC casts, and granular casts in the urine sediment. A 24-h collection of urine showed a total protein of 7.6 g/dL. Serum chemistries—sodium, 139 meq/L; potassium, 5.1 meq/L; chloride, 106 meq/L; bicarbonate, 25 meq/L; BUN, 23 mg/dL; calcium, 8.6 mg/dL; phosphorus, 4.7 mg/dL; creatinine, 1.4 mg/dL; total protein, 5.5 g/dL; albumin, 2.1 g/dL; and cholesterol, 280 mg/dL. Blood counts—Hct, 26 percent; reticulocyte count, 1.6 percent; WBC count, 12,800. Differential: neutrophils, 70 percent; bands, 2 percent; lymphocytes, 21 percent; monocytes, 3 percent; and eosinophils, 3 percent. Serum complement C3, 190 mg/dL; complement C4, 36 mg/dL; antinuclear antibodies test, negative; cryoglobulins, positive; hepatitis B surface antigen test, negative; Coombs' test, negative; and serologic test for syphilis, negative. A renal biopsy was performed, providing six glomeruli for examination by light microscopy. All showed mesangial cell and proliferation necrosis, and five of the six had epithelial crescents. The interstitium showed edema and mononuclear cell infiltrate. There was acute injury to renal tubules and some increase in the thickness of the walls of blood vessels. Electron microscopy showed diffuse increase in mesangial cells and matrix associated with electron-dense deposits. The basement membrane showed occasional subepithelial electron-dense deposits. The foot processes of the glomerular epithelial cells were focally fused, and there were many neutrophils present in the capillary lumens. Immunofluorescence studies showed fine granular staining for IgG, IgA, and C3 in occasional capillary loops and in mesangial areas. Minimal staining for IgM was also present, and there was diffuse staining for fibrin. No staining was seen for C1q and C4. Based on these studies, a diagnosis of rapidly progressive glomerulonephritis secondary to HSP was made and the patient was started on quadruple therapy consisting of azathioprine, 50 mg every 12 h; prednisone, 20 mg every 6 h; dipyridamole,

100 mg every 6 h; and heparin, 1100 units every 6 h. At the same time, coumadin, 4 mg orally, was started for long-term anticoagulation. Four days later, heparin was discontinued and his prothrombin in time was maintained 2 to 2½ times normal. While in the hospital, his hypertension was managed with hydralazine 25 mg every 6 h, hydrocholorothiazide 25 mg once a day, and propranolol 10 mg every 6 h. He was discharged from the hospital approximately 3½ weeks after admission. Although, he continued to have 5 to 6 g proteinuria during hospitalization, his serum creatinine improved and was 0.8 mg at the time of discharge, while the BUN was 25 mg/dL. A repeat renal biopsy was performed approximately 18 months after the onset of HSP, providing 15 glomeruli for study on light microscopy. Most of the glomeruli appeared normal except for minimal mesangial matrix proliferation and segmental sclerosis. The tubules and blood vessels were normal, and there was no interstitial edema or inflammation. Electron microscopy showed a moderate increase in mesangial cells and matrix and an occasional electron-dense deposit was present in the mesangium, but no other abnormalities were seen. On immunofluorescence microscopy, seven glomeruli were available for examination. Only one of these showed the presence of C3, IgA, IgM, C4, C1q, properdin, and fibrin. The staining was predominantly in the mesangium and was most intense for C3 and IgA.

Comment. Clinically, both patients described above had HSP nephritis and the diagnosis was straightforward. Both had heavy proteinuria, depressed serum albumin, elevated cholesterol, and edema, and therefore both had nephrotic syndrome. However, the first patient had essentially normal renal function and normal blood pressure, while the second had a moderate degree of renal failure and was also hypertensive. Although both patients fulfilled the criteria for the diagnosis of nephrotic syndrome, the proteinuria, hypoalbuminemia, and clinical symptomatology in Case History 8–8 was mild. Because of this and lack of evidence for renal failure or hypertension, a renal biopsy was not considered in the first patient. For the same reasons, the patient was managed without corticosteroid or other immunosuppressive therapy. He gradually recovered over a 3-year period.

In contrast to the first patient, the patient in Case History 8–9 had a more severe nephrotic syndrome and also had hypertension and moderate degree of renal failure. Therefore a renal biopsy was performed. Because this showed epithelial crescents in the majority of glomeruli, it was decided to treat the patient with immunosuppressive agents and anticoagulation. Blood pressure was controlled to prevent the risk of cerebral hemorrhage during anticoagulation, and he was switched to every-other-day prednisone after 3½ weeks of daily prednisone. This patient had a complete recovery of renal function. It has, however, been previously reported that despite a clinical recovery of renal function, such patients may demonstrate histologic deterioration on repeat renal biopsies.[290a]

SYSTEMIC LUPUS ERYTHEMATOSUS NEPHRITIS

Systemic lupus erythematosus (SLE) is an immunologically mediated, multisystemic, chronic disease which can present with a host of clinical manifestations of varying severity due to the involvement of various organ systems. Renal involvement in SLE is common and may be present in over 90 percent of patients.[123,292–294] The extent and severity of renal involvement may vary widely, ranging from no overt renal symptoms and a normal urinalysis to rapidly deteriorating renal functions, acute renal failure, and diffuse proliferative crescentic glomerulonephritis. Although the mortality from SLE, particularly of lupus nephritis, has decreased considerably in recent years, morbidity from the disease remains high. Management of children with lupus nephritis is often challenging and frequently a painful problem for the patient, the family, and the physician.

CLINICAL MANIFESTATIONS

As with adults, SLE in children predominantly affects females, with the female:male ratio exceeding 6:1.[123] Most children so affected are over 10 years of age although some as young as 2 years of age are occasionally seen.[293] Because SLE is a multiorgan disease, patients can present with a variety of symptoms. A detailed description of these is beyond the scope of this book. At the onset of the disease, some patients may not fully meet the diagnostic criteria for SLE set by the American College of Rheumatology. Such a clinical manifestation has been termed *incomplete lupus erythematosus.*[294a] A list of common nonrenal manifestations is shown in Table 8–16.

The manifestations of SLE-associated nephritis are varied and differ from patient to patient. Some patients have no identifiable renal symptoms and have normal urinalysis. These are sometimes said to have "silent" lupus nephritis.[293,294,294b,294c] Lupus nephritis is diagnosed only by a renal biopsy, which may range from mild focal proliferative to diffuse proliferative lesions.[293,294,294b] Silent lupus nephritis has been reported to occur in 60 to 80 percent of SLE patients who have no renal manifestations and have a normal urinalysis.[294,294b] Onset of lupus nephritis in other patients is characterized by a sudden development of edema, gross hematuria, acute renal failure, or symptoms of hypertensive encephalopathy such as headaches and seizures. Because the pathologic process can involve all structural components of the kidney (i.e., glomerulus, tubule, and blood vessels), symptoms may involve dysfunction of any or all of these structures. Although glomerular involvement in SLE is well known, some patients may have a prominent tubulointerstitial disease.[295] In fact, almost any clinical presentation of a renal parenchymal disease listed in Table 8–17 may be evident in lupus nephritis.

DIAGNOSIS

The laboratory investigation of a patient suspected of having SLE is geared toward two aims: (1) to confirm the diagnosis and (2) to determine the extent

TABLE 8–16. Extrarenal Clinical Manifestations of Systemic Lupus Erythematosus

General
Fever, weight loss, poor appetite, malaise, etc.
Skin
Butterfly facial rash, discoid skin lesions, tender vasculitis papules, petechiae, purpura, urticaria, etc., alopecia, photosensitivity, Raynaud's phenomenon
Mucous membranes
Oral ulcerations
Joints
Arthralgia, arthritis
Muscles
Myalgia, myositis
Pulmonary
Pleuritis, pneumonitis
Cardiovascular
Pericarditis, myocardial involvement due to vascular involvement of coronary arteries, endocarditis (Libman-Sacks)
Gastrointestinal
Abdominal pain, nausea, vomiting, vasculitis of blood vessels supplying gastrointestinal tract, perforation
Hepatic
Hepatitis
Hematologic
Coombs positive hemolytic anemia, normocytic normochromic anemia, thrombocytopenia, leukopenia, splenomegaly, prolonged prothrombin and partial thromboplastin time (lupus anticoagulant)
Neurologic
Headaches, depression, psychosis, seizures, chorea, hemiparesis/hemiplegia, cranial nerve palsies, coma

and severity of renal involvement. Patients with lupus nephritis usually have several of the extrarenal manifestations of SLE (Table 8–16). Most patients will have elevated titers of antinuclear antibody, antibodies to double-stranded native DNA (dsDNA), and decreased serum complement concentration. However the severity of these laboratory abnormalities fluctuates from time to time,

TABLE 8–17. Renal Manifestations of Systemic Lupus Erythematosus

Hypertension
Asymptomatic hematuria and proteinuria
Gross hematuria
Nephrotic syndrome
Acute renal failure
Rapidly progressive glomerulonephritis
Acute glomerulonephritis
Hyporeninemic type IV renal tubular acidosis
Chronic renal failure
Interstitial nephritis

and in a minority of patients these tests may be normal. This is particularly true of patients with SLE-associated membranous nephropathy.[296,297] Twenty to 50 percent of such patients may have negative ANA titers and normal serum complement concentration.[297–299] Complement C2 deficiency has been reported to be associated with SLE, and this abnormality must be investigated in patients with a positive family history of SLE.[298] Tests for immune complexes may be positive but these tests are generally not necessary for diagnosis.

Urinalysis in patients with lupus nephritis reveals three cardinal features of renal parenchymal involvement: hematuria, proteinuria, and abnormal casts. The urinary sediment of patients with active lupus nephritis may have red and white blood cells, granular casts, red blood cell casts, white blood cell casts, renal tubular cell casts, and waxy casts. Quantitation of proteinuria gives some information about the severity of disease, and it may be in the nephrotic range ($>$40 mg/h/m^2). As pointed out earlier, some patients with morphologic evidence of lupus nephritis may have normal urinalysis. Serum creatinine and creatinine clearance has traditionally been used as a test for clinical estimation of glomerular filtration rate (GFR). However, some recent studies have suggested that estimation of serum creatinine and creatinine clearance in patients with lupus nephritis shows a significant variability in the same patient from time to time. Also, these tests can overestimate GFR in these patients by as much as 40 percent.[299a] The GFR is usually decreased in patients with active nephritis, but it may be normal in others. Complete blood counts may reveal leukocytosis or leukopenia, normal platelets or thrombocytopenia. The erythrocyte sedimentation rate is usually elevated. In patients with anemia, the Coombs test may be positive, and in some patients the serological test for syphilis is falsely positive.

Drug-induced lupus may be confused with idiopathic SLE; therefore a detailed history of all medications recently used by the patient is important. Generally, drug-induced lupus does not lead to clinically evident nephritis and is usually not associated with low serum complement or high levels of anti-dsDNA antibodies, although exceptions occur.[299–301] Drug-induced SLE is characterized by the presence of an antinuclear antibody that is directed against histones[302]; this fact may be useful in differentiating drug-induced SLE from idiopathic SLE. Resolution of disease following discontinuation of the putative drug is a valuable diagnostic clue.

Renal disease may be present in children with mixed connective tissue disease (MCTD), a rare disorder with elevated titer of ANA and overlapping features of SLE, dermatomyositis, scleroderma, and rheumatoid arthritis. This disorder may be confused with lupus nephritis; however, the ANA in MCTD are directed against a ribonucleoprotein and not DNA.[303] Laboratory tests that are helpful in the evaluation of patients with SLE nephritis are listed in Table 8–18.

PATHOLOGY[123,294,294a,304]

Renal histology in SLE nephritis shows a wide variety of patterns, ranging from essentially normal-looking glomeruli to a diffuse proliferative lesion and extensive epithelial crescents. The World Health Organization classification of renal

TABLE 8–18. Laboratory Evaluation of Patients with Systemic Lupus Erythematosus

Urinalysis
Complete blood counts, including erythrocyte sedimentation rate
Quantitation of proteinuria (protein/creatinine ratio on a random urine or 24-h urine protein)
Assessment of renal function (BUN, serum creatinine, creatinine clearance)
Presence of nephrotic syndrome (total serum proteins, serum albumin, cholesterol)
Serologic tests
  Serum complement (CH50, C3, C4)
  Antinuclear antibodies
  Anti-double-stranded (ds) or native DNA antibodies
  LE cell preparation
  Coombs test
  Serologic test for syphilis (false positive)
  Serum immunoglobulins (increased IgG)
  Cryoglobulins
Renal biopsy

morphology classifies lupus nephritis into six categories, as follows: (1) normal glomeruli, (2) mesangial proliferative, (3) focal proliferative, (4) diffuse proliferative, (5) membranous glomerulonephritis, and (6) sclerosing glomerulonephritis.[304a]

Essentially normal glomeruli. Some children have essentially normal glomeruli or show only minimal mesangial matrix increase on light microscopy. The tubules and blood vessels are also normal, and the entire appearance on light microscopy does not differ from that of a normal kidney. However, on immunofluorescence microscopy, granular staining for IgG and C3, C1q, C4, and less often for IgM and IgA is seen. The electron microscopy corroborates these findings and shows electron-dense deposits in the mesangium along with increased mesangial matrix and cellularity. These patients usually have normal renal function and either normal urinalysis or minimal abnormalities. In one large study, nearly 10 to 20 percent of children with lupus nephritis fell into this group.[123]

Mesangial proliferative. The histologic changes on light microscopy in this form are characterized by a definite increase in mesangial matrix and mesangial cellularity. However, the immunofluorescence and electron microscopy findings are similar to those described above for the category with essentially normal glomeruli. This type of morphology is also seen in about 10 to 20 percent of patients.[123] Clinically, a majority of patients have minimal abnormalities of urinalysis and usually normal renal function. However, a small number may develop renal insufficiency and moderate degree (0.1 to 2.5 g) of proteinuria.

Focal proliferative glomerulonephritis. Light microscopy in this type of renal lesion shows focal and segmental proliferation of mesangial and endothelial cells; focal areas of fibroid necrosis, neutrophil infiltration, and thickening of the basement membrane may also be present. Immunofluorescence microscopy shows granular staining for IgG, C3, C1q, and C4 and less often for IgM and IgA in the mesangium and some capillary loops. Electron microscopy shows mesangial and scattered subendothelial and subepithelial electron-dense deposits. This lesion also accounts for 10 to 20 percent of patients.[123]

Diffuse proliferative glomerulonephritis. The histologic changes in this form are severe and consist of diffuse proliferation of mesangial and endothelial cells involving all glomeruli (Fig. 8–17). There may also be proliferation of glomerular epithelial cells and fibroepithelial crescent formation which may affect more than 50 percent of glomeruli. Areas of fibrinoid necrosis associated with neutrophil cell infiltration within the glomeruli, known as *hematoxylin bodies,* may be present. The basement membranes are usually thickened and may show the characteristic eosinophilic "wire loop" lesion, which is the result of large, diffuse subendothelial deposits. Arteritis involving arterioles and interlobular arteries and thrombi in glomerular capillaries may also be observed. Immunofluorescence microscopy shows granular staining in the mesangium and along the capillary loops for IgG, C3, C4, and C1q and less often for IgA and IgM. Epithelial crescents usually stain positive for fibrin. The electron microscopy shows electron-dense deposits, predominantly in the mesangium and subendothelial areas, but some subepithelial deposits may also be seen. The subendothelial deposits are generally large and numerous. Most patients with diffuse proliferative lesions have one or more clinical features of clinically severe dis-

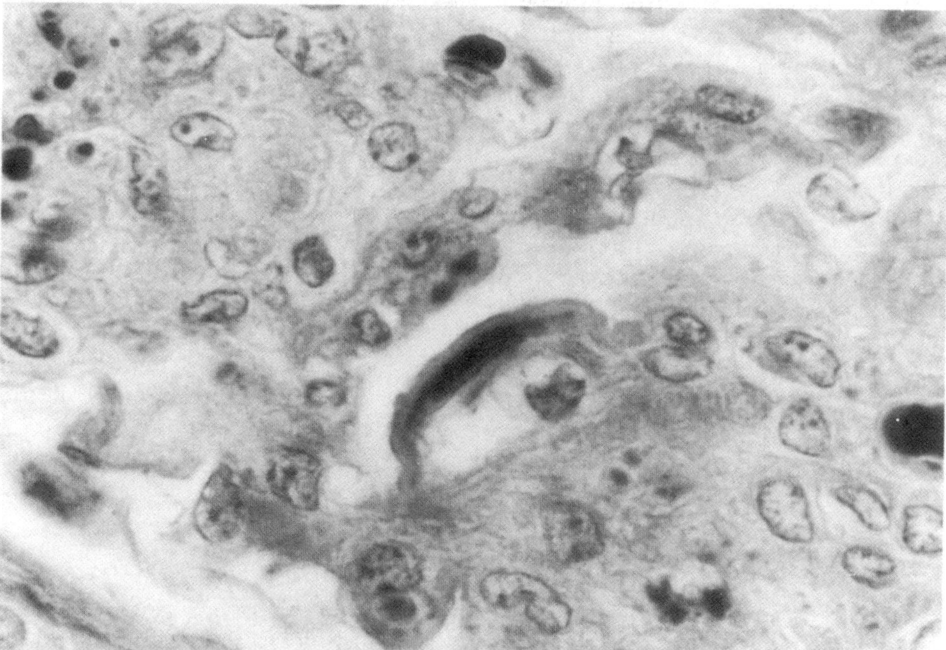

FIG. 8–17. Systemic lupus erythematosus. Light microscopy showing the characteristic wire loop lesion. (Courtesy of Dr. Howard Austin, National Institutes of Health, Bethesda, Maryland.)

ease (i.e., renal failure, nephrotic syndrome, nephritic urinalysis and hypertension). About 10 to 20 percent of children with lupus nephritis present with this type of lesion.[123]

Membranous glomerulonephritis. This lesion is seen in less than 10 percent of cases. On light microscopy the changes may appear similar to those seen in patients with the idiopathic membranous glomerulonephropathy or membranous glomerulonephropathy from other causes. The cellularity in the glomeruli is normal and there is a diffuse thickening of the glomerular basement membrane. The latter is best seen on Jones silver methenamine stain and will usually show the typical spikes. Immunofluorescence microscopy shows granular staining for IgG, C3, C1q, C4, etc., along the glomerular capillary loops. Electron microscopy shows electron-dense deposits in the subepithelial space, but occasional deposits are also seen in the mesangium and sometimes even in the subendothelial areas. All these patients have proteinuria and most of them develop nephrotic syndrome. Microscopic hematuria, hypertension, and mild renal failure may also occur.

Sclerosing glomerulonephritis. Sclerosing glomerulonephritis represents the end result of renal damage seen in lupus nephritis and consists of irreversible chronic changes. These morphologic characteristics include thickening of the mesangial matrix, glomerulosclerosis, tubular atrophy, vascular sclerosis, and interstitial fibrosis.

In addition to the distinct glomerular lesions described above, tubulointerstitial inflammation consisting of mononuclear cell infiltrate, interstitial edema, and thickening of the tubular basement membrane may be the predominant pathology in some cases.[295] Immunofluorescence microscopy in these cases reveals granular[305,306] or linear[285] staining for IgG along the tubular basement membrane. Similar lesions may also be seen along Bowman's capsule.[295] A frequent electron microscopy finding—common to all histologic types of lupus nephritis—is the presence of intraendothelial tubuloreticular structures which look like viral inclusions but may actually be interferon aggregates.[307] This finding is, however, not specific for lupus nephritis and may be seen in other connective tissue diseases.[307,308]

Transformation of one morphologic category of lupus nephritis into another is well known and can occur either spontaneously or following therapy.[308a] For example, the mesangial form may change into a diffuse proliferative lesion spontaneously with clinical worsening, and a diffuse proliferative glomerulonephritis can transform into the membranous or mesangial type following therapy.[309,310]

CLINICOPATHOLOGIC CORRELATION OF RENAL BIOPSY

In general, there is a good correlation between the extent and severity of histological changes on light microscopy and the clinical presentation at onset. Patients with normal urinalysis or minimal urinary abnormalities and no renal failure generally show normal glomeruli or a mesangial proliferative glomerulonephritic lesion. Patients presenting with clinical features of severe nephritis (i.e., nephritic urine, hypertension, and renal failure) will usually show a diffuse proliferative lesion. Patients presenting with nephrotic syndrome and minimal renal dysfunction and hypertension will usually show a membranous lesion. While nephrotic syndrome may also occur with a diffuse proliferative lesion, severe renal failure generally suggests a diffuse proliferative glomerulonephritis with or without crescents.

PATHOGENESIS

Systemic lupus erythematosus is an autoimmune disease in which many of the clinical findings result from the production of autoantibodies to a variety of tissue antigens. Of these, anti-double-stranded or native DNA (dsDNA) antibodies and anti-single-stranded DNA (ssDNA) antibodies have been prominently implicated in the pathogenesis of lupus nephritis. Both these antibodies have been eluted from the glomeruli of patients with lupus nephritis.[311] These eluted antibodies most likely originate from immune complexes present in the diseased glomeruli. The glomerular immune complexes may be formed in circulation from DNA and the anti-DNA antibodies, which are subsequently trapped in the glomeruli. The site of deposition of immune complexes within the glomeruli depends on the size and charge of the immune complexes.[312] Alternatively, these immune complexes may be formed in situ in the glomerulus by binding of circulating dDNA to various glomerular structures followed by binding of anti-dsDNA autoantibodies to dsDNA.[312,313] The in situ mechanism of glomerular immune complex formation may be more applicable to the pathogenesis of the membranous variety of lupus nephritis.[313] Both free DNA and autoantibody to DNA[314,315] and circulating complexes of DNA and anti-DNA antibody have been demonstrated in patients with lupus,[316] but the precise mechanism of glomerular immune complex formation remains poorly understood. Once the immune complexes are deposited or formed in the glomeruli, the complement system is activated. This system is believed, at least in part, to be responsible for the glomerular injury and development of nephritis. The deposition of the membrane attack components (C5b-9) of complement in the kidney correlates with glomerular injury and may be important in the genesis of damage.[317]

The exact cause of SLE is not known. Clearly, there are predisposing genetic factors, as suggested by a 63 percent concordance rate for SLE in identical twins,[318] enhanced incidence of HLA-DR3 and DR-2 genotypes in SLE patients,[319] association of SLE with genetic deficiency of C2 complement,[298] and the increased incidence of SLE and other autoimmune diseases in close relatives of patients with SLE.[320] Hormonal factors may play a role. This is suggested by an increased incidence of SLE in females, particularly in the pubertal and postpubertal age group. Interestingly, this feature is also seen in the animal model of SLE in NZB/W mice; additional evidence for hormonal influence is provided by the observation that administration of androgens to prepubertally castrated female NZB/W mice results in an improvement of SLE. Conversely, when estrogens are given to castrated male animals, SLE worsens and the severity approximates that in the normal female.[321] The mechanism of these hormones' influence in altering the susceptibility to SLE is not clear. A number of immunologic abnormalities have been described in SLE, at the very core of which lies hyperactive B-cell responsiveness. The latter probably results from a form of immune dysregulation.

MANAGEMENT

Management of SLE is dependent upon the severity of extrarenal and renal involvement and the activity of disease. Patients with severe extrarenal involvement generally improve rapidly with corticosteroids. Patients with mild extrarenal involvement may be initially treated with alternative drugs such as salicylates, antimalarials, and nonsteroidal anti-inflammatory agents.

Corticosteroids. The role of corticosteroids in improving the prognosis of patients with lupus nephritis has been known since the early sixties, and they have remained the mainstay of treatment in lupus nephritis.[321a] Corticosteroids may be used either alone or in conjunction with other cytotoxic and immunosuppressive agents.[322–326] Prednisone is generally started at a dosage of 60 mg/m^2/day (maximum 80 mg/day) and is continued until there is a clinical improvement of proteinuria, nephrotic syndrome, renal function, and urinalysis. Additionally, laboratory evidence for improvement in the disease activity—such as normalization of the serum complement and a decrease in the titer of anti-dsDNA antibodies—should also be present. This usually takes 4 to 6 weeks. The dose of corticosteroids can then be tapered gradually to a maintenance dose of nearly 5 to 10 mg/day (0.1 to 0.2 mg/kg, approximately) for an additional 4 to 6 weeks. If the disease activity remains under control, patients can be switched to an alternate-day single-morning-dose prednisone schedule. The goal should be to use the lowest possible dosage needed to control the disease activity. If a patient relapses, daily high-dose prednisone (60 mg/m^2/day) therapy is reinstituted.

In patients with severe lupus nephritis characterized by acute renal failure and with renal biopsy evidence of diffuse proliferative glomerulonephritis and epithelial crescents, intravenous methylprednisolone pulse therapy has been reported to be beneficial.[325] Prednisolone is given intravenously in a dose of 15 mg/kg as an infusion in 50 to 100 mL of 5% dextrose over a period of 30 to 60 min. Such treatments are continued daily for 3 to 6 days, followed by institution of oral prednisone in the dosages indicated above.

Cytotoxic Agents. Treatment with cytotoxic agents, particularly cytoxan, has been shown to increase the median survival of experimental animals with SLE (NZW × NZW,F_1 female mice).[326] Such a therapy has also been shown to be effective in reducing the morphologic progression of the renal disease and improving the outlook for maintaining renal function in human lupus nephritis.[322,323,326–327] Based on these findings, it has generally been recognized that cyclophosphamide may be used as an adjunct in the treatment of lupus nephritis. The circumstances in which cyclophosphamide should be considered in patients with lupus nephritis are less clear; traditionally, this agent has been recommended for patients with severe proliferative glomerulonephritis. Other circumstances where cyclophosphamide therapy may be considered in the treatment of lupus are (1) inability to control the disease activity with corticosteroids alone and (2) the appearance of serious side effects due to corticosteroids, where cyclophosphamide can be used as a steroid-sparing drug. While oral cyclophosphamide therapy has been shown to be effective, pulse cyclophosphamide is considered to be somewhat superior. Pulse cyclophosphamide therapy is administered as an intravenous bolus in the dose of 0.5 to 1.0 g/m^2. In this protocol, the drug is infused over an hour and the patient is kept well hydrated and asked to void frequently in order to reduce the risk of hemorrhagic cystitis. The protocol of cyclophosphamide used by Austin et al. had suggested the use of cyclophosphamide pulses every three months for a total duration of four years, or until at least 18 months of clinical remission of the renal disease.[322] Subsequent studies have reported success of intensive monthly pulse cyclophosphamide treatment for 6 to 12 months in achieving a similar effect on renal function in severe diffuse proliferative lupus nephritis.[326a,326b] In one of the recently reported studies in children, cyclophosphamide boluses given at monthly intervals for 12 months was able to significantly improve the clinical outcome of patients with severe or corticosteroid-nonresponsive lupus nephritis. The dose of cyclophosphamide used in this study was 500 mg/m^2 in the first month, 750 mg/m^2 in the second month, and 1 g/m^2 thereafter.[326b] The only criticism of these otherwise well-conducted studies remains that SLE being a chronic disease, short-term successes of therapy may not necessarily reflect the still unknown long-term prognosis or complications of the therapy. Well-known risks of cyclophosphamide therapy include bone marrow suppression, hemorrhagic cystitis, severe infections, gonadal toxicity, and an increased risk of malignancy in the future. This drug should therefore be used with great caution and the full knowledge of the child and parents.

Other Therapies. Since SLE is an antibody- and immune complex-mediated disease, plasmapheresis has been investigated as an adjunct in the treatment of lupus nephritis. However, a multicenter, randomized, prospective trial with plasmapheresis in diffuse proliferative lupus nephritis has not demonstrated any significant benefit of this treatment modality over conventional immunosuppressive therapy.[328]

SELECTING THE TREATMENT FOR LUPUS NEPHRITIS

The selection of the above-described therapeutic tools and the manner in which they should be used in treating patients with lupus nephritis requires an assessment of the severity, acuteness, and reversibility of the renal lesion and the overall activity of the disease. Focal and proliferative glomerulonephritis, necrosis, cellular crescents, leukocyte infiltration, and interstitial mononuclear cell infiltrate are considered to be acute, potentially responsive, reversible lesions. In contrast, chronic changes (i.e., glomerulosclerosis, tubular atrophy, and interstitial scarring) suggest a less favorable prognosis and irreversibility of the lesion. A patient with a mesangial proliferative lesion with clinical and laboratory evidence of minimal renal involvement (normal renal function, absence of nephrotic syndrome, normal urinalysis, or minimal urine abnormalities) and no laboratory evidence of active disease (normal serum complement, normal anti-DNA antibody titer, etc.) probably need not be given corticosteroids. However, this lesion can transform into a more aggressive diffuse proliferative lesion, and such patients should be closely monitored for signs of disease activity. The treatment of membranous lupus nephritis is unsettled and has ranged from no treatment to the use of alternate-day prednisone with or without cytotoxic drugs. If corticosteroids are used, a dose of 60 mg/m^2 every other day in a single morning dose may be used. Patients with diffuse proliferative glomerulonephritis require an aggressive management strategy which should include daily oral or pulse corticosteroid therapy. Based on currently available data, cytoxan should be considered as an adjunct in the treatment of these patients if they are unresponsive to conventional treatment or develop serious corticosteroid-induced toxicities.[326b,326c]

PROGNOSIS

The overall patient survival of SLE in one large series in children at 1 year was 90 percent, 85 percent at 10 years, and 77 percent at 15 years.[123] The usual causes of death are severe infection as a result of therapeutic interventions and severe central nervous system involvement by the disease. Renal failure is less common in patients with normal or mild mesangial proliferative glomerulonephritis on renal biopsy. On the other hand, diffuse or focal proliferative glomerulonephritis can progresses to renal failure.[328] In addition to the morphologic type of lesion seen on initial renal biopsy, the degree of chronic and irreversible changes (chronicity index) has also been shown to affect the outcome in lupus nephritis.[322] Those who develop end-stage renal failure will need dialysis and renal transplantation. Frequently, the disease "burns out" on dialysis, and patients can undergo renal transplant at this stage. Because of a presumed fear of recurrence of the disease in the transplanted kidney, it has been a common practice to withhold renal transplanation for 1 year after the initiation of dialysis in patients with ESRD due to lupus nephritis. However, in a recent study, duration of dialysis was reported not to affect outcome of transplantation.[328a] Allograft survival in these patients is comparable to that for other patients undergoing renal transplantation. Although recurrent lupus nephritis of the renal transplant has been reported,[328b] the incidence of this complication is low.[328a]

Case History 8–10. A 15-year-old white girl was admitted to the hospital for evaluation of a presumptive diagnosis of SLE. Two months prior to admission she developed pain and swelling of her fingers, which was followed in a few days by swelling of the ankles. She was treated for these complaints with acetaminophen at an outside clinic. In the next few days she developed swelling over her face and feet, a nasal ulcer was noted 2 weeks prior to admission, a malar rash was noted a week before admission, and a generalized rash 2 days prior to admission. Past history was noncontributory, but the family history was significant in that a 23-year-old brother was under treatment for SLE with renal involvement. On physical examination, the patient was alert and in no acute distress. Her blood pressure was 140/92 mmHg and temperature 99.4°F. Her pharynx was congested and she had petechiae on her palate but no oral ulcers. Other positive findings included a diffuse maculopapular rash involving the entire body, including the palms and soles, generalized edema, and swollen, tender finger joints and ankles. The rest of the physical examination was normal. Laboratory data: urinalysis—specific gravity, 1.022; protein, 3+; blood, +; RBCs, 5 to 10; WBCs, 10 to 25; and 10 to 25 granular casts in the sediment; blood counts—Hct, 38.7; WBCs, 4200/mm^3; differential WBC, normal; RBC morphology, normal; adequate platelets and erythrocyte sedimentation rate (ESR) 25 mm/h by the Wintrobe method; prothrombin time, 11 s; partial thromboplastin time, 25 s; serum electrolytes—sodium, 134 meq/L; potassium, 5.5 meq/L; chloride, 107 meq/L; bicarbonate, 22.4 meq/L; calcium, 7.4 mg/dL; phosphorus, 4.7 mg/dL; uric acid, 9.4 mg/dL; BUN, 39 mg/dL; creatinine, 1.2 mg/dL; total proteins, 5.1 g/dL; albumin, 2.4 g/dL; cholesterol, 297 mg/dL. C3 complement, 48.8 mg/dL (normal, 83 to 177); C4 complement, 11.8 mg/dL (normal, 15 to 45); direct Coombs test, positive: 24-h urine protein, 4.6 g; antinuclear antibody test, positive with a titer of 1:1280; anti-dsDNA antibody, 32.0 μg/mL (normal, less than 1.0). A renal biopsy was performed, yielding 23 glomeruli for study on light microscopy. There was diffuse proliferation of mesangial and endothelial cells, but no crescents were seen. The basement membrane was thickened, and occasional fragmented and karyorrhectic nuclei were seen in glomeruli. The interstitium showed mild edema and lymphocytic and plasma cell infiltration. The blood vessels and tubules were unremarkable. Immunofluorescence studies showed granular staining in the mesangium and capillary loops for IgG 4+, C1q 4+, C3 2+, C4+, IgA 3+, IgM 2+, and fibrin 1+. Electron microscopy showed prominent subendothelial deposits with obliteration of capillary loops. The endothelial cells were swollen and tubuloreticular myxoviruslike structures were present in several areas. The mesangial cells were hyperplastic, and many mesangial and occasional subepithelial electron-dense deposits were present. Foot processes of visceral epithelial cells were fused, and reactive hyperplasia of parietal epithelial cells was seen. Bowman's capsule and the tubular basement membrane were normal. A diagnosis of diffuse proliferative glomerulonephritis was made, and the patient was started on oral prednisone 20 mg three times a day. She gradually improved and was discharged 3 weeks later. Her clinical course is summarized in Table 8–19.

Comment. This young girl presented with mild renal failure, nephrotic syndrome, and an active urine sediment as a result of a diffuse proliferative lupus glomerulonephritis. She responded well to daily prednisone, which was gradually reduced to a maintenance dose of 7.5 to 10 mg/day (0.2 mg/kg/day). Although she initially became cushingoid, her appearance later on, while on low maintenance dose of prednisone, was essentially normal. She remained in remission for almost 5 years without any significant side effects. Apparently because she was doing so well, she stopped taking prednisone. She had not taken any medication for 4 to 6 months when she had

TABLE 8–19. Clinical Course of a Patient with Diffuse Proliferative SLE Nephritis (Case History 8–10)

		Urine			Serum Chemistry				
Time	BP	Protein	Blood	24-h Urine Protein, g	BUN, mg/dL	Cr, mg/dL	TP, g/dL	AL, g/dL	Choles-terol, mg/dL
onset	140/92	3+	1+	4.6	39	1.2	5.1	2.4	297
3 weeks	132/88	4+	2+	3.8	25	1.0	4.9	2.9	355
5 weeks	94/60	1+	1+	1.1	23	0.9	5.6	2.8	269
7 weeks	100/60	1+	1+		21	1.1	6.5	3.4	278
3 months	100/60	1+	1+	1.1	19	0.8	6.1	3.9	251
5 months	104/70	1+	3+		9	0.9			
6 months	100/60	1+	1+	0.15	7	0.9	6.5	4.2	247
7 months	100/60	0	tr		8	0.7	7.2	4.9	247
9 months	100/56	1+	0		13	0.8	6.8	4.5	217
1 years	100/60	—	—		11	0.8	6.8	4.8	219
2 years	96/55	—	—		10	0.7	6.8	4.4	175
3 years	110/64	—	tr		8	0.8	6.7	3.9	174
4 years	100/60	—	—		7	0.7			
5 years	108/52	1+	2+		8	0.7	6.5	4.2	

[a]Normal.

Note: BP = blood pressure, mmHg; BUN = blood urea nitrogen; Cr = creatinine; TP = total protein; AL = albumin; ANA = antinuclear antibody; C3 = C3 complement; C4 = C4 complement; ESR = erythrocyte sedimentation rate mm/H (Wintrobe method); P = prednisone; PRO = propranolol; PZ = prazosin; F = furosemide.

a flare-up of the disease and had to be restarted on a higher dose of prednisone. Her clinical course has been quite favorable so far, but not all patients with diffuse proliferative glomerulonephritis do so well.

HEMOLYTIC UREMIC SYNDROME

Hemolytic uremic syndrome (HUS) was first described by Gasser in 1955 as a distinct clinical syndrome characterized by microangiopathic anemia, thrombocytopenia, and acute renal failure that develops acutely in an otherwise healthy child.[329] It is one of the most common causes of acute renal failure in children under 2 to 3 years of age[330,331] and carried much mortality in the past.[332,333] However, with the advent of dialysis and better overall supportive care, the mortality rate is now perhaps less than 5 percent.[334] Many cases are sporadic, but miniepidemics[330,335] occur and the disease seems to be endemic in

Serology					Therapy				
ANA	Anti-DNA Antibody	C3, mg/dL	C4, mg/dL	ESR	P, mg/day	PRO, mg/day	PZ, mg/day	F, mg/day	Comment
1:1280	32	48.8	11.8	25	60	240	12	120	
		36.7	8.7	35	45	240	12	120	
1:160		63.1	15.6	42	30	120	8	80	
		94.3	16.2		30	120	8	80	
		91.8	13.3	37	30	120	8	80	
					20	120	8	40	
					Admitted for pyelonephritis				
	1.0	97.3	16.3	14	20	80	4	40	
	1.0	91	16.9	10	15	80	4	40	
	1.0	82.3	12.9	8	10	—	—	—	
	1.0	75.6	10.3		10	—	—	—	
	255	72.9	12.8		10	—	—	—	Appendectomy
		75.8	12.7		7.5	—	—	—	
	<1:10[a]	115	11.3		7.5	—	—	—	<1:10[a]
		68.1	8		40	—	—	—	Patient stopped prednisone on her own for nearly 6 months

Argentina.[332,333] Hemolytic uremic syndrome can also occur in older children and there is increased incidence of the disease in some families.[336] An increasing incidence of HUS in children has been noted in recent epidemiologic studies done in the United States.[337]

CLINICAL MANIFESTATIONS

Hemolytic uremic syndrome primarily affects infants and children under 3 years of age, although it can occur in the first month of life, in older children, and even in adults.[330–335,338–340] Boys and girls appear to be affected equally.[341] In typical cases there is a prodromal illness, usually gastroenteritis,[330–335,341] but cases have been reported following upper respiratory infections also.[341] The gastrointestinal symptoms include abdominal pain, vomiting, and diarrhea. The latter may be bloody and in severe cases may resemble ulcerative colitis. Patients may also present because of acute abdomen, which may be confused with appendicitis or intussusception. Cases of intestinal perforation and gangrenous bowel have also been reported.[339,342,343]

Symptoms pertaining to the central nervous system (CNS) are also frequently present and may include drowsiness, lethargy, irritability, seizures, cortical blindness, hemiparesis, and coma.[331,333,335,339,344,345] Initially, it was believed that the CNS symptoms were secondary to hypertension, fluid electrolyte disturbances, and uremia. While these factors may be contributory, it has now been well documented that HUS can involve the CNS.[344,345]

Oligoanuria is common at the time of initial presentation. Some patients may be dehydrated due to accompanying gastroenteritis, fever, and poor fluid intake. Other patients may be fluid-overloaded as a result of excessive intravenous fluids administered in the presence of oliguria and deteriorating renal function. Most patients with fluid overload are also hypertensive and may develop congestive heart failure. All patients are pale because of severe anemia, and some patients (15 to 30 percent) may also have jaundice.[335,339,341] Petechiae and ecchymoses are present in 30 to 40 percent of patients.[330–336,338–341] The abdomen is often tender, and bowel sounds may be either normal or infrequent and faint.

LABORATORY FINDINGS

The urinalysis shows hematuria, proteinuria, and cellular casts. All patients have microangiopathic anemia and show typical fragmented and helmet red blood cells on peripheral blood smear (Fig. 8–18). The platelets are diminished in the smear and the absolute counts may go down as low as 5000 to 10,000/ mm^3. Occasionally patients may have a normal platelet count at onset or develop thrombocytopenia only transiently.[339] Reticulocyte count is elevated in established patients due to continued intravascular hemolysis.

Other laboratory findings include normal prothrombin and partial thromboplastin time, negative direct and indirect Coombs' tests, low haptoglobin, high indirect bilirubin, and high plasma lactate dehydrogenase (LDH). Laboratory evidence of acute renal failure—such as elevted BUN and serum creatinine concentrations, hyperkalemia, hypocalcemia, hyperphosphatemia, hyperuricemia, and metabolic acidosis—may be present. The degree of renal failure is variable, from slight elevation of serum creatinine to oligoanuria. Hypocomplementemia may be seen rarely, but its genesis and significance are not clear.[346,347]

PATHOLOGY

The main sites of pathology in the kidney are the glomerular capillaries, arterioles, and small interlobular arteries.[338] The early renal lesion is characterized by platelet and fibrin thrombi in these structures, which may lead to acute cortical necrosis in severe cases.[338] Later in the course of the disease, endothelial cell swelling, separation of the endothelial cell from the basement membrane, and increased mesangial matrix are commonly observed. Separation of the endothelial cell from the underlying basement membrane is better appreciated by electron microscopy, which also shows that the newly created subendothelial space contains a "fluffy" and fibrillar electron-lucent and electron-dense material, fragments of platelets, and parts of mesangial cell extensions.[338,348] Fibrin deposition in these lesions is best revealed by immunofluorescence examination, which may also demonstrate staining for C3 and IgM.[349]

Glomerular capillary lesions are more common in young children, while arteriolar and arterial lesions are more common in older children. The latter are

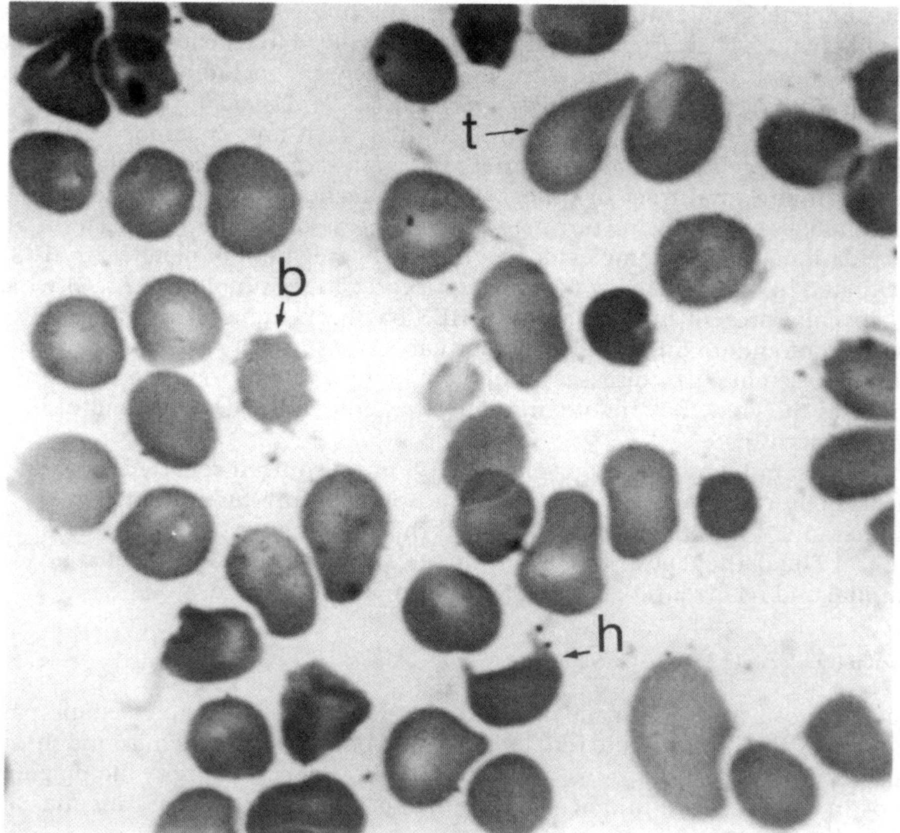

FIG. 8–18. **Hemolytic uremic syndrome. Peripheral smear showing burr red cells (b), helmet-shaped red cells (h), and tear drop red cells (t).**

usually associated with hypertension and poor prognosis for a complete recovery.[338,350]

PATHOGENESIS

The exact pathogenesis of HUS is not known. Thrombocytopenia and the presence of platelets and fibrin in thrombi in glomerular capillaries strongly suggest that there is aggregation and consumption of platelets and local activation of coagulation in the glomerular capillaries and arterioles. Less commonly, similar lesions can be seen in brain, colon, pancreas, heart, lung, and adrenals.[332,333,338,350,351] It must be noted that although there is evidence of coagulopathy within the glomerular capillaries, evidence of disseminated intravascular coagulopathy (DIC) is lacking. Laboratory findings of DIC—such as low levels of fibrinogen, factors V and VIII, and prolonged prothrombin and partial thromboplastin time—are absent in HUS.

What triggers the aggregation of platelet and the local coagulation in HUS is not completely understood. Since HUS usually follows an infectionlike illness, it is likely that a bacterial or viral product is involved in its pathogenesis. It has been reported in association with several infections, including verotoxin-producing *Escherichia coli,*[352] *Shigella,*[353] *Salmonella,*[354] *Yersinia,*[355] *Campylobacter,*[356] enteroviruses[357] involving the gastrointestinal tract, and pneumococcal pneumonia.[358] It is believed that a bacterial toxin gains access to the circulation from the gastrointestinal tract or other areas of infection and injures the vascular endothelial cells. This, in turn, starts the process of platelet aggregation and coagulation. There is some evidence that the aggregation of platelets in HUS is facilitated by the deficiency of a platelet aggregation inhibitor (an IgG) which is normally present in circulation.[359] HUS has been induced in rabbits by the infusion of endotoxin, and the glomerular lesions in this experimental model closely resemble the disease in human beings.[360] This observation further endorses the view that endotoxins play a key role in the development of infection-induced HUS.

Apart from being infection-related, HUS has also been reported to occur in diverse clinical settings such as renal transplantation,[361] use of anticancer chemotherapy,[362] the ingestion of toxins,[363] rhabdomyolysis,[364] and Kawasaki disease.[365] The pathogenesis of HUS in these conditions remains speculative. The familial and recurrent form of HUS has also been described.[366]

DIAGNOSIS AND MANAGEMENT

The diagnosis of HUS is made on the basis of a typical clinical presentation and laboratory findings of acute renal failure, microangiopathic anemia, and thrombocytopenia. Renal biopsy is not necessary in order to confirm the diagnosis and in fact is contraindicated in the presence of severe anemia and thrombocytopenia.

Most children recover spontaneously with appropriate supportive care and management of acute renal failure. This includes strict adherence to fluid balance, management of hypertension, and management of other complications such as hyperkalemia. If the patient is anuric or severely oliguric, peritoneal dialysis should be instituted. Although a variety of other therapeutic modalities have been used in the management of severe HUS, their value remains unproved. Included in these modalities are infusion of fresh frozen plasma,[367] plasma exchange,[368] infusion of prostacyclin,[369] administration of aspirin and dipyridamole,[370] and administration of heparin and streptokinase.[335,339,371]

OUTCOME

Nearly 20 percent of patients recovering from HUS in a study from Argentina have been reported to develop chronic renal failure, and hypertension was noted in 33 percent of such cases during prolonged follow-up.[333] In an analysis of 258 children from western Europe, acute mortality of the disease has been noted to be 9 percent; progression to end-stage renal failure occurred in a further 9 percent.[372] On the other hand, O'Regan et al observed a decrease in GFR in 30 percent of Canadian children with HUS who were followed for 6 to 11 years.[373] Debate about the clinical or laboratory parameters that are predictive of prognosis in HUS is unresolved. Prolonged anuria (>2 weeks),[374] and involvement of multiple organs—such as nervous system, gastrointestinal system, and pancreas (diabetes mellitus)—are indicators of severe disease and are often associated with a poor outcome.[344,351,375] Relationship of age at onset to prognosis is less well established. While some studies have suggested that progression to end-stage renal failure is common in older children,[376] others have not been able to substantiate this observation.[375] Children developing end-stage renal failrue as a result of HUS can undergo renal transplantation, but recurrence of the disease in the transplanted kidney has been reported in several cases.[377]

Case History 8–11. A 3-year-old white girl was transferred from another hospital to the university hospital for the management of acute renal failure. She was well 6 days prior to admission, when she developed watery, yellow diarrhea and a low-grade fever. In the 4 days prior to admission, the mother had noticed streaks of bright red blood in the child's diarrheal stools and she took the patient to her pediatrician. A stool culture was obtained and sulfamethoxazole/trimethoprim was prescribed. However, the patient started to experience vomiting and was not able to take the medicine. The patient was also fussy and sleeping more than usual, and the mother noticed that she was pale and had puffy eyes. She was readmitted by her pediatrician to the hospital, where initial laboratory tests showed the following: Hct, 36 percent; platelets, 78,000/mm^3; BUN, 48 mg/dL; and creatinine, 2.1 mg/dL. Follow-up labs on the second day showed HCT, 26.8 percent; platelets, 41,000/mm^3; BUN, 60 mg/dL; and creatinine, 3.1 mg/dL. The urinalysis showed 3+ blood, 4+ protein, and 0 to 5 coarse granular casts per HPF in the sediment. She passed small amounts of urine twice in the hospital. Past and family history were not contributory except that patient's 15-month-old brother had also had similar diarrhea and vomiting a week earlier but was now well.

The patient's physical examination on admission to the nephrology service showed that she was alert and oriented, but she appeared pale. Her temperature was 99.4°F, pulse 144/min, and blood pressure 120/84 mmHg. She had puffiness over her eyes and pitting edema on both feet. There were multiple petechiae on the dorsa of both feet. Her abdomen was soft but diffusely tender; however, no rebound tenderness was noted. Bowel sounds were normal. The liver was palpable 3 cm below the right costal margin. The rest of the physical examination was normal. Laboratory tests showed the following: HCT, 26 percent; platelets, 20,000/mL, WBC count, 12,700; differential, 68 percent neutrophils, 18 percent bands, 12 percent lymphocytes, and 2 percent monocytes. The peripheral smear showed many fragmented and helmet red blood cells. Reticulocyte count, 1.5 percent; BUN, 75 mg/dL; serum creatinine, 3.6 mg/dL; serum sodium, 131 meq/L; potassium, 4.8 meq/L; chloride, 99 meq/L; CO_2, 20 meq/L; calcium, 8.4 mg/dL; phosphorus, 5 mg/dL; total proteins, 5.0 g/dL; albumin 2.9 g/dL; total bilirubin, 1.5 mg/dL; SGOT, 175 units; SGPT, 126 units; LDH, 3190 units; cholesterol 166 mg/dL; and triglycerides, 328 mg/dL. Prothrombin time and partial thromboplastin time were normal. The stool

TABLE 8–20. Clinical Course of a Child with Hemolytic Uremic Syndrome (Case History 8–11)

Time	Urine Output, mL/day	Urinalysis Protein	Urinalysis Blood	Serum Chemistries BUN, mg/dL	Serum Chemistries Cr, mg/dL	Serum Chemistries Total Bilirubin, mg/dL	Serum Chemistries LDH, Units/L	Blood Counts Hct, %	Blood Counts Platelets, 1 × 1000	Blood Counts Retic, %	Helmet Cells	Comments
Day	>100	4+	3+	48	2.1			36	78			
2 A.M.	Minimal	4+	3+	60	3.1			26.8	41			
2 P.M.	7			75	3.6	1.5	3190	26	20			
3	0			93	5.5	1.0	3310	24.3	108	1.5	+	Dialysis started
4	0			108	6.3	1.0	3750	19.3	30	3.1		
5	0			91	6.4	1.9	4010	15.3	18	7.1	+	Gallop rhythm; blood transfusion
6	420	Tea-colored		87	5.6	2.2	4950	21.7	5	2.9	+	Platelet transfusion
7	0			76	6.2	1.7	2890	17.6	16	6.8	+	
8	330			66	5.7	1.0	1995	15.3	138	9.8	+	
9	330			59	5.0	0.7	1571	14.5	147	13.7	+	
10	660			57	4.3	0.4	989	13.5	212	15.7	+	
11	505	+	+	51	3.4	0.3	899	14.9	342	16.3	+	
12	430	+	+	44	2.7	0.2	686	13.9	403	12.5	+	
13	375			41	2.2	0.2	522	14.1	446	12.1	+	
14	600			38	1.8	0.5	549	16.1	597	10.6	+	
15	300			37	1.7	0.4	465	17.9	676	8.6	+	
16	605			43	1.3	0.3	375	18.4	726	8.1	+	Dialysis discontinued
17	737	Tr	—									Patient discharged
23		—	—	10	0.6	0.4	283	21.1	253		+	Blood pressure 90/60 mmHg
43		—	—	10	0.5							

Note: BUN = blood urea nitrogen; Cr = creatinine; LDH = lactate dehydrogenase, units/L; Retic = reticulocyte; + = positive; — = negative.

culture revealed no pathogens and a rotazyme antigen test was negative. The patient was essentially anuric, and peritoneal dialysis with an indwelling catheter was begun. The clinical course is summarized in Table 8–20.

Comment. The clinical course of this patient is quite typical for HUS in the United States. She made a complete recovery with supportive care and her renal functions recovered completely. Her fluid balance was closely monitored and peritoneal dialysis was started early, as soon as she became oliguric.

Blood transfusions to correct anemia are frequently necessary in patients with HUS (as in this case); such decisions are made on clinical grounds. On the other hand, platelet transfusions[378] have been reported to lead to further coagulopathy and rapid deterioration of neurologic functions and should be avoided.[366,367] Use of anticoagulants and antiplatelet agents has not been found to be of any benefit either.[379,379a]

RAPIDLY PROGRESSIVE GLOMERULONEPHRITIS

The term *rapidly progressive glomerulonephritis* (RPGN), a clinicopathologic entity, is used to describe patients who present with rapidly deteriorating renal function along with diffuse glomerular epithelial crescent formation in their renal biopsies. This clinical and morphologic picture can be seen with a variety of known, well-defined glomerular diseases or may be due to a glomerular disease that does not fit into these morphologic groups and is thus referred to as idiopathic RPGN. The glomerular lesion of RPGN is also sometimes referred to as *crescentic glomerulonephritis.*

CLASSIFICATION

Based on immunofluorescence findings of the renal biopsy, RPGN may be classified into three groups (Table 8–21). The first group is characterized by a linear pattern of immune staining of the glomerular basement membrane (type I), the second group is associated with granular immune deposits along the glomerular basement membrane (type II), and in the third group glomerular immune deposits are absent (type III). RPGN in children is commonly due to one of the following etiologies: poststreptococcal glomerulonephritis, lupus nephritis, HSP purpura nephritis, and the idiopathic variety.

PATHOLOGY

The morphologic hallmark of RPGN is the finding of glomerular epithelial crescents on light microscopy (Fig. 8–19). In an adequate renal biopsy, involvement of more than 60 percent of glomeruli by epithelial crescents is considered as an essential component of the definition of RPGN. The crescents usually fill Bowman's space and encircle the glomerular tuft completely or partially. It appears that both the endogenous proliferating glomerular epithelial cells[384] (visceral and parietal lining of Bowman's capsule) and exogenous infiltrating

TABLE 8–21. Clinicopathologic Classification of Rapidly Progressive Glomerulonephritis

Antiglomerular basement membrane antibody–mediated
- Antiglomerular basement membrane antibody associated with lung hemorrhage (Goodpasture syndrome) or without lung hemorrhage

Immune complex–mediated
- Primary
  - Membranoproliferative glomerulonephritis
  - IgA nephropathy
  - Membranous
  - Idiopathic
- Secondary
  - Infection-related poststreptococcal
    - Shunt nephritis
    - Subacute bacterial endocarditis
    - Others
  - Associated with multisystem disease
    - Lupus nephritis
    - Henoch-Schönlein purpura
    - Other vasculitides[a]—polyarteritis, Wagner's granulomatosis, etc.
    - Mixed cryoglobulinemia

Not immune complex–mediated
- Idiopathic
- Vasculitides[a]—polyarteritis, Wagner's granulomatosis, etc.

[a]Vasculitides may be seen with or without staining.[380–383]

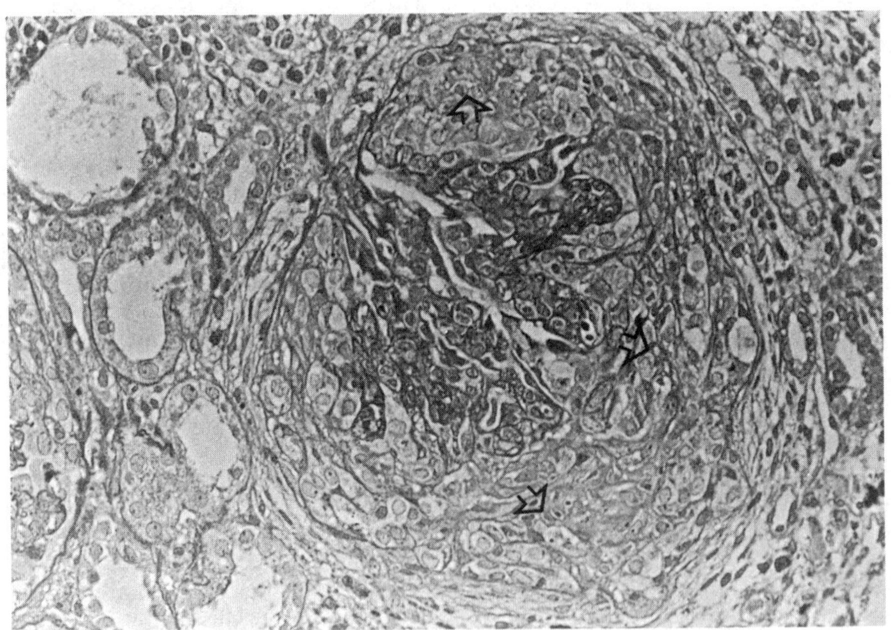

FIG. 8–19. Rapidly progressive glomerulonephritis. Light microscopy showing epithelial crescent *(arrows)*.

macrophages[385] contribute to the cellularity of the epithelial crescents. The glomerular capillaries are compressed and their lumens closed. Other changes in the glomerulus depend on the underlying condition. For example, mesangial proliferation with neutrophil infiltration may be seen in poststreptococcal glomerulonephritis. In the idiopathic variety of RPGN, there may be minimal or no proliferation of mesangial or endothelial cells. Depending upon the severity and the time course when the renal biopsy was performed, there are usually varying grades of interstitial inflammation and tubular dilation. In later stages, the glomerular crescents become fibrotic and eventually hyalinize, and there is more tubular atrophy and interstitial fibrosis.

The immunofluorescence findings, as alluded to earlier, fall into three categories. In the RPGN induced by antiglomerular basement membrane antibody, a smooth, linear staining is seen all along the glomerular basement membrane for IgG and less often for C3. A similar staining may also be seen along the tubular basement membrane. In patients with Goodpasture syndrome, the linear staining is also present along the alveolar basement membrane in the lung. On the other hand, immune complex-mediated RPGN granular staining for IgG and C3 is seen along the capillary loops and in the mesangium. In the third type of RPGN, the immunofluorescence staining for immunoglobulins and complement is negative. However, staining for fibrin in the crescents is seen in all cases of RPGN.

Electron microscopy corroborates the immunofluorescence findings. It may show mesangial, subendothelial, or subepithelial deposits in patients who on immunofluorescence show granular staining for IgG and C3 or may show no deposits in the group that had negative immunofluorescence. Breaks or gaps in the glomerular basement membrane may be present in patients with RPGN and are best appreciated by scanning electron microscopy.[386]

PATHOGENESIS

The origin of epithelial cell crescents is not fully understood. It has been well known that disruptions, or "gaps", in the glomerular basement membrane are common in patients with RPGN.[386] Experimental work suggests that these gaps may be caused by antiglomerular basement membrane antibody,[386–389] activated terminal (membrane attack) components of complement,[390] proteases released by neutrophils,[391] reactive oxygen species, generation of procoagulant by macrophages, and by T cells.[392–395] It appears that plasma, including fibrinogen and other blood cells (especially macrophages), leaks through these gaps and leads to the formation of fibrin and crescents in Bowman's space.[393]

CLINICAL MANIFESTATIONS AND DIAGNOSIS

Since secondary etiologies of RPGN are more common than the idiopathic variety in children, the clinical presentation is dependent upon the underlying glomerular disease. The common underlying conditions associated with RPGN are poststreptococcal glomerulonephritis, lupus nephritis, Henoch-Schönlein purpura nephritis, and membranoproliferative glomerulonephritis. The presentation of these is discussed in detail elsewhere in this chapter. Generally, RPGN

TABLE 8–22. Laboratory Evaluation of Patients with Rapidly Progressive Glomerulonephritis

History
- Recent sore throat, impetigo, symptomatology of Henoch-Schönlein purpura, lupus erythematosus, vasculitis, hemoptysis, etc.

Physical examination
- Hypertension, edema, impetigo lesions, signs of Henoch-Schönlein purpura, lupus erythematosus, etc.

Laboratory
- Urinalysis—proteinuria, hematuria, and cellular casts
- Throat culture—group A beta-hemolytic streptococcus
- Chest x-ray—lung hemorrhage, fluid overload
- Serum chemistries—electrolytes, Ca, P, BUN, creatinine, total proteins, albumin, cholesterol
- Serology—CH50, C3, C4, antinuclear antibody, antibodies to streptococcal proteins (ASO, anti DNase B, antihyaluronidase, streptozyme)
- Antiglomerular basement membrane antibodies (Goodpasture syndrome)
- Antineutrophil cytoplasmic antibodies (vasculitides)
- Renal biopsy

complicating any of these conditions presents with an acute nephritic onset which may consist of gross hematuria, edema, and oliguria. Hypertension is frequently present and urinalysis shows the typical findings of hematuria, proteinuria, and cellular casts. Laboratory evidence of deteriorating renal function is present, and patients may also have features of nephrotic syndrome such as hypoalbuminemia and hypercholesterolemia. A history of a recent upper respiratory infection is not uncommon, and of course arthralgia, rash and other features of HSP or SLE may be present in patients whose RPGN is the result of these conditions. Table 8–22 lists the laboratory tests that are of help in evaluating patients with RPGN.

MANAGEMENT

Management of patients with acute renal failure, fluid overload, and hypertension associated with RPGN is similar to that of other patients with these complications in other clinical circumstances. This is discussed in the chapter on acute renal failure.

If RPGN in a child is due to poststreptococcal glomerulonephritis, the prognosis for complete recovery is generally good. [384,396,397] These children should be given supportive care; use of corticosteroids or other immunosuppressive drugs or anticoagulants is not indicated.

The treatment of all other forms of RPGN is controversial at present. Although in adults various modes of therapy (including plasma exchange, oral corticosteroids, pulse therapy with large intravenous boluses of methylprednisolone, immunosuppressvie agents such as cyclophosphamide and azathioprine, and anticoagulants, etc.) have been used, large, randomized, well-controlled trials have not been performed and no consensus for definitive recommendations has emerged.[398] Until this happens, it may be appropriate to take the following approach.

Patients with Goodpasture syndrome may be treated with plasma exchange and immunosuppression with oral prednisone, cyclophosphamide, and azathioprine.[387] Plasma exchange (approximately equal to 1.5 to 2 times the normal plasma volume) is performed initially every day and continued for 2 weeks or longer, while the serum is monitored for levels of antiglomerular basement membrane antibody. The goal should be to reduce the level of antibody quickly to the lowest possible level. Prednisone is given orally, 1 to 2 mg/kg/day (maximum 60 mg/day), along with cyclophosphamide, 1 to 2 mg/kg/day, and azathioprine, 1 mg/kg/day. Immunosuppression with cyclophosphamide and prednisone is continued for 8 weeks, when cyclophosphamide is discontinued and prednisone tapered gradually.[399,400] The response to this therapy depends upon the severity of the disease when treatment is begun. Significant improvement has been reported in over 80 percent of patients whose serum creatinine is less than 6.5 mg/dL. If serum creatinine is >8 mg/dL and the patient is oliguric and already on dialysis, there is rarely any response.[399,400]

Patients with the idiopathic variety of RPGN may be treated with plasma exchange and immunosuppressive drugs as above, along with corticosteroid pulse therapy.[74,398,401] The latter consists of intravenous administration of methylprednisolone, 15 mg/kg, diluted in 50 to 100 mL of 5% dextrose and given over 30 to 60 min. These boluses are repeated daily for 3 to 6 days, along with the concomitant administration of oral prednisone, 1 to 2 mg/kg/day (maximum 80 mg/day), which is gradually tapered over months. Nearly 50 to 70 percent of such patients respond to pulse therapy, including some patients with oliguria and on dialysis.[74,398,402] The management of RPGN associated with other well-defined glomerular lesions (HSP, lupus nephritis, membranoproliferative glomerulonephritis) is discussed in the management of those entities.

Case History 8–12. An 11-year-old white girl was admitted to the hospital with a 1-day history of passing dark brown urine. She was in good health until a month prior to admission, when she started to have intermittent nausea and vomiting, myalgias, arthralgias, epistaxis, facial swelling, and bruises over the left ankle with swelling. She was seen by various physicians and given suppositories to control her vomiting as well as antibiotics (Augmentin). The parents told of increased lethargy and fatigue in the patient for the preceding month. She also had a sore throat a month prior to admission. Family and past history were noncontributory. On physical examination, the patient's temperature was 97.8°F, BP 120/80 mmHg, and pulse 112/min. Her height was between the 25–50th percentile and weight between the 50–75th percentile. She had minimal facial edema and appeared pale. Her calves were tender and she had old bruises over her knees. The rest of the physical examination was normal.

The laboratory data were as follows: urinalysis—specific gravity, 1.017; protein, 4+; blood, 4+; glucose, +; many RBCs; 1 to 4 WBCs; 5 to 9 granular casts in the sediment; 24-h urine protein of 4.8 g; Hct, 23; WBC count, 9500; neutrophils, 66 percent, lymphocytes, 23 percent; monocytes, 4 percent; basophils, 2 percent; eosinophils, 5 percent; adequate platelets; erythrocyte sedimentation rate (ESR), 123 mm; normal prothrombin and partial thromboplastin time but prolonged bleeding time (>15 min); serum chemistries—sodium, 142 meq/L; potassium, 4.5 meq/L; chloride, 99 meq/L; CO_2, 23 meq/L; glucose, 106 mg/dL; BUN, 120 mg/dL; creatinine, 11.6

mg/dL; calcium, 7 mg/dL; phosphorus, 10.2 mg/dL; uric acid, 6.3 mg/dL; total proteins, 6.7 g/dL; albumin, 2.7 g/dL; cholesterol, 136 mg/dL; serum complement C3, 102 mg/dL; C4, 20 mg/dL; cryoglobulin, negative; Coombs' test, negative; ASO titer, 800 Todd units; antinuclear antibody and DNA antibody tests, negative; hepatitis B surface antigen, negative; rheumatoid factor, negative; anti-DNase B titer, >1360; antiglomerular basement membrane antibody and antineutrophil cytoplasmic antibody tests by ELISA, negative. An abdominal sonogram revealed normal-size kidneys. With supportive care, her renal function improved, with gradual decrease of BUN and serum creatinine. On days 4, 7, and 10 posthospitalization, the serum creatinine values were 8.1, 6.4, and 5.1 mg/dL, respectively. However, she continued to have 4+ proteinuria and hematuria and remained edematous. After 10 days, her creatinine started to rise again; it was 5.8 mg on day 18. A percutaneous renal biopsy was performed, making 12 glomeruli available for study on light microscopy. All of these showed fibroepithelial crescents. Evidence of severe sclerosis was present in all glomeruli as well as in crescents. Silver stain showed increase in mesangial matrix, but the basement membrane was of normal thickness. An occasional neutrophil was seen in the glomeruli. A moderate degree of inflammatory cell infiltrate composed of neutrophils and lymphocytes was present in the edematous interstitium. The interstitium also showed fibrosis. The blood vessels were normal. The immunofluorescence studies were essentially negative, and no electron-dense deposits were seen on electron microscopy. A diagnosis of idiopathic, rapidly progressive glomerulonephritis was made, and she was started on methylprednisolone pulse therapy. She received 6 daily doses of 1 g intravenous methylprednisolone along with 40 mg of oral prednisone daily in 4 divided doses. The daily oral prednisone was continued for another 4 weeks at the same dosage and then gradually reduced. On the day pulse therapy was started, her serum creatinine was 5.6 mg/dL; on day 7, it was 4.7 mg/dL; and on day 12, it was 3.5 mg/dL. The serum creatinine stabilized at this level for 2 to 3 weeks, but it started to rise again and she was started on chronic dialysis. During prednisone therapy she became hypertensive and required furosemide 40 to 80 mg twice a day as well as various antihypertensive drugs (nifedipine, hydralazine, propranolol, etc.) to control blood pressure.

Comment. Based on the classification outlined in Table 8–21, this patient fits into the idiopathic variety of RPGN because the immunofluorescence studies were negative and there was no laboratory or histologic evidence of primary or secondary glomerular diseases. Because of the advanced glomerular damage, her ultimate outcome was poor.

REFERENCES

1. Alport AC: Hereditary familial congenital haemorrhagic nephritis. *Br Med J* 1:504, 1927.

2. Broyer M: Frequence et causes de l'insufficance renale chez l'enfant. In P Royer, R Habib, H Mathieu, M Broyer (eds): *Nephrologie Pediatrique.* Paris, Flammarion Medecine-Sciences, 1983, p 425.
3. Milliner DS, Pierides AN, Holley KE: Renal transplantation in Alport's syndrome: Anti-glomerular basement membrane glomerulonephritis in the allograft. *Mayo Clin Proc* 57:35, 1982.
4. Trachtman H, Weiss RA, Bennett B, et al: Isolated hematuria in children: Indications for a renal biopsy. *Kidney Int* 25:94, 1984.
5. Spear GS, Slusser RJ: Alport's syndrome: Emphasizing electron microscopic studies of the glomerulus. *Am J Pathol* 69:213, 1972.
6. Hinglais N, Grunfeld J-P, Bois LE: Characteristic ultrastructural lesion of the glomerular basement membrane in progressive hereditary nephritis (Alport's syndrome). *Lab Invest* 27:473, 1972.
7. Churg J, Sherman RL: Pathologic characteristics of hereditary nephritis. *Arch Pathol* 95:374, 1973.
8. Yoshikawa N, White RHR, Cameron AH: Familial hematuria: Clinico-pathological correlations. *Clin Nephrol* 17:172, 1982.
9. Rumpelt HJ: Hereditary nephropathy (Alport syndrome): Correlation of clinical data with glomerular basement membrane alterations. *Clin Nephrol* 13:203, 1980.
10. Gubler M, Levy M, Broyer M, et al: Alport's syndrome. *Am J Med* 70:493, 1981.
11. Habib R, Gubler MC, Hinglais N, et al: Alport's syndrome: Experience at Hôpital Necker. *Kidney Int* 21:S20, 1982.
12. Feingold J, Bois E, Chompret A, et al: Genetic heterogeneity of Alport syndrome. *Kidney Int* 27:672, 1985.
13. Evans SH, Erickson RP, Kelsch R, et al: Apparently changing patterns of inheritance in Alport's hereditary nephritis: Genetic heterogeneity versus altered diagnostic criteria. *Clin Genet* 17:285, 1980.
14. Atkin CL, Hasstedt SJ, Menlove L, et al: Mapping of Alport syndrome to the long arm of the X chromosome. *Am J Hum Genet* 42:249, 1988.
15. Brunner H, Schröder C, Van Bennekom C, et al: Localization of the gene for X-linked Alport's syndrome. *Kidney Int* 34:507, 1988.
16. Flinter FA, Abbs S, Bobrow M: Localization of the gene for classic Alport syndrome. *Genomics* 4:335, 1989.
17. Olson DL, Anand SK, Landing BH, et al: Diagnosis of hereditary nephritis by failure of glomeruli to bind anti-glomerular basement membrane antibodies. *J Pediatr* 96:697, 1980.
18. McCoy RC, Johnson HK, Stone WJ, et al: Absence of nephritogenic GBM antigen(s) in some patients with hereditary nephritis. *Kidney Int* 21:642, 1982.
19. Querin S, Noel LH, Grunfeld JP, et al: Linear glomerular IgG fixation in renal allografts: Incidence and significance in Alport's syndrome. *Clin Nephrol* 25:134, 1986.
20. Weislander J, Barr JF, Butkowski RJ, et al: Goodpasture's antigen of the glomerular basement membrane: Localization to noncollagenous regions of type IV collagen. *Proc Nat Acad Sci* 81:3838, 1984.
21. Kleppel MM, Kashtan CE, Butkowski RJ, et al: Alport familial nephritis. Absence of 28 ki-lodalton noncollagenous monomers of type IV collagen in glomerular basement membrane. *J Clin Invest* 80:263, 1987.
22. Antonovych TT, Deasy PF, Tina LU, et al: Hereditary nephritis: Early clinical, functional, and morphological studies. *Pediatr Res* 3:545, 1969.
23. Tishler PV: Healthy female carriers of a gene for the Alport syndrome: Importance for genetic counseling. *Clin Genet* 16:291, 1979.

24. Feingold J, Bois E, Chompret A, et al: Genetic heterogeneity of Alport syndrome. *Kidney Int* 27:672, 1985.
25. Grünfeld J-P, Noel NH, Hafez S, et al: Renal prognosis in women with hereditary nephritis. *Clin Nephrol* 23:267, 1985.
26. Grünfeld, J-P: The clinical spectrum of hereditary nephritis. *Kidney Int* 27:83, 1985.
27. Jordan B, Nowlin J, Remmers A Jr, et al: Renal transplantation and hearing loss in Alport's syndrome. *Transplantation* 38:308, 1984.
28. Hallman N, Hjelt L, Ahvenainen EK: Nephrotic syndrome in newborn and young infants. *Annu Paediatr Fenniae* 2:227, 1956.
29. Hallman N, Hjelt L: Congenital nephrotic syndrome. *J Pediatr* 55:152, 1959.
30. Hallman N, Norio R, Rapola J: Congenital nephrotic syndrome. *Nephron* 11:101, 1973.
31. Norio R: Heredity in the congenital nephrotic syndrome: A genetic study of 57 Finnish families with a review of reported cases. *Annu Paediatr Fenniae* 20:(suppl 27)1, 1966.
32. Kendall-Smith P, Pullon DHH, Tomlinson BE. Congenital nephrotic syndrome in Maori siblings. *NZ Med J* 6:156, 1968.
33. Huttunen NP: Congenital nephrotic syndrome of Finnish type: Study of 75 patients. *Arch Dis Child* 41:344, 1976.
34. Morgan G, Postlethwaite RJ, Lendon M, et al: Postural deformities in congenital nephrotic syndrome. *Arch Dis Child* 56:959, 1981.
35. Harris HW Jr, Umetsu D, Geha R, et al: Altered immunoglobulin status in congenital nephrotic syndrome. *Clin Nephrol* 25:308, 1986.
36. McLean RH, Forsgren A, Bjorksten B: Decreased serum factor B concentration associated with decreased opsonization of *Escherichia coli* in the idiopathic nephrotic syndrome. *Pediatr Res* 11:910, 1977.
37. McLean RH, Kennedy TL, Rosoulpour M, et al: Hypothyroidism in the congenital nephrotic syndrome. *J Pediatr* 101:72, 1982.
38. Martul EV, Cuesta MG, Churg I. Histologic variability of congenital nephrotic syndrome. *Clin Nephrol* 28:161, 1987.
39. Habib R, Bois E: Heterogeneite de syndromes nephrotiques a debut precoce du nourrisson (syndrome nephrotique "infantile"). *Helv Paediatr Acta* 28:91, 1973.
40. Sibley RK, Mahan J, Mauer SM, et al: A clinicopathologic study of forty-eight infants with nephrotic syndrome. *Kidney Int* 27:544, 1985.
41. Huttunen NP, Rapola J, Vilska J, et al: Renal pathology in congenital nephrotic syndrome of Finnish type: A quantitative light microscopic study on 50 patients. *Int J Pediatr Nephrol* 1:10, 1980.
42. Barresi G, Tuccari G, Arena F: Peanut and lotus tetragonolobus binding sites in human kidney from congenital nephrotic syndrome of Finnish type. *Histochemistry* 89:117, 1988.
43. Rapola J, Sariola H, Ekblom P: Pathology of fetal congenital nephrosis: Immunohistochemical and ultrastructural studies. *Kidney Int* 25:701, 1984.
44. Vernier RL, Klein DJ, Sisson SP, et al: Heparin sulfate-rich anionic sites in the human glomerular basement membrane. *N Engl J Med* 309:1001, 1983.
45. Aula P, Rapola J, Karjalainen O, et al: Prenatal diagnosis of congenital nephrosis in 23 high-risk families. *Am J Dis Child* 132:984, 1978.
46. Ryynanen M, Seppala M, Kuusela P, et al: Antenatal screening for congenital nephrosis in Finland by maternal serum alpha-fetoprotein. *Br J Obstet Gynecol* 90:437, 1983.

47. Mahan JD, Mauer SM, Sibley RK, et al: Congenital nephrotic syndrome: Evolution of medical management and results of renal transplantation. *J Pediatr* 105:549, 1984.
48. West CD, McAdams AJ, McConville JM, et al: Hypocomplementemic and normocomplementemic persistent (chronic) glomerulonephritis; Clinical and pathologic characteristics. *J Pediatr* 67:1089, 1965.
49. Gotoff SF, Fellers FX, Vawter GF, et al: The β1C globulin in childhood nephrotic syndrome: Laboratory diagnosis of progressive glomerulonephritis. *N Engl J Med* 273:524, 1965.
50. International Study of Kidney Disease in Children: Nephrotic syndrome in children: Prediction of histopathology from clinical and laboratory characteristics at time of diagnosis. *Kidney Int* 13:159, 1978.
51. White RHR, Glasgow EF, Mills RJ: Clinicopathologic study of nephrotic syndrome in childhood. *Lancet* 1:1353, 1970.
52. Habib R, Kleinknecht C: The primary nephrotic syndrome of children: Classification and clinicopathologic study of 406 cases, in Sommers SC (ed): *Pathology Annual.* Appleton-Century-Crofts, New York, 1971, p 17.
53. Habib R, Kleinknecht C, Gubler MC, et al: Idiopathic membranoproliferative glomerulonephritis in children: Report of 105 cases. *Clin Nephrol* 1:194, 1973.
54. West CS, McAdams AJ: Isolated glomerular diseases: Membranoproliferative glomerulonephritis, in Holliday MA, Barratt TM, Vernier RL (eds): *Pediatric Nephrology.* Baltimore, Williams & Wilkins, 1987, p 420.
55. Strife CF, McAdams AJ, West CD: Membranoproliferative glomerulonephritis characterized by focal, segmental proliferative lesions. *Clin Nephrol* 18:9, 1982.
56. Wyatt RJ, McAdams AJ, Forristal J, et al: Glomerular deposition of complement control proteins in acute and chronic glomerulonephritis. *Kidney Int* 16:505, 1979.
57. Cameron JS, Glasgow EF, Ogg CS, et al: Membranoproliferative glomerulonephritis and persistent hypocomplementemia. *Br Med J* 4:7, 1970.
58. Herdman RC, Pickering RJ, Michael AF, et al: Chronic glomerulonephritis associated with low serum complement activity (chronic hypocomplementemic glomerulonephritis). *Medicine* 49:207, 1970.
59. Donadio JV Jr, Slack TK, Holley KE, et al: Idiopathic membranoproliferative (mesangiocapillary) glomerulonephritis: A clinicopathologic study. *Mayo Clin Proc* 54:141, 1979.
60. Davis AE, Schneeberger EE, Grupe WE, et al: Membranoproliferative glomerulonephritis (MPGN Type I) and dense deposit disease (DDD) in children. *Clin Nephrol* 9:184, 1978.
61. Cameron JS, Ogg CS, White RHR, et al: The clinical features and prognosis of patients with normocomplementemic mesangiocapillary glomerulonephritis. *Clin Nephrol* 1:8, 1973.
62. Charlesworth JA, Williams DG, Sheringtin E, et al: Metabolic studies of the third component of complement and the glycine-rich beta glycoprotein in patients with hypocomplementemia. *J Clin Invest* 53:1578, 1974.
63. Hunsicker LG, Ruddy S, Carpenter CB, et al: Metabolism of the third complement (C3) in nephritis. *N Engl J Med* 287:835, 1972.
64. Davis CA, Marder H, West CD: Circulating immune complexes in membranoproliferative glomerulonephritis. *Kidney Int* 20:728, 1981.
65. Daha MR, Fearon DT, Austen KF: C3 nephritic factor (C3NeF): Stabilization of fluid phase and cell-bound alternative pathway convertase. *J Immunol* 116:1, 1976.

66. Arze RS, Rashid H, Morley R, et al: Shunt nephritis: Report of two cases and review of the literature. *Clin Nephrol* 19:48, 1983.
67. O'Regan S, Makker SP: Shunt nephritis; Demonstration of diphtheroid antigen in glomeruli. *Am J Med Sci* 278:161, 1979.
68. Brzosko WJ, Krawczynski K, Nazarewicz T, et al: Glomerulonephritis associated with hepatitis-B surface antigen immune complexes in children. *Lancet* 2:477, 1974.
69. Droz D, Nabarra B, Noel C-H, et al: Recurrence of dense deposits in transplanted kidneys. *kidney Int* 15:386, 1979.
70. Loirat C, Levy M, Peltier AP, et al: Deficiency of the second component of complement: Its occurrence with membranoproliferative glomerulonephritis. *Arch Pathol Lab Med* 104:467, 1980.
71. Coleman TH, Forristal J, Kosaka T, et al: Inherited complement component deficiencies in membranoproliferative glomerulonephritis. *Kidney Int* 24:681, 1983.
72. McEnery PT, McAdams AJ, West CD: Membranoproliferative glomerulonephritis: Improved survival with alternate day prednisone therapy. *Clin Nephrol* 13:117, 1980.
73. The International Study of Kidney Disease in Children: Alternate day steroid therapy in membranoproliferative glomerulonephritis: A randomized controlled clinical trial (abstract). *Kidney Int* 21:150, 1982.
74. Rose GN, Cole BR, Robson AM: The treatment of severe glomerulonephritis in children using high dose intravenous methylprednisolone pulses. *Am J Kid Dis* 1:148, 1981.
75. Kincaid-Smith P: The treatment of chronic mesangiocapillary (membranoproliferative) glomerulonephritis with impaired renal function. *Med J Aust* II:587, 1972.
76. Cattran DC, Cardella CJ, Roscoe JM, et al: Results of a controlled drug trial in membranoproliferative glomerulonephritis. *Kidney Int* 27:436, 1985.
77. Donadio JV Jr, Anderson CF, Mitchell JC III, et al: Membranoproliferative glomerulonephritis: A prospective clinical trial of platelet inhibitor therapy. *N Engl J Med* 310:1421, 1984.
78. Kim Y, Michael AF: Idiopathic membranoproliferative glomerulonephritis. *Ann Rev Med* 31:273, 1980.
79. Droz D, Noel LH, Barbanel C, et al: Evolution a long terme des glomerulonephrites membranoproliferatives de l'adulte: Remission spontanee durable chez 13 malades avec etude de biopsies renales iteratives dans 5 cas. *Nephrologie* 3:6, 1982.
80. West CD: Childhood membranoproliferative glomerulonephritis: An approach to management. *Kidney Int* 29:1077, 1986.
81. McEnery PT, McAdams AJ, West CD: The effect of prednisone in a high-dose, alternate-day regimen on the natural history of idiopathic membranoproliferative glomerulonephritis. *Medicine* 64:401, 1985.
82. Cameron JS, Turner DR, Hiteman J, et al: Idiopathic mesangiocapillary glomerulonephritis: Comparison of Types I and II in children and adults and long-term prognosis. *Am J Med* 74:175, 1983.
83. Zimmerman SW, Moorthy AV, Dreher WH, et al: Prospective trial of warfarin and dipyridamole in patients with membranoproliferative glomerulonephritis. *Am J Med* 75:920, 1983.
84. Kher KK, Makker SP, Iikawa M, et al. Regression of dense deposits in type II membranoproliferative glomerulonephritis: A case report of clinical course in a child. *Clin Nephrol* 17:100, 1982.
85. Cameron JS, Chantler C, Turner D: Treatment of mesangiocapillary glomerulo-

nephritis in children with combined immunosuppression and anti-coagulation. *Arch Dis Child* 55:446, 1980.

86. Montoliu J, Bergada E, Arrizabalaga P, et al: Acute renal failure in dense deposit disease: Recovery after plasmapheresis. *Brit Med J* 284:940, 1982.
87. Cameron JS: Glomerulonephritis in renal transplants. *Transplantation* 34:237, 1982.
88. Sissons JGP, West RJ, Fallows J, et al: The complement abnormalities of lipodystrophy. *N Engl J Med* 294:461, 1976.
89. Beaufils M, Morel-Maroger L, Sraer JD, et al: Acute renal failure of glomerular origin during visceral abscesses. *N Engl J Med* 295:185, 1976.
90. Strife CF, Chuck G, McAdams AJ, et al: Membranoproliferative glomerulonephritis and $alpha_1$-antitrypsin deficiency in children. *Pediatrics* 71:88, 1983.
91. Cheigh JS, Mouradian J, Susin M, et al: Kidney transplant nephrotic syndrome: Relationship between allograft histopathology and natural course. *Kidney Int* 18:358, 1980.
92. Andrade ZA, van Marck E: Schistosomal nephropathy, in Kibukamusoke JW (ed): *Tropical Nephrology,* Canberra, Citforge Pty, 1984, p 128.
93. Alpers CE, Cotran RS: Neoplasia and glomerular injury. *Kidney Int* 30:465, 1986.
94. Bell ET: A clinicopathological study of subacute and chronic glomerulonephritis, including lipoid nephrosis. *Am J Pathol* 14:691, 1938.
95. Glassock RJ, Cohen AH, Adler SG, et al: Primary glomerular diseases, in Brenner BM, Rector FC Jr (eds): *The Kidney,* 3rd ed. Saunders, Philadelphia, 1986, chap 22.
96. Cameron JS: Histology, protein clearances and responses to treatment in the nephrotic syndrome. *Br Med J* 4:352, 1968.
97. Doi T, Mayumi M, Kanatsu K, et al: Distribution of IgG subclasses in membranous nephropathy. *Clin Exp Immunol* 58:57, 1984.
98. Habib R, Kleinknecht C, Gubler MC: Extramembranous glomerulonephritis in children: Report of 50 cases. *J Pediatr* 82:754, 1972.
99. Couser WG, Steinmuller DR, Stillmant MM, et al: Experimental glomerulonephritis in the isolated perfused rat kidney. *J Clin Invest* 62:1275, 1978.
100. Van Damme BJC, Fleuren GJ, Bakker WW, et al: Experimental glomerulonephritis in the rat induced by antibodies directed against tubular antigen: IV. Fixed glomerular antigens in the pathogenesis of heterologous immune complex glomerulonephritis. *Lab Invest* 38:502, 1978.
101. Makker SP, Moorthy B: In situ immune complex formation in isolated perfused kidney using homologous antibody. *Lab Invest* 42:1, 1981.
102. Makker SP, Kirson I: Immune complex induced nephrotic syndrome (NS) with circulating brush border antibody (BBab) to human Fx1A in an infant immunopathologically similar to Heymann nephritis (HN) of rats (abstract). *Kidney Int* 16:912, 1979.
103. Douglas MFS, Rabideau DP, Schwartz MM, et al: Evidence on autologous immune complex nephritis. *N Engl J Med* 305:1326, 1981.
104. Niles J, Collins B, Baird L, et al: Antibodies reactive with a renal glycoprotein and with deposits in membranous nephritis (abstract). *Kidney Int* 31:338, 1987.
105. Makker SP, Kanalas JJ: Autoantibodies to human gp330 in sera of patients with idiopathic membranous glomerulonephropathy (abstract). *Kidney Int* 35:211, 1989.
106. Couser WG, Baker PJ, Adler S: Complement and the direct mediation of glomerular injury: A new perspective. *Kidney Int* 28:879, 1985.
107. De Heer E, Daha MR, Byakdi S, et al: Possible involvement of terminal complement complex in active Heymann nephritis. *Kidney Int* 27:388, 1985.

108. Dische FE, Swinson DR, Hamilton EB, et al: Immunopathology of penicillamine-induced glomerular disease. *J Rheumatol* 11:584, 1984.
109. Hoorntje SJ, Kallenberg CG, Weening JJ, et al: Immune-complex glomerulopathy in patients treated with captopril. *Lancet.* 1:212, 1980.
110. Textor SC, Gephardt GN, Bravo EL, et al: Membranous glomerulopathy associated with captopril therapy. *Am J Med* 74:705, 1983.
111. Tornroth T, Skrifvars B: Gold nephropathy prototype of membranous glomerulonephritis. *Am J Pathol* 75:573, 1974.
112. Eagen JW, Lewis EJ: Glomerulopathies of neoplasia. *Kidney Int* 11:297, 1977.
113. Kleinknecht C, Habib R: Isolated glomerular diseases: Membranous glomerulonephritis, in Holliday MA, Barratt TM, Vernier RL (eds): *Pediatric Nephrology,* 2nd ed. Baltimore, Williams & Wilkins, 1987, p 462.
114. Antignac C, Hinglais N, Gubler C, et al: De novo membranous glomerulonephritis in renal allografts in children. *Clin Nephrol* 1988;30:1.
115. Combes B, Shorey J, Barrera A, et al: Glomerulonephritis with deposition of Australia antigen-antibody complexes in glomerular basement membrane. *Lancet* 2:234, 1971.
116. Klenknecht C, Levy M, Peix A, et al: Membranous glomerulonephritis and hepatitis B surface antigen in children. *J Pediatr* 95:946, 1979.
117. Southwest Pediatric Nephrology Study Group—Dallas, Texas: Hepatitis B surface antigenemia in North American children with membranous glomerulonephropathy. *J Pediatr* 106:571, 1985.
118. Yoshikawa N, Ito H, Yamada Y, et al: Membranous glomerulonephritis associated with hepatitis B antigen in children: A comparison with idiopathic membranous glomerulonephritis. *Clin Nephrol* 23:28, 1985.
119. Hsu-H-C, Lin G-H, Chang M-H, et al: Association of hepatitis B surface (HBs) antigenemia and membranous nephropathy in children in Taiwan. *Clin Nephrol* 20:121, 1983.
120. Wiggelinkhuizen J, Sinclair-Smith C, Stannard LM, et al: Hepatitis B virus associated membranous glomerulonephritis. *Arch Dis Child* 58:488, 1983.
121. Nagy J, Bajtai G, Brasch H, et al: The role of hepatitis B surface antigen in the pathogenesis of glomerulopathies. *Clin Nephrol* 12:109, 1979.
122. Hirose H, Udo K, Kojima M, et al: Deposition of heptatis B e antigen in membranous glomerulonephritis: Identification by F(ab′)2 fragments of monoclonal antibody. *Kidney Int* 26:338, 1984.
123. Platt JL, Burke BA, Fish AJ, et al: Systemic lupus erythematosus in the first two decades of life. *Am J Kid Dis* 2(suppl 1):212, 1982.
124. Sanchez-Bayle M, Ecija JL, Estepa R, et al: Incidence of glomerulonephritis in congenital syphilis. *Clin Nephrol* 20:27, 1983.
125. Houba V: Immunopathology of nephropathies associated with malaria. *Kidney Int* 16:3, 1979.
126. Southwest Pediatric Nephrology Study Group. Comparison of idiopathic and systemic lupus erythematosus associated membranous glomerulonephritis in children. *Am J Kid Dis* 1986;7:115.
127. Olbing H, Greifer I, Bennet BP, et al: Idiopathic membranous nephropathy in children. *Kidney Int* 3:381, 1973.
128. Latham P, Poucell S, Koresaar A, et al: Idiopathic membranous glomerulopathy in Canadian children: A clinicopathologic study. *J Pediatr.* 101:682, 1982.
129. Ramirez F, Brouhard BH, Travis LB, et al: Idiopathic membranous nephropathy in children. *J Pediatr* 101:677, 1982.

130. Collaborative Study of the Adult Idiopathic Nephrotic Syndrome: A controlled study of short-term prednisone treatment in adults with membranous nephropathy. *N Engl J Med* 301:1301, 1979.
131. Ponticelli C, Zucchelli P, Imbasciati E, et al: Controlled trial of methylprednisolone and chlorambucil in idiopathic membranous nephropathy. *N Engl J Med* 310:946, 1984.
132. Ponticelli C, Zucchelli P, Passerini P, et al: A randomized trial of methylprednisolone and chlorambucil in idiopathic membranous nephropathy. *N Engl J Med* 320:8, 1989.
133. Cattran DC, Delmore T, Roscoe J, et al: A randomized controlled trial of prednisone in patients with idiopathic membranous nephropathy. *N Engl J Med* 320:210, 1989.
134. Berger J, Hinglais N: Intercapillary deposits of IgA-IgG. *J Urol Nephrol* 74:694, 1968.
135. D'Amico G: The commonest glomerulonephritis in the world: IgA nephropathy. *Q J Med* 64:709, 1987.
136. Levy M, Gonzales-Burchard G, Broyer M, et al: Berger's disease in children: Natural history and outcome. *Medicine* 64:157, 1985.
137. Hogg RF, Silva GF: IgA nephropathy: Natural history and prognostic indices in children. *Contrb Nephrol* 40:214, 1984.
138. Yoshikawa N, Ito H, Yoshiara S, et al: Clinical course of immunoglobulin: A nephropathy in children. *J Pediatr* 110:555, 1987.
139. Kusumoto Y, Takebayashi S, Taguchi T, et al: Long-term prognosis and prognostic indices of IgA nephropathy in juvenile and in adult Japanese. *Clin Nephrol* 28:118, 1987.
140. Kher KK, Makker SP, Moorthy B: IgA nephropathy (Berger's disease); A clinicopathologic study in children. *Int J Pediatr Nephrol* 4:11, 1983.
141. Galla JH, Kohaut EC, Alexander R, et al: Racial difference in the prevalence of IgA-associated nephropathies (letter). *Lancet* 2:522, 1984.
142. Michalk D, Waldherr R, Seelig HP, et al: Idiopathic mesangial IgA-glomerulonephritis in childhood: Description of 19 pediatric cases and review of the literature. *Eur J Pediatr* 134:13, 1980.
143. Hattori S, Karashima S, Furuse A, et al: Clinicopathological correlation of IgA nephropathy in children. *Am J Nephrol* 5:182, 1985.
144. Kitagawa T: Lessons learned from the Japanese nephritis screening study. *Pediatr Nephrol* 2:256, 1988.
145. Welch TR, McAdams AJ, Berry A: Rapidly progressive IgA nephropathy. *Am J Dis Child* 142:789, 1988.
146. Valentijn RM, Radl J, Haaijman JJ, et al: Circulating and mesangial secretory component-binding IgA-1-in primary IgA nephropathy. *Kidney Int* 26:760, 1984.
147. Conley ME, Cooper MD, Michael AF: Selective deposition of immunoglobulin A_1 in immunoglobulin A nephropathy, anaphylactoid purpura nephritis, and systemic lupus erythematosus. *J Clin Invest* 66:1432, 1980.
148. Rajaraman S, Goldblum RM, Cavallo T: IgA-associated glomerulonephritides: A study with monoclonal antibodies. *Clin Immunol Immunopathol* 39:514, 1986.
149. Bene MC, Faure G, Duheille J: IgA nephropathy: Characterization of the polymeric nature of mesangial deposits by in vitro binding of free secretory component. *Clin Exp Immunol* 47:527, 1982.
150. Emancipator SN, Gallo GR, Lamm ME: IgA nephropathy: Perspectives on pathogenesis and classification. *Clin Nephrol* 24:161, 1985.

151. Waldherr R, Rambausek M, Rauterberg W, et al: Immunohistochemical features of mesangial IgA glomerulonephritis. *Contrb Nephrol* 40:99, 1984.
152. Levy M, Beaufils H, Gubler MC, et al: Idiopathic recurrent macroscopic hematuria and mesangial IgA-IgG deposits in children (Berger's disease). *Clin Nephrol* 1:63, 1972.
153. Trascasa ML, Egido J, Sancho J, et al: IgA glomerulonephritis (Berger's disease): Evidence of high serum levels of polymeric IgA. *Clin Exp Immunol* 42:247, 1980.
154. Hernando P, Egido J, de Nicholas R, et al: Clinical significance of polymeric and monomeric IgA complexes in patients with IgA nephropathy. *Am J Kid Dis* 8:410, 1986.
155. Hall RP, Stachura I, Cason J, et al: IgA-containing circulating immune complexes in patients with IgA nephropathy. *Am J Med* 74:56, 1983.
156. Levy M, Broyer M, Arsan A, et al: Anaphylactoid purpura nephritis in childhood: Natural history and immunopathology. *Adv Nephrol* 6:183, 1976.
157. Sinniah R, Feng PH: Lupus nephritis: Correlation between light, electron microscopic and immunofluorescent findings and renal function. *Clin Nephrol* 6:340, 1976.
158. Callard P, Feldmann G, Prandi D, et al: Immune complex type glomerulonephritis in cirrhosis of the liver. *Am J Pathol* 80:329, 1975.
159. Bene MC, De Korwin JD, de Ligny BH, et al: IgA nephropathy and alcoholic liver cirrhosis: A prospective necropsy study. *Am J Clin Pathol* 89:769, 1988.
160. Katz A, Dyck RF, Beare RA: Celiac disease associated with immune complex glomerulonephritis. *Clin Nephrol* 11:39, 1979.
161. Shu KH, Lian JD, Yang YF, et al: Glomerulonephritis in ankylosing spondylitis. *Clin Nephrol* 25:169, 1986.
162. Sato M, Kojima H, Koshikawa S: IgA nephropathy in rheumatoid arthritis. *Nephron* 48:169, 1988.
163. Gregory MC, Hammond ME, Brewer ED: Renal deposition of cytomegalovirus antigen in immunoglobulin-A nephropathy. *Lancet* 1:11, 1988.
164. Lai KN, Lai FM, Lo S, et al: IgA nephropathy associated with hepatitis B virus antigenemia. *Nephron* 47:141, 1987.
165. Ramirez G, Stinson JB, Zawada ET, et al: IgA nephritis associated with mycosis fungoides: Report of two cases. *Arch Intern Med* 141:1287, 1981.
166. Pape JF, Mellbye OJ, Oystese B, et al: Glomerulonephritis in dermatitis herpetiformis: A case study. *Acta Med Scand* 203:445, 1978.
167. Lai KN, Lai M, Vallance OJ: A short term controlled trial of cyclosporin-A in IgA nephropathy. *Transplant Proc* 20:297, 1988.
168. Clarkson AR, Seymour AE, Woodroffe AJ, et al: Controlled trial of phentoin therapy in IgA nephropathy. *Clin Nephrol* 13:215, 1980.
169. Southwest Pediatric Nephrology Study Group: Association of IgA nephropathy with steroid-responsive nephrotic syndrome. *Am J Kid Dis* 3:157, 1985.
170. Reuterberg EW, Lieberknecht HM, Wingen AM, et al. Complement membrane attack (MAC) in IgA-glomerulonephritis. *Kidney Int* 1982;31:820.
171. Mihatsch MJ, Imbasciati E, Fogazzi G, et al: Ultrastructural lesions of Henoch-Schönlein syndrome and IgA nephropathy: Similarities and differences. *Contrb Nephrol* 40:255, 1984.
172. Meadow SR, Scott DG: Berger disease: Henoch-Schönlein syndrome without the rash. *J Pediatr* 106:27, 1985.
173. Weiss JH, Bhathena DB, Curtis JJ, et al: A possible relationship between Henoch-

Schönlein syndrome and IgA nephropathy (Berger's disease): An illustrative case. *Nephron* 22:582, 1978.

174. Trygstad CW, Stiehm ER: Elevated serum IgA globulin in anaphylactoid purpura. *Pediatrics* 47:1023, 1971.

175. Levinsky RJ, Barratt TM: IgA immune complexes in Henoch-Schönlein purpura. *Lancet* 2:1100, 1979.

176. Baart de la Faille-Kuyper EH, Kater L, Kuyton RH: Occurrence of vascular IgA deposits in clinically normal skin of patients with renal disease. *Kidney Int* 9:424, 1976.

177. Baart de la Faille-Kuyper EH, Kater L, Kooiker CJ, et al: IgA deposits in cutaneous blood vessel walls and mesangium in Henoch-Schönlein syndrome. *Lancet* 1:892, 1973.

178. Nomoto Y, Sakai H, Arimoris S: Increase of IgA bearing lymphocytes in peripheral blood from patients with IgA nephropathy. *Am J Clin Pathol* 71:158, 1979.

179. Kuno-Sakai H, Sakai H, Nomoto Y, et al: Increase of IgA-bearing peripheral lymphocytes in children with Henoch-Schönlein purpura. *Pediatrics* 64:918, 1979.

180. Bene MC, Hurault De Ligny B, Faure G, et al: Histoimmunological discrepancies in primary IgA nephropathy and anaphylactoid purpura sustain relationships between mucosa and kidney. *Nephron* 43:214, 1986.

181. Nicholls KM, Fairley KF, Dowling JP, et al: The clinical course of mesangial IgA associated nephropathy in adults. *Q J Med* 53:227, 1984.

182. Von Plenciz MA: *Tractatus III de scarlatina.* Vienna, JA Trattner, 1792.

183. Wells WC: *Transactions of a Society for the Improvement of Medical and Chirurgical Knowledge.* London, The Society, 1812, p 3, 194.

184. Sagel I, Treser G, Ty A, et al: Occurrence and nature of glomerular lesions after group A streptococci infections in children. *Ann Intern Med* 79:492, 1973.

185. Fish AJ, Herdman RC, Michael AF, Pickering RJ, Good RA: Epidemic acute glomerulonephritis associated with type 49 streptococcal pyoderma. II. Correlative study of light, immunofluorescent and electron microscopic findings. *Am J Med* 48:28, 1970.

186. Lewy JE, Salinas-Madrigal L, Herdson PB, et al: Clinicopathologic correlations in acute poststreptococcal glomerulonephritis. *Medicine* 50:453, 1971.

187. Dodge WF, Spargo BH, Travis LB, et al: Poststreptococcal glomerulonephritis, a prospective study in children. *N Engl J Med* 286:273, 1972.

188. Inglefinger JR, McCluskey RT, Scheenberger EE, et al: Necrotizing arteritis in acute poststreptococcal glomerulonephritis. *J Pediatr* 91:228, 1977.

189. Michael AF Jr, Drummond KN, Good RA, et al: Acute poststreptococcal glomerulonephritis: Immune deposit disease. *J Clin Invest* 45:237, 1966.

190. Tornroth T: The fate of subepithelial deposits in acute poststreptococcal glomerulonephritis. *Lab Invest* 35:461, 1976.

191. Dodge WF, Spargo BH, Bass JA, et al: The relationship between the clinical and pathologic features of poststreptococcal glomerulonephritis: A study of the early natural history. *Medicine* 47:227, 1968.

192. Barnham M, Thornton TJ, Lange K: Nephritis caused by streptococcus zooepidemicus (Lancefield Group C). *Lancet* 1:945, 1983.

193. Ben-Dov I, Berry EM, Kopolovic J: Poststreptococcal nephritis and acute rheumatic fever in two adults. *Arch Intern Med* 145:338, 1985.

194. Friedman J, van de Rijn I, Ohkuni H, et al: Immunological studies of poststreptococcal sequalae: Evidence for presence of streptococcal antigens in circulating immune complexes. *J Clin Invest* 74:1027, 1984.

195. Vogt A, Batsford S, Rodriguez-Iturbe B, et al: Cationic antigens in poststreptococcal glomerulonephritis. *Clin Nephrol* 20:271, 1983.
196. Rodriguez-Iturbe B, Katiyar VN, Coello J: Neuraminidase activity and free sialic acid levels in the serum of patients with acute poststreptococcal glomerulonephritis. *N Engl J Med* 304:1506, 1981.
197. Rodriguez-Iturbe B: Epidemic poststreptococcal glomerulonephritis. *Kidney Int* 25:129, 1984.
198. Derrick CW, Reeves MS, Dillon HC Jr: Complement and overt asymptomatic nephritis after skin infections. *J Clin Invest* 49:1178, 1970.
199. Lewis EJ, Carpenter CB, Schur: Serum complement levels in human glomerulonephritis. *Ann Intern Med* 75:555, 1971.
200. Cameron JS, Vick RM, Ogg CS, et al: Plasma C3 and C4 concentrations in the management of glomerulonephritis. *Br Med J* 3:668, 1973.
201. Sjoholm AG: Complement components and complement activation in acute poststreptococcal glomerulonephritis. *Int Arch Allergy Appl Immunol* 58:3, 1979.
202. Williams DG, Pteres DK, Fallows J, et al: Studies of serum complement in the hypocomplemententemic nephritides. *Clin Exp Immunol* 18:391, 1974.
203. Nissenson AR, Baraff LJ, Fine RN, et al: Poststreptococcal acute glomerulonephritis: Fact and controversy. *Ann Intern Med* 91:76, 1979.
204. Dillon HC Jr, Reeves MSA: Streptococcal immune response in nephritis after skin infection. *Am J Med* 56:333, 1974.
205. Rammelkamp CH Jr: Acute hemorrhagic glomerulonephritis, in McCarty M, ed: *Streptococcal Infections.* New York, Columbia University Press, 1954.
206. McIntosh RM, Garcia R, Rubio L, et al: Evidence for an autologous immune complex pathogenic mechanism in acute poststreptococcal glomerulonephritis. *Kidney Int* 14:501, 1978.
207. Yoshizawa N, Treser G, McClung JA, et al: Circulating immune complexes in patients with uncomplicated Group A streptococcal pharyngitis and patients with acute poststreptococcal glomerulonephritis. *Am J Nephrol* 3:23, 1983.
208. Stetson CA, Rammelkamp CH Jr, Krause RM, et al: Epidemic acute nephritis: Studies on etiology, natural history, and prevention. *Medicine* 34:431, 1955.
209. Anthony BF, Kaplan EL, Wannamaker LW, et al: Attack rates of acute nephritis after type 49 streptococcal infection of the skin and the respiratory tract. *J Clin Invest* 48:1697, 1969.
210. Makker SP, Kher KK: IgA nephropathy in children. *Semin Nephrol* 9:112, 1989.
211. Habib R, Kleinknecht C, Gubler MC, et al: Idiopathic membranoproliferative glomerulonephritis in children: Report of 105 cases. *Clin Nephrol* 1:194, 1973.
212. Lange K, Azadegan AA, Seligson G, et al: Asymptomatic poststreptococcal glomerulonephritis in relatives of patients with symptomatic glomerulonephritis. *Child Nephrol Urol* 1988–89;9:11.
212a. Fairly C, Mathews DC, Becker GJ: Rapid development of diffuse scents in poststreptococcal glomerulonephritis. *Clin Nephrol* 1987;28:256.
213. Potter EV, Abidh S, Sharrett AR, et al: Two- to six-year follow-up studies of nephritis in Trinidad. *N Engl J Med* 298:767, 1978.
214. Clark G, White RHR, Glasgow EF, et al: Poststreptococcal glomerulonephritis in children: Clinicopathological correlations and long-term prognosis. *Pediatr Nephrol* 1988;2:381.
215. Potter EV, Lipschultz SA, Abidh S, et al: Twelve to seventeen-year follow-up of patients with poststreptococcal acute glomerulonephritis in Trinidad. *N Engl J Med* 307:725, 1982.
216. Baldwin DS: Poststreptococcal glomerulonephritis. *Am J Med* 62:1, 1977.

217. Gallo GR, Feiner HD, Steele Jr JM, et al: Role of intrarenal vascular sclerosis in progression of poststreptococcal glomerulonephritis. *Clin Nephrol* 13:49, 1980.
217a. Ferrario F, Kourilsky O, Morel-Maroger L: Acute endocapillary glomerulonephritis in adults: A histologic and clinical comparison between patients with and without initial acute renal failure. 19:17, 1983.
218. Schachter J, Pomeranz A, Berger I, et al: Acute glomerulonephritis secondary to lobar pneumonia. *Int J Pediatr Nephrol* 8:211, 1987.
219. Neugarten J, Baldwin DS: Glomerulonephritis in bacterial endocarditis. *Am J Med* 77:297, 1986.
220. Danovitch GM, Nord EP, Barki Y: Staphylococcal lung abscess and acute glomerulonephritis. *Isr J Med Sci* 15:840, 1979.
221. Rainford DJ, Woodrow DF, Sloper JC, et al: Postmeningococcal acute glomerular nephritis. *Clin Nephrol* 9:249, 1978.
222. Forrest JW Jr, John F, Milk LR, et al: Immune complex glomerulonephritis associated with *Klebsiella pneumoniae* infection. *Clin Nephrol* 7:76, 1977.
223. Zappacosta AR, Ashby BL: Gram-negative sepsis with acute renal failure: Occurrence from acute glomerulonephritis. *JAMA* 238:1389, 1977.
224. Ebright JR, Komorowski R: Gonococcal endocarditis associated with immune complex glomerulonephritis. *Am J Med* 68:793, 1980.
225. Dunea G, Kark RM, Lannigan R, et al: *Brucella* nephritis. *Ann Intern Med* 70:783, 1969.
226. Sitprija V, Pipatanagul V, Boonpucknavig V, et al: Glomerulitis in typhoid fever. *Ann Intern Med* 81:210, 1974.
227. Vitullo BB, O'Regan S, deChadarevian J-P, et al: Mycoplasma pneumonia associated with acute glomerulonephritis. *Nephron* 21:284, 1978.
228. Griffin RJ, Iseri LT, Boyle AJ, et al: Studies of renal function in Weil's disease. *Am J Med* 10:514, 1951.
229. Weiner ID, Northcutt AD: Leprosy and glomerulonephritis: Case report and review of the literature. *Am J Kid Dis* 13:424, 1989.
230. Johnson RJ, Couser WG: Hepatitis B infection and renal disease: Clinical, immunopathogenetic and therapeutic considerations. *Kidney Int* 37:663, 1990.
231. Minkowitz S, Wenk R, Friedman E, et al: Acute glomerulonephritis associated with varicella infection. *Am J Med* 44:489, 1968.
232. Lin C-Y, Hsu H-C: Measles and acute glomerulonephritis. *Pediatrics* 7:398, 1983.
233. Miller JA: Nephritis complicating mumps. *Med News* 86:585, 1905.
234. Monteiro GE, Lillicrap CA: Case of mumps nephritis. *Br Med J* 4:721, 1967.
235. Woodroffe AJ, Row PG, Meadows R, et al: Nephritis in infectious mononucleosis. *Q J Med* 43:451, 1974.
236. Ozawa T, Stewart JA: Immune-complex glomerulonephritis associated with cytomegalovirus infection. *Am J Clin Pathol* 72:103, 1979.
237. Burch GE, Colcolough HL: Progressive Coxsackie viral pancarditis and nephritis. *Ann Intern Med* 71:963, 1969.
238. Yuceoglu AM, Berkovich S, Minkowitz S: Acute glomerulonephritis associated with Echo virus type 9 infection. *J Pediatr* 69:603, 1966.
239. Wilson CB, Smith RC: Goodpasture's syndrome associated with influenza A2 virus infection. *Ann Intern Med* 76:91, 1972.
240. Strauss J, Abitbol C, Zilleruelo G, et al: Renal disease in children with the acquired immunodeficiency syndrome. *N Engl J Med* 321:625, 1989.
241. Bradford WD, Croker BP, Tisher CC: Kidney lesions in Rocky Mountain spotted fever. *Am J Pathol* 97:381, 1979.
242. Bullock WE, Artz RP, Bhathena D, et al: Histoplasmosis: Association with circu-

lating immune complexes, eosinophilia, and mesangiopathic glomerulonephritis. *Arch Intern Med* 139:700, 1979.

243. Futrakul P, Boonpucknavig V, Boonpucknavig S, et al: Acute glomerulonephritis complicating plasmodium flaciparum infection. *Clin Pediatr* 13:281, 1974.
244. Phanuphak P, Tirawatnpongs S, Hanvanich M, et al: Autoantibodies in falciparum malaria: A sequential study in 183 Thai patients. *Clin Exp Immunol* 53:627, 1983.
245. Wickbom B, Winberg J: Coincidence of congenital toxoplasmosis and acute nephritis with nephrotic syndrome. *Acta Paediatr Scand* 61:470, 1972.
246. Weisinger JR, Pinto A, Velazquez GE, et al: Clinical and histological kidney involvement in human kala azar. *Am J Trop Med Hyg* 27:357, 1978.
247. Goldman M, Lamberg PH: Trypanosomal nephropathy, in Kibukamusoke JW (ed): *Tropical Nephrology.* Canberra, Citforge Pty, 1984, p 142.
248. Malik STA, McHug M, Morley AR, et al: Filariasis (Loa-loa) associated with membranous glomerulonephritis and demonstration of filarial antigen. *Kidney Int* 20:157, 1981.
249. Sitprija V, Keoplung M, Boonpucknavig V, et al: Renal involvement in human trichinosis. *Arch Intern Med* 140:544, 1980.
250. Myers BD, Griffel B, Naveh D, et al: Membranoproliferative glomerulonephritis associated with persistent viral hepatitis. *Am J Clin Pathol* 59:222, 1973.
251. Lai KN, Lai FM, Chan KW, et al: The clinicopathologic features of hepatitis B virus-associated glomerulonephritis. *Quart J Med* 63:323, 1987.
252. Hattori S, Furuse A, Matsuda I: Presence of HBe antibody in glomerular deposits in membranous glomerulonephritis is associated with hepatitis B virus infection. *Am J Nephrol* 8:384, 1988.
253. Takekoshi Y, Shida N, Saheki Y, et al: Strong association between membranous nephropathy and hepatitis-B surface antigenaemia in Japanese children. *Lancet* 2:1065, 1978.
254. Hsu H-C, Wu C-y, Lin C-y, et al: Membranous nephropathy in 52 hepatitis B, surface antigen (HBs B Ag) carrier children in Taiwan. *Kidney Int* 36:1103, 1989.
255. Hirschel BJ, Benusiglio LN, Favre H, et al: Glomerulonephritis associated with hepatitis B: Report of a case and review of the literature. *Clin Nephrol* 8:404, 1977.
256. Lee HS, Choi Y, Yu SH, et al: A renal biopsy study of hepatitis B virus-associated nephropathy in Korea. *Kidney Int* 34:537, 1988.
257. Baehr G: Glomerular lesions of subacute bacterial endocarditis. *J Exp Med* 14:330, 1912.
258. Morel-Maroger L, Sraer JD, Herreman G, et al: Kidney in subacute endocarditis: Pathological and immunofluorescent findings. *Arch Pathol* 94:205, 1972.
259. Williams RC, Kunkel HG: Rheumatoid factor complement and conglutinin aberrations in patients with subacute bacterial endocarditis. *J Clin Invest* 41:666, 1962.
260. Boyer AS, Theophilopoulous AN, Eisenberg R, et al: Circulating immune complexes in infective endocarditis. *N Engl J Med* 295:1500, 1976.
261. Hurwitz D, Quismorio FP, Friow GJ: Cryoglobulinemia in patients with infectious endocarditis. *Clin Exp Immunol* 19:131, 1975.
262. Boulton-Jones JM, Sissons JG, Evans DJ, et al: Renal lesions of subacute infective endocarditis. *Br Med J* 2:11, 1974.
263. Gutman RA, Striker GE, Gilliland BC, et al: The immune complex glomerulonephritis of bacterial endocarditis. *Medicine* 51:1, 1972.
264. Black JA, Challacombe DN, Ockenden BG: Nephrotic syndrome associated with bacteraemia after shunt operations for hydrocephalus. *Lancet* 2:921, 1965.

265. Strife CF, McDonald BM, Ruley EJ, et al: Shunt nephritis: The nature of the serum cryoglobulins and their relation to the complement profile. *J Pediatr* 88:403, 1976.
266. Wyatt RJ, Walsh JW, Holland NH: Shunt nephritis: Role of complement system in its pathogenesis and management. *J Neurosurg* 55:99, 1981.
267. Dobrin RS, Day NK, Quie PG, et al: The role of complement, immunoglobulin, and bacterial antigen in coagulase-negative staphylococcal shunt nephritis. *Am J Med* 59:660, 1975.
268. Bolton WK, Sande MA, Normansell DE, et al: Ventriculojugular shunt nephritis with *Corynebacterium bovis. Am J Med* 59:417, 1975.
269. Dawson KP, Lees H, Smeeton WMI, et al: Glomerulonephritis associated with an infected ventriculo-atrial shunt. *NZ Med J* 91:342, 1980.
270. Schoeneman M, Bennett B, Greifer I: Shunt nephritis progressing to chronic renal failure. *Am J Kid Dis* 2:375, 1982.
271. Schönlein JL: Herisan, literatur-comptoir. *Allgemeine und spezielle Pathologie,* 3rd ed. 2:48, 1837.
272. Frank E: Die essentielle Thrombopenie. *Berlin Klin Wochnschr* 52:454, 1915.
273. Allen DM, Diamond LK, Howell DA: Anaphylactoid purpura in children (Schonlein-Henöch syndrome). *Am J Dis Child* 99:833, 1960.
274. Cameron JS: Henoch-Schönlein purpura: Clinical presentation. *Contrib Nephrol* 40:246, 1984.
275. Stewart M, Savage JM, McCord B: Long term renal prognosis of Henoch-Schönlein purpura in an unselected childhood population. *Eur J Pediatr* 147:113, 1988.
276. Kher KK, Sheth KJ, Makker SP: Stenosing ureteritis in Henoch-Schönlein purpura. *J Urol* 129:1040, 1983.
277. Habib R, Niaudet P: Renal involvement in Schönlein-Henoch purpura, in Tisher CC, Brenner BM (eds): *Renal Pathology with Clinical and Functional Correlations.* Philadelphia, J.B. Lippincott Company, 1989, vol 1, p 409.
278. Simila S, Kouvalainen K, Lanning M: Serum immunoglobulin levels in the course of anaphylactoid purpura in children. *Acta Paediatr Scand* 66:537, 1977.
279. Garcia-Fuentes M, Chantler C, Williams DG: Cyroglobulinaemia in Henoch-Schönlein purpura. *Br Med J* 2:163:165, 1977.
280. Saulsbury FT: IgA rheumatoid factor in Henoch-Schönlein purpura. *J Pediatr* 108:71, 1986.
281. Czerkinsky CM, Koopman WJ, Jackson S, et al: Circulating immune complexes and immunoglobulin: A rheumatoid factor in patients with mesangial immunoglobulin A nephropathies. *J Clin Invest* 77:1931, 1986.
282. Cameron JS: Henoch-Schönlein purpura nephritis: Renal involvement in multisystem and heredofamilial diseases, in Massry SG, Glassock RJ (eds): *Textbook of Nephrology,* 2nd ed. vol 1, p 714. Baltimore, Williams & Wilkins, 1989.
283. Kim CK, Aikawa M, Makker SP: Electron-dense subepithelial deposits in Henoch-Schönlein purpura syndrome. *Arch Pathol Lab Med* 103:595, 1979.
284. Farley TA, Gillespie S, Rasoulpour M, et al: Epidemiology of a cluster of Henoch-Schönlein purpura. *Am J Dis Child* 143:798, 1989.
285. Spitzer RE, Urmson JR, Farnett ML, et al: Alteration of the complement system in children with Henoch-Schönlein purpura. *Clin Immunol Immunopathol* 11:52, 1978.
286. Nyulassy S, Buc M, Sasinska M, et al: The HLA system in glomerulonephritis. *Clin Immunol Immunopathol* 7:319, 1977.
287. Gelfand EW, Clarkson JE, Minta JO: Selective deficiency of the second component of complement in a patient with anaphylactoid purpura. *Clin Immunol Immunopathol* 4:269, 1975.

288. Austin HA III, Balow JE: Henoch-Schönlein nephritis: Prognostic features and the challenge of therapy. *Am J Kid Dis.* 2:512, 1983.

289. Rose GM, Cole BR, Robson AM: The treatment of severe glomerulopathies in children using high dose intravenous methylprednisolone pulses. *Am J Kid Dis* 1:148, 1981.

290. Counahan R, Winterborn MH, White RHR, et al: Prognosis of Henoch-Schönlein nephritis in children. *Br Med J* 2:11, 1977.

290a. Koskimies O, Mir S, Rapola J, et al: Henoch-Schönlein nephritis: Long-term prognosis of unselected patients. *Arch Dis Child* 56:482, 1981.

290b. Levy M, Broyer M, Arsan A, et al: Anaphylactoid purpura nephritis in childhood: Natural history and immunopathology. *Adv Nephrol* 6:183, 1979.

290c. Fogazzi GB, Pasquali S, Moriggi M, et al: Long-term outcome of Schönlein-Henoch nephritis in the adult. *Clin Nephrol* 31:60, 1989.

291. Hasegawa A, Kawamura T, Iti H, et al: Fate of renal grafts with recurrent Henoch-Schölein purpura nephritis in children. *Transplant Proc* 21:2130, 1989.

292. Merslin AG, Rothfield N: Systemic lupus erythematosus in childhood: Analysis of 42 cases, with comparative data on 200 adult cases. *Pediatrics* 42:37, 1968.

293. Leehey DJ, Katz AI, Azaran AH, et al: Silent diffuse lupus nephritis: Long-term follow-up. *Am J Kid Dis* 2(suppl 1):188, 1982.

294. Bennett WM, Boudana EJ, Norman DJ, et al: Natural history of "silent" lupus nephritis. *Am J Kid Dis* 1:359, 1982.

294a. Geer JM, Panush RS: Incomplete lupus erythematosus. *Arch Intern Med* 149:2473, 1989.

294b. Font J, Torras A, Carvera R, et al: Silent renal disease in systemic lupus erythematosus. *Clin Nephrol* 27:283, 1987.

294c. Cavallo T, Cameron WR, Lapenas D: Immunopathology of early and clinically silent lupus nephropathy. *Am J Pathol.* 87:1, 1977.

295. Makker SP: Tubular basement membrane antibody-induced interstitial nephritis in systemic lupus erythematosus. *Am J Med* 69:949, 1980.

296. Lebit SA, Burke B, Michael AF, et al: Extramembranous glomerulonephritis in childhood: Relationship to systemic lupus erythematosus. *J Pediatr* 88:394, 1976.

297. Jennette JC, Iskandar SS, Dalldorf FG: Pathologic differentiation between lupus and nonlupus membranous glomerulonephropathy. *Kidney Int* 24:377, 1983.

298. Provost TT, Arnett FC, Reichlin M: Homozygous C2 deficiency, lupus erythematosus, and anti-Ro (SSA) antibodies. *Arth Rheum* 26:1279, 1983.

299. Shapiro KS, Pinn VW, Harrington JT, et al: Immune complex glomerulonephritis in hydralazine-induced SLE. *Am J Kid Dis* 3:270, 1984.

299a. Petri M, Bockenstedt L, Colman J, et al: Serial assessment of glomeruluar filtration rate in lupus nephropathy. *Kidney Int* 34:832, 1988.

300. Weinstein J: Hypocomplementemia in hydralazine-associated systemic lupus erythematosus. *Am J Med* 65:553, 1978.

301. Bjorck S, Svalander C, Westberg G: Hydralazine-associated glomerulonephritis. *Acta Med Scand* 218:261, 1985.

302. Tan EM, Portanova JP: The role of histones as nuclear-autoantigens in drug-related lupus erythematosus. *Arth Rheum* 24:1064, 1981.

303. Oetgen WJ, Boice JA, Lawless OJ: Mixed connective tissue disease in children and adolescents. *Pediatrics* 67:333, 1981.

304. Platt JL, Burke BA, Fish AJ: Renal manifestations of systemic disease: Systemic lupus erythematosus, in Holiday MA, Barratt TM, Vernier RL (eds): *Pediatric Nephrology*, 2nd ed. Baltimore, Williams & Wilkins, 1987, pp 499–508.

304a. Churg J, Sobin LH: *Renal Disease: Classification and Atlas of Glomerular Disease.* New York, Igaku-Shoin, 1982, p 127.

305. Brentjens JR, Sepulveda M, Baliah T, et al: Interstitial immune complex nephritis in patients with systemic lupus erythematosus. *Kidney Int* 7:342, 1975.

306. Schwartz MM, Fennell JS, Lewis EJ: Pathologic changes in the renal tubule in systemic lupus erythematosus. *Hum Pathol* 13:534, 1982.

307. Grimley PM, Davis GL, Kang Y-H, et al: Tubulorecticular inclusions in peripheral blood mononuclear cells related to systemic therapy with α-interferon. *Lab Invest* 52:638, 1985.

308. Tisher CC, Kelso HB, Robinson RR, et al: Intraendothelial inclusions in kidneys of patients with systemic lupus erythematosus. *Ann Intern Med* 75:537, 1971.

308a. Hill GS, Hinglais N, Tron F, et al: Systemic lupus erythematosus: Morphologic correlation with immunoglogic and clinical data at the time of biopsy. *Am J Med* 64:61, 1978.

309. Ginzler EM, Bollet AJ, Friedman EA: The natural history and response to therapy of lupus nephritis. *Ann Rev Med* 31:463, 1980.

310. Baldwin DS: Clinical usefulness of the morphological classification of lupus nephritis. *Am J Kid Dis* 2(suppl):142, 1982.

311. Agnello V, Koffler D, Kunkel HG: Immune complex systems in the nephritis of systemic lupus erythematosus. *Kidney Int* 3:90–99, 1973.

312. Couser WG, Salant DJ, Madaio MP, et al: Factors influencing glomerular and tubulointerstitial patterns of injury in SLE. *Am J Kid Dis* 2(suppl 1):126–134, 1982.

313. Izui S, Lambert PH, Miescher PA: In vitro demonstration of a particular affinity of glomerular basement membrane and collagen for DNA: A possible basis for a local formation of DNA-anti-DNA complexes in systemic lupus erythematosus. *J Exp Med* 144:428, 1976.

314. Tan EM, Schur PH, Carr RI, et al: Deoxyribonucleic acid (DNA) and antibodies to DNA in the serum of patients with systemic lupus erythematosus. *J Clin Invest* 45:1732, 1966.

315. Raptis L, Menard HA: Quantitation and characterization of plasma DNA in normals and patients with systemic lupus erythematosus. *J Clin Invest* 66:1391, 1980.

316. Emlen W, Ansari R, Burdick G: DNA-anti-DNA immune complexes: Antibody protection of a discrete DNA fragment from DNase digestion in vitro. *J Clin Invest* 74:185, 1984.

317. Biesecker G, Katz S, Koffler D: Renal localization of the membrane attack complex in systemic lupus erythematosus nephritis. *J Exp Med* 154:1779, 1981.

318. Schwartz RS: Immunologic and genetic aspects of systemic lupus erythematosus. *Kidney Int* 19:474, 1981.

319. Fielder AHL, Walport MJ, Batchelor JR, et al: Family study of the major histocompatibility complex in patients with systemic lupus erythematosus: Importance of null alleles of C4A and C4B in determining disease susceptibility. *Br Med J* 286:425, 1983.

320. Reveille JD, Bias WB, Winkelstein JA, et al: Familial systemic lupus erythematosus: Immunogenetic studies in eight families. *Medicine* 62:21, 1983.

321. Roubinian JR, Talal N, Greenspan JS, et al: Effect of castration and sex hormone treatment on survival, antinucleic acid antibodies, and glomerulonephritis in NZB/NZW F_1 mice. *J Exp Med* 147:1568, 1978.

321a. Pollak VE, Pirani CL, Kark RM: Effect of large doses of prednisone on the renal lesions and life span of patients with lupus glomerulonephritis. *J lab Clin Med* 57:495, 1961.

322. Austin HA III, Klippel JH, Balow JE, et al: Therapy of lupus nephritis: Controlled trial of prednisone and cytotoxic drugs. *N Engl J Med* 314:614, 1986.

323. Donadio JV Jr, Holley KE, Ilstrup DM: Cytotoxic drug treatment of lupus nephritis. *Am J Kid Dis* 2(suppl 1):178, 1982.

324. Austin HA III, Muenz LR, Joyce KM, et al: Diffuse proliferative lupus nephritis: Identification of specific pathologic features affecting renal outcome. *Kidney Int.* 25:689, 1984.

325. Ponticelli C, Zucchielli P, Banfi G, et al: Treatment of diffuse proliferative lupus nephritis by intravenous high-dose methylprednisolone. *Q J Med* 51:17, 1982.

326. Balow JE, Austin HA III, Tsokos GC, et al: Lupus nephritis. *Ann Intern Med* 106:79, 1987.

326a. McCune JW, Golbus J, Zeldes W, et al: Clinical and immunologic effects of monthly administration of intravenous cyclophosphamide in severe systemic lupus erythematosus. *N Engl J Med* 318:1423, 1988.

326b. Lehman TJA, Sherry DD, Wagner-Weiner L, et al: Intermittent intravenous cyclophosphamide therapy for lupus nephritis. *J Pediatr* 114:1055, 1989.

326c. McEnery PT, Welch TR, Glass DN: Lupus nephritis in childhood: Cyclophosphamide—yes or no? (editorial). *J Pediatr* 114:993, 1989.

327. Felson DT, Anderson J: Evidence for the superiority of immunosuppressive drugs and prednisone over prednisone alone in lupus nephritis: Results of a pooled analysis. *N Engl J Med* 311:1528, 1984.

328. Lewis E, Lachin J, and Lupus Nephritis Collaborative Study Group (LNCSG): Primary outcomes in the controlled trial of severe lupus nephritis. *Kid Int* 31:208, 1987 (abstract).

328a. Bumgardner GL, Mauer SM, Payne W, et al: Single-center 1-15-year results of renal transplantation in patients with systemic lupus erythematosus. *Transplantation* 46:703, 1988.

328b. Kumano K, Sakai T, Mahimo S, et al: A case of recurrent lupus nephritis after renal transplantation. *Clin Nephrol* 27:94, 1987.

329. Gasser C, Gautier E, Steck A, et al: Hamolytisch-uramisches Syndrome: bilaterale Nieren Rindennekrosen bei akuten erworbenen hamolytischen Anamien. *Schweiz Med Wochenschr* 85:905, 1955.

330. Drummond KN: Hemolytic-uremic syndrome—then and now. *N Engl J Med.* 312:116, 1985.

331. Loirat C, Sonsino E, Varga-Moreno A, et al: Hemolytic-uremic syndrome: An analysis of the natural history and prognostic features. *Acta Paediatr Scand* 73:505, 1984.

332. Gianantonio C, Vitacco M, Mendelaharzu F, et al: The hemolytic-uremic syndrome. *J Pediatr* 64:478, 1964.

333. Gianantonio CA, Vitacco M, Mendilahharzu F, et al: The hemolytic-uremic syndrome: Renal status of 76 patients at long-term follow-up. *J Pediatr* 72:757, 1968.

334. Kaplan BS, Drummond KN: The hemolytic-uremic syndrome is a syndrome. *N Engl J Med* 298:964, 1978.

335. Tune BM, Leavitt TJ, Gribble TJ: The hemolytic-uremic syndrome in California: A review of 28 nonheparinized cases with long-term follow-up. *J Pediatr* 82:304, 1973.

336. Kaplan BS, Chesney RW, Drummond KN: Hemolytic-uremic syndrome in families. *N Engl J Med* 292:1090, 1975.

337. Martin DL, MacDonald KL, White KE, et al: The epidemiology and clinical

aspects of the hemolytic uremic syndrome in Minnesota. *N Engl J Med* 323:1161, 1990.

338. Habib R, Levy M, Gagnadoux M, et al: Prognosis of the hemolytic uremic syndrome in children. *Adv Nephrol* 11:99, 1982.
339. Fong JSC, de Chadaverian JP, Kaplan BS: Hemolytic-uremic syndrome: Current concepts and management. *Pediatr Clin North Am* 29:835, 1982.
340. Morel-Maroger L, Kanfer A, Solez K, et al: Prognostic importance of vascular lesions in acute renal failure with microangiopathic hemolytic anemia (hemolytic-uremic syndrome): Clinicopathologic study in 20 adults. *Kidney Int* 15:548, 1979.
341. Lieberman E: Hemolytic-uremic syndrome. *J Pediatr* 80:1, 1972.
342. Whitington PF, Friedman AL, Chesney RW: Gastrointestinal disease in the hemolytic-uremic syndrome. *Gastroenterology* 76:728, 1979.
343. Smith CD, Schuster SR, Gruppe WE, et al: Hemolytic-uremic syndrome: A diagnostic and therapeutic dilemma for the surgeon. *J Pediatr Surg* 18(6D):597, 1978.
344. Bale JRF, Brasher C, Siegler RL: CNS manifestations of the hemolytic-uremic syndrome. *Am J Dis Child* 134:869, 1980.
345. Crisp DE, Siegler RL, Bale JF, et al: Hemorrhagic cerebral infarction in the hemolytic-uremic syndrome. *J Pediatr* 99:273, 1981.
346. Cameron JS, Vick R: Plasma C3 in haemolytic-uraemic syndrome and thrombotic thrombocytopenic purpura. *Lancet* 2:976, 1973.
347. Kaplan BS, Thomson PD, MacNab GM: Serum complement levels in haemolytic-uraemic syndrome. *Lancet* 2:1505, 1973.
348. Churg J, Goldstein MH, Bernstein J: Thrombotic microangiopathy including hemolytic-uremic syndrome, thrombotic thrombocytopenic purpura, and postpartum renal failure, in Tisher CC, Brenner BM (eds): *Renal Pathology with Clinical and Functional Correlations*. Philadelphia, Lippincott, 1989, vol 2, p 1081.
349. McCoy RC, Abramowsky CR, Kreuger R: The hemolytic uremic syndrome with positive immunofluorescence studies. *J Pediatr* 85:170, 1974.
350. Argyle JC, Hogg RJ, Pysher TJ, et al: A clinicopathological study of 24 children with hemolytic uremic syndrome: A report of the Southwest Pediatric Nephrology Study Group. *Pediatr Nephrol* 4:52, 1990.
351. Upadhyaya K, Barwick K, Fishaut M, et al: The importance of nonrenal involvement in hemolytic-uremic syndrome. *Pediatrics*. 65:115, 1980.
352. Karmali MA, Steele BT, Petric M, et al: Sporadic cases of haemolytic-uraemic syndrome associated with faecal cytotoxin and cytotoxin-producing *escherichia coli* in stools. *Lancet* 1:619, 1983.
353. Koster F, Levin J, Walker L, et al: Hemolytic-uremic syndrome after shigellosis. *N Engl J Med* 298:927, 1978.
354. Baker NMA, Mills E, Rachman I, Thomas JEP: Haemolytic-uraemic syndrome in typhoid fever. *Br Med J* 2:84, 1974.
355. Prober CG, Tune B, Hoder L: *Yersinia pseudotuberculosis* septicemia. *Am J Dis Child* 133:623, 1979.
356. Chamovitz BN, Hartstein A, Alexander SR, et al: *Campylobacter jejuni*-associated hemolytic uremic syndrome in a mother and daughter. *Pediatrics* 71:253, 1983.
357. Austin TW, Ray CG: Coxsackie virus group B infection and the hemolytic uremic syndrome. *J Infect Dis* 127:678, 1973.
358. Moorthy B, Makker SP: Hemolytic-uremic syndrome associated with pneumococal sepsis. *J Pediatr* 95:558, 1979.

359. Monnens L, Van de Meer W, Langenhuysen C, et al: Platelet aggregating factor in the epidemic form of hemolytic-uremic syndrome in childhood. *Clin Nephrol* 24:135, 137, 1985.

360. Misiani R, Appiani AC, Edefonti A, et al: Haemolytic uraemic syndrome: Therapeutic effect of plasma infusion. *Br Med J* 285:1304, 1982.

361. Van Buren D, Van Buren CT, Flechner SM, et al: De novo Hemolytic-uremic syndrome in renal transplant recipient immunosupressed with cyclosporine. *Surgery* 98:54, 1985.

362. Proia AD, Harden EA, Silberman HR. Mitomycin-induced hemolytic-uremic syndrome. *Arch Pathol Lab Med* 108:959, 1984.

363. Granda D, Rhoads M, Bergstrom LB, et al: Acute bromate poisoning associated with renal failure and deafness presenting as hemolytic uremic syndrome. *Am J Nephrol* 4:188, 1984.

364. Andreoli SP, Bergstein JM: Acute rhabdomyolysis associated with hemolytic uremic syndrome. *J Pediatr* 103:78, 1983.

365. Ferrier DM, Wolfsdorf JI: Hemolytic uremic syndrome associated with Kawasaki disease. *Pediatrics* 103:405, 1981.

366. Matto TK, Mahmood MA, Al-Harbi MS, et al: Familial, recurrent hemolytic-uremic syndrome. *J Pediatr* 114:815, 1989.

367. Rizzoni G, Claris-Appiani A, Endefonti A, et al: Plasma infusion for hemolytic-uremic syndrome: Results of a multicenter controlled trial. *J Pediatr* 112:284, 1988.

368. Beattie TJ, Murphy AV, Willoughby MLN, et al: Plasmapheresis in the haemolytic-uraemic syndrome in children. *Br Med J* 282:1667, 1981.

369. Beattie TJ, Murphy AV, Willoughby MLN: Prolonged prostacyclin infusion in haemolytic uraemic syndrome in children. *Br Med J* 283:470, 1981.

370. O'Regan S, Chesney RW, Mongeau J-G, Robitaille P: Aspirin and dipyridamole therapy in the hemolytic-uremic syndrome. *J Pediatr* 97:473, 1980.

371. Monnens L, van Collenburg J, de Jong M, et al: Treatment of the hemolytic-uremic syndrome. *Helv Paediatr Acta* 33:321, 1978.

372. Van Dyck M, Proesmans W, Depraetere M: Hemolytic uremic syndrome in childhood: Renal function ten years later. *Clin Nephrol* 29:109, 1988.

373. O'Regan S, Blais N, Russo P, et al: Hemolytic uremic syndrome: Glomerular filtration rate 6–11 years later measured by ^{99m}Tc DTPA plasma slope clearance. *Clin Nephrol* 32:217, 1989.

374. Trompeter RS, Schwartz R, Chantler C, et al: Hemolytic-uremic syndrome. An analysis of prognostic features. *Arch Dis Child* 58:101, 1983.

375. Robson WLM, Fick GH, Wilson PCG: Prognostic factors in postdiarrhea hemolytic-uremic syndrome. *Child Nephrol Urol* 9:203, 1988–89.

376. Loirat C, Sonsino E, Varga Moreno A, et al: Hemolytic-uremic syndrome: An analysis of the natural history and prognostic features. *Acta Paediatr Scand* 73:505, 1984.

377. Hebert D, Sibley RK, Mauer SM: Recurrence of hemolytic-uremic syndrome in renal transplant recipients. *Kidney Int* 30(suppl):S-51, 1986.

378. Harkness DR, Burnes JJ, Lian E, et al: Hazard of platelet transfusion in thrombotic thrombocytopenic purpura. *JAMA* 246:2931, 1981.

379. Arenson EB Jr, August CS: Preliminary report: Treatment of the hemolytic-uremic syndrome with aspirin and dipyridamole. *J Pediatr* 86:957, 1975.

380. Serra A, Cameron JS, Turner DR, et al: Vasculitis affecting the kidney: Presentation, histopathology and long-term outcome. *Q J Med* 53:181, 1984.

381. D'Agati V, Chander P, Nash M, et al: Idiopathic microscopic polyarteritis nodosa: Ultrastructural observations on the renal vascular and glomerular lesions. *Am J Kid Dis* 7:95, 1986.
382. Ronco P, Verroust P, Mignon F, et al: Immunopathologic studies of polyarteritis nodosa and Wegener's granulomatosis: A report of 43 patients with 51 renal biopsies. *Q J Med* 52:212, 1983.
383. D'Agati V, Appel GB: Polyarteritis nodosa, Wegener's granulomatosis, Churg-Strauss syndrome, temporal arteritis, Takayasu's arteritis, and lymphomatoid granulomatosis, in Tisher CC, Brenner BM (eds): *Renal pathology with Clinical and Functional Correlations.* Philadelphia, Lippincott, 1989, vol II, p 1021.
384. Magil AB: Histogenesis of glomerular crescents: Immunohistochemical demonstration of cytokeratin in crescent cells. *Am J Pathol* 120:22, 1985.
385. Atkins RC, Glasgow EF, Holdsworth SR, et al: The macrophage in human rapidly progressive glomerulonephritis. *Lancet* 1:830, 1976.
386. Bonsib SM: Glomerular basement membrane discontinuities: Scanning electron microscopic study of acellular glomeruli. *Am J Pathol* 119:357, 1985.
387. Couser WG, Stilmant MM, Jermanovich NB: Complement-independent nephrotoxic nephritis in the guinea pig. *Kidney Int* 11:170, 1977.
388. Couser WG, Darby C, Salant DJ, et al: Anti-GBM antibody-induced proteinuria in isolated perfused rat kidney. *Am J Physiol* 249:F241, 1985.
389. Boyce NW, Holdsworth SR: Direct anti-GBM antibody induced alterations in glomerular permselectivity. *Kidney Int* 30:666, 1986.
390. Couser WG, Baker PJ, Adler S: Complement and the direct mediation of immune glomerular injury: A new perspective (editorial review). *Kidney Int* 28:879, 1985.
391. Cochrane CG: Immunologic tissue injury mediated by neutrophilic leukocytes. *Adv Immunol* 9:99, 1968.
392. Rehan A, Johnson KJ, Wiggins RC, et al: Evidence for the role of oxygen radicals in acute nephrotoxic nephritis. *Lab Invest* 51:396, 1984.
393. Tipping PG, Holdsworth SR: The participation of macrophages, glomerular procoagulant activity, and Factor VIII in glomerular fibrin deposition: Studies in anti-GBM antibody induced glomerulonephritis in rabbits. *Am J Pathol* 124:10, 1986.
394. Bhan AK, Collins A, Schneeberger E, et al: A cell mediated reaction against glomerular-bound immune complexes. *J Exp Med* 150:1410, 1979.
395. Bolton WK, Tucker FL, Sturgill BC: New avian model of experimental glomerulonephritis consistent with mediation by cellular immunity. *J Clin Invest* 73:1263, 1984.
396. Anand SK, Trygstad CW, Sharma HM, et al: Extracapillary proliferative glomerulonephritis in children. *Pediatrics* 56:434, 1975.
397. A Report of the Southwest Pediatric Nephrology Study Group: A clinico-pathologic study of crescentic glomerulonephritis in 50 children. *Kidney Int* 27:450, 1985.
398. Couser WG: Rapidly progressive glomerulonephritis: Classification, pathogenetic mechanisms, and therapy. *Am J Kid Dis* 11:449, 1988.
399. Savage CO, Pusey CD, Bowman C, et al: Antiglomerular basement membrane antibody mediated disease in the British Isles 1980–4. *Br Med J* 292:301, 1986.
400. Glassock RJ: Renal involvement in multisystem and heredofamilial diseases: Goodpasture's syndrome, in Massry SG, Glassock RJ (eds): *Textbook of Nephrology,* 2nd ed. Baltimore, Maryland, Williams & Wilkins, 1989, vol 1, pp 719–723.

401. Glockner WM, Sieberth HG, Wichmann HE, et al: Plasma exchange and immunosuppression in rapidly progressive glomerulonephritis. *Clin Nephrol* 29:1, 1988.
402. Bolton WK: Glomerular diseases: Idiopathic crescentic glomerulonephritis, in Massry SG, Glassock RJ (eds): *Textbook of Nephrology*, 2nd ed. Baltimore, Maryland, Williams & Wilkins, 1989, vol 1, pp 651–656.

9

URINARY TRACT INFECTION

Kanwal K. Kher
Heinz E. Leichter

Infections affecting the urinary tract are frequently encountered in both children and adults. Bacterial infection by gram-negative enterococci is the predominant cause of urinary tract infection (UTI), but viral or fungal etiologies may also be operative in some patients. Recurrence of UTI is common in susceptible individuals; early recognition and appropriate treatment of such patients is essential in order to preserve renal function and prevent permanent damage. The diagnostic evaluation of children with UTI has undergone significant evolutionary changes, and noninvasive methods such as ultrasonography and radioisotope imaging are becoming not only more accessible but also more reliable as investigative tools. This chapter will focus on the clinical, pathogenetic, and management aspects of UTI. Asymptomatic bacteriuria (ABU) and vesicoureteral reflux (VUR) in children will also be discussed.

TERMINOLOGY

The term *UTI* denotes infection within the urinary tract and encompasses both renal parenchymal infection and infection of the urinary bladder. Various terms used in the context of UTI are discussed below:

Significant Bacteriuria *Bacteriuria* is an essential feature of UTI, but urine obtained from normal individuals may also exhibit some bacterial growth due to contamination of the specimen by urethal, vaginal, or periurethral flora. In order to distinguish between contaminants in the urine and significant bacteriuria representing true UTI, the presence of >100,000 (10^5) bacterial colonies in a freshly voided clean catch or catheterized urine specimen is used as a cutoff point. However, any bacterial growth in a urine specimen obtained by suprapubic aspiration should be considered significant (Table 9–1).

Symptomatic UTI The presence of significant bacteriuria in a child who presents with clinical symptoms of dysuria, frequency, and urgency of urination with or without fever and flank pain is defined as *symptomatic UTI.* It must be

TABLE 9–1. Criteria for the Diagnosis of UTI in Children

Method of Collection	Colony Count (Pure Culture)	Probability of Infection
Suprapubic aspiration	Gram-negative bacilli: any number	$>99\%$
	Gram-positive cocci: greater than a few thousand	
Catheterization	$>10^5$	95%
	10^4–10^5	Infection likely
	10^3–10^4	Suspicious; repeat
	$<10^3$	Infection unlikely
Clean-voided		
Boy	$\geq 10^4$	Infection likely
Girl	3 specimens: $>10^5$	95%
	2 specimens: $>10^5$	90%
	1 specimen: $>10^5$	80%
	5×10^4–10^5	Suspicious; repeat
	10^4–5×10^4	Symptomatic patient; suspicious; repeat
	10^4–5×10^4	Asymptomatic patient; infection unlikely
	$<10^4$	Infection unlikely

Source: From Hellerstein S: *Urinary Tract Infections in Children.* Chicago, Year Book Medical Publishers, 1982, p.3. Reproduced with permission.

emphasized that symptoms localized to the urinary tract are somewhat determined by the age of the patient and may be minimal in younger infants.

Acute cystitis (or *lower UTI*) denotes an inflammation of the bladder mucosa associated with clinical symptoms referable to the lower urinary tract, such as urgency, dysuria, and frequency of micturition. Fever is not present in these patients.

Acute pyelonephritis represents bacterial infection of the renal parenchyma and is characterized by symptoms of fever, flank pain, vomiting, or other features of systemic toxicity, usually in addition to the manifestations encountered in acute cystitis.

Asymptomatic Bacteriuria During routine screening, significant bacteriuria may be seen in apparently healthy children and adults without any symptoms referable to the urinary tract. This condition is known as *asymptomatic bacteriuria* (ABU). It is particularly common in girls of school age.

Recurrent UTI Recurrent UTI is defined as *repeated symptomatic episodes of UTI with symptom-free intervals.* Recurrent UTI is usually caused by reinfection with a different bacterial species or serotype of the same organism and does not reflect failure to eradicate the organism from the urinary tract.

Relapse of UTI This term denotes persistence of the same bacterial species and strain within the urinary tract despite appropriate antibiotic therapy.

Relapses of UTI are often associated with underlying structural abnormalities of the urinary tract and with renal calculi.

EPIDEMIOLOGY OF UTI

In general, UTI affects females more often than males among children as well as adults. However, in the neonatal period and early infancy UTI is seen more commonly in males (75 to 80 percent) than in females (20 to 25 percent).[1,2] Although a precise reason for increased predilection of the male infant to UTI at this age group is unclear, it may be related to an increased susceptibility to sepsis and other bacterial infections that has been well described in males during early infancy. The prevalence of symptomatic UTI in the neonatal period and early infancy is difficult to assess. When Drew and Acton[3] performed bacterial cultures of urine (by suprapubic aspiration) in 905 ill newborns, UTI was diagnosed in 64 cases (7 percent). Of these, 84 percent were male and 16 percent female. In another study,[4] 7.5 percent of infants less than 8 weeks of age presenting with fever were found to be suffering from UTI. Male predominance in UTI ceases beyond the third month of life[1]; by the first year of life, symptomatic UTI affects girls about three times more often than boys (Fig. 9–1). Dickinson[5] estimated that the risk of symptomatic UTI in children aged 2 to 14 years was 1.6/1000/year in boys and 3.8/1000/year in girls. Studies in Swedish children have shown that the peak incidence of first episode of acute pyelonephritis occurs in the first two years of life and gradually decreases throughout the remainder of childhood.[6] On the other hand, first episodes of cystitis (in boys as well as girls) are usually noted during 2 to 4 years of age (Fig. 9–2).

Classic studies of Kunin and others[7–12] have shown that bacteriuria without any clinical symptoms referable to the urinary tract can occur during childhood, the condition being known as asymptomatic bacteriuria (ABU). Although first reported in school-age girls,[7,8] ABU has been shown to occur in children of all age groups, including infants less than 3 months of age. In a screening study of healthy newborn infants who were followed longitudinally for 1 year, Wettergen et al.[9] found ABU to be present in 1.5 percent of boys and 0.18 percent of girls below 2 months of age. The overall cumulative incidence of ABU during the entire first year of life in this study was, however, found to be 0.9 percent in girls and 2.5 percent in boys. In pre-school-age children (below age 5), Siegel et al.[12] reported the incidence of ABU to be 1.9 percent in females and 0 percent in males.

In children aged 6 to 18 years, ABU affects females almost exclusively; its incidence has been reported to be 1.0 percent among girls in various screening studies.[7,8,10,11] ABU is uncommon in boys, Kunin et al.[9] detected ABU in only 2 of the 7731 school-age male children screened, giving a prevalence of 0.026 percent. In the Newcastle Asymptomatic Bacteriuria Study,[11] the prevalence of asymptomatic bacteriuria in boys 5 to 18 years old was also determined to be only 0.2 percent.

Hospital-acquired (nosocomial) UTI is not uncommon in children and adults. In one study, the rate of such infection was reported to be 14.2 per 1000 pediatric admissions.[13] The presence of a foreign body, especially an indwelling urinary catheter, carries a significant risk for development of nosocomial UTI. The calculated risk of UTI associated with an indwelling urinary catheter is 5 to 10 percent per day of catheterization.[14–16]

MICROBIOLOGY OF UTI

Escherichia coli is the commonest cause of symptomatic UTI as well as ABU in children of all ages, including neonates (Table 9–2).[1–7,17,19] Organisms encountered less frequently are *Klebsiella, Proteus* species, *Staphylococcus saprophyticus,* coagulase-negative staphylococci, *Pseudomonas aeruginosa, Streptococcus faecalis,* and *Streptococcus agalactiae. Proteus* species are often the causative organism of UTI in boys, especially in those with obstructive uropathy or other congenital urinary tract abnormalities.[17–19]

UTI due to *S. saprophyticus* is seen almost exclusively in adolescent girls, especially those who are sexually active.[20] Nosocomial UTI is usually caused by

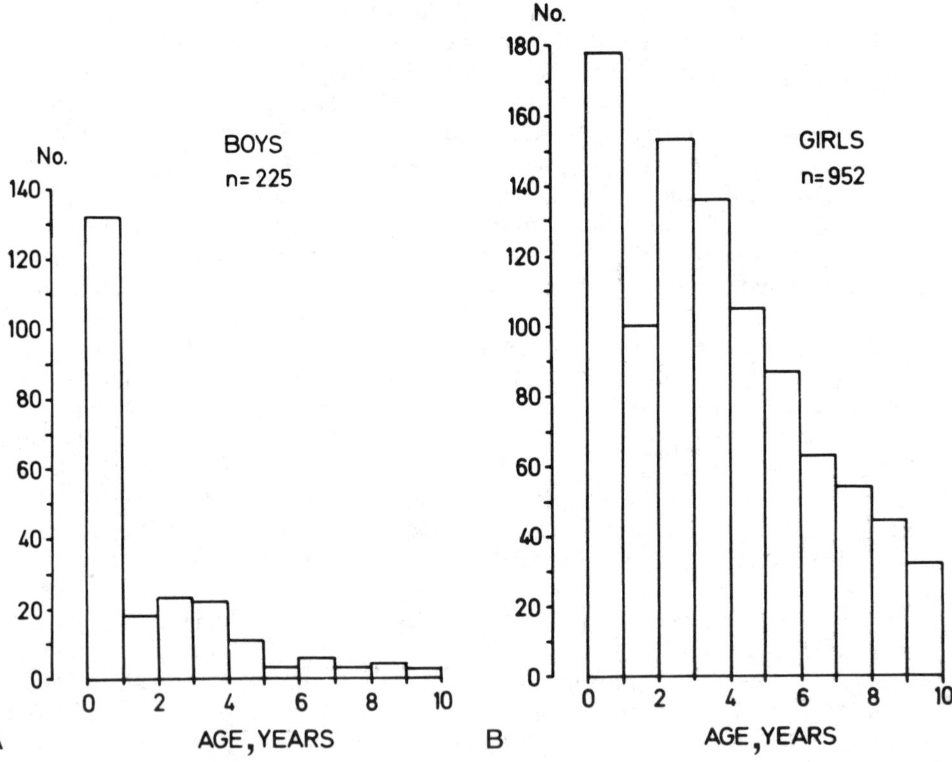

FIG. 9–1. Distribution of age of detection of first symptomatic UTI in boys (*A*) and girls (*B*) in Göteborg, Sweden. The incidence of UTI is highest in the first year in boys and decreases dramatically in the second year and beyond. (Reproduced with permission from Jodal U: The natural history of bacteriuria in childhood. *Infect Dis Clin North Am* 1:713, 1987.)

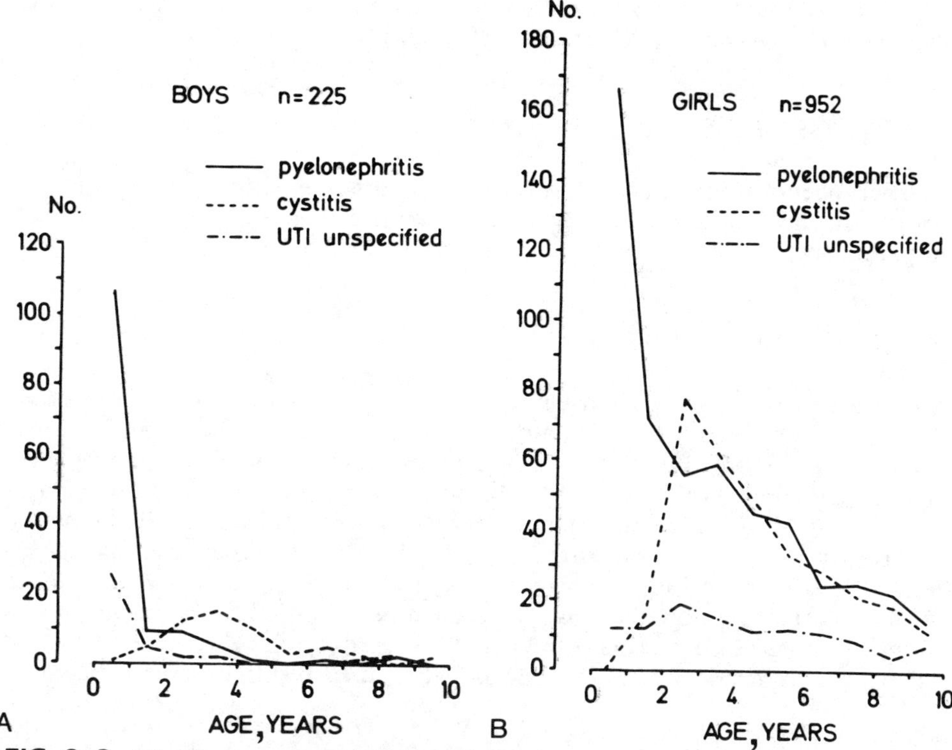

FIG. 9–2. Distribution of age at detection of first symptomatic UTI in boys (*A*) and girls (*B*) in Göteborg, Sweden. There is a dominance of acute pyelonephritis during the first two years of life in children of both sexes. Peak incidence of acute cystitis is seen between 2 and 4 years of age in boys as well as girls. (Reproduced with permission from Jodal U: The natural history of bacteriuria in childhood. *Infect Dis Clin North Am* 1:713, 1987.)

TABLE 9–2. Distribution of Bacterial Species Recovered from Children during First UTI and Recurrences

Species	Total, % (n = 4176)	First Infections, % (n = 1428)	Recurrences, % (n = 2748)
Escherichia coli	79.5	88.6	74.7
Klebsiella	3.5	2.0	4.3
Proteus	3.3	3.4	3.2
Pseudomonas	0.5	0.1	0.6
Enterococcus	2.6	2.9	2.5
Staphylococcus	2.6	0.6	3.6
Others and unknown	8.0	2.4	11.1

Source: Reproduced with permission from Swanborg-Eden C, de Man P: Bacterial virulence in urinary tract infection. *Infect Dis Clin North Am* 1:731, 1987.

E. coli, Pseudomonas species, coagulase-negative staphylococci, *Enterococcus* species, *Klebsiella* species, and *Enterobacter* species.[13]

PATHOGENESIS

The pathogenesis of UTI is complex, involving the interaction of several factors present in the host and in the invading organism (Fig. 9–3). Relevant aspects of pathogenesis and susceptibility are discussed below.

ROUTE OF INFECTION

Bacteria can reach the urinary tract either by a hematogenous route or by ascending from urethral orifice into the urinary bladder, and eventually reaching the kidneys. In general, the hematogenous route is uncommon except perhaps in neonates. Well-documented bacteremia is seen in about 30 percent of neonates and infants less than 3 months of age.[1,2,19] In older children, hematogenous spread of infection to the urinary tract (acute pyelonephritis) is characterized by bacteremia due to virulent organisms such as *S. aureus, P. aeruginosa, Serratia* species, and tuberculosis. Bacteremia developing from a primary focus of infection within the urinary tract is often referred to as *urosepsis*.

In most children and adults, UTI is believed to result from the ascent of

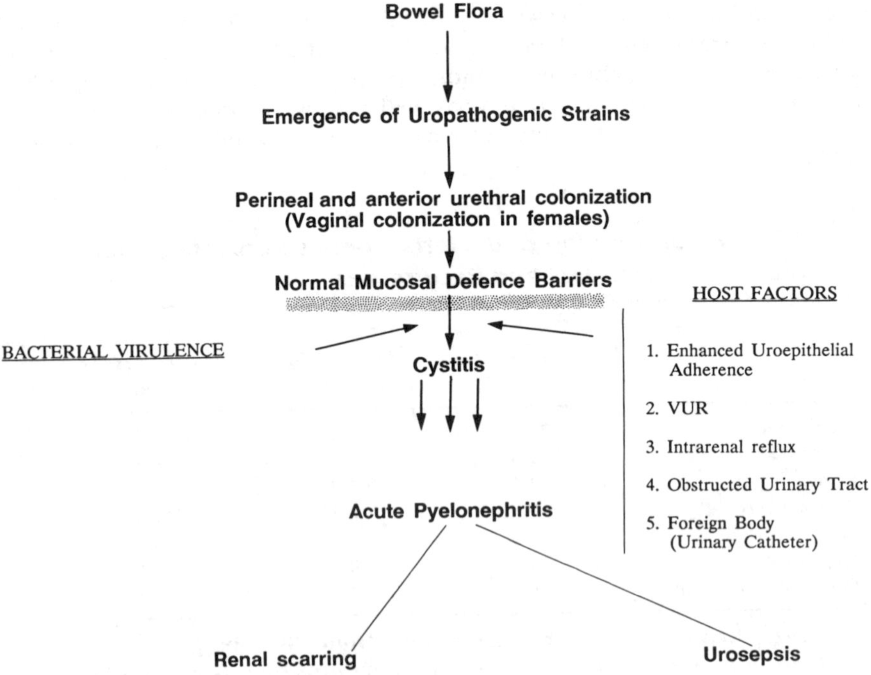

FIG. 9–3. Pathogenesis of ascending UTI.

organisms in a retrograde manner from the urethral orifice to the kidneys (Fig. 9–3). *Escherichia coli* in the colonic flora constitutes a potential reservoir of organisms that can eventually cause ascending UTI.[21] Not all strains of colonic *E. coli* possess the capacity to colonize the urinary tract. Invading bacteria require uropathogenic virulence in order for UTI to occur in an anatomically normal urinary tract. On the other hand, these bacterial virulence factors may not be essential to the pathogenesis of UTI in children with anatomic or neurogenic abnormalities of the urinary tract.[22] An important first step in the pathogenesis of ascending UTI is the appearance of the uropathogenic *E. coli* within the gastrointestinal tract, followed by periurethral and introital colonization in females.[23–25] Periurethral and prepucial colonization has also been shown to occur in boys prior to the development of UTI.[26]

The mechanism by which microorganisms ascend from the periurethral and vaginal region into the urinary bladder is not entirely clear. In some individuals, one or more of the inherited functional disturbances described below may facilitate initial colonization of the urinary bladder. In adult females, sexual activity appears to promote bacterial migration from the periurethral environment into the urinary tract and lead to bacteriuria and UTI. This risk factor may also be operative in sexually active adolescents.[27,28] Several experimental studies have confirmed that bacteria can ascend from the urinary bladder into the kidneys and cause acute pyelonephritis.[29] However, in many of these experimental circumstances, obstruction of the urinary tract is an important prerequisite for the ascending infection to establish itself within the urinary tract. Vesicoureteral reflux is well known to predispose to pyelonephritis by conducting bacteria from the urinary bladder to the renal tissue via the refluxing ureter.

HOST FACTORS AND UTI

While some children are predisposed to UTI because of congenital or developmental anomalies of the urinary tract, such defects are not detectable in others, despite a diligent search. In the latter instances, high bacterial virulence or functional abnormalities of the urinary tract in the host have been postulated. The effect of host factors on the pathogenesis of UTI is discussed below (Table 9–3).

ANATOMIC ABNORMALITIES

In normal individuals, adherence and proliferation of bacteria gaining entrance into the urinary bladder is prevented by the process of bacterial washout during voiding. In addition, several other local and mucosal defense mechanisms may also play a role in preventing UTI (Table 9–4). Congenital and acquired anomalies of the urinary tract may interfere in these local defense mechanisms, and thus enhance the risk of UTI. The overall incidence of radiologically detectable abnormalities of the urinary tract in patients with UTI has been reported to be approximately 40 to 50 percent.[30,31] Vesicoureteral reflux is the most frequently detected anatomic abnormality in patients with UTI, being present in about 30 percent of such patients.[12,30] Vesicoureteral reflux renders children susceptible

TABLE 9–3. Host Factors Predisposing to UTI

Anatomic Factors
Vesicoureteral reflux and intrarenal reflux
Urinary tract obstruction
Foreign body in the urinary tract (e.g., urinary catheter)
Duplicated collecting system
Ureterocele
Increased uroepithelial cell adherence
Nonsecretors with P blood group antigens
Nonsecretors with Lewis blood group Le (a^+ b^-) or recessive Le (a^- b^-) phenotype

to UTI by providing a conduit whereby the infected urine within the urinary bladder can ascend through the ureters and into the renal parenchyma. Additionally, VUR allows bacteria to persist within the refluxing ureter and to provide a constant source of infection within the urinary tract.[30] Stasis due to urinary tract obstruction and presence of residual urine in the urinary tract is another factor that is well known to promote bacterial proliferation.[32] Bladder diverticuli, ureteroceles, poorly draining segments of duplicated collecting systems, and urinary stones similarly predispose to UTI by serving as a nidus where the infection can persist and proliferate within the urinary tract. Presence of a foreign body such as a urinary catheter within the urinary tract also facilitates the development of UTI. The impact of urinary catheterization in predisposing children to UTI is evident from the fact that more than 90 percent of nosocomially acquired UTIs in hospitalized children are associated with catheterization of the urinary bladder.[13]

TABLE 9–4. Host Factors Associated with the Prevention of Bacterial Adherence to the Uroepithelium

Mechanical action of voiding
Tamm-Horsfall protein
Bacterial interference by endogenous periurethral flora
Urinary oligosaccharides
Spontaneous exfoliation of uroepithelial cells
Urinary immunoglobulins
Mucopolysaccharide lining of the bladder wall

Source: Modified and reproduced with permission from Sobel JD: Pathogenesis of urinary tract infection. *Infect Dis Clin North Am* 1:751, 1987.

UROEPITHELIAL ADHERENCE

The absence of anatomically defined defects in the urinary tract of a large number of patients with UTI (50–60%) suggests that other host factors may also be involved in rendering these patients "at risk" for UTI. Of these, the adherence of urinary epithelial (uroepithelial) cells to the invading bacteria has been studied extensively. It has been well established that the uroepithelial adherence of bacteria is an essential prerequisite to colonization of the urinary tract and development of UTI.[24,33–36] Uroepithelial cells in children susceptible to UTI have been shown to possess an increased capacity for binding bacteria,[33,34] possibly due to an increased availability of receptor sites on these cells.[36] Thus, in many children with anatomically normal urinary tracts, increased susceptibility to UTI may be mediated by an increased capacity of the uroepithelium to bind the invading bacteria. Put in a different way, the uroepithelial cells of these patients appear to be "stickier" than normal, thus favoring bacterial persistence and proliferation within the urinary tract. The molecular mechanisms responsible for enhancing uroepithelial bacterial adherence in patients susceptible to UTI are not entirely clear.

Blood group antigens have been recognized as one of the inherited host factors that may determine bacterial adherence to the uroepithelium.[37–41] In addition to their expression on the red blood cell surface, blood group antigens (ABO, P, Lewis) are also present on the uroepithelial cells and are secreted into body secretions of some individuals who are known as "secretors."[42] It has been suggested that women with recurrent UTI are more likely to be "non-secretors".[34] The mechanism by which blood group antigens determine susceptibility to UTI is not fully understood at this time. It has, however, been suggested that presence of blood group antigens on the uroepithelial cell surface possibly obscures or inhibits availability of the uroepithelial receptors for bacterial adhesins in secretors.[36,37,41] Conceivably, absence of blood group antigens on the surface of the uroepithelial cells in non-secretors exposes the surface receptors for bacterial adhesins, permitting a greater degree of direct contact between the invading bacteria and the uroepithelial cell, and inhancing the ability of the bacteria to attach to the uroepithelial cells.[36,37,41]

BACTERIAL VIRULENCE AND UTI

In addition to the role played by the host factors described above, the virulence of infecting organisms also determines the anatomic level to which the infection ascending from the periurethral region will localize. *Escherichia coli* has been studied extensively for various virulence factors that are important in the pathogenesis of UTI.[43–50] One well-characterized observation regarding the uropathogenic virulence of *E. coli* is that strains belonging to a few restricted, serologic OKH types are isolated from patients with acute pyelonephritis.[43,44,50] In contrast, *E. coli* from patients with asymptomatic bacteriuria does not demonstrate any such consistency of serologically determined surface markers.[43,44,50,51] In addition to the OKH serologic characteristics, other bacterial virulence factors associated with the uropathogenicity of *E. coli* are given in Table 9–5. In

TABLE 9–5. Bacterial Factors Associated with Uropathogenic Virulence of *E. coli*

Have P-fimbriae
Adhere to the uroepithelium
Belong to select O and K serotypes
Produce hemolysin
Produce colistin V
Produce aerobactin
Are resistant to the bactericidal action or normal human serum

the absence of these virulence properties, *E. coli* is unable to persist in the urinary tract and/or to induce tissue inflammation. It is, however, unclear if only one or several of these bacterial factors are necessary for *E. coli* to be uropathogenic, since these virulence characteristics are often coexpressed.

The cell adherence property of *E. coli* is essential for the invading organisms to persist in the urinary tract and cause UTI. Adherence between bacteria and uroepithelial cells is mediated through receptors on the uroepithelial cell and protein molecules, known as *adhesins,* present on the bacterial surface. The bacterial adhesins recognize specific receptors present on the uroepithelial cells. In the case of *E. coli,* adhesins are located on the tips of appendages, known as *pili* or *fimbriae,* which radiate from the bacterial surface.[52]

Pili and their corresponding adhesins enable the bacteria to anchor themselves to the host cells. Several types of pili, based on the nature of *adhesin* present, have been described in *E. coli.* Type-1 pili and the accompanying adhesin are characterized by their ability to agglutinate giunea pig red blood cells. This agglutination is, however, inhibited by the presence of mannose. Type-1, or mannose-sensitive, pili are common to many fimbriated (uropathogenic as well as nonpathogenic) *E. coli. Escherichia coli* that adhere to the uroepithelial cells and cause pyelonephritis are able to agglutinate human red blood cells, this agglutination being resistant to the presence of mannose.[52] This adhesin on the pili of uropathogenic *E. coli* interacts with the uroepithelial cells via the glycolipid receptor with the common disaccharide galactose α 1–4 galactose β.[53–55] Pili expressing such receptor-binding characteristics are known as *Gal-Gal pili,* or *P-fimbriae,* named after the P-blood-group antigens which also contain the same glycosphingolipid that is present in the uroepithelial receptors. P-fimbriae are detected in more than 90 percent of *E. coli* isolated from the urine of patients suffering from acute pyelonephritis in a nonobstructive urinary tract.[53–55] On the other hand, P-fimbriae are expressed by only a minority of resident colonic *E. coli.*[49,53] Consequently, the presence of P-fimbriae in *E. coli* is regarded as a recognizable uropathogenic bacterial virulence factor.

Does uroepithelial bacterial adherence promote an inflammatory response within the kidney and/or lead to chronic renal damage and scar formation? This issue is undergoing intensive analysis at present. Marild et al.[44] studied bacterial virulence characteristics and inflammatory response prospectively in children with their first febrile UTI (acute pyelonephritis). Patients infected with adhering *E. coli* had a significantly higher systemic and renal inflammatory response (urinary leukocyte count, serum C-reactive protein, and sedimentation rate) than did those infected with the nonadhering strains. The authors suggest that bacterial adhesion to uroepithelium may promote an inflammatory response by providing bacterial endotoxins and lipopolysaccharides more efficiently and directly to the renal tissues. Although the role of adhering *E. coli* in the pathogenesis of renal scars is not entirely clear, such a link has recently been proposed.[56,57]

CIRCUMCISION AND UTI IN BOYS

In 1975 the ad hoc task force of the America Academy of Pediatrics on circumcision stated that "there was no absolute medical indication for routine circumcision of the newborn."[58] Since then, the rate of circumcision among newborn males has gradually been decreasing.[59] In the last decade, several studies have suggested that the incidence of UTI appears to be higher in uncircumcised males and that circumcision may be beneficial for the young infant. Ginsburg and McCracken[1] demonstrated that 95 percent of male newborns and infants less than 3 months of age who developed UTI were uncircumcised. In their several studies, Wiswell and coworkers[60–62] have reported that circumcision appeared to decrease the risk of UTI in early infancy. Herzog[63] confirmed the findings of Wiswell and coworkers and suggested that circumcision provided protection against UTI not only during the neonatal period but throughout the entire first year of life. A major criticism of these studies describing the relationship of circumcision to UTI in early infancy has been the retrospective nature of their analysis. As pointed out by the Task Force on Circumcision of the American Academy of Pediatrics, prospective studies on the subject are necessary in order to overcome methodologic bias and problems that are inherent in retrospective studies.[64] At present, there appears to be no uniformity of views as to whether or not lack of circumcision poses a risk for UTI in early life. The Task Force suggests that, since there may be potential benefits of circumcision, an informed consent of the parents should be obtained and risk versus benefits of circumcision discussed prior to the procedure in a neonate.[64]

CLINICAL MANIFESTATIONS

Symptoms of UTI vary significantly with the patient's age and the location of the infection within the urinary tract. In the neonatal period, UTI may present with such nonspecific symptoms as slow weight gain, temperature instability, feeding difficulties, irritability, vomiting, abdominal distension, and jaundice. Sepsis is a common accompaniment in neonates, and positive blood cultures with a congruence of urinary and blood bacteriologic isolates are seen in 30 percent of cases.[1–3,19]

Symptoms of UTI in infants less than 1 year of age but beyond the neonatal period are also somewhat nonspecific; they may consist of fever, irritability, a sickly appearance, refusal of food, vomiting, and diarrhea. Jaundice and abdominal distention may also be seen. Preschool and school-aged children with symptomatic UTI generally have symptoms localized to the urinary tract. Dysuria, urgency, and increased frequency are common manifestations of cystitis or lower UTI. Dysuria, however, can also be seen as a manifestation of conditions other than UTI, such as vaginitis, urethritis, or pinworm infection. Day-time or night-time urinary incontinence may be observed in children with UTI, especially in girls.[65] Urinary incontinence in these patients may possibly result from uninhibited bladder contraction. The presence of flank pain, fever, chills, and costovertebral tenderness suggests that the patient has upper urinary tract involvement or acute pyelonephritis.

Macroscopic hematuria is a common manifestation of UTI. Bergström[18] reported that 26 percent of all children (boys and girls) ranging from 1 to 16 years of age with UTI had macroscopic hematuria, which was seen more often in boys (43 percent) than girls (9 percent) in this study. The significance of macroscopic hematuria as a manifestation of UTI is further borne out by the observations of Ingelfinger et al.[66] who noted that UTI was the etiology of macrohematuria in about 25 percent of children investigated in the outpatient clinic at the Children's Hospital of Boston. Hypertension is an uncommon manifestation of cystitis or acute pyelonephritis. Acute renal failure has been reported to be a rare manifestation of acute pyelonephritis.[67] Some patients with recurrent UTI due to *Proteus* species may develop urinary stones (infection stones). Urease produced by these organisms splits urea present in the urine into ammonia and CO_2, which renders the urine alkaline and creates an environment for the precipitation of struvite and the formation of renal stones.

UTI AS A CAUSE OF FEBRILE ILLNESS

Urinary tract infection is often considered in the differential diagnosis of fever in patients seen in the outpatient clinic or emergency room, especially if the focus of infection is not evident on clinical examination. How often does UTI account for fever in children seen in office practice? Bauchner et al.[68] obtained urine cultures in 664 febrile children 1 to 5 years of age. Bacteriuria was documented in only 1.7 percent, a figure similar to that for asymptomatic bacteriuria in this age group. These data suggests that UTI is not a particularly common cause of fever in children 1 to 5 years old who are seen in the office or emergency room. By contast, UTI has been reported to be more common as a cause of fever in infants less than 8 weeks of age. In one study,[12] UTI was the etiology of fever in 7.5 percent of infants in this age group. Another finding of this study was that neither clinical examination nor laboratory findings (urinalysis) were able to predict the presence of UTI as a cause of fever in more than half of these patients.

THE INVESTIGATION OF UTI

The purposes of laboratory investigations of children with UTI are (1) to confirm the diagnosis, (2) to identify patients with urologic malformations, and (3) to localize the site of infection within the urinary tract (pyelonephritis versus cystitis). The series of investigations required to meet these goals may vary from one center to another, depending upon the availability of resources and on institutional preferences.

URINALYSIS

The first and one of the simplest tests to be undertaken in a child with suspected UTI is to perform urinalysis, including examination of the urinary sediment. Pyuria or excretion of an increased number of white blood cells is considered to be presumptive evidence of UTI. Pyuria is defined as the presence of more than 10 white cells per high power field visualized by light microscopy in a centrifuged urinary sediment. This semiquantitative estimation of white cell excretion is influenced by variables such as centrifuge speed, duration of centrifugation time, and volume of urine in which the sediment is resuspended. For these reasons, some have suggested that a white cell count in the urine is more reproducible. A white cell count of more than 250 cells/mm^3 in an uncentrifuged urine sample is suggestive of UTI.[69] While most patients with cystitis as well as pyelonephritis develop pyuria, this test has important diagnostic limitations. Pyuria is an unreliable laboratory finding of UTI in infants below 1 year of age, being absent in over 50 percent of documented cases.[12] Also, pyuria may be caused by several conditions other than UTI (Table 9–6). Hematuria is a frequent finding in patients with UTI. A poorly concentrated (in terms of specific gravity or osmolality) morning urine may be seen in patients with pyelonephritis.

NONCULTURE EVIDENCE OF BACTERIURIA

Several convenient tests designed to detect bacteriuria by nonculture methods are available commercially. These tests are usually used to screen children for asymptomatic bacteriuria and for the evaluation of patients in the office or emergency room. Confirmation of bacteriuria by urine culture is essential as the next step in patients shown to have positive screening tests. Two of the commonly used nonculture tests for bacteriuria used in clinical practice are discussed below.

TABLE 9–6. Clinical Conditions Associated with Pyuria

Dehydration
Vaginitis in girls
Meatal and urethal irritation in boys
Renal stones
Renal tubular acidosis
Interstitial nephritis
Cystic renal disease
Glomerulonephritis
Appendicitis

MICROSCOPIC EXAMINATION OF THE URINE

Two drops of freshly voided, uncentrifuged urine are placed on a glass slide and allowed to dry. The slide is then stained with Gram stain. The presence of one to two bacteria per high power field (oil immersion) is suggestive of significant bacteriuria.

NITRITE, OR GREISS, TEST

It has been well known for over 100 years that the detection of nitrites in the urine indicates UTI.[70] The nitrite, or Greiss, test is based on the fact that bacterial enzyme nitrate reductase can convert the urinary nitrate to nitrite, which can be detected by several available chemical methods. Many of the commercially available dipstick tests for the chemical analysis of urine now incorporate the nitrite detection strip. The urinary nitrite test has been advocated for use primarily as a screening test for detecting bacteriuria; its sensitivity has been reported to be highly variable in several studies.[71,72] In a recent study[73] of 200 children with culture-documented symptomatic urinary tract infection, the nitrite test was positive in only 52 percent. A high rate of false-negative results by the nitrite test for bacteriuria is possibly related to the method of urine collection and the time of day when the test is performed. If urine is not allowed to incubate with infecting bacteria in the urinary bladder, conversion of nitrate to nitrite may be incomplete and thus lead to a falsely negative test. As can be imagined, patients with symptomatic UTI who urinate frequently may be unable to convert nitrate to nitrite, thus producing falsely negative nitrite tests. A negative nitrite test may also be encountered if UTI is caused by bacteria that lack the enzyme nitrate reductase (streptococcal species) and are unable to form nitrite. An early morning specimen is least likely to give false-negative results.

URINE CULTURE

A positive urine culture is the accepted standard laboratory test for the diagnosis of UTI. Although it is an easy test to perform, several aspects must be well understood.

OBTAINING THE SPECIMEN

The method of urine collection has a major impact on the results of urine culture. Urine specimens for culture may be obtained by clean voiding, catheterization, suprapubic bladder aspiration, or urine bag collection (in infants). In older children and adolescents, especially boys, a midstream urine sample obtained after adequate local preparation is usually acceptable. Alternatively, straight catheterization (in and out) may be undertaken. In neonates and infants, suprapubic aspiration or tap is a practical method and is preferred. It is associated with a low rate of complications when done carefully; the failure rate for this procedure is 5 to 10 percent. The superiority of suprapubic aspiration over urine bag collection in infants has been documented in more than one study.[69,74,75] However, negative bacterial culture of a bagged urine specimen can be taken as a reasonable assurance of absence of UTI.

CULTURE TECHNIQUES

Quantitative culture of the urine remains the "gold standard" for confirmation of significant bacteriuria and UTI. Several microbiologic techniques are used to culture urine for quantitative colony counts. In the *pour-plate method* of urine culture, the urine is diluted with broth (1:100), plated on blood agar, and then incubated at 37°C. Although it is an accurate method, the pour-plate technique is cumbersome and has been replaced by the more convenient loop culture method. This technique uses a standard platinum (quantitative) loop which has a volume of 1/1000 mL. Urine is picked up in the loop and streaked thoroughly across a blood agar plate, which is then incubated using standard techniques.

Several convenient urine culture tests suited for office use have been available for some time (Table 9–7). A *dipslide method,* in which an agar-coated slide is dipped into urine and incubated, is cost-effective and convenient (Fig. 9–4).[76] Some of the office culture methods even offer preliminary identification of the organisms by means of a chemical indicator within the culture medium, which changes color in the presence of specific groups of organisms. Confirmatory tests of the bacterial isolates for definitive identification and antibiotic sensitivites must, however, be performed in the laboratory.

The standard criterion for the diagnosis of UTI consists of documenting on culture the growth of 100,000 (or 10^5) bacterial colonies per milliliter of urine from a clean-catch urine specimen. The presence of any bacterial growth in urine samples obtained by suprapubic aspiration or careful bladder catheterization can be interpreted as suggesting infection (Table 9–1).

TABLE 9–7. Commercially Available Bacterial Culture Kits for Office Use

Method	Advantages	Disadvantages
Dipslide	Accurate Preliminary species identification Room temperature incubation possible Sensitivity testing possible	
Filter paper	Compact Sensitivity testing possible Less expensive than dipslide	Inaccurate quantitation if fewer than 10^5 CFU/mL[a] Less accurate than dipslide
Pad culture	Includes nitrite strip	Subculturing not possible
Inverted cup (roll tube)		Subculturing difficult

[a]CFU = colony forming units.

Source: Reproduced with permission from Durbin WA, Peter G: Management of urinary tract infections in infants and children. *Pediatr Infect Dis* 3:564, 1984; © by Williams & Wilkins, 1984.

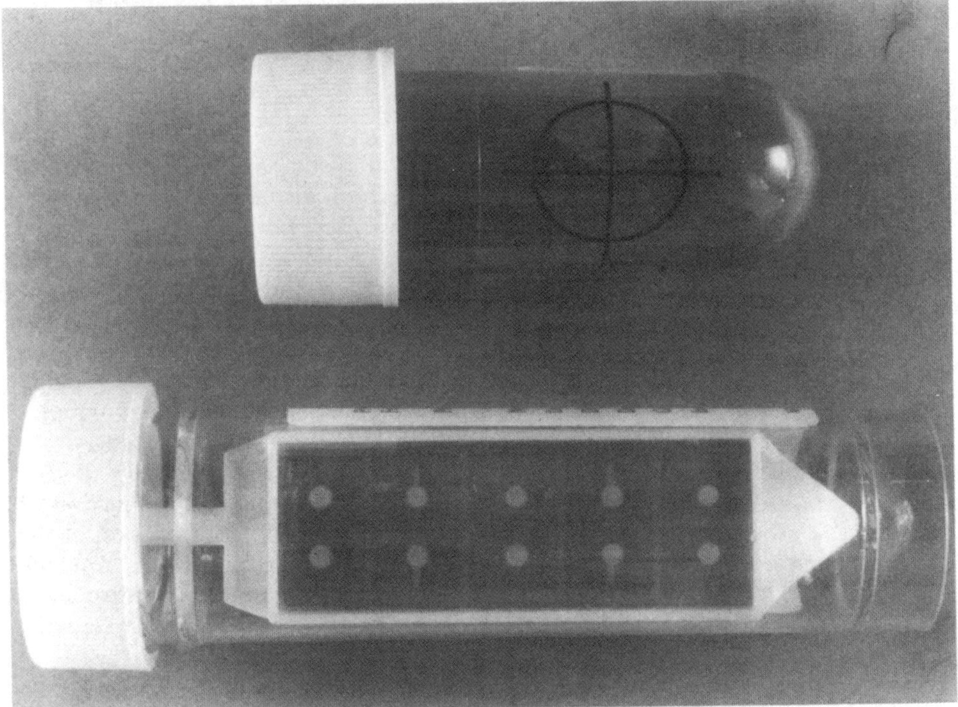

FIG. 9–4. Commercially available office urine culture kits. *A.* Bacturcult (Wampole Labs, N.J.). *B.* Dip N Count (Starplex Scientific, Ontario, Canada).

RADIOLOGIC EVALUATION OF THE URINARY TRACT

The aims of radiologic studies in a patient with UTI are threefold: (1) to uncover any underlying urologic abnormalities, (2) to identify patients in whom chronic renal damage and scarring resulting from previously undiagnosed or untreated UTI may already have developed, and (3) to assist in the diagnosis of acute pyelonephritis. Since urologic anomalies such as vesicoureteral reflux, duplicated collection system, and urinary obstruction can predispose children to chronic renal damage, screening for structural urologic anomalies in patients with UTI is considered essential to the prevention of long-term sequelae. However, there has been no consensus regarding the selection of patients, timing of radiologic evaluation, and types of radiologic tests required for initial screening. While many authors suggest a selective approach based on a child's age and sex, others feel that all children with UTI, especially those below 5 years of age, should undergo diagnostic imaging after their first UTI.[77,78] Remarks listed in Table 9–8 regarding patient selection for radiologic investigation should serve as guidelines for the practicing physician. Radiologically detectable abnormalities of the urinary tract in children with UTI are seen in 40 to 50 percent of cases (Table 9–9).[3,30,31]

TABLE 9–8. Guidelines for Selection of Patients with UTI for Radiologic Investigations

All neonates with first UTI
All males with first UTI at any age
All patients with recurrent UTI
All patients with pyelonephritis

RENAL ULTRASONOGRAPHY

Being a noninvasive test that does not require the injection of any radiocontrast material or radioisotopes, renal ultrasonography is increasingly being advocated as the initial radiologic investigation of choice in children with UTI. The purpose of ultrasonographic evaluation is to detect any renal abnormalities of size and shape as well as obstructive lesions of the urinary tract. The bladder (if full) and ureteral pathways should also be investigated during the initial examination. The disadvantages of ultrasonography are that it requires operator skill, lacks a standard method of representation for record keeping, and is rather poor in detecting renal cortical defects (scars).

INTRAVENOUS PYELOGRAPHY (IVP)

Radiocontrast material injected intravenously is excreted by the kidney, outlining the renal contour in the early nephrogram phase and the urinary collecting system (ureters and urinary bladder) later on. *Intravenous pyelography* provides excellent information about renal size, the presence of renal scars, and the state

TABLE 9–9. Incidence of Radiologic Abnormalities Seen in Children with UTI

	Neonates[a]	0–13 Years[b]
Number	64	572
Normal	45.3%	48%
Vesicoureteral reflux	42.2%	31%
Obstruction	9.4%	7.5%
Duplex system	3.1%	7.0%
Renal scarring with normal studies	—	6.0%
Other renal anomalies (e.g., agenesis, renal cysts)	—	0.5%

[a]Data adapted and reproduced with permission from Drew JH, Acton CM: Radiologic findings in newborn infants with urinary tract infection. *Arch Dis Child* 51:628, 1976.

[b]Data adapted and reproduced with permission from McKerrow W, Davidson-Lamb N, Jones PF: Urinary tract infection in children. *Br Med J* 289:299, 1984.

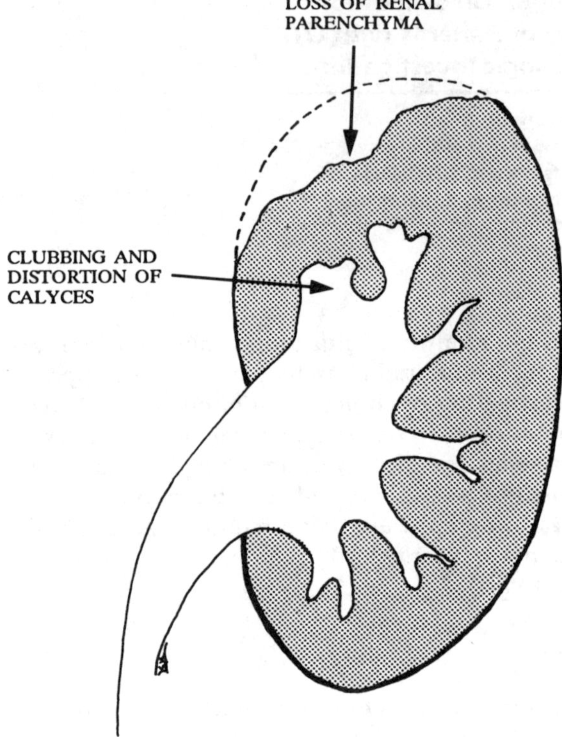

FIG. 9–5. Diagrammatic representation of features of chronic pyelonephritic scars seen in intravenous pyelography.

of pelvicalyceal system. Because of its almost universal availability (even in small medical centers) and a standardized technique for obtaining a permanent radiographic record, IVP has been accepted as the "gold standard" in the evaluation of patients with UTI. In well-established cases, renal scars appear as irregular renal cortical outlines; the corresponding calyx also shows blunting and deformity, especially if there is underlying vesicoureteric reflux (Fig. 9–5). Although IVP provides a better assessment of renal scars than ultrasonography, lesions present on the anterior or posterior aspect may be missed. This is not the radiologic procedure of choice for evaluation of the urinary tract in neonates and children with renal failure, since their inability to concentrate and excrete the contrast material adequately renders interpretation of the results difficult.

VOIDING CYSTOURETHROGRAM (VCUG)

Neither renal ultrasonography nor IVP can diagnose VUR unless it is of severe grade. A voiding cystourethrogram is the definitive method of establishing the diagnosis of VUR and is considered essential in the evaluation of children with UTI. This test can be performed using either conventional radioopaque contrast material or radioisotopes (Figs. 9–6 and 9–7).[79,80] While radioisotope VCUG is becoming popular in many centers, a conventional VCUG using a radiocontrast

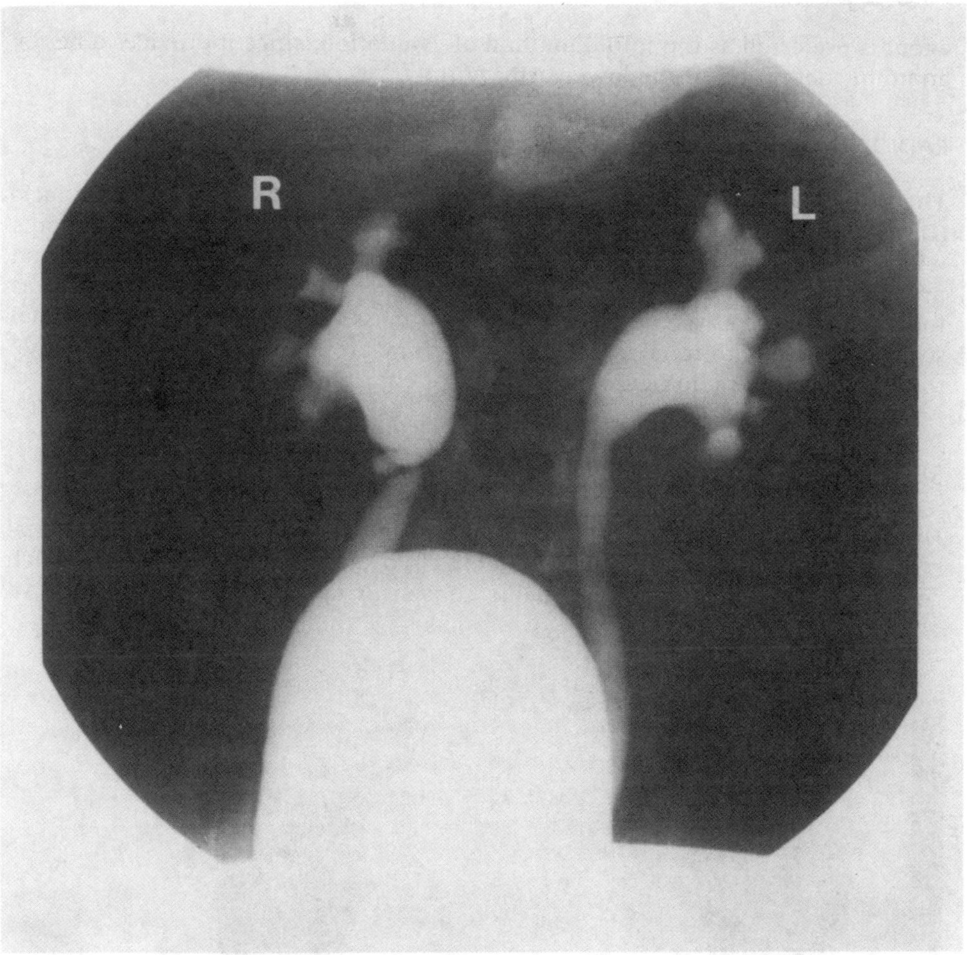

FIG. 9–6. VCUG, grade III reflux on the right side and grade IV reflux on the left side.

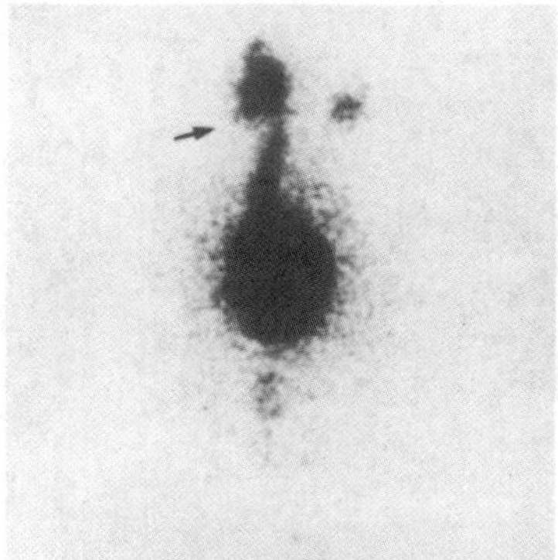

FIG. 9–7. Radioisotope VCUG showing severe reflux on the left side. As can be seen, radioisotope VCUG provides less degree definition of anatomic detail than conventional VCUG using radiocontrast material (Fig. 9–6).

agent is preferred as the initial method of evaluation, since it provides a better anatomic definition of the lower urinary tract.

RADIOISOTOPE SCINTIGRAM

The radioisotope scintigram or scan using ^{99m}Tc dimercaptosuccinic acid (DMSA) can be used as an adjunct in the detection of renal scars in patients with UTI. Radiolabeled DMSA is concentrated in the renal epithelial cells and provides a reasonably well-defined outline of the kidney. Renal scars appear as focal photopenic areas, with loss of cortical mass (Fig. 9–8). The DMSA renal scan combined with renal ultrasonography may provide an effective alternative to the IVP as the radiologic investigation of choice in UTI.[81]

SEQUENCING AND TIMING OF RADIOLOGIC TESTS

Discussions related to the number of radiologic tests required to detect renal scars and anomalies of the urinary tract in children with UTI have evoked much controversy in past, but a reasonable consensus appears to be emerging. An

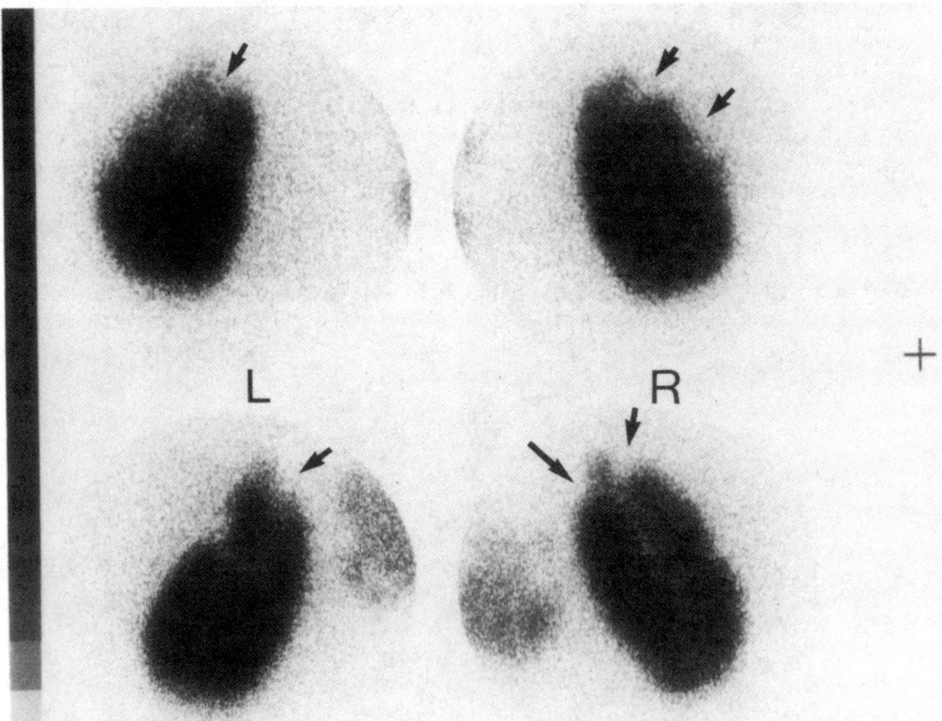

FIG. 9–8. DMSA scan, posterior (*upper panel*) and oblique (*lower panel*) views of the kidney with pyelonephritic scars (*arrows*).

ultrasonographic evaluation of the kidney and a voiding cystourethrogram (VCUG) is regarded as the minimum diagnostic radiologic workup in patients with UTI.[77,78,82] In the past, the IVP has enjoyed a prominent place in the examination of patients with UTI; however, the use of this test has declined as experience with ultrasonography has increased. In most pediatric centers, ultrasonography has replaced IVP as the first radiologic procedure in the evaluation of patients with UTI. However, if renal ultrasonography reveals any abnormality in the renal architecture or if VUR is documented in the VCUG, an IVP may then be considered. As noted earlier, IVP provides a better definition of renal scars than does ultrasonography. The radioisotope renal scan (DMSA scan) is increasingly being employed as one of the initial radiologic investigations in patients with UTI, especially in high-risk patients who are suspected to have renal damage. In conjunction with renal ultrasonography, radioisotope renal scans provide an effective alternative to IVP. Since VUR can be detected only by VCUG, this test constitutes an integral part of the initial radiologic investigation for patients with UTI.

The timing and sequencing of radiologic studies for UTI vary greatly from center to center. In most patients, an ultrasonographic evaluation of the kidney for anatomy and architecture can be undertaken within 10 to 14 days of diagnosis of UTI. A DMSA scan can also be performed at this time for evaluation of renal scarring. If complications of acute pyelonephritis or urinary obstruction are suspected, these radiologic evaluations may be undertaken earlier in the course of the disease. The VCUG can and should be postponed for 4 to 6 weeks following the last episode of UTI.[78] It is well known that ureteral dilatation and mild hydronephrosis without obstruction or VUR can be seen in patients with UTI, particularly those with pyelonephritis.[80,83] This results from atony of the ureteral muscles caused by the infection. A recent study[83] has shown that ureteral dilatation is a common feature of UTI caused by globo-positive *E. coli* (possessing adhesin specific for the globo series of the glycolipid receptors). The authors of the study speculate that this effect on the ureters may be mediated by endotoxins delivered locally by the adhering organisms. On the basis of these observations, it is apparent that radiologic studies performed on an acutely inflamed urinary tract may falsely show a higher incidence of urinary stasis or VUR. Additionally, a VCUG performed when the lower urinary tract is infected may also increase the risk of propagating infection into the kidneys.

USE OF RADIOLOGIC IMAGING IN ACUTE PYELONEPHRITIS

Both ultrasound and radionuclide renal scans can be helpful in providing corroborative evidence of acute pyelonephritis. Ultrasound examination of acute pyelonephritis often shows (1) hypoechoic kidneys with a loss of corticomedullary definition, (2) some dilatation of the renal pelvis, and (3) an increase in renal size.[84,85] Renal cortical scintigraphy using either ^{99}Tc-glucoheptonate or ^{99}Tc-dimercaptosuccinic acid (DMSA) is often helpful in detecting areas of acute inflammation within the renal parenchyma as spherical areas of photopenia (Fig. 9–9) without any loss of cortical mass.[86] Handmaker[87] has described a flare-shaped photopenic area radiating from the pelvicalyceal area toward the cortex

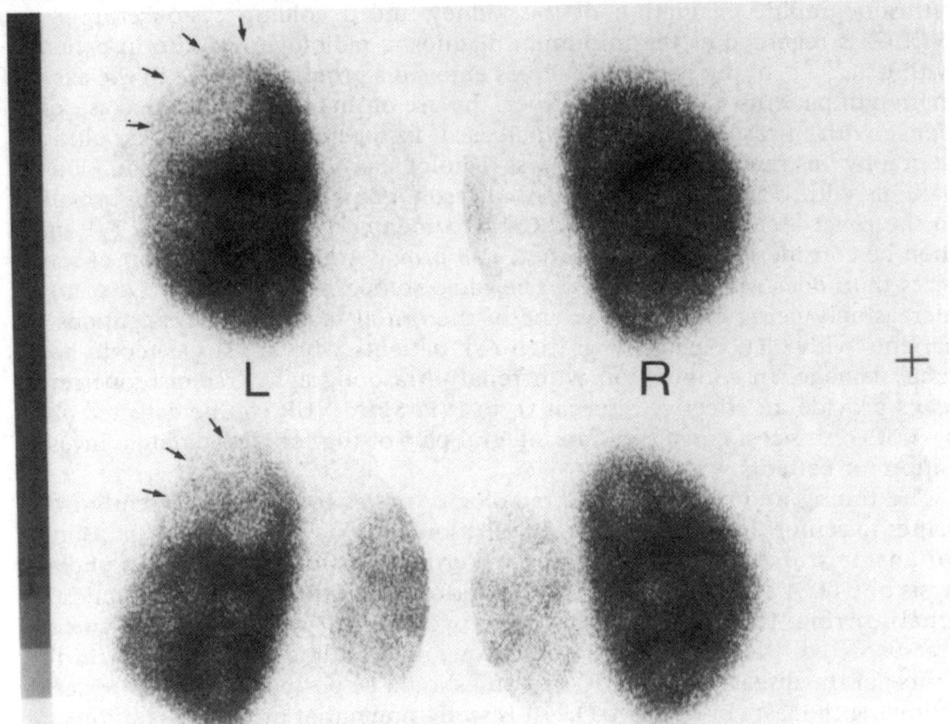

FIG. 9–9. Acute pyelonephritis in a child as seen on DMSA scan. The photopenic area (*arrows*) in the renal parenchyma represents site of inflammatory lesion.

as a common and specific sign for acute pyelonephritis ("flare sign"). It must be pointed out that cortical scintigraphy may fail to differentiate between an established cortical scar and findings associated with acute pyelonephritis. Intravenous pyelography is not a helpful diagnostic test in uncomplicated acute pyelonephritis.

LOCALIZING THE SITE OF INFECTION

Localization of the site of infection has an important bearing on the treatment and prognosis of patients with UTI. While acute pyelonephritis can result in renal damage and scarring, uncomplicated cystitis is not associated with such complications. Moreover, localization of the site of infection is important in choosing therapeutic options. The primary distinction between upper and lower UTI is based on clinical manifestations of the patient. Lower UTI or cystitis is characterized by the clinical features of dysuria, frequency, and urgency of micturition as well as suprapubic tenderness. In contrast, the presence of fever and tenderness of the costovertebral angle in addition to other clinical symptoms of UTI in a patient with pyuria and bacteriuria is suggestive of acute pyelonephritis. While such a clinical differentiation may be easy in most older children, laboratory evidence documenting the location of infection within the urinary tract is sometimes required in younger children, in whom the clinical signs of pyelonephritis may not be as well defined. Several laboratory tests used for localizing the site of infection in the urinary tract are given in Table 9–10. While many of these tests are available in clinical laboratories, some require special equipment and are too cumbersome for widespread clinical application. One commonly available laboratory test is to test the patient's ability to concentrate urine. A low urine specific gravity in the first morning sample is considered presumptive evidence of acute pyelonephritis. Cystitis, on the other hand, is not characterized by a defect in urinary concentrating ability. Other readily available tests for localization of the site of UTI are the erythrocyte sedimentation rate (ESR) and serum C-reactive proteins (CRP). Both these tests are acute-phase reactants that can be elevated in response to an inflammatory process, including infection, and may be elevated (but not always) in instances of acute pyelonephritis.[88,89] The antibody-coated bacteria test which is able to differentiate cystitis from acute pyelonephritis in adults[90] has been reported to be less specific in children.[91]

MANAGEMENT

The management of children with UTI depends largely on the location of the infection within the urinary tract (i.e., pyelonephritis versus cystitis) and the age of the patient (Fig. 9–10). Children of any age who are suspected to have acute pyelonephritis are best treated in the hospital with intravenous antibiotics. Additionally, patients who have UTI complicated by perinephric abscess formation, acute focal pyelonephritis, or urinary tract obstruction should also be hospitalized. Occasionally, patients with severe cystitis who have pain, vomiting, and dehydration should also receive intravenous therapy in the hospital until they demonstrate symptomatic improvement. Patients with uncomplicated cystitis can be managed on an outpatient basis.

TABLE 9–10. Laboratory Tests Indicative of Acute Pyelonephritis in Patients with UTI

Elevated erythrocyte sedimentation rate
Decreased urinary concentrating ability
Pyuria with white cell casts
Increased serum concentration of C-reactive protein
Increased urinary excretion of $beta_2$ microglobulin
Presence of antibody-coated bacteria in urine
Photopenic area in radioisotope (DMSA) renal cortical scintigraphy

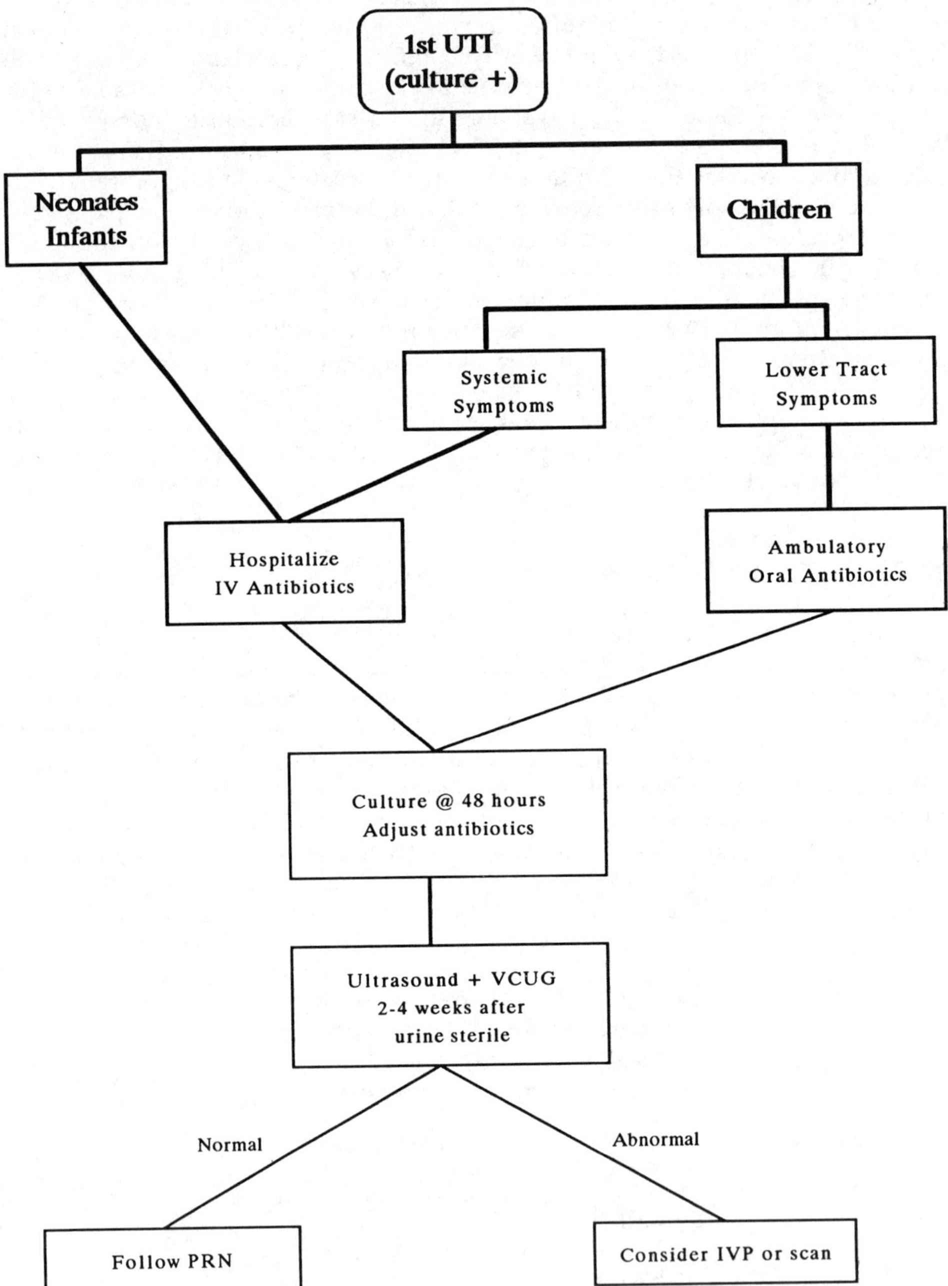

FIG. 9–10. Algorithm for sequencing radiologic studies and managing children with UTI.

ACUTE PYELONEPHRITIS

The treatment of patients with acute pyelonephritis should be initiated with broad antibiotic coverage (i.e., ampicillin and an aminoglycoside) given intravenously. Dosages for the individual drugs are listed in Table 9–11. The potential of aminoglycosides for systemic toxicity and nephrotoxicity should be considered, and serum creatinine and serum aminoglycoside concentrations should be monitored. As a general rule, nitrofurantoin should not be used in the treatment of acute pyelonephritis, because adequate tissue concentration of the drug within the renal parenchyma may not be achieved despite its excellent urinary excretion.[92] A change to a less toxic and appropriate antibiotic can be made once the report of the antibiotic sensitivity of the infecting organism becomes available. Patients usually demonstrate defervescence of fever and an overall improvement within 24 to 48 h of starting antibiotic treatment. Failure to demonstrate such a response is indicative of either antibiotic resistance, an obstructed urinary tract, other urinary tract abnormalities (such as an infected renal cyst), or presence of complications such as perinephric abscess. Urine should be recultured after 48 h of antibiotic therapy to assure the effectiveness of the therapeutic regimen. In most cases parenteral antibiotic therapy may be replaced by oral therapy after 5 days provided that (1) the patient has improved symptomatically, (2) systemic signs of toxicity have disappeared, (3) the patient has been afebrile for 48 h, and (4) the organism is sensitive to an orally administered antibiotic. The recommended duration of antibiotic therapy is 10 to 14

TABLE 9–11. Antibiotic Dosage for Treatment and Prophylaxis of UTI in Children

Drug	Dosage, mg/kg/day	Frequency (Child's Age)	Prophylaxis,[a] mg/kg
Parenteral therapy			
Ampicillin	100	q 12 h (<1 week), q 6–8 h (>1 week)	
Cefotaxime	100	q 8 h	
Gentamicin	5 7.5	q 12 h (<1 week), q 8 h (>1 week)	
Oral therapy (standard course)			
Amoxicillin	20–40	q 8 h	
Ampicillin	50–100	q 6 h	
Augmentin	50	q 8 h	
Cephalexin	50	q 6–8 h	
Nitrofurantoin[b]	5–7	q 6 h	1–2
Sulfisoxazole[b]	120–150	q 6–8 h	50
Trimethoprim[b]	6–12	q 12 h	2
Sulfamethoxazole	30–60	q 12 h	10

[a]Prophylaxis is given by mouth as a single bedtime dose.
[b]Not recommended for newborns or patients with renal insufficiency.

From Feld LG, Greenfield, and Ogra PL: Urinary tract infections in infants and children. *Pediatr Rev* 11: 71, 1989. Reproduced by permission of American Academy of Pediatrics, © 1987.

days. It is recommended to start these patients on low-dose oral prophylactic therapy after treatment for acute pyelonephritis is completed until the results of VCUG are available. If VUR is demonstrated, low-dose antibiotic prophylaxis may be continued for a prolonged period.

CYSTITIS

Children with cystitis can be treated with oral antibiotics and do not require hospitalization. Therapy can begin with either trimethoprim-sulfamethoxazole (Bactrim, Septra) or amoxicillin given in therapeutic doses. Antibiotic therapy must be reevaluated after bacterial sensitivity results become available. Current recommendations are to treat uncomplicated cystitis with 7 to 10 days of antibiotic therapy. In one study resistance of *E. coli* to trimethoprim-sulfamethoxazole has been reported to be 7 percent, but up to 11 percent of patients may exhibit resistance to ampicillin.[94] In communities where the unrestricted use of nonprescription antibiotics is prevalent, a higher rate of antibiotic resistance may be encountered.

UTI IN NEONATES

Since UTI in neonates is commonly associated with sepsis, all such patients require hospitalization. In order to establish the diagnosis with certainty, urine for culture should be obtained by suprapubic aspiration prior to commencing antibiotic therapy. Intravenous antibiotics must be instituted as soon as the diagnosis of UTI is suspected and should be continued until the results of blood and urine culture are available. Adequate coverage for gram-negative organisms *(E. coli)* is necessary in neonates and can be provided by aminoglycosides in conjunction with ampicillin. Dosages of these antibiotics must be adjusted for gestational age in preterm neonates. Renal ultrasonographic evaluation for evidence of urinary tract malformations and obstruction should be considered once the patient is clinically stable. In the absence of any structural malformation or other complications, a 10- to 14-day course of antibiotics should suffice to eradicate the infection.

SHORT-COURSE ANTIBIOTIC THERAPY FOR UTI: USE IN CHILDREN

Several studies in adults during the late 1970s and early 1980s suggested that patients with uncomplicated cystitis could be treated effectively with short courses of antibiotic therapy ranging from 3 to 4 days to single dose therapy.[95–97] The advantages of short-course antibiotic therapy cited by these studies were better patient compliance, lower cost of treatment, potentially decreased change in the bacterial flora of the gastrointestinal tract, and reduced development of antibiotic resistance. Numerous studies in children[97–102] have also evaluated the efficacy of abbreviated antibiotic treatment; while there was early enthusiasm for this approach, reassessment of the published literature and randomized prospective trials have raised concern regarding the effectiveness of such protocols. Although many studies[97–99] found no difference in bacteriologic cure rates between short-course antibiotic therapy and conventional treatment, at least three studies[100–102] have found significant therapeutic drawbacks to the short-course treatment. Avner et al.[100] found that conventional (10-day) treatment of cystitis with amoxicillin resulted in a cure rate (negative urine culture at 4 days) of 92 percent, compared with 63 percent with a single dose of amoxicillin. McCracken et al.[101] compared 10 days of cefadroxil therapy for cystitis to a single day (two doses) of treatment with the same drug.[101] They reported that the reinfection rate (4 to 5 days after discontinuation of the antibiotics) was significantly higher in those treated for a single day than in patients treated with conventional therapy (44.4 percent versus 20.0 percent). Others[102,103] have also reported a higher rate of recurrent UTI following single-dose antibiotic therapy as compared to conventional 7-day treatment protocols. Moffatt et al.[103] recently analyzed the published literature regarding short-course antibiotic therapy and concluded that there was insufficient evidence about the efficacy of abbreviated antibiotic therapy in children with uncomplicated cystitis. The authors recommend that a double-blind controlled study of various antibiotic regimens be undertaken in order to make definitive recommendations. Because of the high risk of renal scarring from undiagnosed or inadequately treated UTI in infants and young children[104] and since clinical differentiation between cystitis and acute pyelonephritis may be difficult at times, short-course antibiotic therapy for UTI can pose additional hazards in them. In view of the conflicting data, it is obvious that short-course antibiotic treatment for UTI cannot be recommended for all children at present. On the basis of available information, such therapy is indicated only for a well-defined group of children with acute cystitis (not acute pyelonephritis), who are older than 5 years of age and who have a urinary tract that is well documented as normal.

PREVENTING RECURRENCE OF UTI

Even in the absence of any urinary tract anomalies, recurrent UTI is common in children, especially girls. About 40 to 50 percent of patients with symptomatic UTI can be expected to have a recurrence of UTI during 2 years of follow-up.[17] Most recurrent UTIs are caused by a different strain of *E. coli* and should be regarded as reinfections, not relapses. Since the risk of renal scarring is higher in patients experiencing recurrent episodes of acute pyelonephritis (Table 9–12),[6] it is essential to undertake measures that will prevent such recurrences. Recurrent UTI as well as renal scarring are particularly common in children with VUR or obstructive uropathy (Table 9–13).[6,104,105] Low-dose antibiotic therapy has been used to prevent recurrences of UTI. In a controlled trial of 45 children with UTI, Smellie et al.[106] showed that low-dose urinary prophylaxis with either trimethoprim-sulfamethoxazole (2 mg trimethoprim and 10 mg sulfamethoxazole per kilogram per day) or nitrofurantoin (1 to 2 mg/kg) prevented UTI in all patients during the treatment period. One year after discontinuation of the low-dose prophylaxis, 68 percent of the treated group and 36 percent of the untreated patients remained free of recurrences. Almost all recurrences came within 6 months of the cessation of prophylactic therapy. In another study, Lohr et al.[107] evaluated the influence of low-dose (1.2 to 2.4 mg/kg/day)

TABLE 9–12. Risk of Renal Scarring in Relation to the Number of Episodes of Acute Pyelonephritis

No. of Attacks	Children, No.	Renal Scarring No.	%
0	141	7	5
1	366	32	9
2	98	15	15
3	35	12	35
≥4	24	14	58
Total	664	80	12

Source: Reproduced with permission from Jodal U: The natural history of bacteriuria in childhood. *Infect Dis Clin North Am* 1:713, 1987.

nitrofurantoin macrocrystals (Macrodantin) on recurrence of UTI and reported that the rate of infection was significantly decreased from 3.8 episodes per patient per year in the placebo group to 0.2 episodes per patient per year in the treated group.

Both nitrofurantoin and trimethoprim-sulfamethoxazole can be used effectively in preventing recurrences of UTI and are given once daily at bedtime. In patients who are either unable to tolerate these two agents or are allergic to them, an oral cephalosporin such as cephalexin (Keflex) may be used as the drug of choice. Nitrofurantoin, which is a urinary antiseptic and not an antibiotic, has a significant advantage over the trimethoprim-sulfamethoxazole combination in that it does not affect the bowel flora.[108] However, its relatively shorter duration of action (8 to 12 h) is a potential disadvantage. The long-term use of trimethoprim-sulfamethoxazole, on the other hand, is well known to encourage development of resistant organisms in the fecal flora.[109] In the event of breakthrough infection, a course of full-dose antibiotic therapy should be

TABLE 9–13. Relationship of Renal Scarring with the Severity of VUR Noted in Children at First UTI

Reflux Grade	Children, No.	Renal Scarring No.	%
0	278	15	5
1	29	3	10
2	99	17	17
≥3	38	25	66
Total	444	60	14

Source: Reproduced with permission from Jodal U: The natural history of bacteriuria in childhood. *Infect Dis Clin North Am* 1:713, 1987.

followed by antibiotic prophylaxis with a drug to which the infecting organism is reported to be sensitive.

In addition to low-dose prophylactic antibiotics, other nonpharmacologic steps may be equally important in preventing recurrent UTI. These measures include adequate fluid intake, frequent voiding during the day, complete voiding (double voiding) at bed time, correction of constipation, and the avoidance of bubble baths.

MANAGEMENT OF ASYMPTOMATIC BACTERIURIA

Bacteriuria in apparently healthy children has been well described and is known as *asymptomatic bacteriuria* (ABU), or *covert bacteriuria.* Although ABU can occur in all age groups, including neonates, infants, and adults, it is more commonly seen in school-age girls. In a study of 3581 unselected infants, Wettergren et al.[9] detected asymptomatic bacteriuria in 2.5 percent of boys and 0.9 percent of girls during the first year of life. Kunin, in his well-known epidemiologic studies,[7,8] noted that 1.1 percent of girls in the first through twelfth grades (5 to 18 years old) had asymptomatic bacteriuria. Other studies have reported a similar prevalence of ABU among school-age girls.[10,12] As in the case of symptomatic UTI, *E. coli* is the most prevalent causative organism in ABU.[7–12,110,111] Less commonly, organisms such as *Klebsiella, Proteus,* and *Staphylococcus* may also be encountered.[111] The *E. coli* organisms causing ABU appear to be less virulent than those recovered from patients with symptomatic UTI. They are often of nontypable O serotype, demonstrate spontaneous bacterial agglutination, and are sensitive to the antibacterial effect of normal human serum.[51] Spontaneous changes in the bacterial serotypes or strain characteristics are not seen in ABU, bacterial virulence characteristics may, however, develop during antibiotic therapy of ABU.[112]

For a considerable time, the management of ABU remained unsettled and the outcome of untreated patients was unknown. Kunin[8] has suggested that the treatment of children with ABU was "clearly justified on the grounds of attempting to reduce morbidity." Savage et al.[111] were the first to evaluate the efficacy of antibiotic/chemotherapeutic prophylaxis in preventing reinfection in children with ABU. They reported that antibiotic treatment did not alter long-term recurrence or eradication rates. Lindberg et al.[113] also found that despite the clearance of bacteriuria by chemotherapeutic intervention (with nitrofurantoin), there was no significant difference in the rate of recurrence between the treated group and the untreated group at the end of 3 years of observation. The Newcastle covert bacteriuria study[114] showed similar results. On the basis of these observations, the current recommendation is that children with ABU should not be treated with antibiotics and, in fact, that children need not be screened routinely for ABU.[110,111,113–116]

Long-term follow-up of children with ABU shows that 40 to 50 percent become culture-negative over 2 to 5 years without any specific antibiotic therapy.[114] The renal function of children with ABU remains well preserved if no underlying urologic abnormalities or renal scars are present[115], renal growth in children with ABU has been reported to be normal and formation of new scars is unusual.[110,113,114] None of the 98 untreated children with ABU in the Cardiff-

Oxford Bacteriuria Study developed new scars over 4 years of follow-up,[110] while only 1 of 106 untreated children in the Newcastle study developed a new renal scar.[114] However, progression of existing renal scars may occur. Asymptomatic bacteriuria detected in infants less than 1 year of age appears to follow the same course noted in older children. In a 6-year follow-up of such infants, Wettergren et al.[116] reported that the condition resolved spontaneously, without any treatment, in 36 of the 50 (72 percent).

VESICOURETERAL REFLUX

Vesicoureteral reflux is defined as *regurgitation of urine from the bladder into the ureter and potentially to the renal parenchyma.* This process exposes the renal pelvis to higher bladder pressure during voiding and also facilitates the passage of bacteria from the bladder to the kidneys. Several studies have demonstrated a causal relationship between VUR, and the development of renal parenchymal scars, or "reflux nephropathy."[30,117,118] Hypertension (in 2.4 to 38 percent of cases), impairment of renal function and endstage renal failure (ESRF) can secondarily result from VUR and reflux nephropathy.[119] An accurate estimate of ESRF due to reflux nephropathy in the United States is difficult, since reflux nephropathy is not classified as a separate diagnostic entity in the annual report of the United States Renal System.[120] In the European studies, reflux nephropathy accounted for about 17 percent of all patients accepted for the care of ESRF.[121] A recent analysis[122] by the North American Pediatric Renal Transplant Cooperative Study indicates that 4.1 percent of children undergoing renal transplantation had reflux nephropathy and an additional 2.9 percent carried the diagnosis of chronic pyelonephritis/interstitial nephritis.

Vesicoureteral reflux can be classified as either primary or secondary. Primary VUR is defined as a congenital incompetence of the valvular mechanism of the vesicoureteral junction. Normal ureter traverses the bladder muscle obliquely and then tunnels between the bladder muscle and mucosa before exiting at the ureteral orifice in the bladder. The submucosal tunnel thus formed serves as a flap valve mechanism, preventing the backward flow of urine from the bladder into the ureter. Absence of the submucosal tunnel in the bladder leads to primary VUR. Secondary VUR, on the other hand, is seen in conditions that are associated with UTI or increased intravesical pressure (neurogenic bladder, posterior urethral valves).

Primary VUR is believed to have a genetic basis, and the mode of inheritance seems to be multifactorial or polygenic. Studies of family members of patients with VUR have shown that about 40 to 50 percent of asymptomatic siblings and first-degree relatives are also affected.[123,124] HLA studies in patients with ESRF secondary to reflux nephropathy revealed an increased frequency of HLA A9-B12 and A2-B8.[125,126]

DIAGNOSIS OF VUR

Vesicoureteral reflux cannot be diagnosed with certainty by either renal ultrasound or IVP; a VCUG with radiocontrast material and fluoroscopy or radioisotopes is required. The radiation exposure is significantly reduced by using the radioisotope method. However, a conventional VCUG is preferred, at least at the time of initial evaluation, since it provides a better definition of the anatomy of the lower urinary tract. Radioisotope VCUG can be used in follow-up studies of patients with documented reflux. The timing of the VCUG in patients with UTI is important and has been discussed earlier. Once the diagnosis of VUR is confirmed, imaging of the upper urinary tract is indicated in order to delineate renal parenchymal damage such as scarring, parenchymal loss, and growth retardation.

GRADING OF VUR

While several schemes have been proposed for grading VUR, the international classification is most widely used.[127] According to it, VUR is divided into five grades on the basis of the severity of the reflux into the ureter, as shown in Fig. 9–11:

Grade I: Contrast material is seen only in the ureter.
Grade II: Ureter, pelvis, and calyces are filled but there is no dilatation and calyceal fornices are normal.
Grade III: The ureter is mildly or moderately dilated; there can be also tortuosity, mild or moderate dilatation of the renal pelvis, but no or slight blunting of the calyces.
Grade IV: Moderate dilatation and/or tortuosity of the ureter and moderate dilatation of the renal pelvis and calyces are seen. There is complete oblit-

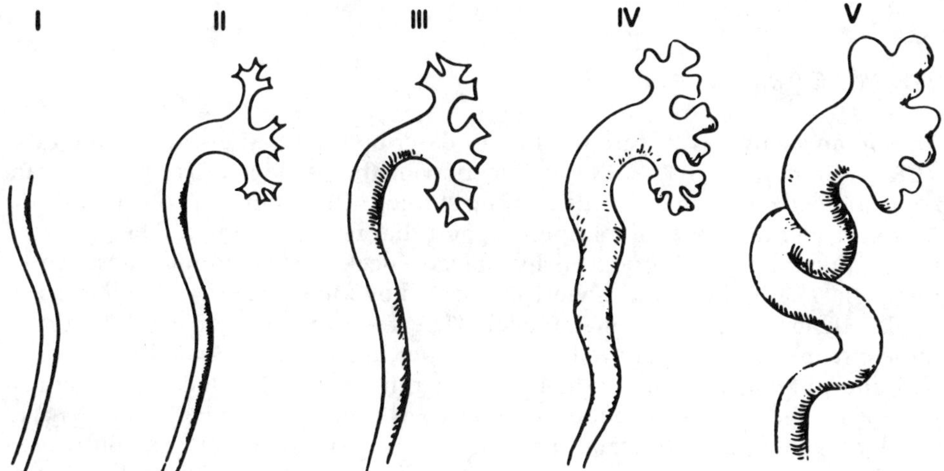

FIG. 9–11. Grading of reflux by the international classification. Details are given in the text. (Reproduced with permission from Report of the International Reflux Study Committee: Medical versus surgical treatment of primary vesicoureteral reflux. *Pediatrics* 67:392, 1981. Copyright © 1981 by American Academy of Pediatrics.)

eration of sharp angles of the fornices, but papillary impressions in the majority of calyces are maintained.

Grade V: There is gross dilatation and tortuosity of the ureter with dilatation of the renal pelvis and the calyces. Papillary impressions are no longer visible in the majority of calyces.

INTRARENAL REFLUX

Intrarenal reflux is defined as the passage of urine from the renal pelvis into the renal tubules through the papillary collecting ducts.[128] During a VCUG study, intrarenal reflux appears as streaks of contrast material extending from the renal pelvis into the parenchyma.

CLINICAL MANIFESTATIONS

By itself, VUR is an asymptomatic disorder and is usually uncovered in the course of investigations of UTI. Smellie et al.[30] reviewed the records of children with UTI and were not able to identify any symptoms that specifically indicated the presence of VUR. Children with severe VUR (grades IV and V) usually present earlier (1 to 3 years), because of symptomatic of UTI or other complications, than do those with mild VUR.[129] In some patients VUR may be detected for the first time when the patient has developed advanced chronic renal failure or during the evaluation of hypertension. As pointed out earlier, a high percentage of asymptomatic siblings of patients with VUR also show this abnormality when studied radiologically.[123,124] Children with lower urinary tract anomalies, particularly hypospadias, have a higher incidence of VUR and should be accordingly studied.[130]

RENAL SCARRING AND VUR

Hodson and Edwards[131] were the first to describe the relationship between the VUR and renal scars. The role of infection in the pathogenesis of these scars has remained somewhat confusing. The studies of Hodson and colleagues[132] in the experimental model of minipigs suggest that renal scarring can be produced by high-pressure VUR (induced by bladder neck obstruction) in absence of infection. These observations were confirmed by Mendoza et al.[133] and Ransley et al.[134] in other experimental models. The renal parenchymal injury under these circumstances is believed to result from intrarenal reflux, which leads to high intratubular pressure; ischemia of the renal medulla induced by compression of the peritubular capillaries; rupture of the renal tubules; and possibly leakage of the Tamm-Horsefall protein into the interstitium.[135] In contrast to the view stated above, Ransley and Risdon,[136] using an experimental model of low-pressure VUR, demonstrated that infection was a necessary component in the pathogenesis of renal scars. Roberts et al.[137] also demonstrated, in primates with low-pressure VUR, that infection was required to produce a decline in renal function. Although the low-pressure VUR probably occurs in clinical conditions such as partial bladder neck obstruction, high-pressure VUR is encountered rarely in clinical practice, since it requires almost complete obstruction of the bladder neck for a prolonged period. However, on the basis of findings by Nielson et al.[138] that high intravesicular pressure (up to 120 cmH_2O) can be generated in patients with a dysfunctional voiding disorder and possibly also in a newly toilet-trained infant (50 to 100 cmH_2O, compared to 25 to 30 cmH_2O in an older child), Arant[139] has recently suggested that sterile reflux may indeed be responsible for renal parenchymal injury and scarring in humans.

Renal scars due to VUR and UTI are generally seen in the polar areas of the kidney, the order of frequency being (1) the upper pole, (2) the lower pole, and (3) the midzone (Fig. 9–12). The susceptibility of the upper pole to scarring probably results from the anatomy of the papillae in this region and the degree of intrarenal reflux permitted by these papillae. A large percentage of upper-pole papillae in children are compound papillae, which have concave surfaces and gaping papillary duct orifices. These openings permit the development of intrarenal reflux and thus expose this region to the harmful effects of VUR.[140] In contrast, the percentage of compound papillae in the lower pole and the midzone is significantly lower. This explains the lower incidence of renal scars in these regions (Fig. 9–13). In advanced stages of reflux nephropathy, however, the entire kidney on the affected side may be small, shrunken, and scarred. The contralateral kidney, if uninvolved by VUR and the scarring process, usually demonstrates compensatory hypertrophy.

It is generally believed that many children with VUR and UTI have already developed renal scars by the time of first evaluation for UTI (usually below age 5).[30,118,141] However, new renal scars can emerge in older children with UTI, particularly in those with VUR.[119] New renal scar formation is particularly common in patients with severe VUR, those who undergo recurrent UTIs, and those who are not treated with antibacterial prophylaxis.[30,119,141]

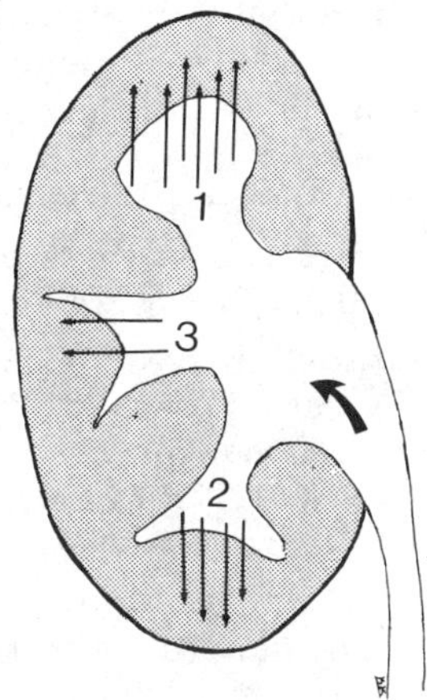

FIG. 9–12. A diagrammatic representation of the areas of the kidney usually affected by scarring due to reflux-associated chronic pyelonephritis.

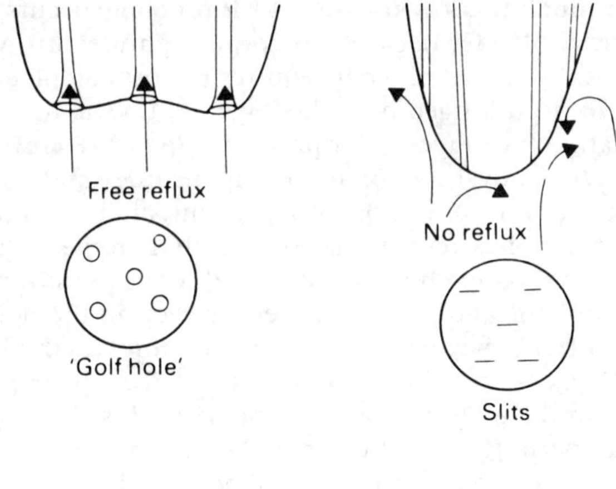

FIG. 9–13. A diagrammatic representation of the mechanism of intrarenal reflux in the compound papillae (*A*) and the features of simple papillae (*B*) that prevent intrarenal reflux in the kidney. (Reproduced with permission from Sweny P, Farrington K, Moorhead JF: *The Kidney and Its Disorders,* London, Blackwell Scientific Publications, 1989.)

MANAGEMENT OF VUR

The goal of therapy for children with VUR is to protect the kidney from scarring, allow maximal renal parenchymal growth, and preserve renal function. In the past, surgical correction was the main mode of treatment, but the last 15 years have seen a gradual shift of emphasis to medical management. This is based on the observation that by keeping the urine of these children sterile by antibiotic prophylaxis, a gradual improvement in the severity of VUR and its eventual disappearance may be promoted.[105,142–144] Nonsurgical or conservative management should be considered for patients with VUR of grades I to III provided that they are willing to undertake prolonged daily antibiotic prophylaxis (Fig. 9–14). Although antibiotic prophylaxis may lessen the severity of VUR in children with reflux of grade IV or above, the cure rate in such patients is low and surgical treatment is generally recommended.[129] Both nitrofurantoin and trimethoprim-sulfamethoxazole are effective as suppressive drugs for prevention of UTI in these patients and are given once daily at bedtime. Apart from antibacterial prophylaxis, efforts should be made to reduce the risk of UTI by encouraging complete bladder emptying (to minimize intravesical pressure) at regular intervals and control of constipation. Constipation can partially obstruct the bladder outlet, causing the retention of residual urine and increasing the risk of UTI.[139] Cooperating children should be taught the technique of double voiding. Urine should be cultured routinely every 3 months to detect bacteriuria, and antibiotic therapy should not be discontinued during this time.

The cure rate of mild to moderate VUR (grades I to III) with long-term antibiotic prophylaxis has been reported to be 30 to 50 percent in patients followed for 5 to 10 years.[129,146,147] In the series of patients reported by Scoog et al.,[129] the mean interval from the start of antibiotic prophylaxis and cure of VUR was 1.69 years and the mean age of resolution was 4.58 years. Surgical antireflux treatment may be considered in patients with severe VUR (grade IV or more). The Birmingham Reflux Study Group,[146] however, did not find that there was any significant difference in the incidence of breakthrough UTIs, renal growth, renal concentrating ability, progression of existing renal scars, and new scar formation between the surgically treated group and those receiving long-term antibiotic prophylaxis.

Follow-up studies in patients with VUR should include an annual VCUG, preferably by the radioisotope method in order to reduce exposure to ionizing radiation. Surveillance for bacteriuria can be relaxed when the VUR has resolved

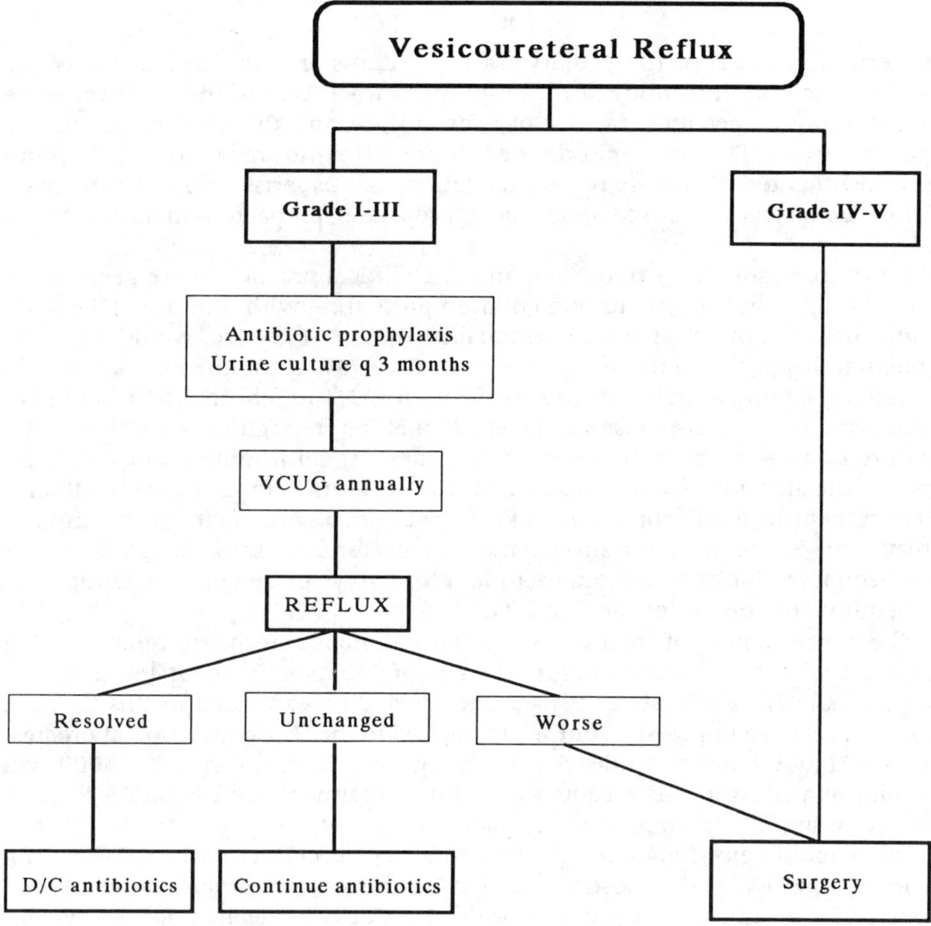

FIG. 9–14. Algorithm for management of children with VUR.

on two consecutive yearly follow-ups. The patient with a renal scar should be monitored for progression of the renal scar by radioisotope renal cortical scintigraphy (DMSA scan) and monitored for the development of hypertension.

A Nephrologist's Perspective of UTI in Children: A Commentary

Billy S. Arant, Jr.

Bacterial infections of the urinary tract in infants are exceeded in frequency only by bacterial infections of the respiratory tract. Due to the inconvenience of obtaining a specimen satisfactory for culture and the absence of specific symptoms for UTI, many episodes of UTI are either not recognized or improperly documented. Disparate recommendations of "experts" also leave the practicing pediatrician confused about the appropriate approach to management of UTI.

If for no reason other than standardizing clinical practice, there needs to be a similar approach to infants and children presenting with their first UTI. Such guidelines, as long as they are reasonable and cost-effective, would have the potential benefit of improving medical care. My recommendations would include 1) having a high index of suspicion for UTI in febrile infants and children with no obvious cause for fever, 2) making a diagnosis of UTI only by culture of an appropriately collected specimen, 3) confirming therapeutic efficacy of the antibiotic by another culture 48–72 hours after initiating treatment, 4) documenting eradication of infection by culture 5–7 days after discontinuing treatment, 5) planning for surveillance for bacteriuria until the urinary tract has been infection-free without treatment for two years and 6) completing radiologic investigation after the first UTI.

The consequences of treating childhood UTI haphazardly are renal scarring (in about 6%), hypertension before the age of 30 years (in about 1%) and end-stage renal disease (in about 0.1%). The morbidity, expressed in this fashion, does not seem so impressive, but when applied to the U.S. population at greatest risk—450,000 children under 5 years of age will have a first UTI—5000 will develop hypertension and 1000 will require treatment for ESRD. These complications are, for the most part, considered preventable.

What radiologic studies should be conducted in children with UTI? In my opinion, a VCUG is the most helpful study. This can be either a conventional contrast or a radionuclide study. Should the VCUG be delayed for 4–6 weeks following a UTI? I do not think so. In fact the only reason to delay the study is to permit the urine to become sterile. There is an advantage, in my opinion, to detecting "transient" reflux because 80% of girls will have a recurrence of UTI, many will be asymptomatic but are at risk of developing pyelonephritis if reflux is present. At the very least, the patient should remain on antibiotic prophylaxis until several days following the VCUG to prevent an interim UTI or one introduced by catheterization at the time of study. If the VCUG is normal, renal ultrasonography can identify an obstruction in the collecting system, but when abnormal, an IVP or DMSA scan is preferable to detect renal parenchymal defects.

How often does radiologic investigation identify an abnormality? On average, 40 percent of young children, boys and girls, with first UTI will have vesicoureteric reflux. Other anatomic lesions increase the number of abnormal findings. Moreover, the incidence of reflux in asymptomatic siblings of children with reflux is about 40% of which many will have evidence for renal scarring. There is probably no other examination done with a greater yield of abnormalities than the radiologic investigation of a child after the first UTI.

While there may be an oral tradition about the clinical management of UTI in children, there is virtually no reference in the remote or recent literature containing data to support any practice other than that outlined above—aggressive detection, treatment, evaluation and systematic follow-up.

A Pediatric Urologist's Perspective of UTI in Children: A Commentary

A. Barry Belman

The risk of a girl having a urinary tract infection during her school career is almost 5%. If all girls with documented infections are evaluated radiographically, one-third or more will be found to have significant anatomic abnormalities of the urinary tract, the most common being vesicoureteral reflux. I have the impression that most primary care physicians think of urinary infections in children as occurring at about three years of age. In view of the fact that the onset of verbalization and expectations for toilet control both peak at this age, that feeling is understandable. However, the risk of urinary infections in children well under three years of age is as high as that for the older group.

It has been generally held that anatomic abnormalities of the urinary tract are the underlying cause of most infections. This has led to a procedure-oriented approach to evaluation and treatment. That is not the case, however, and evaluation in children should be focused toward looking for problems, which, in conjunction with UTI, create a greater risk. Vesicoureteral reflux remains the most serious of these in small children.

UTI appears to be the result of urinary tract invasion by pathogenic organisms against which the host has limited resistance—just like respiratory illnesses. The ability of the pathogen to adhere to and invade the urinary epithelium may primarily be dictated by inherited traits. Additionally, vesicoureteral reflux is known to be a congenitally inherited problem (about one-third of screened siblings have reflux); therefore, the combination of these factors puts some individuals at higher risk than others.

Although many different guidelines exist concerning evaluation, it has become my policy to recommend awake cystography (with voiding films in boys) and sonography in every child in whom a urinary infection has been reliably culture-documented. One must keep in mind that the first culture-documented infection in a child stands a good chance of *not* being her first urinary tract infection. An infection documented in infancy (which may truly be the child's first infection) provides all the more reason to proceed with the evaluation as soon as possible. If reflux is noted or if other upper urinary abnormalities exist, the appropriate isotope renal scan is obtained as further investigation.

It must be noted that the evaluation of the child with infection not responsive to standard treatment becomes more urgent. This holds particularly true for newborns and infants. Performance of the cystogram may not be urgent, but it is essential to rule out ureteral obstruction. Sonography offers a simple, noninvasive means of determining if obstruction exists.

A number of children, primarily girls, have multiple recurrent UTIs. Upon questioning this group in detail, it becomes obvious that many are dysfunctional voiders. They tend to hold off voiding until the last minute, and after getting wet in the process, do not empty their bladders and often are constipated. Some do not void at school, and others may neither void in the morning upon awakening nor at school. A tell-tale symptom in this group is the curtsy sign—these children posture when they have the urge to void, trying to stay dry. Technically, this is a symptom of an uninhibited bladder contraction.

Some children require long-term antibacterial prophylaxis, including those with vesicoureteral reflux, to prevent infection until the reflux resolves, and those with frequently recurring UTIs ($>$ 4 per year). My policy is to recommend continuous medication for at least one year. Experience with either trimethoprim-sulfamethoxazole or nitrofurantoin, administered once or twice daily, has been most gratifying.

Mass screening for UTI is probably not justifiable on the basis of cost. On the other hand, screening as part of well baby care in the pediatrician's office is inexpensive and is recommended. It is becoming apparent that the infant kidney is most susceptible to damage from infection. Whereas older children ($>$ 7 years) and adults with otherwise normal urinary tracts may tolerate renal infection with little or no recognizable damage, the infant has serious potential for scarring and interference with further renal growth from bacterial invasion. If we are to prevent renal damage in the children who are at risk, the diagnosis of urinary tract infection must be made at an early age. If cultures have not been carried out on a routine basis, they become mandatory in all children who present with any sign of possible infection; i.e., poor feeding, diarrhea, weight loss, colic, excessive irritability, or, most commonly, fever.

REFERENCES

1. Ginsburg CM, McCracken GH: Urinary tract infections in young infants. *Pediatrics* 69:409, 1982.
2. Littlewood JM: 66 infants with urinary tract infection in first month of life. *Arch Dis Child* 47:218, 1972.
3. Drew JH, Acton CM: Radiologic findings in newborn infants with urinary tract infection. *Arch Dis Child* 51:628, 1976.
4. Crain EF, Gershel JC: Urinary tract infections in febrile infants younger than 8 weeks of age. *Pediatrics* 86:363, 1990.
5. Dickinson JA: Incidence and outcome of symptomatic urinary tract infection in children. *Br Med J* 1:1330, 1979.
6. Jodal U: The natural history of bacteriuria in childhood. *Infect Dis Clin North Am* 1:713, 1987.
7. Kunin CM, Zacha E, Paquin AJ: Urinary-tract infections in schoolchildren: I. Prevalence of bacteriuria and associated urologic findings. *N Engl J Med* 266:1287, 1962.
8. Kunin CM: A ten-year study of bacteriuria in schoolgirls: Final report of bacteriologic, urologic, and epidemiologic findings. *J Infect Dis* 122:382, 1970.
9. Wettergren B, Jodal U, Jonasson G: Epidemiology of bacteriuria during the first year of life. *Acta Paediatr Scand* 74:925, 1985.
10. Savage DCL, Wilson MI, McHardy M, et al: Covert bacteriuria of childhood. A clinical and epidemiological study. *Arch Dis Child* 48:8, 1973.
11. Newcastle Asymptomatic Bacteriuria Research Group: Asymptomatic bacteriuria in schoolchildren in Newcastle upon Tyne. *Arch Dis Child* 50:90, 1975.
12. Siegel SR, Siegel B, Sokoloff BZ, et al: Urinary infection in infants and preschool children. Five year follow-up. *Am J Dis Child* 134:369, 1980.
13. Lohr JA, Donowitz LG, Sadler JE: Hospital-acquired urinary tract infection. *Pediatrics* 83:193, 1989.
14. Garibaldi RA, Burke JP, Dickman ML, et al: Factors predisposing to bacteriuria during indwelling urethral catheterization. *N Engl J Med* 291:215, 1974.
15. Kunin CM, McCormick RC: Prevention of catheter-induced urinary-tract infections by sterile closed drainage. *N Engl J Med* 274:1155, 1966.
16. Warren JW, Platt R, Thomas RJ, et al: Antibiotic irrigation and catheter-associated urinary-tract infections. *N Engl J Med* 299:570, 1978.
17. Winberg J, Andersen HJ, Bergström T, et al: Epidemiology of symptomatic urinary tract infection in childhood. *Acta Paediatr Scand* 252(suppl):1, 1974.
18. Bergström T: Sex differences in childhood urinary tract infection. *Arch Dis Child* 47:227, 1972.
19. Bergström T, Larson H, Lincoln K, et al: Studies of urinary tract infections in infancy and childhood. XII. Eighty consecutive patients with neonatal infection. *J Pediatr* 80:858, 1972.
20. Jordan PA, Iravani A, Richard GA, et al: Urinary tract infection caused by *Staphylococcus saprophyticus*. *J Infect Dis* 142:510, 1980.
21. Gruneberg RN: Relationship of infecting urinary organisms to fecal flora in patients with symptomatic urinary infection. *Lancet* 2:766, 1969.
22. deMan P, Cläeson I, Johanson I, et al: Bacterial attachment as a predictor of renal abnormalities in boys with urinary tract infection. *J Pediatr* 115:915, 1989.
23. Stamey TA, Sexton CC: The role of vaginal colonization with Enterobacteriaceae in recurrent urinary infections. *J Urol* 113:214, 1975.

24. Fowler JE Jr, Stamey TA: Studies of introital colonization in women with recurrent urinary infections. VII. The role of bacterial adherence. *J Urol* 117:472, 1977.
25. Svanborg-Eden C, Janson GL, Lindberg U: Adhesiveness to urinary tract epithelial cells of fecal and urinary *Escherichia coli* isolates from patients with symptomatic urinary tract infection or asymptomatic bacteriuria of varying duration. *J Urol* 122:185, 1979.
26. Hallett RJ, Pead I, Maskell R: Urinary infection in boys. A three year study. *Lancet* 2:1107, 1976.
27. Buckley RM, McGuckin M, MacGregor RR: Urine bacterial counts after sexual intercourse. *N Engl J Med* 298:321, 1978.
28. Nicolle LE, Harding GKM, Preikasaitis J, et al: The association of urinary tract infection with sexual intercourse. *J Infect Dis* 146:579, 1982.
29. Kaijser B, Larsson P: Experimental acute pyelonephritis caused by enterobacteria in animals. A review. *J Urol* 127:786, 1982.
30. Smellie JM, Normand ICS, Katz G: Children with urinary infection: A comparison of those with and those without vesicoureteric reflux. *Kidney Int* 20:717, 1981.
31. McKerrow W, Davidson-Lamb N, Jones PF: Urinary tract infection in children. *Br Med J* 289:299, 1984.
32. Sobel JD: Pathogenesis of urinary tract infection. *Infect Dis Clin North Am* 1:751, 1987.
33. Kallenius G, Winberg J: Bacterial adherence to periurethral epithelial cells in girls prone to urinary tract infection. *Lancet* 2:540, 1978.
34. Swanborg Eden C, Jodal U: Attachment of *Escherichia coli* to sediment epithelial cells from urinary tract infection and healthy children. *Infect Immun* 27:804, 1980.
35. O'Hanley P, Lark D, Falkow S, et al: Molecular basis of *Escherichia coli* colonization of the upper urinary tract in BALB/c mice. *J Clin Invest* 75:347, 1985.
36. Lomberg H, Cedergren B, Leffler H, et al: Influence of blood groups on the availability of receptors for attachment of uropathogenic *Escherichia coli. Infect Immun* 51:919, 1986.
37. Schoolnik GK: How *Escherichia coli* infect the urinary tract. *N Engl J Med* 320:804, 1989.
38. Swanborg-Eden C, de Man P, Jodal U, et al: Host parasite interaction in urinary tract infection. *Pediatr Nephrol* 1:623, 1987.
39. Lomberg H, Hanson LA, Jacobsson B, et al: Correlation of P blood group, vesicoureteral reflux, and bacterial attachment in patients with recurrent pyelonephritis. *N Engl J Med* 308:1189, 1983.
40. Mulholland SG, Mooreville M, Parson CL: Urinary tract infection and P blood group antigens. *Urology* 24:232, 1984.
41. Sheinfeld J, Schaeffer AJ, Cordon-Cardo C, et al: Association of the Lewis blood-group phenotype with recurrent urinary tract infections in women. *N Engl J Med* 320:773, 1989.
42. Cordon-Cardo C, Lloyd KO, Finstad CL, et al: Immunoanatomic distribution of blood group antigens in the human urinary tract: Influence of secretor status. *Lab Invest* 55:444, 1986.
43. Mabeck CE, Ørskov F, Ørskow I: *E. coli* serotypes and renal involvement in urinary tract infection. *Lancet* 1:1312, 1971.
44. Mårild S, Jodal U, Ørskov I, et al: Special virulence of the *Escherichia coli* O1: K1: H7 clone in acute pyelonephritis. *J Pediatr* 115:40, 1989.
45. Hughes C, Hacker J, Roberts A, et al: Hemolysin production as a virulence marker

in symptomatic and asymptomatic urinary tract infections caused by *Escherichia coli. Infect Immun* 39:546, 1983.

46. Olling S: Sensitivity of gram negative bacilli to the serum bactericidal activity: a marker for host-parasite relationship in acute and persisting infections. *Scand J Infect Dis* 10(suppl):1, 1977.
47. Johnson JR, Moseley SL, Roberts PL, et al: Aerobactin and other virulence factor genes among strains of *E. coli* causing urosepsis: Association with patient characteristics. *Infect Immunol* 56:405, 1988.
48. Davies DL, Falkiner FR, Hardy KG: Colistin V production by clinical isolates of *Escherichia coli. Infect Immun* 31:574, 1981.
49. Hagberg L, Jodal U, Korhonen TK, et al: Adhesion, hemagglutination and virulence of *Escherichia coli* causing urinary tract infections. *Infect Immun* 31:564, 1981.
50. O'Hanley P, Low D, Romero I, et al: Gal-Gal binding and hemolysin phenotypes and genotypes associated with uropathogenic *Escherichia coli. N Engl J Med* 313:414, 1985.
51. Lindberg U, Hanson LA, Jodal U, et al: Asymptomatic bacteriuria in school girls. II. Differences in *Escherichia coli* causing asymptomatic bacteriuria and symptomatic bacteriuria. *Acta Paediatr Scand* 64:432, 1975.
52. Winberg J: P-fimbriae, bacterial adhesion, and pyelonephritis. *Arch Dis Child* 59:180, 1984.
53. Leffler H, Svanborg-Eden C: Chemical identification of a glycosphingolipid receptor for *Eschericia coli* attaching to human urinary tract epithelial cells and agglutinating human erythrocytes. *FEMS Lett* 8:127, 1981.
54. Källenius G, Möllby R, Sevenson S, et al: Occurrence of P-fimbriated *Escherichia coli* in urinary tract infection. *Lancet* 2:1369, 1981.
55. Vaisanen-Rhen V, Elo J, Vaisanen E, et al: P-fimbriated clones among uropathogenic *Escherichia coli* strains. *Infect Immun* 29:801, 1984.
56. Linder H, Engberg I, Baltzer IM, et al: Induction of inflammation by *Escherichia coli* on the mucosal level: Requirement for adherence and endotoxin. *Infect Immun* 56:1309, 1988.
57. Glauser MP, Meylan P, Bille J: The inflammatory response and tissue damage. The example of renal scars following acute renal infection. *Pediatr Nephrol* 1:615, 1987.
58. Thompson HC, King LR, Knox E, et al: Report of the ad hoc task force on circumcision. *Pediatrics* 56:610, 1975.
59. Wiswell TE, Geschke DW: Risks from circumcision during the first month of life compared with those for uncircumcised boys. *Pediatrics* 83:1011, 1989.
60. Wiswell TE, Enzanauer RW, Holton ME, et al: Declining frequency of circumcision: Implications for change in male to female sex ratio of urinary tract infection in early infancy. *Pediatrics* 79:338, 1987.
61. Wiswell TE, Smith FR, Bass JW: Decreased incidence of urinary tract infection in circumcised males. *Pediatrics* 75:901, 1985.
62. Wiswell TE, Roscelli JD: Corroborative evidence for the decreased incidence of urinary tract infections in circumcised male infants. *Pediatrics* 78:96, 1986.
63. Herzog LW: Urinary tract infections and circumcision. A case-control study. *Am J Dis Child* 143:348, 1989.
64. AAP Task Force on Circumcision: Report of the Task Force on Circumcision. *Pediatrics* 84:388, 1989.
65. Sørensen K, Lose G, Nathan E: Urinary tract infection and diurnal incontinence in girls. *Eur J Pediatr* 148:146, 1988.

66. Ingelfinger JR, Davis AE, Grupe WE: Frequency and etiology of gross hematuria in a general pediatric setting. *Pediatrics* 59:546, 1977.
67. Lorentz WB, Iskander S, Browning MC, et al: Acute renal failure due to pyelonephritis. *Nephron* 54:256, 1990.
68. Bauchner H, Philipp B, Dashefsky B, et al: Prevalence of bacteriuria in febrile children. *Pediatr Inf Dis J* 6:239, 1987.
69. Aronson AS, Gustafson B, Svenningsen NW: Combined suprapubic aspiration and clean-voided urine examination in infants and children. *Acta Paediatr Scand* 62:396, 1973.
70. Griess P: Bemerkungen zu der Abhandlung der H. H. Weselsky and Benedikt uber einige Aza verbindungen. *Ber Dtsch Ophthalmol Ges* 12:426, 1879.
71. James GP, Paul KL, Fuller KB: Urinary nitrite and urinary tract infection. *Am J Clin Pathol* 70:671, 1978.
72. Randolph MF, Morris K: Instant screening for bacteriuria in children: Analysis of a dipstick. *J Pediatr* 84:246, 1974.
73. Powell HR, Mccredie DA, Ritchie MA: Urinary nitrite in symptomatic and asymptomatic urinary infection. *Arch Dis Child* 62:138, 1987.
74. Nelson JD, Peters PC: Suprapubic aspiration of urine in premature and term infants. *Pediatrics* 36:132, 1965.
75. Saccharow L, Pryles CV: Further experience with the use of percutaneous suprapubic aspiration of the urinary bladder. Bacteriologic studies in 654 infants and children. *Pediatrics* 43:1018, 1969.
76. Kostiala A, Pylkkänen J: Dipslide cultures in the investigation of suprapubic urinary bladder aspirates of infants and children. *J Clin Pathol* 33:694, 1980.
77. Haycock GB: Investigation of urinary tract infection. *Arch Dis Child* 61:1155, 1986.
78. Hellerstein S, Wald ER, Winberg J, et al: Consensus: roentgenographic evaluation of children with urinary tract infections. *Pediatr Infect Dis* 3:291, 1984.
79. Willi U, Treves S: Radionuclide voiding cystography. *Urol Radiol* 5:161, 1983.
80. Brendstrup L, Carlsen N, Nielsen L, et al: Micturition cystourethrography using x-ray or scintigraphy in children with reflux. *Acta Paediatr Scand* 72:559, 1983.
81. Verber IG, Strudley MR, Meller ST: ^{99m}Tc dimercaptosuccinic acid (DMSA) scan as first investigation of urinary tract infection. *Arch Dis Child* 63:1320, 1988.
82. Hellström M, Jodal U, Marild S, et al: Ureteral dilatation in children with febrile urinary tract infection or bacteriuria. *Am J Radiol* 148:483, 1987.
83. Marild S, Hellström M, Jacobsson B, et al: Influence of bacterial adhesion on ureteral width in children with acute pyelonephritis. *J Pediatr* 115:265, 1989.
84. Edell SL, Bonavita JA: The sonographic appearance of acute pyelonephritis. *Radiology* 132:683, 1979.
85. Johansson B, Troell S, Berg U: Renal parenchymal volume during and after acute pyelonephritis measured by ultrasonography. *Arch Dis Child* 63:1309, 1988.
86. Sty JR, Wells RG, Starshak RJ, et al: Imaging in acute renal infection in children. *Am J Radiol* 148:471, 1987.
87. Handmaker H: Nuclear renal imaging in acute pyelonephritis. *Semin Nucl Med* 12:246, 1982.
88. Jodal U, Lindberg U, Lincoln K: Level diagnosis of symptomatic urinary tract infection in childhood. *Acta Paediatr Scand* 64:201, 1975.
89. Hellerstein S, Duggan E, Welchert E, et al: Serum C-reactive protein and the site of urinary tract infections. *J Pediatr* 100:21, 1982.

90. Thomas V, Forland M: Antibody-coated bacteria in urinary tract infections. *Kidney Int* 21:1, 1982.
91. Hellerstein S, Kennedy E, Nussbaum L, et al: Localization of the site of urinary tract infections by means of antibody-coated bacteria in the urinary sediment. *J Pediatr* 92:188, 1978.
92. Verrier Jones K: Antimicrobial treatment for urinary tract infections. *Arch Dis Child* 65:327, 1990.
93. Durbin WA, Peter G: Management of urinary tract infection in infants and children. *Pediatr Infect Dis* 3:564, 1984.
94. Jodal U, Winberg J; Management of children with unobstructed urinary tract infection. *Pediatr Nephrol* 1:647, 1987.
95. Fang LST, Tolkoff-Rubin NE, Rubin RH: Efficacy of single-dose and conventional amoxicillin therapy in urinary tract infection localized by the antibody-coated technique. *N Engl J Med* 298:413, 1978.
96. Fihn SD, Stamm WE: Interpretation and comparison of treatment studies for uncomplicated urinary tract infections in women. *Rev Infect Dis* 7:468, 1985.
97. Shapiro ED, Wald ER: Single-dose amoxicillin treatment of urinary tract infections. *J Pediatr* 99:989, 1981.
98. Lohr JA, Hayden GF, Kesler RW, et al: Three-day therapy of lower urinary tract infections with nitrofurantoin macrocrystals. A randomized clinical trial. *J Pediatr* 99:980, 1981.
99. Khan AJ, Kumar K, Evans HE: Single-dose gentamycin therapy for recurrent urinary tract infections with normal urinary tracts. *J Pediatr* 110:131, 1987.
100. Avner ED, Ingelfinger JR, Herrin JT, et al: Single-dose amoxicillin therapy for uncomplicated pediatric urinary tract infections. *J Pediatr* 102:623, 1983.
101. McCracken GH, Ginsberg CM, Namasonthi V, et al: Evaluation of short-term antibiotic therapy in children with uncomplicated urinary tract infection. *Pediatrics* 67:796, 1981.
102. Madrigal G, Odio CM, Mohs E, et al: Single dose antibiotic therapy is not as effective as conventional regimens for management of acute urinary tract infections in children. *Pediatr Infect Dis J* 7:316, 1988.
103. Moffat M, Embree J, Grimm P, et al: Short-course antibiotic therapy for urinary tract infections in children: A methodological review of the literature. *Am J Dis Child* 142:57, 1988.
104. Smellie JM, Ransley PG, Normand ICS, et al: Development of new renal scars: A collaborative study. *Br Med J* 290:1957, 1985.
105. Holland NH, Jackson EC, Kazee M, et al: Relation of urinary tract infection and vesicoureteral reflux to scar: Follow-up of thirty-eight patients. *J Pediatr* 116:S65, 1990.
106. Smellie JM, Katz G, Gruenberg RN: Controlled trial of prophylactic treatment in childhood urinary-tract infection. *Lancet* 2:175, 1978.
107. Lohr JA, Nunley DH, Howards SS, et al: Prevention of urinary tract infections in girls. *Pediatrics* 59:562, 1977.
108. Stamey TA, Condy M, Mihara G: Prophylactic efficacy of nitrofurantoin macrocrystals and trimethoprim-sulfamethoxazole in urinary infections. *N Engl J Med* 296:780, 1977.
109. Murray BE, Rensimer ER, DuPont HL: Emergence of high level trimethoprim resistance in fecal *Escherichia coli* during oral administration of trimethoprim or trimethoprim-sulfamethoxazole. *N Engl J Med* 306:130, 1982.

110. Cardiff-Oxford Bacteriuria Study Group: Sequelae of covert bacteriuria in schoolgirls. *Lancet* 1:889, 1978.
111. Savage DCL, Howie G, Adler K, et al: Controlled trial of therapy in covert bacteriuria of childhood. *Lancet* 1:358, 1975.
112. Hansson S, Caugant D, Jodal U, et al: Untreated asymptomatic bacteriuria in girls: I- Stability of urinary isolates. *Br Med* J 298:853, 1988.
113. Lindberg U, Claesson I, Hanson LÅ, et al: Asymptomatic bacteriuria in school girls. VIII. Clinical course during a 3-year follow-up. *J Pediatr* 92:194, 1978.
114. Newcastle Covert Bacteriuria Research Group: Covert bacteriuria in schoolgirls in Newcastle Upon Tyne: 5-year follow-up. *Arch Dis Child* 56:585, 1981.
115. Verrier Jones K, Asscher AW, Verrier Jones ER, et al: Glomerular filtration rate in schoolgirls with covert bacteriuria. *Br Med J* 285:1307, 1982.
116. Wettergren B, Hellstrom M, Stockland E, et al: Six-year follow-up of infants with bacteriuria on screening. *Br Med J* 301:845, 1990.
117. Bailey RR: The relationship of vesico-ureteric reflux to urinary tract infection and chronic pyelonephritis–reflux nephropathy. *Clin Nephrol* 1:132, 1973.
118. Smellie JM, Normand ICS: Bacteriuria, reflux and renal scarring. *Arch Dis Child* 50:581, 1975.
119. Shanon A, and Feldman W: Methodologic limitations in the literature on vesicoureteral reflux: A critical review. *J Pediatr* 117:171, 1990.
120. United States Renal Data System: USRDS 1990 annual data report: The National Institutes of Health, National Institute of Diabetes, Digestive and Kidney Disease, Bethesda, MD, August, 1990, page 12.
121. Tufveson G, Geerlings W, Brunner FP, et al: Combined report on regular dialysis and transplantation in Europe, XIX, 1988. *Nephrol Dial Transpl* 4(suppl 4):5, 1989.
122. North American Pediatric Renal Transplant Cooperative Study: The 1989 report of the North American Pediatric Renal Transplant Cooperative study. *Pediatr Nephrol* 4:542, 1990.
123. Van den Abbeele AD, Treves ST, Lebowitz RL, et al: Vesicoureteral reflux in asymptomatic siblings of patients with known reflux: Radionuclide cystography. *Pediatrics* 79:147, 1987.
124. Aggarwal VK, Verrier Jones K: Vesicoureteric reflux: screening of first degree relatives. *Arch Dis Child* 64:1538, 1989.
125. Torres VE, Moose SB, Kurtz SB, et al: In search of a marker for genetic susceptibility to reflux nephropathy. *Clin Nephrol* 14:217, 1980.
126. Bailey RR: End-stage reflux nephropathy. *Nephron* 27:302, 1981.
127. International Reflux Study in Children: International system of radiographic grading of vesicoureteric reflux. *Pediatr Radiol* 15:105, 1985.
128. Rolleston GL, Maling TMJ, Hodson CJ: Intrarenal reflux and the scarred kidney. *Arch Dis Child* 49:531, 1974.
129. Skoog SJ, Belman BA, Majd M: A nonsurgical approach to the management of primary vesicoureteral reflux. *J Urol* 138:941, 1987.
130. Shafir R, Isur H, Hertz M, et al: Vesicoureteral reflux in boys with hypospadias. *Urology* 20:29, 1982.
131. Hodson CJ, Edwards D: Chronic pyelonephritis and vesicoureteric reflux. *Clin Radiol* 11:219, 1960.
132. Hodson CJ, Maling TMJ, McManaman P, et al: The pathogenesis of reflux nephropathy (chronic atrophic pyelonephritis). *Br J Radiol* 13(suppl):1, 1975.
133. Mendoza JM, Roberts JA: Effects of sterile high pressure vesicoureteral reflux on the monkey. *J Urol* 130:602, 1983.

134. Ransley PG, Risdon RA, Godley ML: High pressure sterile vesicoureteral reflux and renal scarring: An experimental study in the pig and minipig. *Contrib Nephrol* 39:320, 1984.
135. Risdon RA: The small scarred kidney of childhood: A congenital or acquired lesion? *Pediatr Nephrol* 1:632, 1987.
136. Ransley PG, Risdon RA: Reflux and renal scarring. *Br J Radiol* 14(suppl):1, 1978.
137. Roberts JA, Fishman NH, Thomas R: Vesicoureteral reflux in the primate. IV. Does reflux harm the kidney? *J Urol* 128:650, 1982.
138. Nielson JB, Norgaard JP, Sorensen SS, et al: Continuous overnight monitoring of bladder activity in vesico-ureteral reflux patients: II. Bladder activity type. *Neurol Urodynam* 3:7, 1984.
139. Arant BS: Reflux nephropathy, in Ferris TF, Hosstetter TH, Paller MS (eds): *The Kidney.* New York, National Kidney Foundation, 1989, vol 21, page 19.
140. Funston MR, Cremin BJ: Intrarenal reflux–papillary morphology and pressure relationships in children's necropsy kidneys. *Br J Radiol* 51:665, 1978.
141. Shah KJ, Robins DG, White RHR: Renal scarring and vesicoureteric reflux. *Arch Dis Child* 53:210, 1978.
142. Edwards D, Normand ICS, Perscod N, et al: Disappearance of vesicoureteric reflux during long-term prophylaxis of urinary tract infection in children. *Br Med J* 2:285, 1977.
143. Smellie J, Edwards D, Normand ICS, et al: Effect of vesicoureteric reflux on renal growth in children with urinary tract infection. *Arch Dis Child* 56:593, 1981.
144. Steele BT, Robitaille P, DeMaria J, et al: Follow-up evaluation of prenatally recognized vesicoureteric reflux. *J Pediatr* 115:95, 1989.
145. Olbing H: Vesico-uretero-renal reflux and the kidney. *Pediatr Nephrol* 1:638, 1987.
146. Birmingham Reflux Study Group: Prospective trial of operative versus nonoperative treatment of severe vesicoureteral reflux in children: five years observation. *Br Med J* 295:237, 1987.
147. Heale WF: Prolonged follow-up of infants with reflux and reflux nephropathy. *Eur J Pediatr* 140:160, 1983.

10

HYPERTENSION

Kanwal K. Kher

Hypertension is a well-described disorder in adults, and its relationship to increased morbidity and mortality rates due to cardiovascular diseases and stroke is well established.[1,2] On the other hand, the subject of childhood hypertension has received little attention until recently. In part, this has resulted from a lack of consensus regarding normal blood pressure (BP) standards and the definition of hypertension in children. Several recent studies have, however, now established reliable age- and sex-related reference standards for both systolic and diastolic BP in normal children.[3] Although secondary causes of hypertension, particularly renal parenchymal and renovascular diseases, account for most cases of hypertension in the pediatric age group, essential hypertension is also being recognized increasingly among children. Evaluation of BP during routine checkups has improved the detection of hypertension in children in recent years. This chapter addresses issues related to the etiology, pathophysiology, and diagnosis of hypertension in children.

PREVALENCE

Because of a variability in the definition of hypertension in various reported studies in children, precise data related to the prevalence of hypertension in the pediatric age group are lacking. Persistent elevation of BP was recorded in less than 1.0 percent of children aged 5 to 18 years investigated in the Muscatine study,[4] while sustained elevation of systolic and diastolic BP, respectively, was reported by Fixler et al.[5] to be present in 1.2 and 0.37 percent of schoolchildren. This compares with the prevalence rate of hypertension in almost 22 percent of adults of all ages in the United States.[6]

NORMAL BLOOD PRESSURE TREND IN CHILDREN

Blood pressure in normal children varies with age, sex, height, and weight. Following birth, the systolic, diastolic, and mean arterial BP increases gradually during the first week of life (approximately 1 mmHg/day), and a slower upward trend in the systolic BP continues postnatally until 6 to 8 weeks.[7,8] Systolic BP then stabilizes during the first year of life, followed by its gradual increase during the remainder of childhood and adolescence. Diastolic BP, on the other hand, shows a gradual decline in the first 6 to 8 weeks of life and then rises slowly during the first year. Thereafter, the diastolic BP remains relatively stable until the child is between 4 and 5 years of age. Thereafter, it increases gradually throughout childhood and adolescence.[3]

Heavier and/or taller children generally have higher BP than leaner and smaller children of the same age.[3] In children and adolescents, both systolic and diastolic BP during sleep (1 A.M to 8 A.M.) is approximately 10 percent lower than it is during the day (Fig. 10–1).[9] Although hypertension is more common in adult blacks than it is in whites, ethnic origin appears to have little influence on BP in normal children.[3]

DEFINITION OF HYPERTENSION

In adults, hypertension is defined as BP higher than 140/90 mmHg. It is, however, not practical to establish a single numerical level of BP as a cutoff point for the definition of hypertension in children, because the BP of normal children undergoes significant upward readjustments all through childhood. The Task Force on Blood Pressure Control in Children has published reference mean (±SD) BPs of normal, healthy children for different age groups (Figs. 10–2, 10–3, and 10–4). It is recommended that systolic and diastolic BP below the 90th

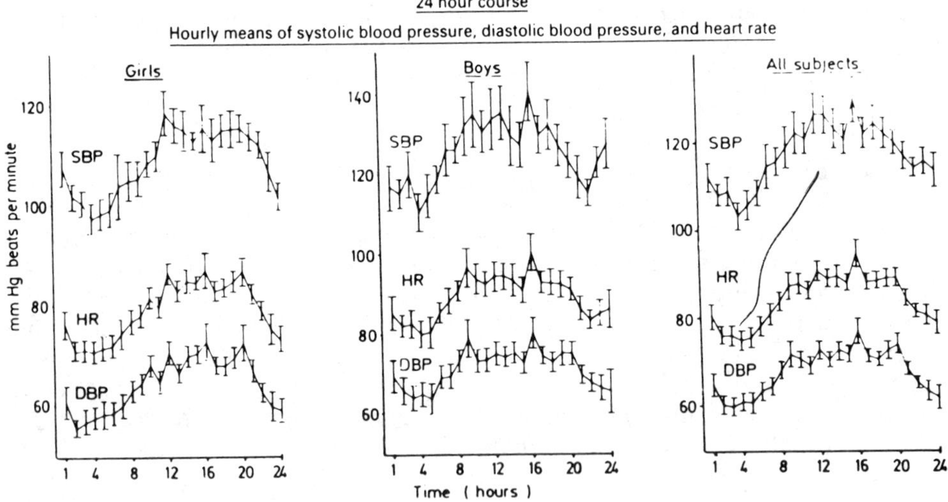

FIG. 10–1. Hourly recordings of BP and heart rate in children, showing variability of BP in 24 h. (Reproduced by permission from Egger M, Bianchetti MG, Gnadinger M, et al: Twenty-four-hour intermittent, ambulatory blood pressure monitoring. *Arch Dis Child* 62:1130, 1987.)

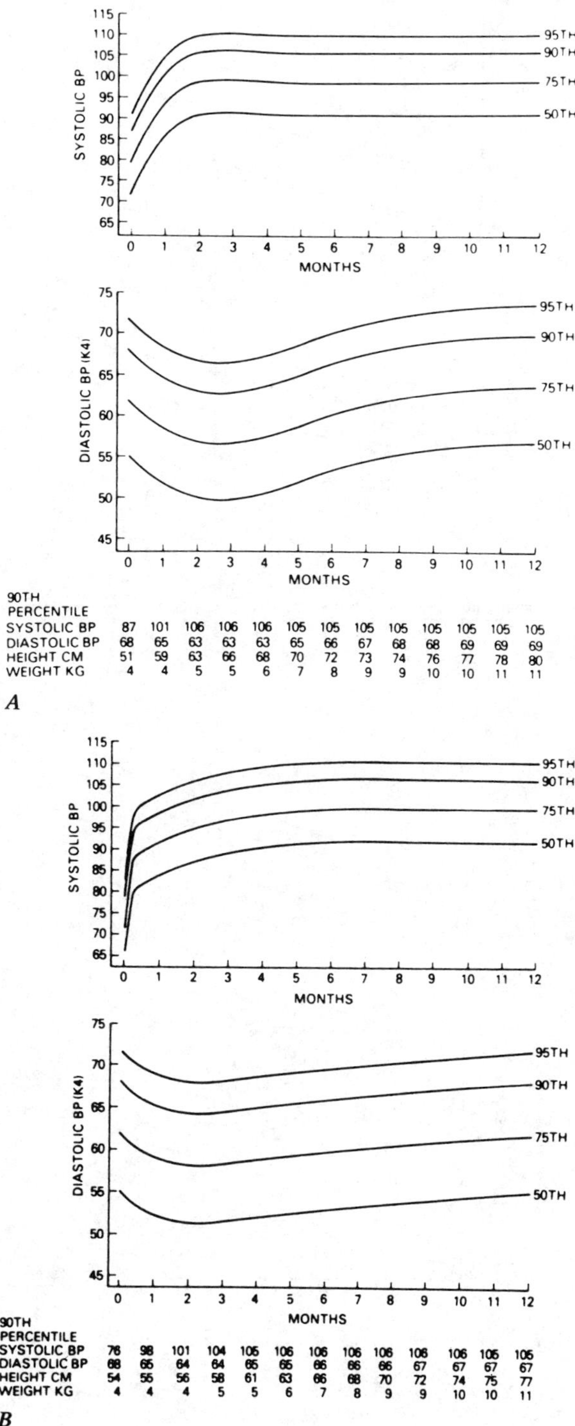

90TH PERCENTILE													
SYSTOLIC BP	87	101	106	106	106	105	105	105	105	105	105	105	105
DIASTOLIC BP	68	65	63	63	63	65	66	67	68	68	69	69	69
HEIGHT CM	51	59	63	66	68	70	72	73	74	76	77	78	80
WEIGHT KG	4	4	5	5	6	7	8	9	9	10	10	11	11

A

90TH PERCENTILE													
SYSTOLIC BP	76	98	101	104	105	106	106	106	106	106	106	105	105
DIASTOLIC BP	68	65	64	64	65	65	66	66	66	67	67	67	67
HEIGHT CM	54	55	56	58	61	63	66	68	70	72	74	75	77
WEIGHT KG	4	4	4	5	5	6	7	8	9	9	10	10	11

B

FIG. 10–2. *A*. Age-specific percentiles of BP measurements in boys—birth to 12 months of age; Korotkoff phase IV (K4) used for diastolic BP. *B*. Age-specific percentiles of BP measurements in girls—birth to 12 months of age. (Report of the Second Task Force on Blood Pressure Control in Children—1987. *Pediatrics* 79:1, 1987. Reproduced by permission of American Academy of Pediatrics, © 1987.)

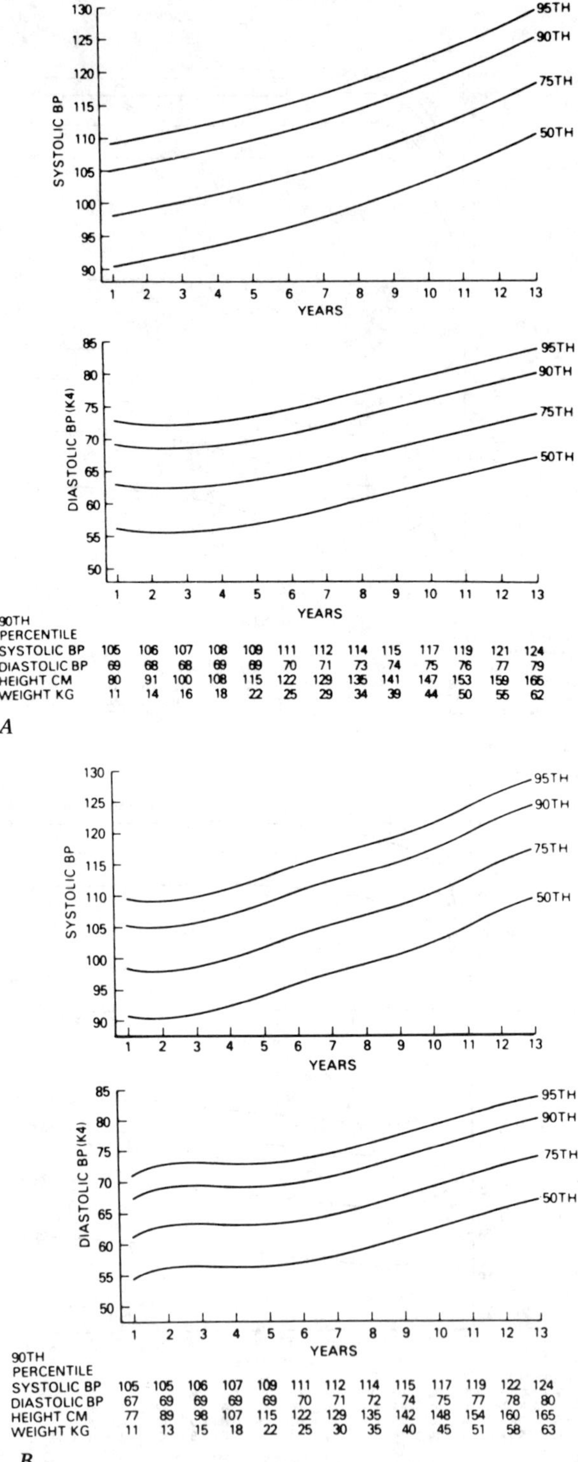

90TH PERCENTILE													
SYSTOLIC BP	105	106	107	108	109	111	112	114	115	117	119	121	124
DIASTOLIC BP	69	68	68	69	69	70	71	73	74	75	76	77	79
HEIGHT CM	80	91	100	108	115	122	129	135	141	147	153	159	166
WEIGHT KG	11	14	16	18	22	25	29	34	39	44	50	56	62

A

90TH PERCENTILE													
SYSTOLIC BP	105	105	106	107	109	111	112	114	115	117	119	122	124
DIASTOLIC BP	67	69	69	69	69	70	71	72	74	75	77	78	80
HEIGHT CM	77	89	98	107	115	122	129	135	142	148	154	160	165
WEIGHT KG	11	13	15	18	22	25	30	35	40	45	51	58	63

B

FIG. 10–3. *A*. Age-specific percentiles of BP measurements in boys—1 to 13 years of age; Korotkoff phase IV (K4) used for diastolic BP. *B*. Age-specific percentiles of BP measurements in girls—1 to 13 years of age; Korotkoff phase IV (K4) used for diastolic BP. (Report of the Second Task Force on Blood Pressure Control in Children—1987. *Pediatrics* 79:1, 1987. Reproduced by permission of American Academy of Pediatrics, © 1987.)

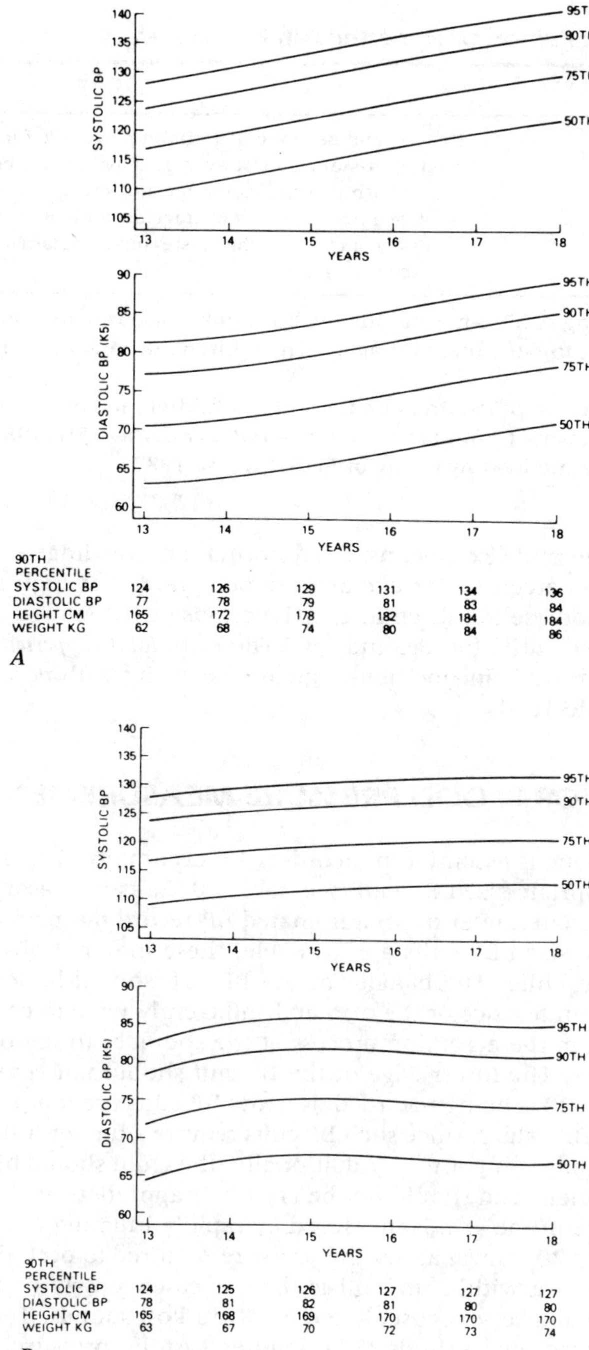

90TH PERCENTILE	13	14	15	16	17	18
SYSTOLIC BP	124	126	129	131	134	136
DIASTOLIC BP	77	78	79	81	83	84
HEIGHT CM	165	172	178	182	184	184
WEIGHT KG	62	68	74	80	84	86

90TH PERCENTILE	13	14	15	16	17	18
SYSTOLIC BP	124	125	126	127	127	127
DIASTOLIC BP	78	81	82	81	80	80
HEIGHT CM	165	168	169	170	170	170
WEIGHT KG	63	67	70	72	73	74

FIG. 10–4. *A*. Age-specific percentiles of BP measurements in boys—13 to 18 years of age; Korotkoff phase V (K5) used for diastolic BP. *B*. Age-specific percentiles for BP measurements in girls—13 to 18 years of age; Korotkoff phase V (K5) used for diastolic BP. (Report of the Second Task Force on Blood Pressure Control in Children—1987. *Pediatrics* 79:1, 1987. Reproduced by permission of American Academy of Pediatrics, © 1987.)

TABLE 10–1. Definition of Hypertension in Children

Term	Definition
Normal BP	Systolic and diastolic BPs <90th percentile for age and sex
High-normal BP[a]	Average systolic and/or average diastolic BPs between 90th and 95th percentiles for age and sex
High BP (hypertension)	Average systolic and/or average diastolic BPs ≥95th percentile for age and sex with measurements obtained on at least three occasions

[a]If the BP reading is high-normal for age but can be accounted for by excess height for age or excess lean body mass for age, such children are considered to have normal BP.

Source: Task Force on Blood Pressure Control in Children: Report of the Second Task Force on Blood Pressure Control in Children—1987. *Pediatrics* 79:1, 1987. Reproduced by permission of American Academy of Pediatrics, © 1987.

percentile for age and sex be considered normal and readings in the range of the 90th to 95th percentile for age and sex be regarded as high normal, especially in taller and well-built children. Hypertension is defined as BP greater than the 95th percentile for age and sex.[3] The term *labile hypertension* describes patients in whom BP is inconsistently greater than the 95th percentile for age and sex (see Table 10–1).

TECHNIQUE OF BLOOD PRESSURE MEASUREMENT

A correct technique is essential in recording BP accurately. This includes selection of an appropriate-sized BP cuff (see Table 10–2) as well as a properly calibrated sphygmomanometer or an automated BP recording machine. Although infant- and child-sized BP cuffs are available, these may not always be appropriate in a given child. The bladder of the BP cuff should be long enough to encircle the circumference of the arm and sufficiently wide to cover two-thirds of the length from the acromion process at the shoulder to the olecranon process of the elbow. The lower edge of the BP cuff should not cover the antecubital fossa while BP is being recorded. Narrow BP cuffs are notorious for giving falsely elevated BP values, since such BP cuffs require a higher inflating pressure to occlude the underlying artery. Additionally, the child should be examined in a quiet environment and should not be crying or apprehensive.

Blood pressure in the arm is measured by rapidly inflating the cuff to a level of approximately 20 mmHg above the pressure required to occlude the brachial artery. The pressure within the cuff is then released slowly (2 to 3 mmHg/s) while the brachial artery is auscultated for Korotkoff sounds. The onset of the first audible interrupted sounds (K1) denotes systolic pressure. The diastolic blood pressure is the level of pressure at which all sounds disappear (K5). In children, however, onset of a low-pitched muffling sound (K4) may be regarded as the diastolic BP if disappearance of all sounds (K5) is difficult to detect. The Task Force-recommended standards have used K4 as the reference for the dia-

TABLE 10–2. Commercially Available Cuff Sizes for the Evaluation of BP in Children

Cuff Name[a]	Bladder Width, cm	Bladder Length, cm
Newborn	2.5–4.0	5.0–9.0
Infant	4.0–6.0	11.5–18.0
Child	7.5–9.0	17.0–19.0
Adult	11.5–13.0	22.0–26.0
Large arm	14.0–15.0	30.5–33.0
Thigh	18.0–19.0	36.0–38.0

[a]Cuff name does not guarantee that the cuff will be appropriate size for a child within that age range.

Source: Task Force on Blood Pressure Control in Children: Report of the Second Task Force on Blood Pressure Control in Children—1987. *Pediatrics* 79:1, 1987. Reproduced by permission of American Academy of Pediatrics, © 1987.

stolic BP in children through age 13 and K5 thereafter.[3] Principles similar to those observed in recording BP in the upper extremities are also necessary for obtaining a proper reading of BP in the lower extremities. While the BP in the lower extremities is being obtained, the patient should be lying down flat so that the popliteal artery can be auscultated adequately. Transient elevation of BP, especially in a crying or apprehensive child, is common. Such abnormal readings call for repeat evaluation of BP on at least three separate occasions before the patient can be considered hypertensive. This is particularly true of children with BP in the high-normal (90th to 95th percentile) range for age and sex. Repeated evaluations in such patients may reveal normal BP and thus avoid costly diagnostic studies. On the other hand, children with severely elevated BP should be investigated promptly.

CLINICAL MANIFESTATIONS

The monitoring of BP in patients with disease known to be associated with hypertension, such as chronic glomerulonephritis or chronic pyelonephritis, is the most frequent mode of detection of hypertension in children (80 to 85 percent).[10] On the other hand, 10 to 15 percent of hypertensive children are detected in the course of routine evaluations of BP not prompted by symptoms.[10,11] Hypertensive crisis characterized by seizures and various neurologic deficits in a previously "well" child is the mode of initial presentation in less than 5 percent of children.[10–12]

Chronic hypertension is often an asymptomatic disorder among children and adolescents, especially if only mild to moderate elevation of BP is present. Gill et al.[11] noted that only about half of the severely hypertensive children they saw had any symptoms. Headache is an important but inconsistent symptom of hypertension during childhood. It has been reported as a presenting symptom in 5 to 30 percent of children with hypertension and is usually seen in patients with severe or rapid elevation of BP.[11–13] While older children are able to identify the symptoms of headache, irritability may be a manifestation of headache in hypertensive infants. When present, the headache is of a throbbing character and can be severe enough to wake the child up from sleep. Abdominal pain, growth failure, and behavioral changes may be seen in some children with hypertension. Congestive cardiac failure may be the sole manifestation of hypertension in neonates and infants. Neurologic deficits such as cortical blindness and isolated facial nerve paralysis (Bell's palsy) have also been reported to result from hypertension in children.[14] Epistaxis is an uncommon symptom of hypertension in childhood, but it can occur. Patients with essential hypertension are usually asymptomatic at the time of their initial detection, and their BP elevation is usually of mild to moderate severity. On the other hand, severe hypertension is generally considered characteristic of secondary hypertension. Symptoms related to the underlying disease causing hypertension in patients with secondary hypertension may at times overshadow those due to hypertension itself.

TABLE 10–3. Etiology of Hypertension as Reported in Various Pediatric Studies

	Gill et al.[11] (1976) n = 100, percent	Uhari and Koskimies[12] (1979) n = 115, percent	Deal et al.[51] (1990) n = 454, percent
Renal			
Chronic glomerulonephritis	35	10	27
Chronic pyelonephritis and reflux nephropathy	14	8	19
Obstructive uropathy	6	6	16
Polycystic kidneys	4	4	5
Renal dysplasia and hypoplasia	5	3	3
Interstitial nephritis	—	1	—
Hemolytic-uremic syndrome	6	1	7
Miscellaneous renal diseases	7	5	—
Renovascular	6	3	8
Cardiovascular			
Coarctation	15	32	2
Other cardiovascular diseases	—	2	—
Endocrine			
Pheochromocytoma	—	1	1
Essential hypertension	1	18	4
Miscellaneous causes	1	6	8

Note: n = number of patients.

ETIOLOGY OF HYPERTENSION

It is well known that secondary hypertension resulting from renal, renovascular, cardiovascular, or endocrine disorders is observed more frequently among children than is primary or essential hypertension. However, since the description of essential hypertension in children by Londe et al.,[15] the existence of essential hypertension has been increasingly recognized in the pediatric population.[16] Several recent studies[10,15] have reported that essential hypertension constitutes the etiology in 12 to 18 percent of all childhood hypertension (Table 10–3). In general, however, hypertension in children, especially in those with severe elevation of BP, should be considered of secondary etiology and investigated more diligently than in adults. Table 10–4 lists the causes of sustained hypertension in children while the causes of transient hypertension are given

TABLE 10–4. Causes of Sustained Hypertension in Children

Secondary Hypertension
- Renal Disease
  - Chronic pyelonephritis and reflux nephropathy
  - Chronic glomerulonephritides
  - Chronic renal failure
  - Hemolytic uremic syndrome
  - Ask-Upmark kidney
  - Renal dysplasia
  - Multicystic kidney disease
  - Polycystic kidney disease
  - Polyarteritis nodosa, systemic vasculitis
  - Wilms tumor
- Renovascular Disorders
  - Fibromuscular dysplasia
  - Congenital renal arterial stenosis
  - Renal arterial thrombosis and embolization
  - Neurofibromatosis
  - Arteritis syndromes affecting aorta and renal blood vessels
  - Renal transplant arterial stenosis
  - External compression on the renal pedicle
- Cardiovascular Diseases
  - Coarctation of the aorta
- Endocrine Diseases
  - Catecholamine-secreting tumors such as pheochromocytoma or neuroblastoma
  - Enzymatic defects in adrenal steroid synthesis
    - 11-hydroxylase deficiency
    - 17-hydroxylase deficiency
  - Conn's syndrome

Essential Hypertension
- Miscellaneous Diseases
  - Sickle cell anemia
  - Williams syndrome
  - Idiopathic arterial calcification of infancy
  - Obesity
  - Closure of abdominal defects in neonates

TABLE 10–5. Causes of Transient Hypertension in Children

Error in reading BP
Drug-induced hypertension
- Corticosteroids
- Sympathomimetic drugs, nasal decongestants
- Oral contraceptive agents
- Sudden withdrawal of some antihypertensive drugs, such as clonidine
- Street drugs

Renal diseases
- Acute poststreptococcal glomerulonephritis
- Henoch-Schönlein purpura nephritis
- Hemolytic uremic syndrome
- Acutely obstructed urinary tract

Hypervolemia resulting from unregulated administration of
- Blood
- IV fluids or plasma

Miscellaneous
- Postrenal transplant
- Urologic surgery
- Hypercalcemia in immobilization
- Orthopedic procedures such as leg traction and placement in tight body casts
- Guillain-Barré syndrome
- Elevated intracranial pressure
- Lead poisoning

in Table 10–5. Common etiologies of hypertension in children, arranged according to various age groups, are listed in Table 10–6.

SECONDARY HYPERTENSION

RENOVASCULAR HYPERTENSION

Stenotic and embolic lesions of the renal artery are potentially correctable causes of secondary hypertension. The single leading etiology of renovascular

TABLE 10–6. Common Causes of Hypertension in Different Pediatric Age Groups

Age Group	Cause
Newborn infants	Renal artery thrombosis, renal artery stenosis, congenital renal malformations, coarctation of the aorta, bronchopulmonary dysplasia
Infancy–6 years	Renal parenchymal diseases,[a] coarctation of the aorta, renal artery stenosis
6–10 years	Renal artery stenosis, renal parenchymal diseases, primary hypertension
Adolescence	Primary hypertension, renal parenchymal diseases

[a]Includes renal structural and inflammatory lesions as well as tumors.

Source: Task Force on Blood Pressure Control in Children: Report of the Second Task Force on Blood Pressure Control in Children—1987. *Pediatrics* 79:1, 1987. Reproduced by permission of American Academy of Pediatrics, © 1987.

hypertension in children is fibromuscular dysplasia (40 to 80 percent).[17–19] Diseases affecting the descending aorta may also result in narrowing of the ostia or lumens of the renal arteries and lead to renovascular hypertension.

Fibromuscular dysplasia of the renal artery is a disease of unknown etiopathogenesis that affects girls more often than boys. The commonest histopathologic feature of the affected renal arteries is extensive thickening of the media (80 percent), resulting in narrowing of the lumen of the blood vessel. Less commonly, perimedial (10 percent) and intimal (10 percent) thickening and dysplasia of the affected artery may also be seen. Fibromuscular dysplasia usually affects the midsection of the main-stem renal artery on one side, but the segmental branches of the renal artery may also be involved. Eventually, the contralateral side may also be affected by the disease process, leading to bilateral renal arterial disease. Areas of arterial thickening are often interspersed with areas of poststenotic aneurysmal dilatation of the blood vessel, resulting in the characteristic beaded appearance of the renal artery on angiographic visualization (Fig. 10–5). This angiopgraphic feature is, however, observed less commonly in children with fibromuscular dysplasia than in adults.[18]

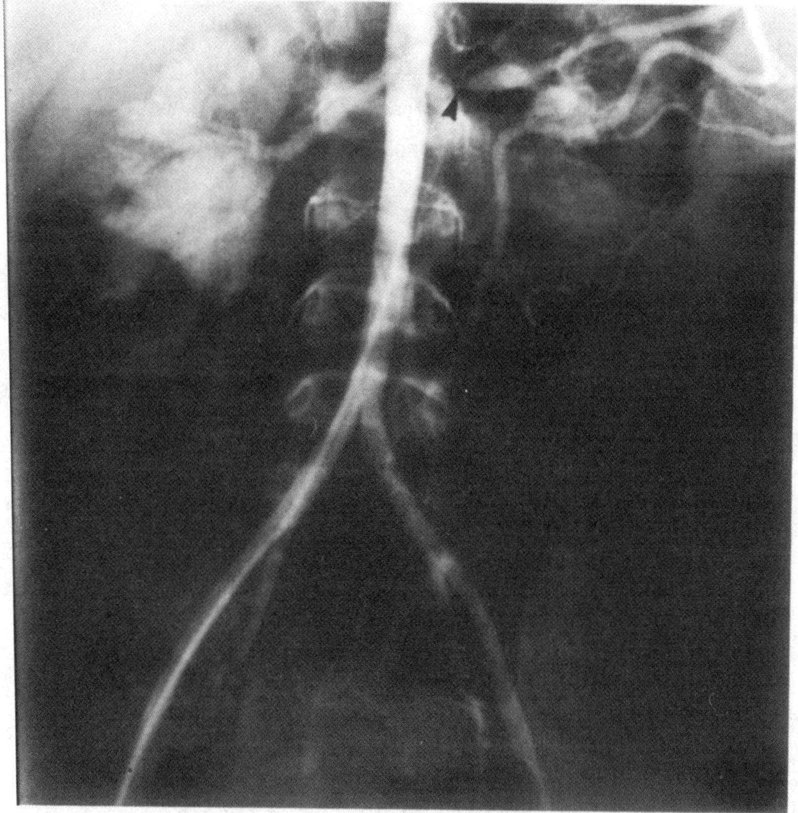

FIG. 10–5. Renal angiogram of a child with renal arterial stenosis due to fibromuscular dysplasia. Arrow points to area of arterial stenosis; poststenotic dilatation of renal artery is also shown.

Diseases other than fibromuscular dysplasia that cause renal arterial stenosis include coarctation of the descending aorta, neurofibromatosis, inflammatory lesions of the aorta (such as Takayasu's disease), and external pressure on the renal artery, as from abdominal tumors or retroperitoneal fibrosis (Fig. 10–6). The stenotic segment of the renal artery in these diseases usually involves the origin of the renal artery from the descending aorta. Renal artery stenosis in neurofibromatosis can be caused by more than one pathologic mechanism, including (1) proliferation of the neural tissue within the vessel wall, (2) fibromas compressing the renal artery, and (3) intimal proliferation of the renal artery. Since patients with neurofibromatosis are at a substantial risk for developing pheochromocytoma, it may also be necessary, in these instances, to rule out this endocrine disorder as a cause of hypertension. Hypertension in neonates is often caused by microembolization of the kidneys by thrombi arising from umbilical arterial catheters. In some patients, however, thrombosis affecting the main renal artery may be the cause of renovascular hypertension. Neonatal hypertension is discussed in further detail in Chap. 24. Renovascular embolization and thrombosis may also be seen in subacute bacterial endocarditis, following cardiovascular surgery or renal angiographic studies.

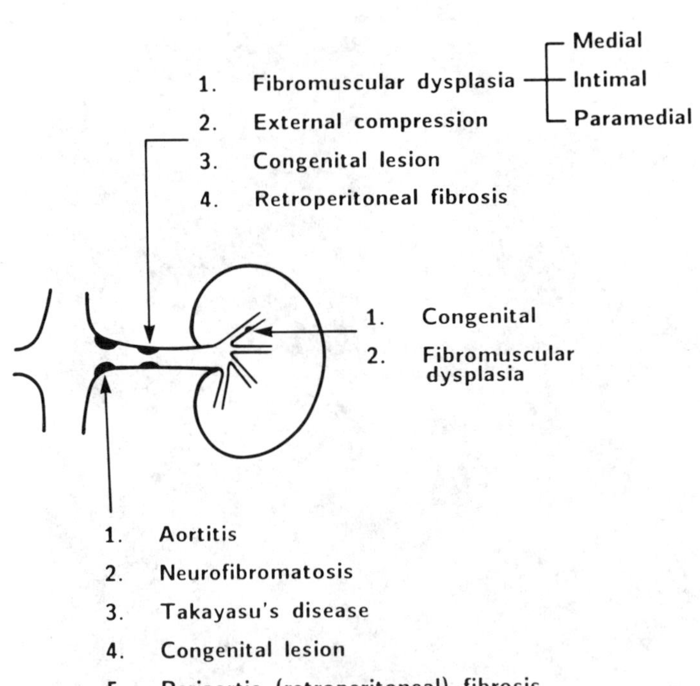

FIG. 10–6. Likely causes of renovascular hypertension based on the level of renal arterial occlusion. Lesions at the origin or renal artery may be due to aortitis, neurofibromatosis, Takayasu's disease, etc., while those affecting the mid-region of the artery usually result from fibromuscular dysplasia, external compression, congenital lesion, or retroperitoneal fibrosis.

TABLE 10–7. Clinical Characteristics of 27 Children with Renovascular Hypertension

Cause	No.	Sex (M/F)	Race: White	Race: Black	Race: Native American	Age (mean year ± SD)	BP, mmHg: Mean	BP, mmHg: Range
Fibromuscular dysplasia	10	4/6	9	0	1	6.0 (3.8)	179/118	140–260/94–140
Arteritis	4	2/2	4	0	0	6.75 (5.2)	177/122	160–200/110–140
Williams syndrome	3	1/2	3	0	0	8.0 (6.2)	147/96	130–170/90–100
Neurofibromatosis	2	1/1	0	2	0	2.0 (1.4)	210/130	180–240/120–140
Congenital	2	1/1	2	0	0	6.0 (5.6)	190/126	190/112–140
Miscellaneous	6	4/2	5	1	0	8.4 (7.2)	149/103	122–180/90–110
Total	27	13/14	23	3	1	6.6 (5.0)	172/114	122–260/90–140

Source: Daniels SR, Loggie JMH, McEnery PT, et al: Clinical spectrum of intrinsic renovascular hypertension in children. *Pediatrics* 80:698, 1987. Reproduced by permission of American Academy of Pediatrics, © 1987.

The symptoms of patients with renovascular hypertension range from none or minimal to severe hypertensive encephalopathy. Most of the 27 children reported by Daniels et al.[17] were detected because of elevated BP recorded during a routine examination (Table 10–7). A similar experience has been reported by Stanley and Fry[18] in 40 pediatric patients with renovascular hypertension. An abdominal bruit heard in the epigastric region and radiating to the flank may be heard in 30 to 50 percent of patients with documented renal arterial stenosis.[19] Some children with renovascular hypertension, especially those with fibromuscular dysplasia, suffer from growth retardation.[19] It has been suggested that hypertension itself is the cause of growth retardation in these patients, since an improved rate of growth has been noted following corrective surgery and normalization of blood pressure in several of these patients.[18,19]

PATHOGENESIS OF RENOVASCULAR HYPERTENSION

Role of the Renin-Angiotensin System. The pathogenesis of hypertension in the renovascular disease has been well linked to excessive renin production from the affected kidney in response to decreased perfusion pressure. Renin elaborated from the underperfused kidney activates the plasma globulin angiotensinogen (also known as renin substrate) in the circulation and converts it to angiotensin I. Angiotensin I is further converted by the angiotensin converting enzyme (ACE) present in the vascular endothelium (primarily in the lungs) to angiotensin II, which is a potent vasopressor agent. Angiotensin II leads to peripheral vasoconstriction and elevation of blood pressure. Additionally,

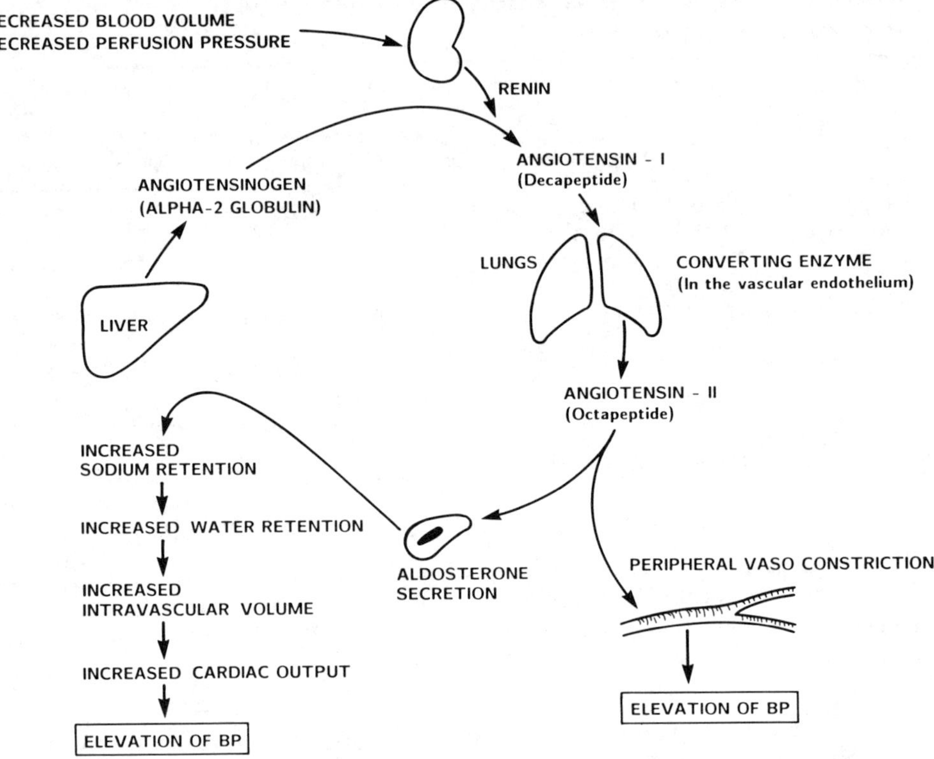

FIG. 10–7. Pathogenesis of renin-mediated hypertension in renal parenchymal and renovascular diseases.

angiotensin II stimulates aldosterone secretion from the adrenals resulting in renal sodium and water retention, which further contributes to elevation of BP (Fig. 10–7). The role played by the renin-angiotensin system in renovascular hypertension is based on the following observations: (1) plasma renin activity (PRA) is elevated in most if not all patients with renovascular disease; (2) removal of the affected kidney, successful surgical revascularization of the affected side, and dilatation of the affected renal artery by percutaneous transluminal angioplasty (PTA) results in a cure of hypertension as well as normalization of PRA in many patients; and (3) angiotensin converting enzyme inhibitors such as captopril are able to lower the blood pressure significantly in patients with renovascular disease.

Role of Intravascular Volume Expansion. While the key role played by the renin-angiotensin system in the pathogenesis of renovascular hypertension cannot be disputed, increased intravascular volume may also play a significant role in the development of elevated BP. Much of the information related to the role of increased intravascular volume in the maintenance of renovascular hypertension has been obtained from studies utilizing Goldblatt models of experimental hypertension in animals. Two experimental models of renovascular hypertension commonly studied deserve some explanation in order to elucidate the pathogenesis of renovascular hypertension. In the first model, the renal artery of one side is clamped with a silver clip, while the contralateral side is left undisturbed. This is the two-kidney-one-clip Goldblatt model. In the second model, one renal artery is clamped but the contralateral kidney is removed. This is the one-kidney-one-clip Goldblatt model. In both models, hypertension is noted soon after the renal arterial clips are applied and increased BP in this initial phase is clearly mediated by the renin-angiotensin system.[20,21] However, after a variable period (depending on the animal species used), PRA in the one-kidney-one-clip Goldblatt model normalizes and hypertension becomes refractory to treatment with the angiotensin II inhibitor saralasin.[20–22] During this chronic phase, the intravascular volume has been shown to be elevated while urinary sodium and water excretion is diminished.[20] Upon volume depletion induced by a low-sodium diet, hypertension in these animals once again becomes responsive to inhibition by saralasin.[22,23] These observations underscore the fact that fluid overload due to diminished renal sodium and water excretion—and not the renin-angiotensin system—plays the leading role in the chronic phase of hypertension in this experimental model of renovascular hypertension.

Even in the two-kidney-one-clip Goldblatt model, intravascular volume expansion has been recognized as an important contributor to hypertension during the chronic phase.[24] Although PRA remains elevated in these animals, they respond suboptimally to the administration of saralasin.[22,24] Also, following sodium restriction and diuretic administration (leading to reduction of intravascular volume), hypertension in these animals becomes responsive to exogenous administration of angiotensin II inhibitor.[24] These two observations support the notion that intravascular volume expansion contributes to the maintenance of hypertension in the chronic phase of hypertension in the two-kidney-one-clip experimental model of renovascular hypertension. Intravascular volume expansion is, however, not as pronounced in the two-kidney-one-clip model as it is in the one-kidney-one-clip model, possibly as a result of pressure natriuresis in the relatively well-perfused contralateral (normal) kidney.[25]

The role of intravascular volume expansion in mediating increased blood pressure in renovascular hypertension in humans is controversial. Based on the Goldblatt models of experimental renovascular hypertension, it can be presumed that in addition to the role of the renin-angiotensin system, intravascular volume expansion is also important in the pathogenesis of human renovascular hypertension. Several lines of evidence may support this. In one clinical study, both cardiac index and stroke index of patients with renovascular hypertension was determined to be elevated, suggesting intravascular volume expansion.[26] Another indirect clinical evidence of fluid volume expansion in patients with renovascular hypertension has been the observation of diuresis that follows correction or repair of the renal arterial stenosis in some patients.[27] It has also been observed that patients with renovascular hypertension who become resistant to treatment with an ACE inhibitor (e.g., captopril) can be made responsive to ACE inhibitor therapy by sodium restriction and diuretic administration, suggesting an expanded intravascular volume in these patients.[28]

RENAL PARENCHYMAL DISEASES

Renal parenchymal diseases are the most frequent (70 to 80 percent) causes of secondary hypertension in children. Chronic glomerulonephritis and renal parenchymal scarring due to chronic pyelonephritis represent the most common acquired renal diseases that lead to chronic hypertension in children.[10–12] Of the developmental anomalies, segmental renal hypoplasia, or Ask-Upmark kidney, is the best-described condition associated with severe hypertension. Traditionally, this condition has been regarded as a congenital malformation of the kidney that affects only a segment of the developing organ. Recent observation, however, suggests that the segmental renal hypoplasia represents an area of renal damage and scarring resulting from intrarenal reflux of urine. Ask-Upmark kidney is now generally considered to be an acquired lesion rather than a congenital developmental anomaly.[29] Polycystic kidney disease of both the autosomal dominant variety (adult type) and the autosomal recessive variety (infantile type) are often associated with hypertension. Hypertension can also be observed in patients with other developmental renal anomalies such as hypoplasia and dysplasia. Acute onset hydronephrosis but not uncomplicated chronic hydronephrosis is often associated with hydronephrosis.[30] Renin-producing tumor of the juxtaglomerular tissue (hemangiopericytoma) is a rare cause of hypertension in children.[31] Occasionally, Wilms tumor will also elaborate renin and thus lead to hypertension.[32] More often, however, Wilms tumor causes compression of the renal tissue and leads to hyperreninemia and hypertension on that pathogenic basis. External compression of the kidney by processes other than a tumor (such as a subcapsular hematoma or retroperitoneal fibrosis) may also cause hypertension, this phenomenon being referred to as the *Page kidney*.

Hypertension is a common accompaniment of chronic glomerulonephritides, being further aggravated by the therapeutic use of corticosteroids. Hypertension is especially common in membranoproliferative glomerulonephritis. Hemolytic-uremic syndrome is also well known to cause chronic hypertension in children as a long-term complication. In a recent study of children with hemolytic-uremic syndrome, chronic hypertension at the end of 10 years of follow-up was reported in 13.1 percent.[33] Other glomerular diseases associated with a high incidence of hypertension include poststreptococcal glomerulonephritis, focal segmental glomerulonephritis, renal involvement by polyarteritis, scleroderma, crescentic glomerulonephritis, and renal infarction. On the other hand, hypertension is relatively less commonly seen in patients with membranous glomerulonephritis and IgA nephropathy.[34]

PATHOGENESIS OF RENAL HYPERTENSION

Hypertension in patients with parenchymal renal diseases can be mediated by more than one mechanism, including (1) hyperreninemia and (2) sodium and fluid overload. Hyperreninemia is the predominant mechanism mediating hypertension in unilateral renal diseases such as acute hydronephrosis, chronic renal scarring, and Ask-Upmark segmental hypoplasia.[30,35,36] On the hand, sodium retention and intravascular fluid overload may be involved in the pathogenesis of hypertension in patients with bilateral renal disease or chronic renal failure due to parenchymal renal diseases.[37,38] It has also been argued that lack of vasodilator substances (prostaglandins and kinins) normally produced by the kidney may also play an important role in the pathogenesis of hypertension in chronic renal parenchymal diseases.[39,40] Hypertension in acute poststreptococcal glomerulonephritis is mediated by sodium and fluid retention rather than by hyperreninemia.[41]

CARDIOVASCULAR DISEASES

COARCTATION OF THE AORTA

Coarctation of the aorta is the leading cardiovascular disease that causes hypertension in children. The reported incidence of coarctation of the aorta as the underlying etiology in hypertensive children ranges from none to 30 percent.[10–13] This variability in the incidence probably reflects referral patterns in individual institutions. The site of coarctation may be either in the thoracic or abdominal aorta; coarctation of the abdominal aorta is, however, relatively uncommon.

Clinical suspicion of aortic coarctation in a hypertensive child is raised by the observation of hypertension in the upper extremities associated with diminished amplitude of the arterial pulses in the lower extremities and a characteristic cardiac murmur. Systolic BP in the upper extremities in coarctation of the aorta usually exceeds the BP in the lower extremities by 20 mmHg. Weak arterial pulse or diminished blood pressure in the lower extremity may not be observed in patients (especially neonates) who have a patent ductus arteriosus or those who have congestive heart failure.[42] Congestive cardiac failure may be the only manifestation of coarctation of the aorta in neonates or young infants. Failure to thrive may be observed in some infants with coarctation, and cold feet, headache, and chest pain have been reported in older children.[43] The diagnosis of coarctation is established by echocardiography, cardiac catheterization, and aortography. The characteristic radiologic features of notching of the ribs by the collateral circulation may sometimes be seen in older children.

The pathophysiology of hypertension in coarctation remains unclear. The role of the kidneys and the renin-angiotensin system in the pathogenesis of hypertension in coarctation of the aorta has been speculated upon, but plasma renin activity is not elevated in all patients.[44,45] The role of the renin-angiotensin system in the pathogenesis of hypertension in coarctation of the aorta is suggested by the clinical observation that the inhibition of angiotensin II with saralasin results in a significant lowering of systolic, diastolic, and mean arterial BP in patients with aortic coarctation.[46] Furthermore, Declusin et al.[47] have shown, in dogs with surgically induced coarctation of the aorta, that plasma renin activity increases while renal perfusion decreases during exercise. These investigators speculate that the hypertensive response in the proximal circulation in this experimental model could result from hyperreninemia. In an alternative hypothesis, Gupta and Wiggers[48] have suggested that hypertension in the upper extremities in coarctation of the aorta results from mechanical factors, such as a decrease in the distensibility (and reduced capacity) of the aorta above the level of coarctation, combined with an enhanced left ventricular systolic discharge.

TAKAYASU'S ARTERITIS

Takayasu's arteritis is a rare form of inflammatory disorder of undetermined etiology that involves large blood vessels such as the aorta. This form of arteritis may affect the entire length of the aorta in a patchy distribution. A single isolated lesion in the aortic arch may simulate coarctation of the aorta, both in hemodynamic effects and clinical presentation. Involvement of the aorta around renal arterial ostia may result in renal arterial stenosis. Systemic symptoms such as malaise and weight loss often accompany this disease, and the erythrocyte sedimentation rate is usually elevated. Autotransplantation of the kidneys or aortorenal bypass surgery may be necessary to relieve hypertension in these patients.

ENDOCRINE CAUSES OF HYPERTENSION

PHEOCHROMOCYTOMA

Pheochromocytoma is a well-recognized but rare etiology of hypertension in children, the reported incidence in various studies being 0 to 3 percent of hypertensive children.[10,11,12,15] Despite its rarity, the significance of considering pheochromocytoma in the evaluation of a hypertensive child lies in the fact that the hypertension is potentially curable upon surgical removal of the causative tumor. Most cases of pheochromocytoma occur in adults; only 10 percent of all such tumors are seen during the childhood years. A majority of pheochromocytomas have been reported in children older than 6 years of age (the mean age of detection of the tumor in the 100 cases reviewed by Stackpole et al.[49] was 11.0 years). However, pheochromocytoma has been reported in infants aged 3 months or less.[50] Boys are affected twice as often as girls. In about 20 percent of these cases, pheochromocytoma has been reported to be familial.[50]

Pheochromocytoma arises from the chromaffin tissue of the adrenal glands or the paraspinal sympathetic ganglia. In approximately half the cases, the tumor is present in one adrenal gland; in another 20 percent, both adrenal glands are involved; and in the remaining 30 percent, the tumor arises from extraadrenal tissues exclusively or may involve these sites in addition to the adrenal gland.[49,50] Childhood pheochromocytomas are generally benign, but in 10 percent of such cases the tumor is malignant. In approximately 20 percent of the affected children, pheochromocytoma is associated with multiple endocrine neoplasia syndrome (MEN).[50] Other conditions associated with a significantly increased risk of pheochromocytoma are tuberous sclerosis, neurofibromatosis, and Von Hippel-Lindau disease.

Headache is the commonest presenting symptom of pheochromocytoma in

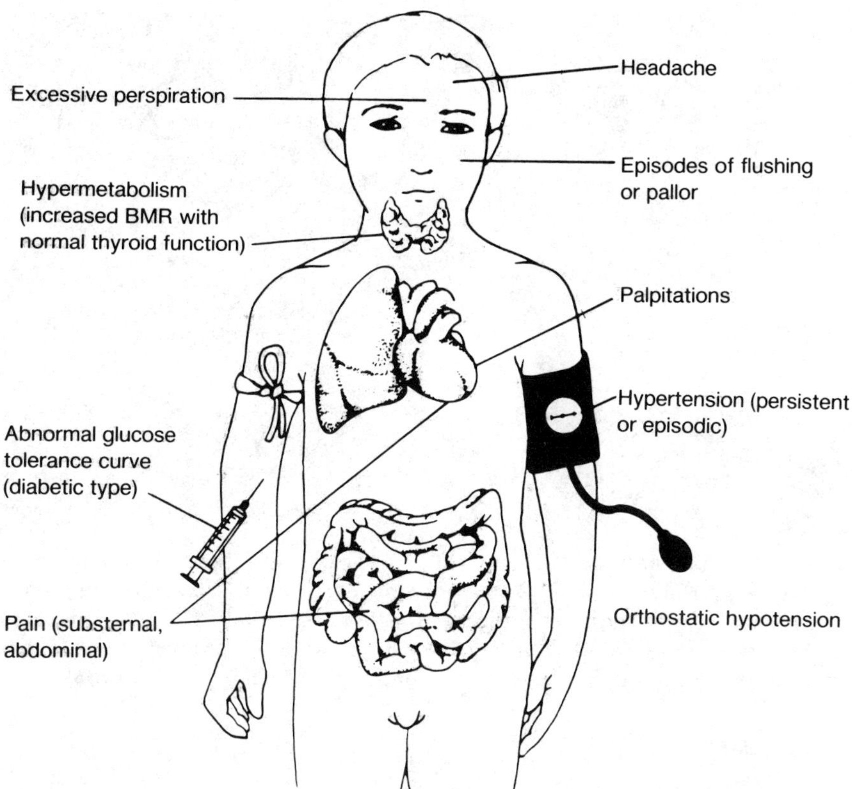

FIG. 10–8. Common clinical manifestations of pheochromocytoma in children. (Reproduced with permission from Ingelfinger JR: *Pediatric Hypertension*. Philadelphia, Saunders, 1982, p 194.)

children and is seen in approximately 80 percent of cases. Hypertension is a consistent finding in patients with pheochromocytoma (100 percent) and is usually of severe degree. Although BP may be elevated intermittently, hypertension is often (in 75 to 80 percent of the cases) sustained in children. Seizures, presumably due to hypertensive encephalopathy, are also commonly seen (20 percent). Hypertensive retinopathy is frequently present in these patients. Other clinical manifestations of pheochromocytoma are those caused by catecholamine excess, such as excessive sweating, weight loss, diarrhea, vomiting, abdominal pain, hyperdynamic precordium, and unexplained resting tachycardia. Since most pheochromocytomas are small (5 to 7 cm), abdominal mass is not a common manifestation of pheochromocytoma.[49–51] In many ways the clinical symptomatology of pheochromocytoma (Fig. 10–8) mimics that of hyperthyroidism except that the thyroid function tests are normal. The rule of six H's is a convenient way to remember the clinical manifestations of pheochromocytoma: hypertension, headache, hyperhidrosis, heart consciousness, hypermetabolism, and hyperglycemia.[52]

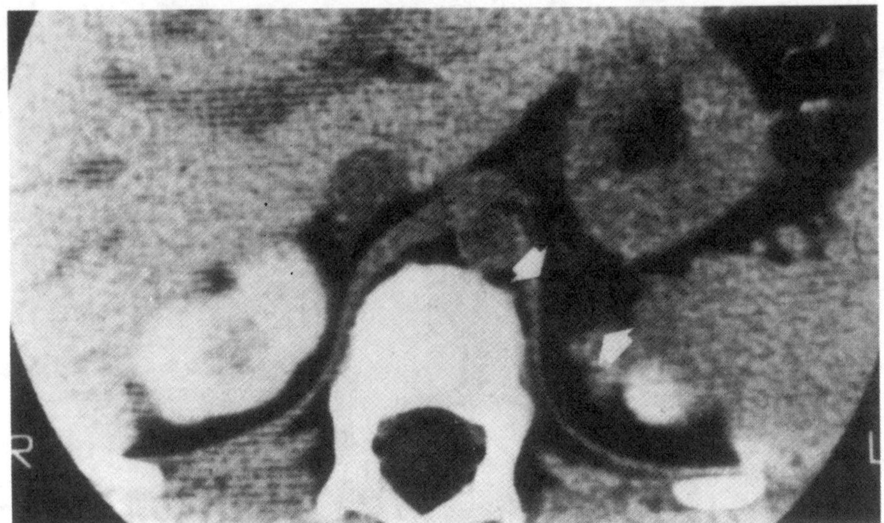

FIG. 10–9. Contrast-enhanced CT scan of a 9-year-old boy, showing an adrenal mass *(arrows)* on the left side. The mass was diagnosed to be an adrenal adenoma. The patient presented with hypertension, polyuria, polydypsia, and muscle weakness. (Reproduced with permission from Dickson BA, Franks RC: Aldosterone-producing adenoma presenting with hypokalemic myopathy. *Clin Pediatr* 27:344, 1988).

RARE ENDOCRINE DISORDERS

Primary Aldosteronism. This rare syndrome is characterized by excess aldosterone production by the adrenal glands (Fig. 10–9). While adrenal adenoma is more common in adults, primary hyperaldosteronism in children is often caused by bilateral adrenal hyperplasia.[53,54] The main symptoms of primary aldosteronism are related to excessive renal loss of potassium and resultant hypokalemia. These include muscular weakness, paresthesia, growth retardation, polyuria (from hypokalemic nephropathy), and polydipsia. Hypertension in primary aldosteronism is caused by renal sodium and water retention in response to excess circulating aldosterone and consequent expansion of the extracellular fluid volume. Plasma renin activity is low because of expanded intravascular volume. Laboratory diagnosis of primary aldosteronism rests on documenting hypokalemia, alkalemia, high renal potassium loss, low plasma renin activity, and a high plasma aldosterone level. Caution, however, must be used in interpreting the serum aldosterone level of a child, since it is affected not only by age but also by posture and salt intake.

Cushing Syndrome. Cushing syndrome is an endocrine disorder caused by an excessive production of adrenal glucocorticoids, often due to an adrenal neoplasm.[55] Exogenous administration of glucocorticoids for the treatment of disorders such as nephrotic syndrome and bronchial asthma can also cause Cushing syndrome and hypertension. The clinical characteristics of this disorder are truncal obesity with "moon facies" and "buffalo hump," hypertension, cutaneous striae, excess hair growth, and wasting of skeletal muscles. Osteoporosis may occur and lead to fractures of the long bones; diabetes mellitus and delayed wound healing may also be seen. Hypertension accompanies approximately 20 to 25 percent of cases with Cushing syndrome caused by exogenously administered glucocorticoids, while it is observed in 80 percent of those with naturally occurring diseases.[55] The precise mechanism of hypertension caused by glucorticoids in Cushing syndrome or by exogenously administered glucocorticoids is not known, but it is believed to be related to (1) sodium retention and plasma volume expansion, (2) potentiation of the vasopressor effects of endogenously available epinephrine, and (3) a poorly defined hypertensinogenic action of glucocorticoids that is distinct from mineralocorticoid action.[55]

Congenital Adrenal Hyperplasia. Enzymatic defects in the biosynthesis of adrenal steroids are rare causes of hypertension in children. The two common enzymatic defects of adrenal steroid biosynthesis that are associated with hypertension are 11-hydroxylase and 17-hydroxylase deficiencies.

11-hydroxylase defect is associated with a deficiency of glucocorticoid production and an increased production of deoxycorticosterone (DOC) and androgens. Because of glucocorticoid deficiency, ACTH production by the anterior pituitary remains uninhibited; the result is an excessive stimulation and an uninterrupted production of androgens and mineralocorticoid (DOC) by the adrenals. Excess DOC production leads to hypokalemia and clinical features similar to those seen in primary aldosteronism, such as muscular weakness, hypokalemia, and hypertension. Genetically female patients are born with ambiguous genitalia and may resemble males with bilateral cryptorchidism. However, the internal sex organs of these newborns are of the normal female type. Genetic males are usually normal at birth but show accelerated somatic growth and development of secondary sexual characteristics. Marked penile hypertrophy is usual, but testes may be of normal size for age. Hypertension is usually of severe degree in these patients and is caused by sodium and fluid retention as a consequence of mineralocorticoid excess.[56,57]

Patients with 17-hydroxylase deficiency are usually not diagnosed until adolescence, when failure of secondary sexual characteristics to develop becomes obvious. At this stage, genetic females lack breast development and axillary hair; their external genitalia appear infantile. The uterus is small and the ovaries show cystic changes. Genetic males are usually raised as girls, since their external genitalia appear to be female. The scrotum is not fused and the testes may be undescended or in the inguinal canal. There is no uterus, but a vaginal pouch with a blind ending may be present.[58] These clinical features result from defective synthesis of both androgen and estrogen. Because of a deficit of glucocorticoid production, ACTH secretion remains elevated and excess synthesis of the mineralocorticoid DOC is present. Sodium and water retention as a result of DOC excess is the cause of hypertension in these patients.

ESSENTIAL HYPERTENSION IN CHILDREN

Prior to the publication of a report by Londe et al.[15] in 1971, essential hypertension was considered an uncommon disorder among children. Many subsequent studies have established the existence of essential hypertension in children, particularly in adolescents. The precise incidence of essential hypertension in children is not well known. In various published studies, essential hypertension has been reported to constitute the etiology of hypertension in 12 to 18 percent of children with sustained elevation of BP.[10–16]

CLINICAL FEATURES

Although essential hypertension has been reported in young children, it is more prevalent in older children and adolescents. A strong family history of essential hypertension is often present but cannot be relied on as a major diagnostic criterion of essential hypertension in children.[16] Obesity is seen in approximately 50 percent of the cases, and elevation of BP is usually of modest degree.[15] Most pediatric patients are asymptomatic at the time of initial detection of essential hypertension; secondary effects of hypertension on target organs, such as retinopathy or hypertensive encephalopathy, are encountered less commonly at the onset of essential hypertension than they are in patients with secondary hypertension. On the other hand, a higher incidence of left ventricular hypertrophy (30 percent) has been reported in children with essential hypertension as opposed to secondary hypertension (15 percent).[16] This observation is suggestive of a longer duration of undetected and asymptomatic hypertension in these children.

The diagnosis of essential hypertension in childhood is established only by exclusion of other secondary causes. As a general rule, hypertension in young children, especially in those with severe elevation of BP, should be presumed to be of secondary etiology, and the diagnosis of essential hypertension should be avoided unless a thorough investigation fails to reveal an etiology. On the other hand, the diagnosis of essential hypertension may be given primary consideration in an asymptomatic adolescent with a modest elevation of BP in whom a family history of essential hypertension is well documented and where tests of renal function and renal ultrasound examination are normal.

PATHOGENESIS

The pathogenesis of essential hypertension is not well understood. Several factors known to be associated with essential hypertension are discussed below.

AGE

Although reported in children as young as 4 years of age, essential hypertension is predominantly a disease of older children and adolescents.[15,16]

RACE

Ethnic background does not seem to determine BP in normal young children,[3] but black adolescents generally have higher BP than do white children.[59,60] Similarly, black adults have a higher incidence of hypertension than do white adults.[61] Whether these racial differences in BP during adolescence and adulthood represent inherited factors or environmental influences is not clear.

SOCIOECONOMIC FACTORS

Several workers have found a positive correlation between BP and socioeconomic factors, particularly among black children. Kotchen et al.[62] documented that black children from the inner-city area of Washington, D.C. had higher BP than those attending schools in middle-class neighborhoods. Gillium et al.[63] also noted that BP in children correlated significantly with mother's occupation, being higher in children from families of unskilled workers than in those of higher socioeconomic status. The mechanism by which socioeconomic status effects BP in children is unclear. Several factors—including high salt intake, a higher incidence of obesity, and lack of exercise in children from socially disadvantaged households—may be involved.

SALT INTAKE

Excess salt (sodium chloride) intake has long been linked to the development of essential hypertension. Most of the evidence is derived from epidemiologic studies of BP in persons from cultures where the dietary intake of salt is high. In analyzing the cardiovascular risk factors in six Solomon Islands societies, Page et al.[64] determined that increased salt intake correlated well with a rising trend of systolic BP seen with advancing age. In contrast, the population subgroups of these islands who were not accustomed to a high-salt diet did not demonstrate an increase of BP with advancing age.[64] Similar epidemiologic studies linking high salt intake to increased incidence of hypertension have been reported in cross-sectional population studies from other geographic areas.[65,66] In one study of third- and tenth-grade children in Massachusetts, Calabrese and Tuthill[67] found that BP was significantly higher in children who lived in communities where the sodium content of the drinking water was high (110 mg/L) as compared to those where the water had a low sodium content (8 mg/L). The role of salt in determining BP in newborns was studied by Hofman et al.[68] Restriction of sodium intake in the formula for the first 6 months of life was shown to result in a lower BP among the infants who received it as compared with infants taking formula that contained a higher (conventional) amount of sodium.[68] Furthermore, salt restriction is well known to decrease BP in hypertensive individuals.[69] All of these epidemiologic and clinical observations suggest that sodium intake plays some role in the regulation of BP and may be important in the pathogenesis of essential hypertension.

Although salt intake is proposed to be an important factor in the pathogenesis of essential hypertension, the mechanism by which sodium induces hypertension is not fully understood. DeWardener and McGregor[70] have hypothesized a pathophysiologic sequence whereby salt may induce essential hypertension in susceptible individuals. They suggest that the kidneys of such individuals are unable to excrete excess dietary sodium, leading to an increased extracellular fluid volume and increased synthesis of a yet unidentified (oua-

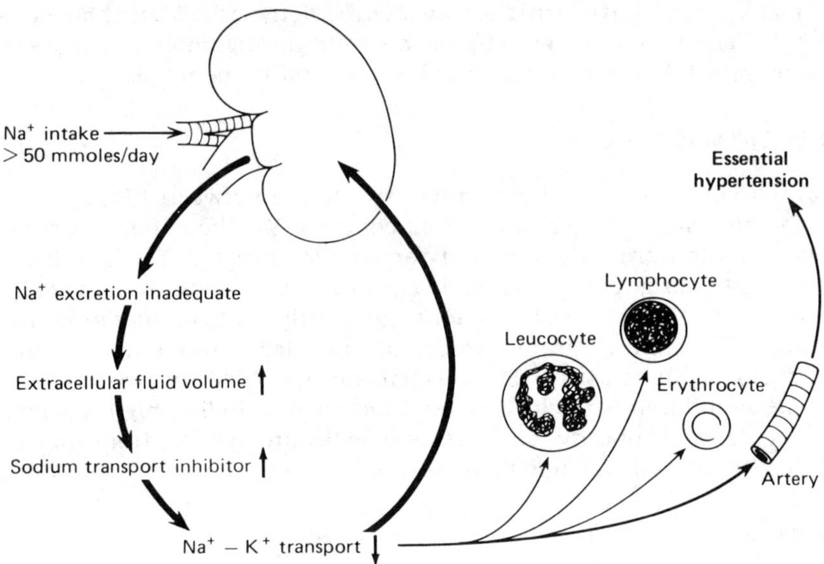

FIG. 10–10. **Hypothesis suggesting the possible role of a circulating sodium-transport-inhibiting factor in the pathogenesis of essential hypertension. (Reproduced by permission from DeWardener HE, MacGregor GA: Dahl's hypothesis that a saluretic substance may be responsible for a sustained rise in arterial pressure: Its possible role in essential hypertension. *Kidney Int* 18:6, 1980.)**

bain-like) sodium transport inhibitor substance (Fig. 10–10). This sodium transport inhibitor supposedly retards renal tubular sodium reabsorption, resulting in renal salt and water excretion and normalization of the extracellular fluid volume. However, the proposed sodium transport inhibitor also reduces sodium transport in other body cells such as the red cells, leukocytes, and arterioles. Consequently, the intracellular sodium and possibly calcium content increases in various tissue cells. Inhibition of cellular sodium transport in the arterioles in this manner is believed to lead to increased vascular reactivity and increased peripheral resistance. Whether patients who develop essential hypertension have a genetic predisposition to produce excess amounts of sodium transport inhibitor is not known. Red cell sodium exchange defect—a marker for this abnormality in cellular sodium transport described in adult patients with essential hypertension—has also been reported in children with essential hypertension.[71]

FAMILIAL AND GENETIC FACTORS

Children in families with a positive history of essential hypertension are at a higher risk of developing essential hypertension. Studies comparing the incidence of hypertension in families with adopted and biologic children suggest a strong genetic influence on the BP of individuals.[72] Miyao and Furusho[73] found that if both parents were hypertensive, the incidence of hypertension in the offspring rose by a factor of 4 to 15 as opposed to families where both parents were normotensive. However, without any known pattern of inheritance, it is difficult assign to any given individual the genetic risk of developing hypertension.

OBESITY

Increased body weight is well known to affect the level of BP in children. Generally, larger children (in both weight and height) have systolic as well as diastolic BP in higher percentile ranges than those who are thin and short.[3] In a recent study, Gutin et al.[74] were able to correlate fatness positively with both systolic and diastolic BP in 5- and 6-year-old boys; the diastolic BP in girls also showed a positive correlation. Weight loss in obese adolescents has also been shown to result in a significant decrease in BP.[75] Increased cardiac output is believed to be the underlying cause of hypertension in obese individuals. Systemic peripheral resistance in obese individuals has been shown to be somewhat decreased.[75]

PERSONALITY AND ENVIRONMENTAL STRESS

Insel et al.[76] have reported a positive correlation between type A personality and BP in children. Working with adolescents who had a borderline high BP (90–95th percentile), Falkner et al.[77] studied cardiovascular response to a mental stress test. They found that those youngsters who progressed to essential hypertension during a 5-year follow-up had had a significantly higher systolic and diastolic BP and heart rate during the test. These findings suggest that personality traits, in addition to other known factors, may contribute to the pathogenesis of essential hypertension.

TRACKING OF BP AND EARLY DETECTION OF ESSENTIAL HYPERTENSION

Lauer et al.[78] have shown that serial monitoring of BP of children may be able to detect patients at high risk of developing essential hypertension later in life. In their observation of a large population of children, they noted that BP may track in one of the four ways shown in Fig. 10–11. In summary, children with BP in the high centiles (group I) or low centiles (group IV) generally follow their respective percentiles; on the other hand, patients in the middle centiles either show an increasing trend (group II) or a decreasing trend (group III). The importance of these findings is in identifying group II patients (increasing BP with age) by periodic BP recordings, since these children appear to be at the greatest risk of developing essential hypertension later in life.

DIAGNOSTIC EVALUATION OF HYPERTENSIVE CHILDREN

As a general rule, it is helpful to consider a few facts in the evaluation of hypertensive children. (1) Hypertension in a majority of children is caused by a secondary etiology, and a thorough evaluation to determine the etiology is required. (2) Severe elevation of BP is often characteristic of secondary hyper-

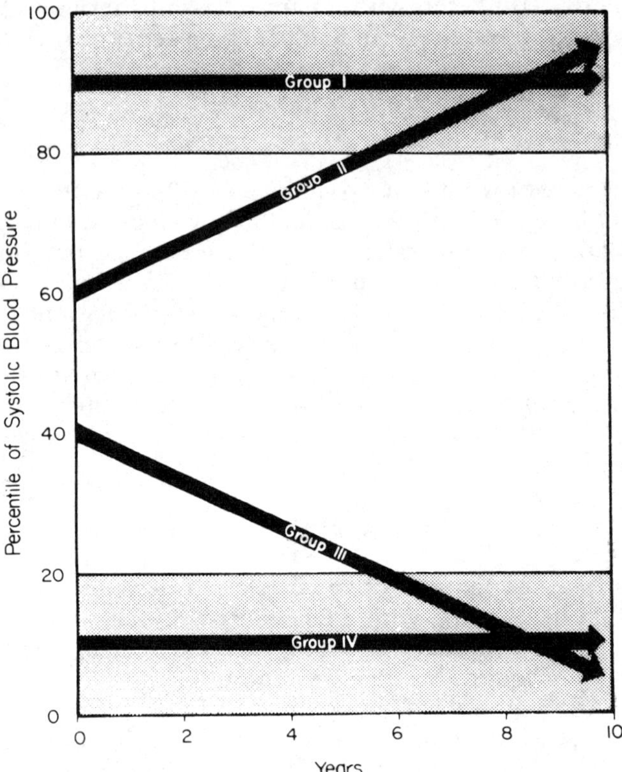

FIG. 10–11. Tracking of blood pressure in childhood, showing the value of monitoring blood pressure. Four graphs of subjects with blood pressure tracking in different ways are shown. Shaded areas represent upper and lower quintiles of blood pressure. Group I (consistently high) maintains lower pressure in the upper quintiles. Group II (increasingly high) tracks upward over time to the upper quintiles. Group III (decreasingly low) tracks downward to the lowest quintiles. Group IV (consistently low) maintains blood pressure in the lowest quintiles. Group II is at highest risk of developing hypertension later in life. (From Lauer RM, Mahoney LT, Clarke WR: Tracking of blood pressure during childhood: The Muscatine Study. *Clin Exp Hyperten* 8:515, 1986. Reproduced by permission of Marcel Dekker, Inc.)

tension rather than essential hypertension. (3) Essential hypertension is usually an asymptomatic disorder and is generally detected in the course of a routine evaluation. Many hypertensive children have known underlying renal diseases such as chronic glomerulonephritis, chronic pyelonephritis, or a congenital renal anomaly. Such patients with a known renal parenchymal disease usually do not need any further diagnostic workup. However, children presenting for the first time with symptomatic or asymptomatic hypertension require detailed laboratory studies in order to arrive at a diagnosis and render appropriate therapy.

A considerable literature has arisen regarding the sequence of diagnostic studies and the extent to which these need to be undertaken in hypertensive patients. Although the basic aims of various proposed investigative protocols are similar, the algorithms advocated by various authors differ. In order to proceed in a systematic manner and avoid costly laboratory investigations, diagnostic tests for hypertensive children have been arbitrarily classed into two categories: initial, or phase I and phase II. Phase I investigations (Table 10–8) should be performed in all hypertensive children. The purpose of these investigations is to obtain preliminary information and determine the organ system that may be responsible for hypertension in the child. Once such information is available, the laboratory tests proposed in phase II (Table 10–9) are done in order to confirm and establish the diagnosis. Obviously, it is not necessary to perform all tests listed in phase II in every patient; laboratory tests must be individualized as indicated. For example, patients suspected of having pheochromocytoma will need confirmation of the tumor by CT scan and scanning with ^{131}I metaiodobenzylguanidine (MIBG scan), while renal angiography will be needed in patients suspected of renovascular hypertension. An algorithm for the diagnostic evaluation of hypertensive children is given in Fig. 10–12. Most laboratory investigations for the evaluation of older children with hypertension can be done in an outpatient setting, but it may be necessary to admit infants and small children to the hospital.

TABLE 10–8. Initial, or Phase I, Diagnostic Evaluation of Hypertensive Children[a]

Test	Purpose of Evaluation
Blood pressure in all four extremities using appropriate-sized cuffs	Coarctation of aorta
Auscultate for abdominal bruits	Renovascular disease
Complete blood cell count	Normocytic normochromic anemia as a feature of chronic renal disease or microangiopathic anemia in hemolytic uremic syndrome
Urinalysis	Renal parenchymal disease such as chronic glomerulonephritis and chronic pyelonephritis
Urine culture	Urinary tract infection
Serum electrolytes, BUN, creatinine, and serum cholesterol	Renal function evaluation Patients with hypokalemia may have hyperaldosteronism Serum cholesterol for cardiovascular risk assessment
Renal ultrasound and radionuclide scan	Evaluate renal size, contour, and other developmental anomalies and determine renal function
Chest radiograph and electrocardiogram or echocardiogram if available	Evaluate secondary effect on the cardiovascular system
Plasma renin activity	Elevated in renovascular or renal disease, decreased in patients with hyperaldosteronism

[a]These clinical and laboratory tests must be performed in all children.

TABLE 10–9. Phase II Diagnostic Evaluation of Hypertensive Children[a]

Test	Purpose
Tests for Renovascular Diseases	
Converting enzyme (captopril) challenge test and radionuclide studies after captopril challenge	For noninvasive diagnostic evidence of renovascular diseases
Renal vein renin	To localize the kidney involved with a renovascular or parenchymal disease; also, evaluate surgical correctability of hypertension
Selective renal angiography	To confirm the diagnosis of renovascular disease
Tests for Pheochromocytoma	
Urinary and plasma catecholamines and metabolites	Initial test for diagnosis of pheochromocytoma
MIGB scan	Localize the site of pheochromocytoma and evaluate if more than one site of origin is present
CAT scan/MRI scan	Confirm the site of origin of pheochromocytoma prior to surgical removal
Angiography and venography	To localize the site of tumor
Tests for Renal Parenchymal Diseases	
Chronic Pyelonephritis	
Renal function tests: BUN, serum creatinine, creatinine clearance	Obtain evidence of renal dysfunction
Renal ultrasound/IVP	Evaluate renal size, renal scars, rule out obstructive uropathy
Vesicocystourethrogram (VCUG)	Rule out underlying reflux as a cause of chronic pyelonephritis
Peripheral plasma renin	Increased values will support the diagnosis of renal parenchymal disease
Selective renal vein renin	May be helpful in evaluating the possibility of a surgical cure for hypertension by unilateral nephrectomy if only one side is involved
Chronic glomerulonephritis	
24-h urine for protein	Significant proteinuria supports the evidence for chronic glomerulonephritis
Renal function tests: BUN, serum creatinine, creatinine clearance	Evaluate renal functions and the the extent of renal parenchymal dysfunction
Serum complement, tests for hepatitis surface and e antigen, serologic tests for SLE	To rule out chronic glomerulonephritis due to hepatitis antigenemia, membranoproliferative glomerulonephritis, and SLE
Renal biopsy	To confirm the diagnosis and classify the chronic glomerulonephritis into its morphologic subtypes for prognosis and appropriate therapy
Tests for Adrenal Enzyme Defects	
Plasma cortisol	Decreased in 17-hydroxylase defect
Plasma deoxycorticosterone (DOC)	Elevated in 11-hydroxylase and 17-hydroxylase enzyme defects
Plasma androgen	Elevated in 11-hydroxylase defect and decreased in 17-hydroxylase defect
Urinary	
17-hydroxysteroids	Both elevated in 11-hydroxylase defect; 17-hydroxysteroids decreased in 17-hydroxylase defect
17-ketosteroids and aldosterone	Decreased in both enzyme defects
Plasma renin activity	Decreased in both enzyme defects

[a]These tests must be individualized depending on the most likely suspected etiology and on the results of the phase I evaluation.

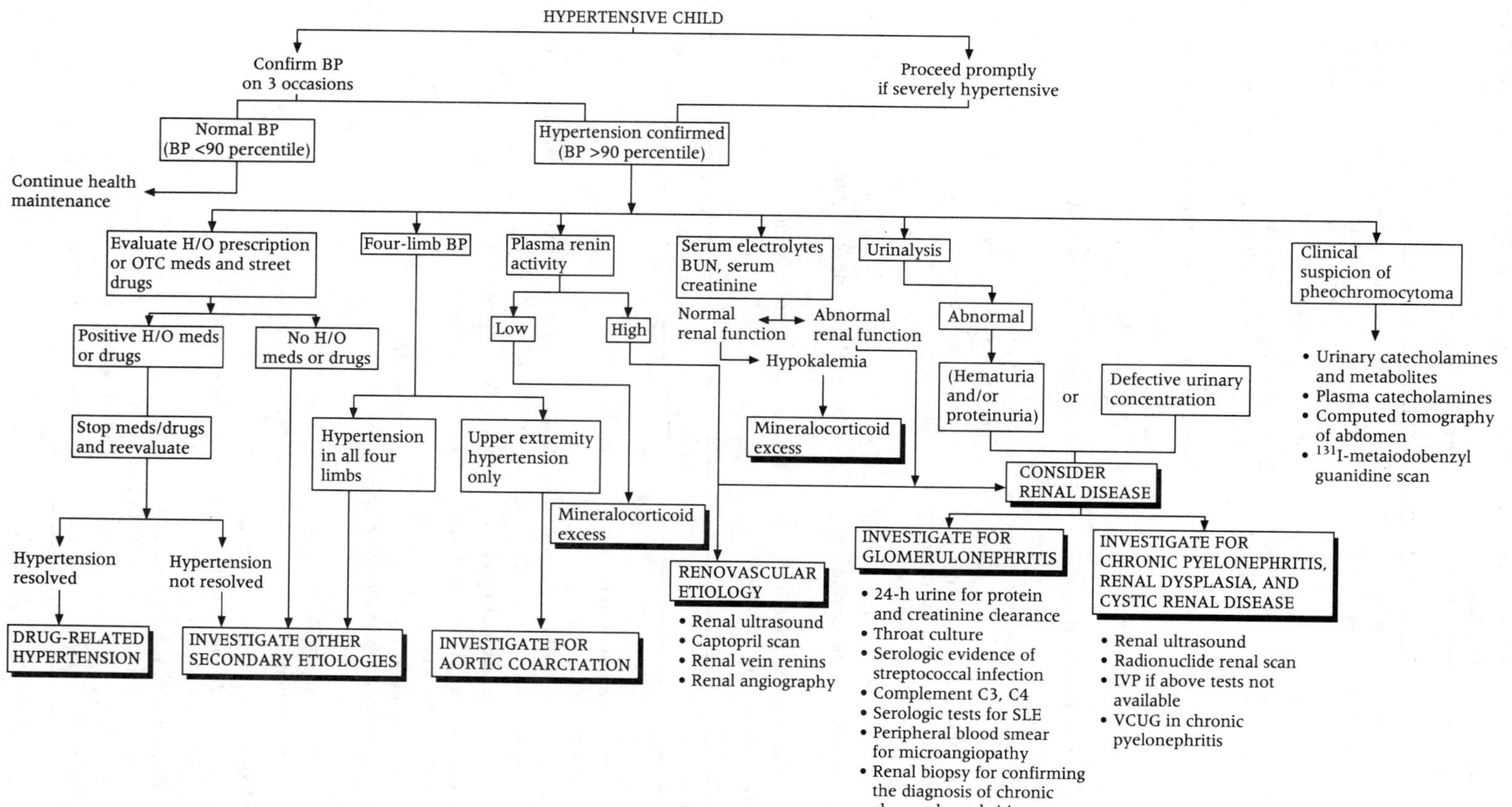

FIG. 10–12. Flowchart for investigating hypertension in children.

TABLE 10–10. Value of History and Physical Examination in the Diagnosis of Hypertension in Children

Historical data	Relevance
Family history of hypertension, preeclampsia, toxemia, renal disease, tumors	Important in essential hypertension, inherited renal disease, and some endocrine diseases (e.g., familial pheochromocytoma with multiple endocrine adenopathy II)
Family history of early complications of hypertension and/or atherosclerosis	Suggests likely course of hypertension and/or presence of other coronary artery disease risk factors
Neonatal history	Use of umbilical artery catheter suggests need to evaluate renal vasculature and kidneys
Headaches, dizziness, epistaxis, visual problems	Nonspecific symptomatology, usually not etiologically helpful
Abdominal pain, dysuria, frequency, nocturia, enuresis	May suggest underlying renal disease
Joint pains/swelling, facial or peripheral edema	Suggests connective tissue disease and/or other forms of glomerulonephritis
Weight loss, failure to gain weight with good appetite, sweating, flushing, fevers, palpitations	In combination, symptoms suggest pheochromocytoma
Muscle cramps, weakness, constipation	May suggest hypokalemia and hyperaldosteronism
Age of onset of menarche, sexual development	May be helpful in suggesting hydroxylase deficiencies
Ingestion of prescription and over-the-counter drugs, contraceptives, illicit drugs	Drug-induced hypertension

Physical Findings	Relevance
General	
Pale mucous membranes, facial or pretibial edema	Renal disease
Pallor, evanescent flushing, increased, sweating at rest	Pheochromocytoma versus hyperdynamic essential hypertension
Café au lait spots, neurofibromas	von Recklinghausen's disease
Moon face, hirsutism, buffalo hump, truncal obesity, striae	Cushing syndrome
Webbing of the neck, low hairline, wide-spaced nipples, wide carrying angle	Turner syndrome
Elfin facies, poor growth, retardation	Williams syndrome
Thyroid enlargement	Hyper- or hypothyroidism
Cardiovascular	
Absent or delayed femoral pulses, low leg pressure relative to arm BP	Aortic coarctation
Heart size, rate, rhythm, murmurs, respiratory difficulty, hepatomegaly	Murmur—coarctation; tachycardia and/or arrhythmia—pheochromocytoma; large heart or heart failure—prolonged or severe hypertension
Bruits over great vessels	Arteritis or arteriopathy

TABLE 10–10 *(Continued)*. **Value of History and Physical Examination in the Diagnosis of Hypertension in Children**

Physical Findings	Relevance
Abdomen	
Epigastric bruit	Renovascular diseases isolated or associated with Williams or von Recklinghausen syndromes, or arteritis
Unilateral or bilateral masses	Wilms tumor, neuroblastoma, pheochromocytoma, polycystic kidneys, other tumors
Neurologic	
Hypertensive funduscopic changes	Chronic hypertension
Bell's palsy	Chronic hypertension
Neurologic deficits (e.g., hemiparesis)	Chronic or severe acute hypertension with stroke

Source: Task Force on Blood Pressure Control in Children: Report of the Second Task Force on Blood Pressure Control in Children—1987. *Pediatrics* 79:1, 1987. Reproduced by permission of American Academy of Pediatrics, © 1987.

INITIAL, OR PHASE I, INVESTIGATIONS

HISTORY

A detailed history is an important first step in the investigation of a hypertensive child (Table 10–10). It is important to consider use of over-the-counter (OTC) medicines that can cause hypertension; these include decongestant nasal sprays or oral decongestants (sympathomimetics) for the common cold; prescribed medicines, such as theophylline preparations; oral contraceptive agents (in adolescent girls); and glucocorticoids or street drugs such as amphetamines and cocaine. A history of symptoms specific to various disorders of the kidney, endocrine system, and cardiovascular system should also be obtained and may lead to the detection of a possible etiology. Pheochromocytoma may be a silent disorder, but the symptom triad of headache, palpitation, and sweating should alert the physician to this diagnosis. Muscular weakness due to hypokalemia may be observed in the rare endocrine disorder of hyperaldosteronism. A family history of hypertension, cardiovascular disease, and stroke may be helpful in the diagnosis of essential hypertension in a child but cannot be overly relied upon.[16]

PHYSICAL EXAMINATION

The physical examination of any hypertensive should include confirmation of elevated BP by an appropriately sized BP cuff under resting conditions. The BP should be recorded in all four extremities. Coarctation of the aorta should be suspected if the BP is elevated in the upper extremities only, i.e., if a systolic BP differential between the upper and lower extremities exceeds 20 mmHg when the BP is recorded with the patient lying down. Other features associated with coarctation of the aorta include weak lower extremity pulses or evidence

TABLE 10–11. Keith-Wagener-Baker Classification of Hypertensive Retinopathy

Grade 1.	Mild narrowing of retinal arteries
Grade 2.	Generalized or localized narrowing of the retinal arteries, arteriovenous compression, and exaggeration of arterial reflex
Grade 3.	Retinal edema, cotton-wool exudates, hemorrhages, and other changes as seen in grade 2 retinopathy
Grade 4.	Diffuse retinal and optic disk edema, narrowing of the retinal arteries

of congestive heart failure in a neonate. The abdomen should be auscultated for bruits (epigastric region and flanks); if bruits are present, it may suggest the diagnosis of renal arterial stenosis. An abdominal mass may be suggestive of either an obstructed urinary tract (hydronephrosis), tumors (such as neuroblastoma or Wilms tumor), or polycystic kidneys. Pheochromocytomas are generally small in children and are not easily palpable. Facial nerve paralysis (Bell's palsy) or hemiplegia sometimes occurs as an isolated complication of severe hypertension in children.[14] Clinical evidence of left ventricular hypertrophy should be looked for. Funduscopic examination by a well-trained clinician or an ophthalmologist is necessary to evaluate the severity and the chronicity of hypertension (Table 10–11).

URINALYSIS

Urinalysis holds an important key to the direction in which further evaluation of children with hypertension must proceed. Detection of proteinuria and hematuria may suggest the diagnosis of glomerulonephritis; further laboratory tests to confirm such a diagnosis are then necessary. Mild to moderate proteinuria (200 mg to 300 mg/24 h) without hematuria may, however, occur as a consequence of hypertension, especially in patients with long-standing hypertension.[79] Low urinary specific gravity or osmolality may suggest renal dysplasia, renal cystic disease, chronic renal failure, or interstitial diseases such as chronic pyelonephritis and interstitial nephritis. A normal urinalysis makes renal disease a less likely etiology. Occasionally, patients with acute poststreptococcal glomerulonephritis may have a minimally abnormal or even normal urinalysis but develop severe elevation of BP. Apart from evidence of mild proteinuria, urinalysis is usually normal in renovascular hypertension.

ROUTINE SERUM CHEMISTRIES

Analysis of serum electrolytes, BUN, and serum creatinine is necessary to evaluate the extent of renal impairment in patients with suspected renal parenchymal disease. Low serum potassium concentration may point toward the diagnosis of hyperaldosteronism. Serum cholesterol and triglyceride concentration should be estimated in children with hypertension in order to define the cardiovascular risk factors. Elevated blood glucose concentration may be seen in pheochromocytoma.

COMPLETE BLOOD CELL COUNT

Complete blood cell count may reveal normocytic, normochromic anemia in patients with chronic renal failure; evidence of microangiopathy (burr cells, fragmented red cells, and teardrop cells) may be seen in patients in the acute phase of hemolytic-uremic syndrome.

CARDIOVASCULAR EVALUATION

In every patient with hypertension, the cardiovascular system should be evaluated either by an electrocardiogram or by echocardiography in order to gauge left ventricular hypertrophy. A chest radiograph is often less informative about cardiac hypertrophy than is echocardiography.[16] These tests are used to judge the severity and chronicity of hypertension, since long-standing hypertension is characterized by left ventricular hypertrophy and other features of cardiac dysfunction. Because cardiac hypertrophy in hypertension often reverses with successful therapy, these tests are also helpful in monitoring patients during follow-up.

RADIOLOGIC STUDIES OF THE KIDNEYS

Since renal parenchymal and renovascular disorders constitute a common etiology of hypertension in children, evaluation of renal anatomy and blood flow by simple radiologic techniques is recommended in patients in whom the etiology of hypertension is undetermined. The type of radiologic investigation that can be recommended for the investigation of hypertensive children is often dictated by the availability of the various diagnostic tests and experience with these tests at the institution. The radiologic studies helpful in the initial evaluation of hypertensive children are discussed below.

Hypertensive Intravenous Pyelogram (IVP). Hypertensive or rapid-sequence IVP has been regarded as the gold standard in the investigation of hypertensive children, largely because of its availability in most diagnostic centers. While a hypertensive IVP is being obtained, the radiocontrast is injected rapidly and radiographs of the kidneys are taken at 1, 2, 3, 4, and 8 min. In this manner, a nephrogram (vascular phase of IVP) is seen in the films obtained at 1 and 2 min, while the calyceal outlines may appear in films taken at 3 min.

The hypertensive IVP is helpful as a preliminary radiologic investigation in identifying patients with renal arterial stenosis. Renal anatomy and the collecting system can also be studied in the delayed radiologic films. Characteristically, the hypertensive IVP in patients with renal arterial stenosis shows a delay in the appearance of the nephrogram on the side that is affected by the arterial stenosis. Delayed excretion of the contrast and a discrepancy in renal size are also suggestive features of renal arterial stenosis. The kidney on the side of renal arterial stenosis is generally smaller in size. A discrepancy in the length of the two kidneys should be greater than 0.5 cm in order to be regarded as significant in children.[79] Abnormalities in the hypertensive IVP are detected in 50 to 60 percent of children with renal arterial stenosis.[80] Renal parenchymal scars in patients with chronic pyelonephritis may also be detected by this technique. A conventional IVP is of little diagnostic help in determining the etiology of hypertension and is not recommended as a routine test.

Radionuclide Renal Scan. Radionuclide renal scans have largely replaced the hypertensive IVP as the initial radiologic study of choice in hypertensive children. The advantages of radionuclide scans are that (1) the patient is exposed to a smaller dose of ionizing radiation; (2) information related to the renal blood flow as well as split renal functions can be obtained; (3) the scans can be performed in patients with compromised renal function; and (4) they are especially informative in neonates, in whom IVP images are generally of poor quality due to the neonate's inability to concentrate the radiocontrast adequately in the kidneys. On the other hand, urinary tract anatomy is not well characterized by radionuclide scans; an examination of the kidneys by ultrasound is recommended to obtain such information.

In patients with renovascular disease, the renal radionuclide (DTPA) scan shows a diminished renal blood flow as well as the glomerular filtration rate (GFR) on the affected side. Since angiotensin converting enzyme inhibitor (captopril) is known to reduce renal blood flow and GFR on the side of renal arterial stenosis (see Chap. 11 for details), this pharmacologic agent has recently been used in conjunction with the radionuclide renal scan to enhance the detection of functionally significant renal arterial stenosis.[81,82] Renal scans are obtained prior to and 1 h after a challenge dose of captopril; the images and the renogram following the captopril challenge show decreased blood flow and GFR on the side of the renal arterial stenosis. Bilateral renovascular disease is difficult to detect with the captopril-enhanced renal scan, since the blood flow is diminished symmetrically on the two sides following this pharmacologic maneuver. Experience of using captopril-enhanced renal scans in the evaluation of children with renovascular hypertension is, however, limited at this time.

Renal Ultrasound Examination. Since ionizing radiation is not involved in an ultrasound study, the latter has largely replaced the IVP for the evaluation of renal anatomy. However, a well-trained physician is needed to provide an adequate interpretation of the results in infants and children. A discrepancy in renal size and renal parenchymal scars should suggest a renal parenchymal or renovascular etiology of hypertension. Anatomic malformations such as renal dysplasia, cystic renal disease, and obstructive uropathy can also be diagnosed by renal ultrasound examination.

PERIPHERAL PLASMA RENIN ACTIVITY

While many investigators advocate the determination of plasma renin activity (PRA) in every hypertensive patient, others differ on its usefulness in view of the fact that several variables—including dietary intake of salt, posture, technique of blood collection and storage, and antihypertensive medications—exert a considerable influence on the PRA. Plasma renin activity is elevated in patients with (1) renovascular hypertension, (2) renal parenchymal diseases, and (3) some of those with essential hypertension. A very low (suppressed) PRA is observed in patients with hypertension caused by mineralocorticoid excess (primary hyperaldosteronism, congenital adrenal hyperplasia). It is useful to measure the PRA in children because of its value in predicting whether renovascular or renal parenchymal disease as an etiology of hypertension should be further investigated.

Plasma renin concentration is not measured directly by the available assay methods. Most available techniques estimate PRA indirectly as the rate of formation of angiotensin I from the renin substrate (angiotensinogen) by the renin present in the patient's plasma. The result of PRA testing is expressed as ng/mL/h of angiotensin I formed. Temperature, pH, and other modifications of the assay methods have a considerable influence on the results and are responsible for the variation in normal standards of PRA from one laboratory to another. In order to provide clinically useful data, PRA in the peripheral blood should be measured using a standardized method of timing, collection, and processing of the blood sample. The blood is collected in a test tube that has been precooled in ice and contains the anticoagulant sodium EDTA. Plasma is separated in a refrigerated centrifuge immediately in order to retard the conversion of renin substrate (angiotensinogen) to angiotensin I at room temperature. Plasma obtained and separated in this manner can be stored for several months at −20°C for assay at a later time. Since peripheral PRA is dependent on posture, being higher when upright posture is assumed, it is also necessary to maintain some uniformity in the patients' postural status. Generally, the supine PRA level is drawn early in the morning after an overnight rest, while 2 to 4 h of ambulation is usually required to obtain the ambulatory PRA. The ambulatory PRA is 1.5 to 2.0 times higher than the supine PRA.

Apart from posture and the techniques of blood collection and processing, other factors—including the child's age, sodium intake, hydration status, and intake of drugs—may also affect the PRA (see Table 10–12). At birth, the PRA is significantly high; it declines rapidly in the first 3 months of life and then gradually decreases during the remainder of childhood.[83,84] Yet throughout childhood, the PRA remains high by comparison with that of adults (Fig. 10–13). The reason for the relatively high PRA in children is not entirely clear. It is important to adhere to the policy of obtaining a PRA in every patient with hypertension before beginning any antihypertensive therapy, since almost all antihypertensive drugs alter PRA and render interpretation of the results difficult. Under most clinical circumstances, it is possible to maintain this policy. The exception would be the rare occurrence of life-threatening complications of hypertension, where urgent treatment is required.

PHASE II INVESTIGATIONS

The tests listed (see Table 10–9) under this subheading are done to confirm the diagnosis of the secondary etiology of hypertension. Accordingly, these tests are not conducted on every hypertensive child but are rather performed selectively, based on the suspected etiology.

TABLE 10–12. Drugs Affecting Plasma Renin Activity (PRA)[a]

Increase	Decrease
Diuretics	Beta blockers
Vasodilators	Alpha agonists
Hydralazine	Clonidine
Minoxidil	Reserpine
Diazoxide	Alpha methyldopa
Nitroprusside	Prazosin
Bupicomide	Labetalol
Beta agonists	Ganglion blockers
Theophylline	Prostaglandin inhibitors
Caffeine	Indomethacin
Alpha blockers	Ibuprofen
Chlorpromazine	Aspirin
Converting enzyme inhibitors	Carbenoxalone
Mineralocorticoid antagonists	Vasopressin
Glucagon	Somatostatin
Anesthetics	Saralasin[b]
Saralasin[b]	
Estrogen[c]	
Glucocorticoids[c]	

[a]These drugs must be discontinued prior to obtaining PRA in hypertensive children, otherwise interpretation of the test is rendered impossible.

[b]Effect depends on renin level and sodium status.

[c]Effect by increasing renin substrate.

Source: Reproduced by permission from Schambelon M, Stockist JR: Pathophysiology of the renin-angiotensin system, in Brenner BM, Stein JH (eds): *Hormonal Functions and the Kidney.* New York, Churchill Livingstone, 1979, pp 1–39.

TESTS FOR RENOVASCULAR DISEASES

RENAL VEIN RENIN ASSAY

The renal vein renin test is used as an adjunct in the diagnosis of renovascular or renal hypertension. The twin aims of this test are to localize the kidney that is responsible for hyperreninemia and to predict whether or not the hypertension is curable by surgery.

The renal vein renin assay is usually performed in conjunction with the renal angiography study (see "Selective Renal Angiography," below) and is done by cannulating the femoral veins under radiologic guidance and obtaining blood samples selectively from each renal vein and from the inferior vena cava, above and below the renal veins. Precautions similar to those mentioned earlier in collecting and storing blood for the measurement of peripheral PRA should be observed in this test also. Normally, renin output from each kidney is almost

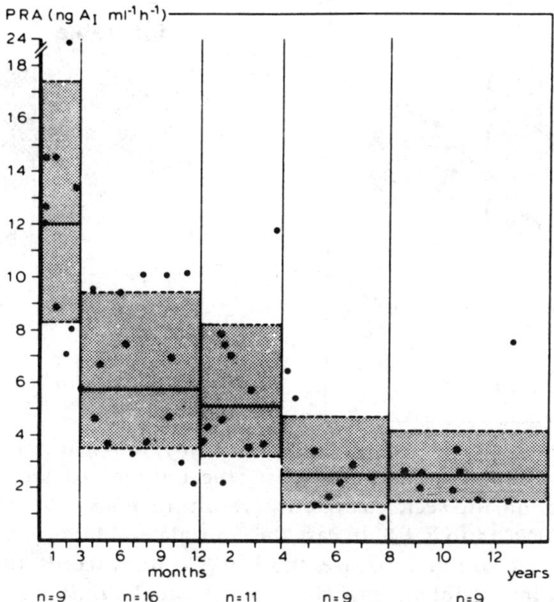

FIG. 10–13. **Plasma renin activity (ng/mL/h of A1 activity) in various pediatric age groups. Model median and one standard deviation range indicated. (Reproduced with permission from Fiselier TJW, Lijnen P, Monnens L, et al: Levels of renin, angiotension I and II, angiotension-converting enzyme and aldosterone in infancy and childhood. *Eur J Paediatr* 141:3, 1983.)**

the same (about 25 percent higher than the peripheral venous PRA). In patients with unilateral renal or renovascular disease, however, the PRA from the affected side is usually exceedingly high, while that from the contralateral (normal) side is suppressed (equal to the PRA in the inferior vena cava). In order to be diagnostic of unilateral renovascular hypertension or a unilateral renal disease, PRA from the diseased side (V_2) should be at least 50 percent higher than PRA in the inferior vena cava (IVC). That is, V_2/IVC renin $\geq$ 1.5 (Fig. 10–14). The renin ratio between the contralateral normal side (V_1) and the IVC is 1.0, since renin synthesis on that side is suppressed. On the other hand, if V_2/IVC is greater than 1.5 and V_1/IVC also exceeds 1.0, it may suggest bilateral renal or renovascular disease. Under these circumstances, a unilateral nephrectomy or correction of renal arterial stenosis by surgery or percutaneous angioplasty will be only partially beneficial in curing the hypertension.[85]

SELECTIVE RENAL ANGIOGRAPHY

Selective renal angiography is done in order to (1) localize the site of renovascular disease and (2) predict the type of disorder causing the renovascular hypertension.[79,80] Fibromuscular dysplasia is a common etiology of renovascular hypertension and is often characterized by stenotic lesions affecting the mid-

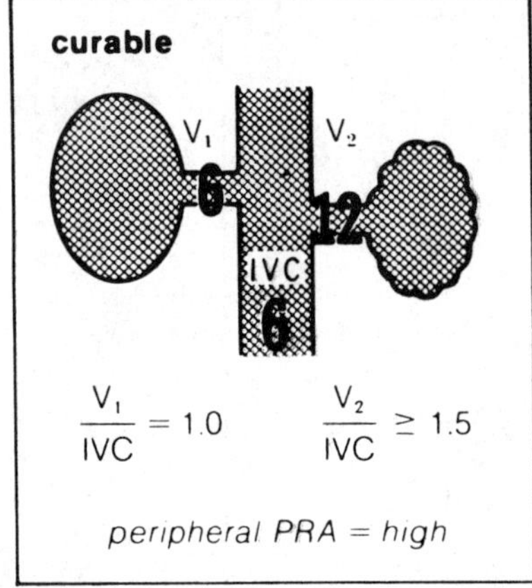

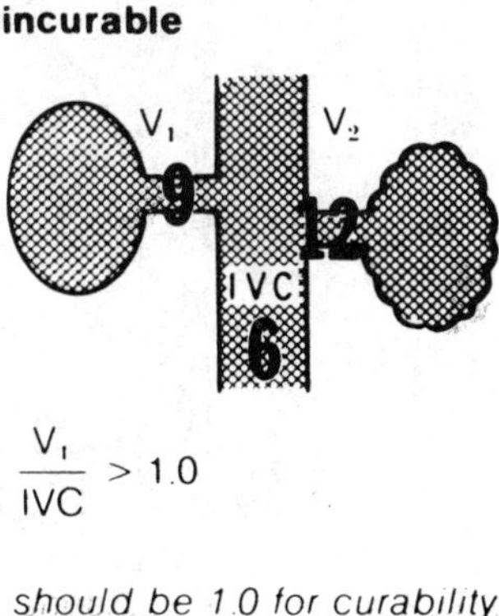

FIG. 10–14. Diagnostic patterns of selective renal-vein renin in patients with renovascular hypertension. In unilateral disease, the uninvolved kidney *(left)* is under endocrine suppression and secretes no renin, resulting in a V_1/IVC ratio of 1.0. On the other hand, the V_2/IVC ratio is 1.5. In case the contralateral kidney *(left)* is also affected by previously undetected renal disease, the V_1/IVC ratio exceeds 1.0. A surgical cure of hypertension is impossible in this situation. (From *J Cardiovasc Med* 2:1065, 1977. Reprinted by permission of Physicians World Communications Group.)

portion of the main renal artery and an aneurysmal poststenotic dilatation. If several segments of the renal artery are affected by fibromuscular dysplasia, this may produce a beaded appearance in the renal artery. Congenital renal arterial stenosis may affect any part of the main or segmental renal artery. Diseases like neurofibromatosis, coarctation of the aorta, and Takayasu's arteritis usually involve the renal arteries at their origin from aorta.

Digital subtraction angiography (DSI) is another alternative to selective angiography. In this test the radiocontrast material is injected intravenously in a large vein and definition of the arterial phase of the renal vasculature is obtained by digital subtraction methodology. However, DSI requires a good deal of cooperation from the patient and the administration of a larger volume of radiocontrast material. DSI is generally regarded as being less useful in demonstrating renal arterial lesions in children (as opposed to adults), probably because of their smaller-sized renal arterial tree.

CONVERTING ENZYME CHALLENGE TEST

Converting enzyme inhibitor (captopril) induces a fall of BP and a marked elevation of peripheral PRA in patients with renovascular hypertension and, to a lesser extent, patients with renal parenchymal diseases. Since it is not an invasive procedure, this therapeutic test is being used increasingly in adults to detect cases of functionally significant renal arterial stenosis. Its sensitivity and specificity in detecting renovascular hypertension in adults has been reported to be almost 95 percent.[86] Before the converting enzyme challenge test is performed, the patient's baseline BP readings are obtained for 2 h at intervals of 30 min.

TABLE 10–13. Sensitivity and Specificity of Common Tests Used in the Diagnosis of Renovascular Hypertension

Test	Sensitivity (%)	Specificity (%)	Comments
Intravenous pyelography	70–80	87–98	False negatives in patients with segmental or bilateral renal artery stenoses
Radioisotopic renography			
Conventional	70	75–80	Same as above
Captopril pretreatment	80	100	Studied in patients with unilateral stenosis; may be predictive of BP response to revascularization
Peripheral venous renin	55–60	65–70	Affected by salt intake, medications, positions, assay, specimen handling
Renal vein renins	63–75	60–100	Interpretation depends on type of ratio used (see text); usually applies only to unilateral stenosis

Source: Modified from Canzanello VJ, Madias NE: A practical approach to renovascular hypertension. *Res Staff Phys.* 53:23, 1989. Reprinted with permission from *Resident and Staff Physician.*

Then a single oral dose of captopril (0.5 to 1.0 mg/kg) is administered and BP is again monitored for 90 to 120 min. Blood samples for estimation of PRA are also obtained at 30-min intervals. For the test to be considered positive (and suggestive of renovascular hypertension), the mean systolic BP (obtained in the test period) should fall to at least 90 percent of the precaptopril mean. The postcaptopril PRA should rise by 150 percent or more, with an absolute rise of at least 10 ng/mL/h from the baseline value. Experience with the converting enzyme challenge test in identifying renovascular hypertension in children has been limited so far, but early studies are promising.[87] Ideally, the test should be performed in conjunction with radionuclide scans in order to enhance the predictability of renovascular disease by this noninvasive test.

The value of various diagnostic tests in the evaluation of patients with renovascular hypertension is given in Table 10–13.

TESTS FOR CATECHOLAMINE-SECRETING TUMORS

URINARY CATECHOLAMINES AND METABOLITES

Urinary excretion of catecholamines (norepinephrine and epinephrine) and products of catecholamine metabolism (vanillylmandelic acid, or VMA, and metanephrines) is elevated in catecholamine-secreting tumors arising from the sympathetic nervous system; these include pheochromocytoma, neuroblastoma, and ganglioneuromas. Tests for measuring VMA in an untimed collection

TABLE 10–14. Drugs Affecting the Urinary Estimation of VMA

Increased Excretion	Decreased Excretion
Epinephrine	Phenobarbital sodium
Norepinephrine	Morphine
Insulin	*p*-hydroxyamphetamine
Histamine	Iproniazid phosphate
Reserpine (initial administration)	Phenelzine sulfate
	Reserpine (long-term administration)
	Chlorpromazine
	Imipramine hydrochloride
	Prenylamine
	Methyldopa

Source: Reprinted by permission from Stewart TC, Freeman JA: Vanillylmandelic acid and catecholamine determination. ©1976 by the American Society of Clinical Pathologists, Chicago.

of urine are available in most clinical laboratories, but a high incidence of false-positives mandates confirmation of the excretion of VMA in a timed urine collection. Ingestion of vanilla, coffee, or tea may cause increased excretion of urinary VMA if calorimetric methods of assay are used, but assays using spectrophotometric methods are not affected by the ingestion of these substances.

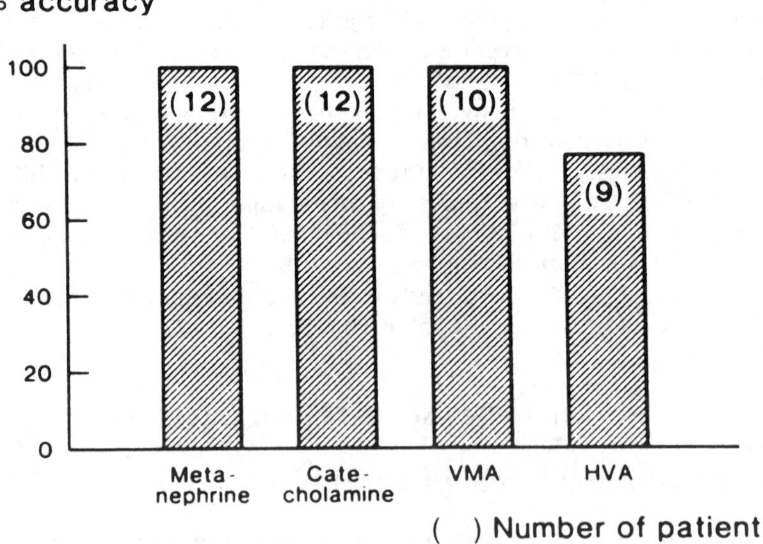

FIG. 10–15. Diagnostic accuracy of estimation of various products of catecholamine metabolism in a timed urinary collection in patients with pheochromocytoma. (Reproduced with permission from Kaufman BH, Telander RL, VanHeerden, et al: Pheochromocytoma in the pediatric age group: Current status. *J Pediatr Surg* 18:879, 1983.)

TABLE 10–15. Normal Values of VMA and Catecholamines (Norepinephrine and Epinephrine) in Children

Age	VMA[a]	Catecholamines (Norepinephrine + Epinephrine[a])
0–12 months	15.0 ±9.9	1.64 ±1.32
1–2 years	13.6 ±8.3	1.68 ±1.13
2–5 years	7.1 ±4.2	1.25 ±0.77
5–10 years	6.7 ±3.36	1.13 ±0.78
10–15 years	4.8 ±2.8	0.60 ±0.48

[a]Values represented as μg/mg creatinine.

Sources: Reprinted by permission from Gitlow SE, Mendlowitz M, Wilk EK, et al: Excretion of catecholamine catabolites by normal children. *J Lab Clin Med* 72:612, 1968. Haymond RE, Knight JA, Bills AC: Normal values of urinary 3-methoxy-4 hydroxymandelic acid (VMA) in children. *Clin Chem.* 24:1853, 1978.

If necessary, they should be excluded from the patient's diet 72 h before urine is collected for this test. Assay of urinary metanephrines is less compromised by the intake of various foods or drugs (Table 10–14), and is also technically easier to perform than the VMA assay. The diagnostic accuracy of tests for urinary catecholamines in patients with pheochromocytoma has been reported to be over 95 percent (Fig. 10–15).[87] Normal values of 24-h urinary excretion of catecholamines and VMA are given in Table 10–15.

PLASMA CATECHOLAMINES

The determination of plasma catecholamines can be a useful adjunct in the diagnosis of pheochromocytoma. Deal et al.[51] reported that plasma catecholamines were diagnostically elevated in 100 percent of patients when this test was employed. Interpretation of plasma catecholamine levels may be difficult if samples are drawn while the child is agitated or crying or other circumstances which will normally increase plasma catecholamine concentrations exist.

COMPUTED TOMOGRAPHY (CT) SCAN

If elevated urinary catecholamine excretion is documented in a hypertensive child, the diagnosis of pheochromocytoma or other catecholamine-secreting tumors as a possible cause of hypertension should be considered. Localization of the tumor site can then be attempted by CT scan or by magnetic resonance imaging (MRI). Since most pheochromocytomas arise from the adrenal glands, these endocrine organs require a close attention in evaluations by CT scan and MRI. Evaluation of the chest and pelvis may also be required in order to rule out an extraadrenal or multifocal origin of pheochromocytoma. Being noninvasive, the CT scan and MRI have become the investigational tests of choice in children suspected of having pheochromocytoma. The diagnostic accuracy of CT scan in children with pheochromocytoma has been reported to be over 80 percent.[50] However, in a recent review[51] of various diagnostic tests for pheochromocytoma in children, the CT scan was unable to localize tumors in 3 of the 5 patients. The authors of this study concluded that the CT scan could localize only the larger tumors.

MIGB SCAN

The agent used for this scan—^{133}I metaiodobenzylguanidine—is a guanethidine analogue of norepinephrine that localizes to the sites of pheochromocytoma when administered to the patients with these tumors. An added advantage of this test is that pheochromocytoma arising from multiple sites and metastatic lesions in malignant pheochromocytoma can also be visualized. The MIGB scan has been reported to be diagnostic in 90 percent of patients with pheochromocytoma.[89] Most false-negatives occur when the tumor is intraadrenal. It has been suggested that the MIGB scan be used as a screening test for pheochromocytoma and that the site of origin can then be confirmed with a CT scan.[90]

ANGIOGRAPHY AND SELECTIVE VENOUS SAMPLING

Because of its invasive nature, angiographic localization of pheochromocytoma is becoming less necessary in centers where CT and other noninvasive investigations are available. The diagnostic accuracy of angiography in localizing the site of origin of pheochromocytoma has been reported to be almost 100 percent (Fig. 10–16).[50] Selective venous sampling of blood along the inferior vena cava and adrenal veins for catecholamine concentration has also been used by some authors to provide information about the site of origin of pheochromocytoma.[51] Although cumbersome, this diagnostic modality may provide valuable information in patients with tumors that are very small or difficult to localize. Selective venous sampling can be performed at the same time as selective angiography.

TESTS FOR RENAL PARENCHYMAL DISEASES

If congenital renal lesions (e.g., cystic diseases or renal dysplasia) are the underlying cause of hypertension, the radiologic investigations (IVP, renal ultrasound) discussed under stage I are likely to indicate the existence of such a pathology. Further diagnostic tests such as renal biopsy are generally not necessary in these cases. On the other hand, if chronic pyelonephritis or glomerulonephritis is considered to be the etiology of hypertension, a detailed workup is required to confirm the diagnosis.

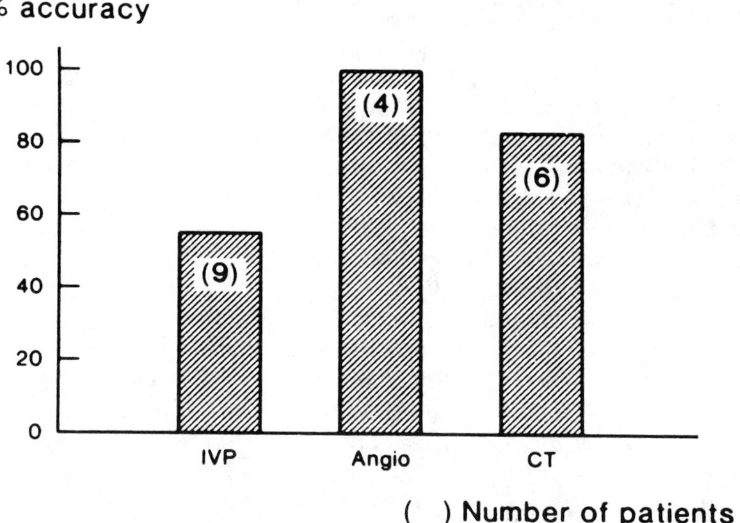

FIG. 10–16. Diagnostic value of various radiologic imaging tests in localizing the site of origin of pheochromocytoma in children. The intravenous pyelogram (IVP) is the least accurate test, while angiography (Angio) and computed tomography (CT) are the most helpful diagnostic aids. The last of these has become the test of choice in localizing pheochromocytoma in children. (Reproduced with permission from Kaufman BH, Telander RL, vanHeerden, et al: Pheochromocytoma in the pediatric age group: Current status. *J Pediatr Surg* 18:879, 1983.)

Tests for renal function and a renal biopsy are necessary in patients suspected of having chronic glomerulonephritis. Patients suspected of having chronic pyelonephritis must undergo evaluation by voiding cystourethrogram (VCUG) to obtain information related to vesicoureteral reflux. If chronic pyelonephritis or reflux nephropathy is suspected to be unilateral, a split renal vein renin assay may be helpful in determining the curability of hypertension by a unilateral nephrectomy.

TEST FOR DEFECTS IN ADRENAL STEROID BIOSYNTHESIS

Diagnostic evaluation of patients suspected of having hypertension due to defects in adrenal steroid biosynthesis is best left to a pediatric endocrinologist. Virilization and accelerated growth are often features of 11-hydroxylase defect, while patients with 17-hydroxylase defect show poor development of secondary sex characteristics. One often encounters amenorrhea (in girls) and evidence of pseudohermaphroditism. Plasma renin activity and urinary aldosterone levels are low in both cases. Further differentiation of the enzymatic defects involves determination of plasma cortisol, deoxycorticosterone (DOC), androgen, and estimation of urinary 17-hydroxysteroids and 17-ketosteroids in a 24-h urinary collection (Table 10–9).

HYPERTENSIVE ENCEPHALOPATHY

Hypertensive encephalopathy is an uncommon but a dramatic complication of uncontrolled hypertension and usually follows severe and sudden elevation of BP. The manifestations of hypertensive encephalopathy include severe headache, visual disturbances, alteration of sensorium, and seizure activity. Seizures may be focal or generalized in nature. Transient neurologic deficits such as aphasia and various cranial nerve deficits may also be seen.[91] Facial nerve paralysis has been reported as a frequent finding in children with hypertensive encephalopathy.[14] Severe hypertensive encephalopathy may result in coma, intracranial bleeding, and lasting neurologic damage.

The pathogenesis of hypertensive encephalopathy is unsettled. Cerebral edema and acute fibrinoid necrosis with perivascular exudates and petechial hemorrhages are the predominant pathologic findings in these patients. Based on these pathologic findings, some have suggested that cerebral vasoconstriction is the primary defect which leads to cerebral ischemia and edema in hypertensive encephalopathy.[92,93] The currently held view, however, is that hypertensive encephalopathy results from a failure of autoregulation of the cerebral blood flow and damage to the blood-brain barrier.[94–96] In normal individuals, cerebral arterioles constrict and dilate with the increase and a decrease of systemic BP; this autoregulatory mechanism ensures an adequate and normal cerebral blood flow during variations of BP (Fig. 10–17). It has been suggested that the acute elevation of BP in patients who develop hypertensive encephalopathy causes a breakdown of this autoregulatory mechanism wherein, instead of constricting, the cerebral blood vessels dilate, causing the cerebral blood flow to increase (Fig. 10–18)[94,95] An additional factor believed to be important in the pathogenesis of hypertensive encephalopathy is an enhanced permeability of

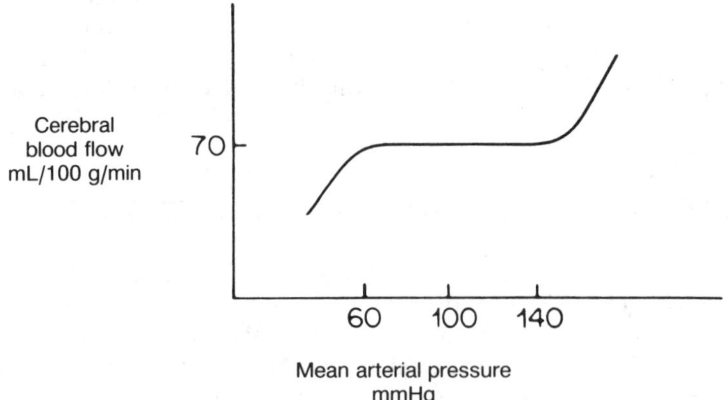

FIG. 10–17. Autoregulation of cerebral blood flow—effect of changes in mean arterial blood pressure on cerebral blood flow in normal persons. Cerebral blood flow is maintained effectively over a wide range of fluctuations of BP. (Reproduced with permission from Reed G, Devous M: Cerebral blood flow autoregulation and hypertension. *Am J Med Sci* 289:37, 1985.)

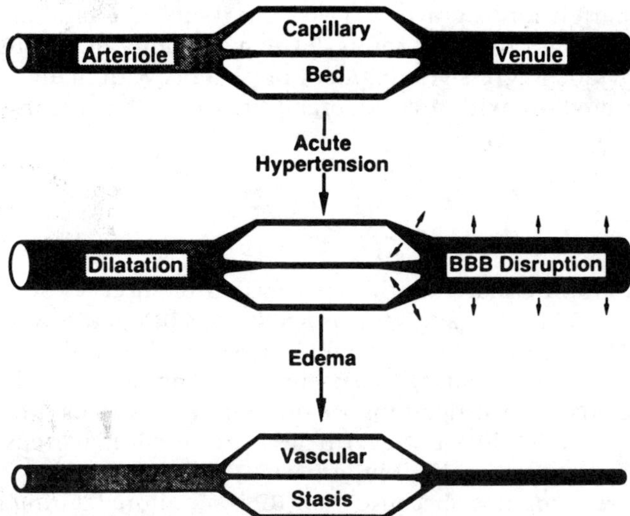

FIG. 10–18. Proposed role of passive dilatation and disruption of the blood-brain barrier in the pathogenesis of hypertensive encephalopathy. Severe hypertension exceeds the body's autoregulatory capacity and produces passive dilatation rather than vasospasm of the cerebral blood vessels. Passive dilatation leads to disruption of the blood-brain barrier (BBB), cerebral edema, and vascular stasis. (From Baumbach GL, Heistadd D: Cerebral circulation in chronic arterial hypertension. *Hypertension.* 12:89, 1988. Reproduced by permission of the American Heart Association, Inc.)

cerebral blood vessels resulting from changes in the blood-brain barrier. The overall effect of these alterations is the development of cerebral edema.[96]

Hypertensive encephalopathy is a potentially life-threatening complication of hypertension, necessitating the aggressive control of BP. Reversal of the clinical symptomatology is generally possible with rapid and appropriate antihypertensive therapy. However, persistent, severe elevation of the BP may lead to intracranial bleeding and irreversible neurologic sequelae.[97]

ACCELERATED AND MALIGNANT HYPERTENSION

Malignant hypertension is a syndrome encountered in patients with severe hypertension and is pathologically characterized by severe fibrinoid necrosis of the arterioles in several organ systems. The clinical hallmark of malignant hypertension is exudative hemorrhages and papilledema on fundoscopic examination (grade IV changes of the Keith-Wagener-Baker classification of hypertensive retinopathy). In addition, multiple organ dysfunctions such as encephalopathy, acute renal failure, cardiac failure and disseminated intravascular coagulopathy are encountered. Accelerated hypertension, on the other hand, is considered to be a premalignant phase of hypertension in which only grade III retinal changes are observed and the clinical symptoms may be somewhat less severe than those seen in malignant hypertension. The prognosis of untreated malignant hypertension is grave. A 1-year mortality rate of almost 90 percent has been recorded in untreated adults.[98] The availability of effective antihypertensive therapy and aggressive treatment of patients with malignant hypertension has been credited with a considerably improved 5-year survival (over 70 percent) in these patients.[99]

SUMMARY

The identification of children with hypertension requires a knowledge of normal standards of BP for sex and various age groups. Proper technique and environment are also essential for obtaining reliable and reproducible readings of BP in children. Since secondary hypertension is commoner in children than it is in adults, extensive investigations are often necessary to identify the etiology of hypertension in children. Nevertheless, essential hypertension is being increasingly recognized in children, especially in adolescents. Most hypertensive children are recognized because their BP is monitored during their workup for various disorders that are usually associated with hypertension; the identification of asymptomatic children during routine examinations, however, is not uncommon. The inclusion of BP measurement as a part of yearly physical examinations of children is highly recommended.

Case History: An Asymptomatic Child With Severe Hypertension. J.A., a 2-year, 10-month-old boy, was seen in the emergency room because he had had fever up to 102°F and emesis for 1 day. The child had no other complaints. He was born at term, and the birthweight was 9.4 lb. His immunizations were up to date. Physical examination in the emergency room revealed an alert child, and vital signs were as follows: temperature, 97.7°F; respiratory rate, 22/min, BP, 204/149 mmHg. His weight was 14.0 kg (50th percentile) and height 104 cm (95th percentile). Except for a mildly injected pharynx, his physical examination was noted to be normal. Because of severely elevated blood pressure, the patient was admitted to the hospital. Further questioning revealed no history of ingestion of any prescribed or over-the-counter drugs. He denied history of headache or nosebleeds, blood in the urine, swelling of the legs, or puffiness of the eyelids. The mother reported that J.A. was usually a happy child who "never stopped running around."

Detailed physical examination showed that the patient was alert and responded to the questions appropriately. The blood pressure remained in the range of 200 mmHg systolic and 100 to 110 mmHg diastolic during the first 24 h of hospitalization. Femoral pulses were normal in amplitude, without any delay from the brachial pulse. The BP in the lower extremities (taken with the patient prone) was similar to that obtained in the upper extremities. No bruits were heard in the abdomen. Funduscopic examination was normal, and the cardiovascular examination revealed clinically detectable left ventricular hypertrophy without evidence of congestive cardiac failure or pulmonary edema. The remainder of the physical examination was unremarkable.

The following laboratory data were obtained on admission. Normal CBC; peripheral smear was also normal. U/A: Specific gravity, 1.009; pH, 7.5; protein, 1+; blood, 3+ (patient was catheterized). Microscopic examination revealed no casts but "too numerous to count" red blood cells. RBCs appeared to be noncrenated. Serum chemistries: sodium, 135 meq/L; potassium, 3.7 meq/L; chloride, 93 meq/L; CO_2, 25 meq/L; BUN, 11 mg/dL; creatinine, 0.3 mg/dL; calcium, 10.4 mg/dL; phosphorous, 3.8 mg/dL; total protein, 7.3 g/dL; and albumin, 4.3 g/dL.

Comment. The history and physical examination of this child with hypertension rule out the possibility of drug-induced hypertension and coarctaton of aorta. The patient exhibits clinical evidence of left ventricular hypertrophy, suggesting that he may have had hypertension for a significant duration of time. The results of the urinalysis raise the suspicion of an acute or chronic glomerulonephritis. However, normal BUN and creatinine make a chronic renal disease such as chronic glomerulonephritis less likely. Mild proteinuria may be due to renal parenchymal disease or result from prolonged hypertension itself. The urinalysis must be repeated to evaluate whether catheterization could account for this laboratory finding. Ask-Upmark kidney or renal scarring resulting from an episode of past unrecognized acute or chronic pyelonephritis may also present with severe hypertension without any significant alteration of renal function. Hypertension due to an acute renal disease, such as acute poststreptococcal glomerulonephritis, cannot be completely ruled out at this point. Normal serum potassium concentration suggests that the diagnosis of primary hyperaldosteronism (wherein hypokalemia should be seen) is unlikely. Further laboratory evaluation of the patient would be necessary in order to identify the etiology of hypertension.

Repeat urinalysis was normal except for 2+ proteinuria. A timed urinary excretion of protein was 377 mg/day. The ASO titer was 222 Todd units (normal), and serum complement C3 was 89 mg/dL (normal). Renal ultrasound examination showed no abnormality of renal anatomy; specifically, renal size was normal on both sides and no renal scars were identified. Radionuclide (DTPA) renal scan showed normal renal perfusion and excretion; DMSA scan also showed normal renal outline bilaterally without any evidence of renal scars. An electrocardiogram showed evidence of left ventricular hypertrophy. The chest radiograph was normal.

Comment. Normal BUN, creatinine, serum complement, and ASO titer as well as resolution of hematuria make acute poststreptococcal glomerulonephritis an unlikely possibility. Left ventricular hypertrophy seen in the ECG further supports the hypothesis that hypertension is not of acute onset but has been present for at least several months. Hematuria was probably the result of urethral catheterization. Mild proteinuria may be due to a secondary effect of hypertension on the kidneys, rather than being due to renal parenchymal disorder, since urinary sediment was otherwise normal. Normal

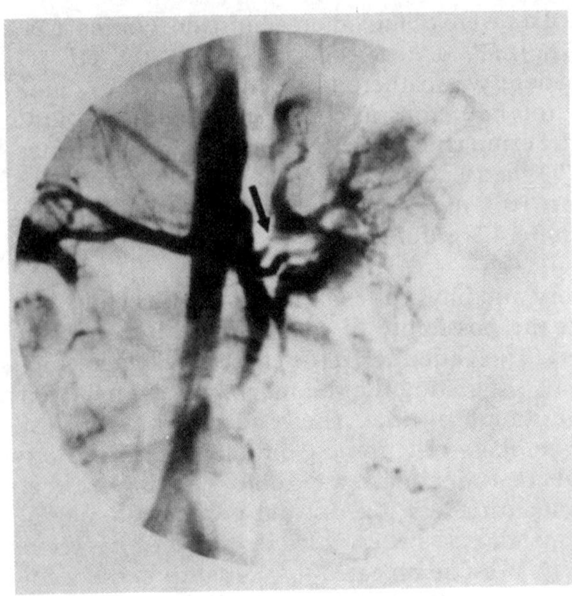

FIG. 10–19. Renal angiogram of patient JA showing stenosis of the left renal arterial branch *(arrow)* and poststenotic dilatation.

radionuclide studies and renal ultrasound examination do not favor the diagnosis of a significant main renal artery stenosis or renal scarring as the etiologies of hypertension. In order to further pursue the evaluation of renovascular hypertension, captopril renal scan may be helpful, but selective renal angiography would be the definitive test. At this point, consideration may also be given to pheochromocytoma as an etiology of sustained hypertension.

Following laboratory tests were then obtained for further evaluation. Peripheral plasma renin activity: 65.5 ng/mL/h (normal mean for age—3.95 ng/mL/h). Urinary catecholamine and VMA: normal for age.

Selective renal angiography revealed a branch stenosis in the upper polar artery of the left kidney (Fig. 10–19). Renal vein renin levels were obtained; the results of these tests were as follows:

$$\begin{aligned}
\text{Right renal vein renin } (V_1) &= 92.8 \text{ ng/mL/h} \\
\text{Left renal vein renin } (V_2) &= 143.6 \text{ ng/mL/h} \\
\text{Inferior vena cava renin} &= 91.6 \text{ ng/mL/h} \\
V_1/\text{IVC} &= 1.013 \\
V_2/\text{IVC} &= 1.5 \\
V_2/V_1 &= 1.5
\end{aligned}$$

Comment. The first clue to renovascular disease as the possible etiology of hypertension in this patient was provided by the elevated PRA while the patient was on a normal diet. A captopril renal scan and captopril challenge test may have been noninvasive tests of choice to perform at this stage, but they were not done. However, it is unlikely that the captopril renal scan would have been able to detect the branch renal arterial stenosis that was diagnosed by selective renal angiography in this patient. The fact that the PRA was suppressed in the right kidney (i.e., PRA was similar to what was observed in the inferior vena cava) and the ratio of PRA on the left side and the right side was 1.5 suggests that the (renovascular) disease was unilateral and was possibly correctable by surgery.

Clinical Course. The patient underwent balloon angioplasty of the stenotic renal branch artery. His BP returned to normal within 12 h, but after 72 h it started to increase once again. He had to be treated with captopril and propranolol. Over the next 8 months, both these antihypertensive drugs were withdrawn slowly, and the patient's BP at the end of 1 year after angioplasty was 100/50 mmHg (normal for age and sex).

Hypertension in Children—View from a Hypertension Clinic: A Commentary

Julie R. Ingelfinger

Even when seeing referred patients in a setting devoted to the evaluation and management of blood pressure elevation in children, one finds that the vast majority of youngsters with documented blood pressure elevation have primary (essential) hypertension. Severe blood pressure elevation in a child or adolescent has a high likelihood of being due to some other cause. Full evaluation of such youngsters is absolutely necessary and is likely to produce a definitive diagnosis. However—and luckily—most blood pressure elevation is either mild in degree or transitory. This has led me to become a staunch advocate of the 95 percent diagnosis—rule out the obvious and then follow the young hypertensive patient, treating as necessary either with nonpharmacologic or pharmacologic intervention. Further diagnostic evaluation may be accomplished later if blood pressure fails to normalize or if new findings develop. This approach is not meant to be cavalier but rather, when approaching any child or adolescent with hypertension, to underscore the real need to consider an individualized approach to an expensive (and sometimes painful) evaluation process and to answer some straightforward questions which then focus the degree and direction of diagnostic evaluation. Some important questions are as follows:

- Is the blood pressure actually elevated for age, body configuration, time of day, situation, and activity? (A substantial number of hypertensive patients will turn out to have had spurious measurements or to have a particular situation, such as physical or mental stress that is being overlooked.)

- Is the blood pressure so high as to constitute a hypertensive emergency or "urgency"? (If so, a diagnostic and therapeutic approach aimed at finding a cause is important.)
- Is there an obvious cause of hypertension (e.g., factitious or iatrogenic hypertension; hypertension related to a renovascular injury, etc.)? If so, attending to the obvious cause and treating it is of utmost importance.
- Is the family or personal history going to be revealing? (One never knows, and it is well worthwhile to ask historical questions more than once.)
- Is there an obvious clue to the cause of hypertension on the physical exam? (It is, for instance, surprising how frequently leg blood pressures are omitted prior to the referral of a hypertensive patient.)

Since the causes of and associated findings in hypertension are protean, a thoughtful approach should be the cornerstone in evaluation of blood pressure elevation. The younger the child and the more severe the hypertension, the more complete the evaluation should be. As time goes by, uncontrolled hypertension of elusive cause demands further investigation. One must also keep in mind that primary or essential hypertension is really a syndrome rather than a single disease entity. In future years it may be possible to distinguish more clearly various forms of primary hypertension in children and adolescents with blood pressure elevation.

REFERENCES

1. Stokes J III, Kannel WB, Wolf PA, et al: Blood pressure as a risk factor for cardiovascular disease: The Framingham Study—30 years of Follow-up. *Hypertension* 13(Suppl I):13, 1989.
2. Kannel WB, Wolf PA, McGee DL, et al: Systolic blood pressure, arterial rigidity and risk of stroke. The Framingham Study. *JAMA.* 245:1225, 1981.
3. Task Force on Blood Pressure Control in Children: Report of the Second Task Force on Blood Pressure Control in Children—1987. *Pediatrics.* 79:1, 1987.
4. Rames LK, Clarke WR, Connor WE, et al: Normal blood pressures and evaluation of sustained blood pressure elevation in childhood: The Muscatine Study. *Pediatrics.* 61:245, 1978.
5. Fixler DE, Laird WP, Fitzgerald V, et al: Hypertension screening in schools: Results of the Dallas Study. *Pediatrics.* 63:32, 1979.
6. Brogan DR, Lakatos E: Hypertension detection, treatment, and control in the United States: Not as bad as it seems. *Am J Epidemiol.* 124:738, 1986.
7. Tan KL: BLood pressure in full-term healthy neonates. *Clin Pediatr.* 26:21, 1987.
8. Earley A, Fayers P, Ng S, et al: Blood pressure in the first 6 weeks of life. *Arch Dis Child.* 55:755, 1980.
9. Egger M, Bianchetti MG, Gnadinger M, et al: Twenty four hour intermittent, ambulatory blood pressure monitoring. *Arch Dis Child.* 62:1130, 1987.
10. Loirat C, Pillion G, Blum C: Hypertension in children: Present data and problems. *Adv Nephrol.* 11:65, 1982.

11. Gill DG, Mendes da Costa B, Cameron JS, et al: Analysis of 100 children with severe and persistent hypertension. *Arch Dis Child.* 51:951, 1976.
12. Uhari M, Koskimies O: A survey of 164 Finnish children and adolescents with hypertension. *Acta Paediatr Scand.* 68:193, 1979.
13. Leumann EP. Blood pressure and hypertension in childhood and adolescence. *Ergeb Inn Med Kinderheilk.* 43:109, 1979.
14. Lloyd AVC, Jewitt DE, Lloyd Still JD: Facial paralysis in children with hypertension. *Arch Dis Child.* 41:291, 1966.
15. Londe S, Bourgoignie JJ, Robson AM, et al: Hypertension in apparently normal children. *J Pediatr.* 78:569, 1971.
16. Ogborn MR, Crocker JFS: Investigation of pediatric hypertension: Use of a tailored protocol. *Am J Dis Child.* 141:1205, 1987.
17. Daniels SR, Loggie JMH, McEnery PT, et al: Clinical spectrum of intrinsic renovascular hypertension in children. *Pediatrics.* 80:698, 1987.
18. Stanely JC, Fry WJ: Pediatric renal artery occlusive disease and renovascular hypertension. *Arch Surg.* 116:669, 1981.
19. Makker SP, Moorthy B: Fibromuscular dysplasia of renal arteries: An important cause of renovascular hypertension in children. *J Pediatr.* 95:940, 1979.
20. Liard JF, Cowley AW Jr, McCaa RE, et al: Renin, aldosterone, body fluid volumes and baroreceptor reflex in the development and reversal of Goldblatt hypertension in conscious dogs. *Circ Res.* 34:549, 1974.
21. Gutmann FD, Tagawa H, Habet E, et al: Renal arterial pressure, renin secretion and blood pressure control in trained dogs. *Am J Physiol.* 24:66, 1973.
22. Miksche LW, Ulrike M, Gross F: Effect of sodium restriction on renal hypertension and renin activity in the rat. *Circ Res.* 27:973, 1970.
23. Garvas H, Brunner HR, Vaughn ED Jr, et al: Angiotension-sodium interaction in blood pressure maintenance of renal hypertensive and normotensive rats. *Science.* 180:1369, 1973.
24. Garvas H, Brunner HR, Thurston H, et al: Reciprocation of renin dependency with sodium volume dependency in renal hypertension. *Science.* 188:1316, 1978.
25. Swales JD, Thurston H, Queiroz FP, et al: Dual mechanism for experimental hypertension. *Lancet.* 2:1181, 1971.
26. Vensel LA, Bevereux RB, Pickering TG, et al: Cardiac structure and function in renovascular hypertension produced by unilateral and bilateral renal artery stenosis. *Am J Cardiol.* 58:575, 1986.
27. Sutters M, Al Kutoubi MA, Mathias CJ, et al: Diuresis and syncope after angioplasty in a patient with one functioning kidney. *Br Med J.* 295:527, 1987.
28. Robertson JIS. Role of renin-angiotension system in hypertension. *Semin Nephrol.* 8:120, 1988.
29. Arant BS Jr, Sotelo-Avila C, Bernstein J: Segmental "hypoplasia" of kidney (Ask-Upmark). *J Pediatr.* 95:931, 1979.
30. Weidmann P, Beretta-Piccoli C, Hirsch D, et al: Curable hypertension in unilateral hydronephrosis: Studies on the role of circulating renin. *Ann Intern Med.* 87:937, 1977.
31. Corvol P, Pinet F, Galen FX, et al: Seven lessons from seven renin secreting tumors. *Kidney Int.* 34(suppl25):38, 1988.
32. Ganguly A, Gribble J, Tune B, et al: Renin-secreting Wilms tumour with severe hypertension: Report of a case and brief review of renin secreting tumors. *Ann Intern Med.* 79:735, 1973.
33. de Jong M, Monnens L: Hemolytic-uremic syndrome: A 10-year follow-up study of 73 patients. *Nephrol Dial Transplant.* 3:379, 1988.

34. Blythe WB: Natural history of hypertension in renal parenchymal disease. *Am J Kid Dis.* 5:A50, 1985.
35. Jacobson SH, Kjellstrand, Lins L-E: Role of hypervolemia and renin in the blood pressure control of patients with pyelonephritic renal scarring. *Acta Med Scand.* 224:224, 1988.
36. Godard C, Valloton MB, Broyer MB: Plasma renin activity in segmental hypoplasia of the kidneys with hypertension. *Nephron.* 11:308, 1973.
37. Tarazi RC, Dustan HP, Frohlich ED, et al: Plasma volume and chronic hypertension: Relationship to arterial blood pressure levels in different hypertensive diseases. *Arch Intern Med.* 125:835, 1970.
38. Brod J: Hypertension and renal parenchymal disease: mechanisms and management. *Cardiovasc Clin.* 9:137, 1978.
39. Mitas JA, Levy SB, Holle R, et al: Urinary kallikrein activity in hypertension of renal parenchymal disease. *N Engl J Med.* 299:162, 1978.
40. Ruilope L, Robles RG, Bernis C, et al: Role of renal prostaglandin E_2 in chronic renal disease hypertension. *Nephron.* 32:202, 1982.
41. Powell HR, Rotenberg E, Williams AL, et al: Plasma renin activity in acute post streptococcal glomerulonephritis and hemolytic-uremic syndrome. *Arch Dis Child.* 49:802, 1974.
42. Perloff MD: Coarctation of aorta, in *The Clinical Recognition of Congenital Heart Diseases.* Philadelphia, Saunders, 1987, p 28.
43. Thoele DG, Muster AJ, Paul MH: Recognition of coarctation of the aorta: A continuing challenge for the primary care physician. *Am J Dis Child.* 141:1201, 1987.
44. Alpert BS, Bain HH, Balfe JW, et al: Role of renin-angiotension-aldosterone system in hypertensive children with coarctation of the aorta. *Am J Cardiol.* 43:828, 1979.
45. Fallo F, Armanini D, Margano I, et al: Plasma renin activity in coarctation of aorta before and after surgical correction. *Br Heart J.* 40:1415, 1978.
46. Ribeiro AB, Krakoff LR: Angiotensin blockade in coarctation of aorta. *N Eng J Med.* 295:148, 1976.
47. Declusin RJ, Boerboom LE, Olinger GN, et al: Hemodynamic and hormonal abnormalities in canine aortic coarctation at rest and during exercise. *J Am Coll Cardiol.* 9:903, 1987.
48. Gupta TC, Wiggers CJ: Basic hemodynamic changes produced by aortic coarctation of different degrees. *Circulation.* 3:17, 1951.
49. Stackpole RH, Melicow MM, Uson AC: Pheochromocytoma in children: Report of 9 cases and review of first 100 published cases with follow up studies. *J Pediatr.* 63:315, 1963.
50. Kaufmann BH, Telander RL, van Heerden JA, et al: Pheochromocytoma in the pediatric age group: Current status. *J Pediatr Surg.* 18:879, 1983.
51. Deal JE, Sever PS, Barrat TM, et al: Pheochromocytoma—investigations and management of 10 cases. *Arch Dis Child.* 65:269, 1990.
52. Manger WM, Giffer RW Jr: Pheochromocytoma, in Laragh JH, Brenner BM (eds): *Hypertension: Pathophysiology, Diagnosis and Managment.* New York, Raven Press, 1990, p 1639.
53. Beglieri EG, Irony I, Kater CE: Adrenocortical forms of human hypertension, in: Laragh JH, Brenner BM (eds), *Hypertension: Pathophysiology, Diagnosis and Management.* New York, Raven Press, 1990, p 1609.
54. Treadwell BLJ, Sever ED, Savage O, et al: Side effects of long-term treatment with corticosteroids and corticotrophin. *Lancet.* 1:1121, 1964.
55. Whitworth JA: Mechanisms of glucocorticoid-induced hypertension. *Kidney Int.* 31:1213, 1987.

56. Rosler A, Leiberman E: Enzymatic defects of steroidogenesis: 11 B-Hydroxylase deficiency congenital adrenal hyperplasia. *Pediatr Adolesc Endocrinol.* 13:47, 1984.
57. Raugh W, Oberfields E: The adrenal cortex in childhood hypertension. *Pediatr Adolesc Endocrinol.* 13:210, 1984.
58. Montero F, Sarconi C: Enzymatic defects of steroidogenesis: 17a Hydroxylase. *Pediatr Adolesc Endocrinol.* 13:83, 1984.
59. Schachter J, Kuller LH, Perfetti C: Blood pressure during the first five years of life: Relation to ethnic group (black or white) and to parental hypertension. *Am J Epidemiol.* 119:541, 1984.
60. Prineas RJ, Gillium RF, Horibe H, et al: Multiple determinants of children's blood pressure: The Minneapolis Children's Blood Pressure Study. *Hypertension.* 2:24, 1980.
61. Gillium RF: Pathophysiology of hypertension in blacks and whites: A review of the bases of racial pressure differences. *Hypertension.* 1:468, 1979.
62. Kotchen JM, Kotchen TA, Schwertman NC, et al: Blood pressure distribution of urban adolescents. *Am J Epidemiol.* 99:315, 1979.
63. Gillium RF, Prineas RJ, Gomez-Martin O, et al: Personality, behavior, family environment, family social status and hypertension risk factors in children: The Minneapolis Children's Blood Pressure Study. *J Chron Dis.* 38:187, 1985.
64. Page LB, Damon A, Moellering RC: Antecedents of cardiovascular disease in six Solomon Islands societies. *Circulation.* 49:1132, 1974.
65. Gleiberman L: Blood pressure and dietary salt in human population. *Ecol Food Nutr.* 2:143, 1973.
66. Oliver WJ, Cohen EL, Neel JV: Blood pressure, sodium intake and sodium-related hormones in Yanomamo Indians, a "no-salt culture." *Circulation.* 52:146, 1975.
67. Calabrese EJ, Tuthill RW: The influence of elevated levels of sodium in drinking water on elementary and high school students in Masschusetts, in Fregly MJ, Kare MR (eds): *The Role of Salt in Cardiovascular Hypertension.* New York, Academic, 1982, p 34.
68. Hofman A, Hazebroek A, Valkenburg H: A randomized trial of sodium intake and blood pressure in newborn infants. *JAMA.* 250:370, 1983.
69. McGregor GA, Markandu N, Bert F, et al: Double-blind randomised crossover trial of moderate sodium restriction in essential hypertension. *Lancet* 1:351, 1982.
70. DeWardener HE, McGregor GA: Dahl's hypothesis that a saluretic substance may be responsible for a sustained rise in arterial pressure: Its possible role in essential hypertension. *Kidney Int.* 18:1, 1980.
71. Uchiyama M, Shah V, Daman Willems CE, et al: Sodium transport in erythrocytes: Differences between normal children and children with primary and secondary hypertension. *Arch Dis Child.* 64:224, 1989.
72. Annest JL, Sng CF, Biron P, et al: Familial aggregation of blood pressure and weight in adoptive families: II Estimation of the relative contribution of genetic and common environmental factors to blood pressure correlations between family. *Am J Epidemiol.* 110:492, 1979.
73. Miyao S, Furusho T: Genetic study of essential hypertension. *Jap Circ J.* 42:1161, 1978.
74. Gutin B, Basch C, Shea S, et al: Blood pressure, fitness, and fatness in 5-year and 6-year old children. *JAMA.* 264:1123, 1990.
75. Rocchini AP, Katch V, Anderson J, et al: Blood pressure in obese adolescents: Effect of weight loss. *Pediatrics.* 82:16, 1988.
76. Insel PM, Fraser GE, Phillips R, et al: Psychosocial factors and blood pressure in children. *J Pschosom Res.* 25:505, 1981.
77. Falkner B, Onesti G, Hamstra B: Stress response characteristics of adolescents with

high genetic risk for essential hypertension: A five year follow up. *Clin Exper Hypertens.* 3:583, 1981.
78. Laur RM, Mahoney LT, Clarke WR: Tracking of blood pressure during childhood: The Muscatine Study. *Clin Exper Hypertens.* A8:515, 1986.
79. Korobkin M, Perloff DL, Palubinskas AJ: Renal arteriography in the evaluation of unexplained hypertension in children and adolescents. *J Pediatr.* 88:388, 1976.
80. Stanley P, Gyepes MT, Olson DL, et al: Renovascular hypertension in children and adolescents. *Pediatr Radiology.* 129:123, 1978.
81. Sfakianakis GN, Jaffe D, and Bourgoignie JJ: Captopril scintigraphy in the diagnosis of renovascular hypertension. *Kidney Int* 34(Suppl 25):S142, 1988.
82. Geyskes GG, Oei HY, Puylaert CBAJ, et al: Renovascular hypertension identified by captopril-induced changes in the renogram. *Hypertension.* 9:451, 1987.
83. Kotchen TA, Strickland AL, Rice TW, et al: A study of the renin-angiotension system in newborn infants. *J Pediatr.* 80:938, 1972.
84. Stalker HP, Holland NH, Kotchen JM, et al: Plasma renin activity in healthy children. *J Pediatr.* 89:256, 1976.
85. Laragh JH, Sealey JE: Renin-sodium profiling: Why, how and when in clinical practice. *Cardiovasc Med.* 2:1053, 1977.
86. Muller FB, Sealey JE, Case DB, et al: The captopril test for identifying renovascular disease in hypertensive patients. *Am J Med.* 80:633, 1986.
87. Willems, CE, Shah V, Uchiyama M, et al: The captopril test: an aid to investigation of hypertension. *Arch Dis Child.* 64:229, 1989.
88. Plouin F, Duclos JM, Menard J, et al: Biochemical tests for diagnosis of pheochromocytoma: Urinary versus plasma determinations. *Br Med J.* 282:853, 1981.
89. Chatal JF, Charbonnel B: Comparison of iodobenzylguanidine imaging with computed tomography in locating pheochromocytoma. *J Clin Endocrinol Metab.* 61:769, 1985.
90. Iodobenzylguanidine for location and treatment of pheochromocytoma. Editorial. *Lancet.* 2:905, 1984.
91. Chester EM, Agamanolis DP, Banker BQ: Hypertensive encephalopathy: A clinicopathologic study of 20 cases. *Neurology.* 28:928, 1978.
92. Byrom FB: The pathogenesis of hypertensive encephalopathy and its relation to the malignant phase of hypertension: Experimental evidence from the hypertensive rat. *Lancet.* 2:2011, 1954.
93. Meyer JS, Waltz AG, Gotoh F: Pathogenesis of cerebral vasospasm in hypertensive encephalopathy: II. The nature of increased irritability of smooth muscles of pial arterioles in renal hypertension. *Neurology.* 10:859, 1960.
94. Farrar JK, Jones JV, Graham DI, et al: Evidence against cerebal vasospasm during acutely induced hypertension. *Brain Res.* 104:176, 1976.
95. Kontos HA, Wei EP, Dietrich WD, et al: Mechanism of cerebral arteriolar abnormalities after acute hypertension. *Am J Physiol.* 240:H511, 1981.
96. Tamaki K, Sadoshima S, Baumbach GL, et al: Evidence that disruption of blood-brain barrier precedes reduction in cerebral blood flow in hypertensive encephalopathy. *Hypertension.* 6(suppl I):I-75, 1984.
97. Woods, JW: Malignant hypertension: Clinical recognition and management. *Cardiovasc Clin.* 9:311, 1978.
98. Keith NM, Wagener HP, Barker NW: Some different types of essential hypertension: Their course and prognosis. *Am J Med Sci.* 197:332, 1937.
99. Guelpa G, Lucsko M, Chaigon M, et al: Hypertension artérielle maligne, aspect sémiologique et pronostique. Etude rétrospective de 140 observations. *Schweiz Med Wochenschr.* 114:1870, 1984.

11

TREATMENT OF HYPERTENSION

Kanwal K. Kher

The beneficial effect of lowering blood pressure (BP) for reducing long-term morbidity and mortality is well known.[1–3] The approach to the treatment of hypertensive children differs somewhat from that to adult patients, even though the general principles remain similar in all age groups. Since hypertension is usually of secondary etiology in children, attention to specific therapy directed toward the underlying disorder is always necessary. In many such children aggressive pharmacotherapy is required for adequate control of elevated BP and to avoid hypertensive catastrophies, such as hypertensive encephalopathy. Essential hypertension, although less common than in adults, also occurs in children. Initial treatment options that may be explored in such hypertensive patients prior to starting drug therapy include nonpharmacologic measures such as decreasing dietary salt load, weight reduction, control of associated hypercholesterolemia, and possibly stress reduction. The treatment of hypertensive patients requires a long-term commitment on the part of both patient and physician to monitor not only BP but also the side effects of treatment.

PHARMACOTHERAPY OF HYPERTENSION

CLASSIFICATION OF ANTIHYPERTENSIVE AGENTS

Blood pressure is determined by the product of cardiac output (CO) and peripheral resistance (PR) and is represented by the formula:

$$\text{Mean BP} = \text{CO} \times \text{PR}$$

Most antihypertensive agents other than diuretics lower BP by reducing peripheral resistance. For the sake of convenience, antihypertensive agents are generally classified according to site of action (Fig. 11–1). Accordingly, antihypertensive drugs can be grouped as those with direct action on the vascular wall (hydralazine, minoxidil) or those which act via the autonomic nervous system and lower the vasoconstrictive tone of the blood vessels (alpha blockers—pra-

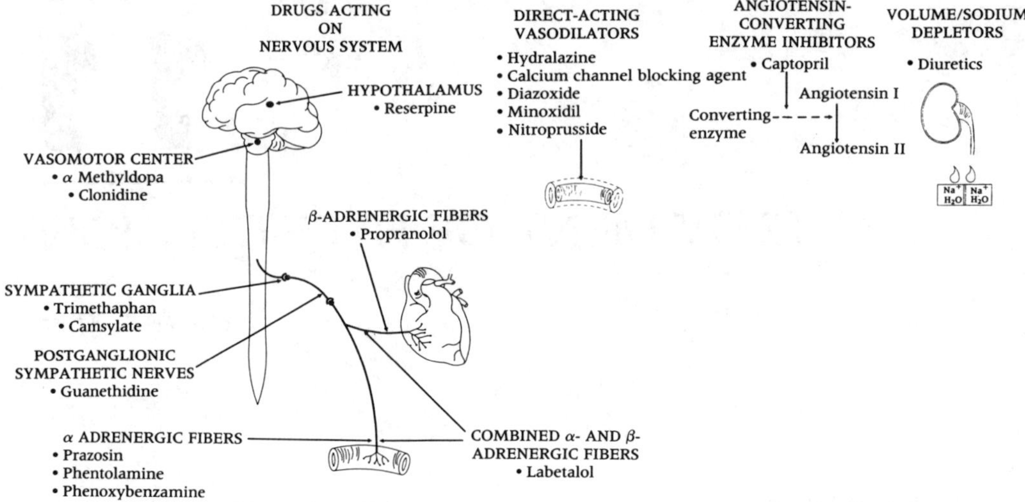

FIG. 11–1. Graphic representation of the site of action of various antihypertensive agents.

zosin; beta blockers—propranolol; or combined alpha and beta blockers—labetalol). Angiotensin converting enzyme (ACE) inhibitors interfere in the generation of angiotensin II and are specifically used in the treatment of patients with high-renin hypertension (renal or renovascular disease). A new class of antihypertensive agents known as calcium channel blockers is increasingly becoming an important therapeutic tool for the treatment of both acute and chronic hypertension. Centrally acting drugs such as clonidine, methyldopa, and guanabenz are rarely used in children at present. Table 11–1 lists the categories of oral antihypertensive agents for use in chronic hypertension.

PRINCIPLES OF THERAPY

The general principles of antihypertensive therapy are listed in Table 11–2. Traditionally a stepped-care approach has been advocated in treating patients with longstanding hypertension. The guidelines for this method were developed from experience with essential hypertension in adults. It involves the use of diuretics (usually thiazides) at first, followed by the addition of beta adrenergic blockers or peripheral vasodilators in sequence. While the stepped-care method offers a general therapeutic plan, the choice of antihypertensive agents in the 1990s should also be guided by (1) the underlying principal mechanism of hypertension—renin-mediated versus volume-mediated; (2) the ease of administration of the drugs—for example, twice a day versus four times a day, (3) the severity and nature of the drug's side effects, and (4) the cost of long-term therapy. Antihypertensive therapy, in children as well as adults, should be individualized in order to meet the needs of a particular patient.

DIURETICS

Thiazide diuretics such as hydrochlorothiazide (Hydrodiuril, Esidrix) are the most widely used agents for the treatment of hypertension. The exact mechanism of action of these drugs remains unknown, but both volume depletion and reduction of peripheral resistance seem to be involved.[4,5] In the initial few weeks of thiazide diuretic therapy, enhanced excretion of sodium and water leads to a decrease in intravascular volume and cardiac output, but peripheral resistance increases (Fig. 11–2). The net hemodynamic effect of these changes, however, is a reduction of BP. After several weeks of continued diuretic use, peripheral resistance begins to fall below the pretreatment level and cardiac output returns to normal while the plasma volume remains somewhat decreased. The long-term antihypertensive effect of thiazide diuretics is believed to be mediated primarily by a reduction in peripheral resistance.[6] Thiazides produce a modest decrease in the BP and are virtually ineffective in patients with moderately severe renal failure. Thiazide diuretics are used primarily in the treatment of essential hypertension. The major side effects of long-term thiazide use are hypokalemia, hypercalcemia, hyperuricemia, hyperglycemia, elevation of serum cholesterol and triglycerides, and a decrease in concentration of the protective high-density lipoprotein (HDL) cholesterol in serum.

Potent "loop" diuretics such as furosemide (Lasix), ethacrynic acid (Edecrin), and bumetanide (Bumex) are also frequently used in the treatment of hypertension. These agents are generally prescribed for patients with compromised renal function, particularly if their hypertension is associated with expanded intravascular volume.

Other less often used diuretics include the potassium-sparing agents such as spironolactone (Aldactone), triamterene (Dyrenium), and amiloride (Midamor). These are primarily used as adjuncts to thiazide or furosemide therapy and to ameliorate urinary potassium loss and hypokalemia. Since hyperkalemia is a potential hazard in patients with renal failure, potassium-sparing diuretics should be avoided in such patients. The site of action of various diuretic agents in the nephron is shown in Fig. 11–3.

BETA BLOCKERS

Alone or in combination with diuretics and peripheral vasodilator drugs, beta blockers are an important group of drugs in the treatment of hypertensive patients. Their antihypertensive action is mediated via (1) reduction in heart rate and cardiac output and (2) blockage of the release of renin from the kidneys in response to adrenergic stimulation. Other possible mechanisms of antihypertensive action of these agents which are likely but have not conclusively been documented in humans are (1) central action on the brain resulting in a decreased efferent sympathetic nerve activity and (2) stimulation of vasodilator prostaglandin synthesis.[7]

Because of its proven record of safety, propranolol (Inderal) is the most com-

TABLE 11–1. Orally Administered Antihypertensive Agents and Their Dose

Site and Mechanism of Action	Agents	Initial Dose, kg/day	Maximum Dose, kg/day	Advantages	Side Effects
DIURETICS	**Hydrochlorothiazide** (Hydrodiuril), 25-, 50-mg tablets	1 mg	4 mg	Mild antihypertensive action	Hypokalemia, hypercalcemia, hyperuricemia, ↓high-density lipoproteins
	Furosemide (Lasix), 20-, 40-mg tablets	0.5–1.0 mg	15 mg		Hypokalemia
	Triamterene (Dyrenium), 50-mg capsule	2 mg	6 mg		
	Bumetanide (Bumex), 0.5-, 1, 2-mg tablets	0.01–0.02 mg	0.4 mg		
	Spironolactone (Aldactone), 25-mg tablet	1 mg	3 mg		Hyperkalemia
DIRECT VASODILATORS	**Hydralazine** (Apresoline), 10-, 25-, 50-, 100-mg tablets	1–2 mg	8 mg	Preferential arteriolar dilation	Tachycardia ↑Renin release Fluid retention Hirsuitism (Minoxidil)
	Minoxidil (Loniten), 2.5-, 10-mg tablets	0.1–0.2 mg	1–2 mg		
ALPHA BLOCKERS	**Prazosin** (Minipress) 1-, 2-, 5-mg capsule	0.05 mg	0.4 mg	Vasodilation	Hypotension Bradycardia
BETA AND ALPHA BLOCKERS	**Labetalol** (Trandate), 100-, 200-, 300-mg tablet	2.0–3.0 mg	10–12 mg	Effective monotherapy	Hypotension Rash
BETA BLOCKERS	**Propranolol** (Inderal), 60-, 80-, 120-, 160-mg tablets	1–2 mg	4–6 mg	↓Renin release	Bronchospasm ↑Triglycerides

	Atenolol (Tenormin), 50-, 100-mg tablets	1 mg	2 mg		↓High-density lipoprotein ↓Cardiac output
	Metoprolol (Lopressor), 50-, 100-mg tablets	1–2 mg	6 mg		
CENTRAL ADRENERGIC AGONISTS	**Clonidine** (Catapres), 0.1-, 0.2-, 0.3-mg tablets	5 μg	30 μg	Less fluid retention	Sedation Dry mouth Hypotension
	Methyldopa (Aldoment), 125-, 250-, 500-mg tablets	5 mg	40 mg		
	Guanabenz, (Wytensin), 4-, 8-mg tablets	0.1 mg	1 mg		
ACE INHIBITORS	**Captopril** (Capoten), 12.5-, 25-, 50-, 100-mg tablet	0.3 mg	5 mg	Vasodilation No sedation	Rash Neutropenia (rare)
	Enalapril (Vasotec), 2.5-, 5-, 10-, 20-mg tablets	0.2 mg	1 mg		Proteinuria Taste impairment
	Lisinopril (Zestril), 5-, 10-, 20-, 40-mg tablets	0.2 mg	1 mg		Hyperkalemia Decreased GFR in renal arterial stenosis Cough (captopril)
CALCIUM CHANNEL BLOCKERS	**Nifedipine** (Procardia), 10-, 20-mg capsules	0.25 mg	1 mg	Vasodilation	Hypotension
	Verapamil (Calan), 80-, 120-mg tablets	3.0 mg	7.0 mg	No sedation ↑Renal salt excretion	AV conduction disturbance ↓Sinus rate (Verapamil)
	Diltiazem (Cardizem), 30-, 60-mg tablets	2.0 mg	3.5 mg		Interferes with cyclosporine metabolism (Verapamil)
	Nifedipine extended release (Procardia-XL) 30-, 60-mg tablets	Unknown	Unknown		

Source: Adapted from Balfe JW, Levin L, Tsuru N, et al: Hypertension in childhood. *Adv Ped* 36:201, 1989; and Hanna JD, Chan JCM, Gill JR, Jr: Hypertension and the kidney. *J Pediatr* 118:327, 1991. Reproduced by permission.

TABLE 11–2. Principles of Treating Chronic Hypertension

- Pharmacologic treatment of hypertension should be used in a stepwise fashion.
- The least toxic drugs should be prescribed first.
- Use the maximum recommended dose of one pharmacologic agent prior to adding another for the control of BP.
- When combination drug therapy is used, the drugs being prescribed should have different sites or modes of action in order to attain an additive effect.

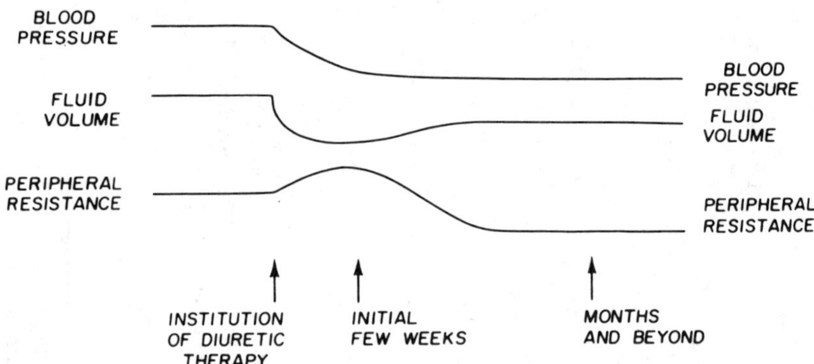

FIG. 11–2. Mechanisms by which thiazide diuretics lower blood pressure at varying times after start of diuretic therapy. [From Kaplan NM: Management strategies in hypertension, in Brenner BM, Stein JH (eds): *Contemporary Issues in Nephrology,* vol 8. New York, Churchill Livingstone, 1981, p 350. Reproduced with permission].

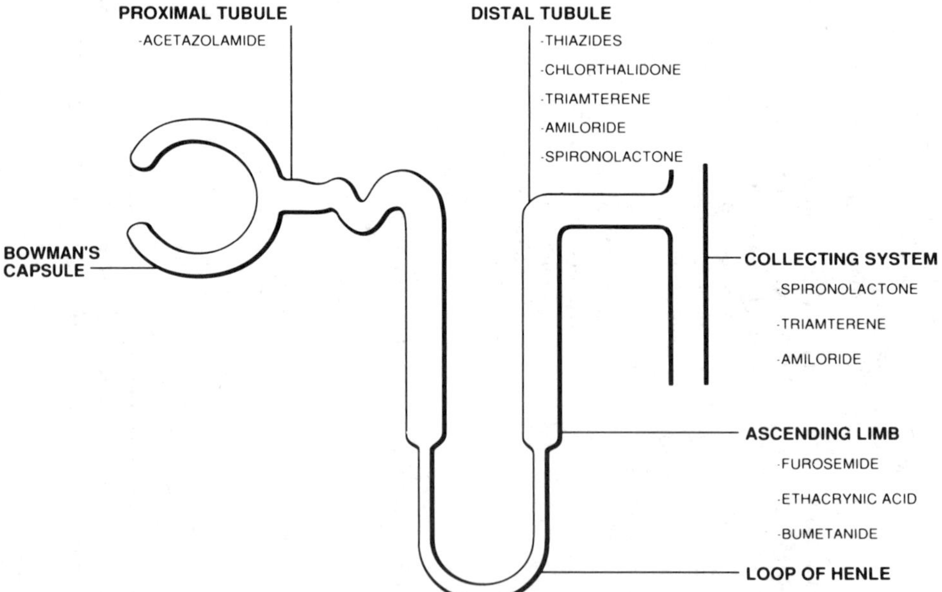

FIG. 11–3. Site of action of various diuretics in the nephron.

monly used beta-blocking agent in children. Extensive experience with longer-acting and more potent beta blockers like atenolol (Tenormin), metoprolol (Lopressor), pindolol (Visken), nadolol (Corgard), and timolol (Blocadren) has not been reported in children. Beta blockers are contraindicated in patients who depend on adrenergic drive for the performance of vital body functions; these include patients with bronchial asthma and congestive heart failure. Beta blockers should also be used with caution in patients with insulin-dependent diabetes mellitus (type I). In these patients, beta blockers can mask the symptoms of hypoglycemia and thus enhance the risks associated with a hypoglycemic crisis.[8] Dosages should be reduced or even discontinued in patients who develop bradycardia during the course of therapy. It is important to note that cardiac output remains low during exercise in patients receiving beta-blocking drugs and that exercise endurance may be reduced in some patients.[9]

ALPHA-ADRENERGIC BLOCKING AGENTS

Until recently, phentolamine (Regitine) and phenoxybenzamine (Dibenzyline) were the main drugs in clinical use in this category, both being used primarily in the preoperative management of hypertension associated with pheochromocytomas. Routine use of this category of antihypertensive agents has largely been hampered by the severe side effects associated with their use. Prazosin (Minipress), a drug with selective $alpha_1$-adrenergic blocking properties, has, however, found a place in the treatment of chronic hypertension in children and adults. Because of its property of reducing peripheral resistance, prazosin was originally thought to be a peripheral vasodilator. But further research on its mechanism of action has shown that its antihypertensive effect stems from its abilities to block the postsynaptic $alpha_1$-adrenergic receptors of the blood vessels.[10] Prazosin is effective in patients with renal insufficiency and may be combined with beta blockers in the treatment of moderately hypertensive patients. Significant hypotension may be noted within 30 to 90 min after the drug is taken for the first time. This, the "first-pass effect," is usually transient and can be avoided by giving the first dose at bedtime and also by initiating therapy with a lower-than-recommended dosage. Doxazosin, a long-acting selective $alpha_1$-blocking agent that is structurally similar to prazosin, is available for clinical use in Europe but has not yet been introduced in this country.[11]

DRUGS WITH ALPHA- AND BETA-BLOCKING PROPERTIES

This unique group of drugs has emerged as a novel treatment for hypertension, particularly in managing hypertensive emergencies. Labetalol (Trandate, Normodyne), the primary drug in this group, has pharmacologic properties of both the adrenergic alpha-blocking drugs (e.g., prazosin) and beta blockers (e.g., propranolol). Labetalol is used primarily in the treatment of hypertensive emergencies. Given acutely, it exerts its antihypertensive effect by lowering total peripheral resistance, heart rate, and cardiac output.[12] Postural hypotension is a frequent side effect of labetalol. Although reports of its use in children have appeared in Europe, pediatric experience with labetalol in the United States is limited.

PERIPHERAL VASODILATORS

Peripheral vasodilator drugs are commonly used for the treatment of hypertension. They reduce blood pressure by acting directly on the smooth muscles of the vascular bed, causing vasodilatation and decreasing peripheral resistance. The side effects of most peripheral vasodilator drugs include reflex tachycardia, increased renin output, and renal sodium and water retention. In order to obtain an additive antihypertensive effect and to counter the side effects of tachycardia and sodium and water retention, vasodilators are often used in combination with beta blockers and/or diuretics.

Hydralazine (Apresoline) is the most frequently used agent in this group. Other vasodilator drugs in clinical use are minoxidil (Loniten), diazoxide (Hyperstat I.V.), and sodium nitroprusside. Diazoxide and sodium nitroprusside are indicated for intravenous administration only and are used exclusively in the treatment of acute hypertensive emergencies. Both hydralazine and minoxidil are administered orally, but hydralazine can also be used parenterally. Hydralazine is well known to result in a positive antinuclear antibody (ANA) test and a lupus-like syndrome. Although a low-titer positive ANA test is noted in 40 to 50 percent of patients taking hydralazine, the risk of developing symptomatic lupus is considerably lower.[13] The overall risk of lupus-like syndrome due to hydralazine increases with the dose of the drug used; patients taking 50 mg or less per day rarely develop this disorder. The incidence of lupus-like syndrome is approximately 5 percent and 10 percent, respectively, in adult patients taking 100 and 200 mg of hydralazine daily.[14] Organ involvement with hydralazine-induced lupus is significantly less than that seen in idiopathic systemic lupus erythematosus.[15]

Minoxidil is significantly more potent in its antihypertensive action than hydralazine. The most unpleasant side effect of prolonged minoxidil therapy is excessive hair growth, particularly around the face and forehead. Minoxidil has also been linked to hirsutism in a newborn child whose mother received minoxidil during pregnancy.[16] Although minoxidil is effective as an antihypertensive agent even in patients with renal insufficiency, it should be reserved only for those with severe and uncontrolled hypertension.

CALCIUM CHANNEL BLOCKING AGENTS

New types of peripheral vasodilators of considerable interest for the treatment of hypertension are calcium channel blockers such as verapamil (Calan), diltiazem (Cardizem), and nifedipine (Procardia). These drugs act on the smooth muscle cells of the blood vessels and inhibit the influx of calcium, which is necessary for muscle contraction. As a consequence, they inhibit the tone of the smooth muscles, causing peripheral vasodilatation and thus reducing peripheral resistance. In contrast to the renal action of other peripheral vasodilators, calcium channel blockers do not lead to the retention of sodium, in fact, they enhance sodium excretion.[17]

Verapamil was the first of the calcium channel blockers to become available for clinical use. Since it depresses cardiac pacemaker activity and can cause severe bradycardia, verapamil should not be used in combination with beta-blocking agents. It also interferes with the metabolism of cyclosporin A, thus raising the plasma concentration of this immunosuppressive agent in renal transplant recipients. Nifedipine, on the other hand, does not affect the conduction system of the heart and results in a significant and sometimes profound decrease in peripheral resistance and BP. Nifedipine is available as a liquid-filled gelatin capsule containing 10 mg of the drug in a volume of 0.34 mL. Older children are asked to bite the capsule in their mouths and either swallow the contents or place it under the tongue. The drug can also be withdrawn from the capsule into a 1 mL syringe and administered sublingually or orally. This is usually done with younger patients. Since the duration of action of nifedipine is unpredictable, ranging from 1 to 4 h, it is useful only in the treatment of episodic acute hypertensive crises.[18] Long-acting nifedipine (Procardia-XL), available for use in adults, can be given once or twice a day. Appropriate dosages of long-acting nifedipine for children remain undetermined at this time.

CENTRALLY ACTING ALPHA STIMULATORS

The two drugs of clinical significance in this group are alphamethyldopa (Aldomet) and clonidine (Catapres). Both these drugs stimulate the $alpha_2$ receptors of the brain stem and thus reduce peripheral adrenergic drive. However, they are used less frequently now than in the past because of their often troublesome side effects as well as the availability of newer, less toxic antihypertensive agents. Clonidine is known to result in rebound hypertension upon sudden withdrawal, sometimes causing hypertensive encephalopathy and seizures. Other results of the withdrawal of clonidine are agitation, restlessness, insomnia, and sweating. These appear 18 to 36 h after the last dose of clonidine has been taken and are believed to be mediated by excessive catecholamine release from the sympathetic nervous system.[19]

Alphamethyldopa achieves a modest reduction of blood pressure in most patients, but it may accumulate in those with compromised renal function. Central nervous system side effects (e.g., sedation and decreased alertness, sleep disturbance, nasal congestion, and gastrointestinal disturbances) may be of concern in school-age children. Rebound hypertension has also been reported, albeit rarely, in patients who have suddenly stopped taking alphamethyldopa.

ANGIOTENSIN CONVERTING ENZYME INHIBITORS

Angiotensin converting enzyme (ACE) inhibitors such as captopril (Capoten) and enalapril (Vasotec) have a specific role in the treatment of high-renin hypertension due to renal parenchymal or renovascular disorders. Such ACE inhibitors block the biotransformation of angiotensin I to angiotensin II. As a consequence, the vasoconstriction, stimulation of aldosterone synthesis, and renal sodium and water retention attributable to angiotensin II are prevented. The significant side effects of this drug include bone marrow depression, skin rash, angioedema, and proteinuria. Captopril has been used successfully in treating renal and renovascular hypertension in neonates as well as in children and adolescents.[20,21] Decreased glomerular filtration rate (GFR) and acute renal failure have been reported in sick hypertensive neonates treated with captopril,[20] and this drug should be used with caution in the newborn period. Renal function tests should be monitored in neonates receiving ACE inhibitors. The intravenously administered ACE inhibitor enalaprilat (Vasotec I.V.) is available for clinical use and may be particularly convenient for patients who cannot be given oral ACE inhibitors. In a recent clinical trial of this drug in neonates, adequate control of hypertension was achieved in a majority of patients, but hypotension was reported in 30 percent.[22] Other side effects of intravenous enalaprilat are similar to those of the orally administered ACE inhibitors.

ACE inhibitors should be used with caution in patients suspected of having renal arterial stenosis in a solitary kidney (such as a congenital single kidney or a renal transplant) or bilateral renal arterial stenosis. Deterioration of renal function or even acute renal failure upon treatment with ACE inhibitors has been reported in such patients.[23] The pathophysiology of acute renal failure in such patients is not fully understood, but alterations in the intrarenal autoregulation of renal perfusion induced by captopril are felt to be responsible. A significant renal arterial stenosis is associated with decreased perfusion pressure in the poststenotic area of the kidney, including in the glomerular capillaries. Under these circumstances, the glomerular filtration rate is believed to be maintained by afferent arteriolar dilatation (autoregulation) and efferent arteriolar constriction mediated by angiotensin II.[24,25] The net effect of these hemodynamic changes is to increase intraglomerular hydrostatic pressure and filtration fraction, thus maintaining the GFR. Upon administration of ACE inhibitors to patients with renal arterial stenosis, the synthesis of angiotensin II is blocked, resulting in dilatation of the glomerular efferent arterioles. As a consequence, the glomerular hydrostatic pressure falls to a critical level, with a concomitant decrease in the GFR (Fig. 11–4). Patients with unilateral renal arterial stenosis and a normal contralateral kidney can compensate for a decreased GFR in the affected kidney by enhancing GFR in the normal kidney. Thus, the overall GFR remains unchanged. In contrast, in patients with bilateral renal arterial stenosis or in those with arterial stenosis in a solitary kidney, reduction in the GFR with captopril therapy may be severe enough to lead to oliguria and acute renal failure (Fig. 11–4). Urinary indices in patients who develop acute renal failure with captopril therapy suggest a prerenal pathophysiology rather than the type seen in acute tubular necrosis. Urine specific gravity and osmolality are elevated and fractional excretion of sodium is low. Preexisting sodium and volume depletion may enhance the acute renal failure resulting from captopril therapy in susceptible patients. An improvement of renal function is usual upon withdrawal of the drug.[23,26]

Treatment with ACE inhibitors is well known to result in hyperkalemic distal renal tubular acidosis (type IV RTA) by virtue of hypoaldosteronism. Hyperkalemia due to this mechanism may be severe and of significant concern in patients with renal disease and those with azotemia.[20,27,28]

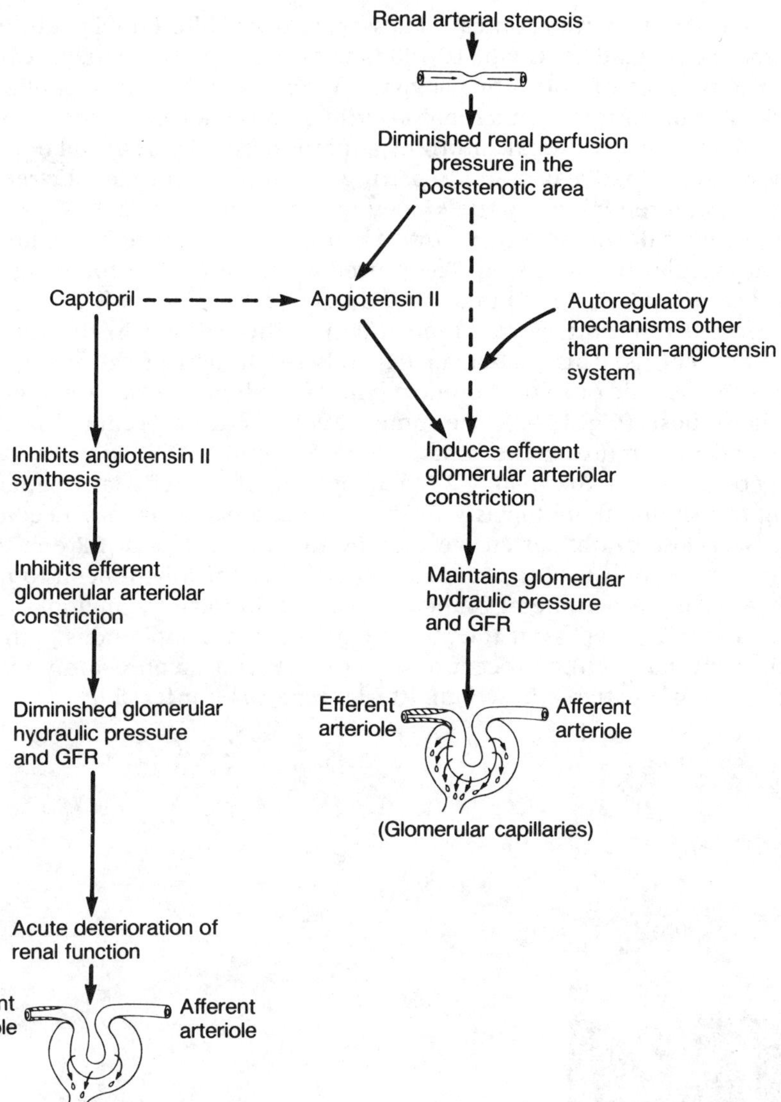

FIG. 11–4. Proposed mechanism of acute renal failure in patients with renal arterial stenosis receiving ACE inhibitors. Details are given in the text.

SURGICAL TREATMENT

Surgery may be necessary and curative in several forms of hypertension in children. These include hypertension caused by renal arterial stenosis, unilateral renal scarring due to pyelonephritis, coarctation of the aorta, and tumors such as pheochromocytoma. Nephrectomy is reserved for patients whose hypertension is believed to result from unilateral renal disease such as scarring due to pyelonephritis, Ask-Upmark renal dysplasia, or whose affected kidney has only limited or residual function. Whether surgical removal of such defective kidneys can cure hypertension can be assessed from differential renin estimation and radiologic studies (Chap. 10). Repair of the stenotic segment can be done by various types of aorto-renal bypass surgeries. Autotransplantation may be considered in patients with renal arterial stenosis affecting the proximal segment of renal artery. Renal autotransplantation involves removal of the affected kidney from its native position, repairing or removing the stenotic renal arterial segment, and reimplanting the kidney in the pelvic area.

Transluminal balloon angioplasty is being used increasingly for the treatment of renovascular hypertension. The procedure consists of introducing a balloon-tipped catheter (Fig. 11–5) under radiologic guidance via a femoral artery into the affected renal artery and then inflating the balloon in the region of the vascular stenosis. This maneuver expands the lumen of the renal artery and breaks the fibrotic or hypertrophic media of the blood vessel, thus relieving the arterial stenosis (Fig. 11–6). The complications of this procedure include thrombosis and/or rupture of the renal artery. Restenosis following balloon angioplasty occurs in approximately 25 to 30 percent of cases.[29] Many patients undergoing transluminal angioplasty for renal arterial stenosis may need continued but lower-dose antihypertensive therapy for the control of BP due to residual stenosis or restenosis of the renal artery. It is technically difficult to relieve stenosis affecting a peripheral branch of the renal artery by angioplasty. In such cases, a surgical bypass of the stenotic area using a saphenous vein or a synthetic graft may be the procedure of choice. Partial nephrectomy may be necessary in some patients in whom arterial repair is not feasible.

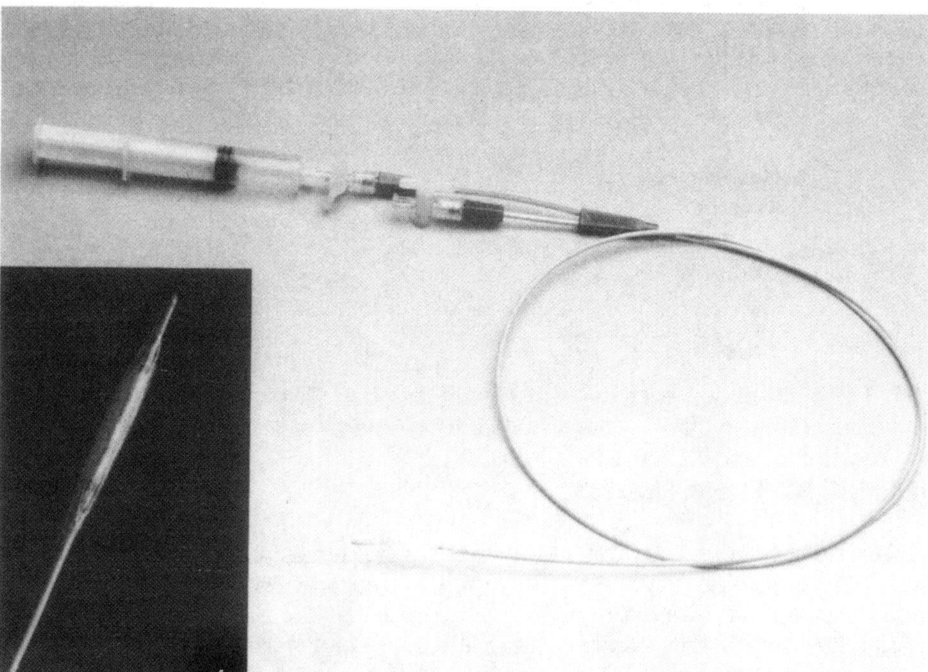

FIG. 11–5. Catheter used for repair of renal arterial stenosis by balloon angioplasty. Inset shows catheter tip with the expanded balloon.

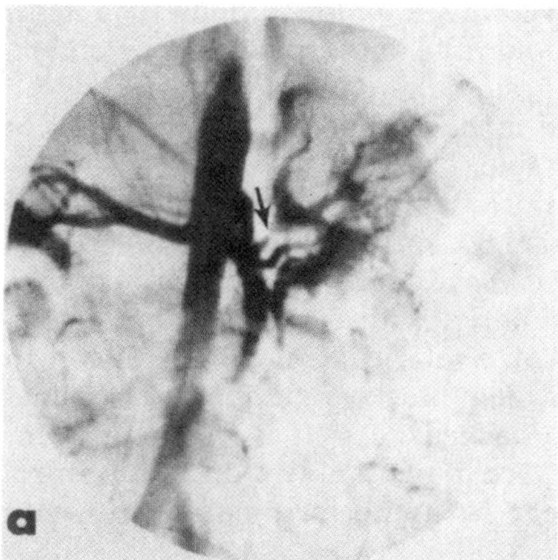

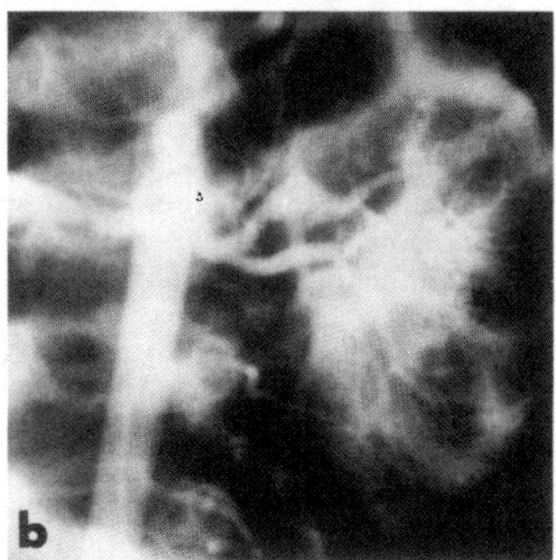

FIG. 11–6. *A*. Angiogram of 2-year-old male child with severe hypertension due to segmental renal arterial stenosis. *B*. Angiogram of same patient following balloon angioplasty.

TREATMENT OF ESSENTIAL HYPERTENSION

Nonpharmacologic therapy should be tried initially in all patients with mild essential hypertension. This includes weight reduction, decreased salt intake, and exercise. However, these measures alone may not suffice to achieve control of BP and the addition of antihypertensive drugs may become necessary. Weight reduction has been reported to lower blood pressure significantly in patients with essential hypertension[30] and should be suggested to those hypertensive patients who are obese. Exercise and the control of caloric intake should be emphasized as part of such weight-reduction strategies. Dynamic exercises (walking, jogging, riding a bike) have been found to be beneficial in hypertensive children, but isometric exercises (weight lifting, "Bull-worker body building") are generally believed to place undue hemodynamic demands on the myocardium and may be harmful.[31] However, Hagberg et al.[32] have shown that even static isometric exercise, such as weight training, is beneficial in reducing both the systolic and diastolic BP in hypertensive adolescents. Blood pressure in a child with moderately severe or severe hypertension may need to be controlled with antihypertensive drugs prior to advising any exercise program. Some children taking beta blockers may not be able to enhance cardiac output during exercise and may develop exercise intolerance. Strenuous exercise should be avoided in such circumstances.

The significance of sodium in the pathogenesis of essential hypertension has been discussed in Chapter 10. Restriction of sodium intake should be advised for all patients with essential hypertension. Hypertensive adolescent patients should attempt to reduce salt (sodium chloride) intake to 40 meq (2.3 g NaCl) per day. Sodium restriction may allow lowering the dose of antihypertensive agents. Most snacks, canned foods, and fast-food items are particularly high in sodium content and should be avoided. Several types of low-sodium food items are now available commercially and can often be substituted for the others. Although it is difficult and often frustrating to adhere to a low-salt diet for a long period of time, an attempt should be made to modify cooking habits at home and also to avoid adding salt at the table.

If nonpharmacologic therapy does not control BP or hypertension is of more than mild degree, antihypertensive drug therapy may be initiated in conjunction with the therapeutic options mentioned above. In general, diuretics or beta blockers may be tried first. Since most children with essential hypertension have normal renal function, mild diuretics like thiazides are quite effective. In patients with a poor response to diuretics, beta blockers, peripheral vasodilators, or calcium channel blockers may be added next. It is uncommon for patients with essential hypertension to require more than two drugs to control their blood pressure. An ACE inhibitor may be useful in some patients with high-renin essential hypertension.

TREATMENT OF HYPERTENSIVE EMERGENCIES

A hypertensive emergency resulting from a sudden and an unexpected rise of BP in children requires immediate medical attention. Two types of hypertensive emergencies commonly encountered in children are hypertensive encephalopathy and intracranial bleeding. Often, these emergencies arise as a result of discontinuation of antihypertensive medications or in the course of disorders with acute onset such as acute poststreptococcal glomerulonephritis or hemolyticuremic syndrome. They may also be due to the intentional or accidental ingestion of drugs (including street drugs). Severe hypertension is also common in the withdrawal syndrome caused by the sudden discontinuation of clonidine and in cases of pheochromocytoma.

Regardless of the underlying etiology, a sudden rise in BP is more likely to lead to hypertensive encephalopathy—and at a lower diastolic BP—than a slow and sustained rise.[33] For this reason BP should be controlled rather aggressively in patients with acute severe hypertension, but the rapidity with which it should be brought down to normal is not well defined. A precipitous reduction of BP to a normal level should, however, be avoided in all cases. Reduction of BP in chronically hypertensive patients should, in general, be undertaken at a slower pace. Decreased cerebral and myocardial perfusion and resultant cerebrovascular accidents and myocardial ischemia have been reported in patients whose BP was normalized too rapidly.[34,35] Similarly, the aim of antihypertensive therapy in a patient with chronic hypertension who develops severe hypertension but is asymptomatic should be a gradual reduction of BP over several hours.[36,37] Of the several drugs available for parenteral administration to severely hypertensive children, hydralazine (Apresoline), diazoxide (Hyperstat), and sodium nitroprusside (Nipride) are the most frequently used. Alpha methyldopa (Aldomet) can also be used parenterally for the treatment of severe hypertension. Table 11–3 lists the drugs that can be used during hypertensive emergencies.

When given parenterally, hydralazine results in a slow (over 10 to 30 min) and unpredictable decline in BP. Diazoxide, on the other hand, acts immedi-

TABLE 11–3. Drugs for the Treatment of Severe Hypertension or Hypertensive Emergencies

Drug	Method of Administration	Dose	Onset of Effect	Duration of Effect	Side Effects: Comments
Hydralazine (Apresoline)	IV or IM	0.1–0.2 mg/kg q 4–6 h	10–30 min	2–6 h	Tachycardia, flushing, headache Not reliable for severe or symptomatic hypertension
Nifedipine (Procardia)	Sublingual or PO (bite and swallow)	0.2–0.5 mg/kg; maximum 10 mg	—	3.5–4.0 h	In sublingual administration, capsule is punctured with 25-gauge needle and contents expressed sublingually
Diazoxide (Hyperstat)	IV (rapid infusion)	1–3 mg/kg; start with 1 mg/kg, gradual increase at 5- to 15 min intervals to 3 mg/kg	3–5 min	4–24 h	Nausea, sodium retention, hyperglycemia
Labetalol (Normodyne, Trandate)	IV infusion, 1 mg/mL; 100 mg (20 mL) labetalol and 80 mL D5W	1 mg/kg/h, maximum 3 mg/kg/h (maximum total daily dose, 300 mg) or 0.25 mg/kg IV over 2 min as a bolus			Absolute contraindications: Congestive heart failure Heart block Sinus tachycardia Relative contraindications: Prior treatment with beta blockers Asthma
Sodium nitroprusside (Nipride)	IV infusion	0.5–8.0 μg/kg/min	Immediate	During infusion	Needs protection from light Requires blood pressure monitoring Thiocyanate blood levels need to be measured if used longer than 48 h
Enalaprilat (Vasotec IV)	IV over 5–10 min	5–25 μg/kg/day in divided doses[a]	15–30 min	6–12 h	Hyperkalemia, hypotension, useful only in high renin hypertension

[a]Dose determined in neonates.[22]

Source: Adapted from Balfe JW, Levin L, Tsuru N, et al: Hypertension in childhood. *Adv Pediatr* 36:201, 1989; and Hanna JD, Chan JMC, Gill JR, Jr: Hypertension and the kidney. *J Pediatr* 118; 327, 1991. Reproduced by permission.

ately upon intravenous administration and is more potent than hydralazine in its antihypertensive action. Both hydralazine and diazoxide are peripheral vasodilators that exert their action by acting directly on the peripheral vasculature. Diazoxide must be administered rapidly as a "push" (over 10 to 30 s), since it quickly binds to the plasma proteins. Tachycardia, renal sodium and water retention, and hyperglycemia are important side effects encountered with the use of diazoxide. These side effects can, however, be mitigated to some extent by concomitant use of diuretics and beta blockers. Diazoxide has been known to cause severe hypotension. Following intravenous administration, the extent to which diazoxide will decrease BP is unpredictable. Therefore care must be taken to use a smaller recommended dose at the beginning of therapy.

Sublingual or orally administered nifedipine, a calcium channel blocking drug, is an effective and safe alternative for conscious patients with severe or symptomatic hypertension. Nifedipine is rapidly replacing diazoxide as the antihypertensive drug of choice for the treatment of severe hypertension and hypertensive emergencies. Nifedipine starts its pharmacologic action within 10 min; peak blood levels and peak hypotensive action are noted at about 30 min. However, the half-life of the drug is short (2 h), and it may have to be administered every 3 to 4 h if BP is to be controlled effectively. Mild reflex tachycardia may be noted in most patients, flushing and sensations of heat may be experienced by about 25 percent of those taking this drug. The degree of hypotensive response is unpredictable and modest; in most patients a decline of 10 to 15 mmHg in systolic and diastolic BP is common. Nifedipine is also effective in patients with renal failure.

Sodium nitroprusside is a potent antihypertensive agent that is often reserved for circumstances when all other agents have been shown to be ineffective. Sodium nitroprusside is unstable in solution and must be reconstituted from its lyophilized form as needed. A significant advantage of this drug is that its rate of infusion can be titrated to achieve the desired degree of BP control. Careful calculation of its dose, administration, and monitoring are necessary in prescribing sodium nitroprusside. This drug should be used with caution in patients with renal insufficiency, since cyanide, a metabolic by-product of nitroprusside, accumulates in these patients, causing cyanide intoxication.[38]

Labetalol is an effective antihypertensive agent for use in hypertensive emergencies; it can be used either as a continuous intravenous infusion or as bolus therapy.[39] However, experience with the use of labetalol in children is limited.

TREATMENT OF HYPERTENSION IN ACUTE POSTSTREPTOCOCCAL GLOMERULONEPHRITIS

Acute poststreptococcal glomerulonephritis may be associated with a symptomatic and sudden elevation of BP, often leading to hypertensive encephalopathy and seizures. Hypertension in such patients is primarily attributed to volume overload, and plasma renin levels are consequently low.[40–42] In addition to hypertension, these patients may show other clinical and radiologic features of intravascular volume expansion (Fig. 11–7). Loop diuretics (furosemide) may be effective in inducing diuresis and reducing BP by volume reduction in a minority of patients. Most will, however, require treatment with other anti-

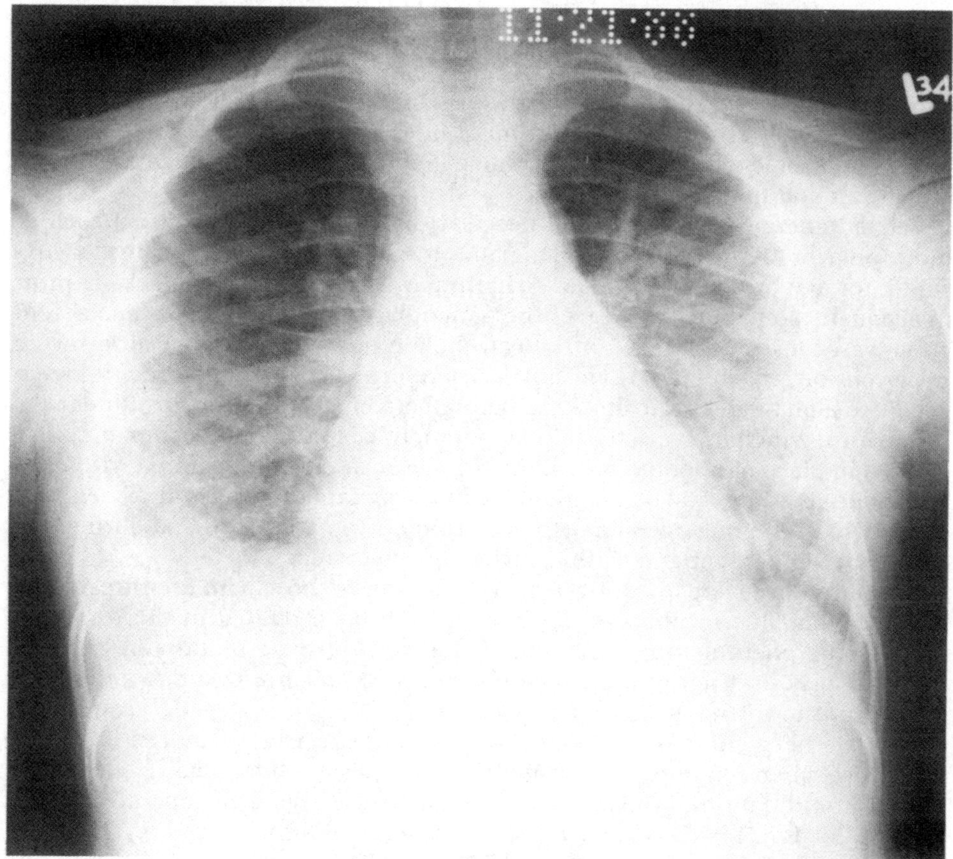

FIG. 11–7. Chest radiogram showing enlarged heart and pulmonary edema in a patient with severe hypertension due to acute poststreptococcal glomerulonephritis.

hypertensive agents.[43] Nifedipine may be prescribed as the drug of first choice for control of BP in these patients. Captopril has also been used in patients with acute poststreptococcal glomerulonephritis with some success but should not be used as the drug of first choice.[44] Blood pressure usually normalizes once the acute phase of fluid retention and intravascular volume overload resolves. It is uncommon for these patients to require antihypertensive treatment beyond 2 weeks.

TREATMENT OF HYPERTENSION IN PHEOCHROMOCYTOMA

Surgical removal of the tumor is the definitive treatment for pheochromocytoma. Surgery should, however, be undertaken in an elective manner so as to minimize risks and complications. Prior to surgery, the patient should be treated with alpha-adrenergic blocking agents in order to prevent hypertensive crises in the intraoperative period. Ideally, the alpha blockade should precede surgery by 10 days to 2 weeks. The drug used traditionally for alpha-adrenergic blockade in pheochromocytoma is phenoxybenzamine (Dibenzyline). The starting dose in children is 2.5 mg, given orally every 12 h.[45] The dose of the drug can be increased every other day (since the maximal drug effect appears only after 2 to 3 days) until adequate control of BP is achieved. Postural hypotension is a common side effect of this drug, and patients should be advised to maintain a high salt and fluid intake.

Beta-adrenergic blockade is not necessary for most patients with pheochromocytoma, but it may be required in patients who demonstrate sustained tachycardia for age or develop cardiac arrhythmias.[46] However, beta blockade prior to adequate alpha blockade leaves the patient with the unopposed alpha adrenergic (vasoconstrictor) effect of the catecholamines, which may lead to severe hypertension and hypertensive crisis. Therefore such patients must undergo adequate alpha-adrenergic blockade before beta blockers can be instituted.

Prazosin, which has selective alpha$_1$-adrenergic blocking properties, may also be used in place of phenoxybenzamine in these patients preoperatively.[47] Labetalol, with its alpha- and beta-adrenergic blocking properties, has also been used effectively in the management of pheochromocytoma prior to and during surgery, especially in patients with associated tachycardia.[48]

Patients with severe uncontrolled hypertension or those with life-threatening complications due to pheochromocytoma have been treated in the past with intravenous phentolamine (Regitine). The starting dose of this drug (given intravenously) is 1 μg/kg/min. It can be adjusted upward (to a maximum of 7 μg/kg/min) until the desired antihypertensive effect is achieved.[45] The use of phentolamine is limited by the severity of side effects experienced with this drug. Also, phentolamine is associated with a persistent hypotensive effect even after discontinuation of the infusion. This can cause severe postoperative hypotension. Sodium nitropruside (Nipride) infusion can also be used for lowering BP in these patients.[49] It presents a therapeutic advantage in that the dose can be titrated to match the desired level of BP control.

Postoperative management of patients in whom pheochromocytomas have been resected requires careful attention to intravascular volume, prevention of hypotension, prevention of hypoglycemia, and treatment of hypoadrenal manifestations in case bilateral adrenalectomy is necessary for removal of the tumor. Intravascular blood volume has been reported to be decreased in patients with pheochromocytoma and their intravascular volume is inversely related to their diastolic pressure.[50] Postoperatively, vasoconstrictor tone (which is maintained by the excess catecholamine secretion by the tumor) suddenly decreases. This effect, combined with preexisting intravascular volume depletion, can lead to severe hypotension. Preoperative blood transfusion[51] and volume expansion[52] have been reported in several studies to be effective in reducing the risk of postoperative hypotension. Volume expansion is the key to overcoming hypotension in the postoperative state.

SUMMARY

Management of hypertensive patients largely depends on the etiology as well as the severity of hypertension. While most children with essential hypertension can be managed initially by instituting nonpharmacologic therapy such as weight reduction, sodium restriction, and exercise, patients with secondary hypertension due to renal or renovascular disease often require aggressive pharmacologic management. Selection of the appropriate antihypertensive agent and the combination of drugs which should be prescribed requires a knowledge of the basic pharmacology and side effects of these drugs. Compliance with long-term antihypertensive therapy remains a common problem, especially in adolescents.

Treatment of Hypertension in Children: A Commentary

Julie R. Ingelfinger

While the general principles of treating hypertension in children are similar to those utilized in treating adults, pediatric considerations are perhaps even more important and override the specifics of therapy of hypertension *per se.* As has been detailed in the above chapter, severe hypertension in childhood is most likely due to secondary causes, and hypotensive therapy must be directed simultaneously both at the underlying cause and at controlling the accompanying hypertension. Yet, as primary hypertension is recognized with increased frequency, we must not overlook the fact that many, if not most, hypertensive youngsters, especially teenagers, have blood pressure elevation of unclear cause and modest degree. The appropriate therapy of such children and adolescents with primary hypertension is still uncertain, but the individual prescribing therapy must keep in mind that the course of blood pressure elevation in early primary hypertension is not infrequently marked by periods of blood pressure lability and by normalization of blood pressure spontaneously. Thus the dictum *primum non nocere* (first do no harm) seems especially relevant. Several caveats concerning therapy in general seem worthwhile recounting in some detail:

1. Pharmacotherapy with any given hypotensive agent has *rarely* been studied prospectively or specifically in children. Pharmacokinetics, toxicity, and patient acceptability of a blood pressure–lowering drug may be different in a pediatric as compared to an adult patient. As prescribing practitioners, we must keep this constantly in mind and should consider
   - Single-drug therapy (monotherapy) to simplify assessing therapy
   - Step-down therapy to see if less drug can still control hypertension
   - Behavioral and general developmental assessment while a child is on drug therapy in order to assess whether there might be unique pediatric side effects from the medication
   - Utilizing those hypotensive agents with which there is, in general, pediatric experience

2. Compliance is a general problem in taking medication and has special importance in childhood and adolescence because
   - Young children may need the help and guidance of parents or caregivers to take medication regularly
   - Adolescence is a time of great change, and adolescents notoriously find it difficult to take medication

   In view of compliance issues, an educational program is essential in the treatment of hypertension, most particularly because hypertension is most often asymptomatic. In contrast, numerous hypotensive agents may cause actual symptoms, so the patient may, especially at the start of therapy, feel worse on medication.
3. Nonpharmacologic therapy, while it is most appealing and, in fact, often efficacious, must be approached in much the same way as pharmacotherapy. Compliance issues, side effects of therapy related to weight loss or mineral balance, and degree of blood pressure control must all be followed prospectively. Patient cooperation and patient education are especially important in this sort of approach.
4. When surgical or interventional therapy (as with radiologic techniques such as transluminal angioplasty) for hypertension is utilized, follow-up is just as important as when pharmacotherapy is used. Recurrence of hypertension after intervention is, unfortunately, not rare. For example, restenosis of a renal artery or development of vascular abnormalities in additional renal vessels may occur in renovascular hypertension.
5. It took large-scale studies to determine that the use of certain hypotensive agents lowered blood pressure yet did not necessarily prolong life in individuals with mild to moderate hypertension. No such studies are available for a pediatric or adolescent population. Thus, it makes sense for those treating hypertension in children and adolescents to exercise continued vigilance concerning each patient's general status as well as blood pressure level.

REFERENCES

1. Hypertension Detection and Follow-up Program Cooperative Group: Persistence of reduction in blood pressure and mortality of participants in the Hypertension Detection and Follow-up Program. *JAMA* 259:2113, 1988.
2. Stokes J III, Kannel WB, Wolf PA, et al: Blood pressure as a risk factor for cardiovascular disease: The Framingham study—30 years of follow-up. *Hypertension* 13(suppl I):13, 1989.
3. Gifford RW: Review of the long-term controlled trials of usefulness of therapy for systemic hypertension. *Am J Cardiol* 63:8B, 1989.
4. Shah S, Khatri I, Freis ED: Mechanism of antihypertensive effect of thiazide diuretics. *Am Heart J* 95:611, 1978.
5. Freis ED: How diuretics lower blood pressure. *Am Heart J* 106:185,1983.
6. Lund-Johansen P: Hemodynamic changes in long-term diuretic therapy of essential hypertension. *Acta Med Scand* 187:509, 1970.
7. Prichard BNC, Owens CWI: β-Adrenoceptor blocking drugs, in Doyle AE (ed): *Handbook of Hypertension*, Amsterdam, Elsevier, 1988, vol 11, pp 187.

8. Lager I, Blohme G, Smith U: The effect of cardioselective and nonselective β-blockade on hypoglycaemic response in insulin-dependent diabetics. *Lancet* 1:458, 1979.
9. Thompson PD, Cullinane EM, Nugent AM, et al: Effect of atenolol or prazosin on maximal exercise performance in hypertensive joggers. *Am J Med* 86(suppl 1B):104, 1989.
10. Graham RM, Oates HF, Stoker LM, et al: Alpha blocking action of the antihypertensive agent, prazosin. *J Pharmacol Exp Ther* 201:747, 1977.
11. Smythe P, Pringle S, Jackson G, et al: Twenty-four hour control of blood pressure by once daily doxazosin: a multicenter double-blind comparison with placebo. *Eur J Clin Pharmacol* 34:613, 1988.
12. MacCarthy EP, Bloomfield SS: Labetalol: A review of its pharmacology, pharmacokinetics, clinical use and adverse effects. *Pharmacotherapy* 3:193, 1983.
13. Mansilla-Tinocor, Harland SF, Ryan PJ, et al: Hydralazine, antinuclear antibodies, and the lupus syndrome. *Br Med J* 284:936, 1982.
14. Cameron HA, Ramsay LE: The lupus syndrome induced by hydralazine: A common complication with low dose treatment. *Br Med J* 289:410, 1984.
15. Cush JJ, Goldings: Southwestern Internal Medicine Conference: Drug induced lupus: Clinical spectrum and pathogenesis. *Am J Med Sci* 290:36, 1985.
16. Kaler SG, Patrinos ME, Lambart GH, et al: Hypertrichosis and congenital anomalies associated with material use of minoxidil. *Pediatrics* 79:434, 1987.
17. Kinoshita M, Kusukawa R, Shimono Y, et al: Effects of diltiazam on renal hemodynamics and urinary electrolyte excretion. *Jpn Circ J* 42:553, 1978.
18. Siegler RL, Brewer ED: Effect of sublingual or oral nifedipine in the treatment of hypertension. *J Pediatr* 112:811, 1988.
19. Hansson L, Hunyor SN, Julius S, et al: Blood pressure crisis following withdrawal of clonidine with special reference to arterial and urinary catecholamine levels and suggestion for acute management. *Am Heart J* 88:608, 1973.
20. Tack ED, Perlman JM: Renal failure in sick hypertensive premature infants receiving captopril therapy. *J Pediatr* 112:805, 1988.
21. Mirkin BL, Newman TJ: Efficacy and safety of captopril in the treatment of severe childhood hypertension: Report of the International Collaborative Study Group. *Pediatrics* 75:1091, 1985.
22. Wells TG, Bunchman, Kearns: Treatment of neonatal hypertension with enalaprilat. *J Pediatr* 117:664, 1990.
23. Hricik DE, Browning PJ, Kopelman R, et al: Captopril-induced functional renal insufficiency in patients with bilateral renal-artery stenosis or renal-artery stenosis in a solitary kidney. *N Engl J Med* 308:373, 1983.
24. Hall JE, Guyton AC, Jackson TE, et al: Control of glomerular filtration rate by renin-angiotensin system. *Am J Physiol* 223:F366, 1977.
25. Steinhausen M, Endlich K, Wiegman DL: Glomerular blood flow. *Kidney Int* 38:769, 1990.
26. Hollenberg NK: The treatment of renovascular hypertension: Surgery, angioplasty, and medical therapy with converting-enzyme inhibitors. *Am J Kid Dis* 10(suppl):52, 1987.
27. Textor SC, Bravo EL, Fouad FM, et al: Hyperkalemia in azotemic patients during angiotensin-converting enzyme inhibition and aldosterone reduction with captopril. *Am J Med* 73:719, 1982.
28. Sakemi T, Ohchi N, Sanai T, et al: Captopril-induced metabolic acidosis with hyperkalemia. *Am J Nephrol* 8:245, 1988.
29. Chevalier RL, Tegtmeyer CJ, Ganez RA: Percutaneous transluminal angioplasty in blood pressure regulation. *Pediatr Nephrol* 1:89, 1987.

30. Rocchini AP, Katch V, Anderson J, et al: Blood pressure in obese adolescents: Effect of weight loss. *Pediatrics* 82:1, 1988.
31. Nelson L, Jennings GL, Esler MD, et al: Effect of changing levels of physical activity on blood pressure and hemodynamics in essential hypertension. *Lancet* 2:473, 1986.
32. Hagberg JM, Ensani AA, Goldring D, et al: Effect of weight training on blood pressure and hemodynamics in hypertensive adolescents. *J Pediatr* 104:147, 1984.
33. Strandgaard S: Autoregulation of cerebral blood flow in hypertensive patients: The modifying influence of prolonged antihypertensive treatment on tolerance to acute drug induced hypotension. *Circulation* 53:720, 1973.
34. O'Mailia JJ, Sander GE, Giles TD: Nifedipine-associated myocardial ischemia or infarction in treatment of hypertensive urgencies. *Ann Intern Med* 107:185, 1987.
35. Bertel O, Marx BE, Connen D. Effects of antihypertensive treatment on cerebral perfusion. *Am J Med* 82(suppl 3B):29, 1987.
36. Zeller KR, Kuhnert LV, Matthews C: Rapid reduction of severe asymptomatic hypertension: A prospective, controlled trial. *Arch Intern Med* 149:2186, 1989.
37. Fagan TC: Acute reduction of blood pressure in asymptomatic patients with severe hypertension: An idea whose time has come—and gone. *Arch Intern Med* 149:2169, 1989.
38. Cottrell JE, Casthely P, Brodie JD, et al: Prevention of nitroprusside-induced cyanide toxicity with hydroxycobalamine. *N Engl J Med* 298:809, 1978.
39. Vidt DG: Intravenous labetalol in the emergency treatment of hypertension. *J Clin Hypertens* 2:179, 1985.
40. Fleisher DS, Voci G, Garfunkel J, et al: Hemodynamic findings in acute glomerulonephritis. *J Pediatr* 69:1054, 1966.
41. Rodriguez-Itrube B, Baggio B, Colina-Chourio J, et al: Studies on the renin-angiotensin system in acute nephritic syndrome. *Kidney Int* 19:47, 1981.
42. Don BR, Schambelan M: Hyperkalemia in acute glomerulonephritis due to transient hyporeninemic hypoaldosteronism. *Kidney Int* 38:1159, 1990.
43. Retan JW, Dillon HC Jr: Furosemide in the treatment of acute post-streptococcal glomerulonephritis. *South Med J* 62:157, 1969.
44. Para G, Rodriguez-Iturbe B, Colina-Chourio J, et al: Short-term treatment in hypertension due to acute glomerulonephritis. *Clin Nephrol* 29:58, 1988.
45. Ingelfinger JR: Pheochromocytoma, in *Pediatric Hypertension.* Philadelphia, Saunders, 1982.
46. Hull CJ: Pheochromocytoma: Diagnosis, preoperative preparation, and anaesthetic management. *Br J Anaesth* 58:1453, 1986.
47. Nicholson JP, Vaughn ED, Pickering TG, et al: Phaeochromocytoma and prazosin. *Ann Intern Med* 99:477, 1983.
48. Navaratnarajah M, White DC: Labetalol and phaeochromocytoma. *Br J Anaesth* 56:1179, 1984.
49. Csansky-Treels JC, Lawick van Pabst L, Brands JWJ, et al: Effects of sodium nitroprusside during excision of phaeochromocytoma. *Anaesthesia* 31:60, 1976.
50. Tarazi RC, Dustan HP, Frohlich ED, et al: Plasma volume and chronic hypertension. *Arch Intern Med* 125:835, 1970.
51. Deoreo GA, Stewart BH, Tarazi RC, et al: Preoperative blood transfusion in the safe surgical management of pheochromocytoma: A review of 46 cases. *J Urol* 111:715, 1974.
52. Pinaud M, Desjars P, Tasseau F, et al: Preoperative acute volume overloading in patients with pheochromocytoma. *Crit Care Med* 13:460, 1984.

12

ENURESIS

H. Gil Rushton

The involuntary voiding of urine beyond the age of anticipated control is defined as *enuresis. Nocturnal enuresis* refers to nighttime wetting, whereas *diurnal enuresis* refers to daytime wetting. A more accurate designation would be *sleepwetting* and *awake wetting,* as recently noted by author Alison Mack.[1] For instance, many otherwise dry children who wet during the night will also wet during a daytime nap. The term *sleepwetting* may eliminate many of the negative connotations associated with the more commonly used *bed-wetting.* Although criteria vary among different authors, a reasonable definition of nocturnal enuresis is persistent sleepwetting more than twice a month past the age of 5 years. *Primary enuresis* is defined as sleepwetting in patients who have never been dry for extended periods. *Secondary enuresis* is the onset of wetting after a continuous dry period of more than 6 months.

The literature is replete with reports concerning the epidemiology, etiology, and management of nocturnal enuresis. Despite this, the causes of and treatment options for enuresis remain controversial. This is not surprising in view of the multiple factors which influence the manifestation and resolution of this perplexing phenomenon.

ATTAINING BLADDER CONTROL

Although the actual details of the neurophysiologic process by which a child acquires urinary control are not completely understood, various developmental stages have been observed.[2–5] Micturition in the newborn period is characterized by reflex voiding occurring at frequent intervals and averaging approximately 20 voids per day.[6] Bladder filling triggers voiding by afferent stimulation of the reflex arc. The efferent response results in detrusor contraction and simultaneous relaxation of the striated muscle (external) urinary sphincter. After 6 months of age, voiding becomes less frequent, but the volume of each void increases. This has been attributed to the development of unconscious inhibition of the voiding reflex.[4]

Based on the observation that bladder capacity increases and the volume of urine per kilogram per day decreases during this time period, some workers have suggested that the decrease in the frequency of voiding after 6 months of age is in part due to a growth of the bladder capacity out of proportion to the increase in the urine volume produced.[6,7] Between 1 and 2 years of age a conscious sensation of bladder fullness develops, setting the stage for voluntary control of voiding.[4] As described by Nash, this process involves three separate developmental events: (1) increase in bladder capacity to allow for adequate storage, (2) voluntary control of the periurethral striated muscle sphincter in order to initiate and terminate voiding, and (3) direct volitional control over the spinal micturition reflex.[8] Voluntary control of micturition involves a complex and as yet incompletely understood interaction of inhibitory and facilitative influences that act on the sacral micturition reflex center.[9] The ability to void or inhibit voiding voluntarily at any degree of bladder filling commonly develops during the second and third year of life, and most children acquire an adult pattern of urinary control by the age of 4 years.[10] The "typical" sequence for the development of bladder and bowel control has been described as follows: (1) nocturnal bowel control, (2) daytime bowel control, (3) daytime control of voiding, (4) nocturnal control of voiding. However, there is considerable interindividual and intercultural variation from this orderly scheme of events.[11]

EPIDEMIOLOGY

The reported prevalence of enuresis varies substantially among different populations, to some extent based on social mores and its definition by different authors (Fig. 12–1).[12] However, it is generally accepted that nocturnal enuresis occurs in 15 to 20 percent of 5-year-old children.[13] An estimated 15 percent of

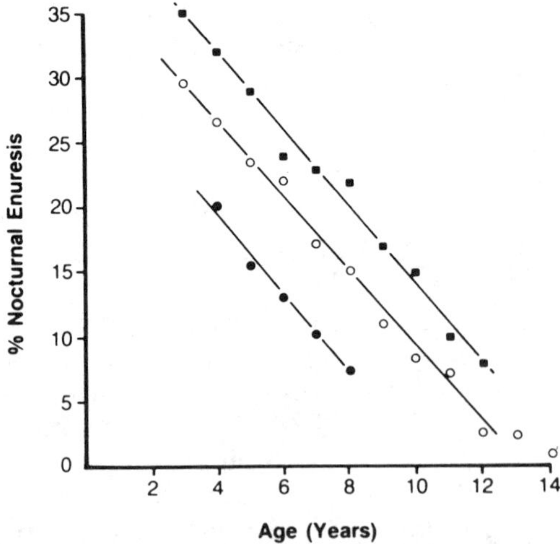

FIG. 12–1. Rates of nocturnal enuresis in children of three disparate populations. ●, children in Christchurch, New Zealand; ○, children in Khartoum, Sudan; ■, children in Baltimore, Maryland. (Reproduced with permission from Crawford JD: Introductory remarks. *J Pediatr* 114:687, 1989.)

sleepwetters will achieve nocturnal control each year and by age 15 years only 1 to 2 percent of adolescents remain enuretic.[13–15] Secondary, or onset, enuresis accounts for approximately 20 to 25 percent of the enuretic population.[13,16,17] Furthermore, approximately 15 to 20 percent of young sleepwetters also have diurnal enuresis (wetting while awake), a prevalence which rapidly decreases in children over 5 years of age.[13] Sleepwetting occurs more commonly in boys, although daytime frequency and wetting tend to be more common in girls.[13] Enuresis is reported to occur more frequently in lower socioeconomic populations and in larger families.[14]

ETIOLOGY

Nocturnal enuresis has been attributed to many diverse causes, including maturational lag and/or developmental delay, abnormal sleep patterns, psychopathology, environmental stress, organic urinary tract disease, and recently to abnormalities of the normal circadian rhythm of antidiuretic hormone (ADH) secretion. Enuresis is best viewed as a symptom rather than disease state. As such, it is a manifestation which can be affected by a number of "etiologic" factors. Efforts to identify the etiology of enuresis in an individual patient are often frustrating and may not always prove beneficial in determining management. Nevertheless, awareness of these etiologic factors is fundamental to understanding the basis of the various treatment options available.

NEUROPHYSIOLOGIC MATURATIONAL LAG

The theory that delayed functional maturation of the central nervous system is a cause of enuresis has remained a popular although not universally accepted explanation.[2,18,19] This hypothesis is largely based on epidemiologic and urodynamic evidence. The most convincing argument in favor of a maturational lag as a cause of enuresis is the observation of a high spontaneous cure rate and eventual gain of urinary control in a majority of these patients. Other indirect evidence for this hypothesis comes from the fact that the sequence of events leading to dryness in enuretic children usually mimics the pattern seen typically in normal children; that is, daytime control develops first and is followed by control during sleep. In many children, this maturational lag may be determined by genetic factors. A positive family history of bed-wetting is one of the most common findings noted by physicians who treat childhood enuresis.[20–22] In one study, the incidence of enuresis in the offspring was noted to be 77 percent when a family history of enuresis was present in both parents. On the other hand, if only one parent had a history of enuresis, 44 percent of the children were enuretic; and when neither parent had a history of enuresis, only 15 percent of the children were affected.[23]

The neurophysiologic defect involved in this maturational lag may be related to an abnormality in pelvic floor activity (urethral sphincteric guarding reflex),[24,25] inadequate central inhibition,[26] or a defect in sensation resulting in inadequate or delayed recognition of bladder filling.[4,27] Urodynamic findings of persistent bladder instability of the infantile type and poorly tolerated bladder filling reported in the majority of enuretics also support the concept of a functional maturational delay. Numerous studies have documented reduced bladder capacities in enuretics compared to normal controls.[7,28–31] The finding that the total bladder capacity in enuretics is actually normal during general anesthesia suggests that the reduced capacity may be functional rather than structural.[26]

Electroencephalography studies in enuretic children have shown an increased incidence of cerebral dysrhythmias.[32–34] Although the actual clinical significance of these minor abnormalities is not known, they have been held by some to represent a delayed functional maturation of portions of the central nervous system.[34,35]

DEVELOPMENTAL DELAY

It has been suggested that enuresis represents a developmental delay that is not the result of a lag in neurophysiological maturation but rather due to deficient learning of a habit pattern.[36] A developmental basis for enuresis is also suggested by a number of epidemiologic studies implicating a role of enviromental factors such as socioeconomic status and stress. Sleepwetting has been reported more frequently in lower socioeconomic populations and larger families.[14,37,38] The prevalence of enuresis also appears to be higher in children from institutions and broken homes, environments where greater stress might be expected.[14,39,40] Conversely, a study of children from upper middle–class neighborhoods in Boston found that 98.5 percent of those raised in low-anxiety, supportive environments achieved bladder control by the age of 5 years.[11]

McKeith has postulated that enuresis is due to developmental delay which may be the result of a transient episode of stress occurring at a critical period of development.[3] He notes that the period from the second to the fourth years of life appears to be a sensitive and perhaps vulnerable one for the acquisition of urinary control. During this time, particularly during the third year as opposed to the periods preceding and following it, there is a high rate of emergence of nocturnal bladder control. A stressful environment or anxiety-provoking episode during this critical period could prevent emergence of the behavioral skills necessary for nocturnal urinary control. This concept is supported by the findings of frequent association of secondary enuresis with a stressful event, such as birth of a new sibling in the family or separation from a parent. It is difficult to attribute secondary onset enuresis to a maturational lag unless one assumes that there is an underlying deficiency in bladder control which is "latent" and susceptible to "exaggerating" or adverse environmental factors.[4] While a higher incidence of stressful events during this sensitive period has been reported in enuretic children in some studies,[41] others have not substantiated this association.[31,22]

ANTIDIURETIC HORMONE

As early as 1952, Poulton considered relative nocturnal polyuria as a pathogenic factor in enuresis.[42] However, little attention was given to this concept until recent studies demonstrated a normal circadian variation in the secretion of antidiuretic hormone (ADH), with an increase during the nighttime.[43] Two

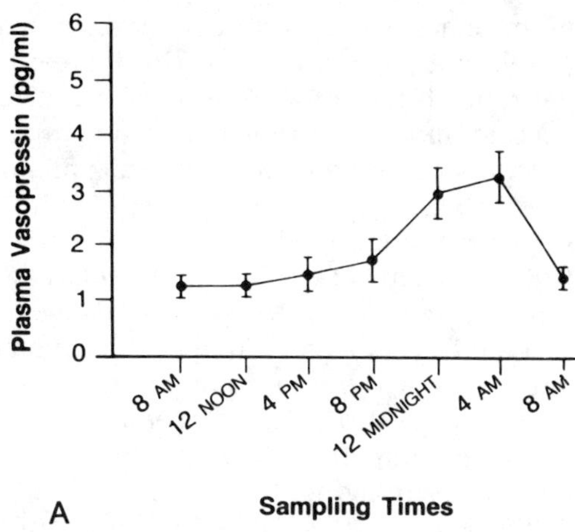

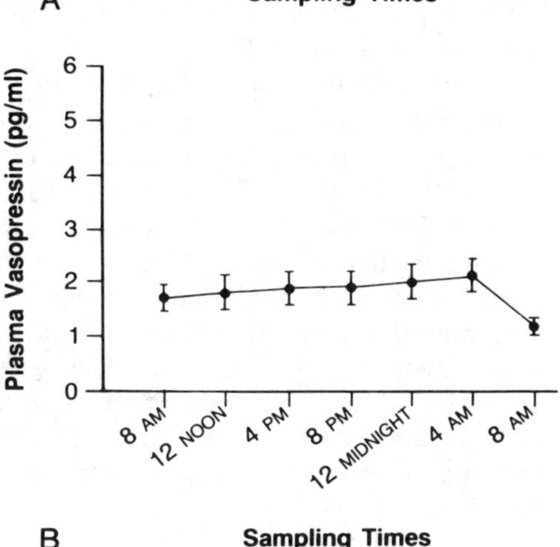

FIG. 12–2. Mean (±SE) plasma levels of vasopressin in 11 normal children (*A*) and 15 enuretic children (*B*). Vasopressin levels are stable in enuretic children throughout the 14-h period, whereas normal children show an increase at night. (Reproduced with permission from Nørgaard JP, Rittig S, Djurhuus JC: Nocturnal enuresis: An approach to treatment based on pathogenesis. *J Pediatr* 114:703, 1989.)

studies in enuretic children failed to demonstrate this increase in nocturnal ADH secretion.[44,45] In a larger controlled study,[46] similar findings of a significantly lower increase in nocturnal mean serum ADH levels was found in a group of enuretic children compared with a group of normal controls (Fig. 12–2). Significantly lower mean nocturnal urine osmolality and a higher mean nocturnal urinary excretion rate were also observed in the enuretic population. However, no difference between enuretic and normal controls was found in the total diurnal urinary volume, osmolality, or tubular capacity for reabsorption of water. Furthermore, the high urinary volume observed during sleep in enuretic children exceeded their daytime functional bladder capacity.[24] Once bladder capacity was exceeded, an enuretic episode occurred. Why these children do not wake up when the bladder is full is unclear.

SLEEP DISORDERS

Historically, bed-wetters have been considered "deep sleepers." Certainly this is one of the most common complaints of parents of enuretic children. This premise has been questioned by some who suggest that it merely reflects a subjective bias resulting from the increased efforts made by parents to awaken enuretic children.[47,48] Others have not found any significant difference in the waking time of enuretic children compared to nonenuretic controls.[22]

The development of electroencephalography in the 1950s made objective studies by sleep monitoring possible. From these studies, two categories of sleep stages were identified: rapid eye movement (REM) and nonrapid eye movement (NREM) sleep. The latter is considered "deep sleep" and is divided into four progressively deeper sleep stages (stages 1 through 4), which are identifiable by specific EEG patterns. Rapid eye movement sleep is associated with increased autonomic activity and dreaming. Normal sleep begins with NREM sleep and consists of cycles of NREM sleep, REM sleep, and occasional awakenings. Children have longer periods of deep sleep (stages 3 and 4), which progressively decrease with aging. In children over 2 years of age and throughout adulthood, REM sleep occupies 20 to 25 percent of total sleep time.[49] A number of studies in enuretics conducted in the 1960s and early 1970s suggested that enuretic events occur primarily during delta or slow-wave sleep (stages 3 and 4).[50–52]

Broughton proposed that bed-wetting was a disorder of arousal, suggesting that enuretic episodes originated in delta sleep and were preceded by arousal signals.[53] Typically, the enuretic event occurred within a few minutes as the child shifted into a lighter stage of sleep. Ritvo identified a small group of patients with psychopathology who wet during arousal or very light sleep.[54] More recent and sophisticated sleep research studies have, however, not substantiated these findings of early reports. In the later studies, enuretic episodes were observed to occur on a random basis throughout the night and in each stage of sleep in proportion to the amount of time spent in that stage.[55,56] These findings suggested that enuresis is independent of sleep stage and that the sleep patterns of enuretics are not appreciably different from those of normal children.

PSYCHOLOGICAL FACTORS

Studies in the literature reporting the prevalence and role of emotional disturbances and psychopathology in enuretics vary considerably, depending on the methodology and study populations. The conclusion of several large reviews is that, although more enuretic children are maladjusted and exhibit measurable behavioral symptoms when compared to nonenuretic controls, only a minority of enuretic children have significant underlying psychopathology.[57–59] Even in those with emotional disturbances, no specific psychiatric or behavioral disorder associated with enuresis can be identified.[22,58] Furthermore, according to psychoanalytic theory, if enuresis were a symptom of underlying emotional problems, successful treatment would result in symptom substitution by another maladaptive behavior. Several investigations of this issue have failed to demonstrate that this actually occurs.[60–64] In summary, the bulk of clinical evidence suggests that the majority of enuretics do not have significant underlying psychopathology.

URINARY TRACT INFECTION

An uncommon but clinically important cause of enuresis is urinary tract infection (UTI). An increased prevalence of bacteriuria has been noted in school-age girls (5.6 percent) with enuresis compared to those without enuresis (1.5 percent).[65] In one study of girls with recurrent infections, 16 of 56 patients with enuresis became dry following successful treatment of the infection. In the remainder, enuresis persisted despite eradiction of the UTI.[66] The increased incidence of bacteriuria in the enuretic population may be related to an underlying bladder instability, particularly in those with daytime voiding symptoms. The mechanism for this is thought to be related to the voluntary contraction of the external striated sphincter that a child makes in response to an unstable bladder contraction in an effort to prevent wetting. This leads to increased intravesical pressures and incomplete emptying, both factors predisposing to UTI. Therefore, UTI must be excluded in all patients who present with enuresis. Urinary tract infection may be found more commonly in patients with secondary enuresis.

EVALUATION

Evaluation and subsequent treatment are contingent upon the pattern of enuresis, physical examination, urinalysis, and urine culture. A careful history noting the severity and type of enuresis, associated daytime voiding problems (diurnal enuresis, intermittent or weak stream, urgency, infrequent voiding), previous episodes of UTI, pertinent psychosocial and family history, and associated constipation or encopresis is the first step. Physical examination should include abdominal and genital examination, observation of the child voiding if the history suggests an abnormal stream, and neurologic evaluation. Neurologic evaluation should include checking peripheral reflexes, evaluation of perineal sensation and anal sphincter tone, observation of gait, and visual inspection of the lower back for evidence of sacral dimpling or cutaneous anomalies suggestive of a spinal abnormality. To rule out renal or metabolic disorders that might produce obligatory polyuria, urinalysis should include determination of urinary glucose, protein, and specific gravity in addition to microscopic examination. A low urine specific gravity (< 1.024) can be further evaluated by testing a concentrated early morning specimen. Bacteriuria should be excluded by culturing the urine.

Based on this initial evaluation, patients can be categorized into (1) uncomplicated or (2) complicated enuresis (Fig. 12–3).[67] Patients with nocturnal enuresis, a normal physical examination, and normal urinalysis and urine culture have uncomplicated enuresis. Frequently, these children will have associated mild daytime frequency or enuresis with a normal urinary stream, a positive family history of enuresis, and perhaps slightly delayed developmental milestones. The incidence of organic uropathology in these children does not appear to be significantly higher than in the normal population.[68,69] No further evaluation is indicated in these patients.

In contrast, patients with a positive urine culture or history of UTI, abnormal

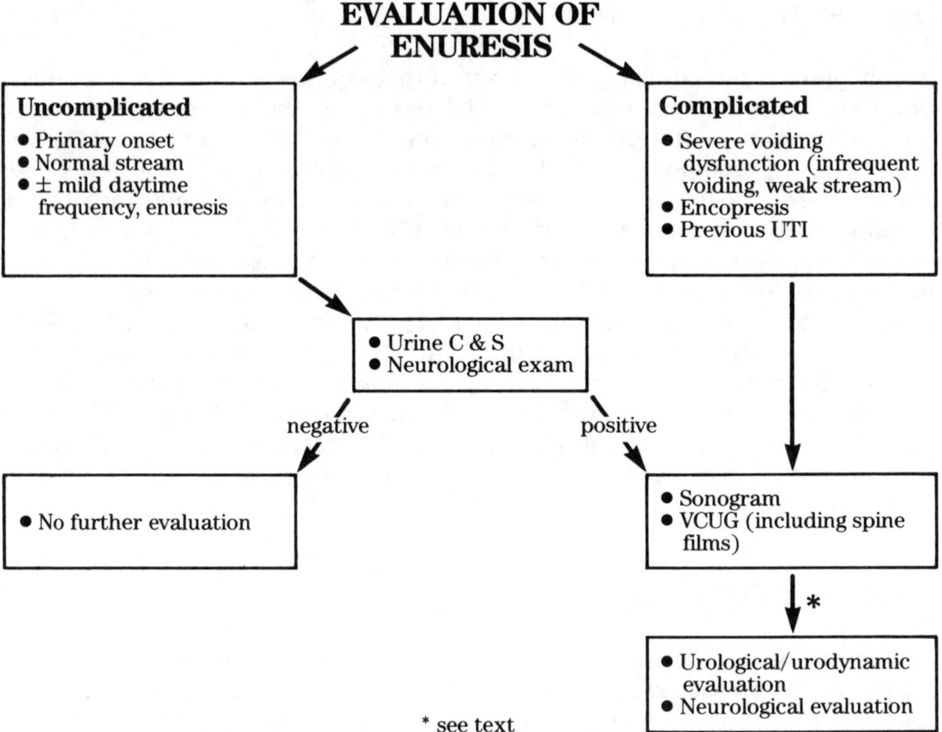

FIG. 12–3. Flowchart for evaluation of uncomplicated and complicated enuresis. C&S–culture and sensitivity; UTI–urinary tract infection; VCUG–voiding cystourethrogram. (Modified and reproduced from Rushton HG: Nocturnal enuresis: epidemiology, evaluation and currently available options. *J Pediatr* 114:691, 1989.)

urinalysis, abnormal neurologic examination, history of significant voiding dysfunction characterized by either infrequent voiding or severe frequency associated with incontinence, poor urinary stream, and/or encopresis have complicated enuresis. These patients constitute a minority of the enuretic population and should be further evaluated with a renal/bladder sonogram and voiding cystogram (with spine films) to exclude vesicoureteral reflux, bladder outlet obstruction, and/or hydroureteronephrosis associated with a thickened, unstable bladder. The latter findings indicate the need for further urologic evaluation, probably including urodynamic evaluation. If the cause is not clearly identified, neurosurgical evaluation is indicated to exclude spina bifida occulta or a tethered spinal cord.

Since many children with tubulointerstitial diseases, polycystic renal diseases, renal dysplasia, and chronic renal failure may also have symptoms of polyuria and may develop enuresis, enuretic patients with polyuria must undergo a study of baseline renal functions such as complete urinalysis and estimation of serum creatinine and blood urea nitrogen (BUN). Most patients with the above-mentioned renal diseases will have poor urinary concentrating ability and evidence of renal insufficiency.

TREATMENT

Therapy for children with enuresis must be individualized and tailored to some extent on the basis of the parents' and child's attitudes toward enuresis, the social structure, and the home environment. For example, if the child shares a room with other siblings, a moisture alarm may not be practical. Furthermore, the family must have appropriate motivation and skills in order to implement behavioral modification. On the other hand, parents may not consider drug therapy as an acceptable form of treatment for enuresis.[70]

The timing of treatment is also important and varies from patient to patient. Treatment should be advocated when wetting becomes a problem to the patient and/or family and is rarely necessary prior to age 5 or 6 years. In younger children, treatment therapy should consist of educating the family as to the causes, commonness, and prognosis of enuresis and suggesting a positive reinforcement program. As the child becomes older, specific therapy may become necessary.

While there is no objective evidence that withholding fluids in the evening, random awakenings of the child to void, or punitive measures result in significant cessation of enuresis, numerous therapeutic options for uncomplicated nocturnal enuresis can be recommended. These include behavioral modification treatment (conditioning therapy, motivational counseling, bladder training exercises), pharmacologic therapy, psychotherapy, diet therapy, and hypnotherapy. The evolution of many different types of therapy clearly suggest that no single therapeutic plan is ideal for all patients.

BEHAVIORAL MODIFICATION

A variety of behavioral modification techniques have been employed in the treatment of enuresis. Although these will be described individually, it is important to recognize that they can often be combined to improve the success of the treatment program. Generally, the behavioral modification approach requires greater commitment and involvement of the parents, the physician, and the child than does pharmacologic therapy. Therefore, motivation is a key element and must be assessed prior to instituting any program of behavioral modification. This approach will usually be more effective in children over 7 years of age who have demonstrated significant interest in becoming dry.

CONDITIONING THERAPY

Conditioning therapy revolves around the use of a signal alarm device which is electrolytically triggered as the child voids. Initially, the child wakens after or during voiding and should be encouraged to get up and void as soon as the alarm sounds. This will usually require initial supervision or direct involvement of the parents. A conditioned response of awakening and inhibition of micturition is gradually evoked by the association with bladder distension. A long-term success rate of about 70 percent has been reported following 4 to 6 months of treatment.[71–74] However, patient dropout may be significant. Some children fail to awaken to the alarm, while others may be frightened by it. In children who fail to awaken to the alarm or who awaken in a confused state, a low dose of imipramine in conjunction with the alarm system may be beneficial.[75] Other adjunctive measures which increase the effectiveness of the alarm system include positive reinforcement programs, with the child receiving a "reward" following a predetermined number of dry nights. The child is encouraged to keep a record of his or her progress, such as placing a star on a calendar for each dry night.

Relapse of enuresis occurs in 20 to 30 percent of patients treated with alarms, but a favorable outcome can be anticipated upon retreatment.[76] Relapses may actually be prevented by overlearning techniques. This involves forcing of fluids prior to bedtime in order to accentuate the conditioning stimulus.[77,78] Relapse is less likely to occur if the electrolytic alarm is discontinued following a 4-week dry period as opposed to a shorter period of dryness.[74] Despite consistently having the highest reported cure rates and lowest relapse rates, conditioning therapy is used by a minority (less than 5 percent) of primary care physicians in the United States for the treatment of enuresis.[70] This contrasts with the 32 to 50 percent of physicians who use drug therapy for enuresis. Perhaps this difference is due to the delayed success of conditioning therapy; the major commitment required by the physician, parents, and child; and the need for instant gratification in our society.

Numerous alarm systems are available at reasonable cost. Occasional complications have been reported with pad and buzzer systems, such as "buzzer ulcers" of the skin or alarm failure if the child is not positioned properly on the pad. Transistorized modifications of the alarm system, such as the Wet-Stop (Palco Labs, Santa Cruz, California) and Nytone (Medical Products, Inc., Salt Lake City, Utah) use a small sensor which is attached to the child's underwear, while the alarm is attached to the child's wrist or pajama collar (Fig. 12–4). These units are compact, safe, and effective; they avoid many of the problems associated with a pad and buzzer.

MOTIVATIONAL THERAPY

Motivational therapy involves a series of counseling sessions during which the child is encouraged to assume responsibility for his or her enuresis and to be an active participant in the treatment program.[79] This involves a combination of approaches, including reassurance, guilt removal, and emotional support by the physician and parents.[71] It also promotes development of a positive relationship between parents and child and provides positive reinforcement, ranging from words of praise to actual material rewards. Reassurance is first provided by the physician concerning both the causes and prognosis of enuresis. It is important to clarify that the child is not at fault, and punishment for bedwetting is discouraged.

One form of this approach is termed *responsibility-reinforcement therapy*.[79] In accord with the principles of "reality therapy" and behavior modification therapy, the child is encouraged to assume responsibility for his or her own learning.[80,81] A progress record is kept by the child (e.g., by means of gold stars on a calendar for each dry night). The development of "sensation awareness"—an

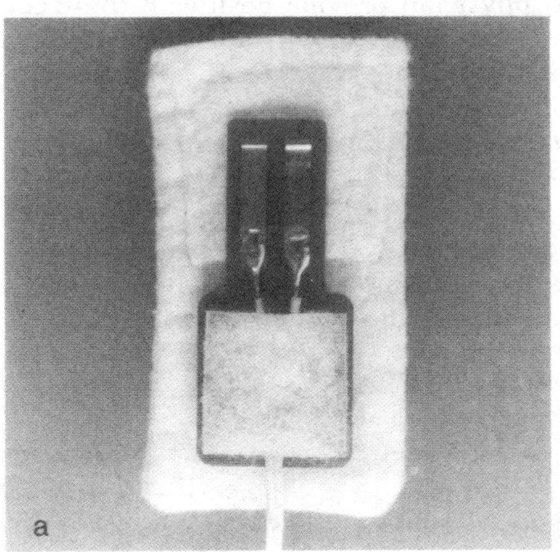

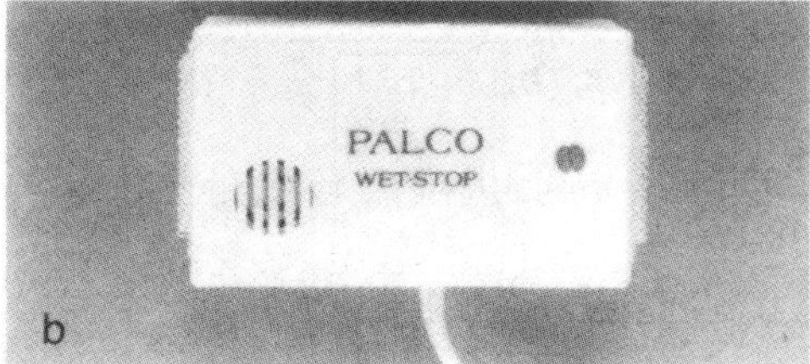

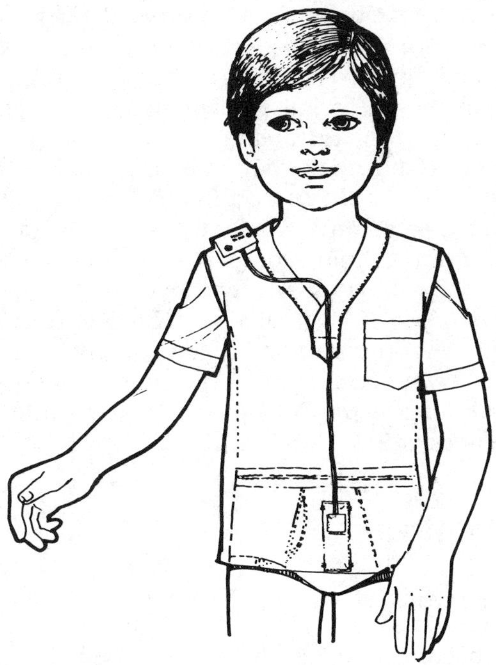

FIG. 12–4. *A*. A miniaturized nocturnal enuresis alarm system showing electrodes that are placed on the underpants. *B*. A battery-powered alarm assembly. *C*. A diagrammatic representation of the alarm assembly on the patient.

improved recognition of the sensation of a full bladder—is another responsibility which the child assumes. As the child progresses stepwise toward the ultimate goal of being dry, the parents and physician provide positive reinforcement as a means of "response shaping." This form of behavior modification obviously requires considerable input by supportive physicians and parents.

The actual cure rate with motivational counseling is unknown, but it is estimated to be about 25 percent.[71] However, "marked improvement" (defined as a decrease in enuresis of 80 percent or more) has been reported in over 70 percent of patients treated with this modality.[79] Although a longer period of treatment is required with this method as opposed to other modes of therapy, the relapse rate is lower. The principles of motivational counseling may be applied along with other treatment programs, including conditioning and pharmacologic therapy.

BLADDER RETENTION TRAINING

Bladder retention training involves conscious attempts at "bladder stretching" by voluntarily prolonging the intervals between voidings. The assumption that improvement in bladder capacity will improve or eliminate enuresis is the basis for this treatment modality. Observations of small bladder capacity and the findings of persistent detrusor instability of infantile type in some patients with enuresis support the utility of this therapy.* Adjunctive measures employed with this technique include conscious stream interruption exercises designed to increase the child's ability to withstand uninhibited bladder contractions. Overtraining by forcing fluids during the daytime may also help to improve bladder capacity although it is often difficult to convince parents of this. An increase in bladder capacity and greater improvement in enuresis have been reported in children treated by forcing fluids compared to those treated either by fluid restriction and random waking or by supportive psychological therapy.[82] In an uncontrolled study of 83 children treated with bladder retention exercises for 6 months, 66 percent demonstrated improvement, including 30 percent who were cured or had only minimal enuresis.[84] Those who responded were found to have a significantly increased bladder capacity (62.4 mL) when compared to children who were not cured (11.25 mL).

PHARMACOLOGIC THERAPY

TRICYCLIC ANTIDEPRESSANTS

A number of pharmacologic agents have been used to treat enuresis. There appears to be no benefit from the use of sedatives, stimulants, or sympathomimetic agents. Tricyclic antidepressants, particularly imipramine (Tofranil), have been studied and used most extensively in the treatment of enuresis. The exact

*Normal bladder capacity in a child can be calculated from the following formula[83]:

$$\text{Bladder capacity (in ounces)} = \text{age in years} + 2$$

pharmacologic mechanism of action of tricyclic antidepressants in enuresis is not well understood. The three theories that have been proposed hinge upon (1) the drugs' antidepressant action, (2) alterations in arousal and sleep mechanisms, and (3) anticholinergic effects.[85]

There is no evidence to suggest that depression plays a significant role as a causative factor in most enuretic children.[57] Furthermore, the antienuretic effects of tricyclic antidepressants are often immediate, whereas the antidepressant effects often take 10 or more days to appear.[86] The theory that tricyclic antidepressants work by altering sleep and arousal mechanisms is based on early sleep research studies reporting that bed-wetting occured during REM sleep and that tricyclic antidepressants decreased the percentage of this in enuretics.[87,88] However, results of recent sleep research studies do not support the existence of a significant relationship between enuretic episodes and sleep stage.[55,56,68] Imipramine has also been demonstrated to exert weak peripheral anticholinergic and antispasmodic effects as well as having a complex effect on sympathetic input to the bladder.[89–91] All this may well explain its efficacy in the treatment of enuresis. Support for this is provided by one study which documented a 34 percent increase in bladder capacity in enuretics treated with imipramine as compared to a 9 percent increase in untreated controls.[92] However, treatment with other pure anticholinergic drugs has not been found to be as effective in controlling nocturnal enuresis.[86,87]

Imipramine is generally not used to treat enuresis in children under 6 to 7 years of age and should be kept out of the reach of small children due to its extreme toxicity in case of overdose and poisoning. The success of imipramine is best noted in older children, in whom complete cessation of enuresis has been reported in up to 40 percent.[85,93,94] Initial success rates on the medication are often higher. Combined data from eight double-blind controlled studies revealed a long-term cure rate of 25 percent.[85] Some who do not respond to imipramine completely nevertheless note a significant improvement. Many children require an increasingly higher dosage of imipramine for effectiveness, and the relapse rate following discontinuation is high, particularly when the drug is stopped abruptly or prematurely.[86,87]

Imipramine is commonly prescribed as a 25-mg tablet to be taken 1 to 2 h prior to bedtime by patients 6 to 8 years of age or as a 50- to 75-mg tablet for older children and adolescents. Clinical response has been shown to correlate with plasma levels.[86,87] On a weight basis, the usual recommended dosage is 0.9 to 1.5 mg/kg/day.[95] In one study, this dosage resulted in a therapeutic plasma level in only 30 percent of patients.[96] It was suggested that a three- to fivefold increase in the dosage would be necessary to achieve therapeutic levels in all children. However, such a dosage would result in nearly toxic levels in a significant number of patients. Other investigators have reported beneficial responses with subtherapeutic plasma levels.[97]

Although the maximal effect of imipramine usually occurs within the first week of therapy,[85] it is best to continue therapy for 1 to 2 weeks before assessing efficacy and adjusting the dosage.[76] The optimal duration of therapy in those patients who respond favorably is uncertain. A reasonable approach would be to treat for 3 to 6 months, at which time the patient should be "weaned" by gradually reducing the dose and/or frequency—that is, every other night over

3 to 4 weeks.[67] Should relapse of enuresis occur, a repeat course of treatment can be started. Often, imipramine will be effective when used on an occasional "as needed" basis, and its use may be reserved for situations when staying dry is particulary important to the child (sleepovers, summer camp).[86]

Side effects from treatment with imipramine are uncommon but include anxiety, insomnia, dry mouth, nausea, and adverse personality changes. Toxic effects have been reported secondary to overdoses. Potentially fatal cardiotoxic effects of imipramine include cardiac arrhythmias, conductive blocks, hypotension, and convulsions.[98,99]

DDAVP THERAPY

Recent studies have reported promising results from the treatment of enuresis with the antidiuretic hormone desmopressin (DDAVP), an analog of arginine vasopressin (AVP). This drug, which has recently been approved for the treatment of nocturnal enuresis, has a highly specific antidiuretic effect, a prolonged half-life, and a long duration of action.[100] It is commercially available in a nasal-spray pump, which delivers a dose of 10 μg of desmopressin per spray. The proposed mechanism of action is a reduction in nocturnal urine output to a volume less than the functional bladder capacity of the enuretic child. This assumes that when a child wets at night, he or she exceeds his or her bladder capacity.[24] The drug is rapidly absorbed from the nasal mucosa, achieving maximal plasma concentrations after 40 to 55 min.[101]

Improvement in enuresis with DDAVP therapy has been reported in several double-blind, randomized trials using a dose of 10 to 40 μg, administered intranasally.[102–108] Complete dryness has been reported in 10 to 30 percent of enuretics treated with DDAVP.[102,106,108] The results of three U.S. multicenter trials demonstrated 24 to 35 percent fewer wet nights in enuretic patients who were taking this drug.[109] Almost all these studies involved children who had failed other forms of treatment. Response to DDAVP appears to be dose-related.[104,109] A significantly better antienuretic response is seen in patients whose early morning urine osmolality during treatment is greater than 1000 mOsm/kg. In one study, 75 percent of patients who had concentrated urine (osmolality greater than 1000 mOsm/kg) had a favorable antienuretic response to DDAVP, compared with only 11 percent of patients who concentrated urine to less than 1000 mOsm/kg.[107]

The relapse rate following discontinuation of DDAVP therapy is high. In one study that compared DDAVP and conditioning therapy, 70 percent of 24 patients given DDAVP improved compared with 86 percent of 22 patients treated with the enuresis alarm.[110] The group given DDAVP was significantly drier during the first week of treatment. After three weeks, however, the group treated with the enuresis alarm was drier, although the difference was not statistically significant. After treatment for 14 weeks, only 1 patient treated with conditioning therapy relapsed, compared with 10 treated with DDAVP.

In all the reported studies, side effects in patients taking DDAVP have been negligible compared with those taking placebo. The selective antidiuretic effect of DDAVP may result in water retention, leading to hyponatremia. However, in the treatment of enuresis, this effect is obviated by the once-nightly use, which allows daytime escape from the effect of the drug by obligatory polyuria.[111] There have been two case reports of symptomatic hyponatremia in children using DDAVP to treat nocturnal enuresis, including one 13-year-old girl who had cystic fibrosis[112] and one healthy 6-year-old boy.[113]

ANTICHOLINERGIC DRUGS

Oxybutynin (Ditropan) and other anticholinergics have been used to reduce or abolish uninhibited bladder contractions; these drugs may be beneficial in patients who have daytime frequency or enuresis that is associated with uninhibited bladder contractions, as manifested by the symptoms of urgency and urge incontinence.[114] However, oxybutynin is rarely beneficial for patients with exclusively nocturnal enuresis. In a recent prospective double-blind crossover study of 30 such children, there was no difference in response to 10 mg oxybutynin compared to placebo.[115] The dose in children over 6 years old is usually 5 mg 2 or 3 times a day. Common side effects include dryness of the mouth and facial flushing. Occasionally, hyperpyrexia may occur, particularly when the child is exposed to hot weather. Excessive dosage may result in blurring of vision.

MISCELLANEOUS TREATMENTS

Varying success has been reported with psychotherapy but it probably does not play a major role in the treatment of most children with uncomplicated nocturnal enuresis who do not also have underlying psychopathology.[116] In those patients with complicated enuresis associated with severe voiding dysfunction, infrequent voiding, and encopresis, a careful family and social history may reveal underlying psychosocial stresses. Treatment of these children is initially directed toward emotional support. Patients with bladder or upper tract damage secondary to severe voiding dysfunction who do not have an organic neurologic or obstructive lesion may also benefit from timed voidings, anticholinergic therapy, and/or biofeedback therapy. Occasionally renal damage may be so severe as to necessitate a program of intermittent catheterization if bladder emptying cannot be achieved by other means. In some of these cases psychotherapy may also be warranted.

Diet therapy may have a role in a minority of enuretic patients. One study reported significant improvement by serially deleting certain foods such as dairy products, chocolate, cola, citrus fruit and juices, and Kool-Aid from the diets of enuretic children.[117] However the success of such a program has not been substantiated by other investigators and may be based on the attention focused on the patient during therapy.

Although not widely practiced, hypnotherapy has reportedly brought about dramatic improvements in children with enuresis. In one study, 31 of 40 children treated by hypnotherapy were cured and an additional 6 were improved.[118] The majority of those cured ceased wetting within the first month of therapy and continued to remain dry during follow-up from 6 to 28 months. Similar success was reported in a group of patients with specific precipitating stresses or high level of family tension at the onset of enuresis.[119] Despite this reported success, hypnotherapy is rarely recommended by physicians for the treatment of enuresis.

SUMMARY

Enuresis is a symptom, not a disease state, and its etiology remains controversial. Evidence supports the theory of a maturational lag and/or developmental delay as a cause of enuresis. Although psychopathology and enuresis may coexist, a majority of enuretic children do not suffer from psychological disorders.

Treatment of childhood enuresis must begin with a careful history, physical examination, urinalysis, and urine culture to determine if one is dealing with uncomplicated or complicated enuresis. The majority of patients will have uncomplicated enuresis, and a number of treatment options are available to the physician which can be tailored to the individual patient. Behavioral modification techniques, specifically conditioning therapy, have the highest reported long-term cure rates, averaging 70 percent. This approach requires greater commitment and involvement of the physician, parents, and child than does pharmacologic therapy. Imipramine has been the most commonly used drug therapy. Recently, desmopressin has shown promising results, with similar reported response rates.

REFERENCES

1. Mack, Alison: *Dry All Night.* Boston, Little Brown, 1989.
2. Muellner SR: Development of urinary control in children: Some aspects of the cause and treatment of primary enuresis. *JAMA* 172:1256, 1960.
3. MacKeith RC, Meadow SR, Turner RK: How children become dry, in Kolvin I, MacKeith RC, Meadow SR (eds): *Bladder Control and Enuresis.* London, Heinemann, 1973, p3.
4. Yeates WK: Bladder function in normal micturition, in Kolvin I, MacKeith RC, Meadow SR (eds): *Bladder Control and Enuresis.* London, Heinemann 1973, p28.
5. Duche DJ: Patterns of micturition in infancy, in Kolvin I, MacKeith RC, Meadow SR (eds): *Bladder Control and Enuresis.* London, Heinemann, 1973, p23.
6. Goellner MH, Ziegler EE, Foman SJ: Urination during the first three years of life. *Nephron* 28:174, 1981.
7. Koff SA: Enuresis, in: *Campbell's Urology,* 5th ed. Philadelphia, Saunders, 1986, p2179.
8. Nash DFE: The development of micturition control with special reference to enuresis. *Ann R Coll Surg Engl* 5:318, 1949.
9. Mahony DT, Laferte RO, Blais DJ: Integral storage in voiding reflexes. *Urology* 9:95, 1977.
10. Stein ZA, Susser MW: Social factors in the development of sphincter control. *Dev Med Child Neurol* 9:692, 1967.

11. Brazelton TB: A child-oriented approach to toilet training. *Pediatrics* 29:121, 1962.
12. Crawford JD: Treatment of nocturnal enuresis: Introductory comments. *J Pediatr* 114:687, 1989.
13. De Jonge DA: Epidemiology of enuresis: A survey of the literature, in Kolvin I, MacKeith RC, Meadow SR (eds): *Bladder Control and Enuresis.* London, Heinemann, 1973, p39.
14. Miller FJW: Children who wet the bed, in Kolvin I, MacKeith RC, Meadow SR (eds): *Bladder Control and Enuresis.* London, Heinemann, 1973, p47.
15. Forsythe WI, Redmond A: Enuresis and spontaneous cure rate: Study of 1129 enuretics. *Arch Dis Child* 49:259, 1974.
16. Hallgren B: Nocturnal enuresis: Aetiologic aspects. *Acta Paediatr* 118(suppl):66, 1959.
17. Notschaele LA: Vedwateren bij kinderen van de kleuter-en lagere school. *Tijdschr Soc Geneesk* 42:226, 1964.
18. Bakwin H: Enuresis in children. *J Pediatr* 58:806, 1961.
19. MacKeith RC: Is maturation delay a frequent factor in the origins of primary nocturnal enuresis? *Dev Med Child Neurol* 14:217, 1972.
20. Hallgren B: Enuresis. A clinical and genetic study. *Acta Psychiatr Neurol Scand (suppl)* 114:1, 1957.
21. Fergusson DM, Hons BA, Horwood LJ, et al: Factors related to the age of attainment of nocturnal bladder control: An 8-year longitudinal study. *Pediatrics* 78:884, 1986.
22. Kaffman M, Elizur E: Infants who become enuretics: A longitudinal study of 161 kibbutz children. *Monogr Soc Res Child Devel* 42(2, serial no 170):1, 1977.
23. Bakwin H: The genetics of enuresis, in Kolvin I, MacKeith RC, Meadow SR (eds): *Bladder Control and Enuresis.* London, Heinemann, 1973, p73.
24. Norgaard JP: Urodynamics in enuresis I: Reservoir function. *Neurol Urol Urodyn* 8:119, 1989.
25. Mahony DT, Laferte RO, Blais DJ: Studies of enuresis: IX. Evidence of a mild form of compensated detrusor hyperreflexia in enuretic children. *J Urol* 126:520, 1981.
26. Troup CW, Hodgson NB: Nocturnal functional bladder capacity in enuretic children. *J Urol* 129:132, 1971.
27. Gillison TH, Skinner JL: Treatment of nocturnal enuresis by the electric alarm. *Br Med J* 2:1268, 1958.
28. Esperanca M, Gerrard JW: Nocturnal enuresis: Studies in bladder function in normal children and enuretics. *Can Med Assoc J* 101:269, 1969.
29. Starfield B, Mellits ED: Increase in functional bladder capacity and improvement in enuresis. *J Pediatr* 72:483, 1968.
30. Hallman N: On the ability of enuretic children to hold urine. *Acta Paediatr* 39:87, 1950.
31. Zaleski A, Gerrard JW, Shokeir MHK: Nocturnal enuresis: The importance of a small bladder capacity, in Kolvin I, MacKeith RC, Meadow SR (eds): *Bladder Control and Enuresis.* London, Heinemann, 1973, p95.
32. Campbell EW Jr, Young JD Jr: Enuresis and its relationship to electroencephalographic disturbances. *J Urol* 96:947, 1966.
33. Fermaglich JL: Electroencephalographic study of enuretics. *Am J Dis Child* 118:473, 1969.
34. Kaijtor S, Ovary I, Zsandanyi O: Nocturnal enuresis: electroencephalographic and cystometric examinations. *Acta Med Acad Sci Hung* 23:153, 1967.
35. Edvardsen P: Neurophysiologic aspects of enuresis. *Acta Neurol Scand* 48:222, 1972.

36. Lovibond SH, Coote MA: Enuresis, in: Costello CG (ed): *Symptoms of Psychopathology.* New York, Wiley, 1970, pp
37. Essen J, Peckham C: Nocturnal enuresis in childhood. *Dev Med Child Neurol* 18:577, 1976.
38. McKendry JBJ, Williams HA, Broughton C: Enuresis—a study of untreated patients. *Appl Ther* 10:815, 1968.
39. Douglas JWB: Broken homes and child behavior. *J R Coll Phys London* 4:203, 1970.
40. Stein ZA, Susser MW: Nocturnal enuresis as a phenomenon of institutions. *Dev Med Child Neurol* 8:677, 1966.
41. Douglas JWB: Early disturbing events in later enuresis, in Kolvin I, MacKeith RC, Meadow SR (eds): *Bladder Control and Enuresis.* London, Heinemann, 1973, p109.
42. Poulton EM: Relative nocturnal polyuria as a factor in enuresis. *Lancet* 2:906, 1952.
43. George CPL, Messerli FH, Genest J, et al: Diurnal variation of plasma vasopressin in man. *J Clin Endocrinol Metab* 41:332, 1975.
44. Norgaard JP, Pedersen EB, Djurhuus JC: Diurnal antidiuretic-hormone levels in enuretics. *J Urol* 1985;134:1029.
45. Puri VN: Urinary levels of antidiuretic hormone in nocturnal enuresis. *Ind Pediatr* 17:675, 1980.
46. Rittig S, Knudsen UB, Nørgaard JP, et al: Abnormal diurnal rhythm of plasma vasopressin and urinary output in patients with enuresis. *Am J Physiol* 256: F664, 1989.
47. Graham P: Depth of sleep and enuresis: A critical review, in Kolvin I. MacKeith RC, Meadow SR (eds): *Bladder Control and Enuresis.* London, Heinemann, 1973, p78.
48. Boyd MM: The depth of sleep in enuretic children and in non-enuretic controls. *J Psychosom Res* 4:274, 1960.
49. Lowy FH: Recent sleep and dream research: Clinical implications. *Can Med Assoc J* 102:1069, 1970.
50. Rechtschaffen A, Kales A: *A Manual of Standardized Terminology, Techniques and Scoring System for Sleep Stages of Human Subjects.* Los Angeles, Brain Information Service/ Brain Research Institute, UCLA, 1968.
51. Evans JI: Sleep of enuretics. *Br Med J* 3:110, 1971.
52. Finley W: An EEG study of the sleep of enuretics at three age levels. *Clin Electroencephalogr* 2:35, 1971.
53. Broughton RF: Sleep disorders: Disorders of arousal? *Science* 159:1070, 1968.
54. Ritvo ER, Ornitz EM, Gottileb F, et al: Arousal and nonarousal enuretic events. *Am J Psychiatry* 126:115, 1969.
55. Mikkelsen EJ, Rapoport JL, Nee L, et al: Childhood enuresis: I. Sleep patterns and psychopathology. *Arch Gen Psychiatry* 37:1139, 1980.
56. Kales A, Kales JM, Jacobson A, et al: Effect of imipramine on enuretic frequency and sleep stages. *Pediatrics* 60:431, 1977.
57. Werry JS: Enuresis—a psychosomatic entity? *Can Med Assoc J* 97:319, 1967.
58. Shaffer D: The association between enuresis and emotional disorder: A review of the literature, in Kolvin I, MacKeith RC, Meadow SR (eds): *Bladder Control and Enuresis.* London, Heinemann, 1973, p118.
59. Moffatt MEK: Nocturnal enuresis: Psychologic implications of treatment and nontreatment. *J Pediatr* 114(suppl):697, 1989.
60. Werry JS, Cohrssen J: Enuresis—an etiologic and therapeutic study. *J Pediatr* 67:423, 1965.
61. Behrle FC, Elkin MH, Laybourne PC: Evaluation of a conditioning device in the treatment of nocturnal enuresis. *Pediatrics* 17:849, 1956.

62. Lovibond SH: Conditioning in enuresis. New York, Pergamon, 1964.
63. Bindelglas PM, Dee G: Enuresis treatment with imipramine hydrochloride: A 10-year follow up study. *Am J Psychiatry* 135:1549, 1978.
64. Oppel WC, Harper PA, Rider RW: The age of attaining bladder control. *Pediatrics* 42:614, 1968.
65. Dodge WF, West EF, Bridgforth EB, et al: Nocturnal enuresis in 6- to 10-year old children: Correlation of bacteriuria, proteinuria and dysuria. *Am J Dis Child* 120:32, 1970.
66. Jones B, Gerrard JW, Shokeir MK, et al: Recurrent urinary infections in girls: Relation to enuresis. *Can Med Assoc J* 106:127, 1972.
67. Rushton HG: Nocturnal enuresis: Epidemiology, evaluation and currently available treatment options. *J Pediatr* 114(suppl):691, 1989.
68. American Academy of Pediatrics, Committee on Radiology: Excretory urography for evaluation of enuretics. *Pediatrics* 65:644, 1980.
69. Redmond JF, Seibert JJ: The uroradiographic evaluation of the enuretic child. *J Urol* 122:799, 1979.
70. Shelov SP, Gundy J, Weiss JC, et al: Enuresis: A contrast of attitudes of parents and physicians. *Pediatrics* 67:707, 1981.
71. Schmitt BD: Nocturnal enuresis: An update on treatment. *Pediatr Clin North Am* 29:21, 1982.
72. Dische S: Management of enuresis. *Br Med J* 2:33, 1971.
73. Wagner W, Johnson SB, Walker D, et al: A controlled comparison of two treatments of nocturnal enuresis. *J Pediatr* 101:302, 1982.
74. Forsythe WI, Redmond A: Enuresis and the electric alarm: A study of 200 cases. *Br Med J* 1:211, 1970.
75. Philpott MG, Flasher MC: The treatment of enuresis: Further clinical experience with imipramine. *Br J Clin Pract* 24:327, 1970.
76. Perlmutter AD: Enuresis, in: *Clinical Pediatric Urology,* 2nd ed. Philadelphia, Saunders, 1985, p 311.
77. Morgan RTT: Relapse and therapeutic response in the conditioning treatment of enuresis: A review of recent findings on intermittent reinforcement, overlearning and stimulus intensity. *Behav Res Ther* 16:278, 1978.
78. Brooshank DJ: The conditioning treatment of bed-wetting in secondary school age children. *J Adolesc* 2:239, 1979.
79. Marshall S, Marshall HH, Lyons RP: Enuresis: An analysis of various therapeutic approaches. *Pediatrics* 52:813, 1973.
80. Glasser W: *Reality Therapy.* New York, Harper & Row, 1965.
81. Skinner BF: *Science and Human Behavior.* New York, Macmillan, 1953.
82. Haaglund TB: Enuretic children treated with fluid restriction or forced drinking: A clinical and cystometric study. *Ann Paediatr Fenn* 11:84, 1965.
83. Koff SA: Estimating bladder capacity in children. *Urology* 21:248, 1988.
84. Starfield B, Mellits ED: Increase in functional bladder capacity and improvement in enuresis. *J Pediatr* 72:483, 1968.
85. Blackwell B, Currah J: The psychopharmacology of nocturnal enuresis, in Kolvin I, MacKeith RC, Meadow SR (eds): *Bladder Control and Enuresis.* London, Heinemann, 1973, p231.
86. Rapoport JL, Mikkelsen EJ, Zavadil A, et al: Childhood enuresis: II. Psychopathology, tricyclic concentration in plasma, and antienuretic effect. *Arch Gen Psychiatr* 37:1146, 1980.

87. Pierce CM, Whitman RM, Mass JW, et al: Enuresis and dreaming: Experimental studies. *Arch Gen Psychiatr* 4:116, 1961.
88. Khazan N, Sulman EG: Effects of imipramine on paradoxical sleep in animals with reference to dreaming and enuresis. *Psychopharmacologia* 10:89, 1966.
89. Sigg EB: Pharmacological studies with Tofranil. *Can Psychiatr Assoc J* 4:75, 1959.
90. Stephenson JD: Physiological and pharmacological basis for the chemotherapy of imipramine. *Psychol Med* 9:249, 1979.
91. Labay P, Boyarsky S: The action of imipramine on the bladder musculature. *J Urol* 109:385, 1973.
92. Haaglund TB, Parkkulainen KV: Enuretic children treated with imipramine (Tofranil): A cystometric study. *Ann Paediatr Fenn* 11:53, 1965.
93. Bindelglas PM, Dee GH, Enos FA: Medical and psychosocial factors in enuretic children treated with imipramine hydrochloride. *Am J Psychiatry* 1124:1107, 1968.
94. General Practitioner Research Group: Imipramine in enuresis. *Practitioner* 203:94, 1969.
95. Poussaint AF, Ditman KS: A controlled study of imipramine (Tofranil) in the treatment of childhood enuresis. *J Pediatr* 67:283, 1965.
96. Jorgenson OJ, Lober M, Christansen J, et al: Plasma concentration and clinical effect in imipramine treatment of childhood enuresis. *Clin Pharmacokinet* 5:386, 1980.
97. Devane C: Concentrations of imipramine and its metabolites during enuresis therapy. *Pediatr Pharmacol* 4:245, 1984.
98. Penny R: Imipramine hydrochloride poisoning in childhood. *Am J Dis Child* 116:181, 1968.
99. Fouron J, Chicoine R: ECG changes in fatal imipramine (Tofranil) intoxication. *Pediatrics* 48:777, 1971.
100. Andersson KE, Arner B: Effects of DDAVP, a synthetic analogue of vasopressin, in patients with cranial diabetes insipidus. *Acta Med Scand* 192;21, 1972.
101. Harris AS, Ohlin M, Lathagen S, et al: Effects of concentration and volume on nasal bioavailability and biological response to desmopressin. *J Pharm Sci* 77:337, 1988.
102. Tuvemo T: DDAVP in childhood nocturnal enuresis. *Acta Paediatr Scand* 67;753, 1978.
103. Aladjem M, Wohl R, Boichis H, et al: Desmopressin and nocturnal enuresis. *Arch Dis Child* 57:137, 1982.
104. Post EM, Richman RA, Blackett PR, et al: Desmospressin response of enuretic children: Effects of age and frequency of enuresis. *Am J Dis Child* 173:962, 1983.
105. Terho P, Kekomaki M: Management of nocturnal enuresis with a vasopressin analogue. *J Urol* 131:925, 1984.
106. Pedersen PS, Hejl M, Kjoller SS: Desamino-D-Arginine vasopressin in childhood nocturnal enuresis. *J Urol* 133:65, 1985.
107. Dimson SB: DDAVP and urine osmolality in refractory enuresis. *Arch Dis Child* 61:1104, 1986.
108. Fjellsted-Paulsen A, Wille S, Harris AS: Comparison of intranasal and oral desmopressin for nocturnal enuresis. *Arch Dis Child* 62:674, 1987.
109. Klauber GT: Clinical efficacy and safety of desmopressin in treatment of nocturnal enuresis. *J Pediatr* 114(suppl):719, 1989.
110. Wille S: Comparison of desmopressin and enuresis alarm for nocturnal enuresis. *Arch Dis Child* 621:30, 1986.
111. Hilton P, Stanton SL: The use of desmopressin (DDAVP) in nocturnal urinary frequency in the female. *Br J Urol* 54:252, 1982.

112. Simmonds EJ, Mahoney MJ, Littlewood JM: Convulsion and coma after intranasal DDAVP in cystic fibrosis. *Br Med J* 297:1614, 1988.
113. Bamford MFM, Cruickshank G: Dangers of intranasal desmopressin for nocturnal enuresis (letter). *JR Coll Gen Pract* 39:345, 1989.
114. Thompson IM, Lauretz R: Oxybutynin in bladder spasm, neurogenic bladder, and enuresis. *Urology* 8:452, 1976.
115. Lovering JS, Tallett SE, McKendry JBJ: Oxybutynin efficacy in treatment of primary enuresis. *Pediatrics* 82:104, 1988.
116. Fraser MJ: Nocturnal enuresis. *Practitioner* 208:203, 1972.
117. Esperanca M, Gerrard JW: Nocturnal enuresis: Comparison of the effect of imipramine and dietary restriction of bladder capacity. *Can Med Assoc J* 101:721, 1969b.
118. Olness K: The use of self-hypnosis in the treatment of childhood nocturnal enuresis. *Clin Pediatr* 14:273, 1975.
119. Collison, PR: Hypnotherapy in the management of nocturnal enuresis. *Med J Aust* 1:52, 1970.

13

CYSTIC RENAL DISEASES

Kanwal K. Kher

A variety of kidney diseases can be associated with cystic lesions in the renal parenchyma, and in some cases renal cysts may constitute one of the primary features of a systemic disease. Accordingly, cystic renal diseases are a heterogenous group of disorders with varing clinical manifestations and prognoses. While early onset of symptoms and renal failure is characteristic in some cystic renal diseases, others may remain essentially asymptomatic throughout life. Most diseases characterized by renal cysts are genetic or developmental in origin, but acquired cystic lesions may be seen in patients with end-stage renal disease (ESRD) undergoing long-term kidney dialysis.[1,2] According to the 1990 report of the United States Renal Data System,[3] cystic renal diseases account for 4.2 percent of children with ESRD in the United States. The pathogenesis of renal cysts remains an enigma. Significant progress has, however, been made toward identifying the genetic defect involved in autosomal dominant polycystic kidney disease, which is a common cause of ESRD in adults. This chapter discusses the classification, diagnosis, and management of cystic renal diseases in children.

CLASSIFICATION

The classification of diseases associated with renal cysts has been a confusing and controversial subject. Most classifications of cystic renal diseases are based on morphologic features of the kidneys in affected individuals.[4,5] Potter and coworkers utilized information gathered from the microdissection of kidneys affected by cystic changes and classified renal cysts into four categories (Table 13–1).[6] A clinicopathologic classification that also recognizes genetic aspects of these diseases has recently been proposed by the Section of Urology of the American Academy of Pediatrics (Table 13–2).[7]

It must be emphasized that the term *polycystic kidney disease* (PKD) should not be used indiscriminately to denote all forms of renal cystic disease. This term is reserved for describing two inherited conditions known as *autosomal recessive (infantile) polycystic kidney disease* and *autosomal dominant (adult) polycystic kidney disease.*

TABLE 13–1. Potter Classification of Renal Cysts

Classification	Microdissection Features	Clinical Equivalent
Type I	Diffuse enlargement of the terminal branches of the collecting tubules, with large diverticula and saccular enlargement of more proximal branches. The pattern of branching of the collecting ducts is normal.	Infantile polycystic kidney disease.
Type II	Collecting tubules have few branches, are enlarged, terminate in large cysts, and have only a few attached glomeruli. Connective tissue content is increased.	Multicystic dysplastic kidney disease
Type III	Local or diffuse enlargement of any segment of the nephron or collecting tubule may be seen. Collecting tubules branch irregularly.	Adult polycystic kidney disease
Type IV	The terminal portions of the collecting tubules are dilated and the nephrons arising from them are abnormal. Other features of obstructive uropathy are present in the neonate.	Renal cysts associated with obstructive uropathy. The condition is not inherited.

AUTOSOMAL RECESSIVE POLYCYSTIC KIDNEY DISEASE

Autosomal recessive polycystic kidney disease (ARPKD) is the most common but not the only type of cystic renal disease encountered in children. Other terms used to describe ARPKD are *infantile polycystic kidney disease* or *Potter type I renal cysts.* The precise incidence of ARPKD is unknown; autopsy data suggest that it is encountered in 1.3 to 5.9 per 1000 pediatric autopsies.[8,9] European reports show that ARPKD accounts for 2.1 percent of children with ESRD.[10] It has been estimated that ARPKD occurs in one out of 40,000 persons in the general population.[11]

PATHOLOGY[6,11,12]

Bilateral enlargement of the kidneys with preservation of their reniform shape is the cardinal pathologic feature of ARPKD. Many cysts are visible to the naked eye on the cortical surface. A cut section of the kidney demonstrates poor differentiation between cortex and medulla, and the renal pyramids are difficult to identify (Fig. 13–1). The kidney tissue is replaced by dilated cystic structures that run perpendicular to the cortical surface. Histologically, these cysts represent dilated collecting tubules lined by well-preserved cuboidal epithelium.

TABLE 13–2. Classification of Renal Cystic Disease Suggested by the Section of Urology of the American Academy of Pediatrics

GENETIC
Polycystic kidney disease
Autosomal recessive (infantile) polycystic kidney disease
Autosomal dominant (adult) kidney disease
Juvenile nephronophthisis/medullary cystic disease complex
Juvenile nephronopthisis (autosomal recessive)
Medullary cystic disease (autosomal dominant)
Congenital nephrotic syndrome (autosomal recessive)
Cysts associated with multiple malformation syndromes:
Meckel's syndrome
Lawrence-Moon-Biedl syndrome
Ivemark syndrome
Zellweger syndrome
Tuberous sclerosis
von Hippel-Lindau disease
NONGENETIC
Multicystic kidney disease (multicystic renal dysplasia)
Multilocular cysts
Simple cysts
Medullary sponge kidney (less than 5 percent are inherited)
Acquired cystic renal disease in chronic dialysis patients
Calyceal diverticulum (pyelogenic cysts)

Source: From Glassberg KI, Stephens FD, Lebowitz RI, et al.: Renal dysgenesis and cystic disease of the kidney: A report on the terminology, nomenclature, and classification. Section on Urology, American Academy of Pediatrics. *J Urol* 138:1085, 1987. Adapted and reproduced by permission. © 1987 by Williams & Wilkins.

Staining with peroxidase-labeled lectins has confirmed that these cysts originate from the distal nephron.[13] Glomeruli are normal in appearance; dysplastic elements such as cartilage, bone, nerve, muscle, etc. are not seen in the renal parenchyma.

GENETICS AND PRENATAL DIAGNOSIS

Transmitted by autosomal recessive inheritance, ARPKD carries a 25-percent probability of recurrence in the pregnancies of the patients. Both parents are free of clinical disease, and their renal sonograms are normal. The genetic defect responsible for ARPKD has not yet been identified. Prenatal diagnosis of ARPKD is difficult but may be considered in a fetus with oligohydramnios and bilaterally enlarged kidneys that show a diffusely increased central renal echo pattern with peripheral hypoechoic areas and poor differentiation of intrarenal structures.[14–16] Renal cysts are usually not visualized by ultrasonography in the

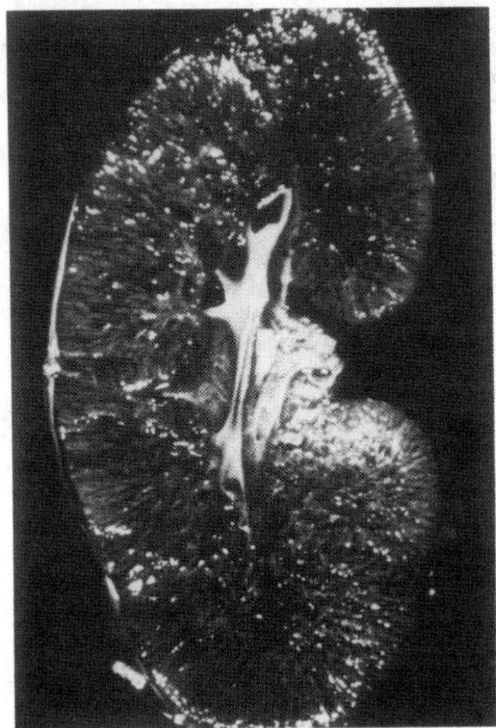

FIG. 13–1. Gross appearance of the kidney in ARPKD. The cysts are delineated by latex injection. (Reproduced by permission from Ault BH, Burton E, Stapleton FB: Cystic kidney disease in infants: A brighter outlook. *Contemp Pediatr* 5:123, 1988. © 1988 by *Contemporary Pediatrics*.)

fetal kidneys. Elevated α-fetoprotein in the amniotic fluid and maternal plasma has been reported in pregnancies where the fetus is affected by ARPKD.[16] The significance of this observation in the prenatal diagnosis of ARPKD is unclear at this time.

CLINICAL MANIFESTATIONS

The clinical onset of ARPKD is not restricted to the neonatal period or early infancy; in fact, many patients remain asymptomatic until late childhood or even adolescence.[17–19] Hepatic fibrosis commonly occurs and is regarded as an integral feature of this disease.[4] The extent of such hepatic involvement is inversely related to the patient's age.[4,11] Accordingly, the clinical manifestations of hepatic fibrosis are less common in neonates and young children but are more often seen in older children with ARPKD (Fig. 13–2). Blythe and Ockenden[4] classified ARPKD—on the basis of age of presentation, clinical manifestations, and prognosis—into the following four clinical categories.

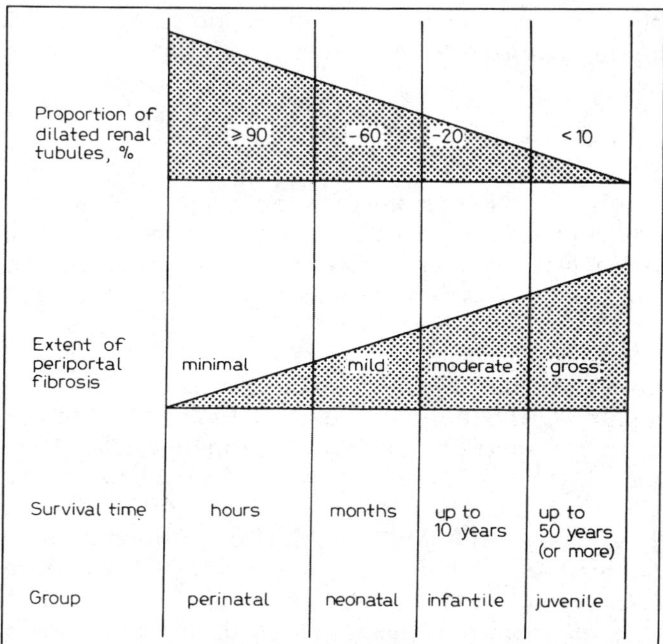

FIG. 13–2. **Manifestations of ARPKD according to age of patient. Based on the classification of Blythe and Ockenden.[4] (Reproduced by permission from Neumann HPH, Zerres K, Fischer CL, et al: Late manifestation of autosomal-recessive polycystic kidney disease in two sisters. *Am J Nephrol* 8:194, 1988. Copyright © 1988 by S. Karger, Basel, Switzerland.)**

PERINATAL

This type of ARPKD is detected at birth. Most of these patients, according to Blythe and Ockenden, have a poor prognosis and rarely survive beyond a few weeks.[4] Marked abdominal distension caused by severely enlarged kidneys is obvious at birth, renal involvement is generally severe, and renal failure occurs early.

NEONATAL

Neonatal ARPKD is diagnosed during the first month of life; renal enlargement is its hallmark. Although renal involvement is severe, kidney failure evolves slowly, with death occurring in 6 to 8 months. Recent studies have, however, suggested a more optimistic outlook for both the perinatal and neonatal varieties of ARPKD.[12,18–20]

INFANTILE

In the infantile variant of ARPKD, the disease is detected between 1 month and 1 year of age, usually between 3 and 6 months. Hepatic enlargement with portal hypertension are common clinical manifestations. Although chronic renal failure develops, progression to ESRD is slow and survival into adolescence is common.

JUVENILE

The juvenile form of ARPKD becomes clinically apparent after the first year of life. Chronic renal insufficiency manifests itself late in these patients; liver disease and portal hypertension are, however, prominent clinical concerns. The juvenile variant of ARPKD is also described sometimes as *congenital hepatic fibrosis with renal cysts.*

About 45 to 60 percent of patients with ARPKD are diagnosed during the neonatal period.[12,18] In the future, however, routine fetal ultrasonography will probably increase its detection during intrauterine life. The classic manifestation of ARPKD in neonates consists of severe bilateral enlargement of the kidneys.[4,12,18–20] Labor and delivery may be difficult for some of the patients because of their abdominal enlargement and oligohydramnios. Stillbirth and early neonatal death are common among severely affected fetuses, the usual cause of death being pulmonary insufficiency due to hypoplastic lungs. In one study, autopsy evidence of pulmonary hypoplasia and atelectasis was observed in 48 of the 54 neonates with ARPKD who died in the first month of life.[19] Respiratory problems are compounded in these patients by poor respiratory excursions due to compression of the diaphragm by the enlarged kidneys and recurrent episodes of pneumothorax.[18–20] Compression of the gastrointestinal tract often leads to poor gastric emptying and frequent vomiting, both of which have an adverse effect on nutrition.

Hypertension has been reported in 60 to 65 percent of patients with ARPKD and develops early in the course of the disease.[4,12,18,20] Its pathogenesis is unclear. Plasma renin activity has been reported to be either normal or suppressed for patient's age, suggesting expansion of the intravascular volume.[18] Yet in the author's own experience as well as that of others,[12] angiotensin converting enzyme (ACE) inhibitors such as captopril are very effective in treating such hypertension. Hyponatremia is common in neonates with ARPKD and has been reported in 40 to 80 percent of them.[18,19] In the patients studied by Kaplan et al.,[18] hyponatremia was believed to be dilutional in origin. Although inadequate sodium intake and excessive renal sodium excretion in a neonate can also result in hyponatremia, these were not considered to be contributing factors in this study. Renal function may be compromised at birth, but oliguria is uncommon.[12,19] Transient improvment of GFR is well known to occur in patients with ARPKD who survive the neonatal period, but decline of renal function may begin in survivors unpredictably, usually during the second year of life.[12,19–22] Poor urine concentrating ability is a prominent feature of ARPKD and does not improve significantly with age, as would be expected normally. Urinary osmolality is generally in the range of 120 to 220 mosmol/L in the neonates,[18] and maximal urine concentrating ability does not usually exceed 500 mosmol/L in older children.[12,19,21] Mild proteinuria and microscopic hematuria have been reported in some series,[19,20] while others have reported these urinary findings to be uncommon.[12]

Enlargement of the kidneys is the predominant clinical symptom of children presenting in infancy and childhood. Hepatomegaly has been reported to occur in about 35 percent and splenomegaly in 23 percent of infants in whom ARPKD was diagnosed during the first year of life.[20] Kääriäinen et al.[19] reported hepatic enlargement in 50 percent of infants that survive the neonatal period or present for the first time in childhood. Although hepatocellular failure does not usually occur in patients with uncomplicated ARPKD, abnormalities in hepatic enzymes may be present in some.[19] Portal hypertension manifesting as splenomegaly and esophageal varices is a common clinical problem in older children with ARPKD, but it may also be seen in children less than 5 years of age.[19,20,23] Pancytopenia may result from hypersplenism in such patients. Urinary tract infection may be the initial presenting feature of ARPKD in some patients, but sterile pyuria may be observed in others.[12] Growth failure is a consistent feature in these patients; it is probably the result of poor caloric intake, renal failure, and hypertension.

DIAGNOSIS

The diagnosis of ARPKD may be suggested by a positive family history of the disorder in siblings. As pointed out earlier, the pattern of inheritance of ARPKD is autosomal recessive. Therefore the kidneys of both parents should be normal by clinical examination as well as by ultrasound study. Radiologic study is the primary mode of diagnosing ARPKD. Such studies include ultrasonography, axial computed tomography (CT), and intravenous pyelography (IVP). High-resolution ultrasonography in experienced hands provides a reasonably accurate diagnosis of ARPKD. Intravenous pyelography and renal biopsy are necessary only if the diagnosis cannot be confirmed by ultrasonography. Renal biopsy has been reported to be of help in determining prognosis but is not essential for diagnosis.[24]

Ultrasonography in neonates demonstrates bilaterally enlarged kidneys with poor differentiation between the renal cortex and the medulla (Fig. 13–3). The renal parenchyma demonstrates increased echogenicity. Cysts are small and may not always be detected in neonates and are better characterized in older patients. The collecting system is not distended, but it may be distorted because of the renal cysts. Increased hepatic echogenicity may be demonstrated in children with hepatic fibrosis. The CT scan demonstrates bilaterally enlarged kidneys; small cysts are distributed throughout the renal parenchyma, and corticomedullary differentiation is poor. Intravenous pyelography is no longer considered to be the gold standard in the diagnosis of ARPKD. Findings on IVP include poor excretion of the contrast medium as a result of poor renal function. Delayed films (12 to 24 h) are of diagnostic value and show pooling of the contrast material within the cystic collecting system, giving rise to the characteristic radiologic feature of radial streaks perpendicular to the renal cortex. Radionuclide imaging demonstrates features similar to those on IVP, such as renal enlargement, poor excretion of the radionuclide, and pooling of the radioisotope in the kidney in delayed films (Fig. 13–4*A* and *B*).

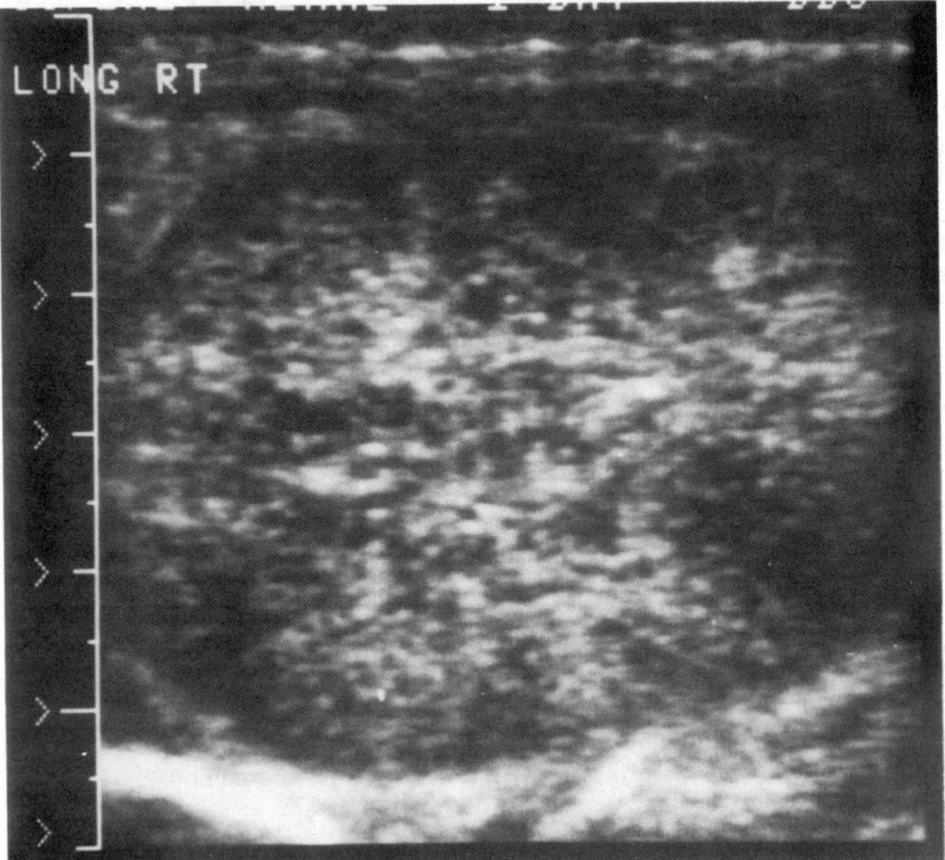

FIG. 13–3. Ultrasonography features of ARPKD in a newborn infant. Lack of differentiation of the renal parenchyma into cortex and medulla is obvious. Small cysts are distributed throughout the kidney.

PROGNOSIS

The mortality rate of patients with severe ARPKD presenting in the neonatal period is high, primarily due to complications of pulmonary hypoplasia.[19] However, those surviving the neonatal period have been reported to have a more optimistic outcome than had previously been expected. First-year mortality in 61 patients in three recent studies was only 18 percent.[12,20,24] Gagnadoux et al.[12] projected the 10-year survival to be 78 percent in patients who survive the neonatal period. A somewhat lower 10-year survival (51 percent) has been projected by Kaplan et al.[18] One of the morphologic indicators of prognosis reported by Gang and Herrin[24] is the severity of cystic changes in the kidneys: in a cross-sectional microscopic study, prognosis was found to be poor if 90 percent or more of the renal parenchyma was affected by cystic dilatation. None of the patients with this degree of parenchymal involvement survived beyond 20 days, while those with 20 to 75 percent of renal parenchyma affected by

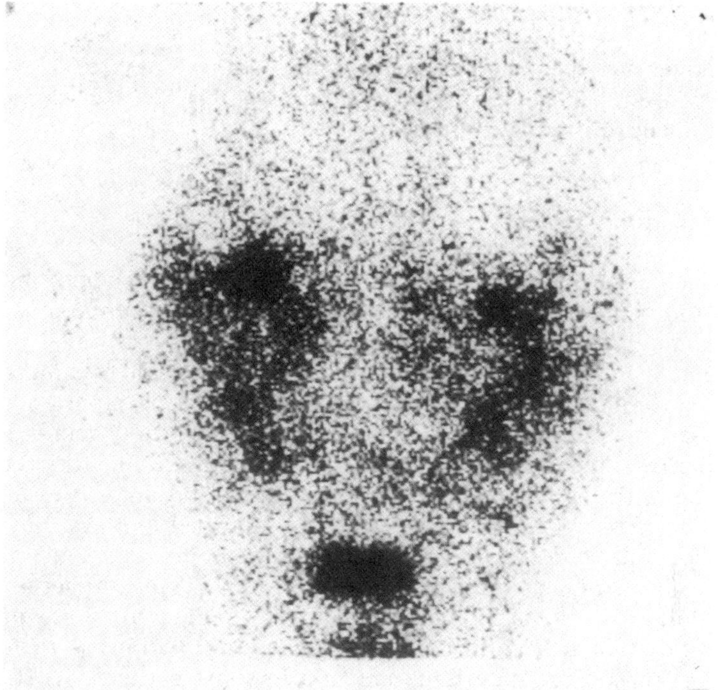

A

B

FIG. 13–4. *A*. Radionuclide scan (2½h after injection) in the patient with ARPKD shown in Fig. 13–3. Large renal uptake area suggests renal enlargement. *B*. Renal scan in another patient with ARPKD showing renal enlargement and pooling of the radionuclide material in the cysts of the kidney (12h after injection)—negative image.

cystic changes survived the first year of life, one of them to 21 years. Time course for onset of ESRD in surviving patients with ARPKD is variable. In one study it ranged from 8 to 197 months.[20]

MANAGEMENT ISSUES

The management of patients with ARPKD is a challenge for both the neonatalogist and the nephrologist. Pulmonary hypoplasia, poor ventilatory excursion, and recurrent pneumothorax are responsible for early neonatal mortality in these patients. Pulmonary complications require prompt treatment and may necessitate prolonged ventilatory support. Other issues of importance that must be addressed are abnormalities in fluid, electrolyte, and acid-base balance. Many patients with ARPKD are polyuric and may have obligatory renal sodium loss. For them, the provision of additional sodium and fluids is essential. Since compression of the gastrointestinal tract by enlarged kidneys may limit oral intake of formula, continuous nasograstric daytime or nighttime feeding may be attempted. Other patients may require intravenous hyperalimentation. Hypertension can be a difficult management problem in these patients. As pointed out earlier, ACE inhibitors such as captopril will usually control blood pressure but may precipitate hyperkalemia in some patients. As suggested by Kaplan et al.,[18] expansion of the intravascular fluid volume may be the etiology of hypertension in some patients with ARPKD. For them, therefore, appropriate diuretic therapy and management of fluids will be essential.

Early preemptive renal transplantation may be attempted if an organ donor is available and the surgical procedure is technically feasible. Bilateral nephrectomy is usually necessary in order to provide intraabdominal space for the allograft and may be performed at the time of transplantation. As patients grow older, portal hypertension and bleeding from esophageal varices may occur, and some of these patients will require surgical portocaval shunting procedures.

AUTOSOMAL DOMINANT POLYCYSTIC KIDNEY DISEASE

Autosomal dominant polycystic kidney disease (ADPKD) is also known as *adult polycystic kidney disease* or *Potter type III cystic renal disease.* The term *adult polycystic kidney disease* is a misnomer, since this condition has also been described in children, including neonates.[25–30] The incidence of ADPKD in children is not well established, but in the general population it has been estimated to be one per 1000 individuals.[31]

PATHOLOGY

Both kidneys are usually affected by ADPKD and are enlarged,[11] but unilateral disease has also been reported.[4,32] In adults, examination by the naked eye reveals the surface of the kidney to be covered by cysts of varying sizes (Fig. 13–5*A*). In neonates and children, the cysts are generally smaller.[4,6] The cut

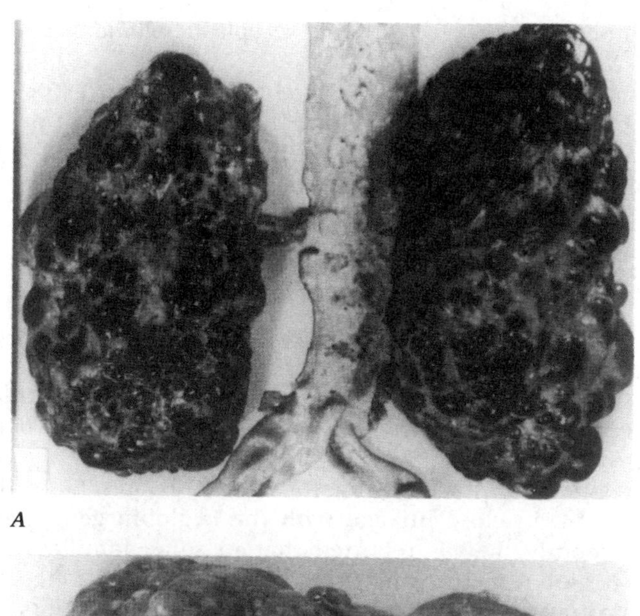

A

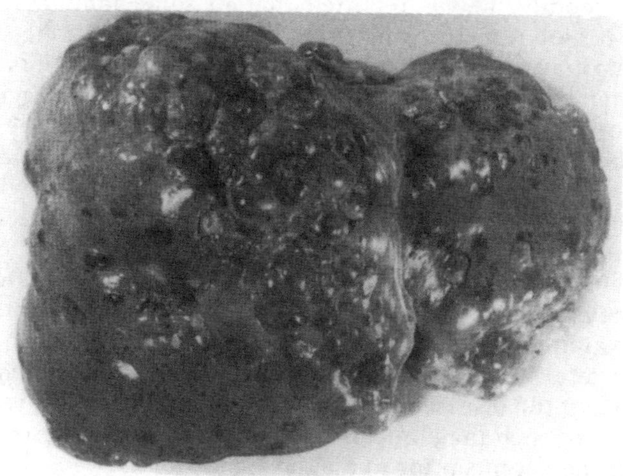

B

FIG. 13–5. *A*. Gross appearance of the kidney in ADPKD. *B*. Hepatic cysts in ADPKD. (From Zerres K, Volpel MC, Weiss H: Cystic kidneys: Genetics, pathologic anatomy, clinical picture, and prenatal diagnosis. *Hum Genet* 68:104, 1984. Copyright © 1984 by Springer-Verlag. Reproduced by permission.)

surface of the kidney demonstrates poor corticomedullary differentiation and cysts replacing renal parenchyma give it a honeycomb appearance.[6,11]

Renal cysts in ADPKD may arise from any segment of the nephron, the most common area being the loop of Henle.[6] The epithelial lining of the cysts is heterogenous, being a single layer of well-defined tubular epithelium in some segments and phenotypically undefined cells (84 percent) in other areas.[32a] On scanning electron microscopy, epithelial cell hyperplasia may sometimes give the appearance of polyps within the cysts. Glomerular cysts with enlargement of the Bowman capsule may be present.[6] Dysplastic elements such as cartilage are not seen.

Hepatic cysts may also be seen in patients with ADPKD (Fig. 13.5*B*). Such hepatic cysts have been reported in 30 to 40 percent of adult patients.[33,34] The incidence of hepatic cysts in children with ADPKD is not well known. Portal hypertension and splenomegaly are not seen in children or adults with ADPKD.

GENETICS AND PRENATAL DIAGNOSIS

Inherited in an autosomal dominant fashion, ADPKD carries a 50-percent chance of inheritance in the subsequent pregnancies of the parents. Often, one of the parents is known to have ADPKD. At other times, the children may be first to be diagnosed as having the disease, which may then be detected in one of the parents on screening.[27,32]

In 1985 it was shown that the gene for ADPKD is present on the short arm of chromosome 16, in close linkage with the α globin gene complex (PKD1 locus).[35] Subsequently, it was reported that in some families ADPKD is not linked to the α globin gene complex, suggesting genetic hetergeneity of the disease.[36,37] This may mean that more than one gene abnormality is responsible for the phenotypic expressions of ADPKD. The actual gene or gene product for ADPKD has not yet been isolated. Association of ADPKD with the α globin gene complex on the short arm of chromosome 16 has been used as a gene marker for the diagnosis of asymptomatic family members of patients with ADPKD[36,37] as well as in the prenatal diagnosis of this disease.[38] Another tool used for prenatal diagnosis is fetal ultrasonography. Bilateral enlargement of the kidneys with discernible cysts is usually seen in the affected fetus.[25,28] However, ultrasonography may not reveal enlargement of the fetal kidneys (as it does in infantile polycystic kidney disease) until late in the third trimester.[39] Since ADPKD is not always fatal, especially in childhood, prenatal knowledge about the genetic carriage of the disease may be of limited value. Ethical issues regarding the termination of such pregnancies have not yet been addressed and must be discussed with the parents prior to diagnostic testing.

CLINICAL MANIFESTATIONS

A bimodal distribution of the age at which ADPKD is detected has been described, the first peak occurring in the neonatal period and the second in later childhood (after age 6).[40] A flank mass has been reported to be the most common (100 percent) manifestation of ADPKD in children below 1 year of age.[20] Clinical manifestations of ADPKD reported by Sedman et al.[27] include flank mass (22 percent), gross hematuria (26 percent), hernias (22 percent), hypertension (22 percent), urinary tract infection (13 percent), and headache (13 percent). The incidence of hypertension has been reported to be higher (75 percent) in some recent studies and is usually present even before the onset of renal failure.[41] The pathogenesis of hypertension in ADPKD remains controversial. It has been suggested that the renin-angiotensin system plays an important role.[42] Hyperreninemia is believed to result from renal ischemia developing from distortion of the renal parenchymal architecture by the renal cysts.[42]

Hematuria has been reported to be a prominent presenting feature by Kaplan et al.[25] It may occur spontaneously or following minor trauma, as in sports. Proteinuria is seen in a minority of patients and is usually not severe.[25] Urinary tract infection, often resulting in acute pyelonephritis, may develop in patients with ADPKD. Complications of acute pyelonephritis, such as sepsis and perinephric abscess formation have been reported more frequently.[43] Infection localizing into the renal cysts (pyocysts) may not be associated with bacteriuria. Cyst puncture has been advocated for diagnosis and isolation of the infecting organism in such patients.[44]

Intracranial aneurysms are a common extrarenal manifestation of ADPKD, having been reported in 10 to 41 percent of patients.[45–47] Rupture of these aneurysms can lead to a catastrophic neurologic outcome in adults as well as in children.[27] There is some indication that intracranial aneurysms may be more prevalent in some families with ADPKD than in others.[45] A high incidence of mitral valve prolapse, mitral valve incompetence, and other heart valve dysfunctions have been reported in adult patients with ADPKD.[48] Although hepatic cysts are a common feature of ADPKD, liver dysfunction and portal hypertension are unusual.

DIAGNOSIS

Often the diagnosis of ADPKD is suspected because of a positive family history of the disease and its autosomal dominant pattern of inheritance. Accordingly, one of the parents is expected to be affected by ADPKD, but other siblings may or may not be involved. At times, parents may be unaware of their own disease and are first found to have an abnormal renal ultrasonogram on screening after the disease has been diagnosed in an offspring. Ultrasound examination remains the primary method of diagnosis of ADPKD. The characteristic ultrasound findings in such patients are bilaterally enlarged kidneys with poor corticomedullary differentiation and large cysts that are distributed throughout the renal parenchyma. A CT scan will confirm nephromegaly with cystic changes throughout the renal parencyhma (Fig. 13–6). Intravenous pyelography may also sometimes be used to diagnose ADPKD in patients with normal renal function; an outline of the large parenchymal cysts can be detected in the nephrogram phase of the IVP. Distortion of the collecting system produced by the cysts is another characteristic IVP finding in ADPKD. Features distinguishing ARPKD from ADPKD are listed in Table 13–3.

Despite the fact that the mutant gene responsible for ADPKD has not yet been isolated, the use of genetic linkage analysis for the detection of ADPKD in asymptomatic family members and in the fetus has been available for some time. By this technique, DNA probes are used to study DNA flanking the PKD1 region on chromosome 16 in the affected patients within a family. The asymptomatic members of the family are also studied using identical techniques. Chromosome 16 carrying the PKD1 gene is identified in the affected individuals, and its presence or absence in the asymptomatic family members is noted.

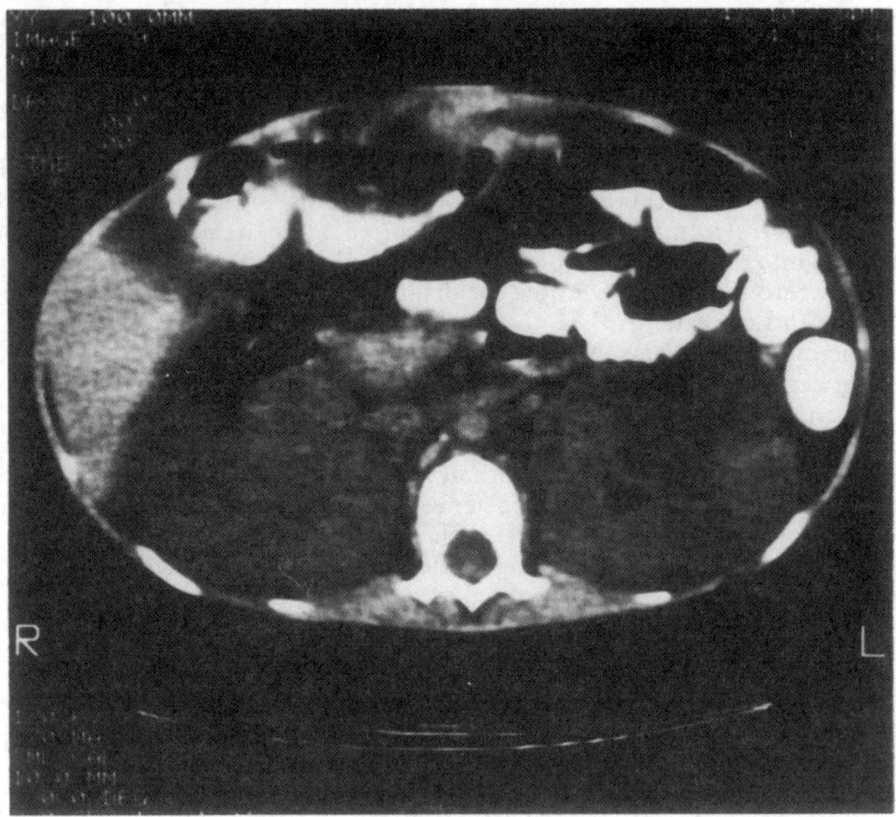

FIG. 13–6. **CT scan in a child with ADPKD. Gross bilateral enlargement of the kidneys is evident; cystic lesions are distributed throughout both the kidneys.**

Family members bearing the PKD1 gene are expected to have inherited the gene for the disease (Fig. 13–7). At least one, and preferably two, affected members of the family are required for genetic linkage analysis, which is carried on blood samples. Genetic linkage analysis for the PKD1 locus is available commercially.* Since there is sufficient evidence to suggest the genetic heterogeneity of APKD,[37,49] further work regarding the reliability of genetic diagnostic tests for this disease must be undertaken.

PROGNOSIS

The prognosis of ADPKD in children has not been well studied. Death may occur during the neonatal period due to respiratory insufficiency, and features of Potter syndrome have been described. Of the four patients followed by Sed-

*Collaborative Research, Inc., 1365 Main Street, Waltham, Massachusetts 02154. Telephone: (617) 894-5807.

TABLE 13–3. Clinical and Genetic Features Distinguishing ARPKD from ADPKD

	Autosomal Recessive PKD	Autosomal Dominant PKD
Mode of inheritance	Autosomal recessive	Autosomal dominant
Family History		
Parents	Normal; kidneys normal by ultrasound	One parent affected, renal ultrasound abnormal
Siblings	May be affected	May be affected
Clinical Features		
Common age of onset	Neonates	Older children, can be seen in neonates
Usual presentation	Renal mass	Renal mass
Hypertension	Common	Common
Hepatic disease	Fibrosis, portal hypertension	Asymptomatic hepatic cysts
Intracranial aneurysms	No	Yes
Mitral valve prolapse	No	Yes
Genetic Diagnosis	Not yet possible	Possible to identify affected family members by linkage analysis
Recurrence in transplants	None reported	None reported

man et al.[27] who presented before one year of age, two developed ESRD at 3.5 years and 15 years of age. The other two patients had stable renal function at last follow-up (4 years and 5 years). ADPKD detected in adults leads to chronic renal failure; the need for renal replacement therapy arises by about the fifth decade of life.

MANAGEMENT ISSUES

Hypertension is a common clinical problem in children with ADPKD and may be an important factor in the progression of their disease. Hypertension may also predispose some of these patients to bleeding from intracranial berry aneurysms. Because of the suggested role of the renin-angiotensin system in the pathogenesis of hypertension, ACE inhibitors such as captopril may be considered as the drugs of choice for the treatment of hypertension in children with ADPKD. Additional diuretic therapy may be required in some patients to achieve adequate control of blood pressure. As chronic renal insufficiency evolves, patients will need supportive care in order to maintain fluid, electrolyte, divalent ion, and acid-base metabolism. Renal transplantation should be considered for the treatment of ESRD in patients with ADPKD, although bilateral nephrectomy may be required in some young children in order to provide the intraabdominal space needed for an allograft. In a recently reported series of 54 adult patients with ADPKD who underwent renal transplantation, no unusual complications or recurrence of the cystic disease was reported.[50] Others have, however, reported increased incidence of infections (acute pyelonephritis) in the native kidneys of these patients following transplantation.[51]

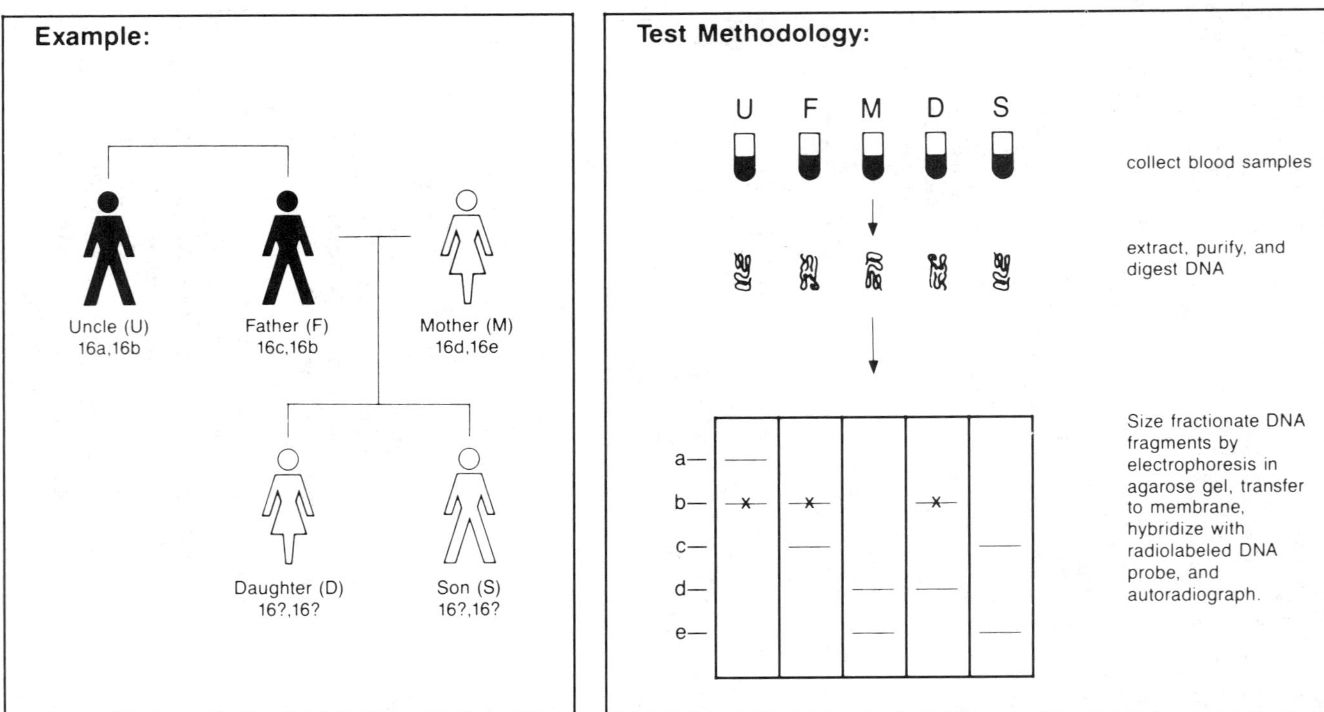

FIG. 13–7. Presymptomatic diagnosis of ADPKD using linkage analysis. In this example *(left panel)*, the father (F) and his brother (U) had been diagnosed to have ADPKD and are affected by the PKD1 gene. Blood samples are collected from unaffected family members for linkage analysis. Results *(right panel)* indicate that the father (F) and his brother (U) have only chromosome 16b in common. Thus chromosome 16b can be presumed to be the carrier of the PKD1 gene. The affected father's daughter (D) also has inherited chromosome 16b and would be affected with PKD1, but the son (S) is not affected by the disease. (From an informational pamphlet on the presymptomatic diagnosis of adult polycystic kidney disease using DNA probes. Collaborative Research, Inc., Waltham, Massachusetts. Reproduced by permission.)

Hematuria and flank pain in ADPKD should be treated symptomatically; severe uncontrolled hematuria may call for blood transfusion therapy in some patients. Because of the greater danger of renal trauma, children with ADPKD should be advised to avoid contact sports. A CT scan and an MRI of the head may be advised for the detection of unruptured intracranial aneurysms; carotid angiography, however, remains the definitive test for detection of such angiomatous malformations. Whether all patients with ADPKD should undergo carotid angiography is controversial. Some groups have recommended the procedure,[47] while others do not see any significant benefit from it.[52] As technology and noninvasive methods of investigations evolve, screening for intracranial aneurysms may become a routine procedure for these patients.

MEDULLARY CYSTIC DISEASE COMPLEX

Two cystic kidney diseases included in the category of medullary cystic disease complex are *juvenile nephronophthisis* (JN) and *medullary cystic disease* (MCD). These diseases are similar in their clinical manifestations and pathologic features but differ in the age of onset and mode of inheritance. While JN is exclusively seen in children and usually has its onset at age 8 to 10 years, MCD is a disease of adults, often beginning in the mid to late twenties. The mode of inheritance is autosomal recessive in JN[53] and autosomal dominant in MCD.[54] JN is an important etiology of ESRD in children in Europe. Garel et al.[55] reported its incidence to be 15 percent in all children undergoing renal transplantation at the Hôpital des Enfants Malades in Paris. In Germany, its incidence as a cause of ESRD has been reported to be 10 percent.[56] Both JN and MCD appear to be less common in the United States.

CLINICAL MANIFESTATIONS

Both JN and MCD remain asymptomatic until late in the course. Renal masses are neither visible nor palpable; by the time renal failure develops, the kidneys are usually moderately shrunken in size.[55] Anemia, which is characteristically out of proportion to the degree of renal failure, is a common feature of JN. In a family with a strong history of either disease, the detection of unexplained normocytic normochromic anemia may be the initial clue to the diagnosis of renal disease. Growth failure, inability to concentrate urine, a tendency torward renal sodium wasting, polyuria, and enuresis are the other features of this disease.[57,58] Once chronic renal failure develops, progression to ESRD is generally rapid.[59] In one study of 39 children,[60] ESRD developed within 27 ± 8 months of initial detection of JN. An identical rate of deterioration of renal function and renal death has been reported in twins with JN.[61]

Several skeletal, neurologic, and ophthalmic abnormalities and syndromes have been described in patients with JN.[57] Such disorders are rare in patients with MCD, but a few reports of neurologic abnormalities in MCD have, in fact, appeared in the literature recently.[62]

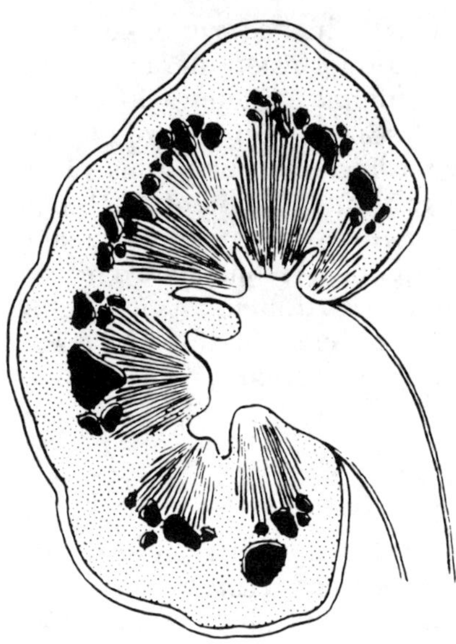

FIG. 13–8. Schematic drawing of distribution of cysts in medullary cystic disease. (From Spence HM, Singleton R: What is sponge kidney disease and where does it fit in the spectrum of cystic disorder? *J Urol* 107:176, 1972. © 1972 by Williams & Wilkins. Reproduced by permission.)

PATHOLOGY

The pathologic features of JN and MCD are strikingly similar. The kidneys are shrunken in size; on cut section, small cysts are seen in the corticomedullary junction (Fig. 13–8). The location of these cysts in the corticomedullary junctional area is confirmed by low-power light microscopy. The characteristic microscopic feature of juvenile nephronophthisis is the presence of interstitial disease with significant tubular atrophy. Cysts in these two disorders involve the collecting ducts, distal convoluted tubule, and the loop of Henle.[63]

DIAGNOSIS

Normocytic normochromic anemia which is out of proportion to the degree of renal failure is a common indicator of the JN-MCD complex. Urinalysis is usually unremarkable except for the a low urine specific gravity. Diagnosis can be established by demonstration of characteristic small cysts in the corticomedullary area by ultrasonography or CT scan. The IVP shows typical streaking of contrast in the renal medulla. Since the histologic features of interstitial disease and tubular atrophy can be seen in many renal diseases, renal biopsy is not always diagnostic, especially if cysts cannot be demonstrated.

MANAGEMENT ISSUES

The treatment of patients with MCD complex consists of symptomatic management of chronic renal failure. Dialysis and transplantation can be considered when ESRD is reached.

MULTICYSTIC DYSPLASTIC KIDNEY

Multicystic dysplastic kidney is a nongenetic disorder characterized by renal cysts and poor renal function in the affected kidney. Other terms used interchangeably to describe this condition are *Potter type II renal cysts, multicystic kidney, and multicystic renal dysplasia.* In the neonate, multicystic dysplastic kidney usually manifests itself as a unilateral renal mass;[64] some patients may, however, remain asymptomatic and undetected well into adulthood.[65] Bilateral disease is seen less commonly and may simulate polycystic kidney disease. Patients with bilateral disease may manifest oligohydramnios and features of Potter facies; prognosis is usually unfavorable in such cases.[64] Unilateral enlargement of the affected kidney may sometimes be so severe as to result in respiratory and gastrointestinal compromise.[66]

Hypertension is frequently seen in patients with multicystic dysplastic kidneys.[67] Renal failure is uncommon unless the disease is bilateral or the contralateral kidney demonstrates obstruction. When detected in the fetus, multicystic kidney may demonstrate regression and sometimes result in renal agenesis on the affected side.[64]

PATHOLOGY

Kidneys with multicystic dysplasia demonstrate an irregular and cystic surface on macroscopic examination, with poor organization of renal parenchyma and large cystic areas on cut section (Fig. 13–9). Microscopic examination reveals islands of disorganized cellular elements and poorly formed, primitive nephron

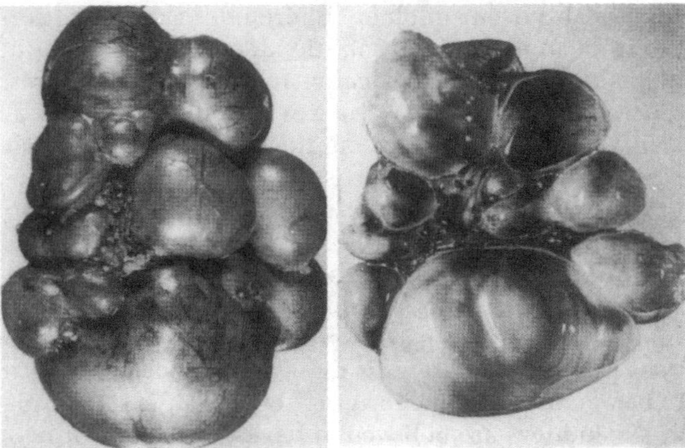

FIG. 13–9. Gross appearance of multicystic dysplastic kidney (*A*). The right panel (*B*) shows the cut section of the kidney; large cysts with little normal renal tissue are obvious. (From Zerres K, Volpel MC, Weiss H: Cystic kidneys: Genetics, pathology, anatomy, clinical picture, and prenatal diagnosis. *Hum Genet* 68:104, 1984. Copyright © 1984 by Springer-Verlag. Reproduced by permission.)

structures. Primitive tubular structures, cartilage, blood vessels, nerves, and even bone are seen in such poorly formed organs.[6] Cysts are distributed throughout the mass of tissues and are derived from the terminal portions of the collecting tubules. Erythropoiesis has been reported in the tissues of multicystic dysplastic kidneys.[6] The presence of these dysplastic elements is essential to the diagnosis of multicystic dysplastic kidney. Abnormalities in the contralateral kidney can be present in as many as 50 percent of cases; these include agenesis, dysplasia, and obstructive lesions.[64]

MANAGEMENT ISSUES

There is a continuing debate in the literature as to the best mode of treatment of multicystic dysplastic kidneys. Those who advocate removal of the affected kidney base their argument on cure of hypertension[67] and reducing the risk of malignant transformation in the dysplastic kidney.[68] The risk of malignant transformation is, however, low in such patients. In a recently reported study involving 60 cases of multicystic dysplastic kidneys, nephroblastomatous lesions were noted in 6.7 percent of cases.[68] Conservative therapy consisting of antihypertensive therapy and periodic ultrasonographic monitoring of the affected kidney can be an alternative method of managing these patients.

MULTILOCULAR CYSTS

Multilocular cystic renal disease is an uncommon disorder characterized by a unilateral renal mass with large cysts in it. The disease is most commonly seen in neonates but can also occur in older children.[69,70] Differentiation of multilocular renal cysts from multicystic dysplastic kidney disease may be difficult by ultrasonography alone. Characteristically, renal function is preserved in the noncystic parenchyma of the kidney and can be demonstrated by a radionuclide scan or IVP. This contrasts with the multicystic dysplastic kidneys, which do not demonstrate any functional renal tissue by radionuclide scans. Pathologic criteria for the diagnosis of multilocular cysts are as follows: (1) the cysts should be unilateral, (2) they should not communicate with the renal pelvis, (3) they should not communicate with each other, (4) they should have an epithelial lining, and (5) dysplastic elements should not be present in the noncystic parenchyma (some immature tubules can be seen between the intervening septae of the cysts).[71] Cysts in multilocular cystic disease have been demonstrated, by lectin staining, to be of collecting duct origin.[70] Like multicystic dysplastic kidneys, multilocular cystic kidneys are believed to have a potential for neoplastic transformation.[72,73] However, the incidence of such malignancies has not been defined and is probably very low. Because of the increased risk of malignancy, nephrectomy has been recommended by some as the treatment of choice for multilocular renal cysts.[72]

SIMPLE RENAL CYSTS

Simple renal cystic disease is an uncommon disorder in children, but its incidence has been reported to be as high as 50 percent in adults above age 50.[74] Using ultrasound screening, McHugh and coworkers reported the incidence of simple renal cysts among the children they studied to be 0.22 percent.[75] Age and sex distribution of simple cysts was even in this study. Simple cysts are usually small in size (a few centimeters), and a high percentage have been reported in the upper poles of the kidney (especiallly the right side).[75,76] Simple renal cysts are usually asymptomatic and are generally detected on routine ultrasound examination of the abdomen. Simple cysts do not require surgical removal.

MEDULLARY SPONGE KIDNEY

Medullary sponge kidney is an unusual type of renal cystic disease that is more common in adults but will be seen rarely in children.[77,78] Renal cysts are present in the papillae of kidneys in a cut section (Fig. 13–10). Medullary sponge kidney may be associated with hemihypertrophy syndromes in childhood.[78,79] Although medullary sponge kidney disease can remain asymptomatic, it characteristically presents because of the formation of kidney stones, which may lead to urinary tract obstruction or urinary tract infection. Hematuria and hypercalciuria are also common manifestations in children.[77] Renal function (glomerular filtration rate) is normal, but urine concentrating defect may be present. Renal tubular acidosis and growth failure may also occur in some children.[80] Hypercalciuria has been observed in patients with medullary sponge

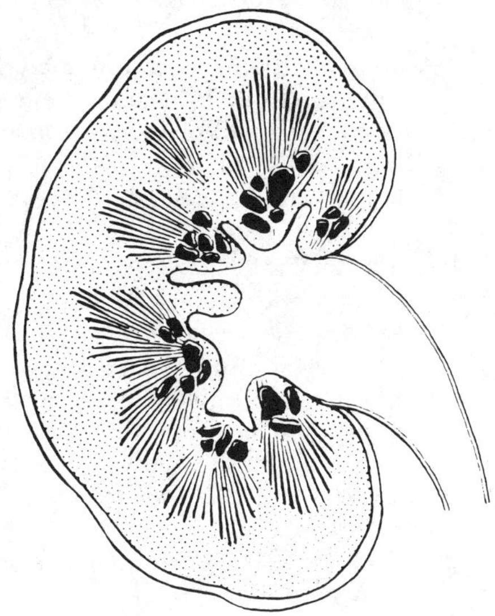

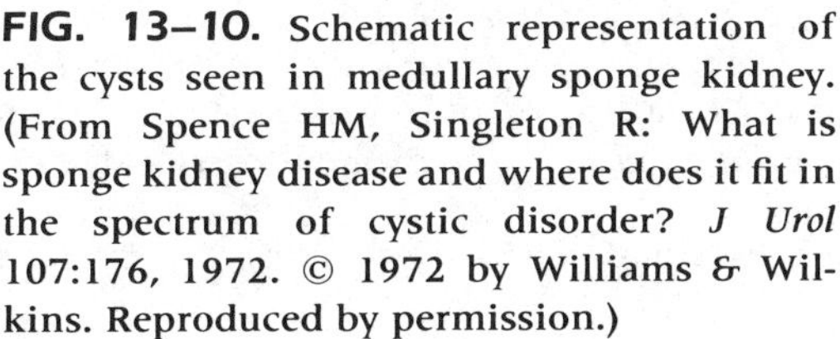

FIG. 13–10. Schematic representation of the cysts seen in medullary sponge kidney. (From Spence HM, Singleton R: What is sponge kidney disease and where does it fit in the spectrum of cystic disorder? *J Urol* 107:176, 1972. © 1972 by Williams & Wilkins. Reproduced by permission.)

kidney[81] but is not seen all patients.[82] The pathogenesis of hypercalciuria in medullary sponge kidney is unclear. The diagnosis of medullary sponge kidney is established by IVP, which shows linear striation of the dye in the region of the papillae. Renal ultrasonography is of limited diagnostic value.

ACQUIRED RENAL CYSTS

The development of renal cysts in patients with ESRD who were being treated with long-term hemodialysis was first described in 1977.[83] Since then, it has become well established that nonfunctioning kidneys frequently develop cystic changes. The incidence in a review of 601 adult patients was 44 percent.[1] Leichter et al.[2] reported the incidence of acquired renal cystic disease in 33 percent of children undergoing long-term dialysis. Although this condition is commonly seen in patients who are treated by hemodialysis, acquired renal cysts have also been reported in patients undergoing peritoneal dialysis,[2,84] in the native kidneys of renal allograft recipients, and in patients with poorly functioning renal allografts.[85] Many patients remain asymptomatic, but hemorrhage into the cysts and hematuria can occur. Neoplasia has been described in adult patients with acquired renal cystic disease.[86] Patients at the highest risk for the development of acquired renal cysts are those who have received dialysis therapy for more than 3 years.[1] Diagnosis can be established by utlrasound or CT scan.

REFERENCES

1. Grantham JJ, Levine E: Acquired cystic disease: Replacing one kidney disease with another. *Kidney Int* 28:99, 1985.
2. Leichter HE, Dietrich RB, Salusky IB, et al: Acquired cystic kidney disease in children undergoing long term dialysis. *Pediatr Nephrol* 2:8, 1988.
3. United States Renal Data System: *USRDS 1990 Annual Report.* National Institutes of Health, National Institute of Diabetes and Digestive and Kidney Disease, Bethesda, Maryland, 1990, p. A46.
4. Blythe H. Ockenden BG: Polycystic disease of the kidney and liver presenting in childhood. *J Med Genet* 8:257, 1971.
5. Bernstein J: A classification of renal cysts, in Gardner KD Jr (ed): *Cystic Disease of the Kidneys.* New York, Wiley, 1976, pp 7–30.
6. Potter EL: *Normal and Abnormal Development of the Kidney.* Year Book Medical Publishers, Chicago. 1972, pp 141–220.
7. Glassberg KI, Stephens FD, Lebowitz RI, et al: Renal dysgenesis and cystic disease of the kidney: A report on the terminology, nomenclature and classification. Section on urology, American Academy of Pediatrics. *J Urol* 138:1085, 1987.
8. Larroche JC: *Development Pathology of the Neonate.* Amsterdam, Excerpta Medica, 1977, p. 96.
9. Uhari M, Herva R: Polycystic kidney disease of perinatal type. *Acta Paediatr Scand* 68:443, 1979.

10. Broyer M, Brunner FP, Brynger H, et al: Demography of dialysis and transplantation in children in Europe. *Nephrol Dial Transplant* 1:9, 1986.
11. Zerres K, Volpel MC, Weiss H: Cystic kidneys: Genetics, pathologic anatomy, clinical picture, and prenatal diagnosis. *Hum Genet* 68:104, 1984.
12. Gagnadoux M-F, Habib R, Levy M, et al: Cystic renal diseases in children. *Adv Nephrol* 18:33, 1989.
13. A report of the Southwest Pediatric Nephrology Study Group: Renal cystic disease of infancy: results of histochemical studies. *Pediatr Nephrol* 3:37, 1989.
14. Romero R, Cullen M, Jeanty P, et al: The diagnosis of congenital renal anomalies with ultrasound: II. Infantile polycystic kidney disease. *Am J Obstet Gynecol* 150:259, 1984.
15. Fong KW, Rahmani MR, Skidmore MB, et al: Fetal renal cystic disease: Sonographic-pathologic correlation. *Am J Roentgen* 146:767, 1986.
16. Townsend RR, Goldstein RB, Filly RA, et al: Sonographic identification of autosomal recessive polycystic kidney disease associated with increased maternal serum/amniotic fluid alpha-fetoprotein. *Obstet Gynecol* 71:1008, 1988.
17. Neumann HPH, Zerres K, Fischer CL, et al: Late manifestation of autosomal-recessive polycystic kidney disease in two sisters. *Am J Nephrol* 8:194, 1988.
18. Kaplan BS, Shah V, Dillon MJ, et al: Autosomal recessive polycystic kidney disease. *Pediatr Nephrol* 3:43, 1989.
19. Kääriäinen H, Koskimies O, Norio R: Dominant and recessive polycystic kidney disease in children: Evaluation of clinical and laboratory data. *Pediatr Nephrol* 2:296, 1988.
20. Cole BR, Conley SB, Stapleton B: Polycystic kidney disease in the first year of life. *J Pediatr* 111:693, 1987.
21. Anand SK, Chan JC, Lieberman E: Polycystic disease and hepatic fibrosis in children: Renal function studies. *Am J Dis Child* 129:810, 1975.
22. Anand SK, Alon U, Chan JCM: Cystic diseases of the kidney in children. *Adv Pediatr* 31:371, 1984.
23. Alvarez F, Bernard O, Brunelle F, et al: Congenital hepatic fibrosis in children. *J Pediatr* 99:370, 1981.
24. Gang DL, Herrin TH: Infantile polycystic disease of the liver and kidneys. *Clin Nephrol* 25:28, 1986.
25. Kaplan BS, Rabin I, Drummond KN: Autosomal dominant polycystic renal disease in children. *J Pediatr* 90:782, 1977.
26. Bear JC, McManamon P, Morgan J, et al: Age at clinical onset and at ultrasonographic detection of adult polycystic kidney disease: Data for genetic counselling. *Am J Med Genet* 18:45, 1984.
27. Sedman A, Bell P, Manco-Johnson M, et al: Autosomal dominant polycystic kidney disease in childhood: A longitudinal study. *Kidney Int* 31:1000, 1987.
28. Chevalier RL, Garland TA, Buschi AJ: The neonate with adult-type autosomal dominant polycystic kidney disease. *Int J Pediatr Nephrol* 2:73, 1981.
29. Proesman W, Van Damme B, Casaer P, et al: Autosomal dominant polycystic kidney disease in the neonatal period: Association with cerebral arteriovenous malformation. *Pediatrics* 70:971, 1982.
30. Zerres K, Weiss H, Bulla M, et al: Prenatal diagnosis of an early manifestation of autosomal dominant adult-type polycystic kidney disease. *Lancet* 2:988, 1982.
31. Dalgaard OZ: Bilateral polycystic disease of the kidney: A follow-up of two hundred eighty-four patients and their families. *Acta Med Scand* 158(suppl 328):1, 1957.

32. Porch P, Noe N, Stapleton FB: Unilateral presentation of adult-type polycystic kidney disease in children. *J Urol* 135:744, 1986.
32a. Grantham JJ, Geiser JL, Evan AP: Cyst formation and growth in autosomal dominant polycystic kidney disease. *Kidney Int* 31:1145, 1987.
33. Multinovic J, Fialkow PJ, Rudd TG, et al: Liver cysts in patients with autosomal dominant polycystic kidney disease. *Am J Med* 68:741, 1980.
34. Gabow PA, Ikle DW, Holmes JH: Polycystic kidney disease: Prospective analysis of nonazotemic patients and family members. *Ann Intern Med* 101:238, 1984.
35. Reeders ST, Breuning MH, Davies KE, et al: A highly polymorphic DNA marker linked to adult polycystic kidney disease on chromosome 16. *Nature* 317:542, 1985.
36. Reeders ST, Breuning MH, Ryynanen MA, et al: A study of genetic linkage heterogeneity in adult polycystic kidney disease. *Hum Genet* 76:348, 1987.
37. Kimberling WJ, Fain PR, Kenyon JB, et al: Linkage heterogeneity of automsomal dominant polycystic kidney disease. *N Engl J Med* 319:913, 1988.
38. Reeders ST, Zerres K, Gal A, et al: Prenatal diagnosis of autosomal dominant polycystic kidney disease using a DNA probe. *Lancet* 1:1, 1986.
39. Main D, Mennuti M, Cornfeld D, et al: Prenatal diagnosis of adult polycystic kidney disease. *Lancet* 2:337, 1983.
40. Taitz LS, Brown CB, Blank CE, et al: Screening for polycystic kidney disease: Importance of clinical presentation in the newborn. *Arch Dis Child* 62:45, 1987.
41. Geberth ST, Zeier M, Schmidt C, et al: Blood pressure in children with autosomal dominant polycystic kidney disease (ADPKD). *J Am Soc Nephrol* 1:299, 1990 (abstract).
42. Chapman AB, Johnson A, Gabow PA, et al: The renin-angiotensin-aldosterone system and autosomal dominant polycystic kidney disease. *N Engl J Med* 323:1091, 1990.
43. Sklar AN, Caruana RJ, Lammers JE, et al: Renal infections in autosomal dominant polycystic kidney disease. *Am J Kidney Dis* 10:81, 1987.
44. Schwab SJ, Bander SJ: Cyst infection in autosomal dominant polycystic kidney disease. *Am J Med* 82:714, 1987.
45. Gabow PA: Autosomal dominant polycystic kidney disease—more than a renal disease. *Am J Kidney Dis* 16:403, 1990.
46. Bigelow NH: The association of polycystic kidneys with intracranial aneurysms and other related disorders. *Am J Med Sci* 225:485, 1953.
47. Wakabayashi T, Fujuita S, Ohbora Y, et al: Polycystic kidney disease and intracranial aneurysms: Early angiographic diagnosis and early operation for unruptured aneurysm. *J Neurosurg* 58:488, 1983.
48. Hossack KF, Leddy CL, Johnson AM, et al: Echocardiographic findings in autosomal dominant polycystic kidney disease. *N Engl J Med* 319:907, 1988.
49. Parfrey PS, Bear JC, Morgan J, et al: The diagnosis and prognosis of autosomal dominant polycystic kidney disease. *N Engl J Med* 323:1085, 1990.
50. Fitzpatrick PM, Torres VE, Charboneau JW, et al: Long-term outcome of renal transplantation in autosomal dominant polycystic kidney disease. *Am J Kidney Dis* 15:535, 1990.
51. Rayner BL, Cassidy JD, Jacobsen JE, et al: Is preliminary binephrectomy necessary in patients with autosomal dominant polycystic kidney disease undergoing renal transplantation? *Clin Nephrol* 34:122, 1990.
52. Levey AS, Pauker SG, Kassirer JP: Occult intracranial aneurysms in polycystic kidney disease: When is cerebral arteriography justified? *N Engl J Med* 308:986, 1983.

53. Mangos J, Opitz JM, Lobeck CC, et al: Familial juvenile nephronophthisis: An unrecognized renal disease in the United States. *Pediatrics* 34:337, 1964.
54. Kyle VN: Medullary cystic disease of the kidneys: Report of a family. *Can J Surg* 16:121, 1973.
55. Garel LA, Habib R, Pariente D, et al: Juvenile nephronophthisis. *Radiology* 151:93, 1984.
56. Waldherr R, Lennert T, Weber HP, et al: The nephronophthisis complex: A clinicopathologic study. *Virchows Arch* (*Pathol Anat*)394:235, 1982.
57. Donaldson MD, Warner AA, Trompeter RS, et al: Familial juvenile nephronophthesis, Jeune's syndrome and associated disorders. *Arch Dis Child* 60:426, 1985.
58. Brouhard BH, Srivastava RN, Travis LB, et al: Nephronophthisis. *Nephron* 19:99, 1977.
59. Gretz N, Schärer K, Waldherr R, et al: Rate of deterioration of renal function in juvenile nephronophthisis. *Pediatr Nephrol* 3:56, 1989.
60. Arbeeitsgemeinschaft für pädiatrische Nephrologie: Children with chronic renal failure in the Federal Republic of Germany: II. Primary renal diseases, age and intervals from early renal failure to renal death. *Clin Nephrol* 23:278, 1985.
61. Makker SP, Grupe WE, Perrin F, et al: Identical progression of juvenile hereditary nephronophthisis in monozygotic twins. *J Pediatr* 82:773, 1973.
62. Green A , Kinirons M, O'Meara YO, et al: Familial adult medullary cystic disease with spastic quadriparesis: A new disease association. *Clin Nephrol* 33:237, 1990.
63. Sherman FM, Studnicki FM, Fetterman GH: Renal lesions of familial juvenile nephronophthisis examined by microdissection. *J Clin Pathol* 55:391, 1971.
64. Dungan JS, Fernandez MT, Abbitt P, et al: Multicystic dysplastic kidney: Natural history of prenatally detected cases. *Prenat Diagn* 10:175, 1990.
65. Ambrose SS, Gould RA, Trulock TS, et al: Unilateral multicystic renal disease in adults. *J Urol* 128:366, 1982.
66. Middleton AW, Melzer RB: Neonatal multicystic kidney with associated respiratory distress, obstruction of the contralteral ureter, and gastric compromise. *Urology* 34:36, 1989.
67. Susskind MR, Kim KS, King LR: Hypertension and multicystic kidney. *Urology* 34:362, 1989.
68. Dimmick JE, Johnson HW, Coleman GU, et al: Wilms tumorlet, nodular renal blastema and multicystic renal dysplasia. *J Urol* 142:484, 1989.
69. Thomas DFM, Androulakakis PA, Ransley, PG: Conservation of the kidney following an unusual presentation of multilocular cyst in a 7-year-old child. *J Urol* 128:363, 1981.
70. Friedman GC, Verani R, Rosenberg H, et al: Collecting duct origin of multilocular renal cysts by peroxidase-labelled lectin studies. *Am J Nephrol* 8:255, 1988.
71. Powell T, Schackman R, Johnson HD: Multiocular cysts of the kidney. *Br J Urol* 23:142, 1951.
72. Takeuchi T, Tanaka T, Tokuyama H, et al: Multilocular cystic renal adenocarcinoma: A case report and review of the literature. *J Surg Oncol* 25:136, 1984.
73. Sherman ME, Silverman ML, Balogh K, et al: Multilocular renal cyst: A hamartoma with potential for neoplastic transformation? *Arch Pathol Lab Med* 111:732, 1987.
74. Kissane JM: The morphology of renal cystic disease, in Gardner KD (ed): *Cystic Diseases of the Kidney*. New York, Wiley, 1976, p 31.
75. McHugh K, Stringer DA, Hebert D, et al: Simple renal cysts in children: Diagnosis and follow-up with US. *Radiology* 178:383, 1991.

76. Kramer SA, Hoffman AD, Aydin G, et al: Simple cysts in children. *J Urol* 128:1259, 1982.
77. Patriquin HB, O'Regan S: Medullary sponge kidney in childhood. *Am J Roentgenol* 145:315, 1985.
78. Chesney RW, Kaufman R, Stapelton FB, et al: Association of medullary sponge kidney and medullary dysplasia in Beckwith-Wiedmann syndrome. *J Pediatr* 115:761, 1989.
79. Harris RE, Ruch EF, Kaempf MJ: Medullary sponge kidney and congenital hemihypertrophy: Case report and literature review. *J Urol* 126:676, 1981.
80. Sluysmans T, Vanoverschelde JP, Malvaux P: Growth failure associated with medullary sponge kidney due to incomplete renal tubular acidosis. *Eur J Pediatr* 146:78, 1987.
81. Higashihara E, Nutahara K, Niijina T: Renal hypercalciuria and metabolic acidosis associated with medullary sponge kidney: Effect of alkali therapy. *Urol Res* 16:95, 1988.
82. Parks JH, Coe FL, Strauss AL: Calcium nephrolithiasis and medullary sponge kidney in women. *N Engl J Med* 306:1088, 1982.
83. Dunhill MS, Millard PR, Oliver D: Acquired cystic disease of the kidneys: A hazard of long-term intermittent maintenance haemodialysis. *J Clin Pathol* 30:868, 1977.
84. Beardsworth SF, Goldsmith HJ, Ahmad R, et al: Acquisition of renal cysts during peritoneal dialysis. *Lancet* 2:1482, 1984.
85. Ishikawa I, Shikura N, Kitada H, et al: Severity of acquried renal cysts in native kidneys and renal allograft with long-standing poor function. *Am J Kidney Dis* 14:18, 1989.
86. Houghson MD, Buchwald D, Fox M: Renal neoplasia and acquired cystic kidney disease in patients receiving long-term dialysis. *Arch Pathol Lab Med* 110:592, 1986.

14

OBSTRUCTIVE UROPATHY

Kanwal K. Kher

Urinary tract obstruction is an important cause of acute and chronic renal failure in children. Recovery of renal function in the obstructed urinary tract depends on prompt diagnosis and the prevention of renal parenchymal damage. Not only does unresolved or chronic obstruction predispose to a poor recovery of renal function, but it also leads to recurrent infections and renal stones associated with stasis. Obstructive uropathy in children usually results from developmental anomalies of the urinary tract, but acquired lesions may also occasionally be seen. Congenital urinary tract obstruction, despite early and adequate surgical therapy, can lead to chronic renal failure and end stage renal disease (ESRD). Tejani et al.[1] report that obstructive uropathy was the underlying etiology in 45 percent of children receiving care for ESRD at their center. According to the 1990 report of U.S Renal Data Systems, 11 percent of the reported cases of ESRD in the United States had the primary diagnosis of obstructive uropathy.[2] This chapter focuses primarily on the alterations of renal function that result from urinary tract obstruction.

EFFECTS OF OBSTRUCTION ON KIDNEY FUNCTION

Apart from preventing the flow of urine, obstruction of the urinary tract leads to several alterations in renal function. The severity of these derangements is determined not only by the duration of obstruction but also by whether one or both kidneys are affected. Studies performed in the last decade suggest that the host immune response, the renin-angiotensin system, and prostaglandins are intimately involved in the pathogenesis of abnormalities of renal function observed in an obstructed kidney. Most investigative work regarding the effects of urinary tract obstruction on renal function has been conducted in experimental animals; although species differences may exist, these observations can be considered relevant to human beings as well.

EFFECT ON INTRARENAL PRESSURE

Acute ureteral obstruction is characterized by an increase in hydrostatic pressure within the urinary tract proximal to the site of obstruction. Elevated hydrostatic pressure is transmitted to the renal tubules and the Bowman capsule, neutralizing the net filtration pressure across the glomerular capillaries and thereby diminishing the glomerular filtration rate (GFR).[3,4] However, with continued obstruction, the intratubular pressure does not remain elevated indefinitely. In unilateral ureteral obstruction (UUO), the hydrostatic pressure increases within minutes of ureteral ligation and peaks in 1 to 6 h. The intratubular pressure begins to decline thereafter, and normalizes by 24 h (Fig. 14–1).[5–8] Acute bilateral ureteral obstruction (BUO) also results in a prompt elevation of intrarenal pressure, but it is considerably higher at the end of 24 h in BUO than in UUO and its normalization is also significantly slower than in UUO.[4,6,7] The mechanisms invoked for the decline of intraureteral and intratubular pressure in chronic ureteral obstruction are (1) decreased GFR, (2) increased reabsorption of tubular fluid, and (3) dilatation and increased compliance of the renal pelvis.[7]

EFFECTS ON RENAL HEMODYNAMICS

Within a few minutes of ureteral obstruction, the renal blood flow to the ipsilateral kidney increases and remains high for 2 to 3 h.[6,9–12] The initial renal vasodilatory response in the obstructed kidney is, however, followed by renal vasoconstriction, which continues for a variable period even after the relief of ureteral obstruction.[10] Moody et al.[6] have broken this response down into three phases. Phase I starts at the onset of ureteral obstruction and extends for 2 to 3 h. Renal blood flow increases during this period, despite increasing intratu-

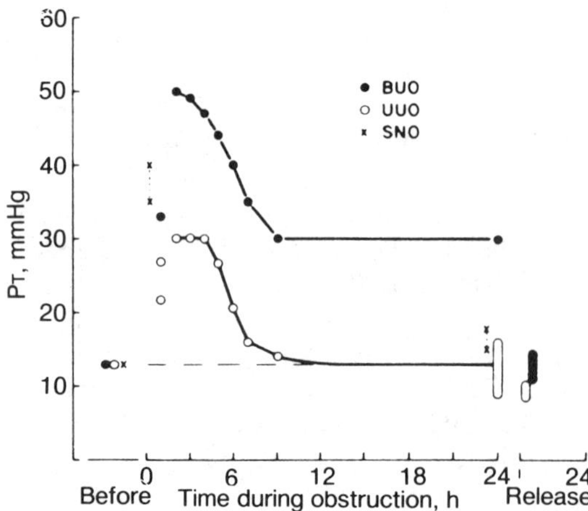

FIG. 14–1. Pressure changes observed in the proximal tubule (P_T) before, during, and after release of complete obstruction of one ureter (UUO, *open circles*), both ureters (BUO, *closed circles*), and single nephrons (SNO, x's). (From Wright FS: Effects of urinary tract obstruction on glomerular filtration rate and blood flow. *Semin Nephrol* 2:5, 1982. Reproduced by permission.)

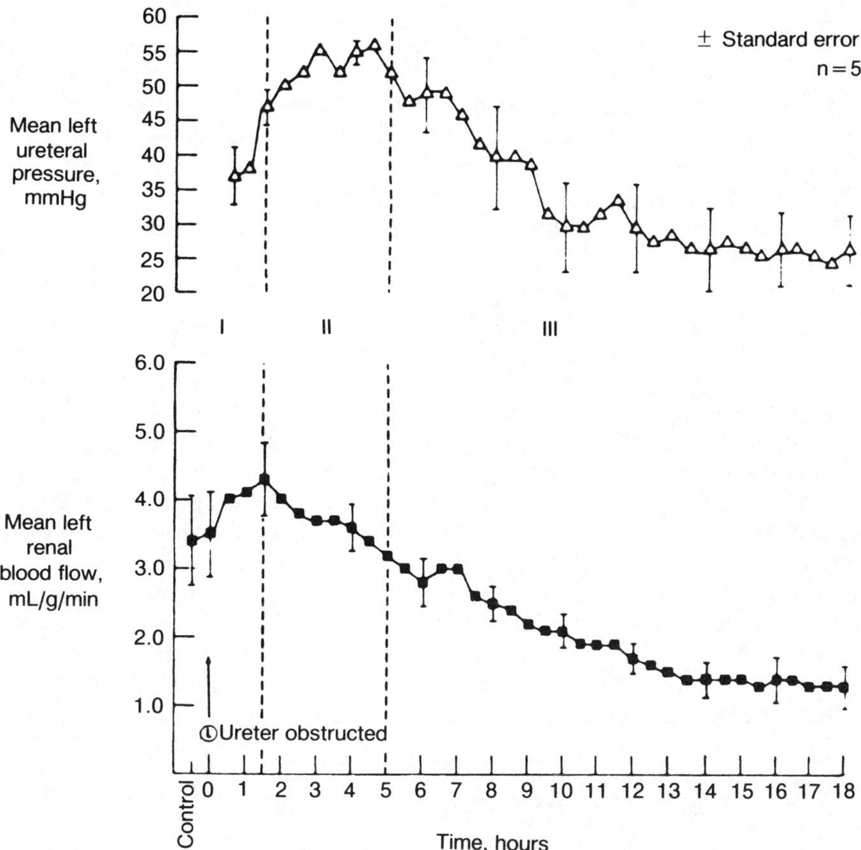

FIG. 14–2. Hemodynamic and ureteral pressure changes during 18 h of left ureteral obstruction. An initial increase in ipsilateral renal blood flow until 1½ h, then a progressive fall in blood flow reaching a steady state at about 13 h postobstruction is observed. Ureteral pressure rises steeply over the first 1½ h with a continued but less steep rise in pressure, reaching a peak at 4½ h. This is followed by a decline in pressure which stabilizes at 13 h. (From Moody TE, Vaughn ED, Gillenwater JY: Relationship between renal blood flow and ureteral pressure during 18 h of total unilateral ureteral occlusion. *Invest Urol* 13:246, 1975. Copyright © 1975 by Williams & Wilkins. Reproduced by permission.)

hydrostatic pressure. In phase III, the intratubular hydrostatic pressure declines steadily despite continued ureteral obstruction, yet the renal blood flow continues its downward trend (Fig. 14–2).

The initial renal vasodilatory response in ureteral obstruction is believed to be mediated by afferent arteriolar dilatation caused by locally synthesized vasodilator prostaglandins in the kidney.[11,13] Although the stimulus for renal vasodilator prostaglandin synthesis in early ureteral obstruction is not clearly understood, the activity of the enzymes phospholipase and cyclooxygenase (which are necessary for the synthesis of prostaglandins) has been shown to be increased in obstructed kidneys.[14,15] The decreased renal blood flow observed with continued ureteral obstruction is characterized by an increase in the afferent arterial tone.[3,4] Factors mediating renal vasoconstriction during this phase of obstruction have been a subject of considerable study. Experimental evidence implicates the vasoconstrictor hormones angiotensin II and thromboxane A_2.[15–17] Pretreatment with angiotensin converting enzyme (ACE) inhibitors as well as inhibitors of thromboxane synthesis prevent the expected decrease in renal blood flow and GFR in kidneys that have undergone ureteral obstruction.[16,17]

The role of immunologic factors in mediating renal vasoconstriction in obstructive uropathy has recently attracted considerable attention. Infiltration of the interstitial mononuclear cells is a characteristic feature of kidneys that undergo ureteral obstruction,[18] and this infiltration diminishes when the obstruction is relieved.[19] The mononuclear cell infiltrate of the obstructed kidney consists mostly of macrophages and to a lesser extent of suppressor T cells.[20] It has been proposed that the leukocytes infiltrating the kidney are responsible for hemodynamic alterations in the obstructed kidney, perhaps by producing thromboxane A_2 locally in the renal tissue.[20] This conclusion is based on the observation in experimental animals that leukocyte depletion by total body irradiation prior to ureteral obstruction diminishes the expected decline in renal blood flow.[21] A second leukocyte-independent vasoconstrictor mechanism—possibly involving thromboxane A_2 synthesis by intrinsic renal cells—may also be operative,[22] since leukocyte depletion does not completely abrogate the diminished renal blood flow in the affected kidneys.[20–21]

EFFECT ON GLOMERULAR FILTRATION RATE

Diminished GFR is an expected result of ureteral obstruction. The pathogenesis of diminished GFR varies with the stage of urinary obstruction. In the initial phase, increased intratubular hydrostatic pressure is the primary factor impeding glomerular filtration.[10] In UUO, however, the intratubular hydrostatic pressure diminishes significantly by the end of 24 h of obstruction yet the GFR remains low, suggesting that other factors are also operative. On the other hand, intratubular hydrostatic pressure remains elevated for a longer time in BUO and can constitute an important factor in the pathogenesis of diminished GFR for a prolonged period. Once the intratubular pressure normalizes, renal vasoconstriction and decreased renal blood flow appear to be the main factors involved in diminishing GFR in the obstructed kidneys.[10] During this phase, afferent and efferent arteriolar constriction, possibly in response to vasoactive hormones, reduces glomerular blood flow as well as intraglomerular capillary hydrostatic pressure.[10,20] Both these factors diminish the net glomerular capillary filtration pressure and glomerular ultrafiltration, thereby reducing GFR. Renal vasoconstriction following urinary obstruction is brought about by the pathophysiologic mechanisms discussed previously. In addition to afferent arteriolar constriction, the vasoactive hormone angiotensin II, generated in the obstructed kidney, may also diminish GFR by decreasing the ultrafiltration coefficient (K_f) of the glomeruli in the affected kidney, thus further reducing GFR.[15,23]

EFFECT ON TUBULAR FUNCTIONS

Urinary tract obstruction has profound implications for renal tubular function. Derangements in tubular functions are commonly observed following relief of urinary obstruction. Fractional excretion of sodium is increased in kidneys affected by obstruction.[24] However, in UUO, the absolute amount of sodium excreted by the affected kidney may be comparable to that of the contralateral normal kidney because of diminished GFR on the involved side. On the other hand, relief of bilateral ureteral obstruction is characterized by increased absolute as well as fractional excretion of sodium in both kidneys.[24] The significance of these observations is that because of the renal salt-wasting state in the postobstructive phase, patients may develop hyponatremia and require sodium supplementation.

Urinary obstruction is associated with impaired urinary concentrating ability.[24] Consequently, the postobstructive state is characterized by excretion of a low-specific-gravity urine, and by an obligatory renal water loss. Postobstructive diuresis can lead to profound volume depletion in some patients. The pathogenesis of postobstructive diuresis is not precisely understood, but the following factors are implicated: (1) osmotic diuresis due to elevated blood urea nitrogen,[25] (2) expanded intravascular volume due to diminished urine output during urinary obstruction, and (3) elevated plasma atrial natriuretic factor (ANF).[26,27] Plasma ANF concentration is elevated in patients with a single obstructed kidney as well as in those with bilaterally obstructed urinary tracts.[27] In experimental UUO, on the other hand, plasma ANF concentration has not been reported to be increased.[26] The reason for this discrepancy is not clear. It is conceivable that BUO is associated with sodium and fluid retention and an increased intravascular volume, leading to elevated plasma concentration of ANF.

Most but not all patients with obstructive uropathy, despite systemic acidosis, are unable to excrete an acidic urine in the postobstructive state,[28] suggesting the presence of renal tubular acidosis (RTA). Currently available evidence suggests that RTA is of the distal type (type 1) in these patients.[20,28] Proximal tubular bicarbonate reabsorption has been reported to be normal in experimental chronic urinary obstruction.[28,29] Hyporeninemic hypoaldosteronism associated with hyperchloremic metabolic acidosis, hyperkalemia, normal anion gap, and impaired distal renal tubular functions (type 4 RTA) may also be seen in humans.[30] RTA seen in the postobstructive state resolves gradually over a few days to a few weeks.

Hyperkalemia is a common clinical feature in patients with obstructive uropathy and can arise from both diminished GFR and decreased renal tubular potassium excretion. Possible mechanisms by which the tubular handling of potassium may be impaired include (1) hyporeninemic hypoaldosteronism and (2) defective tubular transport of potassium. It has been proposed that hypoaldosteronism associated with obstructive uropathy results in decreased tubular resorption of sodium in the distal nephron, which, in turn, leads to a decreased potential difference between the tubular lumen and the cell itself. The consequence of these alterations is diminished potassium as well as hydrogen ion transport in this segment of the nephron.[30] There is some experimental evidence to suggest that a defect in the Na-K pump is induced by ureteral obstruction in the cortical collecting tubules; this may also contribute to diminished tubular excretion of potassium and lead to hyperkalemia.[31] This pump defect is reversible in brief obstruction, but with prolonged urinary tract obstruction recovery may be only partial.[31] Following relief of the obstruction, however, excretion of potassium in urine increases during the diuretic phase and can lead to a negative potassium balance.[24]

EFFECTS OF URINARY TRACT OBSTRUCTION ON THE DEVELOPING FETUS

It is well known that congenital urinary tract obstruction can lead to renal dysplasia (Fig. 14–3*A* and *B*) and pulmonary hypoplasia.[32] Pulmonary hypoplasia is a common cause of early neonatal mortality in the severely affected fetuses and is believed to result from oligohydramnios, which induces a mechanical restriction of growth in the fetal chest.[33] Histologic examination of the hypoplastic lungs in fetal lambs reveals normal histology,[34] but the number of airway branchings is commonly reduced in human fetuses.[35] The manner in which fetal obstructive lesions lead to renal dysplasia is not well settled. Experimental observations suggest that the timing of urinary tract obstruction in relation to gestation is an important factor in determining whether or not renal dysplasia will develop. Ureteral obstruction induced late in the gestation of fetal sheep (equivalent to 22 to 29 weeks in humans) only produces hydronephrosis without any evidence of renal dysplasia.[36,37] On the other hand, urinary obstruction in early gestation produces renal dysplasia, and relief of urinary obstruction in utero prevents such changes.[38,39] Intrauterine lower urinary tract obstruction has also been implicated in the pathogenesis of prune-belly syndrome (also known as Eagle-Barrett syndrome), which consists of the following triad: loose hypoplastic musculature of the abdominal wall; urogenital abnormalities, such as megaureters; and undescended testes in males.[40] As a consequence of these experimental observations, fetal surgery and intrauterine decompression of the urinary tract obstruction has been attempted in human fetuses with obstructive uropathy with a view to preventing developmental renal damage.[32] An international registry for monitoring the outcome of such fetal surgical procedures has also been established.[32] Data on long-term survival and renal function in surviving children who have undergone intrauterine decompression of the urinary tract are not yet available.

LOWER URNARY TRACT OBSTRUCTION

The lower urinary tract is designated as the segment that extends from the ureterovesicular junction to the urethral meatus. Developmental lesions of the lower urinary tract are frequently the etiology of lower urinary tract obstruction in children, but acquired lesions—such as bladder stones, extrinsic or intrinsic compression from a mass lesion, postoperative states, and side effects of medications—can also lead to obstruction of the lower urinary tract. Table 14–1 lists the anatomically classified lesions that lead to lower urinary tract obstruction.

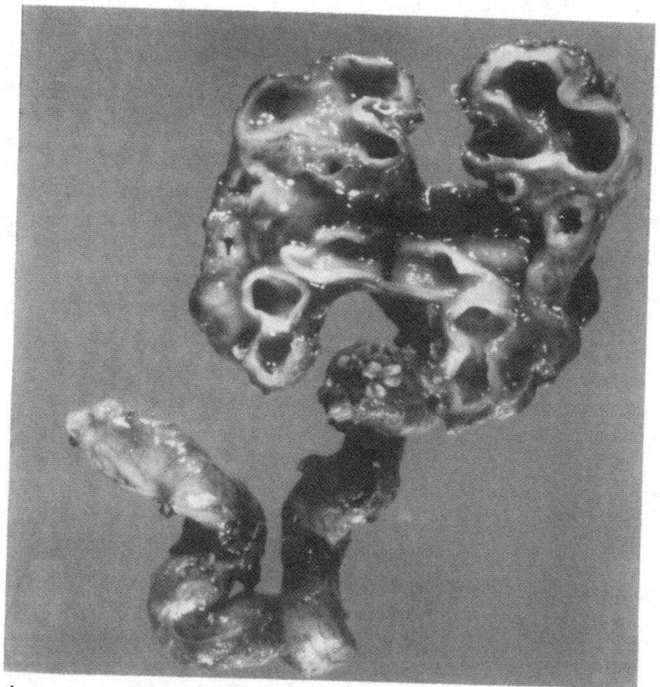

A

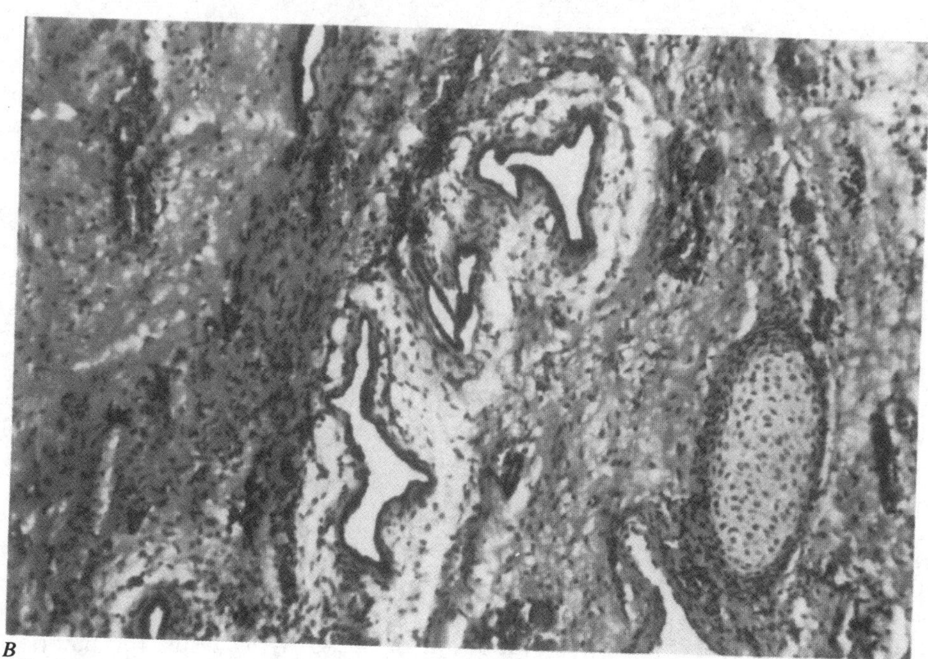

B

FIG. 14–3. *A*. Nephroureterectomy specimen of a 4-day-old neonate with posterior urethral valves, showing dilated ureter and deformed kidney with dilatation affecting the pelvicalyceal system. No clear demarcation of renal cortex and medulla was seen in the kidney. *B*. Light microscopy section of the kidney showing dysplasia characterized by the presence of cartilage. [Photographs courtesy of Dr. Kathleen Patterson, Department of Pathology, Children's National Medical Center, Washington, D.C.]

TABLE 14–1. Causes of Lower Urinary Tract Obstruction in Children

Anatomic	Functional
Urethra	
Posterior urethral valves	Dysfunctional voiding
Urethral stricture	Detrusor-sphincter dyssynergia
Urethral polyps	
Anterior urethral valves	
Meatal stenosis	
Urethral aplasia	
Bladder	
Ureterocele	Neurogenic bladder
Primary bladder neck obstruction	Neurogenic-nonneurogenic bladder
Bladder stones	Postoperative state
	Medications
Ureterovesical Junction	
Primary obstructive megaureter	High-grade reflux
Detrusor hypertrophy	Postoperative state
Ureterocele	
Ectopic ureter	
Postoperative state	

Source: From Rink RC, Mitchell MC: Physiology of lower urinary tract obstruction. *Urol Clin North Am* 17:329, 1990. Reproduced by permission.

POSTERIOR URETHRAL VALVES

Posterior urethral valves (PUV) are the commonest etiology of lower urinary tract obstruction in male children. Of the 130 male children reported in one study, PUV was the etiology of lower urinary tract obstruction in 91 cases (69.2 percent).[41] PUV are located in the posterior urethra, which constitutes the urethral passage extending for a few centimeters below the bladder neck. Young and coworkers[42] have classified PUV into three anatomic categories (Fig. 14–4*A* and *B*). According to this classification, the type 1 valve, the commonest form of PUV, consists of membranous folds that are present below the verumontanum and obstruct the flow of urine from the bladder (Fig. 14–5). The type 3 valve is the next most frequent form of PUV and consists of a membranous diaphragm below the level of verumontanum with a central hole. The least common clinical variety of PUV is type 2, which consists of membranous folds above the level of verumontanum.

CLINICAL MANIFESTATIONS

Clinical manifestations of PUV can be varied, ranging from almost none to severe urinary obstruction, parenchymal renal damage, and renal failure. With increasing prenatal ultrasound evaluation of the growing fetus, the diagnosis of PUV is often suspected prior to birth. Ultrasonographic features suggestive of PUV in the fetus consist of an enlarged urinary bladder (which may demonstrate a thickened wall) and bilateral hydronephrosis. At birth, a palpable bladder with or without abdominal distension and enlargement of the kidneys

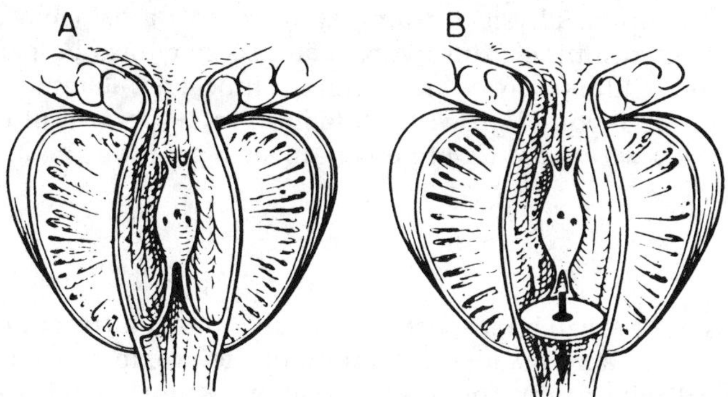

FIG. 14–4. Diagrammatic representation of type 1 (*A*) and type 3 (*B*) posterior urethral valves. Type 1 posterior urethral valves usually arise like a pair of spinnakers from the crista distal to the verumontanum. Type 3 posterior urethral valves are diaphragmlike, with a central opening. [From Colodny A: Urethral lesions in infants and children, in Gillenwater JY, Grayhack JT, Howards SS, Duckett JW (eds): *Adult and Pediatric Urology*. St. Louis, Missouri, Mosby Year Book, 1991, p. 1995. Reproduced by permission.]

is a usual finding. Oligohydramnios and pulmonary hypoplasia may be prominent clinical features of some neonates born with severe obstructive uropathy due to PUV. Ascites may be seen at times in infants with severe lower urinary tract obstruction due to PUV. In others, urinary tract infection or sepsis may be the initial manifestation of PUV. In patients in whom PUV are not detected at birth, symptoms related to poor urinary stream, dribbling, and urinary tract

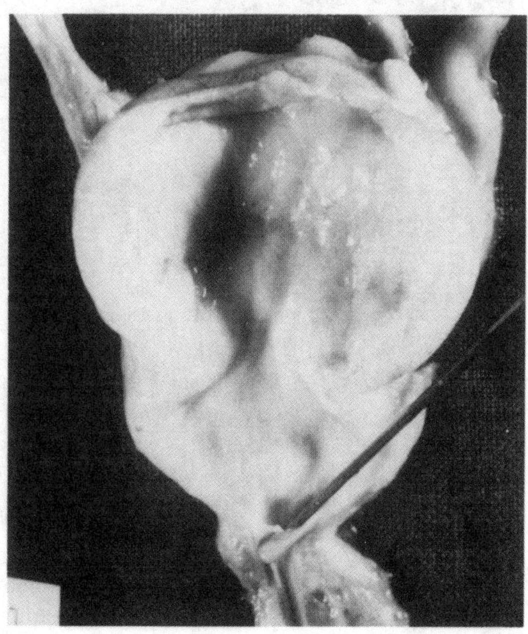

FIG. 14–5. Autopsy specimen showing bladder and urethra. Type 1 posterior urethral valve is indicated by the position of probe. (Photograph courtesy of Dr. A. Barry Belman, Department of Urology, Children's National Medical Center, Washington, D.C.)

infection are common. Physical examination reveals a palpable urinary bladder; renal masses resulting from hydronephrosis may also be palpable. Renal dysfunction and failure to thrive are common clinical problems in children with PUV. Tejani et al.[1] reported growth retardation in 40 percent of children with PUV, while ESRD was noted in 44 percent of such cases during a mean follow-up of 9 years.

DIAGNOSIS

The diagnosis of PUV can be suspected by an abdominal ultrasound demonstrating a thick-walled, large bladder. Dilatation of the proximal urethra can sometimes be visualized by ultrasound examination. Kidneys and ureters may be enlarged bilaterally due to vesicoureteral reflux. Severe urinary obstruction may be associated with cystic renal dysplasia.[43] The diagnosis of PUV is confirmed by voiding cystourethrography (VCUG), which demonstrates the area of obstruction in the urethra and dilatation of the posterior urethra (Fig. 14–6). The capacity of the bladder is usually decreased in older children due to hypertrophy of the muscle wall, which also gives rise to the trabeculated appearance

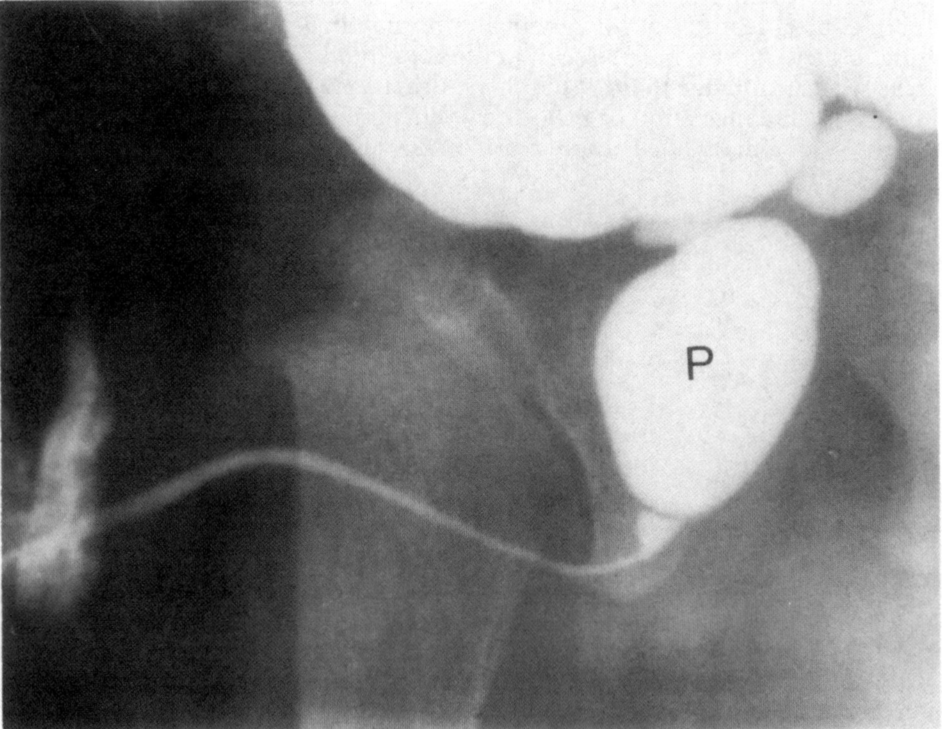

FIG. 14–6. Voiding cystourethrogram of neonate with posterior urethral valves (type 1). Dilated posterior urethra (P) is a characteristic radiologic sign. (Photograph courtesy of Dr. A. Barry Belman, Department of Urology, Children's National Medical Center, Washington, D.C.)

of the bladder. Renal functions should be assessed by analysis of blood urea nitrogen (BUN), and serum creatinine as well as by radionuclide renal scan. Dysplastic kidneys seen in patients with severe PUV demonstrate poor renal perfusion and function by radionuclide scan.

MANAGEMENT

Management of PUV is determined by the age of the patient and the severity of the obstruction. Temporary relief of urinary obstruction in a neonate may be essential until the patient is fit to undergo surgery. This can be provided by indwelling urethral catheter drainage. In neonates with renal insufficiency and severe urinary obstruction, the placement of a urinary catheter can also provide information about the potential for reversibility of renal dysfunction. A decline in serum creatinine and BUN during 4 to 5 days of urethral catheterization may suggest that the renal parenchymal damage is minimal, while failure of serum creatinine to decline or its actual rise indicates poor prognosis for renal function even after surgical correction or drainage procedure.[44]

Several types of surgical procedures can be undertaken in patients with PUV.[45] Bilateral cutaneous ureterostomy is performed by some centers as the procedure of choice in patients with severe PUV, vesicoureteral reflux, and a dilated urinary tract. Others prefer surgical drainage of the bladder by a vesicostomy. With the availability of small-caliber endoscopes, cystoscopic ablation of the PUV is increasingly becoming a practical option, even in neonates. Postobstructive diuresis associated with increased urinary volume and electrolyte loss can be expected following relief of obstruction by either catheter drainage or surgery. Resection of the valves is the treatment of choice in older children. Management of chronic renal failure involves control of fluid and electrolyte balance, attention to divalent ion metabolism, growth, and treatment of anemia by recombinant erythropoietin therapy, as outlined in Chap. 16. Patients with PUV must be monitored by the urologist-nephrologist team for the development of chronic renal failure and hypertension.

PROGNOSIS

In a study of infants undergoing surgical intervention for PUV during the first year of life, Warshaw et al.[44] determined that patients achieving a serum creatinine nadir of 0.8 mg/dL by 12 months of age were able to maintain their serum creatinine below or equal to 1.1 mg/dL at a mean follow-up period of 5.8 years. However, it is a common clinical observation that even with early and appropriate surgical therapy, patients with PUV may develop chronic renal failure.[1] These impressions were confirmed in a recent long-term study of 98 boys followed for a mean period of 15 years.[46] Twenty-six percent of the children in this study developed chronic renal failure or ESRD during follow-up. Recurrent urinary tract infection, vesicoureteral reflux, and hypertension may be involved in ongoing renal parenchymal damage, scarring, and the development of chronic renal failure. A delay in the diagnosis of congenital obstructive uropathy and vesicoureteral reflux is associated with a poor outcome for renal function.[1] It remains unclear whether the underlying renal dysplasia noted in patients with obstructive uropathy contributes to chronic renal failure.[43]

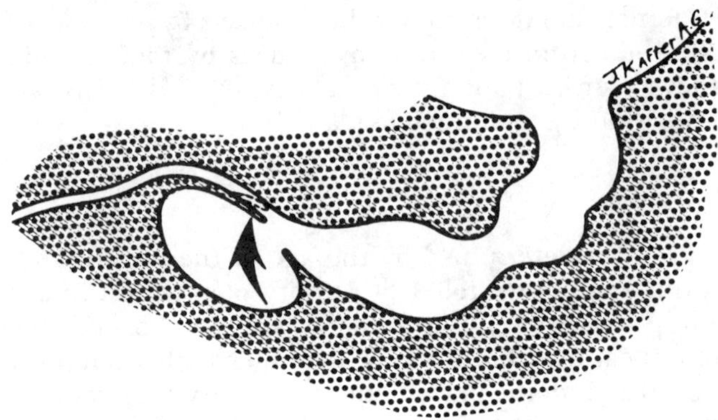

FIG. 14–7. Diagrammatic representation of an anterior urethral diverticulum. When the diverticulum fills with urine, the anterior lip acts as an obstructing one-way flap valve. [From Colodny A: Urethal lesions in infants and children, in Gillenwater JY, Grayhack JT, Howards SS, Duckett JW (eds): *Adult and Pediatric Urology*. St. Louis, Missouri, Mosby Year Book, 1991, p. 1995. Reproduced by permission.]

ANTERIOR URETHRAL VALVES AND DIVERTICULA

Anterior urethral valves are often seen in association with a urethral diverticulum; therefore they are considered together here. The diverticulum affecting the anterior urethra manifests as a bulge in the penoscrotal area, and the patient may have symptoms of dribbling. Pressure over the bulge may lead to the expression of urine. The anterior lip of the diverticulum can act as a valve and obstruct the outward flow of urine (Fig. 14–7). Valves not associated with a diverticulum can also be seen in some patients.[47]

The diagnosis of anterior urethral diverticulum and valves can be established by VCUG. Resection of the valve using an endoscope may be curative in those who do not have an associated diverticulum. Surgical resection is necessary in the patient with a large diverticulum. In neonates with severe obstructive features, vesicotomy may be essential as the initial step in the surgical correction of the defect.[48]

URETHRAL POLYPS

Urethral polyps are an uncommon cause of lower urinary tract obstruction in young infants and children. They are benign growths that usually arise in the posterior urethra, in the region of verumontanum, and may be either sessile or pedunculated (Fig. 14–8).[49] Common clinical manifestations of urethral polyps are intermittent urinary obstruction, macroscopic hematuria, and urinary frequency. Diagnosis is established by VCUG, which demonstrates a filling defect in the posterior urethra. Treatment consists of surgical removal of the polyp. Recurrence of urethral polyps is uncommon but can occur.[50]

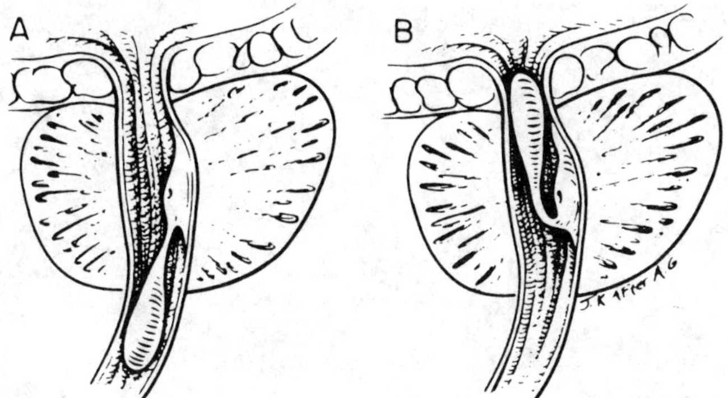

FIG. 14–8. A pedunculated urethral polyp on a relatively long stalk arising from the distal end of the verumontanum. If the stalk is long enough, the polyp may lie in the bulbous urethra (*A*), at the bladder neck (*B*), or completely within the bladder. [From Colodny A: Urethral lesions in infants and children, in Gillenwater JY, Grayhack JT, Howards SS, Duckett JW (eds): *Adult and Pediatric Urology*. St. Louis, Missouri, Mosby Year Book, 1991, p. 1995. Reproduced by permission.]

FUNCTIONAL DISORDERS OF THE URINARY BLADDER

The normal voiding process involves two essential events that occur in sequence. The first is the phase of urine storage during which the detrusor muscle, which forms the bulk of bladder wall, undergoes relaxation and both the internal and external urethral sphincters remain closed. During the voiding phase, the detrusor muscles contract while the internal and external urethral sphincters relax, allowing the passage of urine from the urinary bladder into the urethra and the initiation of voiding. Intact neurologic innervation is essential for proper bladder function and a normal voiding response. Many neurologic disorders, generally grouped under the category of *neurogenic bladder*, can be associated with abnormalities of innervation of the urinary bladder and result in voiding dysfunctions. The commonest cause of neurogenic bladder in children is meningomyelocele.

The clinical consequences of neurogenic bladder resulting from meningomyelocele are complex. Based on the functional classification proposed by Raezer et al.,[51] patients with neurogenic bladder may have either failure of bladder emptying or failure of urine storage within the bladder. Even without any evidence of anatomic urinary tract obstruction, patients with neurogenic bladder can manifest increased intravesicular pressure due to dysfunctional voiding patterns. This, combined with vesicoureteral reflux, can lead to ongoing renal scarring and deterioration of renal function.

Another form of bladder and voiding dysfunction, described by Hinman and Bauman,[52] is characterized by the clinical features of urinary incontinence, recurrent urinary tract infections, radiologic evidence of a large urinary bladder associated with thickened trabeculated muscle wall, and a variable degree of upper urinary tract dilatation and damage. No anatomically identifiable obstructive lesions can be demonstrated by detailed urologic evaluation, and neurologic examination of these children is entirely normal (Fig. 14–9). This

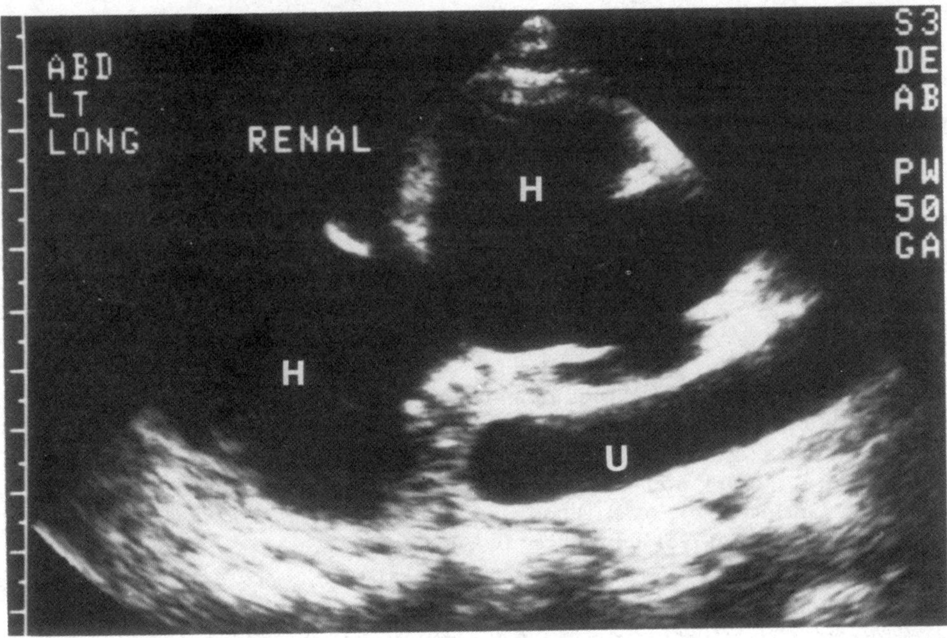

A

FIG. 14–9. This 8-year-old boy presented with a history of urinary incontinence, urinary tract infection, and elevated serum creatinine. Bilateral hydronephrosis (H) with large ureters (U) and an enlarged bladder was noted on ultrasound examination (*A*). DTPA renal scan (*B*) demonstrated poorly functioning kidneys bilaterally. Voiding cystourethrogram (*C*) demonstrated an enlarged bladder with no evidence of anatomically defined obstruction. Cystoscopy was also unable to demonstrate any urethral or bladder neck abnormality. Neurologic examination of the patient was entirely within normal limits. A diagnosis of nonneurogenic neurogenic bladder was made. End-stage renal failure developed one year later.

condition is often described as *nonneurogenic neurogenic bladder*. Recently, it has been recommended that this disorder be referred to as *Hinman syndrome.*[53] Other terms used to describe it are *unstable bladder, dysfunctional bladder, lazy bladder, pseudoobstructed bladder,* and *occult neurogenic bladder.*

It has been suggested that nonneurogenic neurogenic bladder develops from excessive and uninhibited contraction of the detrusor muscle and failure to relax the external sphincter or pelvic diaphragm, leading to incoordination between these two essential neuroanatomic events involved in voiding. These children are apparently unaware of the sensation of bladder distension and keep themselves dry by contracting the external sphincter. However, increased pressure within the bladder eventually leads to hypertrophy of its wall as well as the development of back pressure into the ureters and kidney. Chronic renal failure may develop in some patients. The diagnosis is established by ruling out anatomic obstructive lesions of the lower urinary tract by VCUG and cystoscopy and by demonstrating uninhibited detrusor contractions via cystometrogram. Treatment of nonneurogenic neurogenic bladder consists of bladder retraining,

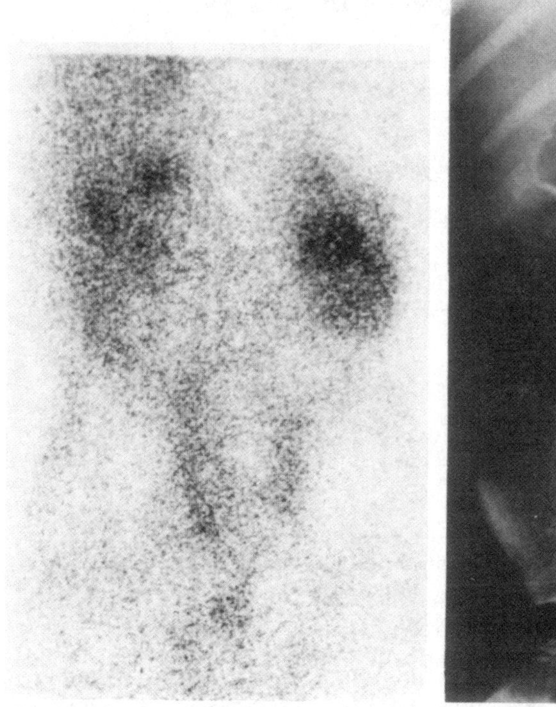

B

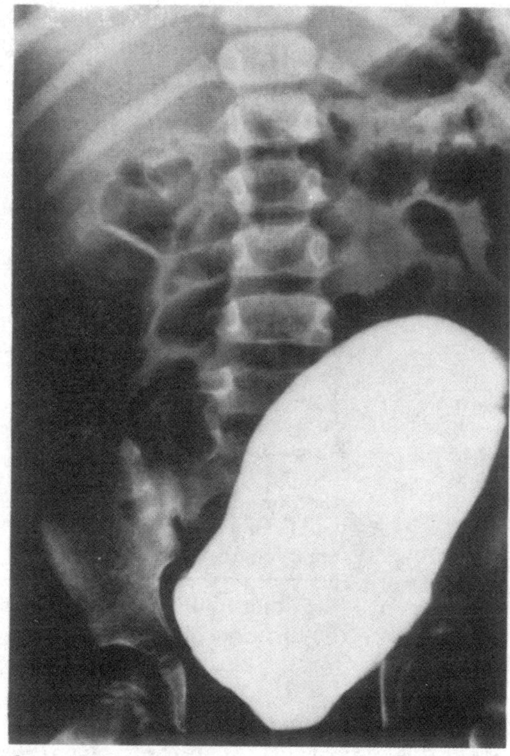

C

FIG. 14–9 (*Continued*).

biofeedback, and hypnosis as well as pharmacotherapy with anticholinergic drugs to inhibit detrusor contraction.[53]

UPPER URINARY TRACT OBSTRUCTION—HYDRONEPHROSIS

Obstruction involving the upper urinary tract or kidneys and ureters results in dilatation of the ureters and pelvicalyceal system, or hydronephrosis. Bilateral upper urinary tract obstruction is caused by lesions affecting the urinary bladder or urethra, while unilateral obstruction is caused by lesions affecting the ipsilateral collecting system. The etiology of upper urinary tract obstruction in children is given in Table 14–2.

DIAGNOSIS

The diagnosis of upper urinary tract obstruction and hydronephrosis is established by ultrasonography and, if necessary, intravenous pyelography. Sonography reveals dilatation of the ureters and pelvicalyceal system as well as renal

TABLE 14–2. Causes of Upper Urinary Tract Obstruction Affecting the Ureters, Ureteropelvic Junction, and Kidneys

Ureterovesical Junction
Ureterovesical junction stricture
Congenital ureteral valves
Ureteral Length
Vascular compression of ureter
Compression by bladder diverticulum
Extrinsic compression by a pelvic tumor, fecal mass
Ureteral stricture
Ureteral stones
Ureteral kinks
Ureteropelvic junction stricture
Periureteric fibrosis
Fungus ball[a]
Renal Pelvis
Aberrant blood vessel crossing renal pelvis
Renal stone
Renal tumor

[a]Fungus balls can lead to obstruction anywhere along the urinary collection system.

enlargement. Renal cortical thickness may be reduced in chronic hydronephrosis and is indicative of a poor reserve of renal function. Radionuclide renal scans have generally replaced intravenous pyelography in the diagnosis of obstruction affecting the urinary tract. The radionuclide renal scan is especially helpful in neonates, in whose kidneys intravenous contrast material is poorly concentrated and satisfactory images of the kidney and the collecting system are not always produced. It is important to note that not all patients showing dilated urinary tracts and hydronephrosis have obstructive uropathy. Many such children will have severe vesicoureteral reflux as the etiology of urinary tract dilatation. This diagnosis must be considered if an obstructive lesion cannot be documented in a dilated urinary tract by ultrasonography or radionuclide renal scan.

The Whitaker test[54] or perfusion-pressure study, which involves placement of a nephrostomy catheter percutaneously, is helpful in the evaluation of patients in whom an obstruction to the flow of urine in the upper urinary tract is suspected but for whom an anatomic site of obstruction cannot be localized by conventional investigative techniques. In this test, the kidney is perfused via the nephrostomy catheter at a constant rate of 10 mL/min, and a pressure tracing is simultaneously made. A positive Whitaker test shows of a rise in intrarenal pressure to 22 cmH_2O or more and suggests an obstruction on the ipsilateral side. The test is not always helpful, since equivocal results characterized by a rise in pressure between 16 and 21 cmH_2O are difficult to interpret with certainty.[55] Diuretic radioisotope scintigraphy, a noninvasive procedure for the diagnosis of upper urinary tract obstruction, can be conducted in place of the Whitaker test and is discussed in Chap. 3.

TREATMENT

The treatment of upper urinary tract obstruction is always surgical correction, and the choice of procedure is guided by the level of the lesion and the underlying etiology of the obstruction. A detailed discussion of surgical correction of upper urinary tract obstruction is beyond the scope of this chapter. Since chronic renal failure, hypertension, and recurrent urinary tract infections are commonly associated clinical problems, these issues must be appropriately addressed.

SUMMARY

This chapter has described the functional changes seen in the kidney following obstruction of the urinary tract (UT). The mechanisms involved in decreasing GFR in the obstructed UT have been better elucidated in the last two decades, and the role played by the renin-angiotensin system and the prostaglandins in diminishing GFR is well accepted. Evidence implicating the involvement of the immune system in affecting renal function in urinary obstruction has been presented recently. Preventing ongoing renal parenchymal damage and preserving renal function are the primary objectives that drive the need to better delineate anatomic and functional alterations induced by UT obstruction. In order to provide the reader with some familiarity with the subject, common clinical conditions that cause UT obstruction in children have been discussed briefly in this chapter. The scope of such discussions has, however, been entirely limited to the medical aspects, and the reader should consult a urology textbook for further details.

REFERENCES

1. Tejani A, Butt K, Glassberg K, et al: Predictors of eventual end stage renal disease in children with posterior urethral valves. *J Urol* 136:857, 1986.
2. U.S. Renal Data Systems: *USRDS 1990 Annual Data Report*. The National Institutes of Health, National Institute of Diabetes, Digestive and Kidney Diseases, Bethesda, Maryland, 1990, p A46.
3. Dal Canton A, Corradi A, Stanziale R, et al: Effect of 24-hour unilateral ureteral obstruction on glomerular hemodynamics in rat kidney. *Kidney Int* 15:457, 1979.
4. Dal Canton A, Corradi A, Stanziale R, et al: Glomerular hemodynamics before and release of 24-hour bilateral ureteral obstruction. *Kidney Int* 17:491, 1980.
5. Yarger WE, Griffith LD: Intrarenal hemodynamics following chronic unilateral obstruction in the dog. *Am J Physiol* 227:816, 1974.
6. Moody TE, Vaughn ED, Gillenwater JY: Relationship between renal blood flow and ureteral pressure during 18 hours of unilateral ureteral occlusion. *Invest Urol* 13:246, 1975.
7. Wilson DR: Pathophysiology of obstructive nephropathy. *Kidney Int* 18:281, 1980.
8. Jaenike JR: The renal response to ureteral obstruction: A model for the study of factors which influence glomerular filtration pressure. *J Clin Lab Med* 76:373, 1970.

9. Vaughn ED Jr, Sorenson EJ, and Gillenwater JY: The renal hemodynamic response to chronic unilateral complete ureteral occlusion. *Invest Urol* 8:78, 1970.
10. Wright FS: Effects of urinary tract obstruction on glomerular filtration rate and renal blood flow. *Semin Nephrol* 2:5, 1982.
11. Navar LG, Bear PG: Renal autoregulatory and glomerular filtration response to gradual ureteral obstruction. *Nephron* 7:301, 1970.
12. Suki WN, Guthrie AG, Martinez-Maldonado M, et al: Effect of ureteral pressure elevation on renal hemodynamics and urine concentration. *Am J Physiol* 220:38, 1971.
13. Morrison AR, Benabe JE: Prostaglandins and vascular tone in experimental obstructive nephropathy. *Kidney Int* 19:786, 1981.
14. Morrison AR, Pascoe N, Needleman P: Perfusion dependent induction of de novo synthesis of renal phosphatide acyl hydrolase in ureter-obstructed rabbit kidney. *J Biol Chem* 225:20, 1980.
15. Klahr S, Harris K, Purkerson ML: Effects of obstruction on renal functions. *Pediatric Nephrol* 2:34, 1988.
16. Yarger WE, Shocken DD, Harris RH, et al: Obstructive nephropathy in the rat: Possible role for renin-angiotensin system, prostaglandins and thromboxane in postobstructive renal function. *J Clin Invest* 65:400, 1980.
17. Purkerson ML, Klahr S: Prior inhibition of vasoconstrictors normalizes GFR in postobstructed kidney. *Kidney Int* 35:1306, 1989.
18. Nagle RB, Johnson ME, Jervis HR: Proliferation of renal interstitial cell following injury by ureteral obstruction. *Lab Invest* 35:18, 1976.
19. Schreiner G, Harris KPG, Purkerson ML, et al: The immunologic aspects of acute ureteral obstruction: Immunology of cell infiltrate in the kidney. *Kidney Int* 34:487, 1988.
20. Klahr S: Pathophysiology of obstructive nephropathy: A 1991 update. *Semin Nephrol* 11:156, 1991.
21. Harris KPG, Schreiner GF, Klahr S: Effects of leukocyte depletion on the function of postobstructed kidney in the rat. *Kidney Int* 36:210, 1989.
22. Yanagisawa H, Morrissey J, Morrison A, et al: Eicosanoid production by isolated glomeruli of rats with unilateral ureteral obstruction. *Kidney Int* 37:1528, 1990.
23. Mitchell KD, Navar LG: Interactive effects of angiotensin II on renal hemodynamics and tubular reabsorptive function. *Kidney Int* 38(suppl 30):S69, 1990.
24. Yarger WE, Buerkert J: Effect of urinary tract obstruction on renal tubular function. *Semin Nephrol* 2:17, 1982.
25. Harris RH, Yarger WE: The pathogenesis of postobstructive diuresis: The role of circulating natriuretic and diuretic factors, including urea. *J Clin Invest* 56:880, 1975.
26. Purkerson ML, Blaine EH, Stokes TJ, et al: Role of atrial natriuretic peptide in natriuresis and diuresis that follows relief of obstruction in rats. *Am J Physiol* 256:F583, 1989.
27. Gulmi FA, Mooppan UMM, Chou S-Y, et al: Atrial natiruetic peptide in patients with obstructive uropathy. *J Urol* 142:268, 1989.
28. Berlyne GM: Distal tubular function in chronic hydronephrosis. *Q J Med* 30:339, 1971.
29. Walls J, Buerkert JE, Purkerson ML, et al: Nature of acidifying defect after relief of ureteral obstruction. *Kidney Int* 7:304, 1975.
30. Batlle DC, Arruda JAL, Kurtzman NA: Hyperkalemic distal renal tubular acidosis associated with obstructive uropathy. *N Engl J Med* 304:373, 1981.
31. Kimura H, Mujais SK: Cortical collecting duct Na-K pump in obstructive nephropathy. *Am J Physiol* 258:F1320, 1990.
32. Manning FA, Harrison MR, Rodeck C, et al: Catheter shunts for fetal hydronephrosis

and hydrocephalus: Report of the International Fetal Surgery Registry. *N Engl J Med* 315:336, 1986.

33. Nakayama DK, Glick PL, Harrison MR, et al: Experimental pulmonary hypoplasia due to oligohydramnios and its reversal by relieving thoracic compression. *J Pediatr Surg* 18:347, 1983.
34. Adzick NS, Harrison MR, Glick PL, et al: Fetal urinary tract obstruction: Experimental pathophysiology. *Semin Perinatol* 9:79, 1985.
35. Wigglesworth JS, Dejai R, Guerrini P, et al: Fetal lung hypoplasia: Biochemical and structural variations and their possible significance. *Arch Dis Child* 56:606, 1981.
36. Beck AD: The effect of intra-uterine urinary obstruction upon the development of fetal kidney. *J Urol* 105:784, 1971.
37. Harrison MR, Ross N, Noall R, et al: Correction of congenital hydronephrosis in utero: I. The model: Fetal urethral obstruction produces hydronephrosis and pulmonary hypoplasia in fetal lambs. *J Pediatr Surg* 18:247, 1983.
38. Glick PL, Harrison MR, Noall R, et al: Correction of congenital hydronephrosis in utero: III. Early and mid-trimester ureteral obstruction produces renal dysplasia. *J Pediatr Surg* 18:681, 1983.
39. Glick PL, Harrison MR, Adzick NS, et al: Correction of congenital hydronephrosis in utero: IV. In utero decompression prevents renal dysplasia. *J Pediatr Surg* 19:649, 1984.
40. Moerman P, Fryns J-P, Goddeeris P, et al: Pathogenesis of the prune-belly syndrome: A functional urethral obstruction caused by prostatic hypoplasia. *Pediatrics* 73:470, 1984.
41. Tsinglolou S, Dickson JAS: Lower urinary obstruction in infancy: A review of lesions and symptoms in 165 cases. *Arch Dis Child* 47:215, 1972.
42. Young HH, Fronz WA, Baldwin JC: Congenital obstruction of posterior urethra. *J Urol* 3:289, 1919.
43. Hoover DL, Duckett JW: Posterior urethral valves, unilateral reflux and renal dysplasia: A syndrome. *J Urol* 128:994, 1982.
44. Warshaw BL, Hymes LC, Trulock TS, et al: Prognostic features in infants with obstructive uropathy due to posterior urethral valves. *J Urol* 133:240, 1985.
45. Egami K, Smith ED: A study of the sequelae of posterior urethral valves. *J Urol* 127:84, 1982.
46. Parkhouse HF, Barratt TM, Dillon MJ, et al: Long-term outcome of boys with posterior urethral valves. *Br J Urol* 62:50, 1988.
47. Golimbu M, Orca M, Al-Askari S, et al: Anterior urethral valves. *Urology* 12:343, 1978.
48. Rushton HG, Parrot TS, Woodward JR, et al: The role of vesicotomy in the management of anterior urethral valves in neonates and infants. *J Urol* 137:123, 1987.
49. Youssif M: Posterior urethral polyps in infants and children. *Eur Urol* 11:69, 1985.
50. Frates R, DeLuca FG: Urethral polyps in male children. *Radiology* 89:289, 1967.
51. Raezer DM, Benson GS, Wein AJ, et al: The functional approach to the management of the pediatric neuropathic bladder: A clinical study. *J Urol* 117:649, 1977.
52. Hinman F Jr, Bauman FW: Vesical and ureteral damage in boys without neurological or obstructive disease. *J Urol* 109:727, 1973.
53. Hinman F Jr: Nonneurogenic neurogenic bladder (the Hinman syndrome)—15 years later. *J Urol* 136:769, 1986.
54. Whitaker RH: Methods of assessing obstruction in dilated ureters. *Br J Urol* 45:15, 1973.
55. Whitaker RH, Buxton-Thomas MS: A comparison of pressure-flow studies and renography in equivocal upper urinary tract obstruction. *J Urol* 131:446, 1985.

RENAL FAILURE

15

ACUTE RENAL FAILURE

Glenn H. Bock

Acute renal failure (ARF) is defined as a sudden decline of renal function, with resultant retention of nitrogenous waste products, such as blood urea nitrogen (BUN) and creatinine. Although diminished urine output is a common feature of ARF in many patients, urinary volume may be normal or even increased in others. Normal renal function depends on intact nephron perfusion, adequate glomerular ultrafiltration, appropriate tubular functions, and an unimpaired urine outflow. Consequently, ARF can result from disturbances in any of the elements involved in this physiologic sequence. The etiology of ARF in children varies from one geographic region of the world to another. While diarrheal dehydration is a common cause of ARF in the underdeveloped countries, post-surgical and nephrotoxic etiologies are more prevalent in the industrialized world. The management of children with ARF necessitates careful monitoring for fluid and electrolyte abnormalities, institution of dialysis therapy at an appropriate time, and prevention of complications. The availability of modern methods of dialysis and hemofiltration has made the care of these children easier and improved their outlook for survival.

TERMINOLOGY

Oliguria In adults, oliguria is defined as urine ouput below 400 mL/1.73 m^2/24 h.[1] In older children, oliguria is considered to be present when urine output is below 200 mL/m^2/24 h.[2] The generally accepted definition of oliguria in neonates and young children is a urine output below 1 mL/kg/h.[3]
Anuria Anuria is defined as complete cessation of urinary output. However, a nominal urinary volume (some few millimeters voided per 8-h nursing shift) should also be considered within the broader definition of anuria.
Polyuria In the context of ARF, polyuria is defined as a normal or excessive urinary output (>2 mL/kg/h) in the presence of an acutely rising BUN or serum creatinine.

CLASSIFICATION

On the basis of the clinical criteria of urine output, ARF can be classified into oliguric (classic) or nonoliguric subtypes. *Nonoliguric ARF* is characterized by acutely rising BUN and serum creatinine concentrations despite excretion of a normal or even an increased urinary volume. *Oliguric ARF,* on the other hand, is associated with curtailed daily urinary excretion and evidence of renal dysfunction. Possibly as a result of an increasing awareness of its existence in the last two decades, nonoliguric ARF has been reported to be the more common clinical variety of ARF.[4]

Alternatively, ARF can be categorized on the basis of its pathophysiologic mechanism into (1) prerenal azotemia, (2) intrinsic or parenchymal ARF, and (3) postrenal ARF. *Prerenal azotemia* is defined as a transient disturbance of renal function caused by hypoperfusion of the kidney. Complete recovery of renal function is expected upon the return of normal renal perfusion. *Intrinsic* or *parenchymal ARF* results from intrinsic renal damage caused by a variety of etiologies, such as prolonged and severe hypoperfusion, nephrotoxic renal injury, and intrinsic renal disease. *Postrenal ARF* implies an underlying acute urinary tract obstruction as the factor responsible for renal dysfunction. In relating the pathophysiologic classification to clinical settings, one must remain both cautious and flexible, since many etiologies of ARF will manifest abnormalities which cross these traditional boundaries of categorization. For example, hypovolemia and renal hypoperfusion can lead to prerenal azotemia, but if the renal ischemic episode is of severe degree or prolonged duration, intrinsic renal failure can develop.

PRERENAL AZOTEMIA

Prerenal azotemia is caused by diminished blood flow to an otherwise functionally intact kidney. In its truest sense, prerenal azotemia may not be regarded as a state of "renal failure" but should be considered an appropriate renal response to hypoperfusion. Although diminished urine output, elevation of BUN, and—to a lesser degree—increased serum creatinine concentration are observed in prerenal azotemia, normalization of renal function upon therapeutic intervention is an essential hallmark of this disorder. Oliguria observed in prerenal azotemia constitutes an attempt by the kidneys to preserve intravascular volume in the presence of hypotension or intravascular volume depletion. However, when these renal compensatory mechanisms are exceeded, as in prolonged or repeated episodes of severe hypotension, intrinsic renal damage and parenchymal ARF can develop. Total body fluid depletion, diminished intravascular volume, or reduced effective intravascular volume are the common clinical conditions that lead to prerenal azotemia in children (Table 15–1).

PATHOPHYSIOLOGY

Hypovolemia and decreased renal perfusion evoke several protective systemic and intrarenal responses, all of these being directed toward normalizing intra-

TABLE 15–1. Etiology of Prerenal Azotemia

Total Body Volume Depletion
Gastrointestinal (vomiting and/or diarrhea)
Osmotic diuresis (e.g., diabetes mellitus)
Diabetes insipidus
Burns
Intravascular Volume Depletion
Hemorrhage
"Third spacing" of fluid following shock, surgery, trauma
Nephrotic syndrome
Diminished Effective Circulating Volume
Shock
Diminished cardiac output
Pharmacologic vasodilation
Renal Vasoconstriction
Prostaglandin synthetase inhibitors
Cyclosporine
Other pharmacologic vasoconstrictors, such as high-dose dopamine and epinephrine therapy for shock
Hepatorenal syndrome

vascular blood volume, systemic blood pressure, and renal perfusion. Adaptive renal responses to hypoperfusion are mediated by (1) renal autoregulation and (2) alteration of renal tubular sodium and water reabsorption.

RENAL AUTOREGULATION

Renal autoregulatory responses that follow renal hypoperfusion are geared toward maintaining the glomerular filtration rate (GFR) and include (1) the myogenic reflex, (2) glomerulotubular feedback, and (3) angiotensin II (Fig 15–1). The myogenic reflex involves the unique ability of the afferent arteriole to dilate or constrict in response to the stretch of its own walls. This reflex operates independently of the neurogenic innervation of kidney.[5] As a result of the myogenic reflex, the afferent arteriole dilates and helps maintain glomerular blood flow in the event of renal hypoperfusion. Tubuloglomerular feedback is an autoregulatory response (constriction or dilatation) elicited in the afferent arteriole by a variation in chloride delivery to the macula densa region of the corresponding nephron.[6] Diminished sodium and chloride delivery to the distal nephron in prerenal azotemia activates tubuloglomerular feedback, resulting in dilatation of the corresponding afferent arteriole.[7] Tubuloglomerular feedback provides an additional protective mechanism for maintaining glomerular blood flow in prerenal azotemia.

The role of endogenous angiotensin II in regulating GFR in renal hypoperfusion is complex. In general, angiotensin II exhibits vasoconstrictor properties and increases the vascular resistance of both the afferent and the efferent arterioles, but the efferent arteriolar tone is affected to a greater extent than the afferent.[8,9] Angiotensin II also diminishes the glomerular coefficient of filtration (K_f), possibly through its actions on the mesangial cells.[10,11] Elevated afferent

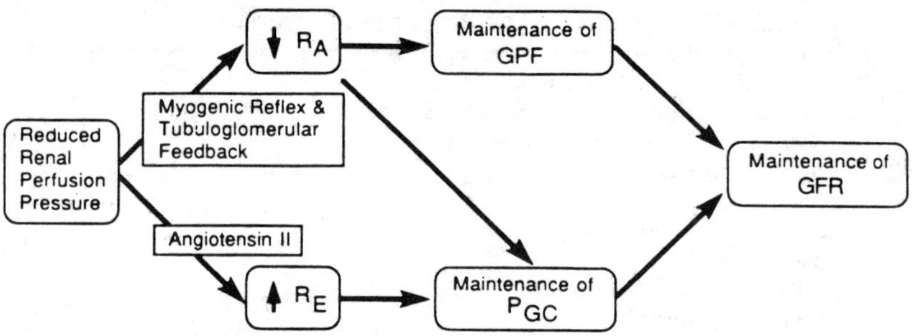

FIG. 15–1. Mechanism for intrarenal autoregulation. When an otherwise normal person faces a hypotensive episode, a highly efficient mechanism (autoregulation) comes into play to maintain the glomerular filtration rate (GFR). This is accomplished by a marked reduction in afferent arteriolar resistance (R_A), by virtue of both myogenic reflex and tubuloglomerular feedback mechanisms, and an increase in efferent arteriolar resistance (R_E) in response to locally released angiotensin II. By maintaining the glomerular plasma flow rate (GPF) and glomerular capillary hydraulic pressure (P_{GC}), these arteriolar adjustments successfully maintain GFR. (From Badar KF, Ichikawa I: Prerenal failure: A deleterious shift from renal compensation to decompensation. *N Engl J Med* 319:623, 1988. Reproduced by permission.)

arteriolar resistance and diminished K_f affect the GFR negatively, but increased efferent arteriolar resistance enhances intraglomerular pressure and maintains glomerular filtration while increasing the filtration fraction.[7] The net effect of endogenous angiotensin II on glomerular circulation in prerenal azotemia is to help preserve GFR.

Other factors that also play a significant role in the intrarenal autoregulatory system during renal hypoperfusion are neural sympathetic stimulation, renal prostaglandin synthesis, and circulating vasopressin concentration.[7]

SODIUM AND WATER REABSORPTION

Prerenal azotemia is characterized by renal sodium and water avidity, which is mediated by an increased circulating concentration of aldosterone and vasopressin. Renal hypoperfusion stimulates the release of renin from kidneys, which in turn leads to the generation of angiotensin and increased aldosterone synthesis.[12] Elevated plasma osmolality provides the primary stimulus for vasopressin release from the posterior pituitary gland, but moderate hypovolemia (more than 5 percent dehydration) can also promote vasopressin secretion.[13] While aldosterone enhances sodium reabsorption from the glomerular filtrate in the distal nephron segment, vasopressin increases renal tubular water reabsorption (Fig. 15–2). The overall effect of these two compensatory renal responses is to decrease urine volume and reduce urinary sodium content. Also, as explained above, prerenal azotemia is associated with an increase in filtration fraction,[7] as a consequence of which blood emerging from the glomerular capillary at the efferent arteriolar end contains a significantly increased plasma

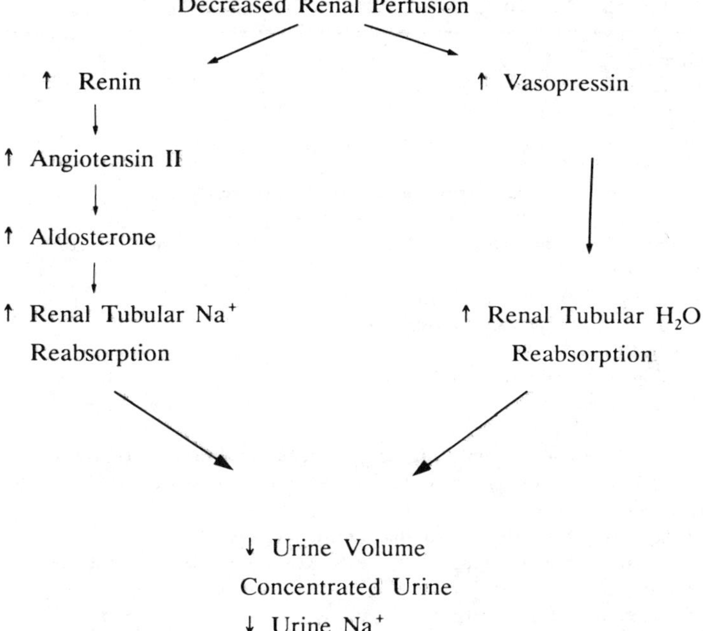

FIG. 15–2. Mechanisms by which sodium and water conservation are affected in prerenal azotemia.

protein concentration. Since the proximal renal tubules are perfused by postglomerular blood, increased oncotic pressure due to high protein concentration within the peritubular capillaries provides an additional stimulus for proximal tubular sodium and water reabsorption.[14]

It must be emphasized that the renal compensatory mechanisms that maintain GFR in prerenal azotemia cannot be expected to operate indefinitely. Failure to provide therapeutic intervention in the form of volume repletion and correction of hypotension in patients with prerenal azotemia can be detrimental and result in intrinsic ARF and even permanent renal damage.

INTRINSIC ARF

A wide array of renal disorders may lead to intrinsic or parenchymal ARF in children. It is useful to place these disorders into three broad etiologic categories: (1) ischemic or hemodynamic, (2) nephrotoxic, and (3) vascular/glomerular (Table 15–2). Such a classification is useful in considering the pathophysiology, clinical manifestations, and management of various forms of intrinsic ARF. The term *acute tubular necrosis* (ATN) is sometimes used to denote the clinical and morphologic manifestations of parenchymal ARF resulting from ischemic or nephrotoxic damage.

TABLE 15–2. Etiology of Parenchymal ARF

Ischemic
- Shock syndromes
- Respiratory distress syndromes
- Severe heart failure

Nephrotoxic
- Antibiotics (especially aminoglycosides, amphotericin)
- Heavy metals
- Organic solvents (glycols, carbon tetrachloride, methanol, toluene)
- Salicylates
- Fluorinated hydrocarbon anesthetics
- Prostaglandin synthetase inhibitors
- Cisplatin
- Radiographic contrast media
- Rhabdomyolysis
- Massive hemolysis
- Uricosuric/hyperuricemic agents (pancreatic enzymes, loop diuretics, salicylates, radiographic contrast media, antineoplastics)

Vascular/Glomerular
- Renal artery occlusion (embolus, vasculitis, thrombus)
- Renal artery stenosis (especially with converting enzyme inhibitors)
- Renal vein thrombosis
- Acute glomerulonephritis
- Rapidly progressive glomerulonephritis
- Microvascular
  - Vasculitis
  - Hemolytic-uremic syndrome
  - Malignant hypertension

Other
- Fulminant pyelonephritis
- Acute interstitial nephritis

MORPHOLOGY

The damage to the nephrons in ischemic and nephrotoxic ARF is confined primarily to the renal tubules; the glomeruli are relatively well preserved. The tubular damage in ischemic ARF is patchy in distribution (Fig. 15–3), but the proximal tubule, especially the portion residing in the outer medulla (straight segment), appears to be particularly vulnerable to such injury.[15–18] The affected tubular segments demonstrate epithelial cell degeneration and disruption of the basement membrane (tubulorrhexis). Casts formed by the damaged and denuded tubular cells are also present within the tubular lumens.

Like ischemic ARF, the glomerular morphology in most models of nephrotoxic ARF also appears relatively intact, but the tubular damage is often extensive and affects segments of the nephron in a patchy manner (Fig. 15–3). The tubular basement membrane is usually intact in nephrotoxic ARF (unlike ischemic ATN); the tubular cells are swollen, necrotic, and denuded from the basement membrane itself (tubulolysis). Cellular debris fills the tubular lumen extensively (Fig. 15–4).

Intrinsic ARF caused by glomerular diseases such as acute or rapidly progressive glomerulonephritis or hemolytic uremic syndrome is characterized by the

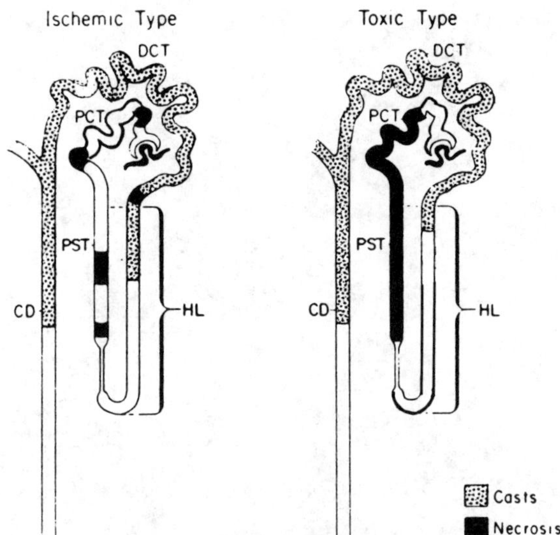

FIG. 15–3. A diagrammatic representation of the tubular damage seen in ischemic and nephrotoxic types of intrinsic ARF. In ischemic ARF, necrosis is patchy. Short lengths of tubules are affected, the straight segments of the proximal tubule being most vulnerable. Rupturing of the necrotic tubular segments may occur (tubulorrhexis). In nephrotoxic ARF, extensive necrosis is present along the proximal tubule and tubulorrhexis does not occur. (From Kreisberg JI, Venkatachalam MA: Morphologic factors in acute renal failure, in Brenner BM, Lazarus JM (eds): *Acute Renal Failure*. New York, Churchill Livingstone, 1988, p 45. Reproduced by permission.)

respective glomerular morphologic changes of these conditions, with minimal tubular involvement.

PATHOPHYSIOLOGY

HEMODYNAMIC/NEPHROTOXIC DISEASES

The initial response to renal hypoperfusion is characterized by compensatory renal and systemic hemodynamic changes, as outlined above in the discussion of prerenal azotemia. Severe and prolonged renal hypoperfusion, however, commonly evolves into the syndrome of intrinsic ARF. The pathogenesis of ARF under these circumstances has been the subject of intense discussion. It is likely that more than one factor is involved in the pathogenesis of diminished GFR in ischemic ARF. Three potential mechanisms that have been proposed to explain the pathogenesis of ischemic ARF are (1) decreased renal blood flow and glomerular K_f, (2) tubular obstruction, and (3) tubular back leak (Fig. 15–5).

It has been well described that renal blood flow is decreased modestly (40 to 50 percent of normal) during the maintenance phase of ARF, cortical blood flow being affected more severely than the medullary circulation.[19–21] Factors considered as possible mediators of renal vasoconstriction and diminished renal perfusion in ischemic ARF include the presence of angiotensin II,[22] lack of vaso-

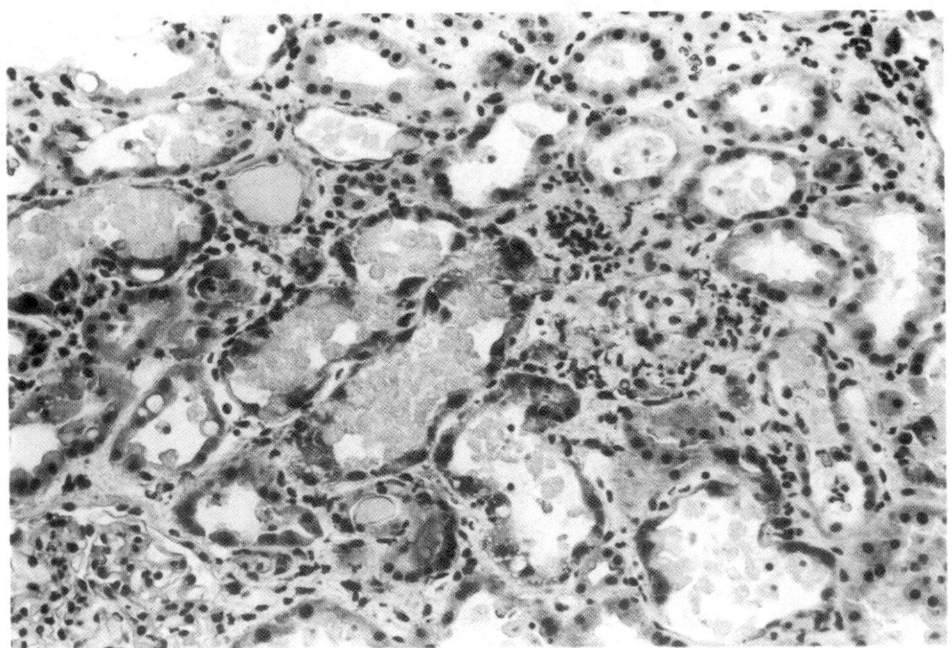

FIG. 15–4. Renal biopsy of a patient with ARF that followed the use of multiple nephrotoxic antibiotics used to treat severe pneumonia. (Photograph courtesy of Sudesh Kapur, M.D., Department of Pathology, Children's National Medical Center, Washington, DC.)

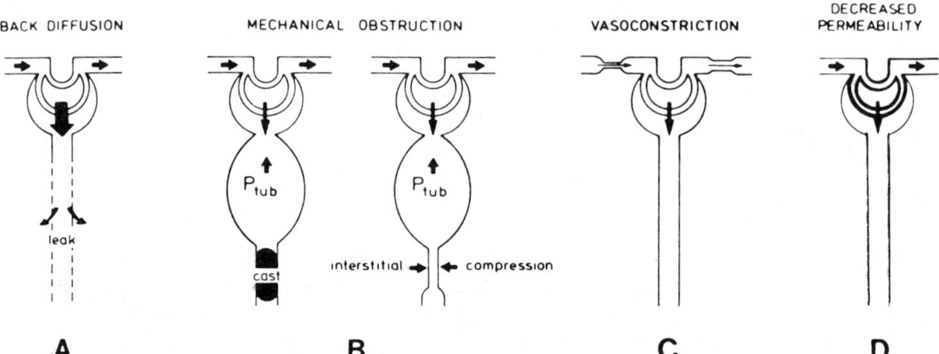

FIG. 15–5. Proposed pathophysiologic mechanisms responsible for the excretory dysfunction of the kidney during ARF. *A.* Filtered fluid and solutes are lost from the tubular system back into the circulation. *B.* Reduced glomerular filtration due to increased tubular pressure caused by intratubular cast formation or tubular compression. *C.* Reduced glomerular filtration due to preferential afferent arteriolar vasoconstriction. *D.* Reduced glomerular filtration due to decreased filtering area and/or permeability of glomerular capillaries. P_{tub} = hydrostatic pressure in the tubules and Bowman's capsule. (From Thuru K, Mason J, Gstraunthaler G: Experimental acute renal failure, in Seldin DW, Giebisch G (eds): *The Kidney, Physiology and Pathophysiology.* New York, Raven Press, page 1885, 1985. Reproduced by permission.)

dilator prostaglandins,[23] sympathetic neural stimulation,[24] vasopressin,[25] and endothelin.[26] However, renal vasoconstriction alone cannot explain the failure of glomerular filtration in ischemic ARF, since the decrease in GFR is disproportionately greater than the degree to which renal perfusion is diminished.[21,27,28] In recent years attention has been focused on abnormalities of the glomerular filtration membrane in ischemic ARF. The glomerular K_f has been shown to be decreased in experimental ischemic ARF.[28] Since mesangial cells possess contractile properties and respond to angiotensin II,[10] K_f may be diminished by a reduction of the glomerular surface area available for filtration by the effects of endogenous angiotensin II on the mesangial cells.[11,27] Morphologic changes noted in the glomeruli of animals with ischemic ARF include a reduction in endothelial fenestration and flattening of the epithelial foot processes.[18,29] Whether these anatomic changes can be linked to a decrease in K_f has not been clearly established.

Tubular obstruction as a contributing factor in the pathogenesis of ischemic as well as nephrotoxic ARF has also received considerable attention. Evidence for renal tubular obstruction comes from the examination of renal tissue in humans and in experimental models of ARF, wherein the tubular lumens have been shown to be filled with cellular debris.[15–18] Tubular obstruction is further aggravated by swelling and necrosis of renal tubular cells. Not only does intratubular obstruction prevent the outflow of filtrate formed by the glomeruli but it also diminishes glomerular filtration by increasing the hydrostatic pressure within Bowman's capsule as a result of back pressure.

Another factor that deserves attention as a potential contributor to the decreased GFR in ischemic ARF is the ''back leak'' of glomerular filtrate. As a result of disruption in the tubular basement membrane, tubular cell necrosis, and obstruction within the tubular lumen, the filtrate formed at the glomerulus diffuses back (back leak) from the renal tubular lumen into the renal interstitium.[27,30,31] An additional consequence of tubular back leak is that calculated GFR, as determined by standard clearance techniques, is lower than the actual GFR. Under these circumstances the filtered marker (endogenous creatinine or inulin) for GFR estimation leaves the tubular lumen and reaches the renal interstitium rather than being excreted in the urine, thus reducing the excretion of the entire quantity of the marker filtered in the glomeruli and diminishing the calculated GFR. Although the phenomenon of back leak has been well established in ischemic and nephrotoxic ARF, the degree of its contribution to diminishing GFR remains unclear and, in itself, may not explain the profound decrease in GFR in these circumstances.[32]

The mechanism by which GFR is reduced in nephrotoxic ARF varies with the nephrotoxin used. While a reduction in the K_f of the glomerular capillaries plays a significant role in some models of nephrotoxic ARF, tubular obstruction by necrotic debris is a prominent feature of all forms of nephrotoxic ARF.[27,33] Reduction in K_f in ARF may be mediated by angiotensin II.

VASCULAR/GLOMERULAR DISEASES

Renal arterial and/or venous occlusion leading to ARF is uncommon beyond the neonatal period. The former may arise as a complication of umbilical artery catheterization and the latter is seen in diverse disease states, including maternal diabetes mellitus, birth asphyxia, and cyanotic congenital heart disease. In older infants and children, bilateral renal artery stenosis can result in ARF, especially during a period of accelerated hypertension or following treatment with angiotensin converting enzyme (ACE) inhibitors. Decrease of GFR in renal arterial disease is a direct consequence of diminished renal blood flow (Chap. 11). Reports of recovery of renal function after prolonged periods of arterial occlusion[34] suggest that complete parenchymal necrosis may not occur due to the development of a collateral blood supply. Renal vein thrombosis may accompany hyperosmolar dehydration or states of hypercoagulability, as in nephrotic syndrome, or polycythemia.[35] In one series, renal vein thrombosis was the underlying etiology for ARF in 8 percent of infants below 1 year of age.[36] Renal vein thrombosis is associated with hemorrhagic necrosis and venous congestion, although the necrosis may be patchy. Partial recovery of renal function in ARF due to renal vein thrombosis is common.[36]

Another form of vascular occlusive disease which is invariably associated with ARF is the hemolytic uremic syndrome (HUS), which primarily affects children under 5 years of age and typically follows a gastrointestinal or respiratory illness. Familial and recurrent forms of HUS have been described. A simplistic version of the pathophysiologic schema for ARF is one in which microvascular endothelial cell injury results in intraluminal deposition of platelet-fibrin thrombi. This process leads to the consumption of platelets, injury of passing red blood cells by fibrin strands, and reduction or obliteration of glomerular capillary blood flow and filtration surface area. Other clinical aspects of HUS are discussed in Chap. 8.

Last, microvascular disease affecting the glomerular capillaries, as seen with renal vasculitis, may also result in ARF. Although the clinical syndromes associated with these diseases may vary widely, the renal lesion is most commonly an exudative glomerulitis, often associated with crescent formation. The reduction of GFR is a result of several factors: reduced renal blood flow (RBF) due to increased resistance of injured vasculature, direct injury to the glomerular capillary wall, and net loss of filtration surface area.

POSTRENAL ARF

In pediatric patients, the occurrence of ARF as a result of urinary tract obstruction is uncommon beyond the newborn period. The significance of postrenal ARF lies in its potential reversibility. There are few clinically relevant data to indicate the duration of total or partial urinary obstruction which can be sustained and yet permit complete functional recovery of the kidney. However, as with many of the prerenal causes of ARF, accurate diagnosis and prompt correction of the cause of postrenal ARF can result in the return of renal function.

Postrenal obstruction is commonly considered in terms of structural disease distal to the nephron (e.g., ureteropelvic junction obstruction). However, intrarenal causes of tubular obstruction (e.g., intratubular precipitation of uric acid and possibly xanthines during tumor lysis) must be considered in the appropri-

TABLE 15–3. Etiology of Obstructive ARF

Urinary Tract Structural/Functional Abnormalities
Urethral valves
Obstruction of the ureteropelvic junction
Ureteroceles
Neuropathic bladder
Phimosis/urethral stricture
Acquired Nonstructural Abnormalities
Blood clot (e.g., posttraumatic or postbiopsy)
Retroperitoneal or intraabdominal tumor
Calculus (upper urinary tract or bladder)
Drugs causing pharmacologic urinary retention

Note: Obstruction to urine flow proximal to the bladder neck may cause ARF in patients with a solitary functioning kidney.

ate clinical setting.[37,38] In children, the postnephron causes of urinary tract obstruction most commonly have a chronic component and usually occur as a result of a congenital structural abnormality of the urinary tract. However, the degree of antecedent renal injury from chronic obstructive uropathy can be extremely variable. Causes of urinary tract obstruction are listed in Table 15–3.

The sudden development of anuria should strongly suggest the possibility of total urinary obstruction (either bilateral, distal to the urinary bladder, or in a solitary kidney). However, incomplete urinary obstruction of variable duration may be associated with extremely variable urine volume and electrolyte concentrations. Furthermore, unilateral obstruction may remain undiagnosed, since the contralateral kidney can quickly compensate for the acute loss of function. In those clinical settings where the cause of ARF is not evident, urinary tract obstruction must be considered.

PATHOPHYSIOLOGY[39–41]

Complete ureteral obstruction in experimental models is characterized by a rise in hydrostatic pressure within the ureters and Bowman's capsule, which usually falls slowly after the initial 24 h, especially in unilateral obstruction. RBF shows a biphasic response in ureteral obstruction, rising early in the course (first few hours) and followed by a progressive decline, which persists with continued obstruction. The increase in RBF noted in the first few hours of obstruction is probably mediated by the intrarenal synthesis of vasodilator prostaglandins. The GFR in ureteral obstruction declines progressively—a phenomenon that appears to be of multifactorial origin. The rise of hydrostatic pressure within Bowman's capsule may prevent glomerular filtration, but this alone cannot explain the decrease in GFR, especially since hydrostatic pressure in these locations improves beyond 24 h. Renal vasoconstriction and a decrease in RBF appear to be the most probable reasons for declining GFR in acute urinary tract obstruction.

Progressive distal tubular dysfunction may lead to diminished responsiveness to antidiuretic hormone (ADH) as well as impaired acidification and potassium excretion. The latter two may present as hyperkalemic distal tubular acidosis. It should be understood from this simplified version of a rather complex, multifactorial process that urinary composition and volume can be variable, especially in partial obstruction, and are rather poor indicators of urinary tract obstruction. Pathophysiology of acute urinary tract obstruction is discussed further in Chap. 14.

CLINICAL MANIFESTATIONS

In clinical practice, ARF manifests itself as a syndrome of varying severity and pathophysiologic disturbances. The clinical manifestations of ARF are varied and result primarily from the underlying condition; however, secondary clinical concerns due to fluid overload, hypertension, and disturbances of electrolyte metabolism predominate in most instances. Since ARF may be superimposed on preexisting chronic renal insufficiency, the clinical presentation of these patients may be confusing. In some patients, ARF is of the nonoliguric variety, while in others it is characterized by severe oliguria or anuria. In patients with hemodynamically mediated ARF, the transition from prerenal azotemia to well-established ARF may be marked by an intermediate stage also known as *incipient ARF.*

OLIGURIC ARF

Traditional teaching proposes that the clinical course of ischemic or nephrotoxic ARF goes through two contiguous but distinct stages: (1) an oliguric phase and (2) a polyuric phase. The oliguric phase is characterized by oliguria of variable severity or anuria. The clinical problems of ARF at this stage include fluid overload, cardiorespiratory compromise, and hypertension, in addition to the associated metabolic disturbances. Accordingly, patients at this stage may have clinical evidence of edema, pulmonary edema, or even congestive heart failure. Hypertension in these patients is usually due to fluid overload, but in some cases intrinsic renal disease (such as hemolytic uremic syndrome or other types of chronic glomerulonephritides) may also be contributory. Hypertension in the latter group of patients can be severe; in them, a sudden rise of blood pressure may lead to hypertensive encephalopathy or even intracranial hemorrhagic complications. The oliguric phase of ARF usually lasts up to 2 weeks and is followed by a slow transition into the polyuric phase. The beginning of the polyuric phase is heralded by a gradual increase in the daily urinary output, which may reach excessive proportions. The serum creatinine and BUN may remain elevated early in this phase, but they begin to decline slowly. The polyuric phase generally lasts for 7 to 14 days but may continue as long as a month in some patients. Dehydration and excessive losses of urinary electrolytes remain clinical concerns during this phase.

ARF is accompanied by numerous metabolic derangements such as hyperkalemia, hypocalcemia, and hyperphosphatemia, in addition to uremia. Hyperkalemia is the most frequently seen metabolic abnormality in ARF and results from the kidney's inability to excrete the ingested and endogenous load of potassium. Factors which promote and accelerate the development of hyperkalemia include excessive intake in the form of blood transfusions and potassium salts of various antibiotics and hypercatabolism induced by infection, ischemic tissue damage, and cell death (e.g., sepsis, burns, abscess, hemolysis, acidosis, rhabdomyolysis, tumor lysis, and poor nutritional status). In acute poststreptococcal glomerulonephritis, hyperkalemia may also result from a hyporeninemic hypoaldosteronemic state.[42] Unfortunately, hyperkalemia is not recognizable clinically until the serum concentration reaches a cardiotoxic level. Surveillance is the key to early detection of this derangement. A rise in serum potassium concentration leads to a progressive and recognizable electrocardiographic finding of elevated T waves (also known as tented or peaked T waves) and diminution in the amplitude of R waves. In severe hyperkalemia (>7.5 meq/L), the electrocardiogram additionally demonstrates a widened QRS complex and absent P wave. Cardiac arrest in asystole should be considered incipient at this stage.

Hyperphosphatemia caused by diminished renal phosphate excretion in ARF does not usually lead to any clinically detectable symptoms. However, hypocalcemia, resulting from microprecipitation of calcium and phosphorus complexes (discussed in Chap. 16), often leads to the manifestations of neuromuscular irritability such as muscular twitching, carpopedal muscle spasms, and even seizures. Hyponatremia, as a result of excessive urinary losses, may occur during the polyuric phase of ARF or in patients with nonoliguric ARF. Hyponatremia manifests itself as lethargy, irritability, and generalized seizures, especially when it evolves rapidly (hours).

Uremic symptoms are not generally seen in patients with ARF until renal dysfunction reaches an advanced stage (BUN >100 mg/dL), usually when patients cannot or are unwilling to undergo dialysis therapy.

NONOLIGURIC ARF

In many patients, ARF can occur without any well-documented oliguric phase. This clinical form of ARF is designated as *nonoliguric ARF* and is particularly common in patients with nephrotoxic renal injury. Nonoliguric ARF has been recognized as a common form of ARF in both adults[4] and children.[43] In the pediatric age group, nonoliguric ARF is particularly common in neonates, in whom it has been reported to be the clinical presentation in almost 50 percent of patients with ARF.[43] Possible explanations for an apparent increase in recognition of nonoliguric ATN during the last two decades are (1) routine biochemical monitoring of renal function of hospitalized and other at-risk patients, (2) prompt fluid resuscitation of traumatized patients, and (3) increased use of diuretics, vasodilators, and volume expanders in high-risk (especially surgical)

TABLE 15–4. Disorders Commonly Associated with Nonoliguric ARF

Nephrotoxins
Aminoglycosides
Cisplatin
Radiocontrast material
Rhabdomyolysis
Burns
Postsurgery
Cardiac surgery
Aortic repair
Renal hypoperfusion
Dehydration
Shock
Use of mannitol or furosemide early in the course of acute tubular necrosis, intraoperatively in cardiac surgery
Posttrauma

patients.[4] The clinical conditions that are commonly associated with nonoliguric ARF are listed in Table 15–4.

DIAGNOSTIC EVALUATION

Morbidity and mortality rates in patients with ARF are high, often as a consequence of the underlying condition leading to ARF. Early recognition of ARF, implementation of an effective diagnostic plan, and expeditious therapeutic intervention are essential to optimal patient management. Accurate interpretation of clinical and laboratory information may be difficult when there is an underlying serious systemic illness, and access to diagnostic radiographic procedures may be limited by the condition of the patient. Figure 15–6 outlines a diagnostic tree that may be of help in evaluating patients in whom ARF is suspected.

CLINICAL CONSIDERATIONS

A thorough history and clinical examination are important in determining the etiology of ARF. History of a recent diarrheal illness and/or vomiting may suggest the diagnosis of prerenal azotemia or hemolytic uremic syndrome. A streptococcal pharyngitis or impetigo preceding the onset of ARF may point to poststreptococcal glomerulonephritis. A history of fever, rash, arthritis, or pulmonary symptoms suggests multisystem inflammatory diseases, such as systemic lupus erythematosus or vasculitis. Careful questioning regarding accidental or intentional intake of toxic agents or medications must be undertaken in all patients with unexplained ARF. Hospitalized patients often develop ARF following a surgical procedure, especially cardiovascular surgery, or administration of nephrotoxic drugs (antibiotics, chemotherapeutic agents, or radiographic contrast media). Evaluation of the details of the circumstances under

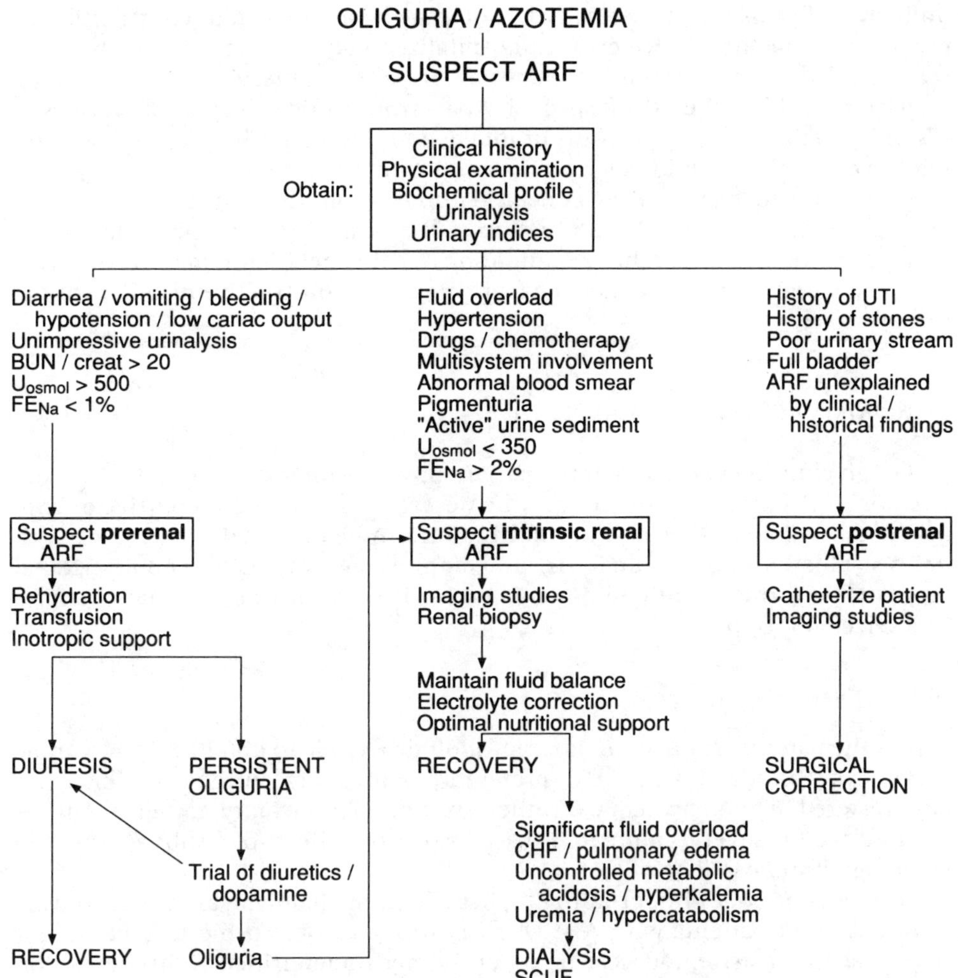

FIG. 15–6. A diagnostic tree that may be used for the management of patients with oliguria/anuria. (Modified from Ruley EJ, Bock GH: Acute renal failure in infants and children, in Shoemaker WC, Ayres S, Grenvik A, Holbrook AP, Thompson WL (eds): *Textbook of Critical Care*. Philadelphia, W.B. Saunders, 1989, p 721. With permission.)

which ARF developed is usually helpful in determining the etiology of the disorder.

Physical examination of a patient with ARF is essential in order to determine two important facts: (1) the patient's fluid status and intravascular volume and (2) whether there is clinical evidence of any systemic illness. An assessment of the patient's intravascular volume and state of hydration is helpful in determining whether prerenal azotemia must be considered in the diagnosis. An acutely ill child with oliguria, tachycardia, dry mucous membranes, and orthostatic hypotension may have prerenal azotemia, while the oliguric child with tachycardia and jugular venous distension whose blood pressure is elevated is unlikely to fit this diagnosis. Dehydration may be an important contributing or precipitating factor in ARF even in hospitalized patients (e.g., those who have received radiographic contrast material or, after surgery, those with fluid sequestered within the "third space"). Apart from clinical evaluation of the status of hydration, hospital records of intake and output are helpful in determining the dynamics of fluid balance in such patients.

In addition to historical evidence, features of multisystem diseases should also be sought on physical examination of the skin, joints, lymph nodes, abdomen, and so on. A careful examination of the abdomen may also reveal enlarged kidneys or a distended bladder, suggesting obstructive disorders of the urinary tract.

LABORATORY ASSESSMENT

Although clinical evaluation of the patient provides important clues to the diagnosis of ARF, laboratory studies may be necessary to provide supportive or confirmatory evidence. A wealth of information can be obtained from routine urinalysis, blood chemistry analysis, and noninvasive radiologic studies. Renal biopsy is performed rarely in patients with ARF but may be extremely helpful in a selected group.

URINALYSIS

Unless the patient is anuric, an attempt should be made to obtain a urine sample for analysis as soon as possible, preferably before any diuretics or fluids are administered. This may require catheterization. The urinary catheter may be left in place for several hours in order to assess the effects of a subsequent fluid challenge if indicated.

Urinalysis provides important and virtually immediately available diagnostic information in patients with ARF. A rusty or tea-colored urine may be indicative of acute poststreptococcal or other glomerulonephritides. Pink urine, on the other hand, can be seen in hemoglobinuria or myoglobinuria. These two conditions can be differentiated by the methods outlined in Chap. 2 (Table 2–2). A maximally concentrated urine (specific gravity above 1.020) is highly suggestive of prerenal azotemia. It must be pointed out that patients with acute poststreptococcal glomerulonephritis also elaborate a concentrated urine. Diminished maximal urine concentrating ability may rarely be seen in some patients with prerenal azotemia.[44] Poor urinary concentrating ability in patients with ARF is indicative of established parenchymal ARF. Inability to concentrate urine may be the first indication of impending intrinsic ARF in a patient with profound shock or intravascular volume depletion. Mild proteinuria (2+ or less) and minimal hematuria (1+ to 2+) may be seen in prerenal azotemia or early acute tubular necrosis. Heavy proteinuria, on the other hand, is indicative of glomerulonephritis. Microscopic examination of the urinary sediment should be performed in every patient with ARF. Dysmorphic red blood cells (RBCs) in the urinary sediment indicate a glomerular disease, while eosinophiluria is seen in acute interstitial nephritis. Hyaline casts and fine granular

TABLE 15–5. Urinary Indices Used in Differentiating Prerenal Azotemia from Established Parenchymal ARF

Test	Prerenal Azotemia	Established ARF
Urine specific gravity	>1.020	<1.020
Urine osmolality	>500	<350
Urine/plasma osmolality	>1.3	<1.3
Urine sodium (meq/L)	<20	>20
FE_{Na}	<1.0	>2.0

casts are commonly seen in prerenal azotemia. Coarse granular and/or RBC casts are suggestive of glomerulonephritis, while casts composed of renal tubular cells are seen in nephrotoxic or ischemic renal parenchymal injury.

URINARY INDICES IN ARF

Over the years, many tests determining the integrity of renal tubular function have been used in an attempt to differentiate parenchymal ARF from prerenal azotemia (Table 15–5). In general, the principle on which the commonly used urinary indices are based is the fact that prerenal azotemia is associated with normal and appropriate renal tubular function, while established intrinsic ARF results in disturbances of these functions. Although these data are helpful in many patients, indeterminate values may render interpretation difficult in some.[45]

Urine/Serum Osmolality. Urine in patients with prerenal azotemia is highly concentrated and both specific gravity and urine osmolality are elevated. In contrast, isotonic urine specific gravity and osmolality are features of established intrinsic ARF. Accurate interpretation of urine specific gravity may be substantially limited by the abnormal appearance of various solutes in the urine, including protein, radiographic contrast media, glucose, and mannitol. Osmolality is a more useful (although less accessible) measure of urinary concentration, since its value is minimally affected by the appearance of such materials in their usual concentrations. Urine osmolality greater than 500 mosmol/kg/H_2O suggests prerenal azotemia; that less than 350 mosmol/kg/H_2O indicates established intrinsic ARF. A considerable overlap of values between the two conditions, however, limits the absolute usefulness of this test.[45] The ratio between the urine (U_o) and serum osmolality (S_o) can also be used to differentiate between prerenal azotemia and parenchymal ARF.[45] A U_o/S_o ratio of greater than 1.3 suggests prerenal azotemia.[47]

Urinary Sodium. Because of renal tubular dysfunction, patients with established parenchymal ARF tend to produce urine with a U_{Na} concentration greater than 40 meq/L. Patients with prerenal azotemia, in contrast, have avid tubular Na^+ reabsorption, which is generally associated with a urinary Na^+ concentration below 20 meq/L. Urinary sodium can be obtained in an untimed spot sample of urine.

Fractional Excretion of Sodium. Fractional excretion of Na^+ (FE_{Na}) has been shown to have greater discriminatory value in distinguishing prerenal azotemia from parenchymal ARF than urinary sodium excretion.[45,48,49] The FE_{Na} represents the fraction of filtered Na^+ which is excreted in urine. Since the amount of Na^+ excreted is equal to the urine [Na] × urine volume and the total amount filtered is equal to the serum [Na] × GFR (or UV/P creatinine), then the FE_{Na} is calculated as

$$([U/P]\ Na)/([U/P]\ Cr) \times 100$$

The FE_{Na} is determined by measuring the concentration of sodium and creatinine in a simultaneously obtained spot serum and urine sample. FE_{Na} below 1 percent (or more than 99 percent tubular Na^+ reabsorption) indicates prerenal azotemia, while a FE_{Na} greater than 2 percent (or less than 98 percent tubular Na^+ reabsorption) indicates ATN. When the test is conducted appropriately, FE_{Na} can correctly distinguish prerenal ARF from oliguric ATN in a majority of patients. However, the predictive value of FE_{Na} is low in diagnosing ARF due to acute glomerulonephritis, where FE_{Na} as well as urinary Na^+ are low.[50,51] Although interpretation of urinary Na^+ following diuretic therapy has been considered to invalidate FE_{Na}, a value of less than 1 percent still strongly suggests a prerenal etiology. Finally, a higher cutoff value for FE_{Na} has been suggested for premature infants with oliguric ARF in view of their greater obligate urinary sodium losses.[52,53]

BUN/Creatinine Ratio. While creatinine is excreted in the urine primarily by glomerular filtration (and to a lesser but significant extent by tubular excretion), urinary excretion of urea is determined by the net balance between glomerular filtration and tubular reabsorption. In patients with intravascular volume depletion and other causes of prerenal azotemia, large amounts of urea are reabsorbed in the proximal renal tubule passively in response to sodium and water reabsorption in that segment of the nephron. As a result, the serum concentration of BUN rises out of proportion to the concentration of creatinine and the ratio exceeds the normal value of 10:1.

RADIOLOGIC ASSESSMENT

The goals of radiologic assessment in a patient with ARF of unknown etiology are to (1) determine whether both kidneys are present, (2) evaluate renal size, (3) rule out any urinary tract obstruction, and (4) establish the adequacy of renal blood flow. A plain radiograph of the abdomen is usually of limited help in providing the required information under these circumstances. Since there is a substantial risk of augmenting renal parenchymal damage from radiocontrast material in patients with underlying renal damage or in those with prerenal ARF, intravenous pyelography is not recommended. In addition, visualization of the parenchymal and collecting systems is often inadequate in the presence of impaired GFR. Sonography, on the other hand, is noninvasive, can be performed at the bedside of a critically ill patient, and provides useful information about the general parenchymal architecture and collecting system drainage. For these reasons sonography has replaced intravenous pyelography as the initial radiographic evaluation of choice in patients with ARF. Clinically useful evaluation of renal blood flow and urinary drainage can be obtained by the technetium 99m diethylenetriaminepentacetic acid (DTPA) renal scan. Recently, Doppler flow ultrasonography has evolved as a promising radiologic tool for evaluating renal arterial and venous blood flow. Doppler flow ultrasonography, however, requires significant operator skill to be an effective diagnostic procedure.

RENAL BIOPSY

A renal biopsy is not usually required in the diagnostic evaluation of patients with ARF unless an underlying rapidly progressive glomerulonephritis or acute interstitial nephritis is suspected. Renal biopsy is of considerable diagnostic help in differentiating ATN from acute allograft rejection in renal transplant patients who develop primary nonfunction of the organ following renal transplantation.

MANAGEMENT

Most forms of renal dysfunction result in disturbances of homeostasis, the restoration of which requires therapeutic intervention. The goals of therapy in a patient with established ARF are (1) to correct preexisting biophysiologic abnormalities and (2) to provide anticipatory management so as to prevent the development of secondary complications due to ARF. Both of these aims must be pursued simultaneously in order to achieve the desired results.

DISTURBANCES OF FLUID BALANCE

The goal in patients with ARF is to correct any existing fluid and electrolyte imbalance and provide replacements of appropriately constituted fluids at a rate that is likely to maintain a stable clinical state. Conventional nomograms for the determination of maintenance fluid requirements are not generally applicable to children with ARF, since such estimates are often excessive in the setting of disturbed urine production. The fluid requirements of a patient with established ARF consist of an aggregate of insensible and measurable losses (e.g., from urine, stool, nasogastric drainage, and any other type of drainage). An estimate of the insensible water requirement is derived from the patient's caloric intake, being calculated at rate of about 45 mL for each 100 calories provided.[54] An estimate of the insensible water requirement can be calculated from the data given in Table 15–6. It may be emphasized that the estimate of insensible water loss must be altered in the presence of fever, highly humidified air (respirator support), infections, etc. Finally, since acutely ill patients with ARF are hypercatabolic,[55] inadequate caloric replacement will lead to the utilization of endogenous lean body mass and fat stores for energy. This can result

TABLE 15–6. Insensible Water Requirements in Children

	Neonate	2-year-old	5-year-old	10-year-old	15-year-old
Weight,kg	3.5	12.5	18.8	32.6	54.5
Calories/kg	125	85	75	65	55
Calculated IWL, mL/kg[a]	56.25	38.25	33.75	29.25	24.75
Practical generalization of IWL, mL/kg	40–50	40	35	30	25

[a]IWL= Insensible water loss.

Note: Calculation of IWL based on the formula that 45 mL water is required for each 100 calories provided. Accordingly, in the neonate, IWL/kg= 45 $\times$125/100 or 56.25 mL. Age-dependent caloric requirement may be calculated with any of the conventional formulas.

in a daily weight loss of as much as 0.5 percent of lean body mass. The corollary of this statement is that stable patient weight may represent slowly evolving fluid overload in a child with ARF.

DISTURBANCES OF ELECTROLYTE METABOLISM

In general, patients with nonoliguric ARF should receive replacement fluids whose sodium content is determined by daily urinary losses of this ion. Insensible losses should be replaced with sodium-free solutions if possible. This may not always be practical, since patients frequently require medications, colloid, and blood products containing large amounts of sodium salts, but attempts to this effect should be made. The composition of replacement fluid for measurable water loss is largely dictated by the composition of the fluids that need to be replaced. Analysis of urine electrolytes provides an important guide in this respect. Nonoliguric patients or those in the polyuric phase of classic ARF usually excrete large amounts of sodium and may require additional sodium supplementation. The most common disturbance of sodium balance observed in ARF is hyponatremia, and this is usually a result of fluid overload.

Hyperkalemia is a common and potentially fatal complication of ARF, usually as a result of dysfunction of cardiac rhythm. Hyperkalemia occurs most typically in oliguric patients, often despite early K^+ restriction. The mode of treatment of hyperkalemia is guided by the severity of the disorder which, based on serum potassium concentration, is classified as follows: mild, $K^+ <$ 6.5 meq/L; moderate, K^+ 6.5 to 7.5 meq/L; severe, $K^+ >$7.5 meq/L. The aggressiveness with which hyperkalemia is treated is dictated by the severity of the abnormalities seen in the ECG. Several types of therapies for the treatment of hyperkalemia, as well as their mechanisms of action, are listed in Table 15–7. Calcium, glucose/insulin, and bicarbonate infusions are only temporizing measures that either sequester K^+ intracellularly or counteract its cardiotoxic effects. Whenever such measures are implemented, thought must also be given to correcting the underlying total body K^+ excess by either dialysis or the use of sodium polystyrene sulfonate (Kayexalate). If the patient has no sign of

TABLE 15–7. Therapeutic Agents Used in the Treatment of Hyperkalemia

Agent	Action	Dose	Onset/Duration
Calcium gluconate (10%)	Stabilization of membrane potential	0.5 mg elemental Ca^{++}/kg IV over 2–4 min	Rapid (min)/ transient (h)
Glucose (50%) and insulin	Promotes cellular uptake of K^+	1 mL/kg of glucose with 0.1 U regular insulin/kg IV by slow push or rapid drip	Rapid (30 min)/ transient (h)
Sodium bicarbonate (7.5%)	Promotes cellular uptake of K^+	2.5 meq/kg (approx. 3 mL/kg) by slow push or rapid drip	Rapid (30 min)/ transient (h)
Sodium polystyrene sulfonate	Cation exchange resin	1 g/kg PO (with 3–4 mL of 70% sorbitol/g of resin) or PR (with 10 mL of 70% sorbitol/g of resin)	Hours/days

Source: From Ruley EJ, Bock GH: Acute renal failure in infants and children, in Shoemaker WC, Ayres S, Grenvik A, Holbrook AP, Thompson WL (eds): *Textbook of Critical Care.* Philadelphia, W. B. Saunders, 1989, p 728. With permission.

impending K^+ toxicity or the degree of hyperkalemia is mild, treatment may be as simple as better control of acidosis and use of cation exchange resins. Sodium polystyrene sulfonate is administered in a 70% sorbitol solution when given orally and in a 30% solution rectally. Given sufficient time for maximal exchange, each gram of the resin can bind approximately 1 meq of K^+. While oral administration is generally more effective, rectal administration has a more rapid onset of action. In addition, if there is an obvious source of excess K^+ (e.g., hematoma, necrotic wound), this should be dealt with promptly.

Under circumstances of more severe or unresolving hyperkalemia, institution of dialysis is necessary. When urgent K^+ reduction by dialysis is required, peritoneal dialysis will not generally provide a sufficiently rapid decrease of the serum K^+ concentration.[56] On the other hand, hemodialysis (HD) can reduce the serum K^+ level quickly.[57] In patients for whom HD is not feasible, hemofiltration alone or with dialysis may provide a less efficient alternative.[58,59]

Other biochemical disturbances of ARF include metabolic acidosis, hypocalcemia and hyperphosphatemia. Under ordinary circumstances, metabolic processes generate approximately 1 meq/kg/day of hydrogen ions. In the infected or otherwise catabolic patient, this value may be significantly higher. Hydrogen ion excretory capacity in many forms of parenchymal ARF is frequently inadequate to maintain acid-base balance. The resulting acidemia is nonetheless generally mild because of the nonbicarbonate buffering systems. In the patient with a more severe degree of acidemia, sodium bicarbonate must be administered cautiously, since it may exacerbate intravascular volume overload and hypocalcemia. Hypocalcemia can arise because of multiple factors, including phosphate retention, diminished calcium intake, and decreased gastrointestinal calcium absorption. Acute hyperphosphatemia can be effectively treated with oral phosphate binders such as calcium carbonate or calcium acetate. While providing calcium supplementation, an attempt must be made to keep the calcium $\times$ phosphorus product below 70.

NUTRITION DURING ARF

Multiple factors predispose patients with ARF to severe catabolism, two of the most important being inadequate caloric intake and infection.[55] Although studies comprising mainly postoperative patients indicate that early nutritional support can reduce morbidity and mortality rates,[60,61] such data have been more equivocal for patients with ARF.[55,62] In addition, some experimental observations have suggested that a high protein intake may potentiate renal injury in ARF.[63,64] Avoidance of catabolism in the severely ill patient with ARF is particularly difficult, since nutritional efforts are often restricted by fluid intolerance and the risk of worsening the degree of azotemia. Previously published data from children with ARF suggest that protein catabolism can be minimized if nonprotein caloric intake (glucose) is increased to as much as 50 to 60 kcal/kg/day while restricting protein, as a mixture of essential and nonessential amino acids, to approximately 0.5 mg/kg/day.[65]

DIALYSIS

In the last two decades technology and equipment have developed to the point where all forms of peritoneal and extracorporeal dialysis therapy can be offered to virtually all patients regardless of size. The indications for dialysis given in Table 15–8 can serve as general guidelines. At times, the decision to initiate dialysis is based on an overall clinical impression of its potential benefits in a patient who may not present an absolute indication for dialysis. For example, the severely undernourished patient with limited fluid tolerance may require prospective ultrafiltration to facilitate hyperalimentation.

Selection of the type of dialysis is based on several factors: (1) the patient's cardiopulmonary stability, (2) whether there has been recent intraabdominal surgery, (3) the availability of an adequate vascular access, (4) the specific goals of the dialysis therapy, and (5) the technical support available. Acute, potentially dangerous metabolic disturbances and dialyzable poisonings are best treated with the more efficient HD procedure. Peritoneal dialysis (PD), while less efficient than HD, is generally less destabilizing hemodynamically. Peritoneal dialysis can occasionally accentuate cardiac instability by diminishing left ventricular function in patients with marginal cardiac reserve.[66] Peritoneal dialysis using small-volume fluid exchanges is probably the method of choice in these patients.

TABLE 15–8. Indications for Dialysis in Children with ARF

The treatment of symptomatic volume overload unresponsive to more conservative management
Serious, life-threatening, or medically uncontrollable metabolic disturbances (e.g., hyperkalemia, intractable acidosis, hyperuricemia, hyperphosphatemia)
The adjunctive management of fluid-mediated hypertension
Acute tubular necrosis associated with poisoning due to dialyzable or hemofilterable compounds

HEMOFILTRATION

Hemofiltration is a technique by which plasma can be ultrafiltered in order to remove excess fluid volume. The primary utility of hemofiltration is as an adjunct in the treatment of fluid overload in patients with ARF.[58,59,67] This procedure has, however, also been used effectively in the treatment of metabolic derangements in the tumor lysis syndrome[68] as well as in rhabdomyolysis.[69]

Hemofiltration can be performed by way of an arterial and a venous access (usually through femoral vessels), utilizing the patient's own blood pressure as the hydraulic force. This procedure is technically known as continuous arteriovenous hemofiltration (CAVH). However, many children, particularly neonates, may have hypotension associated with ARF, making CAVH difficult. The rate of ultrafiltration by CAVH under these circumstances may be slow and unpredictable. In these patients, hemofiltration may be conducted by interposing a blood pump (and an air-foam detector) in the extracorporeal circuit in order to provide hydraulic pressure within the hemofilter. Pump-assisted hemofiltration (Fig. 15–7) using venovenous accesses instead of arterial and venous lines is equally effective. This technique is known as *continuous venovenous hemofiltration* (CVVH).[59,70] Another modification of the basic hemofiltration system used for immediate or anticipatory fluid management is slow continuous ultrafiltration (SCUF).[71]

The single most important issue determining the success of CVVH or CAVH is the type of vascular access available in the patient. In neonates, especially in those who are premature, a large-bore vascular catheter with a double lumen is difficult to place, since it usually obstructs the entire lumen of the femoral blood vessel. In our institution, where CVVH is preferred over CAVH, we use a single-lumen venous catheter (at least 4 French in size) placed in the femoral vein on each side, one side being used as the designated "arterial" port to draw blood from the patient and the other serving as the venous return line. Beyond the second month of life, a dual-lumen 7 French vascular-access catheter usually provides adequate blood flow for CVVH.

Heparinization of the CVVH/CAVH circuit is necessary (10 units/kg/h), but patients with high activating clotting time (ACT) prior to the start of the procedure may be monitored without heparin administration. Heparin can, however, be instituted if ACT falls below 180 s. Clotting of the hemofilters is a common problem with both CAVH and CVVH; its incidence is especially high when the rate of blood flow is low. Adequate preparation of the hemofilter using heparinized saline is also essential in prolonging the life of this device. In small neonates, it is usually necessary to prime the system with whole blood in order to prevent complications that may result from a large extracorporeal circulating blood volume.

Finally, dialysis may be added to continuous hemofiltration. This involves infusing the dialysate through one side port of the hemofilter (counter to the flow of blood) and draining it through the other port in a large bag. Both the inflow and the outflow of the dialysate are modulated through a controller pump. Unless there is a specific contraindication, standard (sterile) peritoneal dialysis solution containing 1.5 g/dL dextrose can be used. The dialysate flow rate in this procedure need rarely exceed 15 mL/min, or 999 mL/h, which is

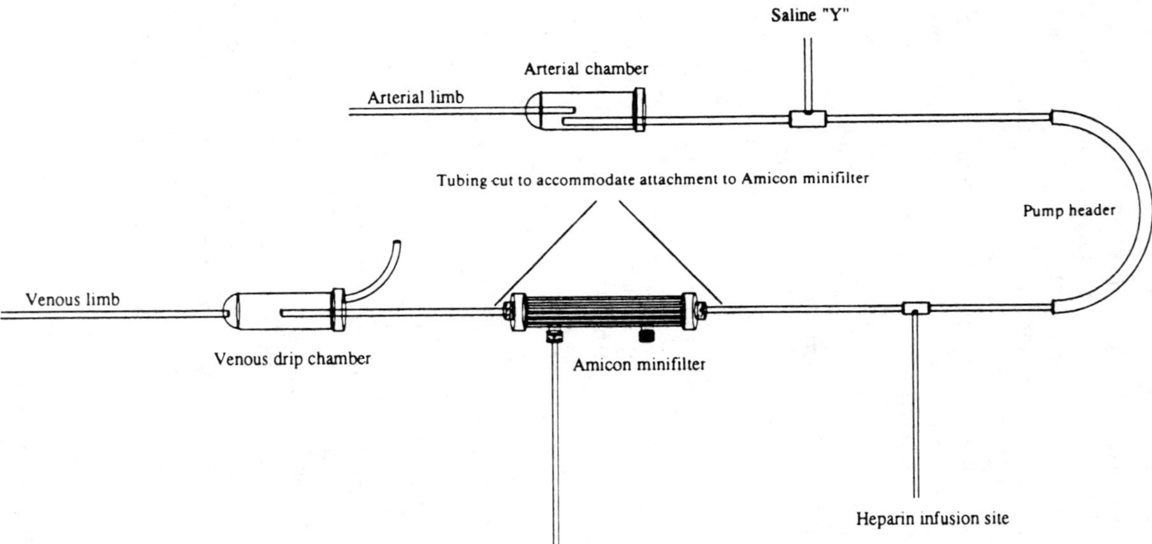

FIG. 15–7. Apparatus setup for conducting pump-assisted hemofiltration. The system is constructed using available hemodialysis blood lines. Several sizes of the hemofiltration device are available from various manufacturers. This figure shows the Amicon Minifilter in use as a hemofiltration device. For performing CVVH, one side port of the hemofilter is "capped off"; for CVVH-D, the dialysate flows into the hemofilter via one side port and exits through the other. (From Yorgin PD, Krensky AM, Tune BM: Continuous venovenous hemofiltration. *Pediatric Nephrol* 4:640, 1990. Reproduced by permission.)

the maximum flow rate that most controller pumps will permit. This rate contrasts with the dialysate flow rate of 500 mL/min in conventional HD. At this time, tubing designed specifically for the purpose of CVVH and CVVH plus dialysis (CVVH-D) is not available and must be constructed in a sterile fashion locally by the dialysis staff. We use Imed-Gemini pump for controlling the inflow as well as the outflow rate of the dialysate. The inflow rate of the dialysate must be set at a rate lower than the outflow rate in order to accommodate the amount of fluid that must be removed by ultrafiltration. Use of CAVH-D or CVVH-D results in a significant increase of the rate of small solute clearance.[58,72]

OTHER TREATMENT ISSUES

Fluid overload in oliguric patients makes them especially liable to develop hypertension. Another cause of hypertension in patients with ARF can be an underlying renal disease such as hemolytic uremic syndrome or acute glomerulonephritis. Since the renal response to diuresis is diminished during established ARF, it is often difficult to correct hypervolemia rapidly and conservatively in these patients. This is particularly true of critically ill patients who require considerable quantities of fluids so that blood pressure can be maintained and medications administered. The use of vasodilatory antihypertensive agents (nifedipine, diazoxide) may normalize blood pressure temporarily, but institution of dialysis is the treatment of choice in such cases.

Bleeding diatheses are common in patients with ARF. Erosive gastritis and upper gastrointestinal hemorrhage are frequently seen in these patients. The persistence of serious bleeding complications may call for the infusion of blood or blood products such as clotting factors and platelets. Some patients with ARF may warrant correction of uremia with dialysis or administration of desmopressin acetate (DDAVP) for treatment of bleeding disorders associated with uremia.[73]

While no systematic pediatric study has been done, infections generally occur more commonly in adult patients who have traumatic and postoperative causes underlying their ARF as opposed to the nephrotoxic etiologies.[74] Infectious complications of ARF are a significant cause of morbidity and mortality, occurring in more than half of these patients.[75] Not surprisingly, the urinary tract is the most common site of primary infection, accounting for more than one-third of the total infections, especially in patients undergoing frequent or prolonged bladder catheterization.[75] The bacterial organisms commonly isolated from the urinary tracts of these patients are of colonic and cutaneous origin. Sepsis, often associated with colonization of central venous lines, accounts for a further significant portion of the infectious events subsequent to ARF.

The principles of preventing infectious complications in ARF are the same as those generally recommended in the care of other high-risk patients. They include careful aseptic techniques and minimizing the period of single-site intravascular cannulation. Particular attention must be paid to the use of urinary catheters. Bladder catheterization should be minimized or even avoided, if possible; there are few legitimate reasons for a prolonged catheterization. Finally, there is a general agreement against the use of prophylactic antibiotics to prevent infection, both urinary and otherwise, during ARF.

USE OF DRUGS DURING ARF

Drug selection and drug dosing must be carefully monitored during ARF. The possibility of amplifying the renal injury by the use of drugs with potential nephrotoxicity must be considered in drug selection. Consider alternative, safer agents if available. Many aspects of drug metabolism and elimination are altered in the presence of renal failure. This includes the rate of biotransformation, plasma protein binding, and volume of distribution as well as altered drug excretion as a result of abnormal glomerular filtration and/or tubular secretion. Compendiums of drug dosing information during renal failure exist,[76] although there is little specific pediatric information. Many of the dosing guidelines depend on an estimate of creatinine clearance. Generally, it is sufficient to estimate creatinine clearance using previously described formulas based on the patient's height or on nomograms developed for this purpose (Chap. 1).[77–79] These estimates of renal function provide information which is useful in making drug dosing changes. However, there are many potential sources for misestimation. Therefore, whenever possible, actual drug levels should be measured.

PREVENTION OF ARF

As is the case with many illnesses, the best treatment for ARF is its prevention. It is essential that the physician recognize both the clinical conditions that are associated with a high risk for the development of ARF (e.g., shock, asphyxia, severe heart failure, etc.) as well as those circumstances which could contribute to renal dysfunction (e.g., use of potentially nephrotoxic drugs, maintenance of a volume-depleted state, use of radiographic contrast media, etc.). In many of these settings preservation of a high urinary flow rate and hence a diminished stimulus for proximal tubular reabsorption can prevent or ameliorate the ARF. The manner in which this may be accomplished will vary from patient to patient, depending on the underlying condition. For example, volume expansion is considered an essential part of initial therapy for conditions such as dehydration, rhabdomyolysis, and early tumor lysis. By contrast, pharmacologically increased myocardial contractility and afterload reduction is the general approach for patients with cardiac dysfunction.

The adjunctive roles of a variety of pharmacologic agents in preventing or ameliorating ARF remain, in most cases, controversial. The three most commonly advocated drugs for the prevention of ARF are mannitol, furosemide, and low-dose dopamine. Mannitol has been reported to be of benefit in the prevention of ARF.[80] Potential mechanisms by which mannitol may exert its beneficial effects in ARF are (1) a vasodilatory effect on the postischemic kidney; (2) maintenance of ultrafiltrate flow rate as an osmotic diuretic, thereby possibly diminishing both intratubular obstruction and proximal tubular resorptive work; (3) diminution of proximal tubular swelling because mannitol is a nonabsorbable solute; and (4) diminution of tubular cell damage by scavanging of oxygen free radicals.

A number of laboratory and clinical studies have now demonstrated that mannitol can ameliorate the anticipated decline in renal function following an acute renal injury, in ischemic as well as nephrotoxic insults.[80] However, it must be emphasized that the available evidence indicates that the potential benefit, if any, occurs when mannitol is administered prophylactically or in the very early phase of ARF. Mannitol should not be given casually to the at-risk patient, since the increases of serum osmolality can result in intravascular volume overload. Overenthusiastic use of mannitol in patients with prerenal azotemia can volume-deplete these patients even further and put them at risk for developing parenchymal ARF.[81]

Loop diuretics (furosemide, bumetanide) have also been reported to be of benefit in preventing ARF in several experimental models.[80] The benefits of loop diuretics in preventing or ameliorating ARF are primarily mediated by their renal vasodilatory effects and the enhancement of ultrafiltrate flow rate (see above). Some workers have found furosemide to be of limited use in reducing the overall morbidity and mortality rates of patients with ARF.[82–84] Nonetheless, others have shown that both mannitol and loop diuretics can attenuate the oliguric phase of ATN and possibly decrease the requirement for dialysis.[80,85,86]

Recently, the constant intravenous infusion of dopamine (1 to 3 μg/kg/min) in patients with oliguric ARF has been shown to help reverse oliguria and, in some cases, to be associated with improved renal function.[87,88] In addition, a number of studies have investigated the possible salutary effect of combined treatment with furosemide and low-dose dopamine in patients with early oliguric ARF.[89–91] This approach is based upon the anticipated synergistic effects of these two drugs on renal vascular resistance and redistribution of intrarenal blood flow as well as the increase in urine flow.

Numerous novel pharmacologic approaches to the prevention or reversal of ARF are currently being investigated in the laboratory. These studies include the use of combined norepinephrine/low-dose dopamine therapy in experimental shock to preserve renal blood flow during pressor therapy as well as the use of agents (e.g., calcium channel blockers, modulators or analogs of prostanoids, antagonists of platelet-activating factor, xanthine compounds, and *p*-chlorophenylalanine) to prevent parenchymal injury. None of these experimental therapies can be recommended for clinical application until more extensive experimental data are available. However, the potential benefits and minimal risks of the judicious use of either mannitol or a loop diuretic in combination with a low-dose dopamine infusion seem justified in the patient at high risk for ARF.

COURSE AND PROGNOSIS

The time course to the recovery of renal function in ARF is often difficult to predict, since the etiology and degree of underlying renal parenchymal injury may vary considerably from patient to patient. However, certain clinical observations are useful. Among survivors, patients with oliguric ATN should be expected to have signs of improving renal function within several weeks, and the vast majority of these patients will recover renal function within a month.

Patients with nonoliguric renal failure may have a somewhat shorter course to recovery. If oliguria persists beyond this period of time, it is advisable to reconsider the diagnosis. A diuretic phase frequently follows the oliguria and immediately precedes the progressive improvement of renal function. However, it is important to realize that GFR at the onset of the diuretic phase is still quite low. In fact, serum creatinine may continue to rise in the early part of the diuretic phase. Therefore, a premature false sense of security may lead to potentially avoidable complications, including the misdosing of drugs and excessive or inadequate fluid and electrolyte replacement. However, once diuresis is well under way and the BUN has declined to below 60 to 70 mg/dL, most older patients will reacquire the ability to autoregulate, particularly if they can drink liquids freely.

As mentioned, the mortality rates of patients with ARF relate, to a great degree, to complications of their underlying conditions.[92,93] The severity of ARF and the need for dialysis is not a major factor in determining mortality rates.[92] Poorer outcomes generally occur in postsurgical patients, those with serious underlying medical illnesses, those who are poorly nourished, and younger patients.[94–99]

SUMMARY

The acute renal failure syndrome usually occurs in the setting of serious or complex underlying disease. The unfavorable morbidity and mortality associated with ARF underscore the importance of vigilant observation and prompt preventive measures for the patient at high risk. Proper management of the patient with ARF involves a great deal more than management of fluid and solute homeostasis. Consideration must be given to clinical stability, anticipatory nutritional and fluid needs, evolving infectious illnesses, drug treatment regimens, and possible sources of further renal injury. It is only after these and other clinical factors are considered that a proper treatment plan can be formulated.

REFERENCES

1. Basil CP, Rudnick MR, Narins RC: Diagnostic approaches to acute renal failure, in Brenner BM, Stein JH (eds): *Acute Renal Failure.* New York, Churchill Livingstone, 1980, p. 17.
2. Reimold EW, Don TD, Worthen HG: Renal failure during the first year of life. *Pediatrics* 59:987, 1977.
3. Norman ME, Assadi FK: A prospective study of acute renal failure in the newborn infant. *Pediatrics* 63:475, 1979.
4. Dixon BS, Anderson RJ: Nonoliguric acute renal failure. *Am J Kid Dis* 6:71, 1985.
5. Steinhausen M, Blum M, Fleming JT, et al: Visualization of renal autoregulation in the split hydronephrotic kidney of rats. *Kidney Int* 35:1151, 1989.
6. Moore LC, Casellas D: Tubuloglomerular feedback dependence of autoregulation in rat juxtamedullary afferent arterioles. *Kidney Int* 37:1402, 1990.

7. Badar KF, Ichikawa I: Prerenal failure: A deleterious shift from renal compensation to decompensation. *N Engl J Med* 319:623, 1988.
8. Hall JE: Control of sodium excretion by angiotensin II: Intrarenal mechanisms and blood pressure regulation. *Am J Physiol* 150:R960, 1986.
9. Steinhausen M, Kucherer H, Parekh N, et al: Angiotensin II control of the renal microcirculation: Effect of blockade by saralasin. *Kidney Int* 30:56, 1986.
10. Ausiello DA, Kreisberg JJ, Roy C, et al: Contraction of cultured rat glomerular mesangial cell after stimulation with angiotensin and argenine vasopressin. *J Clin Invest* 65:754, 1980.
11. Blantz RC, Konnen KS, Tucker BJ: Angiotensin II effects upon the glomerular microcirculation and ultrafiltration coefficient of the rat. *J Clin Invest* 57:419, 1976.
12. Brown JJ, Lever AF, Morton JJ, et al: Raided plasma angiotensin II and aldosterone during dietary sodium restriction. *Lancet* 2:1106, 1972.
13. Johnson JA, Zahr JE, Moore WW: Effects of separate and concurrent osmotic and volume stimuli on plasma ADH in sheep. *Am J Physiol* 218;1273, 1970.
14. Weinman EJ, Kashgarian M, Hayslett JP: Role of peritubular protein concentration in sodium reabsorption. *Am J Physiol* 221;1521, 1971.
15. Olsen S, Solez K: Acute renal failure in man: Pathogenesis in light of new morphologic data. *Clin Nephrol* 27:271, 1987.
16. Kreisberg JI, Venkatachalam MA: Morphologic factors in acute renal failure, in Brenner BM, Lazarus JM (eds): *Acute Renal Failure.* New York, Churchill Livingstone, 1988, p. 45.
17. Oliver J, McDowell M, Tracy A: The pathogenesis of acute renal failure associated with traumatic and toxic injury: Renal ischemia, nephrotoxic damage and the ischemuric episode. *J Clin Invest* 30:1305, 1951.
18. Solez K, Morel-Maroger L, Sraer JD: The morphology of "acute tubular necrosis" in man: Analysis of 57 renal biopsies and a comparison with glycerol model. *Medicine* 58:362, 1979.
19. Hollenberg N, Epstein M, Rosen R, et al: Acute oliguric renal failure in man: Evidence for preferential renal cortical ischemia. *Medicine* 47:455, 1968.
20. Reubi FC, Vorburger C: Renal hemodynamics in acute renal failure after shock in man. *Kidney Int* 10:S137, 1976.
21. Myers BD, Miller C, Mehigan JT, et al: Nature of the renal injury following total renal ischemia. *J Clin Invest* 73:329, 1984.
22. Semple P, Brown JJ, Lever A, et al: Renin, angiotensin II, and III in acute renal failure: Note on the measurement of angiotensin II and III in rat blood. *Kidney Int* 10:S169, 1976.
23. Held E: Protective effects of renomedullary autotransplants upon the course of postischemic acute renal failure in rabbits. *Kidney Int* 10:S201, 1976.
24. Kon V, Yared A, Ichikawa I: Role of renal sympathetic nerves in mediating hypoperfusion of renal cortical microcirculation in experimental heart failure and acute extracellular fluid volume depletion. *J Clin Invest* 76:1913, 1985.
25. Goldsmith SR: Vasopressin as a vasopressor. *Am J Med* 82:1213, 1987.
26. Firth JD, Ratcliffe PJ, Raine AEG, Ledingham JGG: Endothelin: An important factor in acute renal failure? *Lancet* 2:1179, 1988.
27. Kon V, Ichikawa I: Research seminar: Physiology of acute renal failure. *J Pediatr* 105:351, 1984.
28. Williams RH, Thomas CE, Navar LG, et al: Hemodynamic and single nephron function during maintenance phase of ischemic acute renal failure in the dog. *Kidney Int* 19:503, 1981.

29. Barnes JL, Osgood RW, Reinecke HJ, et al: Glomerular alterations in an ischemic model of acute renal failure. *Lab Invest* 45:378, 1981.
30. Donohoe JF, Venkatachalam MA, Bernard DB, et al: Tubular leakage and obstruction after renal ischemia: Structural-functional correlation. *Kidney Int* 3:208, 1978.
31. Myers BD, Moran MS: Hemodynamically mediated acute renal failure. *N Engl J Med* 314:97, 1986.
32. Oken DE: The pathogenetic significance of tubular leakage in acute renal failure (vasomotor nephrophathy). *Renal Failure* 10:125, 1988.
33. Brezis M, Rosen S, Epstein FH: Acute renal failure, in Brenner BM, Rector FC (eds): *The Kidney.* Philadelphia, Saunders, 1991, p 993.
34. Patterson LT, Bock GH, Guzzetta PC, Ruley EJ: Restoration of kidney function after prolonged renal artery occlusion. *Pediatr Nephrol* 4:163, 1990.
35. Cameron JS: Coagulation and thromboembolic complications in the nephrotic syndrome. *Adv Nephrol* 13:75, 1984.
36. Barratt TM: Renal disease in the first year of life. *Recent Adv Renal Med* 2:197, 1982.
37. Conger JD, Falk SA, Guggenheim SJ, et al: A micropuncture study of the early phase of acute urate nephropathy. *J Clin Invest* 58:681, 1976.
38. Andreoli SP, Clark JH, McGuire WA, Bergstein JM: Purine excretion during tumor lysis in children with acute lymphocytic leukemia receiving allopurinol: Relationship to acute renal failure. *J Pediatr* 109:292, 1986.
39. Wilson DR: Pathophysiology of obstructive nephropathy. *Kidney Int* 18:281, 1980.
40. Awazu M, Barakat AY, Chevalier RL, et al: The cause of uremia in obstructed kidneys. *J Pediatr* 114:179, 1989.
41. Klahr S: Pathophysiology of obstructive nephropathy: A 1991 update. *Semin Nephrol* 11:156, 1991.
42. Don BR, Schambelan M: Hyperkalemia in acute glomerulonephritis due to transient hyporeninemic hypoaldosteronism. *Kidney Int* 38:1159, 1990.
43. Chevalier RL, Campbell F, Brenbridge ANAG: Prognostic factors in neonatal acute renal failure. *Pediatrics* 74:265, 1984.
44. Miller PD, Krebs RA, Neal BJ, McIntyre DO: Polyuric prerenal failure. *Arch Intern Med* 140:907, 1980.
45. Miller TR, Anderson RJ, Linas SL, et al: Urinary diagnostic indices in acute renal failure: A prospective study. *Ann Intern Med* 89:47, 1978.
46. Eliahou HE, Bata A: The diagnosis of acute renal failure. *Nephrology* 2:287, 1967.
47. Bidini A, Churchill PC: Acute renal failure. *DM* 35:63, 1989.
48. Espinal CH: The FE_{Na} test: Use in the differential diagnosis of acute renal failure. JAMA 236:579, 1976.
49. Espinal CH, Gregory AW: Differential diagnosis of acute renal failure. *Clin Nephrol* 13:73, 1980.
50. Zarich S, Fang LST, Diamond JR: Fractional excretion of sodium: Exceptions to its diagnostic value. *Arch Intern Med* 145:108, 1980.
51. Saha H, Mustonen J, Helin H, Pasternack A: Limited value of the fractional excretion of sodium test in the diagnosis of acute renal failure. *Nephrol Dial Transplant* 2:79, 1987.
52. Shaffer SE, Norman ME: Renal function and renal failure in the newborn. *Clin Perinatol* 16:199, 1989.
53. Ellis EN, Arnold WC: Use of urinary indices in renal failure in the newborn. *Am J Dis Child* 136:615, 1982.
54. Weil WB Jr, Bailie MD: *Fluid and Electrolyte Metabolism in Infants and Children: A Unified Approach.* New York, Grune and Stratton, 1977, chap. 1.

55. Teschner M, Heidland A: Hypercatabolism in acute renal failure: Mechanisms and therapeutical approaches. *Blood Purif* 7:16, 1989.
56. Chan JCM: Peritoneal dialysis of renal failure in childhood: Clinical aspects and electrolyte changes as observed in 20 cases. *Clin Pediatr* 17:349, 1978.
57. Sargent JA, Gotch FA: Principles and biophysics of dialysis, in Maher JF (ed): *Replacement of Renal Function by Dialysis.* Dordrecht, Kluwer Academic, 1989, p 87.
58. Yorgin PD, Kersky AM, Tune BM: Continuous venovenous hemofiltration. *Pediatr Nephrol* 4:640, 1990.
59. Zobel G, Kuttnig M, Ring E: Continuous arteriovenous hemodialysis in critically ill infants. *Child Nephrol Urol* 10:196, 1990.
60. Mullen JL: Consequences of malnutrition in the surgical patient. *Surg Clin North Am* 61:465, 1981.
61. Starker PM, LaSala PA, Askanazi J, et al: The influence of postoperative TPN on morbidity and mortality. *Surg Gynecol Obstet* 162:569, 1986.
62. Feinstein EI, Kopple JD, Silberman H, Massry SG: Total parenteral nutrition with high or low nitrogen intakes in patients with acute renal failure. *Kidney Int* 24 (suppl):S319, 1983.
63. Zager RA, Venkatachalam MA: Potentiation of ischemic renal injury by amino acid infusion. *Kidney Int* 24:620, 1983.
64. Andrews PM, Bates SB: Dietary protein prior to renal ischemia dramatically affects postischemic kidney function. *Kidney Int* 30:299, 1986.
65. Abitbol CL, Holliday MA: Total parenteral nutrition in anuric children. *Clin Nephrol* 5:153, 1976.
66. Franklin JO, Alpert MA, Twardowski ZJ, et al: Effect of increasing intraabdominal pressure and volume on left ventricular function in continuous ambulatory peritoneal dialysis (CAPD). *Am J Kid Dis* 12:291, 1988.
67. Lieberman KV, Nardi L, Bosch JP: Treatment of acute renal failure in an infant using continuous arteriovenous hemofiltration. *J Pediatr* 106:646, 1985.
68. Heney D, Essex-Cater A, Brocklebank JT, et al: Continuous arteriovenous hemofiltration in the treatment of tumour lysis syndrome. *Pediatr Nephrol* 4:245, 1990.
69. Winterberg B, Tenschert W, Rolf N, et al: CAVH in myorenal syndrome. *Adv Exp Med Biol* 252:385, 1989.
70. Canaud B, Garred LJ, Christol J-P, et al: Pump assisted continuous venovenous hemofiltration for treating acute uremia. *Kidney Int* 33(suppl):S154, 1988.
71. Paganini EP, Nakamoto S: Continuous slow ultrafiltration in oliguric acute renal failure. *Trans Am Soc Artif Intern Organs* 26:201, 1980.
72. Schneider NS, Geronemus RP: Continuous arteriovenous hemodialysis. *Kidney Int* 33(suppl):S159, 1988.
73. Mannucci PM, Remuzzi G, Pusineri F, et al: Deamino-8-D-arginine vasopressin shortens the bleeding time in uremia. *N Engl J Med* 308:8, 1983.
74. McMurray SD, Luft FC, Maxwell DR, et al: Prevailing patterns and predictor variables in patients with acute tubular necrosis. *Arch Intern Med* 138:950, 1978.
75. Zech P, Bouletreau R, Moskovtchenko JF, et al: Infection in acute renal failure, in Hamburger J, Crosnier J, Maxwell MH (eds): *Advances in Nephrology from the Necker Hospital,* vol 1. Chicago, Year Book Medical Publishers, 1971, p 231.
76. Bennett WM, Aronoff GR, Golper TA, et al: *Drug Prescribing in Renal Failure.* Philadelphia, American College of Physicians, 1987.
77. Schwartz GJ, Feld LG, Langford DJ: A simple estimate of glomerular filtration rate in full-grown infants during the first year of life. *J Pediatr* 104:849, 1984.
78. Schwartz GJ, Haycock GB, Edelmann CM Jr, Spitzer A: A simple estimate of glo-

merular filtration rate in children derived from body length and plasma creatinine. *Pediatrics* 58:259, 1976.

79. Hallynck T, Soep HH, Thomis J, et al: Prediction of creatinine clearance from serum creatinine concentration based on lean body mass. *Clin Pharmacol Ther* 30:414, 1981.
80. Levinsky NG, Bernard DB, Johnston PA: Mannitol and loop diuretics in acute renal failure, in Brenner BM, Lazarus JM (eds): *Acute Renal Failure.* Philadelphia, Saunders, 1973, p 712.
81. Horgan KJ, Ottaviano YL, Watson AJ: Acute renal failure due to mannitol intoxication. *Am J Nephrol* 9:106, 1989.
82. Kleinknecht D, Ganeval D, Gonzalezz-Duque LA, Fermanian J: Furosemide in acute oliguric renal failure: A controlled trial. *Nephron* 17:51, 1976.
83. Lucas CE, Zito JG, Carter KM, et al: Questionable value of furosemide in preventing renal failure. *Surgery* 82:314, 1977.
84. Fink M: Are diuretics useful in the treatment or prevention of acute renal failure? *South Med J* 75:329, 1982.
85. Cantarovich F, Galli C, Benedetti L, et al: High dose furosemide in established acute renal failure. *Br Med J* 4:449, 1973.
86. Brown CB, Ogg CS, Cameron JS: High dose furosemide in acute renal failure: A controlled trial. *Clin Nephrol* 15:90, 1981.
87. Polson RJ, Park GR, Lindop MJ, et al: The prevention of renal impairment in patients undergoing orthotopic liver grafting by infusion of low dose dopamine. *Anaesthesia* 42:15, 1987.
88. Henderson IS, Beattie TJ, Kennedy AC: Dopamine hydrochloride in oliguric states. *Lancet* 2:827, 1980.
89. Lindner A: Synergism of dopamine and furosemide in diuretic-resistant oliguric renal failure. *Nephron* 33:121, 1983.
90. Graziani G, Cantaluppi A, Casati S, et al: Dopamine and furosemide in oliguric acute renal failure. *Nephron* 37:39, 1984.
91. Baquero A, Morris M, Om A, et al: Dopamine and furosemide infusion for prevention of post-transplant oliguric renal failure. *Dial Transpl* 16:327, 1987.
92. Hodson EM, Kjellstrand CM, Mauer SM: Acute renal failure in infants and children: Outcome of 53 patients requiring hemodialysis treatment. *J Pediatr* 93:756, 1978.
93. Rigden SPA et al: Acute renal failure complicating cardiopulmonary bypass surgery. *Arch Dis Child* 57:425, 1982.
94. Chaudhry VP, Srivastava RN, Vellodi A, et al: A study of acute renal failure. *Indian J Pediatr* 17:405, 1980.
95. Niaudet P, Haj-Ibrahim M, Gignadous MF: Outcome of children with acute renal failure. *Kidney Int* 28(suppl):S148, 1985.
96. Anand SK: Acute renal failure in the neonate. *Pediatr Clin North Am* 29:791, 1982.
97. Chevalier RL, Campbell F, Brenbridge AN: Prognostic factors in neonatal renal failure. *Pediatrics* 74:265, 1984.
98. Jones AS, James E, Bland H, Groshong T: Renal failure in the newborn. *Clin Pediatr* 18:286, 1979.
99. Ellis D, Gartner JC, Galvis AG: Acute renal failure in infants and children: Diagnosis, complications, and treatment. *Crit Care Med* 9:607, 1981.

16

CHRONIC RENAL FAILURE

Kanwal K. Kher

Chronic renal failure (CRF) is defined as an *irreversible loss of renal function with a resultant decrease in the glomerular filtration rate* (GFR). Since kidneys maintain a large functional reserve, renal damage must exceed 50 percent of the nephron population for CRF to develop. Accordingly, renal diseases associated with loss of half or less of the renal mass or surgical removal of one kidney, such as by donating one kidney for renal transplantation, do not lead to CRF, provided the remaining kidney is normal. Nephron loss induces compensatory hypertrophy in the surviving nephrons thus promoting increased function in individual nephrons.[1] However, these compensatory changes can by themselves lead to glomerular damage and are considered important in causing progressive deterioration of renal function in patients with renal diseases.[1,2] This chapter discusses the pathophysiology of CRF and provides guidelines for the evaluation of children with compromised renal function. The management of CRF is discussed in detail in Chap. 17.

DEFINITIONS

Although in its broadest sense CRF denotes an irreversible loss of renal function, the severity of such renal dysfunction is variable and can range from mild to profound deterioration of the GFR. Accordingly, CRF is arbitrarily classified into the following clinical categories, which are used to define the severity of disease:

- *Early renal failure (ERF).* Decreased renal function with residual GFR of 50 to 80 percent of normal.
- *Chronic renal insufficiency (CRI).* Decreased renal function with residual GFR between 25 to 50 percent of normal.
- *Chronic renal failure (CRF).* Strictly speaking, this term implies a GFR ranging from 10 to 25 percent of normal for age, but it is often applied broadly to all patients with chronically deteriorating renal function. The term *CRF* is used in this sense throughout this chapter.

- *End-stage renal disease (ESRD).* This term applies when the GFR is 10 percent or less of normal for age.
- *Uremia.* Uremia is a syndrome that develops as a result of compromised renal function, usually when the GFR is 10 percent or less of normal for age. Uremic syndrome is characterized by symptoms such as lack of appetite, nausea, vomiting, hiccups, fatigue, manifestations of uremic pericarditis, seizures, and coma. Because of their inability to maintain fluid and electrolyte balance, these patients may also develop edema, hyperkalemia, hypocalcemia, and hyponatremia, with attendant clinical manifestations. Terminally, uremia is associated with coma and death; dialysis therapy is required to sustain life at this point.

INCIDENCE

It is difficult to ascertain the true incidence of CRF in children. Potter et al.[3] reported that the incidence of CRF in northern California was 1.6 patients per million population per year. However, these data clearly underestimate the incidence of CRF, since only children who developed ESRD were considered in this study, which did not include others with CRF who had not yet undergone dialysis therapy or renal transplantation. European studies report detection of five to six new cases of ESRD per million children per year.[4–6]

ETIOLOGY

Two leading causes of CRF in children are the congenital urologic abnormalities and chronic glomerulonephritis (Table 16–1). The most prevalent etiologies of CRF in the first 6 years of life are congenital malformations and developmental anomalies of the urinary tract, such as obstructive uropathy, renal hypoplasia, dysplasia, and polycystic kidneys. Despite the fact that children born with urologic malformations may develop CRF early in life, ESRD may be delayed until they reach 8 to 12 years of age. Some European studies have reported a high incidence of pyelonephritis as a cause of ESRD in children; most such cases, however, are associated with congenital malformations of the urinary tract, such as vesicoureteral reflux or obstructive uropathy.[3,7] The incidence of chronic glomerulonephritis as a cause of CRF increases with age, and this category of renal diseases constitutes a leading etiology of CRF during the later years of childhood and in adolescence.

UREMIC TOXINS

The term *uremia* means "urine in the blood" and accurately conveys the impression of failing kidneys. Chronic renal failure and the uremic state are characterized by the accumulation of a variety of substances that are normally excreted through or metabolized by the kidneys. Of these, creatinine, blood urea nitrogen (BUN), uric acid, and phosphate are commonly assessed in the clinical laboratories. In addition, several other metabolic products (Table 16–2)

TABLE 16–1. Etiology of CRF in Children[a]

Disease Group	Habib et al.,[b] n = 270	Potter et al.,[c] n = 154	Zilleruelo et al.,[d] n = 81	Pistor et al.,[e] n = 623
Congenital malformations, including obstructive uropathy	116 (43.0)	45 (29.2)	46 (56.8)	209 (33.5)
Primary and secondary chronic glomerulonephritis, including that secondary to systemic disorders	71 (26.3)	59 (38.4)	22 (27.1)	122 (19.6)
Interstitial nephritis and pyelonephritis not associated with obstructive uropathy	—	12 (7.8)	—	74 (11.9)
Hereditary disorders	61 (22.5)	20 (13.0)	2 (2.5)	119 (19.1)
Vascular nephropathies, including hemolytic uremic syndrome	11 (4.1)	9 (5.8)	5 (6.2)	27 (4.3)
Others	11 (4.1)	9 (5.8)	6 (7.4)	72 (11.6)

[a]Numbers in parentheses represent percentages; n = number of patients.

[b]Habib R, Broyer M, Benmaiz H: Chronic renal failure in children. Causes, rate of deterioration and survival. *Nephron* 11:209, 1973.

[c]Potter DE, Holliday MA, Piel CF et al: Treatment of endstage renal disease in children: A 15-year experience. *Kidney Int* 18:103, 1980.

[d]Zilleruelo G, Andia J, Gorman HM et al: Chronic renal failure in children: Analysis of main causes and deterioration in 81 children, *Int J Pediatr Nephrol* 1:30, 1980.

[e]Pistor K, Scharer K, Olbing H et al: Children with chronic renal failure in the Federal Republic of Germany: II. primary renal diseases, age and intervals from early renal failure to renal death. *Clin Nephrol* 23:278, 1985.

accumulate in CRF and have been incriminated as the toxic compounds responsible for the multiorgan dysfunction encountered in this condition. Some manifestations of CRF, such as anemia and renal osteodystrophy result from the lack of hormones that are normally synthesized in the kidneys.

During the 1970s, uremic manifestations were largely attributed to the retention of "middle-molecule" uremic toxins. These toxins have a molecular mass of 300 to 2000 Da (possibly up to 4000 Da)[8] and consist of several heterogenous chemical substances[9] rather than a single toxic molecule. Bergstrom,[10] in a reevaluation of the issue, has argued that with the development of newer artificial dialysis membranes—which can remove substances of larger molecular weight than did the membranes used in early dialysis—middle-molecule toxins probably assume a lesser role in the development of dysfunctions observed in uremic patients undergoing chronic dialysis. Currently available evidence suggests that these toxins represent only some of the several toxic products retained in CRF that contribute to uremic manifestations.

PATHOPHYSIOLOGY OF CRF

The clinical manifestations of CRF result from a combination of (1) failure to maintain fluid and electrolyte balance; (2) the accumulation of toxic metabolites, usually referred to as uremic toxins; (3) lack of renal hormones such as

TABLE 16–2. Some of the Compounds (Uremic Toxins) Implicated in the Toxicity of Uremia

Organic metabolites
Urea (cyanate)
Creatinine
Guanidine compounds
Aliphatic amines
Phenols and aromatic amines
Uric acid
Oxalic acid
Myoinositol
2,3-Butylene glycol
Peptides and protein degradation products
Middle molecules
Amino acids
β_2-Microglobulin
Enzymes
Renin
Ribonuclease
Lysozyme
Hormones
Parathyroid hormone
Glucagon
Growth hormone
Calcitonin
Natriuretic hormone

Source: Reproduced by permission from Blanchley JD, Konchel JP: Biochemistry of uremia, in Brenner BM, Stein JH (eds.): *Chronic Renal Failure.* New York, Churchill Livingstone, 1981, p. 30.

erythropoietin and the bioactive form of vitamin D—1,25-dihydroxyvitamin D_3 (1,25-$(OH)_2D_3$), and (4) abnormalities in end-organ response to endogenous hormones (growth hormone). A greater understanding of the pathophysiology of the metabolic disturbances in CRF has encouraged the development and application of newer and more effective therapeutic modalities such as the use of recombinant erythropoietin and growth hormone.

GROWTH

Children with CRF are unable to achieve normal growth and are short in stature. Problems of growth encountered by children suffering from CRF are illustrated in Fig. 16–1. The risk of growth failure is highest in patients who develop CRF at birth or early in infancy and those with a GFR below 40 mL/min/1.73 m^2 (Fig. 16–2).[11–13] Bone age is usually delayed in such children.[13,14] Although the pubertal growth spurt is observed, its timing is usually delayed and corresponds more to bone age than to chronologic age.[15]

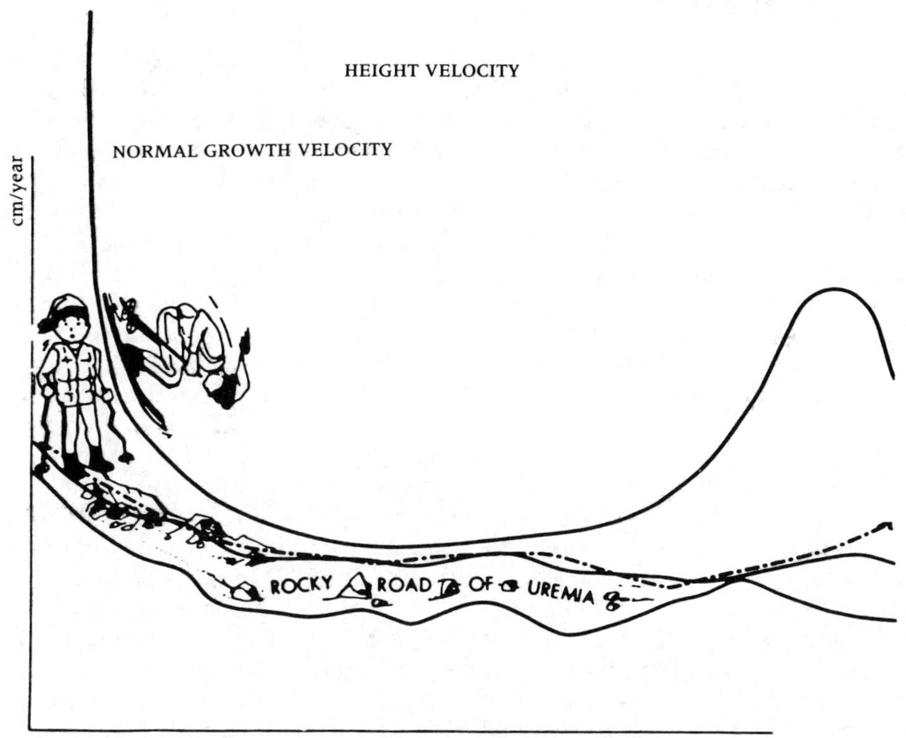

FIG. 16–1. A diagrammatic representation of the problems of growth encountered by children with CRF. The growth velocity of these children generally remains subnormal throughout the course of uremia. (Reproduced by permission from Abitbol C, Zilleruelo G, Strauss J: Renal-genitourinary disorders: Progression, replacement, therapy, growth, in Strauss J (ed): *Pediatric Nepheology: Current Concepts in Diagnosis and Management*. Miami, Florida, University of Miami Press, 1986, p 14.)

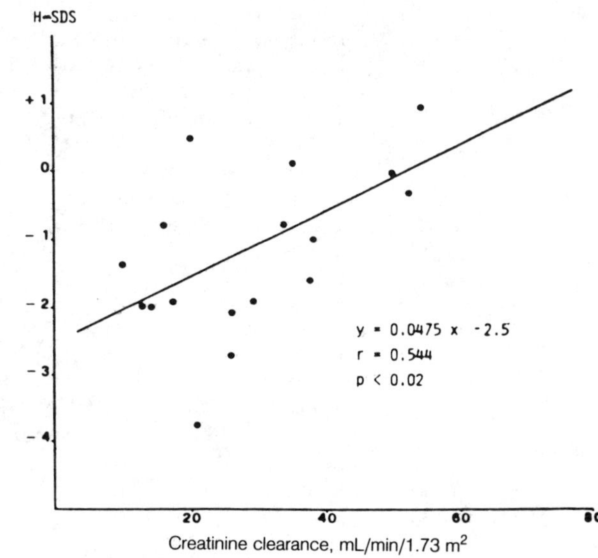

FIG. 16–2. Correlation between GFR and height standard deviation score (H-SDS). (Reproduced by permission from Claris-Appiani A, Bianchi ML, Bini P, et al: Growth in young children with chronic renal failure. *Pediatr Nephrol* 3:301, 1989.)

The etiology of growth failure in children with CRF is complex and poorly understood (Table 16–3). Initial investigative attention centered on the role of growth hormone (GH) in the pathogenesis of growth retardation. However, it has been determined that plasma GH concentration is either elevated or normal in both children[16] and adults[17] with CRF. Derangements in the synthesis and metabolic activity of somatomedins or insulinlike growth factors (IGF) have received considerable attention. These IGFs are peptides that mediate the metabolic effects of GH on the cartilage and have insulinlike effects on the nonskeletal tissues.[18] The two somatomedins of primary relevance to skeletal growth failure are insulinlike growth factor 1 (IGF-1) and insulinlike growth factor 2 (IGF-2). The results of plasma IGF-1 and IGF-2 assay in CRF have been somewhat conflicting, possibly because of the variability in assay methodology used by various investigators. The bioassayed plasma concentration of somatomedins, which measures the total biologic activity of IGF-1 and IGF-2, has been shown to be either normal[19] or low.[20] As measured by radioreceptor assay, IGF-2 concentration has generally been found to be elevated in CRF.[21–24] On the other hand, the circulating IGF-1 concentration determined by radioimmunoassay has been reported to be low,[22] normal,[23] or high[24] in these patients. Upon subjecting the serum of uremic children to acid chromatography (in order to separate substances that may interfere in the assay of IGFs), however, the concentration of IGF-1 determined by radioimmunoassay has been reported to be similar to that of normal age-matched controls.[21] This has led Powell and coworkers[21] to believe that the apparently low serum concentration of IGF-1 encountered in other studies may be an artifact due to the presence of unsatu-

TABLE 16–3. Factors Involved in the Pathogenesis of Growth Failure in CRF

Hormonal imbalance
GH-IGF axis
Hypothalamic-pituitary-thyroid axis
Hypothalamic-pituitary-gonadal axis
Energy malnutrition
Uremic toxins and inhibitors of hormone action
Renal osteodystrophy
Sodium bicarbonate wasting
Sodium chloride wasting
Hyposthenuria
Prednisone therapy
Psychosocial dysfunction
Hypertension
Anemia

Source: Reproduced by permission from Powel DR: Renal diseases and growth retardation, *Growth, Genetics and Hormones* 6:1, 1988.

rated somatomedin carrier protein in the uremic serum. Based on the available evidence that growth hormone and IGFs are present in adequate concentration in children with CRF, growth retardation in these patients may be accounted for by peripheral resistance to the IGFs, possibly caused by circulating uremic toxins.[16,21] Conclusive proof of this hypothesis has, however, yet to be provided.

Renal osteodystrophy resulting from disturbances in phosphorus, calcium, parathyroid hormone (PTH), and vitamin D metabolism leads to deformities of bones and can also contribute to short stature in patients with CRF. Prevention and treatment of renal osteodystrophy by administration of 1,25-$(OH)_2D_3$ has been shown to accelerate linear growth in children with CRF.[25] Metabolic acidosis, which accompanies CRF, also contributes to poor growth in these patients. Although the precise mechanism by which acidosis in CRF leads to growth failure is poorly defined, resumption of a normal growth pattern in other diseases associated with chronic metabolic acidosis upon treatment of acidosis is well known.[26] Decreased caloric intake due to altered taste and anorexia—which is compounded by the poor palatability of food low in sodium, potassium, and protein as well as by fluid restriction—is common in patients with CRF. Many children with CRF show evidence of energy malnutrition. Support for the view that energy malnutrition contributes to growth failure in CRF comes from the fact that the provision of supplemental calories promotes growth in these children.[27–29]

Other factors—such as anemia, hypertension, and psychosocial problems—have also been incriminated as contributing to growth failure in children with CRF. Prior to the development of CRF, corticosteroid treatment of a variety of renal diseases (such as chronic glomerulonephritis) can also affect the growth potential of such patients.[30] The cumulative dose and the regimen of corticosteroid therapy are important determinants of the extent to which growth suppression occurs. Alternate-day corticosteroid therapy has been shown to be less growth-suppressive than daily treatment.[31]

ASSESSING GROWTH IN CHILDREN WITH CRF

Plotting of height and weight percentiles on a standard chart provides a convenient and a generally satisfactory representation of the nutritional status and growth of normal children. However, other than providing an impression of trends, such graphic representations offer little help in the quantitative monitoring of linear growth in children with CRF who are below the 5th percentile. Two methods of quantifying linear growth in such children involve using (1) a height standard deviation score (Ht-SDS) and (2) a growth velocity standard deviation score (GV-SDS).[32,33] These indexes are calculated as follows:

$$\text{Ht-SDS} = \frac{\text{Observed height} - \text{mean height for age}}{\text{standard deviation of height for age}}$$

$$\text{GV-SDS} = \frac{\text{Observed growth velocity} - \text{mean growth velocity for age}}{\text{standard deviation of growth velocity for age}}$$

Ht-SDS expresses the height of the individual child relative to the mean height of same-age normal children; GV-SDS provides similar information about the velocity of growth. Both these indexes provide a quantitative measurement of linear growth in children, especially those who exhibit growth retardation. Thus, a child at height SDS of −1.5 would be considered to have improved with therapy over time if the same score 6 months earlier was −1.9; in contrast, his growth would have deteriorated if the earlier score had been only −1.2.

Standards of age-related length[34] to be used in calculating Ht-SDS for American children are given in the appendix at the end of this chapter. Standards for growth velocity can be calculated from Ref. 35.

RENAL OSTEODYSTROPHY

The term *renal osteodystrophy* (ROD), or uremic bone disease, denotes the characteristic histologic and radiologic alterations observed in the bones of patients suffering from CRF. Essentially, two interrelated but distinct pathophysiologic events lead to renal osteodystrophy: (1) secondary hyperparathyroidism and (2) derangements in vitamin D metabolism (Fig. 16–3.). In addition to these met-

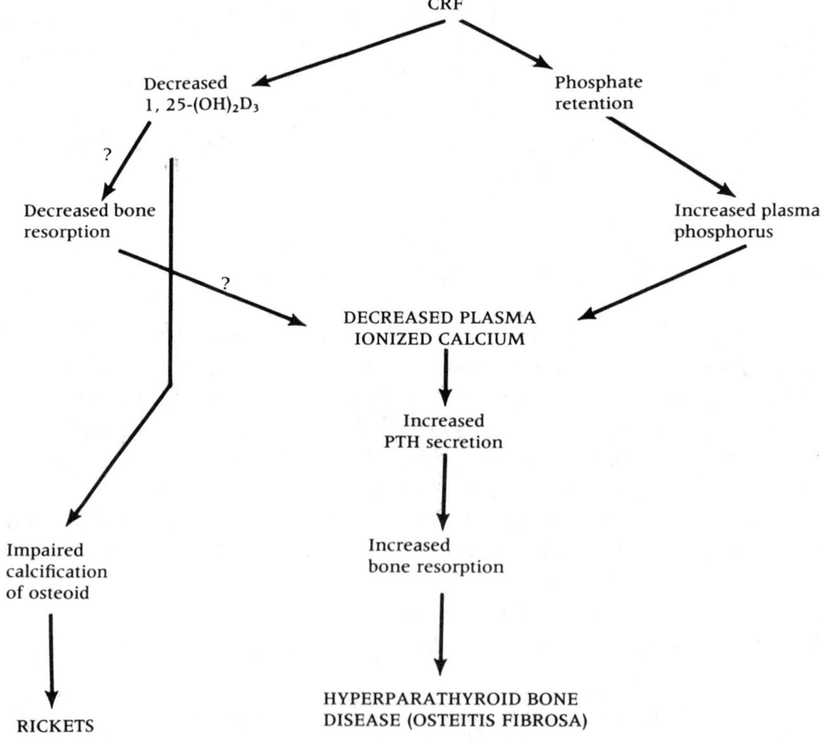

FIG. 16–3. Pathogenesis of renal osteodystrophy in chronic renal failure.

abolic problems, the use of aluminum-containing phosphate binders to control hyperphosphatemia may also lead to the development of osteomalacia (due to aluminum toxicity) in many patients with CRF and may aggravate existing ROD.[36]

HYPERPARATHYROIDISM IN CRF

Secondary hyperparathyroidism associated with declining renal function plays a central role in the development of ROD. Hypocalcemia is considered to be the primary underlying stimulus for hyperparathyroidism associated with CRF, but the mechanism by which hypocalcemia is produced in these patients is unclear. The traditionally accepted view or "trade-off hypothesis" proposes that reduced GFR (even in early stages) is characterized by diminished renal phosphorus excretion, leading to the retention of this ion and an eventual increase in serum phosphorus concentration.[37,38] Retained inorganic phosphorus is believed to complex with plasma calcium and give rise to $CaHPO_4$, resulting in a lowered plasma ionized calcium concentration.[37–40] This physiochemical sequence possibly occurs transiently during the postprandial period, especially early in the course of CRF.[39] Hypocalcemia thus induced evokes an increased parathyroid hormone (PTH) response, which increases renal phosphate excretion by inhibiting renal tubular phosphate reabsorption in the surviving nephrons. However, in order to maintain this new steady state of increased renal phosphate excretion, PTH secretion must be maintained at a new high concentration as a trade-off.[38] As a consequence of progressive nephron loss in CRF, phosphate retention continues despite elevated PTH concentration, requiring an even higher PTH secretion and eventually resulting in hypertrophy of the parathyroid glands. Thus, a state of persistently elevated PTH level or secondary hyperparathyroidism becomes established in patients with CRF.

The trade-off hypothesis discussed above, although widely accepted as an explanation for the pathogenesis of hyperparathyroidism in CRF, is not without criticism. First, transient hyperphosphatemia as envisioned by this hypothesis in early CRF has been difficult to document, even in children with moderately advanced CRF (GFR 25 to 50 $mL/min/1.73\ m^2$).[41,42] Second, in vitro observations have shown that in order to produce chemical complexing of calcium and phosphorus in an aqueous solution and simulate hypocalcemia of the degree that can evoke a compensatory PTH response (at least a change of serum calcium concentration by 0.1 mg/dL),[43] the phosphorus concentration must increase by at least 3.7 mg/dL.[44] Based on these observations, minor elevations of serum phosphorus as proposed by the trade-off hypothesis would be unable to induce a decrease in the serum calcium concentration. Last, it has been shown in experimental animals with CRF that hyperparathyroidism develops despite the maintenance of serum calcium within a normal or hypercalcemic range, suggesting that hypocalcemia alone, as proposed by the trade-off hypothesis, may not be the sole determinant in the pathogenesis of hyperparathyroidism of CRF.[45] Supplementation of $1,25\text{-}(OH)_2D_3$ in these normocalcemic animals with CRF, on the other hand, was able to prevent the development of hyperparathyroidism. These observations suggest that factors other than hyperphosphatemia and calcium-phosphorus complexing may be involved in the pathogenesis of hyperparathyroidism in CRF.

In summary, the trade-off hypothesis suggests a potential mechanism by which hyperparathyroidism may develop in CRF, but several other factors may be equally important, especially in the early phase of the disease.

VITAMIN D METABOLISM IN CRF

Vitamin D metabolism is intimately related to kidney function and is deranged in patients with CRF. Vitamin D reaches the body via two sources: (1) synthesis in the skin, by the action of sunlight on the provitamin D_3 (7-dehydrocholesterol), and (2) dietary intake of vitamin D (cholecalciferol). Following its absorption from exogenous or endogenous sources, vitamin D undergoes hydroxylation in the liver to 25-hydroxyvitamin D (25-OHD_3).[46] Further hydroxylation of 25-OHD_3 to the compound 1,25-$(OH)_2D_3$ occurs in the kidney, most likely in the renal proximal tubular cells.[47] 1,25-$(OH)_2D_3$ is the most important bioactive metabolite of vitamin D and is essential in exerting the physiologic influence of vitamin D on the gastrointestinal tract, bones, and the parathyroid glands as well as in the regulation of calcium homeostasis.[48] In the gastrointestinal tract (mainly the small intestine), 1,25-$(OH)_2D_3$ enhances absorption of both calcium and phosphorus.[48–50] The action of 1,25-$(OH)_2D_3$ on bones leads to bone resorption and aids in the maintenance of serum calcium concentration.[51] Seemingly paradoxically, 1,25-$(OH)_2D_3$ is also essential for the mineralization of bone. It is believed that osseous mineralization by 1,25-$(OH)_2D_3$ is induced by a greater availability of calcium and phosphorus ions to the bone (as a result of enhanced gastrointestinal absorption) rather than by any specific effect of vitamin D on the bone itself.[52,53]

Serum concentration of the vitamin D metabolite 1,25-$(OH)_2D_3$ is reduced in children with CRF.[41,42,54] The circulating level of 1,25-$(OH)_2D_3$ is not much reduced from normal controls in children with a GFR above 75 mL/min/1.73 m^2,[54] but it is significantly reduced in those with a GFR below 50 mL/min/1.73 m^2.[41,42,54]

BONES IN RENAL OSTEODYSTROPHY[55,56]

Bone morphology in ROD is consistent with the combined effects of hyperparathyroidism (increased bone turnover) and lack of 1,25-$(OH)_2D_3$ (deficient mineralization). Morphologically, hyperparathyroidism is characterized by a high rate of bone turnover, increased osteoclast and osteoblast population of the bone, and laying of excess osteoid, which consists mostly of poorly organized woven collagen rather than the well laid lamellar collagen present in healthy bones. Fibrosis of the marrow cavity, or endosteal fibrosis, also occurs in uremic patients as a result of hyperthyroidism. The pathologic changes in the bones caused by hyperparathyroidism are collectively referred to as *osteitis fibrosa*.

After the laying of the osteoid or collagenous matrix of the bone, the next step in the formation of mature bone consists of its mineralization. Patients with CRF are unable to mineralize the osteoid adequately, leaving the bones soft and pliable, which may result in the deformities of the long bones sometimes seen in these children. This increase in the nonmineralized or poorly mineralized osteoid is termed *rickets* (also known as *osteomalacia* in adults). Defective mineralization, or rickets, of CRF appears to result from an inadequate supply of calcium to the bones rather than from any specific defect induced in the bone tissue by lack of the vitamin D metabolite 1,25-$(OH)_2$-D_3.[52,53]

Other factors that may aggravate or contribute to the pathogenesis of bone disease in children with CRF include overzealous phosphate restriction or use of phosphate binders,[57] aluminum overload resulting from the use of aluminum-containing phosphate binders,[36,58] and acidosis.[59]

Bordier et al.[60] have suggested that ROD evolves in four overlapping stages (Fig. 16–4). In stage I, the serum calcium and phosphorus concentrations are normal while the serum PTH level is elevated. Progression of ROD results from the combined effects of persistent secondary hyperparathyroidism and a lack of circulating 1,25-$(OH)_2D_3$. During stage II ROD, despite a rising PTH level, renal phosphate excretion cannot be maintained within normal limits and serum phosphorus concentration rises progressively, while serum calcium concentration declines. Bone morphology shows evidence of PTH hypersecretion as well as defective mineralization of osteoid (rickets or osteomalacia). Progression to stage III ROD is characterized by normalization of serum calcium associated with excessively elevated serum PTH and phosphorus concentrations. Worsening of bone morphology due to hyperparathyroidism (osteitis fibrosa) is noted, while normalization of serum calcium is the consequence of mobilization of bone mineral due to the hyperparathyroid state. Stage IV is characterized by hypercalcemia in the presence of hyperparathyroidism and hyperphosphatemia as a consequence of an autonomous hyperparathyroid gland. As a result of ele-

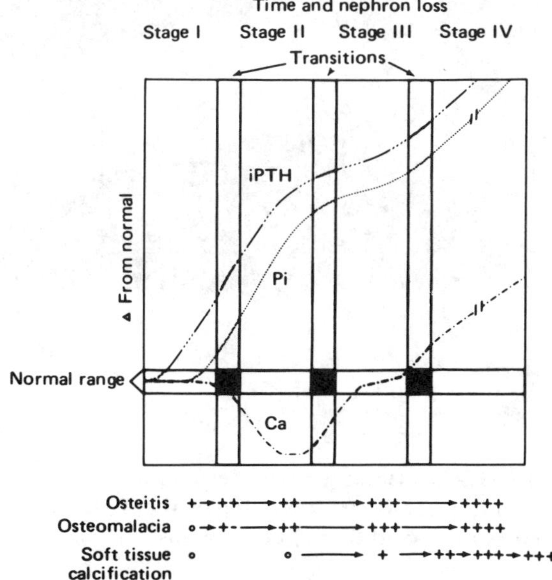

FIG. 16–4. Schematic drawing of the progression and staging of biochemical and osseous abnormalities in renal osteodystrophy as a function of time and nephron loss. (Reproduced by permission from *Kidney Int* 7(suppl 2): S102, 1975.)

vated serum calcium × phosphorus product, patients with stage IV renal osteodystrophy are vulnerable to metastatic calcifications in various organs and soft tissues.

DIAGNOSIS OF RENAL OSTEODYSTROPHY

CLINICAL FEATURES

Renal osteodystrophy is a common problem in children with CRF and somewhat more so in those who develop this condition early in life.[61,62] The most recognized manifestation of ROD consists of deformities of the skeletal system (Fig. 16–5), but other clinically detectable features include growth retardation, bone pain, myopathy, slipped epiphyses, and pathologic fractures. However, by the time ROD becomes clinically overt, the disease has already reached an advanced stage. Therefore, attempts must be made to recognize and treat ROD in its early stages and, even better, to prevent its development entirely.

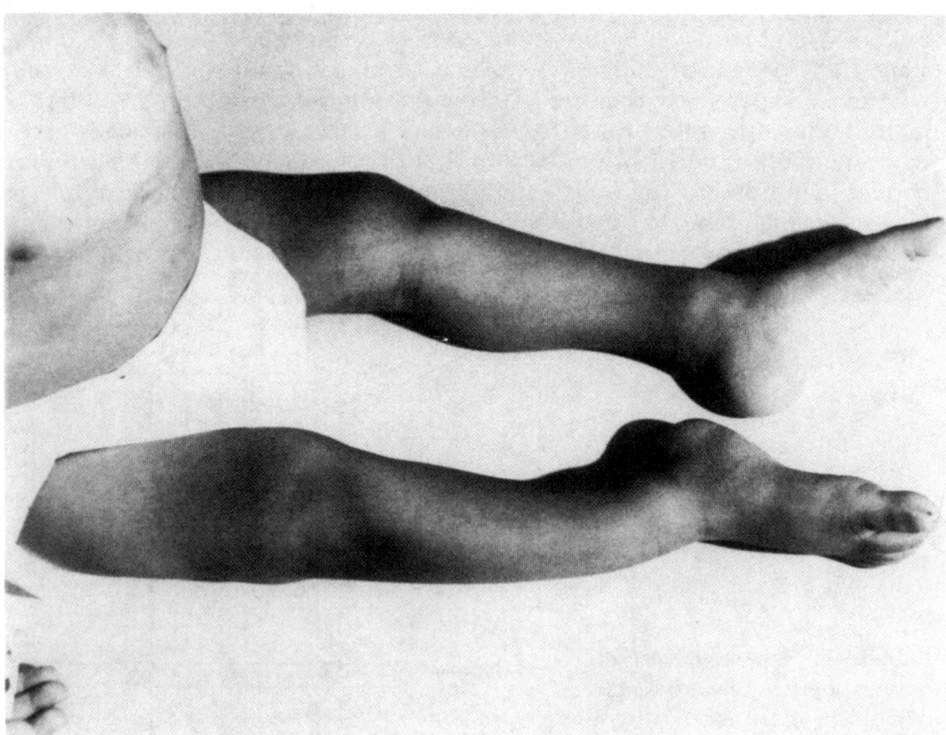

FIG. 16–5. Deformities of legs due to renal osteodystrophy in a child with chronic renal failure. Anterior bowing of the right leg and widening of the lower ends of the bones (tibia and fibula) are obvious.

SERUM CHEMISTRIES

Determinations of serum calcium and phosphorus are usually normal in early CRF and correlate poorly with both radiographic evaluation and bone morphology.[60] Serum alkaline phosphatase and PTH are elevated and are helpful in assessing the degree of hyperparathyroidism. Both these tests should be done as part of the initial patient workup. Later in the course of CRF (GFR below 25 percent of normal), hyperphosphatemia and hypocalcemia are usually evident, in addition to elevated alkaline phosphatase activity and PTH concentration. Hypercalcemia, appearing either spontaneously or upon administration of very small doses of vitamin D analogues, is indicative of either aluminum-related bone disease or severe hyperparathyroidism (stage IV of Bordier's classification).[56] An increasing serum alkaline phosphatase level (especially the bone fraction) is reflective of worsening of ROD. Serum concentrations of vitamin D metabolites 25-OHD_3, 1,25-$(OH)_2D_3$, and 24,25-$(OH)_2D_3$ are low in children with CRF, but their determination is rarely helpful in the management or follow-up of these patients.

RADIOLOGIC STUDIES

Radiologic evaluation of the bones shows three distinct patterns in children with ROD: (1) evidence of hyperparathyroidism, (2) evidence of rickets or osteomalacia, and (3) evidence of osteosclerosis (Fig. 16–6). Hyperparathyroidism is characterized by subperiosteal resorption of bones, which can be best seen in the radial aspect of the middle and proximal phalanges (Fig. 16–7) but may also be evident at other sites such as the femoral neck and medial aspect of the proximal tibia.[63] The degree of bone resorption increases with the extent of hyperparathyroidism. Erosion and loss of alveolar septi of the jaw is also considered a characteristic radiologic finding in secondary hyperparathyroidism.[64]

Renal rickets in children, or osteomalacia in adults, is characterized by a lack of mineralization of osteoid. It is best seen radiologically in the ends of long bones, particularly in the wrists and knees. Widening of the nonmineralized osteoid in the epiphyseal ends of the long bones is the hallmark of renal rickets. Bowing of the long bones may also be seen. Osteosclerosis, a common feature of hyperparathyroidism in adults, is observed less often in children. Characteristically, osteosclerosis affects the cancellous bone of the vertebrae resulting in the so-called "rugger-jersey spine." Delayed bone age is a common feature of CRF. Cundall et al.[14] noted that bone age trailed chronologic age by a mean of 2.6 years in children with CRF.

BONE MINERAL CONTENT

Determination of bone mineral content (BMC) by the noninvasive method of single-beam photon absorptiometery is a useful method of following mineral status in bones. This test involves determining the degree of attenuation of a photon beam generated from a low-intensity radioactive source as it passes through tissues. The degree to which the photon beam is attenuated by passage

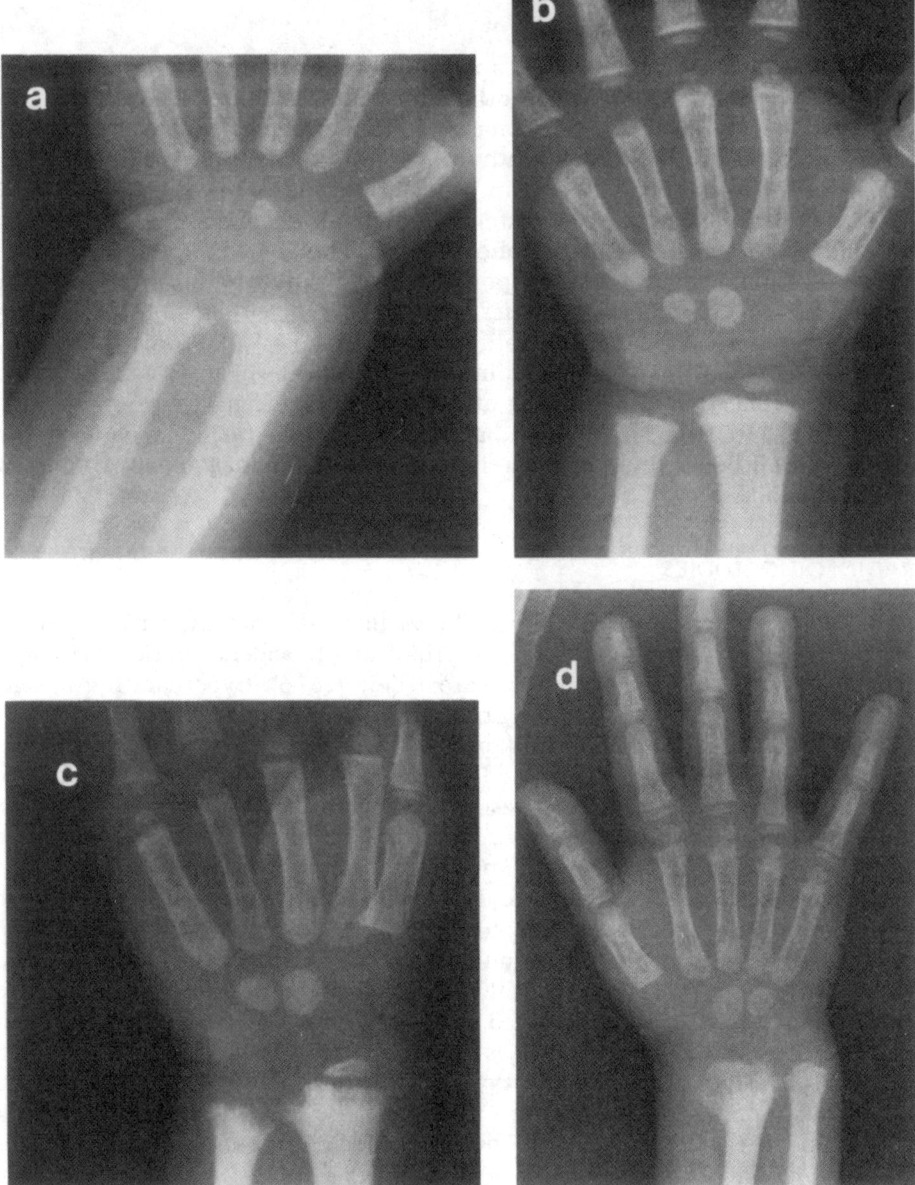

FIG. 16–6. Sequential radiographs of hands of a child with bilateral renal dysplasia, showing progression of renal osteodystrophy and effects of treatment with 1,25-$(OH)_2D_3$ and renal transplantation. *A*: Frontal projection of wrists at 6 months of age, showing fraying and widening of the metaphysis of the distal radius and ulna, suggestive of rickets. *B*: Frontal projection of wrist at 3 years of age. Bone age is delayed (2 years). Ricketic changes noted in *A* have mostly healed upon treatment with 1,25-$(OH)_2D_3$. *C*: Frontal projection of wrists at 6 years of age. Bone age is severely delayed (2 years, 8 months). Subperiosteal resorption of the middle phalanges suggestive of secondary hyperthyroidism is seen. Note the deformed and irregularly ossified distal radius. *D*: Frontal projection of wrist at 7 years of age. The patient had developed ESRD by now. Note worsening of ricketic changes in the distal ends of radius and ulna.

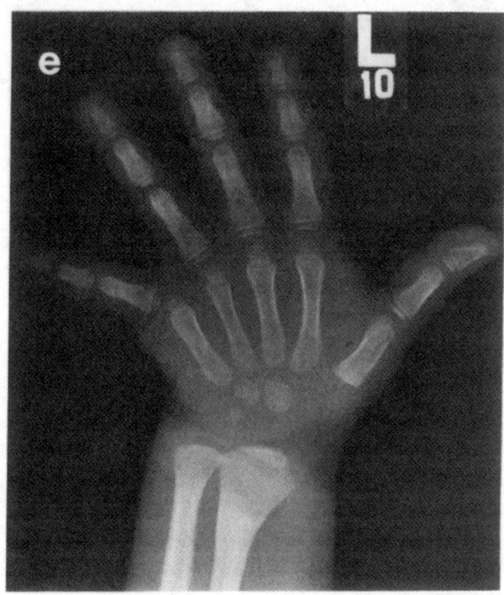

FIG. 16–6 *(Continued)*. *E*: Frontal projection of wrist at 8 years of age, 1 year following renal transplantation. Delayed bone age (3.5 years) persists. Subperiosteal resorption of bones has improved. Distal metaphyses of radius and ulna are better ossified.

through bones depends on the mineral content of the bones, which can be measured.[65] The value of this test in diagnosis and follow-up of ROD remains undetermined. A correlation between BMC and the stature of children with CRF has, however, been established in one recent study.[66] BMC remains subnormal following renal transplantation, possibly due to the use of corticosteroids for immunosuppression.[67]

BONE BIOPSY

Bone biopsy after dual tetracycline labeling is the most accurate method of assessing the type and degree of ROD in patients with CRF. In experienced

FIG. 16–7. A semiquantitative grading of subperiosteal resorption of bones by hyperparathyroidism in radiographs of the hand in CRF. Grade 0 = normal; grade 1 = serration or fuzziness of the basal third of the phalanges, may be a normal variation sometimes; grade 2 = serrations or fuzziness involving middle or distal phalangeal surfaces; grade 3 = involvement of bones other than the middle and distal phalanges by subperiosteal or subchondral resorption. s = serrations, h = haziness or fuzziness of bone outline. (Reproduced by permission from Meema HE, Meidok M, Oreopoulos DG: Radiology of renal osteodystrophy, in Brenner BM, Stein JH (eds): *Divalent Ion Homeostasis*. New York, Churchill Livingstone, 1983, p 261.)

GRADE: 0 1 + 2 + 3 +
PHALANGES
middle
proximal
s
h

hands, iliac crest bone biopsies can be performed with ease in children too. However, most centers still confine the use of bone biopsies in children to research purposes.

ANEMIA

Normocytic, normochromic anemia is universally seen in patients with advanced CRF, and a hematocrit of 20 to 25 percent is considered usual in these patients. Anemia bears an approximate correlation to the degree of renal CRF (Fig. 16–8). The principal cause of anemia in CRF is lack of erythropoietin, a glycoprotein hormone that is produced in the kidneys (90 percent)[68] and to a minor extent (10 percent) by extrarenal sources such as the liver.[69] Significant serum concentration of erythropoietin can be detected in anephric children.[70]

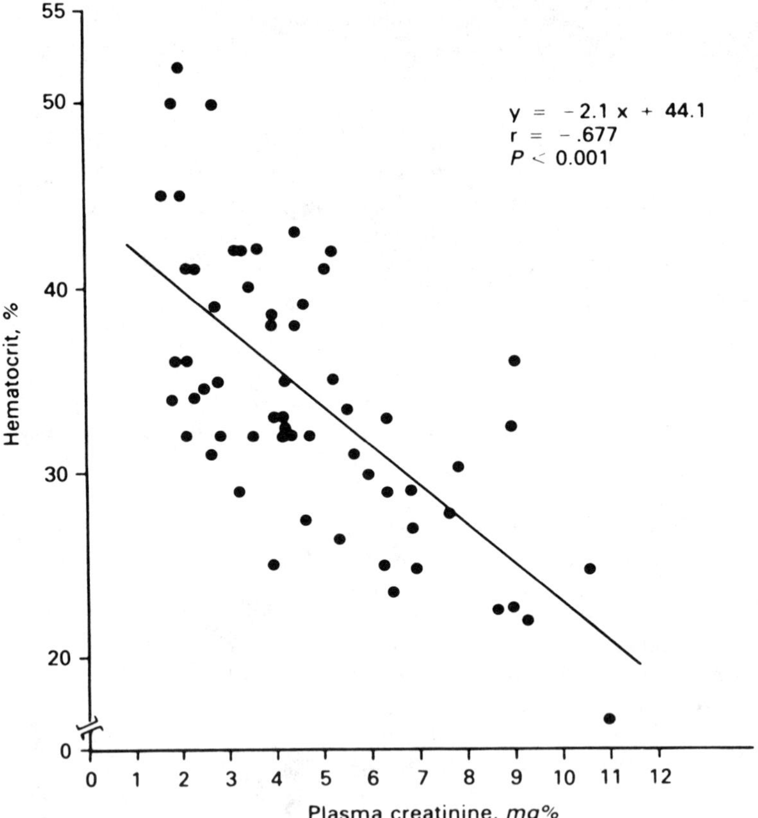

FIG. 16–8. Relationship between hematocrit and plasma creatinine concentration in patients with varying degree of CRF. Higher plasma creatinine, reflecting a greater degree of renal insufficiency, is associated with a lower hematocrit. (Reproduced by permission from McGonigle RJS, Wallin JD, Shadduck RK, et al: Erythropoietin deficiency and inhibition of erythropoiesis in renal insufficiency. *Kidney Int* 25:437, 1984.)

However, the kidney does not appear to be a predominant site of erythropoietin production during human fetal life.[71] Serum erythropoietin level is significantly decreased in children with advanced CRF, but correlation between serum erythropoietin concentration and renal function is poor when GFR is greater than 20 mL/min/1.73 m^2.[72] Erythropoietin exerts its action on the bone marrow erythroid colony-forming cells through a specific receptor present on the surface of these cells.[73] Anemia of CRF can be successfully corrected by exogenous administration of recombinant human erythropoietin.[74–76] Response to this treatment in patients with CRF is dose-dependent.[74] Improvement in exercise tolerance, cognitive functions, and overall quality of life has been reported in adults and children treated with recombinant erythropoietin.[76–79]

Mechanisms other than erythropoietin deficiency that may be operative in the pathogenesis of anemia in patients with CRF are (1) shortened red cell survival—to two thirds of normal—possibly because of uremic toxins;[80,81] (Fig. 16–9) (2) aluminum toxicity associated with the use of aluminum-containing phosphate binders;[82] (3) iatrogenic blood loss during hemodialysis or frequent blood sampling; and (4) folic acid deficiency in CRF patients undergoing dialysis.

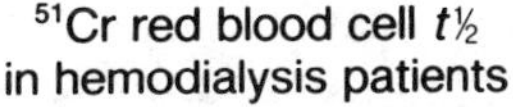

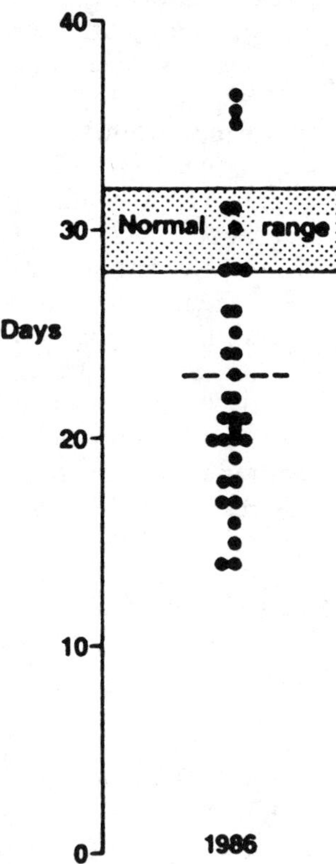

FIG. 16–9. Red blood cell survival ($t½$) in anemic hemodialysis patients as determined by chromium 51 labeling. (Reproduced by permission from Eschback JW, Adamson JW: Recombinant human erythropoietin: Implications for nephrology. *Am J Kid Dis* 11:203, 1988.)

The hemopoietic toxicity resulting from the use of aluminum-containing phosphate binders is now well recognized. The anemia that results from aluminum toxicity is of the microcytic, hypochromic type, similar to that seen in iron deficiency. However, serum iron, iron-binding capacity, and ferritin levels are normal in these patients. Bone marrow examination shows elevated or normal iron stores and absent or severely reduced sideroblasts, suggesting that aluminum probably interferes with the incorporation of iron into heme pigment. Treatment of aluminum intoxication by deferoxamine reverses anemia due to aluminum intoxication.[82]

METABOLIC ACIDOSIS

Metabolic acidosis is commonly observed in patients with established CRF (usually GFR below 25 percent of normal) and is characterized by (1) a lowered plasma bicarbonate concentration (tCO_2) and (2) an elevated anion gap.[83] Patients with CRF often run a tCO_2 of 12 to 15 meq/L. Metabolic acidosis in CRF results from the inability to excrete hydrogen ions or the endogenous acid load due to insufficient ammonium synthesis in the distal nephron segment, while titratable acid excretion is normal in most cases.[83,84] Increased anion gap develops from the retention of anions such as sulfates, phosphate, urates, and hippurates in the plasma; these are normally excreted by glomerular filtration and are retained in CRF due to reduction in GFR.[83] Additionally, some evidence also points to renal bicarbonate loss as a contributing factor to the development of acidosis in these patients.[85]

Metabolic acidosis in early CRF (GFR 30 to 50 percent of normal) may be of the normal anion gap (hyperchloremic) type rather than the high anion gap variety (Fig. 16–10).[86] Normal anion gap acidosis in early CRF is as common in patients with CRF due to glomerular diseases as in those with tubulointerstitial diseases such as pyelonephritis.[87] Severe renal failure (GFR below 20 mL/min/1.73 m^2), on the other hand, is universally characterized by a high anion gap type of metabolic acidosis.[83,86]

Apart from being involved in the pathogenesis of growth retardation and aggravation of existing hyperkalemia in patients with CRF, acidosis has also recently been shown to be important in inducing a protein catabolic state in experimental animals[88] as well as in humans.[89] Correction of acidosis by sodium bicarbonate has been shown to lower blood urea concentration (BUN) in adult patients with CRF, possibly by reducing catabolism.[89]

ELECTROLYTE BALANCE

SODIUM

With a progressive decline in GFR, kidneys in patients with CRF maintain sodium balance by increasing sodium excretion in the surviving nephron population. In the absence of such adaptation, sodium retention will result, producing a net positive sodium balance and causing significant deleterious effects

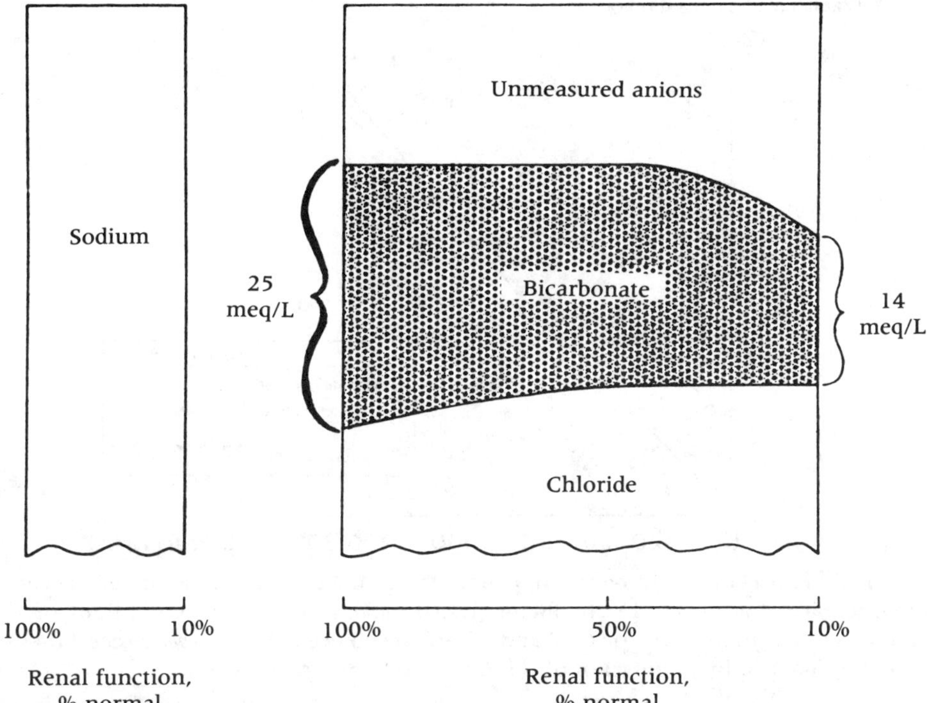

FIG. 16–10. Changing pattern of serum electrolyte composition and anion gap with progression of chronic renal failure. Note that the concentration of serum sodium does not change appreciably during decline of renal function. By contrast, the anion composition changes considerably. Early in development of CRF, decrease in serum bicarbonate is compensated by an increase in serum chloride, unmeasured anions remaining constant. When renal function falls below 30 to 50 percent of normal, this pattern of hyperchloremic acidosis gives way to the more familiar "anion-gap" acidosis of azotemia. (Reproduced by permission from *Arch Intern Med* 139:1099, 1979. Copyright © 1979 by American Medical Association.)

on the body. Increased sodium excretion by the surviving nephrons in CRF results from an increased tubular rejection of the filtered sodium, leading to an increased fractional excretion of sodium (FeNa).[90] The process of increased sodium excretion per nephron in patients with CRF has been termed the *magnification phenomenon* by Bricker et al.[91] Factors prompting the surviving nephrons to increase FeNa in CRF are poorly understood. Suda et al.,[92] in a study of adult patients with CRF (GFR 11 to 66 mL/min/1.73 m^2), reported that the plasma immunoreactive ANF level is high in such patients and that these levels correlate closely with FeNa (Fig. 16–11). This suggests that increased atrial natriuretic factor production may be involved in enhancing sodium excretion by the surviving nephrons in patients with CRF.

Despite these adaptive changes in sodium handling by the nephrons, however, patients with CRF cannot eliminate sodium load rapidly. Ghani and coworkers[93] showed that patients with subnormal GFR (mean GFR 34 mL/min/

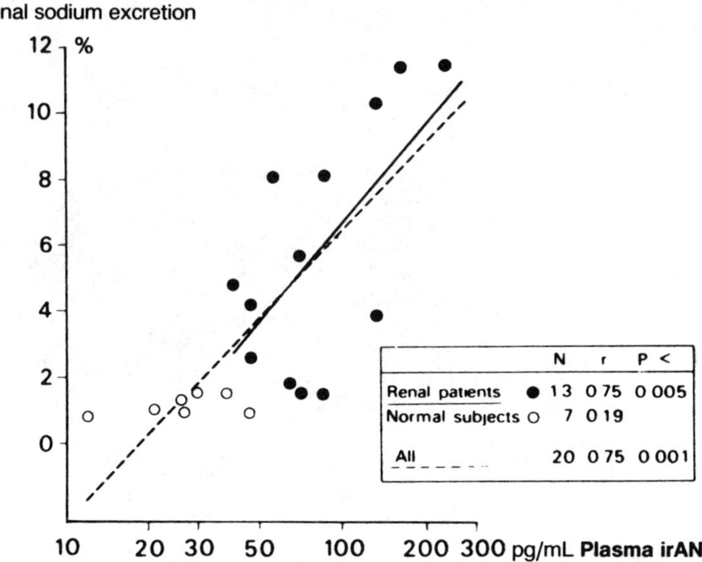

FIG. 16–11. Relationship between urinary fractional sodium excretion and plasma immunoreactive atrial natriuretic factor (IrANF) levels under basal conditions in 13 patients with mild to moderate CRF and 7 normal subjects. (From *Hypertension* 11:483, 1988. Reproduced by permission of the American Heart Association.)

1.73 m^2) were able to excrete only half as much sodium as normal individuals over 2 hours when given an infusion of saline. Blunted natriuretic response and sodium retention upon excess salt administration in CRF have been further documented in experimental animals and appear to be independent of the route by which the salt is administered (PO versus IV).[94] The implication of these observations is that despite the magnification phenomenon, a sudden increase in sodium intake is poorly tolerated by patients with CRF and can lead to increased extracellular volume and consequent complications.

In the face of sodium restriction, normal kidneys can decrease urinary sodium excretion almost to zero. However, patients with CRF are unable to lower their daily urinary sodium excretion adequately when placed on a sodium-restricted diet. The minimum urinary sodium concentration achieved by patients with mild to moderate CRF is around 25 to 30 meq/L. The mechanism of obligatory renal salt wasting in CRF has been thought to be due to an inability of the distal nephron to increase sodium reabsorption in view of increased sodium delivery from the proximal tubular segment.[95] Thus, patients with CRF behave as obligatory renal salt losers, and sudden and profound salt restriction in these patients can lead to a reduced extracellular fluid volume and a decrease in renal perfusion and GFR. Patients with CRF due to interstitial renal diseases, renal dysplasia, and various cystic renal disorders, are particularly prone to excessive renal sodium loss and are highly susceptible to sudden alterations in sodium intake. Distal tubular unresponsiveness to endogenous aldosterone (pseudohypoaldosteronism) is also noted in patients with CRF due to underlying obstructive nephropathy; this may further exacerbate renal salt wasting in these patients.[96,97] Consequently, sudden and profound sodium restriction in such patients can be detrimental and may result in hyponatremia, shock, and further deterioration of renal function.

POTASSIUM

Serum potassium concentration is relatively well regulated in most patients with CRF until the GFR falls below 10 mL/min/1.73 m^2, but most patients are unable to handle excess potassium intake effectively. Potassium homeostasis in CRF is maintained by increased renal and extrarenal excretion of potassium. Dietary intake is the major source of potassium accumulation in the body. In normal individuals as well as in patients with CRF, renal excretion is the primary route for the elimination of potassium. In CRF renal potassium excretion is achieved by an enhanced fractional excretion (by the process of renal tubular secretion of potassium) of potassium in the surviving nephrons.[98] Enhanced extrarenal potassium elimination, primarily through fecal excretion, is well known to occur in patients with CRF. While normal subjects excrete less than 20 percent of their dietary potassium intake via the gastrointestinal route, patients with CRF may excrete as much as 75 percent by this route.[99] Despite these metabolic adjustments, hyperkalemia poses a constant threat to patients with CRF. It can develop rapidly in these patients if they receive an acute load of potassium, as by dietary intake, blood transfusion, or the mobilization of intracellular potassium in catabolic states such as sepsis and acidosis.

FLUID BALANCE

CRF is characteristically associated with a defect in elaborating a concentrated urine. While normal individuals can concentrate urine up to 1500 mosmol/L under circumstances of water restriction, patients with CRF are commonly unable to concentrate urine above 300 mosmol/L. The urinary specific gravity and osmolality are often equal or similar to that of plasma. It is believed that with increasing nephron loss, the burden of excreting daily osmotic load falls on the surviving nephron population. Each nephron is thus faced with more osmotically active molecules in the tubular lumen than under normal circumstances; this leads to decreased tubular water reabsorption in a manner similar to that seen with the use of osmotic diuretics. Since the glomerular ultrafiltrate does not undergo significant reabsorption in the tubular lumen, the osmolality of the resulting urine is similar to that of plasma (300 mosmol/L or specific gravity 1.010—*isosthenuria*). The urinary concentration in patients with CRF changes little from day to day (fixed osmolality or specific gravity). Isosthenuria in CRF is resistant to exogenously administered pitressin, suggesting that a defect in tubular responsiveness to the antidiuretic hormone, in addition to osmotic diuresis, contributes to the concentrating defect in CRF.[100] The circulating level of the antidiuretic hormone arginine vasopressin (AVP) is usually elevated in advanced CRF in both children[101] and adults.[102] Other factors such as decreased medullary osmotic gradient and deranged vascular and tubular architecture resulting from renal disease may also significantly contribute to defective urinary concentrating ability in CRF.

These observations are significant because some children with CRF may develop polyuria and secondary enuresis as a result of the urinary concentrating defect. This is particularly common in patients whose CRF is due to obstructive uropathy, renal dysplasia, cystic renal diseases, and interstitial disorders like chronic pyelonephritis. Such patients can easily develop dehydration if their water intake is inadequate or restricted. Recurrent episodes of dehydration and shock may lead to a further reduction of GFR. The parents of such children should be advised to provide a liberal fluid intake at home and instructed to seek medical attention early if their children develop gastroenteritis or other conditions leading to abnormal fluid losses.

Children with CRF also cannot produce a maximally diluted urine or eliminate a sudden water overload effectively. Such patients need a longer time to eliminate excess fluid and are at risk for developing serious symptoms of fluid overload. Fluid retention is usually a significant problem with children whose GFR is below 10 percent for age and in those with chronic glomerular diseases.

METABOLIC DISTURBANCES

CARBOHYDRATE METABOLISM

Glucose intolerance, despite elevated basal immunoreactive insulin level, is characteristic of uremia.[103–105] This is believed to result from peripheral resistance to endogenous insulin. Dialysis improves glucose intolerance in uremic patients, suggesting that a dialyzable factor or uremic toxin may be responsible for insulin resistance in uremia.[106] Some studies have identified a low molecular weight peptide (uremic toxin) in uremic serum as being responsible for mediating insulin resistance in uremia.[107] Other factors such as elevated levels of glucagon[108] and growth hormones[105] may also contribute to the abnormality in carbohydrate metabolism. Despite these metabolic derangements in carbohydrate metabolism, children with CRF rarely develop frank diabetes mellitus.

PROTEIN METABOLISM

Abnormalities in protein metabolism exist in almost all cases of CRF. Overt protein malnutrition is, however, uncommon. Serum albumin and transferrin concentrations are normal in most children with CRF unless an associated urinary or gastrointestinal protein loss is also present.[109] Abnormalities in the serum amino acid profile have commonly been reported in CRF. Fasting serum concentrations of valine, leucine, isoleucine, lysine, histidine, tyrosine, and serine are lower than normal, while those of glycine, citrulline, proline, and methyl histidine are elevated.[110] Dialysis does not significantly improve the amino acid profile in children with CRF.[109] The mechanism responsible for alterations in plasma amino acid distribution in CRF is not well understood. Low levels of essential amino acids may suggest the need for routine supplementation in patients with CRF, especially those who are being treated with a restricted protein diet.

LIPID METABOLISM

Hyperlipidemia is a common feature of patients with CRF and is characterized by hypertriglyceridemia, normal cholesterol level, elevated triglyceride carrying plasma very low density lipoproteins (VLDL), and low cholesterol carrying plasma high-density lipoproteins (HDL).[111] Hypertriglyceridemia in CRF can arise from (1) increased hepatic triglyceride synthesis or (2) decreased triglyceride catabolism. Although enhanced hepatic synthesis of triglycerides and VLDL has been considered, available evidence does not support such an abnormality as the underlying cause of uremic lipemia. Current thinking is that the main defect in the lipid metabolism in uremia lies in the catabolic pathway of triglycerides. Decreased clearance of exogenously administered triglycerides (e.g., Intralipid) is common and supports the concept of a decreased triglyceride clearance in uremia.[112] Such a defect may result from reduced lipoprotein lipase[113] and hepatic lipase activity.[114] Whether decreased lipase activity is caused by an inhibitor or a uremic toxin in CRF is not entirely settled. Dialysis does not improve hyperlipidemia in patients with CRF. This could be due to the failure of adequate removal of presumed uremic toxins involved in the pathogenesis of hyperlipidemia or to an adverse effect of high glucose dialysis.[115]

ALTERATIONS IN HORMONE METABOLISM

Changes in the growth hormone, insulinlike growth factors (somatomedins), and insulin have been outlined above. The plasma concentration and metabolism of other hormones are also affected significantly by uremia. These hormonal alterations are listed in Table 16–4.

TABLE 16–4. Hormonal Changes in CRF

	Plasma Level	Possible Cause
Pituitary		
Growth hormone	Elevated	Decreased renal excretion
Insulinlike growth factor 1	Low/Normal	Interference in assay by uremic toxins
Insulinlike growth factor 2	Elevated	Decreased renal degradation
Prolactin	Elevated	Increased secretion and decreased degradation
ACTH	Normal	
Thyroid		
TBG	Normal	—
TSH	Normal	—
T_3	Decreased	Decreased peripheral conversion of T_4 to T_3
T_4	Normal	
Parathyroid	Elevated	Hyperphosphatemia
Insulin	Elevated	Decreased catabolism as well as renal excretion
Glucagon	Elevated	Decreased degradation
Adrenal		
Cortisol	Normal	

CARDIOVASCULAR SYSTEM DYSFUNCTION

HYPERTENSION

Hypertension in patients with CRF is often mediated by high renin output from the diseased kidneys. However, as GFR declines and urine output diminishes, fluid retention evolves as an important cofactor in the pathogenesis of hypertension.

PERICARDITIS

Pericarditis has generally been considered to be an uncommon complication of CRF, often developing in undialyzed patients with advanced uremia and in those who may be underdialyzed.[116] However, recent studies in adults have shown that pericarditis, diagnosed by echocardiographic evidence of fluid in the pericardial sac, occurs more frequently than had been suggested earlier. Yoshida et al.[117] have demonstrated pericardial effusion in 62 percent of undialyzed patients with CRF. Uremic pericarditis is characteristically of the fibrinous or serofibrinous exudative variety and is usually associated with mild pericardial effusion. Occasionally, pericarditis and hemorrhagic effusion develop in uremic patients despite adequate dialysis. Patients dialyzed by peritoneal dialysis have been reported to have a lower incidence of pericarditis than those receiving hemodialysis.[118]

The pathogenesis of uremic pericarditis is not well understood. Although the retention of undefined uremic toxins in the predialytic uremic state has traditionally been incriminated,[116,117] some have argued that fluid overload may play a role in the development of pericardial effusion.[119] Infectious agents have been difficult to isolate in the uremic pericardial fluid, even though many patients have been noted to have preceding infections, particularly due to viruses.[120] Use of anticoagulants in the process of dialysis has been etiologically linked to the pathogenesis of hemorrhagic pericarditis in uremic patients.[121]

Clinical manifestations of uremic pericarditis include chest pain, fever, and pericardial effusion.[117,122] Upon accumulation of a significant pericardial effusion, the pericardial rub disappears and the heart sounds become faint and distant in intensity. Such findings are of ominous significance in patients with advanced uremia. Cardiac tamponade may also occur in patients with uremic pericarditis, particularly those who develop hemorrhagic pericardial effusion. The clinical features of cardiac tamponade are hypotension, elevated jugular venous pulse, pulsus paradoxus, diminished apical cardiac impulse, distant cardiac sounds, hepatomegaly, and in some cases peripheral edema. Pulsus paradoxus is characterized by a decrease in systolic blood pressure of more than 10 mmHg during a slow inspiration. In severe tamponade, pulsus paradoxus may be detected by a weakening or complete disappearance of the peripheral pulse during inspiration. The cardiac silhouette is enlarged in a chest radiograph in patients with tamponade. Chronic constrictive pericarditis may develop as a long-term complication of uremic pericarditis and effusion.[123]

MYOCARDIAL FUNCTION AND RESPONSE TO EXERCISE

Exercise tolerance has been noted to be lower in children with CRF and is inversely related to its severity.[124] Diminished aerobic working capacity in patients with CRF and end stage renal disease (ESRD) on chronic hemodialysis has been reported to correlate well with reduced hemoglobin concentration in some studies,[124,125] while other studies have been unable to document such a relationship.[126] Improvement of exercise tolerance has been reported to occur following correction of anemia with recombinant erythropoietin therapy.[127]

Uremic cardiomyopathy often involves cardiac dysfunction, which may be associated with congestive heart failure and is usually observed in patients with advanced CRF or ESRD.[128–131] Such uremic cardiomyopathy has been attributed to fluid overload,[128] anemia, hypertension, and possibly uremic toxins.[125] Removal of fluid during hemodialysis improves cardiac function in a large percentage of patients with CRF. Clearly, fluid overload constitutes an important element in the myocardial dysfunction of these patients.[128] In some patients, myocardial function improves following hemodialysis independent of fluid status. These findings have been interpreted to show that uremic toxins may also contribute to the myocardial dysfunction observed in uremic patients. A distinct congestive cardiomyopathy characterized by concentric left ventricular hypertrophy and thickening of the interventricular septum may also be seen in uremic patients.[131]

NEUROLOGIC COMPLICATIONS

PERIPHERAL NEUROPATHY

Mixed motor and sensory neuropathy, mainly affecting the distal segments of the limbs, is an uncommon complication of CRF in children. In a recent study, Beaufort et al.[132] did not find evidence of clinical neuropathy in any of their 12 patients undergoing hemodialysis, and none of them showed electrophysiologic evidence (abnormality in peripheral nerve conduction velocity) suggestive of peripheral neuropathy. However, other investigators had earlier reported significant electrophysiologic alterations in the peripheral nerves of uremic children and claimed that these abnormalities improve upon dialysis.[133] Abnormal nerve conduction velocity has been reported in approximately 75 percent of adults with CRF.[134]

Uremic peripheral neuropathy manifests itself as paresthesias and muscle cramps usually referred to as *restless-leg syndrome.* Tenderness and swelling of the feet may also be seen and is known as *burning-foot syndrome.* Loss of sensation distally and diminution of deep tendon reflexes are characteristic of uremic neuropathy. Nerve conduction velocity, an objective method of assessing uremic peripheral neuropathy, correlates well with the degree of renal failure. The effect of dialysis on peripheral neuropathy is variable, often leading to a slow or partial recovery. Renal transplantation may result in a dramatic improvement of symptoms.[133]

HYPERTENSIVE ENCEPHALOPATHY

A sudden and severe elevation of blood pressure can result in intracranial arteriolar necrosis and cerebral edema, causing headache, alterations of the sensorium, and seizures. Such hypertensive crises often occur in patients with advanced CRF and can be aggravated by corticosteroid therapy. Prompt reduction of blood pressure generally results in a reversal of symptoms without any residual effects. Intracerebral or intraventricular hemorrhage during a hypertensive crisis can, however, lead to neurologic deficits or even death. Hypertensive encephalopathy and its management are discussed in Chaps. 10 and 11.

NEURODEVELOPMENT IN YOUNG UREMICS

Several recent studies suggest that significant problems in neurodevelopment are encountered in children with CRF, particularly when uremia sets in during the neonatal period or in early infancy. Even though the head circumference may be normal at the onset of CRF, growth in head circumference is uniformly subnormal in infants who develop uremia early in life.[135] Gross motor delay along with global developmental retardation and a lack of maturation on electroencephalography are common in children who develop CRF as neonates or young infants.[136] Progressive encephalopathy characterized by myoclonic seizures, regression of developmental milestones, cerebellar dysfunction, and motor retardation has also been described in nondialyzed young infants.[137,138]

The etiology of neurodevelopmental dysfunctions in young children with CRF remains unknown, but is probably multifactorial in origin. Malnutrition in infants with CRF has long been considered a significant cause of neurodevelopmental delay in such children as they grow older. Warady et al.[139] have reported some success in improving developmental scores in infants with CRF by aggressive nutritional support. The direct effect of uremic toxins on the developing brain and a possible lack of neurotransmitters arising from deficiency of their amino acid precursors may also play a role in causing delayed neurodevelopment in infants with CRF. Aluminum, a toxin well known to induce a progressive encephalopathy in adults,[140] has been considered in the pathogenesis of neurologic dysfunction in children with CRF, but the relationship has not been established firmly.[138]

BLEEDING DISORDER IN UREMIA

Advanced CRF is usually complicated by a hemorrhagic tendency. While platelet count is generally normal, bleeding time is prolonged in uremia. This has been attributed to a defect in platelet function.[141] Laboratory evaluation of platelet function in CRF suggests defective platelet aggregation and reduced generation of thromboxane B_2 in response to exogenous adenosine diphosphate, collagen, and epinephrine.[142] Availability of platelet factor 3 for the process of clotting and clot retraction is also decreased in CRF.[143] A partial correction of these defects occurs with dialysis, suggesting that a dialyzable factor may be responsible for deranged platelet function in uremia.[144]

A defect in the clotting factor VIII, or von Willebrand factor, has also been postulated as a cause of the bleeding tendency in uremia. Correction of prolonged bleeding time in uremia by cryoprecipitates[145] and desmopressin (DDAVP),[146] a synthetic analogue of antidiuretic hormone that stimulates the release of von Willebrand factor, is suggestive of a possible defect in the synthesis or function of this clotting factor in uremia. Some investigators have also implicated an abnormality in prostaglandin I_2 (PGI_2) metabolism as a contributory factor in the enhanced bleeding tendency in uremia. Prostaglandin I_2 is involved in the inhibition of platelet aggregation, and uremic serum has been shown to enhance the synthesis of PGI_2 in endothelial cells cultured in vitro.[147] Aspirin further increases bleeding time in uremic patients.[148]

IMMUNITY IN CRF

Multiple defects in the immune system have been described in patients with CRF. However, these immunologic defects do not generally appear until the GFR declines to less than 25 mL/min/1.73 m^2.[149] Most of the immune abnormalities associated with CRF have been described in patients undergoing dialysis therapy. The most common finding observed in these patients is lymphopenia,[150] but $T4^+$ (helper cells) and $T8^+$ (suppressor) cells are generally normal in number and ratio.[151] Some studies have shown a reduction in the $T4^+$ and $T8^+$ cells with a normal ratio.[152] Reports dealing with the response of the T cells to mitogen stimulation have been conflicting. While some have reported normal mitogenic responses,[151] others have found profound diminution of the proliferative response.[150] Antibody response to tetanus toxoid, *Salmonella typhi* antigens, and hepatitis B vaccine has been noted to be lower in patients with CRF-ESRD than in normal, healthy patients.[152–154] It has been suggested that uremic patients undergoing dialysis therapy demonstrate an impaired neutrophil response to acute bacterial infection.[155] While this may be true in uremic patients on dialysis, experimental animals with CRF, in another study, showed an appropriate neutrophilic response to infection, suggesting that uremia per se may not be responsible for any dysfunction of neutrophils.[156] An impairment in the macrophage Fc_{γ}-receptor function has also been demonstrated in patients with ESRD undergoing hemodialysis.[157] This defect causes a poor clearance of IgG-coated particles from the systemic circulation by the reticuloendothelial system and has been implicated in excessive bacterial infections in these patients.[157]

PREDICTING THE ONSET OF ESRD

Monitoring the serum concentration of metabolic products retained in the blood—such as BUN and creatinine (Scr)—or obtaining creatinine clearance at periodic intervals is the traditional method of evaluating the rate of decline of renal function in CRF. A rising serum concentration of creatinine or declining creatinine clearance is indicative of deteriorating renal function. Using the plot of reciprocal of Scr (1/Scr) over time in months, Mitch et al.[158] observed that the regression line of such a plot followed a straight line, as opposed to the curvilinear pattern seen if unaltered serum creatinine was used (Fig. 16–12).

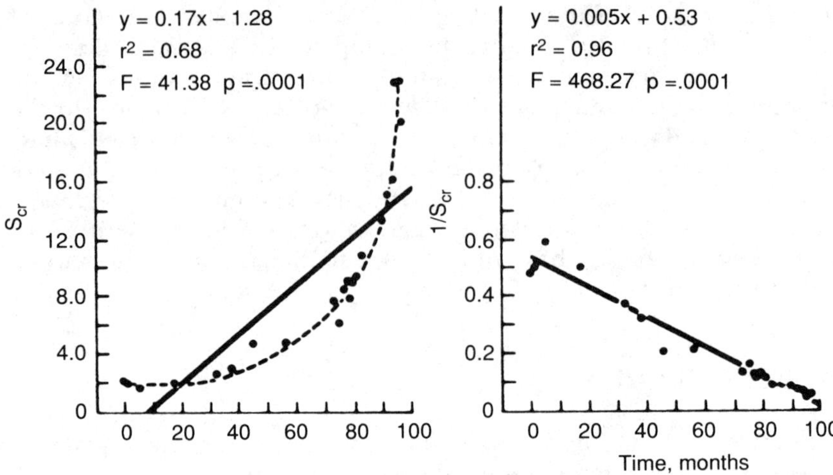

FIG. 16–12. Predicting the progression of CRF by the reciprocal of serum creatinine (Scr). This graph shows the regression lines of Scr formed by untransformed Scr on the left and the reciprocal of Scr (1/Scr) on the right plotted during a 100-month follow-up of a patient with CRF. (Reproduced by permission from *Am J Dis Child* 135:1039, 1981. Copyright 1981, American Medical Association.)

These authors suggested that this technique could be used to predict the time it would take to develop ESRD. These observations have been confirmed in both adults[159] and children,[160] and the method is increasingly used to follow the course of patients with CRF and predicting the onset of ESRD, dialysis, and transplantation. This approach can also be used to judge the effect of various therapeutic interventions on the course of CRF. A rapid downturn of the regression line suggests quicker deterioration of GFR, while an upturn of this line would indicate a slowing of deterioration of renal function (also see Chap. 1).

EVALUATION OF PATIENTS WITH CHRONIC RENAL FAILURE

The purpose of investigations in children with CRF is fourfold: (1) establishing the diagnosis of CRF, (2) investigating the etiology of CRF, (3) evaluating residual renal function, and (4) diagnosing and preventing complications of CRF.

ESTABLISHING THE DIAGNOSIS

Patients with diminished renal function may have either acute renal failure (ARF) or CRF. From a diagnostic and prognostic point of view, it is essential that these conditions be differentiated and that the diagnosis of CRF be established firmly. This can be achieved by history, physical examination, and laboratory studies. Children with undiagnosed CRF who present for the first time may have a history suggestive of recurrent urinary tract infections (chronic pyelonephritis), long-standing body swelling, complaints of a slow decrease in appetite, diminished physical activity, fatigue, a decline in academic performance, polyuria and secondary enuresis, polydypsia, and short stature. Less commonly, such patients may present initially because of a complication of CRF, such as bony deformities (renal rickets), bone fractures upon only minimal trauma, or full-blown uremic syndrome with vomiting, coma, or pericarditis.

On the other hand, patients with ARF often manifest a sudden onset of symptoms, and a history suggestive of preexisting conditions associated with ARF can be documented. These may include administration of nephrotoxins, documented hypovolemia, and hypoperfusion. Acute glomerular and tubulointerstitial diseases can also present with acute deterioration of renal function and may be suspected from the clinical manifestation of recent onset of macroscopic hematuria, development of edema due to proteinuria, and secondary effects of acute hypertension (headache or seizures due to hypertensive encephalopathy).

The physical examination of patients with CRF may confirm growth failure and presence of ROD, both features being suggestive of chronicity of the disorder. The presence of normocytic normochromic anemia in a patient with renal failure also favors the diagnosis CRF rather than an acute renal disease provided that microangiopathic hemolytic anemia (hemolytic uremic syndrome) can be ruled out. Determination of renal size by an ultrasound examination is also helpful in clarifying the nature of renal failure. While patients with CRF may have small (and scarred) kidneys or other obvious developmental malformations or defects (hypoplasia, dysplasia, polycystic disease, medullary cystic disease, etc.), those with ARF or acute glomerular and tubulointerstitial disorders usually have normal or even enlarged kidneys. The presence of hyperparathyroidism and ROD on bone radiographs also favors the diagnosis of CRF.

ESTABLISHING THE ETIOLOGY OF CRF

Since many patients with CRF will present for the first time with advanced CRF or even ESRD, it may be impossible to determine the underlying disease that caused CRF or ESRD. Kidney size is generally small by ultrasound examination and renal biopsy reveals chronically scarred kidneys with glomerular sclerosis, interstitial fibrosis, and tubular atrophy. Establishing a morphologic diagnosis is difficult under these circumstances. Attempts should, however, be made to determine the etiology of CRF in those patients who, when first seen, show only a mild to moderate compromise of renal function. A careful history may reveal information related to hereditary disorders such as Alport syndrome or polycystic renal disease in other members of the family. A history of recurrent urinary tract infection may suggest pyelonephritis, while well-documented proteinuria with or without hematuria points to a diagnosis of chronic glomerular or tubulointerstitial diseases as the etiology. Urinalysis may provide an essential clue to the etiology in CRF, since patients with glomerular diseases will show proteinuria, hematuria, and an active urinary sediment (red cell or granular casts); in contrast, urinalysis in developmental or congenital urologic disorders is usually unremarkable other than indicating a low urinary specific gravity. Patients believed to have CRF due to glomerular or tubulointerstitial disorders (other than pyelonephritis) should undergo further diagnostic evaluation, including renal biopsy (Chap. 8). Those who are considered to have chronic pyelonephritis or developmental renal diseases should also be investigated by renal ultrasound. In selected cases a voiding cystourethrogram will establish whether or not the urinary tract is anatomically normal.

EVALUATING RENAL FUNCTION

Renal function can be determined by serum creatinine, creatinine clearance, or several of the formulas based on the relationship of serum creatinine to body length (Chap. 1). It may be recalled that creatinine clearance overestimates GFR in patients with CRF because of the tubular secretion of creatinine. In young children and infants, a radioisotope GFR may provide reasonably accurate information. Apart from determining renal function, the patient's serum electrolytes and acid base status must also be evaluated for evidence of such abnormalities as acidosis, hyperkalemia, hyperphosphatemia and hypocalcemia. Hyponatremia is also a common problem in children (unlike adults) with CRF who manifest high urine output states such as renal dysplasia, cystic renal diseases, and obstructive uropathies.[96]

DIAGNOSIS OF COMPLICATIONS

Initial and periodic follow-up examinations should focus on detecting and treating the complications of CRF. Growth should be monitored by the parameters already discussed. Progress of ROD can be assessed by evaluating serum calcium, phosphorus, alkaline phosphatase, and PTH as well as by radiologic evaluation. Periodic evaluation of serum electrolytes should also be undertaken to assess hyperkalemia, disturbances of serum sodium concentration, and acid base status. Hematocrit and hemoglobin should also be monitored for the purpose of possible therapeutic intervention with recombinant erythropoietin therapy. Such treatment is recommended when the hematocrit falls below 30 percent. The frequency of these tests is dictated by the severity of CRF and the patient's clinical condition.

SUMMARY

CRF is a complex disorder characterized by the malfunction of multiple organ systems. To provide appropriate care and treatment plans for these patients, it is essential to understand the pathogenic mechanisms involved in the evolution of these malfunctions. Once diagnosed, patients with CRF must be followed up periodically and monitored for the effects of uremia. Steps must then be taken to correct and prevent the resulting clinical dysfunctions.

Renal Osteodystrophy in Children: A Commentary

Russell W. Chesney

Renal failure associated with skeletal deformities and marked growth retardation in childhood has been recognized since the description reported by Lucas, an English physician, in 1883. Childhood renal osteodystrophy is best defined as the *bone disease which affects children with moderate or severe chronic renal failure.* Pathologic changes in the skeleton of these uremic children include several histologic lesions. The most common is osteitis fibrosa cystica, which reflects the reabsorptive effects of heightened osteoclastic activity due to secondary hyperparathyroidism. Osteomalacia is also quite common and relates usually to a defect in bone trabecular mineralization secondary to alterations in vitamin D metabolism induced by the reduction in renal mass. Less common is osteosclerosis or osteoporosis. These lesions may appear singularly or in combination.

Although the causes of growth failure in children with chronic renal failure are multifactorial, renal osteodystrophy is an important cause of a reduction in stature. Impaired renal function that develops in infancy or early childhood also has a more deleterious influence on linear growth as compared to its occurrence in older children. Severe growth delay is found in children who show evidence of epiphyseal slippage. The pattern of epiphyseal slipping is usually age-related. Infants and young children tend to have upper and lower femoral epiphyseal slipping, while school-aged children tend to exhibit radial and ulnar slipping and adolescents forearm slipping. Failure of calcification of the growth plate as well as fibrosis of this region result in a weakening of the metaphyseal-epiphyseal region. Because growth involves mineralization at the ends of bone, a failure of this mineralization greatly impairs linear growth. Hence, the strategy to increase the growth of uremic children must include an attempt to enhance growth plate bone mineralization and reduce PTH-induced bone resorption and osteoid fibrosis.

It should also be noted that these children generally have a marked secondary hyperparathyroidism and hypocalcemia. Because children often do not follow dietary advice, the incidence of secondary hyperparathyroidism is also higher in children than in adults. This disorder in adults has a pathogenesis similar to childhood renal osteodystrophy. However, children show unique or different features of osteodystrophy. Already mentioned are growth retardation and epiphyseal slipping. Because the bones of children are growing and becoming mineralized, e.g., carpal and tarsal ossification centers are becoming mineralized, the radiologic representation is often more pronounced in children than in uremic adults. This poor mineralization and epiphyseal slippage cause overt skeletal deformities in children. Uremic children also demonstrate a myopathy, especially common in proximal muscles.

The pathogenesis of renal osteodystrophy involves two main seemingly confounding variables. As renal mass decreases to 30 to 50 percent of normal mass and as the glomerular filtration rate (GFR) decreases to less than 35 percent of normal, filtered phosphate (P) cannot be excreted adequately and the synthesis of 1,25-dihydroxyvitamin D_3 (1,25-$(OH)_2D_3$) from 25 hydroxyvitamin D_3 (25-OHD_3) is reduced. At first, parathyroid hormone (PTH) increases in uremic children to overcome this P excretory defect. As renal function further declines, a threshhold is reached at which no further increase in PTH secretion can result in phosphaturia; PTH levels are massive and considerable gland hypertrophy has taken place. Hypocalcemia is also found along with hyperphosphatemia. Simultaneously, the decline in renal mass limits the availability of the mitochondrial enzyme 25-hydroxyvitamin D-1-α-hydroxylase. At a GFR level under 50 mL/min/1.73 m^2, a significant reduction in circulating 1,25-$(OH)_2D_3$ is evident. At GFR values under 15 to 20 mL/min/1.73 m^2, serum 1,25-$(OH)_2D_3$ values are reduced by 80 to 90 percent, despite hypocalcemia and elevated PTH concentrations, which normally stimulate α-hydroxylase activity. The end result of the above-mentioned pathogenic sequence is hypocalcemia, hyperphosphatemia, secondary hyperparathyroidism, impaired intestinal calcium absorption, and reduced mineralization.

Various laboratory and radiologic studies are useful in the diagnosis of renal osteodystrophy. For example, serum calcium is low, phosphate is elevated, and alkaline phosphatase activity is raised. PTH values are increased: *N*-terminal portion of the molecule, midmolecule, "intact" molecule, and the large inactive fragment *C*-terminal PTH. Radiographs can reveal widened metaphyses, epiphyseal slipping, coarse trabecular markings of long bones, varies or valgus deformities of the legs, bone age delay, and Looser zones or pseudofractures. Subtle reductions in bone mineral are not evident in roentgenograms of long bones; single and/or dual-beam photon absorptiometry is highly accurate and reproducible in defining the extent of demineralization. Newer imaging techniques including quantitative computer tomography of the lumbar spine and dual energy x-ray absorptiometry will also help define the degree of undermineralization.

The differential diagnosis of bone disease in a uremic child is limited. Children with oxalosis may have extensive skeletal deposition of calcium oxalate, which results in lacunar lesions and frequent fractures. The use of aluminum hydroxide as a phosphate sequestering agent or, more infrequently, as a contaminant of water used for hemodialysis can result in osteomalacia with stainable aluminum at the bone formation surface. Osteoporosis is a component of several syndromes of which chronic renal disease is a feature. Among these are Lowe's syndrome and cystinosis. Finally, malnutrition, which is often found in the uremic child, may contribute to bone disease as the calcium, phosphorus, and protein intake is reduced.

Appendix: Length of Boys and Girls from Birth through 18 Years

	Boys		Girls			Boys		Girls	
Age years	Length	Std Dev	Length	Std Dev	Age years	Length	Std Dev	Length	Std Dev
0	50.5	2.29	49.9	2.17	9.25	133.5	5.77	133.7	6.61
.25	61.1	2.65	59.5	2.49	9.5	134.8	5.88	135.2	6.69
.5	67.8	2.69	65.9	2.64	9.75	136.1	5.99	136.8	6.77
.75	72.3	2.65	70.4	2.73	10	137.5	6.11	138.3	6.83
1	76.1	2.70	74.3	2.84	10.25	138.9	6.25	139.9	6.88
1.25	79.4	2.85	77.8	2.95	10.5	140.3	6.39	141.5	6.92
1.5	82.4	3.04	80.9	3.07	10.75	141.8	6.54	143.1	6.94
1.75	85.1	3.23	83.8	3.18	11	143.3	6.71	144.8	6.94
2	87.6	3.37	86.5	3.28	11.25	144.8	6.89	146.5	6.93
2.25	90.0	3.42	89.0	3.35	11.5	146.4	7.08	148.2	6.90
2.5	92.3	4.43	91.3	3.41	11.75	148.0	7.29	149.9	6.86
2.75	94.5	3.45	93.5	3.48	12	149.7	7.51	151.5	6.82
3	96.5	3.53	95.6	3.57	12.25	151.3	7.72	153.1	6.78
3.25	97.0	3.93	96.0	3.84	12.5	153.0	7.92	154.6	6.74
3.5	99.1	4.05	97.9	3.89	12.75	154.8	8.11	155.9	6.70
3.75	101.0	4.16	99.8	3.95	13	156.5	8.28	157.1	6.68
4	102.9	4.26	101.6	4.02	13.25	158.2	8.42	158.2	6.67
4.25	104.8	4.36	103.3	4.10	13.5	159.9	8.51	159.0	6.67
4.5	106.6	4.44	105.0	4.20	13.75	161.5	8.57	159.8	6.67
4.75	108.3	4.52	106.7	4.30	14	163.1	8.56	160.4	6.69
5	109.9	4.60	108.4	4.41	14.25	164.7	8.51	160.8	6.70
5.25	111.5	4.67	110.0	4.53	14.5	166.2	8.40	161.2	6.72
5.5	113.1	4.74	111.6	4.66	14.75	167.6	8.24	161.5	6.73
5.75	114.6	4.80	113.1	4.79	15	169.0	8.06	161.8	6.74
6	116.1	4.86	114.6	4.92	15.25	170.3	7.85	162.0	6.74
6.25	117.5	4.92	116.2	5.06	15.5	171.5	7.63	162.1	6.73
6.5	119.0	4.98	117.6	5.20	15.75	172.6	7.41	162.3	6.70
6.75	120.3	5.04	119.1	5.35	16	173.5	7.19	162.4	6.66
7	121.7	5.10	120.6	5.49	16.25	174.4	6.99	162.6	6.60
7.25	123.0	5.16	122.1	5.63	16.5	175.2	6.81	162.7	6.52
7.5	124.4	5.22	123.5	5.77	16.75	175.8	6.67	162.9	6.44
7.75	125.7	5.28	124.9	5.91	17	176.2	6.57	163.1	6.40
8	127.0	5.35	126.4	6.04	17.25	176.5	6.52	163.2	6.24
8.25	128.3	5.42	127.8	6.17	17.5	176.7	6.52	163.4	6.14
8.5	129.6	5.50	129.3	6.29	17.75	176.8	6.54	163.6	6.05
8.75	130.9	5.59	130.8	6.40	18.00	176.8	6.60	163.7	5.96
9	132.2	5.68	132.2	6.51					

Source: Data derived from Ref. 34. Computed data kindly provided by Dr. Steven Wassner, Penn State College of Medicine, University Hospital, Hershey, Pennsylvania.

REFERENCES

1. Brenner BM, Meyer TW, Hostetter TH: Dietary protein intake and progressive nature of kidney disease: The role of hemodynamically mediated glomerular injury in the pathogenesis of progressive glomerular sclerosis in aging, renal ablation and intrinsic renal disease. *N Engl J Med* 307:652, 1982.
2. Klahr S, Schreiner G, Ichikawa I: The progression of renal disease. *N Engl J Med* 318:1657, 1988.
3. Potter DE, Holliday MA, Piel C, et al: Treatment of end stage renal disease in children: A 15 year experience. *Kidney Int* 18:103, 1980.
4. Broyer M, Rizzoni G, Brunner FP, et al: Combined report on regular dialysis and transplantation of children in Europe, XIV, 1984, *Proceedings of the European Dialysis and Transplant Association—European Renal Association, Twenty-second Congress, Brussels, Belgium, 1985.* London, Bailliere Tindall, 1985, p 55.
5. Esbjorner E, Aronson S, Jodal U, et al: Children with chronic renal failure in Sweden, 1978–1985. *Pediatr Nephrol* 4:249, 1990.
6. Arbeitsgemeinschaft für Padiatrische Nephrologie: Children with chronic renal failure in the Federal Republic of Germany: I. Epidemiology, modes of treatment, survival. *Clin Nephrol* 23:272, 1985.
7. Arbeitsgemeinschaft für Padiatrische Nephrologie: Children with chronic renal failure in the Federal Republic of Germany: II. Primary renal diseases, age, and intervals from early renal failure to renal death. *Clin Nephrol* 23:278, 1985.
8. Babb AL, Farrell PC, Uvelli DA, et al: Hemodialyzer evaluation by examination of solute molecular spectra. *Trans Am Soc Artif Intern Organs* 18:98, 1972.
9. Bergstrom J, Furst P: Uremic middle molecules. *Clin Nephrol* 5:143, 1976.
10. Bergstrom J: Uremia is an intoxication. *Kidney Int* 28(suppl 17):S2,1985.
11. Betts PR, Magrath G: Growth pattern and dietary intake of children with chronic renal insufficiency. *Br Med J* 2:189, 1979.
12. Kleinknecht C, Broyer M, Hout D, et al: Growth in children with chronic renal failure on conservative treatment. *Kidney Int* 24:40, 1983.
13. Claris-Appiani A, Bianchi ML, Bini P, et al: Growth in young children with chronic renal failure. *Pediatr Nephrol* 3:301, 1989.
14. Cundall DB, Brocklebank JT, Bucker JMH: Which bone age in chronic renal insufficiency and end-stage renal disease? *Pediatr Nephrol* 2:200, 1988.
15. Rizzoni G, Bano T, Setari M: Growth in children with chronic renal failure on conservative treatment. *Kidney Int* 26:52, 1984.
16. Schaefer F, Hamill G, Stanhope R, et al: Pulsatile growth hormone secretion in peripubertal patients with chronic renal failure. *J Pediatr* 119:568, 1991.
17. Samaan NA, Freeman RM: Growth hormone levels in severe renal failure. *Metabolism* 19:102, 1970.
18. Schoenle E, Zapf J, Hauri C, et al: Comparison of in vivo effects of insulin-like growth factors I and II and of growth hormone in hypophysectomized rats. *Acta Endocrinol (Copenh)* 108:167, 1985.
19. Arnold WC, Uthne K, Spencer EM, et al: Somatomedin in children with chronic renal insufficiency. *Int J Pediatr Nephrol* 6:29, 1983.
20. Schwalbe SL, Betts PR, Rayner DH, et al: Somatomedin in growth disorders and chronic renal insufficiency in children. *Br Med J* 1:679, 1977.
21. Powell D, Rosenfeld R, Sperry J, et al: Serum concentrations of insulin-like growth factor (IGF)-1, IGF-2 and unsaturated somatomedin carrier proteins in children with chronic renal failure. *Am J Kid Dis* 10:287, 1987.

22. Goldberg AC, Trivedi B, Delmez JA, et al: Uremia reduces serum insulin-like growth factor I, increases insulin-like growth factor II, and modifies their serum binding. *J Clin Endocrinol Metab* 55:1040, 1982.
23. Powell DR, Rosenfeld RG, Baker BK, et al: Serum somatomedin levels in adults with chronic renal failure: The importance of measuring insulin-like growth factor I (IGF-1) and IGF II in acid chromatographed uremic serum. *J Clin Endocrinol Metab* 63:1186, 1986.
24. Engberg G, Hall K: Immunoreactive IGF-II in serum of healthy subjects and patients with growth disturbances and uraemia. *Acta Endocrinol (Copenh)* 107:164, 1984.
25. Chesney RW, Moorthy AV, Eisman JA, et al: Increased growth after long term oral 1-alpha-25 vitamin D in childhood renal osteodystrophy. *N Engl J Med* 287:481, 1978.
26. McSherry E, Morris RC: Attainment and maintenance of normal stature with alkali therapy in infants and children with classic renal tubular acidosis. *J Clin Invest* 61:509, 1978.
27. Arnold WC, Danford D, Holliday MA: Effects of caloric supplementation on growth in children with uremia. *Kidney Int* 29:205, 1983.
28. Warady BA, Kriley M, Lovell H, et al: Growth and development of infants with end-stage renal disease receiving long-term dialysis. *J Pediatr* 112:714, 1988.
29. Ray PE, Holliday M: Growth rate in infants with impaired renal function. *J Pediatr* 113:594, 1988.
30. Preece MA: The effect of administered corticosteroids in the growth of children. *Postgrad Med J* 52:625, 1976.
31. Polito C, Oporto MR, Totino SF, et al: Normal growth of nephrotic children during long-term alternate day prednisone therapy. *Acta Paediatr Scand* 75:245, 1986.
32. Barrett TM, Broyer M, Chantler C, et al: Assessment of growth. *Am J Kid Dis* 7:340, 1986.
33. Abitbol C, Foreman JW, Strife F, et al: Quantitation of growth deficits in children with renal diseases. *Semin Nephrol* 9:31, 1989.
34. Hamill PVV, Drizd TA, Johnson CL, et al: NCHS growth curves for children birth–18 years, United States. Washington, DC: US Government Printing Office, 1977. [Vital and health statistics, series 11, no 165; DHEW publication no (PHS) 78-1650.]
35. Baumgartner RN, Roche AF, Himes JH: Incremental growth tables: Supplementary to previously published charts. *Am J Clin Nutr* 43:711, 1986.
36. Andreoli SP, Bergstein JM, Sherrard DJ: Aluminum intoxication from aluminum-containing phosphate binders in children with azotemia not undergoing dialysis. *N Engl J Med* 310:1079, 1984.
37. Slatopolsky E, Calgar S, Pennel JP, et al: On the pathogenesis of hyperparathyroidism in chronic renal insufficiency in the dog. *J Clin Invest* 50:492, 1971.
38. Bricker NS: On the pathogenesis of the uremic state: An exposition of the "trade-off hypothesis." *N Engl J Med* 286:1093, 1972.
39. Slatopolsky E, Rutherford WE, Hruska K, et al: How important is phosphate in the pathogenesis of renal osteodystrophy? *Arch Intern Med* 138:848, 1978.
40. Herbert LA, Lemann J Jr, Petersen JR, et al: Studies of the mechanism by which phosphate infusion lowers serum calcium concentration. *J Clin Invest* 45:1886, 1966.
41. Portale AA, Booth BE, Tsai HC, et al: Reduced plasma concentration of 1,25-dihydroxyvitamin D in children with renal insufficiency. *Kidney Int* 21:627, 1982.
42. Portale AA, Booth BE, Halloran BP, et al: Effect of dietary phosphorus on circulat-

ing 1,25-dihydroxyvitamin D and immunoreactive parathyroid hormone in children with moderate renal insufficiency. *J Clin Invest* 73:1580, 1984.

43. Blum JW, Fischer JA, Schwoerer D, et al: Acute parathyroid hormone response: Sensitivity, relationship to hypocalcemia and rapidity. *Endocrinology* 95:753, 1974.
44. Adler AJ, Ferran N, Berlyne GM: Effect of inorganic phosphate of serum ionized calcium concentration in vitro: A reassessment of the "trade-off hypothesis." *Kidney Int* 28:932, 1985.
45. Lopez-Hilker S, Galceran T, Chan Y, et al: Hypocalcemia may not be essential for the development of secondary hyperparathyroidism in chronic renal failure. *J Clin Invest* 78:1097, 1986.
46. DeLuca HF: The vitamin D story. A success of basic science in the treatment of disease, in Castells S, Finberg L (eds): *Metabolic Bone Diseases in Children.* New York, Marcel Dekker, 1990, p 1.
47. Brunette MG, Chan M, Ferriere C, et al: Site of 1,25-$(OH)_2$ vitamin D_3 synthesis in the kidney. *Nature* 276:287, 1978.
48. Reichel H, Koeffler P, Norman AW: The role of the vitamin D endocrine system and disease. *N Engl J Med* 32:890, 1989.
49. DeLuca HF, Schnoes HK: Vitamin D: Recent advances. *Ann Rev Biochem* 52:411, 1983.
50. Haussler MR, McCain TA: Basic and clinical concepts related to vitamin D metabolism and action. *N Engl J Med* 297:974, 1977.
51. Raisz LG, Trummel CL, Holick MF, et al: 1,25-dihydroxycholecalciferol: A potent stimulator of bone resorption in tissue culture. *Science* 175:768, 1972.
52. Underwood JL, DeLuca HF: Vitamin D is not directly necessary for bone growth and mineralization. *Am J Physiol* 246:E493, 1984.
53. Holtrop ME, Cox KA, Carnes DL, et al: Effect of serum calcium and phosphorus on skeletal mineralization in vitamin D-deficient rats. *Am J Physiol* 251:E234, 1986.
54. Chesney RW, Hamstra AJ, Mazess RB, et al: Circulating vitamin D metabolite concentration in childhood renal disease. *Kidney Int* 21:65, 1982.
55. Malluch H, Faugere M-C: Renal bone disease 1990: An unmet challenge for the nephrologist. *Kidney Int* 38:193, 1990.
56. Malluche HH, Ritz E, Lange HP, et al: Bone histology in incipient and advanced renal failure. *Kidney Int* 9:355, 1976.
57. Cooke ND, Titelbaum S, Avioli LV: Antacid-induced osteomalacia and nephrolithiasis. *Arch Intern Med* 138:1007, 1978.
58. Andreoli SP, Aluminum and bone diseases in children, in Castells S, Finberg L (eds): *Metabolic Bone Diseases in Children.* New York, Dekker, 1990, p 231.
59. Cunningham J, Fraher LJ, Clemens TL, et al: Chronic acidosis with metabolic bone disease: Effect of alkali on bone morphology and vitamin D metabolism. *Am J Med* 73:199, 1982.
60. Bordier PJ, Marie PJ, Arnaud CD: Evaluation of renal osteodystrophy: Correlation of bone histomorphometry and serum mineral and immunoreactive parathyroid hormone values before and after treatment with calcium carbonate or 25-hydroxycholecalciferol. *Kidney Int* 7 (suppl 2):S102, 1975.
61. Norman ME, Mazur AT, Borden S, et al: Early diagnosis of juvenile renal osteodystrophy. *J Pediatr* 97:226, 1980.
62. Hsu AC, Kooh SW, Fraser D, et al: Renal osteodystrophy in children with chronic renal failure: An unexpectedly common and incapacitating complication. *Pediatrics* 70:742, 1982.

63. Kirks DR: Skeletal System, in *Practical Pediatric Imaging.* Boston, Little Brown, 1984, p 314.
64. Bublitz A, Alacht E, Scharer K, et al: Changes in dental development in pediatric patients with chronic kidney disease. *Proc Eur Dial Transplant Assoc* 18:517, 1981.
65. Chesney RW, Shore RM: The noninvasive determination of bone mineral content by photon absorptiometry. *Am J Dis Child* 136:578, 1982.
66. Chesney RW, Rose P, Mazess RB, et al: Long-term follow-up of bone mineral status in children with renal disease. *Pediatr Nephrol* 2:22, 1988.
67. Chesney RW, Rose PG, Mazess RB: Persistence of diminished bone mineral content following renal transplantation in childhood. *Pediatrics* 73:459, 1984.
68. Lacombe C, Da Silva JL, Bruneval P, et al: Peritubular cells are the site of erythropoietin synthesis in the murine hypoxic kidney. *J Clin Invest* 81:620, 1988.
69. Meyrier A, Simon P, Boffa G, et al: Uremia and the liver: I. The liver and erythropoiesis in chronic renal failure. *Nephron* 29:3, 1981.
70. Beckman BS, Brookins JW, Garcia MM, et al: Measurement of erythropoietin in anephric children: A report of the Southwest Pediatric Nephrology Study Group. *Pediatr Nephrol* 3:75, 1989.
71. Widness JA, Phillips AF, Clemons GK: Erythropoietin levels and erythropoiesis at birth in infants with Potter syndrome. *J Pediatr* 117:155, 1990.
72. Chandra M, Clemons GK, McVicar MI: Relation of serum erythropoietin levels to renal excretory function: Evidence for lowered set point for erythropoietin production in chronic renal failure. *J Pediatr* 113:1015, 1988.
73. Swada K, Krantz SB, Dai CH, et al: Purification of human blood burst-forming units-erythroid and demonstration of the evolution of erythropoietin receptors. *J Cell Physiol* 142:219, 1990.
74. Eschbach JW, Egrie J, Downing MR, et al: Correction of the anemia of end stage renal disease with recombinant human erythropoietin: Results of a combined phase I and clinical trial. *N Eng J Med* 316:73, 1987.
75. Sinai-Trieman L, Salusky IB, Fine RN: Use of subcutaneous recombinant human reythropoietin in children undergoing continuous cycling peritoneal dialysis. *J Pediatr* 114:550, 1989.
76. Montini G, Zacchello G, Baraldi E, et al: Benefits and risks of anemia correction with recombinant human erythropoietin in children maintained on hemodialysis. *J Pediatr* 117:556, 1990.
77. Marsh JT, Brown WS, Wolcott D, et al: rHuEPO treatment improves brain and cognitive function of dialysis patients. *Kidney Int* 39:155, 1991.
78. Johnson WJ, McCarthy JT, Tanagihara T, et al: Effects of recombinant human erythropoietin on cerebral and cutaneous blood flow and blood coagulation. *Kidney Int* 38:919, 1990.
79. Evans RW, Rader B, Manninen DL, et al: The quality of life of hemodialysis recipients treated with recombinant human erythropoietin. *JAMA* 263:825, 1990.
80. Shaw AB: Hemolysis in chronic renal failure. *Br Med J* 2:213, 1967.
81. Eschbach JW, Adamson JW: Anemia of end stage renal disease (ESRD). *Kidney Int* 28:1, 1985.
82. Kaiser L, Schwartz KA: Aluminum-induced anemia. *Am J Kid Dis* 6:348, 1985.
83. Warnock DG: Uremic acidosis. *Kidney Int* 34:278, 1988.
84. Goodman DA, Lemann J, Lennon EJ, et al: Production, excretion and net balance of fixed acid in patients with renal acidosis. *J Clin Invest* 44:495, 1965.
85. Schwartz WB, Hall PW, Hays RM, et al: On the mechanism of acidosis in chronic renal disease. *J Clin Invest* 38:39, 1959.

86. Widmer B, Gerhardt RE, Harrington JT, et al: Serum electrolyte and acid base composition: The influence of graded degrees of chronic renal failure. *Arch Intern Med* 139:1099, 1979.
87. Wallia R, Greenberg A, Piraino B, et al: Serum electrolyte patterns in end stage renal disease. *Am J Kid Dis* 8:98, 1986.
88. May RA, Kelley RA, Mitch WE: Mechanisms for defects in muscle protein metabolism in rats with chronic uremia: Influence of metabolic acidosis. *J Clin Invest* 79:1099, 1987.
89. Jenkins D, Burton PR, Bennett SE, et al: The metabolic consequences of the correction of acidosis in uraemia. *Nephrol Dial Transplant* 4:92, 1989.
90. Slatopolsky E, Elkan IO, Weerts C, et al: Studies on the characteristics of the control system governing sodium excretion in uremic man. *J Clin Invest* 47:521, 1968.
91. Bricker NS, Fine LG, Kaplan M, et al: "Magnification phenomenon" in chronic renal disease. *N Engl J Med* 299:1287, 1978.
92. Suda S, Weidmann P, Saxenhofer H, et al: Arterial natriuretic factor in mild to moderate chronic renal failure. *Hypertension* 11:483, 1988.
93. Ghani M, Kahn T, Stein RM: Effects of saline loading in hypertensive and normotensive azotemic man (abstract). *Clin Res* 20:603, 1972.
94. Bourgoigne JJ, Kaplan M, Cavellas G, et al: Sodium homeostatis in dogs with chronic renal failure. *Kidney Int* 21:820, 1982.
95. Coleman AJ, Aeias M, Carter NW, et al: The mechanism of salt wastage in chronic renal disease. *J Clin Invest* 45:1116, 1966.
96. Marra G, Goy V, Appiani A, et al: Persistent tubular resistance to aldosterone in infants with congenital hydronephrosis corrected neonatally. *J Pediatr* 110:868, 1987.
97. Terzi F, Assael BM, Claris-Appiani A, et al: Increased sodium requirement following early postnatal surgical correction of congenital uropathies in infants. *Pediatr Nephrol* 4:581, 1990.
98. Schultze RG, Taggart DD, Shapiro H, et al: On the adaptation in potassium excretion associated with nephron reduction in the dog. *J Clin Invest* 50:1061, 1971.
99. Hayes CP, McLeod MC, Robinson RR, et al: An extrarenal mechanism for the maintenance of potassium balance in severe chronic renal failure. *Trans Assoc Am Phys* 80:207, 1967.
100. Holliday MA, Egan TJ, Morris CR, et al: Pitressin-resistant hyposthenuria in chronic renal disease. *Am J Med* 42:378, 1967.
101. Rauh N, Hund E, Sohl G, et al: Vasoactive hormone in children with chronic renal failure. *Kidney Int* 24 (suppl 15):S27, 1982.
102. Horkey K, Sramkova J, Lachmanova J, et al: Plasma concentration antidiuretic hormone in patients with chronic renal insufficiency on maintenance dialysis. *Horm Metab Res* 11:241, 1979.
103. DeFronza RA, Andres R, Edger P, et al: Carbohydrate metabolism in uremia: A review. *Medicine (Baltimore)* 52:469, 1973.
104. Mak RH, Haycock GB, Chantler C: Glucose intolerance in children with chronic renal failure. *Kidney Int* 24(suppl 15):S22, 1982.
105. El-Bishti MM, Counahan RC, Bloom SR, et al: Hormonal and metabolic responses to intravenous glucose in children and hemodialysis. *Am J Clin Nutr* 31:1865, 1978.
106. McCaleb ML, Izzo MS, Lockwood DH: Characterization and purification of a factor from uremic human serum that induces insulin resistance. *J Clin Invest* 75:391, 1985.

107. DeFronzo RA, Tobin JD, Rowe JW, et al: Glucose intolerance in uremia. Quantification of pancreatic beta cell sensitivity to glucose and tissue sensitivity to insulin. *J Clin Invest* 62:425, 1978.
108. Bilbery GL, Faloona GR, White MC, et al: Hyperglucagonemia in uremia reversal by transplantation. *Ann Intern Med* 82:525, 1975.
109. Conley SB, Rose GM, Robson AM, et al: Effects of dietary intake and hemodialysis on protein turnover in uremic children. *Kidney Int* 17:837, 1980.
110. Counahan R, El-Bishti M, Cox BD, et al: Plasma aminoacids in children and adolescents on hemodialysis. *Kidney Int* 10:471, 1976.
111. Heuck C, Ritz E: Hyperlipoproteinemia in renal insufficiency. *Nephron* 25:1, 1980.
112. Attman PO, Gustafson A, Alaupovic P, et al: Lipid metabolism in patients with chronic renal failure in predialytic phase. *Contr Nephrol* 65:29, 1988.
113. Bagdade JD: Uremic lipemia. An unrecognized abnormality in triglyceride production and removal. *Arch Intern Med* 120:875, 1970.
114. Mordasin R, Frey F, Flury W, et al: Selective deficiency of hepatic triglyceride lipase in uremic patients. *N Engl J Med* 297:1362, 1977.
115. Swamy AP, Cestero RVM, Campbell RG, et al: Dialysate glucose and hyperlipidemia. *Dialysis Transplant* 6:52, 1977.
116. Wray TM, Stone WJ: Uremic pericarditis: A prospective echocardiographic and clinical study. *Clin Nephrol* 6:295, 1976.
117. Yoshida K, Shina A, Asamo Y, et al: Uremic pericardial effusion: Detection and evaluation of pericardial effusion by echocardiography. *Clin Nephrol* 13:260, 1980.
118. Silverberg S, Oreopoulos DG, Wise DJ, et al: Pericarditis in patients undergoing long-term hemodialysis and peritoneal dialysis: Incidence, complications, and management. *Am J Med* 63:879, 1977.
119. Suki WN: Pericarditis. *Kidney Int* 33(suppl 24):S-10, 1988.
120. Osanloo E, Shaloub RJ, Cioffi RF, et al: Viral pericarditis in patients receiving hemodialysis. *Arch Intern Med* 139:301, 1979.
121. Alfrey AL, Goss JE, Ogden DA, et al: Uremic hemopericardium. *Am J Med* 45:391, 1968.
122. Luft TC, Gilman JK, Weyman AE: Pericarditis in patients with uremia: Clinical and echocardiographic evaluation. *Nephron* 25:160, 1980.
123. Kumar S, Lesch M: Pericarditis in renal disease. *Progr Cardiovasc Dis* 22:357, 1980.
124. Ulmer HE, Greiner H, Schuler HW, et al: Cardiovascular impairment and physical working capacity in children with chronic renal failure. *Acta Paediatr Scand* 67:43, 1978.
125. Zanconato S, Baraldi E, Montini G, et al: Exercise tolerance in end-stage renal disease. *Child Nephrol Urol* 10:26, 1990.
126. Painter P, Messer-Rehak DL, Hanson P, et al: Exercise capacity in hemodialysis, CAPD, and renal transplant patients. *Nephron* 42:47, 1986.
127. Baraldi E, Montini G, Zanconato S, et al: Exercise tolerance after anemia correction with recombinant human erythropoietin in end-stage renal disease. *Pediatr Nephrol* 4:623, 1990.
128. Prosser D, Parsons V: The case for a specific uremic myocardiopathy. *Nephron* 15:4, 1975.
129. Hung J, Harris PJ, Uren RF, et al: Uremic cardiomyopathy—effect of hemodialysis on left ventricular function in end-stage renal failure. *N Engl J Med* 302:547, 1980.
130. O'Regan S, Villemand D, Revillon L, et al: Effects of hemodialysis on myocardial function in pediatric patients. *Nephron* 25:214, 1980.

131. Renger A, Muller M, Jutzler GA, et al: Echocardiographic evaluation of left ventricular dimensions and function in chronic hemodialysis patients with cardiomegaly. *Clin Nephrol* 21:164, 1984.
132. de Beaufort CE, Andre J, Heimans JJ, et al: Peripheral nerve function in children with end stage renal failure. *Pediatr Nephrol* 3:175, 1989.
133. Arbus GS, Barnor NA, Hsu AC, et al: Effect of chronic renal failure, dialysis and transplantation on motor nerve conduction velocity in children. *Can Med Assoc J* 113:517, 1975.
134. Thomas PK, Hollinrake K, Lascelles RG, et al: The polyneuropathy of chronic renal failure. *Brain* 94:761, 1971.
135. McGraw ME, Haka-Ikse K: Neurologic-developmental sequelae of chronic renal failure in infancy. *J Pediatr* 106:579, 1988.
136. Bock GH, Conners K, Ruley J, et al: Disturbances of brain maturation and neurodevelopment during chronic renal failure in infancy. *J Pediatr* 114:231, 1989.
137. Bale JF, Siegler RL, Bray PF: Encephalopathy in young children with moderate chronic renal failure. *Am J Dis Child* 134:581, 1980.
138. Geary DF, Fennel RS, Andriola M, et al: Encephalopathy in children with chronic renal failure. *J Pediatr* 97:41, 1980.
139. Warady BA, Kriley M, Lovell H, et al: Growth and development of infants with end-stage renal disease receiving long-term peritoneal dialysis. *J Pediatr* 112:714, 1988.
140. Alfrey AC, LeGendre GR, Kaehaney WD: The dialysis encephalopathy syndrome, possible aluminum intoxication. *N Engl J Med* 294:184, 1976.
141. Eknoyan G, Wacksman SG, Glueck M, et al: Platelet function in renal failure. *N Engl J Med* 280:677, 1969.
142. Minno GD, Martinez J, Dela Rosa J, et al: Platelet dysfunction in uremia. Multifaceted defect partially corrected by dialysis. *Am J Med* 79:552, 1985.
143. Rabiner SF, Hrodeck O: Platelet factor-3 in normal subjects and patients with renal failure. *J Clin Invest* 47:901, 1968.
144. Remuzzi G, Livio M, Marchiaro G, et al: Altered platelet function in chronic uremia only partially corrected by hemodialysis. *Nephron* 22:347, 1978.
145. Janson PA, Jubelirer SJ, Weinstein MJ, et al: Treatment of the bleeding tendency in uremia with cryoprecipitate. *N Engl J Med* 303:1318, 1980.
146. Mannucci PM, Remuzzi G, Pusineri F, et al: Deamino-8-D-arginine vasopressin shortens the bleeding time in uremia. *N Engl J Med* 308:8, 1983.
147. Defreyn G, Vergara DM, Machin SJ, et al: Plasma factor in uremia which stimulates prostacyclin release from cultured endothelial cells. *Thromb Res* 19:695, 1980.
148. Gaspari F, Vigano G, Orisio S, et al: Aspirin prolongs bleeding time in uremia by a mechanism distinct from platelet cyclooxygenase inhibition. *J Clin Invest* 79:1788, 1987.
149. Drukker A, Schlesinger M: The immune system in uremia. *Child Nephrol Urol* 10:61, 1990.
150. Kurtz P, Kohler H, Meuer S, et al: Impaired cellular immune response in chronic renal failure: Evidence for a T cell defect. *Kidney Int* 29:1209, 1986.
151. Drachman R, Schlesinger M, Shapira H, et al: The immune status of uremic children/adolescents with chronic renal failure and renal replacement therapy. *Pediatr Nephrol* 3:305, 1989.
152. Byron PR, Mallick NP, Taylor G: Immune potential in human uremia: I. Relation-

ship of glomerular filtration rate to depression of immune potential. *J Clin Pathol* 29:765, 1976.

153. Stevens CE, Alter HJ, Taylor PE, et al: Hepatitis B vaccine in patients receiving hemodialysis. *N Engl J Med* 311:496, 1984.
154. van Gleen JA, Schalm SW, de Visser EM, et al: Immune response to hepatitis vaccine in hemodialysis patients. *Nephron* 45:216, 1987.
155. Perescenschi G, Blum M, Aviram A, et al: Impaired neutrophil response to acute bacterial infection in dialyzed patients. *Arch Intern Med* 141:1301, 1981.
156. Nelson J, Ormrod DJ, Miller TE: Host immune status in uraemia: VI. Leucocytic response to bacterial infection in chronic renal failure. *Nephron* 39:21, 1985.
157. Ruiz P, Gomez F, Schreiber AD: Impaired function of macrophage Fc_γ receptors in end-stage renal disease. *N Engl J Med* 322:717, 1990.
158. Mitch WE, Walser M, Buffington GA, et al: A simple method of estimating progression of chronic renal failure. *Lancet* 2:1326, 1976.
159. Rutherford WE, Blondin J, Miller JP, et al: Chronic progressive renal disease: Rate of change of serum creatinine. *Kidney Int* 11:62, 1977.
160. Reimold EW: Chronic progressive renal failure: Rate of progression monitored by change of serum creatinine concentration. *Am J Dis Child* 135:1039, 1981.

17

CONSERVATIVE MANAGEMENT OF CHRONIC RENAL FAILURE

Kanwal K. Kher

The management of children with chronic renal failure (CRF) should involve a team consisting of a pediatric nephrologist, a nutritionist, a social worker, and a psychologist. As renal failure progresses to end-stage renal disease (ESRD), dialysis and transplantation staff must also be included in the management team. It is helpful to organize periodic meetings with the entire management team in order to assess progress and problems and develop plans for the patient's continued care. The need for therapeutic intervention in the management of CRF is variable and depends on the degree of renal failure, volume of urine produced daily, and evidence of any complications arising from CRF, such as hypertension and renal osteodystrophy (ROD). The management strategy is aimed at minimizing the metabolic side effects of uremia, maintaining a normal fluid and electrolyte balance, preventing long-term complications, and treating complications that may have already developed (Fig. 17–1).

NUTRITION

Because of anorexia, dietary restrictions (to curtail intake of fluid, salt, potassium, and protein), and possibly some alteration of taste, reduced caloric intake is common among patients with moderately severe CRF—that is, those with a glomerular filtration rate (GFR) 25 to 30 percent of normal. The adverse effects of caloric deprivation on growth, particularly in patients with CRF, are well known.[1] Short stature and decreased growth velocity in children with CRF may be due partly to decreased caloric intake (Fig. 17–2). Arnold et al.[2] have observed that a caloric intake of less than 75 percent of the recommended daily allowance (RDA) was universally associated with poor growth in children with CRF. Caloric supplementation in such children, on the other hand, has been shown to enhance the rate of growth.[2,3] It has been suggested that in order to maintain an acceptable rate of growth in children with CRF, caloric intake should be maintained above 75 percent of RDA, preferably in the range of 100

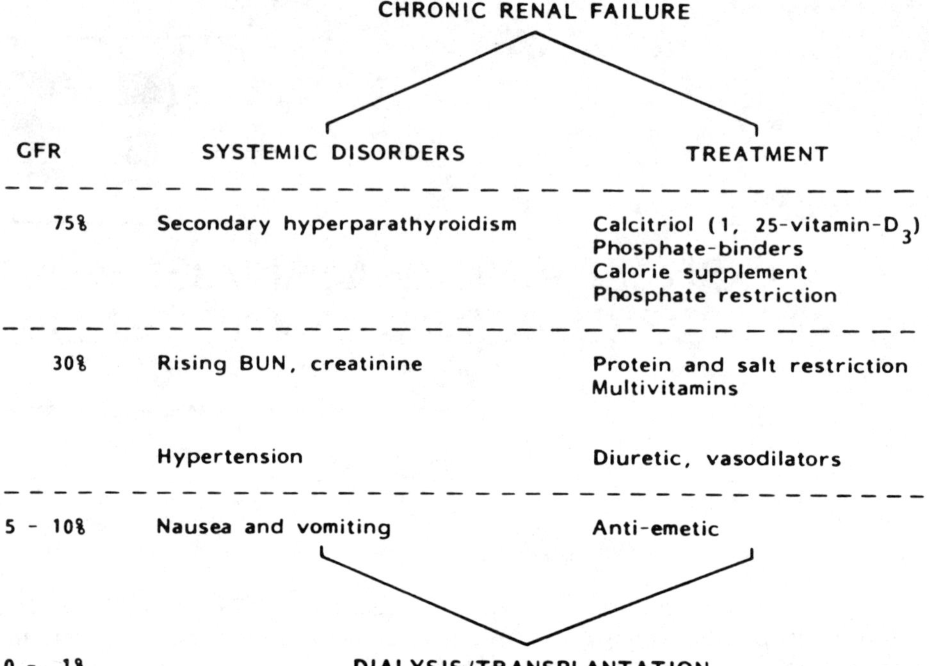

FIG. 17–1. Sequence of initiation of treatment modalities in relationship to progressive decline of glomerular filtration rate (expressed as percent of normal). (Reproduced by permission from *Int J Pediatr Nephrol* 7:161, 1986.)

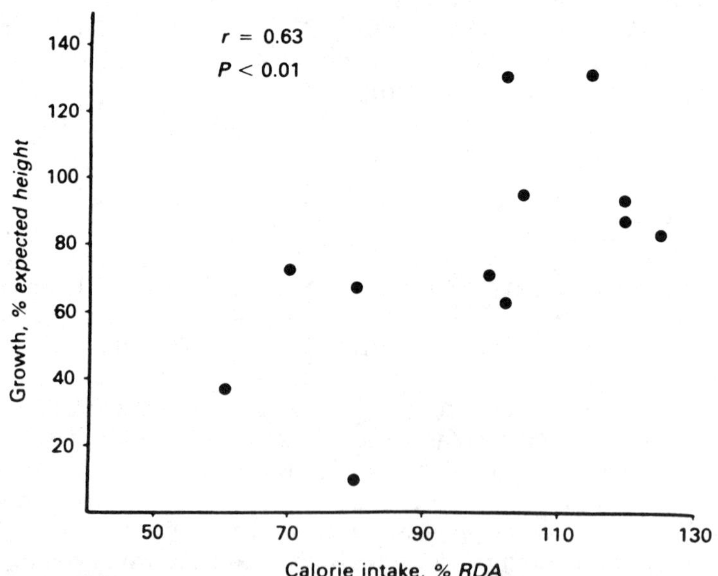

FIG. 17–2. Correlation of caloric intake and growth rate in infants. Growth rates are expressed as percent of normal. Nearly normal growth is achieved if caloric intake of 100 percent is maintained. (Reproduced by permission from Rizzoni G, Basso T, Setari M: Growth in children with chronic renal failure on conservative treatment. *Kidney Int* 26:52, 1984.)

TABLE 17–1. Recommended Daily Dietary Allowances for Calories and Protein in Children and Adolescents

Category	Age years	Weight kg	Weight lb	Height cm	Height in.	Energy Needs with Range kcal	Energy Needs range	Protein, g
Infants	0.0–0.5	6	13	60	24	kg × 115	(95–145)	13
	0.5–1.0	9	20	71	28	kg × 105	(80–135)	14
Children	1–3	13	29	90	35	1300	(900–1800)	16
	4–6	20	44	112	44	1700	(1300–2300)	24
	7–10	28	62	132	52	2400	(1650–3300)	28
Males	11–14	45	99	157	62	2700	(2000–3700)	45
	15–18	66	145	176	69	2800	(2100–3900)	59
Females	11–14	45	101	157	62	2200	(1500–3000)	46
	15–18	55	120	163	64	2100	(1200–3000)	44

Source: Based on the recommendations of the Nutrition Board, National Academy of Sciences—National Research Council, revised 1989. Reproduced by permission from Recommended Dietary Allowances, 10th edition. Published by National Academy Press, Washington, D.C. © 1989 by National Academy of Sciences.

to 110 percent[3]. Table 17–1 lists the RDA for calories and proteins in normal children.

Maintaining appropriate caloric intake for growth in children with CRF requires the coordinated efforts of the patient, the parents, and the nutritionist. Periodic reassessment of food intake by recall or by prospectively registered dietary history reinforces compliance and has been noted to be an effective tool in the nutritional management of these patients.[3] When caloric supplementation is necessary, it may be achieved by increasing the caloric density of the food by adding easily digestible carbohydrates such as Polycose, an unflavored polymer of glucose. Caloric intake may also be enhanced by providing nutritional supplements in addition to diet. Most commercially available nutritional supplements for use in CRF (Table 17–2) are prepared as a flavored drink and are well accepted by children. In infants, whose daytime food intake cannot be further increased, caloric supplementation may be attempted by nocturnal continuous nasogastric feeding. Parents need to be educated and adequately trained as to the proper method of placing a nasogastric tube as well as the care of the mechanical device needed to maintain a continuous infusion. The caloric density and volume of the formula or nutritional supplement to be prescribed is largely determined by the patient's gastrointestinal tolerance and adequacy of urine output. Oliguric patients need a formula or supplement with a higher caloric density, while polyuric patients are somewhat easier to manage, in that the necessary calories may be provided by increasing their net intake of the formula or diet. The supervision of a nutritionist is necessary to promote and ensure an adequate nutritional status.

The role of protein restriction in treating patients with renal failure is well known. However, a renewed interest in the use of protein restriction in CRF has been generated by the observation—in experimental animals—that protein intake in the presence of renal injury, renal failure, or renal ablation promotes further glomerular injury in the surviving nephrons.[3,4] Such glomerular damage is believed to stem from the elevated glomerular blood flow and pressure, and

TABLE 17–2. Commercially Available Nutritional Supplements for Treating Patients with Chronic Renal Failure

	Tolerex	Amin-Aid	Polycose	
			Liquid	Powder
How supplied	Powder pack; flavor packs available	Powder pack	4-fl-oz bottles, unflavored	12.3-oz cans
Reconstituted volume	300 mL	340 mL	—	—
Protein (as free aminoacids)	6.18 g/300 mL	0.8 g	0	0
Calories	1 cal/mL	2 cal/mL	2 cal/mL	8 cal/level teaspoon (2 g)
Fats	0.435 g/300 mL	15.7 g/340 mL	0	0
Sodium	20.4 meq/L	5 meq/340 mL	3 meq/100 mL	4.8 meq/100 g
Potassium	30.0 meq/L		0.15 meq	0.3 meq/100 g
Osmolality	550 mOsm/kg	700 mOsm/kg	900 mOsm/kg	

hyperfiltration resulting from the kidney's efforts to maintain an adequate glomerular filtration rate and excrete the metabolic waste products. The end result of hyperfiltration is glomerular hyalinization and sclerosis (Fig. 17–3). Protein restriction in humans has been reported to be helpful in retarding the progression of the renal disease and CRF.[5,6] Restriction of protein to 0.5 g/kg/day in adults with CRF has been shown to slow decline of renal function in these patients.[6] The extent to which protein should be restricted in children with CRF is not well established. In a recent study conducted in children with CRF, a low protein diet (0.8 to 1.1 g/kg/day) was, however, found to have no significant influence on growth, weight gain, or progression of CRF.[7] Since growth and development are of significant concern in children, severe protein restriction is not recommended until the risks and benefits of such a therapy are better defined. In the absence of well-established guidelines, the author prescribes the lower limit of the RDA of protein for age and weight in these children. The source of dietary protein should be from foods of high biologic value, such as dairy products and meats. Because of its low phosphorus content, Similac PM 60/40 is the preferred feeding formula for infants with CRF. Since this formula is also low in sodium content, many patients with renal sodium wasting will require sodium supplements.

Schloerb,[8] in a clinical study, demonstrated that, in patients with CRF, it was possible to achieve an anabolic state and reduce BUN by providing a low-protein diet supplemented with L-essential amino acids. An improved nitrogen balance in patients with CRF has also been shown to result from the supplementation of a low-protein diet with essential amino acids (EAA) and their alpha and alpha hydroxyketoanalogues (KA).[9–12] However, the beneficial effect of EAA and KA on the rate of progression of renal failure, though reported in some studies,[9,12] has not been reproduced consistently in children with CRF.[10,11] Some authors have demonstrated an improvement in growth velocity and

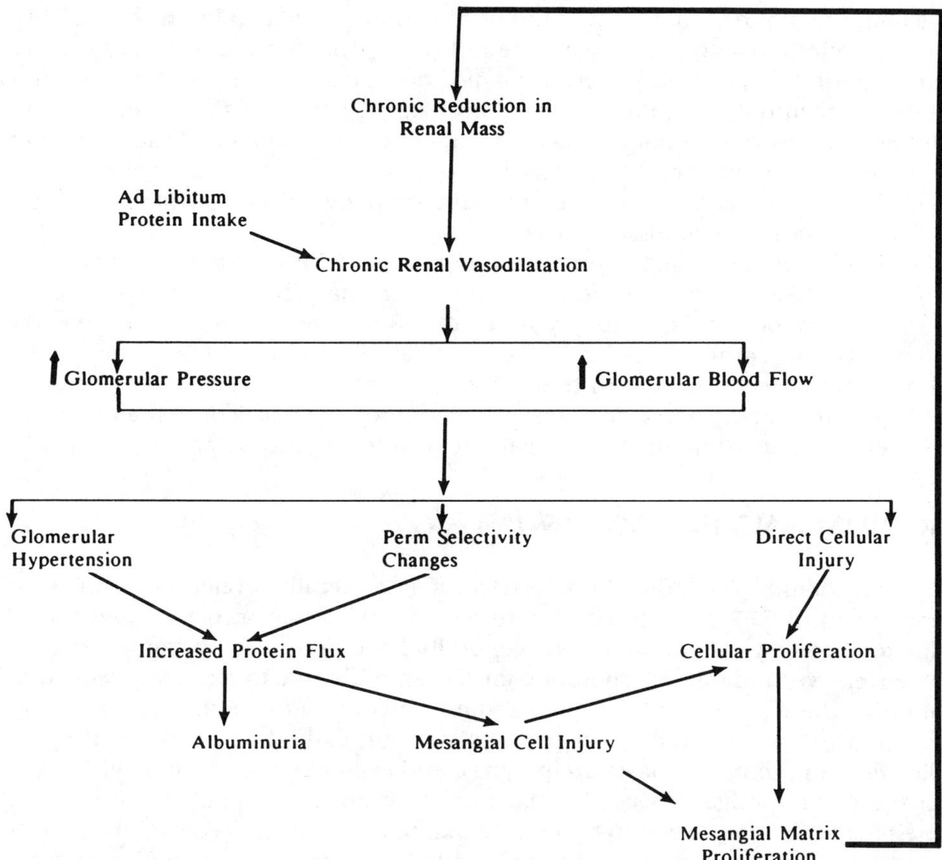

FIG. 17–3. Proposed mechanism of progressive glomerulosclerosis in patients with renal disease on ad libitum protein intake. (Modified and reproduced with permission from *N Engl J Med* 307:652, 1982.)

nutritional status in children with CRF whose diet was supplemented with EAA and KA,[10] but others were unable to find such a favorable effect on growth in infants.[11] Although BUN and BUN/creatinine ratio generally improve in patients supplemented with EAA/KA,[9,10] suggesting an anabolic effect in uremia, the abnormalities in the plasma amino acid distribution seen in CRF persist.[10] In essence, despite a possible anabolic action, the role of EAA/KA supplementation in the nutritional management children with CRF is not entirely clear.

FLUID INTAKE

It is erroneous to presume that all patients with CRF are oliguric. In fact, most children with mild to moderate CRF (GFR 30 to 40 mL/min/1.73 m^2)—especially those with interstitial diseases such as pyelonephritis, renal dysplasia, and cystic renal diseases—are polyuric and need supplemental fluids to maintain adequate hydration. Obviously, fluid intake in most such children must be liberal; in circumstances of excess fluid loss or inability to ingest adequate amounts of fluid (as in gastrointestinal disorders), careful attention to hydration status is required. Hospitalization to provide intravenous fluid therapy may even be necessary in some instances. An approximate estimate of the daily fluid requirements of patients with polyuria would be a sum of insensible water requirement, replacement of the approximate daily urinary volume, and volume of abnormal fluid loss, if any.

Patients with CRF due to chronic glomerulonephritis or those who have progressed to ESRD often manifest oliguria or anuria. The fluid intake of such patients must be handled with great caution, since they are at a significant risk of developing complications of fluid overload. Their total daily fluid intake should not exceed the sum of their insensible water requirement and the volume of urine excreted in a day. Because of severe fluid restriction, the provision of adequate nourishment to these patients is often a considerable problem.

SODIUM AND POTASSIUM INTAKE

Dietary sodium and potassium restriction is generally unnecessary in most patients until GFR reaches 10 percent of normal. However, patients with CRF due to chronic glomerulonephritis generally have poor urine output, are often hypertensive, and tolerate sodium poorly even with mild to moderate reduction of GFR. These patients will require sodium restriction to about 1 to 2 meq/kg/day. On the other hand, most patients with interstitial diseases, renal cystic disorder, and renal dysplasia are polyuric and excrete large amounts of sodium in the urine (obligatory salt losers). In the absence of supplemental sodium, these patients often develop hyponatremia. Such patients need sodium supplementation, which can be provided by adding extra salt to foods or offering sodium in the form of a medicinal supplement such as hypertonic 3 percent saline (which provides 0.5 meq sodium/mL). The requirement for additional sodium in such patients varies from 1 to 3 meq/kg/day.*

Hyperkalemia is an uncommon problem in patients with mild to moderate CRF; on the other hand, it is a serious threat in patients with severely compromised renal function. Patients with interstitial renal disease or hyporeninemic hypoaldosteronism and those taking beta blockers (propranolol or atenolol) or angiotensin converting enzyme inhibitors (captopril or enalapril) are at higher risk of developing hyperkalemia. In general, children with CRF tolerate excess potassium poorly and should avoid foods with high potassium content, such as citrus fruits, bananas, chocolate, tomatoes, and potatoes. Vegetables should be soaked in water to reduce their potassium content. If hyperkalemia persists despite dietary restriction of potassium, sodium polystyrenesulfonate (Kayexalate) should be prescribed. Kayexalate is a cation exchange resin that removes potassium in exchange for sodium in the gastrointestinal tract (mainly the colon) and is administered orally as a powder or suspension in a flavored syrup

*The following equation may be used to convert salt (NaCl) content in the diet to sodium (Na) content: NaCl (in milligrams) × 0.40 = milligrams of Na. To convert sodium in milligrams to milliequivalents: Na in milligrams ÷ 23 = Na in milliequivalents. To convert sodium in milliequivalents to milligrams: Na in milliequivalents × 23 = Na in milligrams.

(5 percent sorbitol). Fresh suspension should be made every 24 h in order to maintain the efficacy of the drug. Depending on the degree of hyperkalemia and the response obtained, the dose of Kayexalate may vary from 0.5 to 1.0 g/kg of body weight divided into three or four doses, given orally. One gram of Kayexalate contains 4.1 meq (100 mg) of sodium; about 25 to 30 percent of it is available for exchange in vitro. Therefore, for practical purposes, 1 g of Kayexalate can be expected to remove 1 meq of potassium and provide an equal load (1 meq) of sodium to the body. Kayexalate should be used with caution in patients who cannot tolerate additional sodium. Constipation is a usual side effect of this drug, but it can be managed by the concomitant use of stool softeners and by suspending Kayexalate in sorbitol.

PREVENTION OF RENAL OSTEODYSTROPHY

Maintaining a positive calcium balance, normal serum phosphorus level, and PTH concentration are essential in preventing renal osteodystrophy. As the GFR falls below 75 percent of normal, elevation of serum phosphorus, alkaline phosphatase activity, and parathyroid hormone (PTH) is first noted. Restriction of dietary phosphate intake (as in milk, milk products, and meats) may be enough to normalize the divalent ion metabolism at this stage. As GFR falls further, additional measures to control serum phosphorus in the form of phosphate binders are necessary. The phosphate binders reduce serum phosphorus by complexing with the dietary phosphorus and reducing its availability for absorption in the gastrointestinal tract. Therefore these agents are most effective when taken with meals or soon thereafter. Aluminum hydroxide is an effective phosphate binder, but because of the risk of aluminum toxicity, is rarely used today. Calcium carbonate is being used increasingly as the phosphate binder of choice in children with CRF. For best results, calcium carbonate should be taken with the meals. When given between meals, it acts largely as a calcium supplement. The dose of calcium carbonate should be titrated to each patient's requirements and usually varies from 100 to 300 mg/kg/day. Hypercalcemia may be a side effect in some patients. The several types of calcium preparations available for use in children are listed in Table 17–3.

Since bioavailable vitamin D is essential for the prevention of renal osteodystrophy, supplementation with metabolically active vitamin D preparations becomes necessary when the GFR reaches 50 percent. The two preparations of vitamin D used widely in CRF are 1,25-(OH)-D_3 and dihydrotachysterol. The dosages of various bioactive vitamin D preparations for use in CRF are given in Table 17–4. In addition to improving calcium absorption from the gastrointestinal tract and maintaining serum calcium concentration, supplementation with 1,25-$(OH)_2$-D_3 and other analogues of vitamin D also improves bone mineralization and decreases circulating PTH. The major side effect of such therapy is hypercalcemia; therefore serum calcium level should be monitored periodically. Hyperphosphatemia should be controlled prior to prescribing vitamin D analogues, since dangerously high calcium $\times$ phosphate product ($>$70) can cause widespread soft tissue calcifications. Decline of serum alkaline phosphatase and serum PTH concentration is a good indicator of improving bone turnover and healing of the renal osteodystrophy.

TABLE 17–3. Various Commercially Available Preparations of Calcium Containing Phosphate Binders

	Available Size	Elemental Calcium
CALCIUM CARBONATE		
Chewable Tablets		
Oscal, 500 mg (Marion)	1250 mg/tablet	500 mg
Suplical (Parke-Davis)	1500 mg/tablet	600 mg
Biocal Chewable, 250 mg (Miles)	625 mg/tablet	250 mg
Tablets		
Tums (Norcliff Thayer)	500 mg/tablet	200 mg
Tums Extra Strength (Norcliff Thayer)	750 mg/tablet	300 mg
Biocal, 500 mg (Miles)	1250 mg/tablet	500 mg
Cal Sup, 300 mg (3M Company)	750 mg/tablet	300 mg
Oscal, 500 mg (Marion)	1250 mg/tablet	500 mg
Liquid		
Calcium Carbonate Suspension (Roxane Laboratories)	1250 mg/5 mL	500 mg
Powder		
Cal Carb–HD (Lafayette Pharmacals)	6.5 g/packet	370 mg/g
CALCIUM ACETATE		
PhosLo (Braintree Laboratories)	667 mg	169 mg
Phos-Ex-167 (Vitaline Corp.)	668 mg	167 mg
Phos-Ex-250	1000 mg	250 mg

TABLE 17–4. Preparations of Vitamin D Available for Use in Chronic Renal Failure

Vitamin D Compound	Trade Name	Available Size	Dose
$1,25(OH)_2D_3$	Rocaltrol (Roche)	0.25 μg/capsule	0.25 μg/day (15–40 ng/kg/day)
Dihydrotachysterol	DHT (Roxane)	0.125 mg tablet	0.125 mg (15–45 μg/kg/day)
	Intensol (Roxane)	0.2 mg/ml	—
1α-hydroxyvitamin D_3[a]	One Alpha (Leo Pharmaceuticals, U.K.)	0.25 μg/mL	0.5 to 3 μg/day

[a] 1α-Hydroxyvitamin D_3 is not yet commercially available in the United States.

TABLE 17–5. Alkali Therapy for Correction of Acidosis

Brand Name	Amount of Sodium, meq	Amount of Potassium, meq	Amount of Alkali, meq	Comment
LIQUID				
Polycitra (sodium citrate, potassium citrate)	1 meq/mL	1 meq/mL	2 meq/mL	Do not use in patients with hyperkalemia or chronic renal failure
Bicitra (sodium citrate, citric acid)	1 meq/mL	0	1 meq/mL	Ideal for infants
TABLETS				
Sodium bicarbonate				
325 mg	4 meq/tab	0	4 meq/tab	Useful in older children
650 mg	8 meq/tab	0	8 meq/tab	
POWDER				
Baking soda	20 meq per ½ tsf		20 meq per ½ tsf	

CORRECTION OF ACIDOSIS

Chronic acidosis is one of the significant causes of bone disease and stunted growth in children with CRF. The precise development of these disorders from acidosis is unclear. Some recent evidence indicates that acidosis may also be involved in increased protein degradation and may therefore contribute to an increased formation of "uremic toxins" derived from protein catabolism.[13] Aggressive correction of acidosis should be attempted in every patient with CRF at the earliest opportunity. Sodium bicarbonate can be used safely in most patients with CRF; the dosage may vary from 1 to 5 meq/kg/day. For an adequate growth pattern, serum bicarbonate concentration should be maintained at 23 to 25 meq/L. Table 17–5 lists the composition of some of the alkali supplements used for correction of acidosis.

TREATMENT OF ANEMIA

Most patients with CRF develop anemia that is resistant to iron and vitamin therapy. The primary cause of anemia in CRF is a deficiency in erythropoietin. Iron deficiency may, however, develop in patients who have low iron reserves or undergo blood loss, such as follows surgery or frequent laboratory studies. Recombinant human erythropoietin (r-HuEPO) has been used extensively for the treatment of anemia in patients with ESRD who are undergoing dialysis therapy.[14,15] It has also recently been approved for use in patients with chronic renal failure who are not undergoing dialysis therapy. Clinical studies in adults have confirmed the efficacy of r-HuEPO in treating the anemia of CRF.[16,17] The rise of hematocrit following r-HuEPO therapy in these patients is dose-dependent, as also demonstrated previously in patients undergoing dialysis. The dose of r-HuEPO used varies from 50 to 150 units/kg and is given three times a week. Target hematocrit of 30 percent can usually be reached in 4 to 6 weeks in most children provided that iron deficiency does not coexist. It may be possible to decrease the frequency of r-HuEPO injection to after a week once the patient has reached a stable target hematocrit. The commonest causes of failure to respond to r-HuEPO therapy are either a low dose of the drug or iron deficiency. Aluminum toxicity can also result in the failure of therapy in patients undergoing dialysis. Iron status must be evaluated in all patients prior to and during such therapy. Supplemental iron should be prescribed in those with low body stores. Hematocrit and reticulocyte count should be obtained on a weekly basis, at least initially, in order to monitor response. An increased sense of well-being and improved exercise tolerance have been reported in CRF patients receiving r-HuEPO therapy. Its major side effects are hypertension and seizures. Erythropoeitin therapy has not so far been shown to be of benefit in patients with CRF and sickle cell anemia. These patients will unfortunately remain transfusion-dependent for treatment of anemia, and may need to be hypertransfused in order to prevent the complications of sickle cell disease.

TREATMENT OF HYPERTENSION

Progression of renal disease by events unrelated to the primary parenchymal disease is well known. Of these, uncontrolled hypertension has been well documented to be one of the major factors causing further renal damage and reduction in GFR.[18] Additionally, long-term hypertension leads to a higher risk of cardiovascular morbidity and mortality. Since hypertension in many patients with CRF is renin-mediated, the angiotensin converting enzyme inhibitor (ACE inhibitor) captopril (Capoten) is particularly effective in these patients. Hyperkalemia is a potentially serious sideeffect of ACE inhibitor therapy, especially in patients with compromized renal function. Fluid overload may also be a signficant factor in the pathogenesis of hypertension in some patients with CRF or those who have progressed to ESRD. Sodium restriction and appropriate limitation of fluids is necessary in such patients. Potent diuretics (furosemide) are sometimes helpful in these patients, while mild diuretics (thiazides) are usually ineffective. Most other antihypertensive agents can be used in usual dosage to control blood pressure.

PROVIDING PSYCHOSOCIAL SUPPORT

Being a potentially life-threatening chronic illness, CRF results in significant psychosocial stress for the patient as well as the parents. Disruption of family life, often resulting in marital problems among parents, is common in the families where children are undergoing dialysis and transplantation.[19] The need for frequent hospitalization and hence separation from school, friends, and siblings is also stressful for the children themselves. Children with mild to moderate CRF, as well as those undergoing dialysis therapy for ESRD, exhibit definite difficulties in school adjustment; experience feelings of loneliness and anxiety;

and tend to show depressive symptoms.[20] Prolonged hospitalization may necessitate in-hospital schooling. Those undergoing dialysis should be encouraged to attend school. If dialysis is being undertaken in the hospital, it may be scheduled after school hours so as to minimize loss of school time. Parents of children with CRF should be given access to the social service–psychiatry team, which can suggest helpful interventions for decreasing the family's stress level. In some situations, offering the parents some "time off" from the daily monotony of life can be helpful. This may be particularly important for parents who are undertaking home dialysis for their children.

PREPARING FOR DIALYSIS AND TRANSPLANTATION

The preparation of CRF patients for dialysis and transplantation is an important aspect of their management and care. As CRF progresses toward ESRD, the parents and the patients themselves (older children and adolescents) should be advised about the options available for further treatment. This can best be achieved in a conference where both the dialysis staff and the renal transplant surgical services are represented. This gives the parents an opportunity to be introduced to all the members of the team that may be involved in taking care of their child. A tour of the dialysis facility, especially while a child is actually being dialyzed, is usually helpful for the parents. A follow-up meeting is generally necessary to answer the parents' questions. Since renal transplantation is the preferred method of treating chldren with ESRD, workup of potential living related donors should also be suggested. Preemptive renal transplantation (without preceding dialysis therapy) is becoming an important practical alternative in pediatric patients and should be explored in families where a living donor from the family (usually a parent) is available. In some cases, living nonrelated donors (such as stepparent or a step-grandparent) may be also considered if related donors are either not available or are medically unsuitable for donation or for the surgery involved.

OTHER MANAGEMENT ISSUES

ALUMINUM TOXICITY

Aluminum is increasingly becoming an element of considerable significance in the long-term management of patients with CRF. It has been implicated in the pathogenesis of progressive encephalopathy, osteomalacic bone disease, and anemia.[21,22] Most of the orally administered aluminum is excreted in feces; only 1 to 2 percent is absorbed; and most of the absorbed aluminum is excreted through the kidney.[23] Patients with CRF who ingest large amounts of aluminum as aluminum hydroxide are particularly at risk of accumulating aluminum in various tissue sites. Drinking water and water used during dialysis may be another important source of aluminum load, even in patients who are not receiving aluminum-containing phosphate binders, since aluminum sulfate (alum) is used in the process of water purification in many municipal water treatment plants. Freundlich et al.[22] have reported that infant formulas can be a potential source of aluminum intoxication in infants with CRF. Commercially available albumin has also been incriminated as a possible source of aluminum load for patients with CRF, particularly those who have undergone plasmapheresis (for the treatment of various types of chronic glomerulonephritis) where the plasma fractions removed during the procedure have been replaced with albumin-containing solutions.[24]

Suspicion is the key to the diagnosis of aluminum intoxication. A triad consisting of microcytic anemia, disabling bone disease (osteomalacia), and progressive neurologic symptoms in a patient with CRF should point to the possibility of aluminum intoxication. A plasma aluminum concentration higher than 100 μg/L indicates that a patient is at high risk of aluminum intoxication.[21] Bone histomorphology and staining for aluminum may also aid in the diagnosis of aluminum-associated bone disease.

Prevention is essential to decreasing the incidence of aluminum toxicity in patients with CRF. Aluminum hydroxide should not be used as a phosphate binder in children with CRF. Calcium carbonate or calcium acetate is presently recommended as the phosphate binder of choice. Desferoxamine has been sucessfully used to treat aluminum intoxication in several patients, but clear guidelines for patient selection are lacking at this time.[25,26]

GROWTH

Impaired growth is a well-known feature of CRF and appears to be of multifactorial etiology. Although the improvement of nutritional status improves growth velocity, the stature of these children remains subnormal even following transplantation.[27] Mehls et al.[28] have described an improvement of growth and food utilization by rats with CRF when they were given human recombinant growth hormone. Lippe et al.,[29] in preliminary study in children with CRF, reported accelerated growth following treatment with recombinant human growth hormone. In another recent study, Fine et al.[30] have further confirmed the beneficial effect of recombinant human growth hormone on the linear growth of children with CRF. Bone age was not reported to be adversely affected by such therapy in this study. However, it needs to be further determined whether such a therapy can improve the long-term outlook and adult height of children with CRF.

REPRODUCTIVE FUNCTIONS

Pregnancy rarely occurs in uremic women, but patients with moderate and severe CRF have been reported to conceive.[31] Although the infants may be born prematurely, they are usually of appropriate size for gestation.

In peripubertal uremic boys, serum testosterone and follicle stimulating hormone levels are usually normal, but luteinizing hormone (LH) levels are elevated.[32] The elevated levels of LH in uremia correlate with the degree of renal failure. In view of normal testosterone level, elevated LH concentration may suggest testicular insensitivity to LH. Similar abnormalities have been reported in adult males.[33] Spermatogenesis in adult uremic males is subnormal.[34]

UREMIC BLEEDING

Prolonged bleeding time is a characteristic feature of CRF. Although gastrointestinal and mucosal bleeding is less common in the present-day care of patients with CRF, it may still be of concern in an occasional patient. Cryoprecipitate infusions have been successfully used in uremic patients with bleeding[35]; bleeding time remains normal for 24 to 36 h following such therapy. Recently, desmopressin (DDAVP), which induces the release of endogenous von Willebrand factor in the body, has also been used effectively in the treatment of uremic patients with bleeding. The dose of such therapy is 0.3 μg/kg intravenously as an infusion and 3.0 μg/kg for intranasal administration.[36]

FINANCIAL PLANNING FOR ESRD

Although medicare underwrites a significant cost involved in dialysis and renal transplantation of children in the United States, it does not cover all expenses involved. Information regarding medicare coverage for patients with ESRD can be obtained from the U.S. Department of Health and Human Services.* In brief, patients who elect self-care dialysis (home dialysis such as CAPD, CCPD, etc.) will be covered by Medicare from the time dialysis therapy begins. On the other hand, for patients electing institutional dialysis (e.g., outpatient hemodialysis), Medicare coverage begins 3 months after the initiation of dialysis. Patients undergoing home dialysis must be trained by an approved dialysis facility and offered continuous support and supervision. Medicare covers the cost of supplies and equipment involved in home dialysis. Current Medicare rules do not allow for the purchase of dialysis equipment by the patient; necessary equipment can, however, be provided by the facility supervising such care (method I) or be leased from an independent supplier who is willing to accept Medicare-assigned reimbursement rates. Medicare coverage for renal transplantation begins in the month such surgery is performed. Investigations for preemptive or planned transplantation will usually be covered if the transplant is undertaken within a total of 3 months after the beginning of such investigations. Medicare covers all costs involved in the hospitalization of a kidney donor, and there is no deductible charge involved. Purchase of organs is prohibited and is not covered by Medicare, but the cost involved in acquiring a kidney from a cadaveric donor is fully covered.

SUMMARY

Children with CRF are best managed by a team of medical and paramedical experts. Maintaining adequate growth by providing the required caloric intake, correcting acidosis, and preventing disabling renal osteodystrophy are the essential aims of management prior to dialysis. As the time for dialysis and

**Medicare Coverage of Kidney Dialysis and Kidney Transplant Services: A Supplement to Your Medicare Handbook.* HCFA Publication No 10128. U.S. Department of Health and Human Services, Health Care Financing Administration, 6325 Security Blvd., Baltimore, Maryland 21207.

renal transplantation approaches, these children and their families require significant social and psychologic support to help them endure the problems associated with such therapeutic interventions. Use of newer treatment modalities, such as therapy with recombinant human erythropoietin and human growth hormone, are bound the change the outlook for growth and development in many children with CRF in the near future.

Management of Renal Osteodystrophy: A Commentary

Russel W. Chesney

Renal bone disease therapy focuses on dietary restriction of phosphate and replacement of active vitamin D metabolites. Dietary phosphate restriction is difficult because phosphate is ubiquitous in our diet and because children prefer high phosphate-containing foods such as milk, cheese, soft drinks, and snack foods. The infant with moderate-to-severe renal insufficiency should be placed on a low phosphate formula such as PM-60/40 or human milk. Many young children with chronic renal failure due to obstructive uropathy have relative urinary salt wasting and hence crave salt. Cheese, corn-containing snack foods, and soups high in sodium also have a high phosphate content. Thus, the child with obstructive uropathy as a cause for renal failure frequently has an extremely high dietary phosphate intake.

The use of aluminum hydroxide as a phosphate-binding agent should be avoided. Recent evidence from Salusky's research team suggests that even low doses (30 mg/kg/24 h) of aluminum hydroxide result in bone aluminum deposition. Calcium carbonate (1 to 2 tablets with meals) is an effective phosphate-binding agent and is the preferred agent. Calcium acetate (1 to 2 tablets with meals) is also an effective binding agent. The appropriate dose of calcium carbonate or acetate should be derived by titration of the individual patient. In addition, monthly serum calcium and phosphate measurements should be obtained.

The most appropriate vitamin D metabolites to use are either $1,25(OH)_2D_3$ at 10 to 15 ng/kg/24 h or dihydrotachysterol (DHT) at a dose of 100 to 200 μg daily. Studies to date do not indicate a superiority of $1,25(OH)_2D_3$ over DHT, although the shorter half-life of $1,25(OH)_2D_3$ may indicate that this agent is safer than DHT. Because a 0.25-μg capsule of $1,25(OH)_2D_3$ equals a dose in excess of the recommended amount when administered to small children, the intravenous calcitriol product (Calcijex, Abbott Laboratories, North Chicago, Illinois) can be taken orally. Serum calcium and phosphate values should be measured in patients who are treated with active vitamin D metabolites at least monthly and possibly as often as every 2 weeks during the first 3 months of therapy.

The most appropriate means of treating children for renal bone disease is actually to prevent the development of osteodystrophy. As the creatinine clearance falls under 30 mL/min/1.73 m^2, it is advisable to start phosphate restriction, calcium supplements, and vitamin D metabolites. Perhaps the most appropriate means of following these patients is to measure N-terminal or intact PTH values over time with the aim of maintaining these values in the normal range. If this can be accomplished, severe renal osteodystrophy should not develop.

REFERENCES

1. Betts GS, Magrath G: Growth pattern and dietary intake of children with chronic renal insufficiency. *Br Med J* 2:189, 1974.
2. Arnold WC, Danford D, Holliday MA: Effects of caloric supplementation on growth in children with uremia. *Kidney Int* 29:205, 1983.
3. Rizzoni G, Basso T, and Setari M: Growth in children with chronic renal failure on conservative treatment. *Kidney Int* 26:52, 1984.
4. Brenner BM, Meyer TW, Hostetter TH; Dietary protein intake and progressive nature of kidney disease: The role of hemodynamically mediated glomerular injury in the pathogenesis of progressive glomerulosclerosis in aging, renal ablation and intrinsic renal disease. *N Engl J Med* 307:652, 1982.
5. Alverstrand A, Ahlberg M, Bergstrom J: Retardation of progression of renal insufficiency in patients with low-protein diets. *Kidney Int* 24(suppl 16):S:268, 1983.
6. Barsotti G, Morelli A, Giannoni A, et al: Restricted phosphorus and nitrogen intake to slow the progression of chronic renal failure: A controlled study. *Kidney Int* 24(suppl 16):S-278, 1983.
7. European Study Group for Nutritional Treatment of Chronic Renal Failure in Childhood: Low-protein diet in children with chronic renal failure—1-year results. *Pediatr Nephrol* 5:496, 1991.
8. Schloerb PR: Essential L-amino acids administration in uremia. *Am J Med Sci* 252:650, 1966.
9. Jureidini KF, Hogg RJ, Van Renen MJ, et al: Evaluation of long-term aggressive dietary management of chronic renal failure in children. *Pediatr Nephrol* 4:1, 1990.
10. Jones R, Dalton N, Turner C, et al: Oral essential amino acid and ketoacid supplements in children with chronic renal failure. *Kidney Int* 24:95, 1983.
11. Broyer M, Guillot M, Naidet P, et al: Comparison of three low-nitrogen diets containing essential amino acids and their alpha analogues for severely uremic children. *Kidney Int* 24(suppl 16):S-290, 1983.
12. Walser M: 1988 Herman Award lecture: Effect of ketoanalogues in chronic renal failure and other disorders. *Am J Clin Nutr* 49:17, 1989.
13. Jenkins D, Burton PR, Bennet SE, et al: Metabolic consequences of correction of acidosis in uremia. *Nephrol Dial Transplant* 4:92, 1989.
14. Eschbach JW, Egrie J, Downing MR, et al: Correction of the anemia of end-stage renal disease with recombinant human erythropoietin: Results of combined phase I and clinical trial. *N Engl J Med* 316:73, 1987.
15. Sinai-Triman L, Salusky IB, Fine RN: Use of subcutaneous recombinant human erythropoietin in children undergoing chronic continuous cycling peritoneal dialysis. *J Pediatr* 114:550, 1989.

16. Lim VS, DeGowin RL, Zavala D, et al: Recombinant human erythropoietin treatment in pre-dialysis patients: A double-blind placebo-controlled trial. *Ann Intern Med* 110:108, 1989.
17. Stone WJ, Graber SE, Krantz SB, et al: Treatment of anemia of predialysis patients with recombinant human erythropoeitin: A randomized, placebo-controlled trial. *Am J Med Sci* 296:171, 1988.
18. Rostand SG, Brown G, Kirk KA, et al: Renal insufficiency in treated essential hypertension. *N Engl J Med* 320:684, 1989.
19. Reynolds JM, Garralda ME, Jameson RA, et al: How parents and families cope with chronic renal failure. *Arch Dis Child* 63:82, 1988.
20. Garralda ME, Jameson RA, Reynolds JM, et al: Psychiatric adjustments in children with chronic renal failure. *J Child Psychol Psychiatry* 29:79, 1988.
21. Andreoli SP, Bergstein JM, Sherrord DJ: Aluminum intoxication from aluminum containing phosphate binders in children with azotemia not undergoing hemodialysis. *N Engl J Med* 310:1079, 1984.
22. Freundlich M, Zilleruelo G, Abitbol C, et al: Infant formula as a cause of aluminum toxicity in neonatal uremia. *Lancet* 2:527, 1985.
23. Alfrey AC: Aluminum. *Adv Clin Chem* 23:69, 1983.
24. Milliner DS, Shinaberger JH, Shuman P, et al: Inadvertent aluminum administration during plasma exchange due to albumin containing replacement solutions. *N Engl J Med* 312:165, 1985.
25. Hood SA, Clark WF, Hodsoman AB, et al: Successful treatment of dialysis osteomalacia and demention, using desferoxamine infusions and oral 1-alpha-hydroxycholecalciferol. *Am J Nephrol* :369, 1984.
26. Freundlich M, Zilleruelo, Faugere M, et al: Treatment of aluminum toxicity in infantile uremia with desferoxamine. *J Pediatr* 109:140, 1986.
27. Ress L, Greene SA, Adlord P, et al: Growth and endocrine function after renal transplantation. *Arch Dis Child* 63:1326, 1988.
28. Mehls O, Ritz E, Hunziker E, et al: Improvement of growth and food utilization by human recombinant growth hormone in uremia. *Kidney Int* 33:45, 1988.
29. Lippe B, Fine RN, Kock VH, et al: Accelerated growth following treatment of children with chronic renal failure with recombinant human growth hormone (somafrem): A preliminary report. *Acta Paediatr Scand (suppl)* 343:127, 1988.
30. Fine RN, Pyke-Grimm K, Nelson PA, et al.: Recombinant human growth hormone treatment of children with chronic renal failure: Long-term (1–3-year) outcome. *Pediatr Nephrol* 5:477, 1991.
31. Brem AS, Singer D, Anderson L, et al: Infants of azotemic mothers: A report of three live births. *Am J Kid Dis* 12:299, 1988.
32. Marder HK, Srivastava LS, Burnstein S: Hypergonadotropism in peripubertal boys with chronic renal failure. *Pediatrics* 72:386, 1983.
33. Van Kammen E, Thijssen JHH, Schwarz F: Sex hormones in male patients with chronic renal failure: I. The production of testosterone and of androstenedione. *Clin Endocrinol* 8:7, 1978.
34. deKrester DM, Atkins RD, Hudson B, et al: Disordered spermatogenesis in patients with chronic renal failure undergoing maintenance hemodialysis. *Aust NZ J Med* 4:178, 1978.
35. Janson PA, Jubelires SJ, Weinstein MJ, et al: Treatment of bleeding tendency in uremia with cryoprecipitate. *N Eng J Med* 303:1318, 1980.
36. Mannucci PM, Remuzzi G, Pusinen F, et al: Deamino-8-D-arginine vasopressin shortens the bleeding time in uremia. *N Engl J Med* 308:8, 1983.

18

MANAGEMENT OF END-STAGE RENAL FAILURE—DIALYSIS THERAPY

Heinz E. Leichter
Kanwal K. Kher

The care of children with end-stage renal disease (ESRD), especially neonates and young infants, has always been more challenging than that of adult patients. Technical advances made in the last decade, such as the development of low-compliance and low-priming-volume dialyzers, automated peritoneal dialysis machines capable of delivering small dialysate volumes, and continuous ambulatory peritoneal dialysis (CAPD) for infants have facilitated the care of infants and children with ESRD. Additionally, the availability of a wider array of immunosuppressive agents has also contributed to an improved survival among children with ESRD undergoing renal transplantation.

INCIDENCE OF ESRD IN CHILDREN

End-stage renal disease is considerably less common in children than in adults and is an uncommon cause of morbidity and mortality during childhood. Potter et al.[1] estimated that the yearly incidence of ESRD among children in San Francisco was 1.6 new patients per million population. An average of 819 new pediatric ESRD patients obtained entitlement for Medicare coverage in the United States in each year from 1978 to 1987.[2] The European Dialysis and Transplantation Association (EDTA) has reported that 3.9 new patients per million children in the population were accepted for renal replacement therapy (including dialysis and transplant treatments) in Europe in 1987.[3] According to data from the U.S. Renal Data Systems report (1990), approximately 2.5 percent of the total ESRD population in the United States is composed of children (newborn to age 19 years).[4]

THE ETIOLOGY OF ESRD IN CHILDREN

Inherited and congenital diseases of the urinary tract account for almost half the cases of ESRD during childhood. Chronic glomerulonephritides and vascu-

TABLE 18–1. Etiology of ESRD in Children

Etiology	Avner et al.[5]	Potter et al.[1]
Chronic Glomerulonephritis	(35.8%)	(38.4%)
Primary	41	55
Secondary	2	4
Congenital/Hereditary		
Renal Diseases	(46.7%)	(37.0%)
Renal hypoplasia/dysplasia	25	16
Obstructive uropathy	18	20
Polycystic renal disease	1	2
Cystinosis	3	3
Congenital nephrosis	0	3
Prune belly syndrome	2	0
Nephronophthisis	4	0
Medullary cystic disease	0	9
Alport syndrome	3	4
Pyelonephritis/Interstitial Nephritis	8 (6.7%)	12 (7.8%)
Vascular Renal Disease	(5.0%)	(5.8%)
Hemolytic uremic syndrome	1	9
Renal vein thrombosis	2	0
Polyarteritis nodosa	1	0
Hypertensive glomerulosclerosis	2	0
Renal Tumors	(1.6%)	(5.8%)
Wilms tumor	2	9
Hereditary Syndromes and Miscellaneous Causes	5(4.2%)	8(5.2%)
Total number of patients	120	154

lar renal diseases make up the remaining half.[1,4–6] A majority of congenital and inherited diseases leading to ESRD fall under the categories of renal dysplasia, hypoplasia, obstructive uropathies, cystic renal diseases, cystinosis, and Alport syndrome. Rarely, bilateral nephrectomy for the treatment of Wilms tumor or congenital nephrotic syndrome may be encountered as an underlying cause of ESRD. A list of causes of ESRD in children is given in Table 18–1.

CARE OF CHILDREN WITH ESRD—A TEAM APPROACH

In order to optimize treatment and improve outcome, the management of children with ESRD should involve a multidisciplinary team approach. Ideally, the ESRD management team should consist of a pediatric nephrologist, renal transplant surgeon, dialysis nurse, social worker, and dietitian. Since many children with ESRD have underlying urologic disorders, the services of a pediatric urologist should also be available. The management aims of the ESRD team are (1) to ameliorate life-threatening clinical effects of uremia by dialysis and other available therapies and (2) to prepare the patient for renal transplantation.

A close follow-up of children with chronic renal failure is necessary when the GFR reaches between 15 and 20 mL/min/1.73 m^2. A conference between the ESRD team and the patient's family should be arranged to provide an overview of therapeutic options. Such a planned discussion should specifically focus on the types of dialysis therapies available, dietary restrictions imposed on dialysis patients, and the lifestyle of these patients and their families while on dialysis. The subject of renal transplantation should also be introduced during the meeting, and the advantages of renal transplantation over long-term dialysis in a growing child should be outlined. Often, a follow-up meeting is necessary to clarify the questions that may arise as a result of the discussions that the patient's family may engage in at home. The social worker's evaluation of the family, their response to stress, and their coping mechanisms is immensely helpful at this stage; the social worker also helps to provide support during later stages of patient care. A "walk-through" of the dialysis facility may also be arranged for the patient and family.

With progression of chronic renal insufficiency, a follow-up meeting between the patient, his or her family, and the ESRD team should be held in order to decide upon the most appropriate mode of treatment for the patient. All options, including renal transplantation, must be discussed in detail, and the patient's (and his or her family's) choice of therapy must be well documented. Since it may take 6 to 9 weeks or longer to create an arteriovenous fistula that is ready for clinical use, surgery for vascular access must be arranged ahead of time in patients who choose hemodialysis as the treatment modality. In patients considering peritoneal dialysis, surgical placement of a peritoneal dialysis catheter should be arranged 10 to 15 days before the anticipated day of dialysis. Such a policy allows proper healing of the abdominal wound and decreases the chances of dialysate leaking around the catheter.

Infants who suffer from chronic renal failure during the first year of life frequently develop progressive encephalopathy characterized by developmental delay, microcephaly, and seizures.[7] The etiology of these neurologic lesions is not well delineated, but an adverse impact of uremia on brain growth during the first 2 years of life has been hypothesized.[8] To minimize the impact of uremia on physical and neurologic development of young infants, preemptive renal transplantation prior to the onset of progressive encephalopathy has been suggested. Short-term results indicate that improvement in cognitive and psychomotor functions is possible if renal transplantation is performed early in children with ESRD.[9,10] When patients are being considered for preemptive renal transplantation, potential transplant donors must be selected and evaluated. However, prior to renal transplantation, some children may require bilateral nephrectomy for the treatment of severe uncontrolled hypertension or a severely malformed and chronically infected urinary tract. These patients will need dialysis in order to tide them over the anephric phase prior to transplantation. Such issues must be discussed with the family and appropriate arrangements made.

The approximate time when a patient with chronic renal failure may develop ESRD and need dialysis/transplant therapy can be calculated by plotting the reciprocal relation of serum creatinine to time (Chaps. 1 and 16).[11]

INDICATIONS FOR CHRONIC DIALYSIS THERAPY

The indications for initiating chronic dialysis therapy in children are not as well defined as they are for adults. Although residual renal function is an important and measurable criterion for judging the need for dialysis therapy, clinical observations—such as the impact of chronic renal failure on growth, bone disease, neurologic development, and the general health of the patient—must also be considered in timing the start of treatment. A decline in the glomerular filtration rate (GFR) to 5 to 10 mL/min/1.73 m^2 is associated with early uremic manifestations such as lethargy, decreased exercise tolerance, nausea, and vomiting. Additionally, hypertension, edema, and electrolyte abnormalities such as hyperkalemia and metabolic acidosis can pose significant management concerns at this low level of GFR. Failure to provide renal replacement therapy at this stage may lead to serious uremic complications such as pericarditis, peripheral neuropathy, encephalopathy, and hemorrhagic diathesis. Dialysis should be initiated before any major metabolic derangements caused by uremia occur and before compromise of the cardiovascular system by fluid overload develops. It is generally done when the GFR reaches the range of 5 to 10 mL/min/1.73 m^2. Dialytic therapy may be initiated earlier in the course of chronic renal failure in infants and children if growth, development, and nutrition cannot be effectively managed by conservative therapy alone. Clinical settings considered to be absolute indications for initiating dialysis in a child with chronic renal failure are fluid overload, congestive heart failure, uncontrolled hyperkalemia, pericarditis, uremic encephalopathy, and uremic peripheral neuropathy.

CHOOSING THE DIALYSIS MODALITY

Although renal transplantation is considered to be the optimal renal replacement therapy for children with ESRD, many patients will require short- or long-term dialysis prior to transplantation. The choice of dialysis modality in such instances must be individualized and should be based on the patient's age, developmental status and underlying renal disease as well as whether the parents are willing and able to perform the dialysis procedure at home.[12]

AGE

While short-term and acute hemodialysis therapy is technically feasible in infants and young children, chronic hemodialysis is generally avoided in this age group because of the problems associated with long-term vascular access. Additionally, hemodialysis (HD) in infants requires technical know-how and specialized dialysis equipment which is usually available only in tertiary-care pediatric facilities. This fact limits the use of chronic HD to the larger pediatric centers. On the other hand, peritoneal dialysis (PD) done at home minimizes hospital visits, allows the patient to remain in the home environment, and promotes the parents' participation in the treatment process. These benefits make

PD the modality of choice in infants and young children. Additional reported benefits of PD in comparison to HD include better control of hypertension, reduction in the transfusion requirements, and an improvement in bone disease.[13] Both continuous ambulatory peritoneal dialysis (CAPD) and continuous cycling peritoneal dialysis (CCPD) are effective and technically feasible forms of PD in children with ESRD in this age group.

Peritoneal dialysis is also the preferred modality in preschool children with ESRD. The choice between CAPD and CCPD is usually dictated by the family's preference. Peritoneal dialysis, especially CCPD, presents very little interference in the daily activities of children of this age. Hemodialysis is feasible without any significant technical difficulties in school-age children and adolescents (6 to 15 years). However, hospital-based outpatient hemodialysis three times a week makes it impossible for these patients to attend school regularly. Home hemodialysis can facilitate attendance at school, but the high level of technical training and participation it requires of parents has rendered home hemodialysis for children a rarity in the United States. Even in this age group, PD (CAPD or CCPD) is generally attractive to patients, since it does not interrupt school, play, or social activities.

OTHER CONSIDERATIONS IN CHOOSING DIALYSIS THERAPY

Patients who have undergone previous abdominal surgical procedures may not be good candidates for PD, since peritoneal scarring and adhesions may decrease the peritoneal surface area available for dialysis. In such instances, hemodialysis may be the only possible treatment modality. The presence of an ileostomy or ureterostomy makes PD difficult but does not constitute an absolute contraindication.[14] Peritoneal dialysis is usually not considered a treatment option for patients with ventriculoperitoneal shunts for the treatment of hydrocephalus; however, one recent report has described successful PD in such patients.[15] Patients who undergo bilateral nephrectomy for Wilms tumor are often dialyzed by HD rather than PD. If there is no evidence of tumor recurrence, the child may then be considered for PD or renal transplantation.[16] Poorly motivated patients are at a significantly higher risk of developing peritonitis while on PD; HD may be an acceptable alternative for such patients. Fig. 18–1 shows the relative distribution of hemodialysis and peritoneal dialysis in children with ESRD undergoing dialysis therapy in the United States.

HEMODIALYSIS

Since the first clinical report of HD in a preadolescent patient with chronic renal failure in 1966,[17] enormous technical progress has been made in adapting HD for children of all ages. These advances include developments in the field of vascular surgery and techniques in vascular access for dialysis, availability of low-priming-volume hollow fiber dialyzers, and small blood lines for dialysis. Hemodialysis can now be carried out in patients of any age, including newborns.

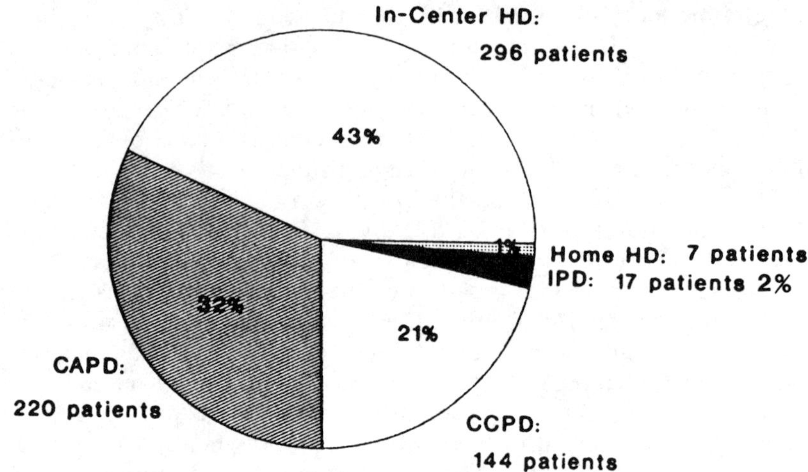

FIG. 18–1. Maintenance dialysis modalities of 684 children in the United States under 15 years of age who were undergoing dialysis on December 31, 1987. [Reproduced by permission from Alexander SR, Lindbald AS, Nolph KD, et al: Pediatric CAPD/CCPD in the United States: New concepts and applications, in Twardowski ZJ, Nolph KD, Khanna R (eds): *Peritoneal Dialysis*. New York, Churchill Livingstone, 1990, p 231.]

VASCULAR ACCESS FOR HEMODIALYSIS IN CHILDREN

Hemodialysis is an extracorporeal procedure, requiring a vascular access in order to remove the blood from the patient and return it back after it is circulated through the "artificial kidney" or dialyzer. Several types of vascular access can be used for HD in children, ranging from vein-to-vein vascular catheters to arteriovenous shunts and arteriovenous fistulas. The choice of vascular access is strongly influenced by the urgency of providing dialysis, the anticipated time for which the access will be required, and the state of patient's blood vessels.

VEIN-TO-VEIN VASCULAR CATHETERS

Vein-to-vein HD catheters are used to provide HD access in patients who need dialysis for a short time as in acute renal failure. Such catheters may also be used in ESRD patients to provide temporary vascular access if the patients do not have an established vascular access or if the access is not yet fully ready for clinical use. Vein-to-vein dialysis is performed by inserting a double-lumen cannula in a large vein such as the femoral vein or subclavian vein by way of the Seldinger technique. Short catheters of at least 7 French size can be used in small children (less than 15 kg in weight) as an access through the femoral vein, while longer catheters may be necessary for access through the subclavian vein. Several types of double-lumen HD catheters, including Hickman catheters, are

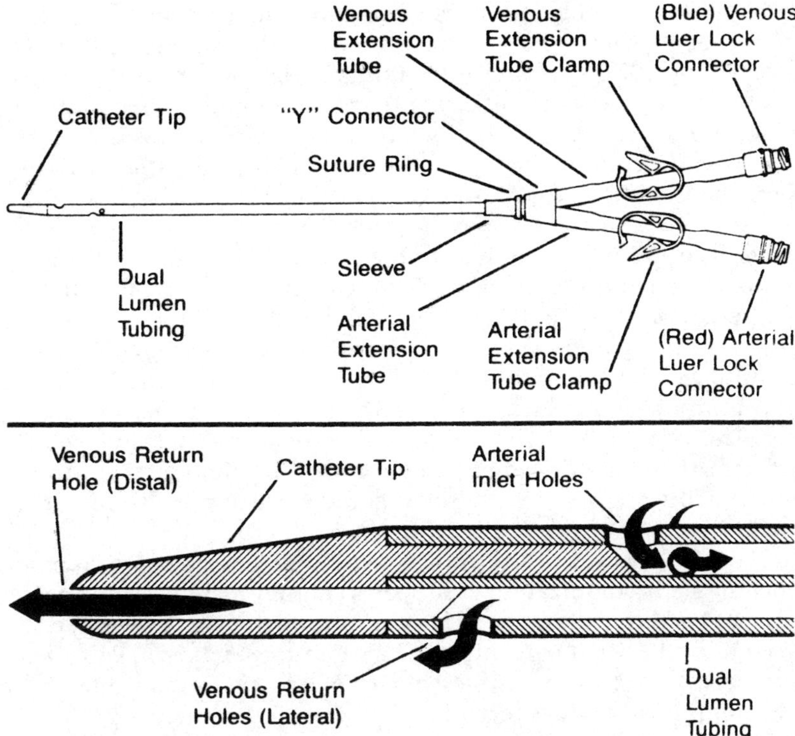

FIG. 18–2. Mahurkar dual-lumen subclavian hemodialysis catheter. (Reproduced from instruction package by permission of Quinton Instruments Co., Seattle, Washington.)

available commercially.[18] If double-lumen catheters are used for dialysis, one lumen is used to withdraw blood from the patient while the other serves to return dialyzed blood back to the patient. The two lumens of these catheters are usually arranged so as to minimize recirculation of blood. A diagrammatic representation of one of the commercially available dual-lumen HD catheters is shown in Fig. 18–2. Sometimes a single-lumen venous catheter placed in the subclavian vein or right atrium is the only vascular access available for HD. Under these circumstances, HD can be accomplished by using a single-needle uniclamp apparatus (Cobe-Gambro-Hospal, Williamsburgh, Virginia); alternatively, the centrally placed catheter may be used to draw the patient's blood for dialysis (arterial line), the dialyzed blood being returned to the patient through another large peripheral vein (venous line).

Most manufacturers of venous HD catheters recommend that they not be left in place for more than a few days, especially in the femoral location. However, in one study,[18] the mean duration for use of venous catheters in the subclavian location was reported to be 60 days (range: 13 to 135 days), and a mean of 17 HD procedures (range: 4 to 34) were performed with each catheter.

Apart from the surgical risks associated with the insertion of the venous catheter, other major complications involving venous catheters used for HD are obstruction of the blood flow, displacement of the catheter, bleeding around the catheter insertion site, and infection.[18,19] Obstruction to the flow of blood through the catheter may result either from a clot in the catheter lumen or from adherence of the catheter's distal lumen to the vessel wall. A high incidence of residual thrombosis in the blood vessels used for venous catheterization for HD has been reported by some authors.[19] It has been speculated that the use of large-size catheters may predispose to such thrombosis.

In order to prevent clotting within the lumen of the dialysis catheter during the interdialytic period, each port of the catheter is injected with 100 to 500 units of heparinized saline three times daily as long as the patient remains in the hospital. After patient's discharge from the hospital, handling of the catheter is minimized by instillation of 3000 to 5000 units of heparin (10,000 units/mL concentration) diluted in normal saline into each port of the double-lumen catheter. The volume (usually 1.0 mL) of the heparinized saline solution to be injected into the catheter lumen is determined by the length of the catheter. The heparin concentrate is withdrawn and discarded prior to the next dialysis treatment.

Bacterial colonization of the subclavian HD catheter occurs commonly; the incidence of such colonization has been reported as high at 50 percent. The incidence of bacteremia as a result of colonization of the HD catheter has been estimated to be 17 to 20 percent.[20,21] Skin flora *(Staphylococcus epidermidis, Staphylococcus aureus)* are the commonest microbial agents responsible for catheter-related colonization and bacteremia. The life of HD catheters can be enhanced by meticulous attention to sterile and aseptic techniques during their use. In order to reduce the risk of infection, the use of subclavian dialysis catheters for the purpose of intravenous therapy or drawing blood should be discouraged. Changing the subclavian HD catheters once a week over a guide wire has not been shown to decrease the risk of dialysis-catheter related infection.[22] It has also been suggested that HD catheters with subcutaneous cuffs may help reduce the risk of infection.[19]

ARTERIOVENOUS SHUNTS

The arteriovenous (A-V) shunt, first developed by Quinton, Dillard, and Scribner, has been used extensively in the past as the vascular access for HD in children, especially in infants with body weights of less than 20 kg.[23] The A-V shunt consists of two clear Silastic tubes connected by a removable connector sleeve in the middle. The proximal end of each tube has an adapter tip that can fit into a blood vessel. These tubes are surgically placed into an adjacent artery and vein; when they are connected outside the body through the connector sleeve, the blood flows from the artery into the vein via the shunt tubing. At the time of performing HD, the shunt is disconnected at the connector sleeve and its arterial and venous ends are connected to the dialyzer via a connection tubing. After the dialysis, the arterial and venous tubings of the A-V shunt are reconnected in order to establish the blood flow.

Clotting is the most frequent complication of external shunts; 50 percent of A-V shunts in children have been reported to be so affected.[24] The average life of an A-V shunt in a large series was found to be only 113 days.[25] Anticoagulation or antiplatelet therapy may be tried in an effort to prolong shunt life. Infection is the second most common complication of shunts, usually being caused by *S. aureus.* The infection rate can be reduced by using sterile technique when the shunt must be manipulated. Also, the shunt should be covered by a dressing in the interdialytic period so as to prevent the child from manipulating the tubing. Accidental disconnection of the shunt at the connector sleeve may lead to hemorrhage; therefore parents must be educated about the procedure of applying bulldog clamps to the shunt to prevent exsanguination.

ARTERIOVENOUS FISTULAE

The arteriovenous fistula (AVF) initially described by Brescia and Cimino[26] is the most convenient and safest long-term blood access for chronic HD. The AVF for HD is created surgically by anastomosing an adjacent artery and vein either using an end-to-side or side-to-side anastomosis. The ideal site for the construction of an AVF is between the radial artery and cephalic vein in the patient's nondominant arm. When the radial artery cannot be utilized, other arteries (brachial, ulnar) can be used. Whenever possible, an AVF should be created 2 to 3 months prior to its projected use, usually when the serum creatinine concentration is between 6 to 7 mg/dL. This allows the venous limb of the fistula to become thicker (arterialization) and to enlarge in size—a process termed as *maturation of the fistula.* Maturation of the AVF can be accelerated by instructing the patient to exercise the arm, as by squeezing a soft rubber ball. Eventually, as blood flow through the arm improves, a lightly applied tourniquet above the fistula may be incorporated during the arm exercises.

Because of the small size of children's blood vessels, an AVF can be technically difficult to construct and may be slower to mature in a child than in an adult. However, experience from a large pediatric center suggests no difference in survival rate of fistulas in children weighing less than 20 kg and those weighing more than 20 kg.[27] If it is not possible to construct an AVF using the patient's own blood vessels, a synthetic vascular graft made of polytetrafluorethylene (PTFE), marketed as Goretex or Impra, or an autologous saphenous vein transplant may be used to bridge the vessels. Bovine arterial heterografts are less popular. An increased incidence of thrombus formation, infections, and hematomas is seen with an AVF made of synthetic or autologous graft material as compared to an AVF created from native adjacent blood vessels.[28]

Needles specially designed for the purpose of HD (usually 18-gauge) are inserted into the enlarged and arterialized venous segment of the AVF to remove the patient's blood for dialysis (designated as the *arterial line*). The dialyzed blood is returned to the patient through another venipuncture at a more proximal site of the fistula (designated as the *venous line*). The arterial needle is directed toward the distal end of the fistula in order to capture the arterial blood flow, while the venous needle is directed somewhat proximally in order to permit the flow of dialyzed blood centrally and to minimize admixture or recirculation of the dialyzed and nondialyzed blood in the fistula (Fig. 18–3).

Clotting is much less a problem in the Cimino fistula than in external A-V shunts, but the risk is enhanced if saphenous or bovine heterografts are

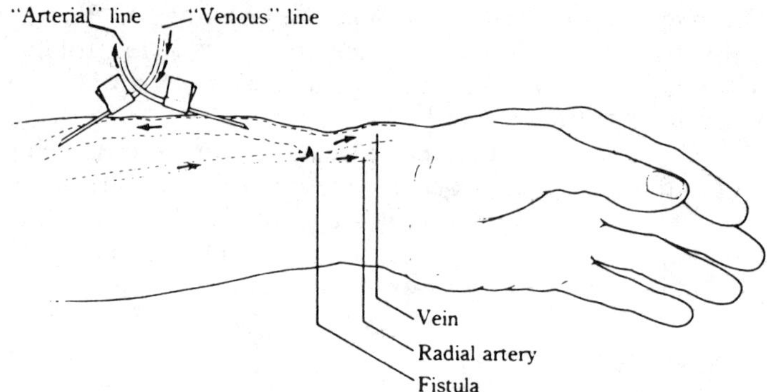

FIG. 18–3. Diagrammatic representation of radiocephalic A-V fistula showing blood flow and usual position of access needles. [Reproduced by permission from Raja RM: Vascular access for hemodialysis, in Daugridas JT, Ing TS (eds): *Handbook of Dialysis*. Boston, Little, Brown, 1988, p 53.]

used.[28,29] Use of an AVF before it has fully matured leads to missed punctures, thrombosis, and hematoma formation due to poor hemostasis in the thin-walled fistula. Although alterations in cardiac function have been noted to result from AVF, especially in patients with rates of high blood flow, overt cardiac failure is rare.[30]

BASIC PRINCIPLES OF HEMODIALYSIS

In its essence, HD involves removal of the patient's blood from the body via the arterial end of an AVF, achieving exchange of water and solutes in the dialyzer, and returning the blood to the patient through the venous needle inserted in the AVF. All HD systems are composed of three basic elements: (1) a closed-loop blood delivery system, (2) the dialyzer, and (3) a dialysate delivery system (Fig. 18–4).

BLOOD DELIVERY

During HD the patient's blood is removed from the body by inserting a large-bore needle into the arterialized vein or AVF, and connecting it to special dialysis tubing. The blood tubing is placed in a pumping device that generates enough pressure to overcome resistance to the blood flow in the dialyzer and promote ultrafiltration. In order to reduce the risk of spontaneous coagulation in the extracorporeal system, the patient's blood is also anticoagulated before its entry into the dialyzer. The blood exiting the dialyzer is returned to the patient via blood lines connected to a large-bore needle inserted into the AVF. An air and foam alarm is placed in the path of the blood returning to the patient in order to detect air that may find its way in the returning blood, thus ensuring patient safety (Fig. 18–4).

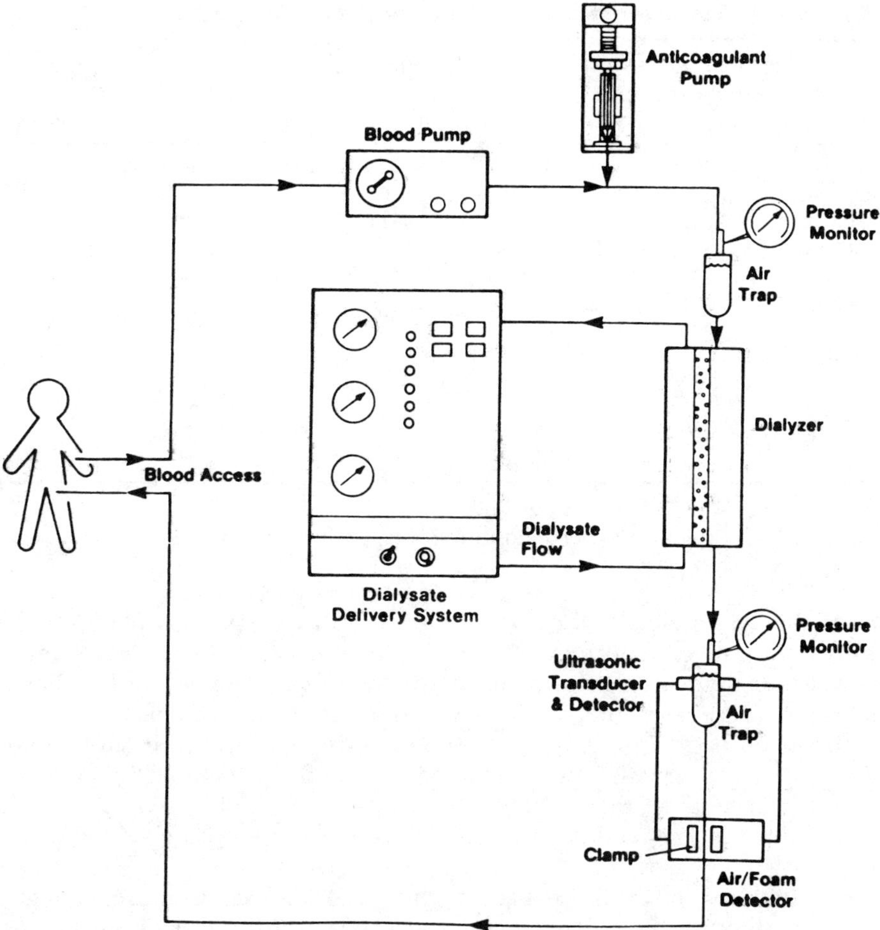

FIG 18–4. Schematic representation of central dialysate delivery system and extracorporeal blood circuit in hemodialysis. [Reproduced by permission from Keshaviah P: Equipment for hemodialysis and peritoneal dialysis, in Nissenson AR, Fine RN, Gentile DE (eds): *Clinical Dialysis*. Norwalk, Connecticut, Appleton and Lange, 1990, p 45.]

THE DIALYZER

The dialyzer is a device made of a semipermeable membrane through which the patient's blood flows within a designated path. The blood path is enclosed by the semipermeable membrane and is bathed by the dialysate solution on the outside; this configuration allows the exchange of water and solute (dialysis) between the two separate compartments. The semipermeable membranes used in most dialyzers are made of chemically altered cellulose or synthetic materials such as polyacrylonitrile (PAN) or polysulfone. Two different types of dialyzers

TABLE 18–2. Characteristics of Commonly Used Dialyzers

Dialyzer	Priming Volume, mL	Compliance, mL/100 mmHg	Surface Area, m^2	Type	Urea Clearance, mL/min[a]	Ultrafiltratiron Coefficient, mL/mmHg/h
Mini Minor (Gambro)	20	6	0.20	PF	61	0.5
Lundia Minor (Gambro)	33	10	0.41	PF	100	1.4
CA-50 (Baxter)	38	0	0.5	HF	128	2.4
CA-70 (Baxter)	51	0	0.7	HF	153	3.4
CA-90 (Baxter)	64	0	0.9	HF	169	4.3
CA-110 (Baxter)	80	0	1.1	HF	176	5.3

PF = parallel flow; HF = hollow fiber.
[a]Measured at 200 mL/min perfusion flow rate, TMP = 160 mmHg.

are available commercially for clinical use; these are (1) parallel-plate dialyzers and (2) hollow-fiber dialyzers. The parallel-plate dialyzer consists of one or more thin, baglike chambers (or plates) made of the semipermeable dialyzer membrane; these are interconnected and housed in a single casing. The patient's blood flows into and out of the dialysis chambers through two ports while the dialysate circulates around the blood column separated by the dialysis membrane. Because of the problems associated with the high-compliance and high-ultrafiltration capability of plate dialyzers, these are rarely used in children today.

The hollow-fiber or capillary dialyzer consists of thousands of thin capillaries made of semipermeable membrane that are encased in a clear plastic housing. Both ends of the capillaries are open and are brought together and compacted in a way that the patient's incoming blood flows into the lumen of the capillaries, traverses them through the length of the dialyzer, and exits from the opposite end. The dialysate is pumped into the dialyzer through a separate port and bathes the outside of the dialyzer capillaries. A clear advantage of the hollow-fiber dialyzer is that it usually requires lesser priming volume and is less compliant during dialysis. However, a slightly higher blood loss is common in hollow-fiber dialyzers due to microclotting in the dialyzer capillaries. Characteristics of several types of dialyzers available commercially for use in children are given in Table 18–2.

DIALYSATE DELIVERY

The dialysate consists of purified water and electrolytes and resembles plasma in constitution. Municipal water must be purified prior to being used for the purpose of dialysis and must meet the standards of the Association for the Advancement of Medical Instrumentation (AAMI) given in Table 18–3. Water

TABLE 18–3. Standards for Hemodialysis Water Quality

Contaminant	Suggested Maximum Level, mg/L
Calcium	2 (0.1 meq/L)
Magnesium	4 (0.3 meq/L)
Sodium	70 (3 meq/L)
Potassium	8 (0.2 meq/L)
Fluoride	0.2
Chlorine	0.5
Chloramines	0.1
Nitrate (N)	2
Sulfate	100
Copper, barium, zinc	each 0.1
Aluminum	0.01
Arsenic, lead, silver	each 0.005
Cadmium	0.001
Chromium	0.014
Selenium	0.09
Mercury	0.0002

Source: Reproduced by permission of American Association for the Advancement of Medical Instrumentation, Arlington, Virginia, 1990.

purification for dialysis is done by a stepwise passage through a water softener, carbon filter, sediment filters, and reverse osmosis. This purification process removes virtually all particulate and chemical impurities from municipal water. After purification, the water is mixed with electrolyte concentrate to provide the desired dialysate electrolyte concentration. This process can be done in a central plant or individually at each dialysis station if dialysis machines with proportioning capabilities are used. The sole advantage of a central dialysate delivery system is a reduction in operating costs, but it means that all patients must receive the same dialysate prescription, since changes to fit the needs of individual patients cannot be made. On the other hand, the composition of dialysate can be altered according to each patients' requirements (e.g., potassium concentration, bicarbonate bath, etc.) if the dialysate is reconstituted by individual dialysis machines.

The dialysate is pumped at a high flow rate (500 mL/min) into the dialyzer in such a manner that it runs counter to the direction of the blood flow. Within the dialyzer the dialysate is separated from the blood column by the semipermeable dialysis membrane. The dialysate exiting from the dialyzer is discarded in a drain (single-pass system). The typical dialysate composition for chronic HD is shown in Table 18–4. Most nephrologists agree that bicarbonate dialysate offers significantly greater advantages in patient management on HD than acetate dialysate; therefore the former is increasingly being used for chronic HD in

TABLE 18–4. Composition of Standard Acetate and Bicarbonate Dialysate

Component	Acetate-containing, meq/L	Bicarbonate-containing, meq/L
Sodium	135–145	135–145
Potassium	0–4.0	0–4.0
Calcium	2.5–3.5	2.5–3.5
Magnesium	0.5–1.0	0.5–1.0
Chloride	100–119	100–124
Acetate	35–38	2–4
Bicarbonate	0	30–38
Dextrose	11	11
P_{CO_2}, mmHg	0.5	40–100
pH	Variable	7.1–7.3

Source: Reproduced by permission from Van Stone JC: Hemodialysis apparatus, in Daugridas JT, Ing TS (eds): *Handbook of Dialysis.* Boston, Little Brown, 1988, p 21.

patients with ESRD.[31,32] Some HD machines that use proportioning systems to make dialysate "on line" allow the dialysate sodium concentration to be varied from 125 to 140 meq/L and bicarbonate concentration to vary from 25 to 35 meq/L. On the other hand, the potassium concentration of the dialysate can be changed only by altering the potassium concentration of the electrolyte concentrate that is used.

TECHNICAL DETAILS OF DIALYSIS

SELECTION OF DIALYZER AND BLOOD LINES

Priming volume, clearance efficiency, and ultrafiltration characteristics are taken into account in selecting a dialyzer for patients undergoing HD. Clinical experience has shown that the total extracorporeal blood volume (blood volume of the dialyzer and the blood lines) should not exceed 10 percent of the child's estimated blood volume.[33] Since the blood volume of a child is approximately 80 mL/kg, the extracorporeal blood volume should not exceed 0.8 percent of the child's body weight. As an example, extracorporeal circulating blood volume in a child weighing 25 kg should not exceed 200 mL. Because of this limitation, a dialyzer with a low priming volume is a requirement for undertaking HD in children, particularly in infants and neonates. Small caliber blood lines that require considerably less priming blood volume than the adult blood lines are available commercially. Pediatric blood lines with tubing 3 mm in diameter may, however, restrict blood flow to <75 mL/min. If small blood lines are not available, the dialyzer may be primed with blood in order to conduct safe dialysis. For neonates and children weighing less than 10 kg, the Gambro Mini-Minor Dialyzer (Cobe-Gambro-Hospal, Williamsburg, Virginia) is very useful. Dialyzers with a priming volume of about 50 mL (Baxter CA-50) are suitable for children weighing 15 kg or more.

The urea clearance of the dialyzer must also be adequate for the acceptable

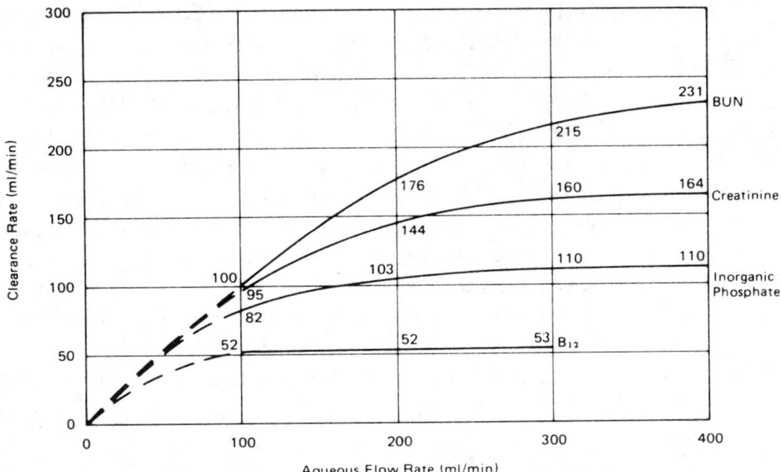

FIG. 18–5. Clearance data for urea, creatinine, inorganic phosphate, and vitamin B_{12} for model CA-70 hollow-fiber dialyzer. (Reproduced from the package insert.)

removal of BUN and other solutes during dialysis. The urea clearance of most currently available dialyzers is well within the "adequate" range. Highly efficient dialysis will obviously remove urea and other uremic toxins effectively and quickly, but such a rapid change in body composition and osmolality is often associated with dialysis disequilibrium syndrome (DDS).[33] Commercially available dialyzers differ in their urea clearance capability because of their variability in membrane characteristics and surface area. Clearance of urea, creatinine, vitamin B_{12},, and phosphorus for each type of dialyzer in relation to blood flow is available from the manufacturers of these devices (Fig. 18–5). In addition to the dialyzer's inherent characteristics, clearance of various solutes is also a direct function of the rate at which blood flows through the dialyzer. Therefore, an alteration in the blood flow will effectively change the urea clearance. The blood flow rate required to obtain a defined urea clearance can be calculated from the graphs supplied by the manufacturer of the dialyzer.

Present-day dialyzers are able to achieve a high ultrafiltration rate without disrupting the dialyzer membrane. Apart from blood flow, the degree of ultrafiltration also depends on the transmembrane hydrostatic pressure (TMP) applied to enhance the movement of water from the blood column and on the inherent permeability or coefficient of ultrafiltration (K_{uf}) of the dialyzer. Because of a potential risk of excessive fluid removal during dialysis and volume depletion, dialyzers with a high K_{uf} are unsuitable for use in small children.

BLOOD FLOW

The rate at which the patient's blood must be pumped into the dialyzer depends on how rapidly the solute exchange and water removal must take place during dialysis. Although high-efficiency HD (a blood flow rate of >400 mL/min) is becoming the trend in adult patients (since it saves time), it is generally recommended that children be dialyzed at a relatively low blood flow rate in order to minimize the risk of dialysis disequilibrium syndrome. Urea is considered a surrogate for the uremic toxins, and its clearance during dialysis is equated with the clearance of uremic toxins. The general principles of HD developed by Kjellstrand, using the urea clearance rates of dialyzers, are helpful guides in prescribing blood flow rate for HD in children.[33] In order to minimize the risk of DDS, urea clearance during dialysis should not exceed 3mL/kg/min. For example, in a patient weighing 20 kg, the blood flow during dialysis should be such as not to exceed the urea clearance of 60 mL/min. Information on the relationship of blood flow to urea clearance is available from the manufacturers; it should be consulted for an accurate determination of the blood flow rate required (Fig. 18–5). In practical terms, however, a blood flow rate of 3 mL/kg/min will correspond to the value of calculated urea clearance (3 mL/kg/min) for most dialyzers used in children and may be used as an approximate parameter.

ANTICOAGULATION DURING DIALYSIS

The patient's blood must be anticoagulated in order to prevent spontaneous coagulation in the extracorporeal circuit. Heparin is used as the anticoagulant for most patients undergoing HD. It must be pointed out that sensitivity to heparin varies from patient to patient and the potency of heparin (at the same dose) may also vary from one preparation to another and from batch to batch. Heparinization for HD is usually done by administering a heparin bolus (dose, 40 to 50 units/kg) at the start of dialysis and monitoring the activated clotting time (ACT) during the treatment session. Smaller additional doses of heparin may be necessary during dialysis in order to maintain the ACT within the recommended range of 180 to 200 percent of the baseline predialysis value. In patients at risk of bleeding, the heparinization can be managed by a smaller initial bolus (dose, 15 units/kg), followed by an infusion of heparin at a dose of 10 units/kg/h. Under these circumstances the ACT should be maintained at 140 to 150 percent of baseline value (tight heparinization). Obviously, ACT should be checked more frequently during tight heparinization and the dialyzer inspected for evidence of blood clotting. The high hematrocrit in the dialysis patient, as in patients receiving recombinant erythropoeitin therapy, predisposes to dialyzer clotting; a higher dose of heparin is advocated in such patients.[34]

PRIMING THE SYSTEM

Generally, the dialyzer and the blood lines are primed with isotonic saline in order to remove air from the system. If the child is fluid-overloaded, it is safe to "bleed" the patient into the dialyzer and connect the venous blood line when the patient's blood column reaches the venous end of the dialyzer. In this manner a significant portion of the saline used for priming the extracorporeal circuit is not infused into the patient. Blood or 5% albumin may be used to prime the dialyzer and tubing if the patient is anemic or hypovolemic. At the end of dialysis, the extracorporeal blood is transfused back into the patient. Only small amounts of saline (<50 mL) are used for the dialyzer washback procedure.

MONITORING THE PATIENTS

Careful monitoring of the patient's blood pressure and other vital signs during dialysis is mandatory. In order to estimate fluid removed during dialysis, the patient's dialysis chair or bed may be placed on an electronic bed scale. Many of the newer hemodialysis machines are able to provide continuous electronic read-out of the volume of fluid removed during hemodialysis. The purpose of such monitoring is to prevent excessive fluid removal and hypotension during dialysis. For small children and infants, a nurse-patient ratio of one-to-one is often required during the length of dialysis. Small children are very active, so that there is a risk of dislodging the needle or accidentally disconnecting the tubing. Special attention must be paid to symptoms such as yawning, restlessness, nausea, staring, or changes in skin color, which often precede episodes of hypotension, dialysis disequilibrium syndrome, and vomiting.

ACUTE COMPLICATIONS ASSOCIATED WITH HEMODIALYSIS

HYPOTENSION

Hypotension occurs commonly during dialysis and can be caused by dialyzers that are too large and compliant, by rapid removal of large fluid volumes, and by decreased cardiac output or total peripheral resistance. Symptoms of nausea, vomiting, dizziness, headache and tachycardia, sweating, and fainting are often seen in patients who develop hypotension on HD. Excessive ultrafiltration during dialysis is the most common cause of dialysis-associated hypotension, but other factors such as accumulation of acetate, decrease in serum osmolality, rise of body temperature, and hypoxemia have all been incriminated.[35] Use of the dialyzer and blood line to match the patient's blood volume is essential in order to avoid hypotension during dialysis. At no point should the blood in the extracorporeal circuit (dialyzer and blood lines) exceed 10 percent of the patient's blood volume. Continuous monitoring of weight during dialysis helps to prevent excessive fluid removal and development of hypotension, especially in neonates, infants, and young children. Treatment of hypotension during dialysis consists of placing the patient in a recumbent posture by tilting the dialysis chair and infusing normal saline (5 to 10 mL/kg) rapidly. Infusion of colloid (25% albumin) may be required in some instances to maintain blood pressure. Concomitantly, the rate of blood flow through the dialyzer must be reduced and ultrafiltration discontinued in order to prevent further loss of intravascular volume. Because of obligatory fluid loss during dialysis, some patients who often develop hypotension during HD may benefit from periodic replacement of volume during the entire dialysis procedure. Some patients with excessive fluid gain in the inter-dialytic period tolerate sequential ultrafiltration followed by dialysis better than concurrent ultrafiltration and dialysis. Although ultrafiltration prior to HD leads to a decrease in cardiac output, a concomitant increase in peripheral resistance prevents any fall of systemic blood pressure. In contrast, ultrafiltration during HD is not associated with any concomitant rise of peripheral resistance and leads to a decline of BP.[35] Cooling of blood during HD (by circulating cooled dialysate) has been advocated by some as a method of reducing the incidence of dialysis-associated hypotension.[36] Henderson and coworkers[37] have proposed that the antihypotensive effect of cooling results from inhibition of interleukin-1 activation. Others, however, contend that the norepinephrine concentration in plasma rises during cooling and may be responsible for preventing a fall of the systemic blood pressure.[38] Hemodialysis machines capable of cooling the dialysate are now available commercially. Patients who are unable to tolerate acetate dialysis may benefit from switching to a bicarbonate dialysis bath.

MUSCLE CRAMPS

Muscle cramps are a common symptom in hemodialysis, having been noted to occur in approximately 20 percent of adult patients.[39] Although such cramps are painful, they are not life-threatening. Several hypotheses have been advanced for their pathogenesis, including rapid decrease in plasma osmolality relative to muscle tissue and rapid ultrafiltration.[39,40] Frequent occurrence of dialysis-related muscle cramps may signal that the patient's targeted "dry weight" needs upward revision. Specific treatment includes a transient decrease in the ultrafiltration rate and intermittent administration of 0.9% or hypertonic sodium chloride (3%) solution.

DIALYSIS DISEQUILIBRIUM SYNDROME

Neurologic complications from hemodialysis are collectively known as the *dialysis disequilibrium syndrome* (DDS). Early manifestations of DDS include irritability, headache, disorientation, muscle cramps, and nausea. If left untreated, drowsiness, seizures and coma can ensue.[41] DDS usually occurs towards the end of dialysis or within the 24 h thereafter. It is more common in children than in adults and is practically unknown in patients undergoing peritoneal dialysis.[41] DDS is especially common during initial HD treatments in uremic patients and in children with high BUN (>150 mg/DL).

Based on the works of Arieff and colleagues,[42] DDS is believed to result from brain swelling. Hemodialysis is characterized by removal of urea and other osmotically active solutes from the plasma at a slightly higher rate than can occur across the blood-brain barrier and the brain tissue. This results in the development of an osmotic gradient between brain tissue and blood. Generation of idiogenic molecules in the brain tissue has also been suggested as an additional factor for the development of a brain-blood osmotic gradient in uremic patients undergoing HD.[43,44] Consequently, water enters brain tissue and leads to its swelling and subsequent symptomatology. These changes are especially pronounced during high-efficiency and rapid HD.

Dialysis disequilibrium can be prevented by intentionally reducing the efficiency of dialysis. This can be achieved by using a small sized (in terms of surface area) dialyzer and by reducing the blood flow rate during the procedure. Kjellstrand[33] has suggested that a blood flow rate that equals a urea clearance of 2 to 3 mL/kg/min reduces the risks of dialysis disequilibrium. Another measure that may be helpful in preventing a decline in serum osmolality during HD is infusion of an osmotically active substance like mannitol. The dose of mannitol is 1 g/kg body weight given intravenously during the first 1 to 2 h of HD. Since DDS is common during the initial dialysis treatments, continued administration of mannitol during subsequent HD treatments is usually not required.

COMPLICATIONS RELATED TO ANTICOAGULATION

Patients undergoing chronic hemodialysis are at an increased risk of bleeding due to the platelet dysfunction associated with uremia and also as a result of the heparinization that is necessary during the procedure.[45] Those who have undergone or need to undergo a surgical procedure within the 24 to 48 h period of HD are at a higher risk of hemorrhagic complications. Patients who have a history of gastrointestinal bleeding are especially at risk for redevelopment of hemorrhagic episodes. A careful low-dose heparin infusion along with close monitoring of ACT during dialysis may lessen but not completely eliminate the risk of hemorrhage in susceptible patients.[46] Others have recently attempted to minimize the risk hemorrhagic complications in such patients by using a small amount of systemically administered heparin (500 units) and periodic rinsing of the dialyzers with normal saline in order to prevent the dialyzer from clotting.[34] In the rare circumstance that the patient has received excess heparin during dialysis, protamine sulfate may be used to reverse the anticoagulant effect of heparin. The dose of protamine to be used depends on the amount of excess heparin that must be neutralized. Each milligram of protamine neutralizes approximately 100 units of heparin. Active bleeding associated with dialysis may have to be treated by the transfusion of blood or cryoprecipitate. Deamino-8-arginine vasopressin (DDAVP) may also be used to control uremic bleeding that is unrelated to anticoagulation during HD.[47]

PERITONEAL DIALYSIS

Peritoneal dialysis was first performed by Ganter in 1923 and was exclusively used during the 1940s until it fell into disfavor with the introduction of HD.[48] However, with the introduction of CAPD in 1976, PD once again became an efficient alternative to HD in the treatment of patients with ESRD.[49] Revival of automated PD and development of modern PD cycler machines in the 1980s—along with the availability of smaller dialysate bags—has made PD a practical modality for the treatment of children with ESRD. According to the report of the European Dialysis and Transplant Association (EDTA),[3] by the end of 1987, 30 percent of patients below 15 years of age with ESRD and 62 percent of children below 2 years of age were undergoing PD.

THE PERITONEUM AS A DIALYZER

The peritoneum consists of a thin membrane which lines the abdominal organs and the inner aspect of the abdominal wall. The peritoneal lining is continuous and encloses a potential space known as the peritoneal cavity. The peritoneal surface consists of a mesh of fine capillaries encased in interstitial tissue and lined by mesothelial cells. Total peritoneal surface in relation to body weight is larger in children than in adults. Mean calculated peritoneal surface area in children has been reported to be 383 cm^2/kg (range, 281 to 488); this compares to a mean peritoneal surface area of 177 cm^2/kg (range, 131 to 206) in adults.[50] However, all of the peritoneal surface is not believed to be available for dialysis.[51]

Solute exchange between the dialysate fluid in the peritoneal cavity and the blood circulating through the peritoneal membrane occurs by two separate but concurrent processes: (1) diffusion and (2) convective transport. Diffusion of solutes across the peritoneal membrane is mediated by the concentration gradient of solutes existing across the two sides of the peritoneal membrane. The process of diffusive solute transport is bidirectional, since urea and other uremic toxins as well as electrolytes (such as potassium) flow from blood into the peritoneal fluid while glucose, calcium, and lactate move from the dialysate fluid into the blood. Since the dialysate fluid is hypertonic in relation to plasma, it promotes the movement of water from blood into the dialysate in the peritoneal cavity (ultrafiltration). Removal of solutes as a result of cotransport with ultrafiltered water is known as *convective transport of solutes.* The net exchange of solutes during PD is an arithmetic sum of the diffusive and convective processes. Removal of solutes of larger molecular weight, including proteins, is favored in the convective transport. Enhanced peritoneal protein loss is known to be associated with an increased ultrafiltration rate.[52] Transfer of solutes from plasma into the dialysate fluid occurs at varying rates. Exchange of urea is achieved rapidly and reaches a point of equilibration by 240 min, while that of creatinine is slower and *does not* reach this point even by the end of 8 hours (Fig. 18–6).[53] Ultrafiltration of fluid during PD is governed by both the dialysate volume and the concentration of the osmotic agent (dextrose) used (Fig. 18–7).[54] Accordingly, a 4.2% dextrose dialysate is more efficient than a 1.5% dextrose dialysate in removing fluid from the patient, and use of a 40 mL/kg/exchange volume achieves greater ultrafiltration than a 30 mL/kg/exchange volume of dialysate.

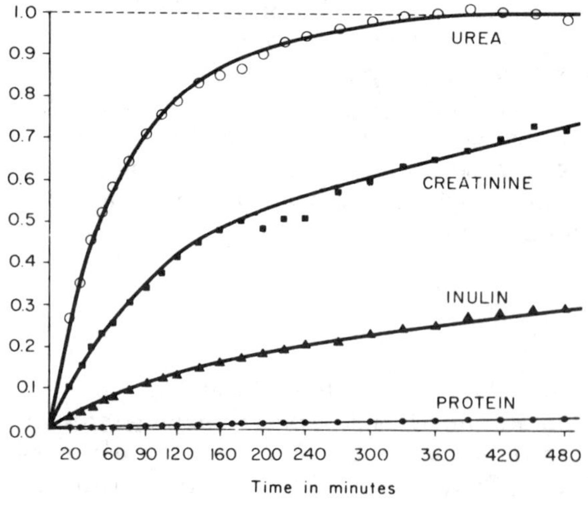

FIG. 18–6. Dialysate/plasma concentration ratios for urea, creatinine, inulin, and protein in patients undergoing CAPD. (Reproduced with permission from Popovich RP, Moncrief JW, Nalph KD, et al: Continuous ambulatory peritoneal dialysis. *Ann Intern Med* 88:449, 1978. ©1978 Am College of Physicians.)

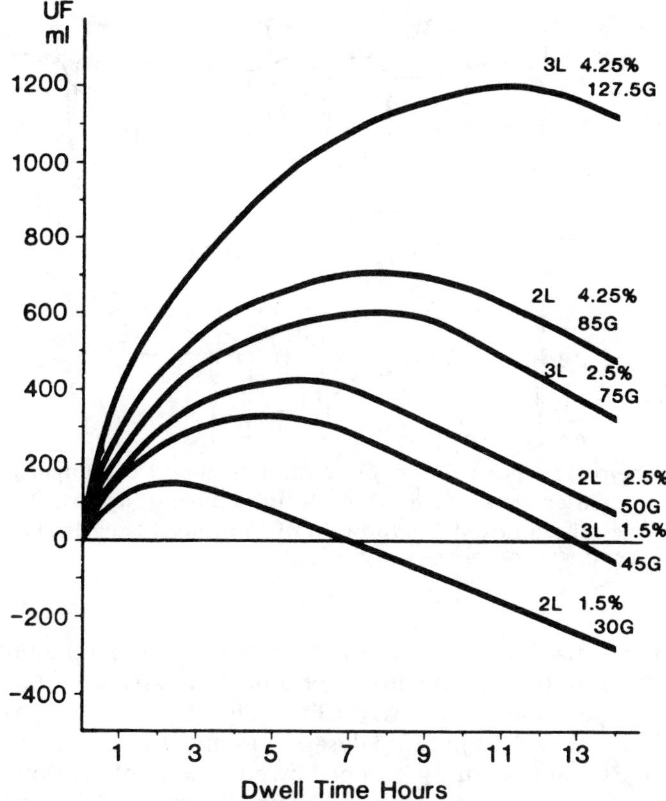

FIG. 18–7. Ultrafiltration profiles during peritoneal dialysis exchanges to show the influence of dialysate volume and varying dialysate dextrose concentrations. (From Twardowski ZJ, Khanna R, Nolph KD: Osmotic agents and ultrafiltration in peritoneal dialysis. *Nephron* 42:92, 1986. Reproduced by permission from S. Karger AG, Basel, Switzerland.)

TERMINOLOGY

Peritoneal dialysis uses the peritoneal membrane as a naturally available dialyzer for the purpose of exchanging solutes and water. The dialysate is instilled in the peritoneal cavity, allowed to equilibrate with the blood flowing through the capillaries within the peritoneal membrane, and then drained out and discarded. In order to improve its efficacy and practical clinical application, the technique of PD has undergone several significant modifications since its original description. It can be performed manually or by an automated cycler machine and the therapy may be prescribed in a continuous or intermittent manner, as discussed below.

CONTINUOUS DIALYSIS TECHNIQUES

The continuous techniques for PD are designed to improve its efficacy and require instillation of dialysate continuously during the 24-h cycle and through-

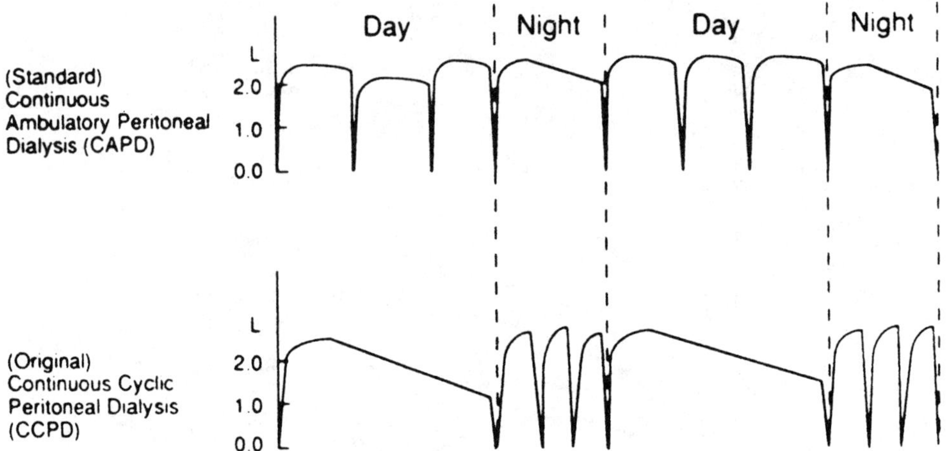

FIG. 18–8. Schematic representation of continuous-flow PD regimens. The peritoneal cavity of the patient remains filled at all times during the day, 7 days a week. (Reproduced by permission from Twardowski ZJ: Peritoneal dialysis glossary III. *Perit Dial Int* 10:173, 1990. ©1990 Pergamon Press plc.)

out the 7 days of the week. Two distinct modifications of the continuous PD method are (1) continuous ambulatory peritoneal dialysis (CAPD), and (2) continuous cycling peritoneal dialysis (CCPD) (Fig. 18–8). The CAPD method involves the manual exchanges of dialysate into and out of the peritoneal cavity. Three such exchanges with prolonged dwell time (4 h) are done during the daytime hours and the last exchange (the fourth) is allowed to dwell overnight and is drained in the morning, when another cycle is begun. The chief advantage of CAPD is the simplicity of the technology and the fact that dialysis machines are not required. This reduces the yearly operating cost of dialysis and also allows patients and their parents greater mobility. CAPD is an especially a good dialysis option for infants and young children in their preschool years who are dialyzed by their parents and for adolescents who can perform dialysis exchanges while at school.

The technique of CCPD is a hybrid between CAPD and the intermittent method of dialysis and requires an automated dialysis machine. The patient undergoes exchanges by an automated machine during the night, while sleeping, and the final exchange is allowed to dwell in the peritoneal cavity during the day. As is obvious, CCPD is best suited for patients who do not want or are unable to undertake the daytime dialysis exchanges required for CAPD.

INTERMITTENT DIALYSIS TECHNIQUE

Intermittent peritoneal dialysis (IPD) has been in use since PD was first described in patients with ESRD. The original method recommended a 40-h-per-week dialysis, usually done in four 10-h sessions, each dialysis cycle lasting 1 h (inflow, dwell, and drain). As it was in its original form, IPD is rarely used at present; however, two of its modified forms are frequently prescribed: (1)

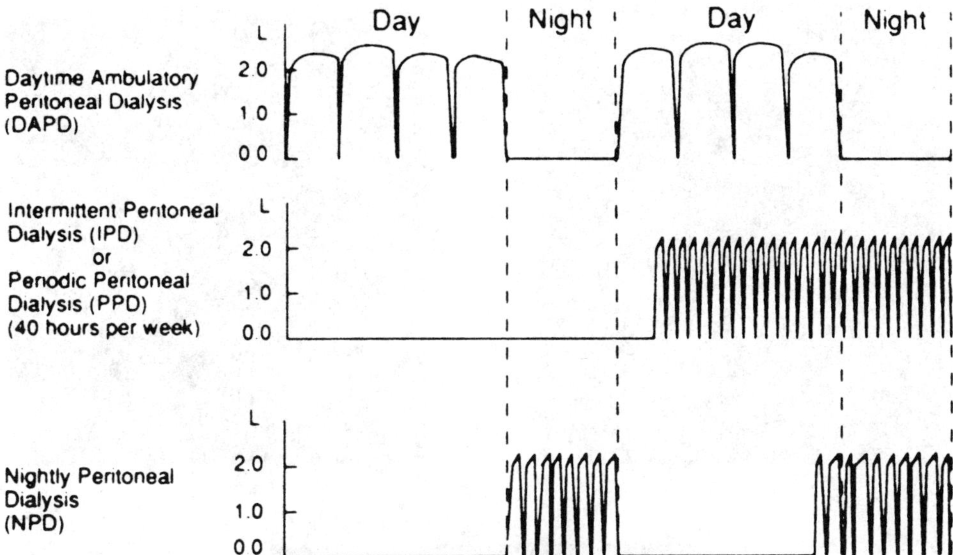

FIG. 18–9. Schematic representation of intermittent PD regimens. The peritoneal cavity of the patient remains empty during a part of the 24-h cycle. (Reproduced by permission from Twardowski ZJ: Peritoneal dialysis glossary III. *Peri Dial Int* 10:173, 1990. ©1990 Pergamon Press plc.)

nightly peritoneal dialysis (NPD) and (2) daytime ambulatory peritoneal dialysis (DAPD) (Fig. 18–9). The DAPD involves performing four exchanges during the day, as is done in CAPD, but nighttime dwell of the dialysate is not undertaken. This method (DAPD) can only be recommended in patients who have a very high peritoneal clearance rate of solutes. The NPD involves dialysis with an automatic cycler at night using 8 to 10 hourly exchanges. The peritoneal cavity is completely drained in the morning prior to disconnecting from the cycler. The dialysis is reinstituted at night.

PERITONEAL DIALYSIS TECHNIQUE

DIALYSIS CATHETERS

Access to the peritoneal cavity via a PD catheter is required in order to accomplish PD. Early PD technology required repeated insertions of the PD catheters each time the dialysis was to be performed. Tenckhoff and Schecter,[55] however, revolutionized chronic PD by developing a Silastic PD catheter which could be left in place indefinitely if proper technique in its placement and aftercare were practiced. The Tenckhoff PD catheter consists of a Silastic tube that has multiple side holes toward its peritoneal end to allow flow of the dialysate into the peritoneal cavity. Two Dacron cuffs anchor the catheter along its path in the abdominal wall, and scar tissue formed around these cuffs prevents entry of infection around the catheter into the peritoneal cavity. Several other catheters

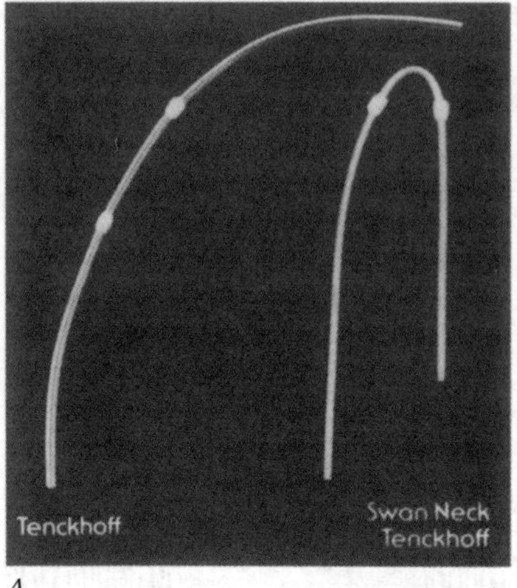

A

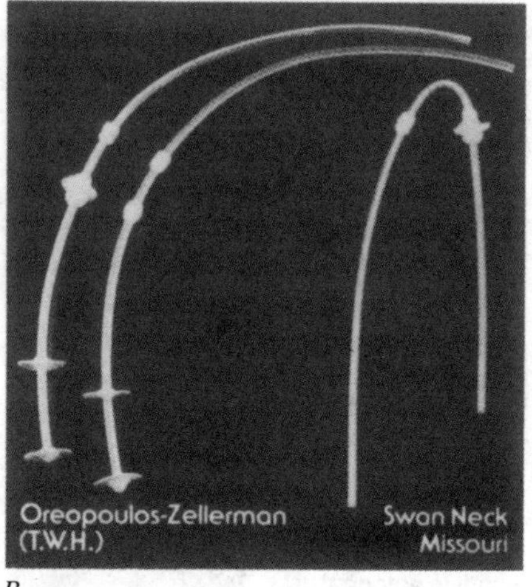

B

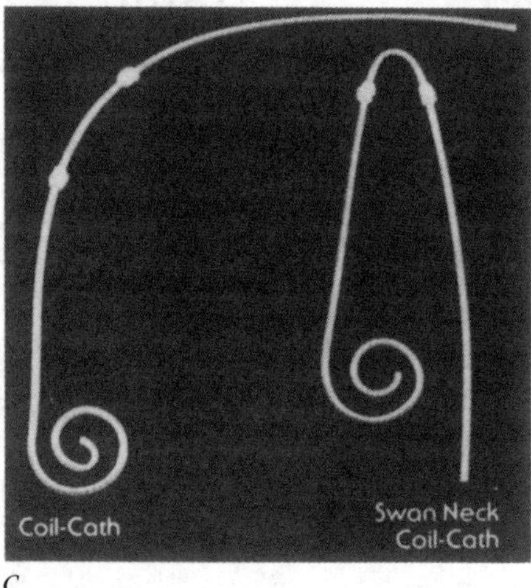

C

FIG. 18–10. **Various peritoneal dialysis catheters available for use in children. (Photographs coutesy of Accurate Surgical Instruments Corp., Toronto, Ontario, Canada.)**

that interpose barriers to infection along the catheter path or "tunnel" are now available for clinical use (Fig. 18–10). It has been argued that only one Dacron cuff on the PD catheter may not be an adequate barrier to infection; we generally prefer double-cuff catheters, since the rate of infection with the use of these seems to be less. An adult-sized catheter can be used for children >30 kg body weight; for patients between 10 and 30 kg weight, the pediatric-sized PD catheter is appropriate; and for infants <10 kg, an infant PD catheter can be used.

TABLE 18–5. Guidelines for Dialysis after PD Catheter Insertion

- Upon patient's return from the OR, infuse 10 mL/kg of 1.5% dextrose concentration with heparin (500 units/L) dialysis solution into the peritoneal cavity. Drain the dialysate after 5 to 10 min. Send specimen for cell count, Gram stain, and culture.
- Continue dialysis for the first 24 h with a dwell time of 2 to 4 h. The purpose of these exchanges is to remove blood, fibrin, and debris from the peritoneal cavity.
- If the fluid clears during the first 24 h, the dialysis can be discontinued.
- If the dialysate fluid does not clear, dialysis may be continued for another 24 h. Some centers advocate addition of antibiotics (250 mg/L of cefazolin) to the dialysate at this stage.
- Heparin is discontinued if cellular debris, blood, or fibrin are no longer present in the returning dialysate.
- The dialysis catheter is capped with heparinized saline and the patient is discharged home.
- Training for CAPD or CCPD starts 2 weeks after the catheter has been inserted.

CATHETER INSERTION

Insertion of a chronic PD catheter in children is done surgically under anesthesia and requires special attention in smaller children who may have a thin abdominal wall. If a double-cuff catheter is used, the cuffs are placed just above the peritoneum and just below the skin. In the single cuff catheter, the outer cuff (just below the skin) is eliminated. A partial or total omentectomy is often necessary in children, especially in infants, because of higher risk of developing outflow obstruction when the omentum wraps around the catheter. The inserted PD catheter should be directed toward the right or left pelvic fossa for optimal functioning. Before the patient leaves the operating room, catheter function is checked by irrigation and gravity drainage.

CATHETER CARE

If the patient requires dialysis urgently for treatment of uremia or other complications of ESRD, it may be undertaken soon after insertion of the PD catheter. In circumstances where the PD catheter has been placed electively, the first dialysis may be postponed until the surgical wounds have healed and fibrosis around the peritoneal dialysis cuffs has taken place to provide a seal against infection. Postponement of the first dialysis also reduces the chance of leakage of the dialysate around the catheter that may otherwise occur. Even if the first PD is postponed, the peritoneal cavity must be lavaged with the dialysate until the returning fluid is clear. The protocol for postinsertion care of the dialysis catheter used at our institution is given in Table 18–5. Heparinized dialysate (1 unit/mL) is then used to flush the catheter once or twice a week.

DIALYSIS PRESCRIPTION AND PROCEDURE FOR CAPD AND CCPD

The dialysate volume prescribed per exchange should be 20 to 40 mL/kg body weight and is determined by the patient's tolerance of the procedure. For CAPD,

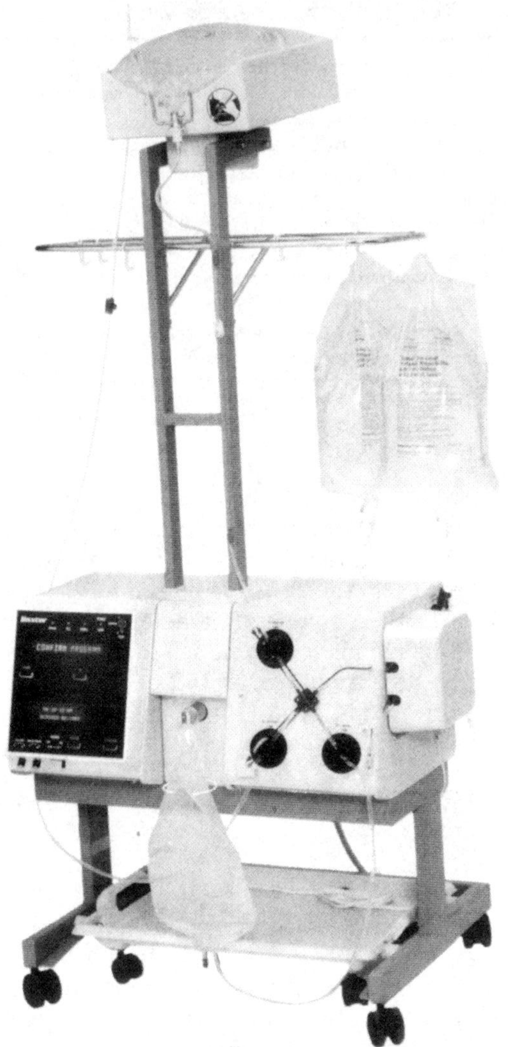

FIG. 18–11. The Pac-Xtra peritoneal dialysis cycler machine. (Photograph courtesy of Baxter Healthcare Corp., Deerfield, Illinois.)

four exchanges per day, of which three are conducted during the daytime and the fourth is allowed to dwell overnight, are sufficient to attain good biochemical control of uremia.[56] It is not necessary to add potassium to the dialysate during CAPD. The glucose concentration of the dialysate is adjusted to satisfy clinical requirements of achieving ideal dry weight and blood pressure. Last dwell is generally of a higher dextrose concentration dialysate than the daytime dwell. The CAPD exchanges are performed in a clean environment at school or home; dusty places should be avoided. In preparation for the exchange, face masks are worn by both the patient and the helper, if any. The scrub tray (or on-off tray) is opened and the dialysate bag and the transfer set are placed on a handling area or a table nearby. The catheter connector is scrubbed with Betadine for at least 2 min. The transfer set is opened and its proximal end is spiked

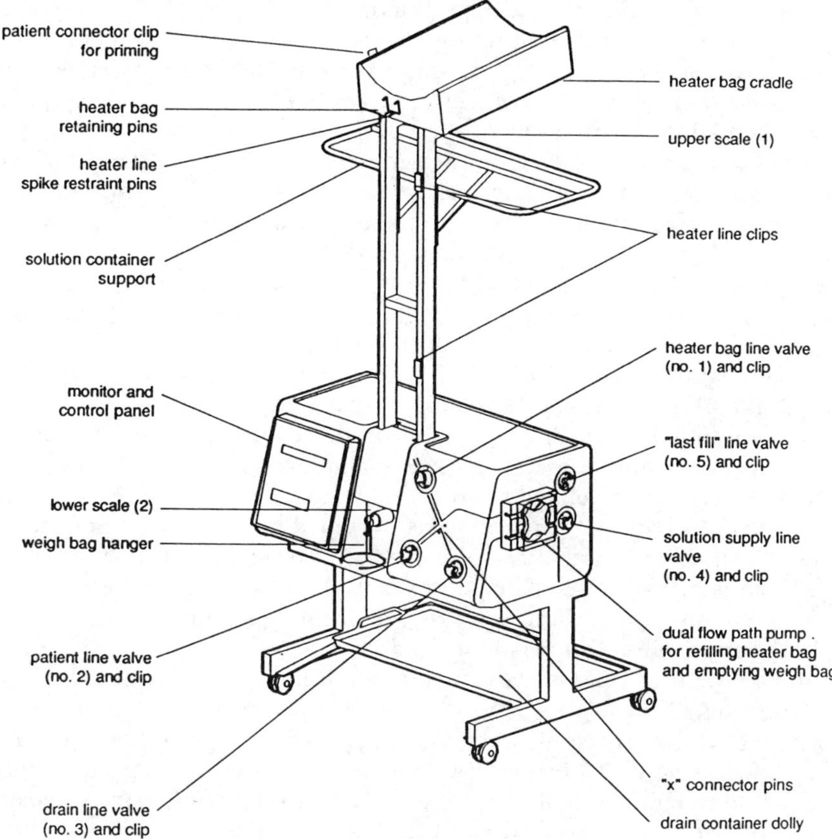

FIG. 18–12. Schematic representation of parts of Pac-Xtra cycler machine. (Photograph courtesy of Baxter Healthcare Corp., Deerfield, Illinois.)

into the dialysate bag aseptically. The distal end of the transfer set is connected to the previously cleaned PD catheter connector. The dialysate is allowed to flow by gravity into the peritoneal cavity. The connection between the transfer set and the PD catheter is wrapped with a Betadine-soaked gauze Connection Shield-III (Baxter Healthcare Corporation, Deerfield, Illinois) in order to lessen the chances of bacterial migration into the dialysate via this junction. The tubing and the empty PD bag are placed in a dressing pouch over the abdomen. Upon completion of the designated dwell time (usually 4 h), the dialysate in the peritoneal cavity is drained into the empty bag by gravity, the bag being then discarded and another cycle initiated.

Continuous cycling peritoneal dialysis requires the use of an automated peritoneal dialysis machine (Fig. 18–11 and 18–12). In general, these machines deliver prewarmed and premixed dialysate from a PD bag to the patient and also drain the dialysate at the end of a preset interval. The cycle is then repeated automatically for the number of times programmed into the cycler machine. One such machine introduced recently for clinical use (Pac-Xtra, Baxter Healthcare Corporation, Deerfield, Illinois) can deliver a minimum volume of 50 mL dialysate, which can be increased by increments of 10 mL. This assures the utility of the machine in CCPD therapy in a wide spectrum of pediatric patients, including neonates and young infants. Most of the automated PD cycler machines are monitored electronically; in case of malfunction, the apparatus activates an audible alarm and stops the cycler until corrective action is taken. The patient undergoing CCPD is connected to the automated PD machine in the evening, using the same precautions as outlined for CAPD. The volume and dextrose concentration of the dialysate to be used and the length of dwell time are determined by patient's clinical requirements. After the last fill in the morning, the patient is disconnected from the machine and the dialysate is allowed to dwell in the peritoneal cavity for the entire day. This is then drained in the evening, prior to the start of next dialysis cycle.

In a recent study, several CCPD dialysis regimens were evaluated to delineate the optimal dialysis therapy. Ten pediatric patients were assigned to undergo dialysis according to five different dialysis protocols. Over a 10-h period at night, the patients had 10 exchanges, 5 exchanges, or only 3 exchanges with or without a daytime dwell. Urea and creatinine clearances were measured for each protocol. Hourly nightime dialysis provided the best solute clearance. A daytime dwell further enhanced the total solute clearance and was recommended in anuric patients.[57] Alliapoulus et al.[56] found little difference in serum chemistry (sodium, potassium, total CO_2, chloride, phosphorus, calcium, alkaline phosphatase, albumin) between children who were treated with CAPD and those treated with CCPD. Only the mean creatinine value was significantly elevated (10.8 mg/dL versus 9.7 mg/dL) in CCPD patients when compared with CAPD patients. Blood urea nitrogen values are comparable in both groups. The primary advantage of CCPD over CAPD is that it allows the patient to undergo dialysis while sleeping and obviates the need for exchanges during the day. For vacations or out-of-town trips, the CCPD patients can be switched to CAPD temporarily by utilizing a special tubing set.

OTHER MEDICAL THERAPIES IN CHILDREN WITH ESRD

Dialysis as the renal replacement therapy for the management of ESRD cannot normalize all symptoms and signs of uremia. These patients suffer from significant biochemical derangements that need to be addressed in order to minimize the effects of toxins that accumulate as a result of chronic renal failure. The patients' nutrition, fluid and electrolyte balance, calcium and phosphorus balance, vitamin D requirements, anemia, and growth failure need to be evaluated periodically and addressed appropriately (Chap. 17). Of note is the fact that patients undergoing HD and PD lose folate during the procedures and need supplemental folic acid as long as dialysis therapy is required.

COMPLICATIONS OF PERITONEAL DIALYSIS

EXIT-SITE AND TUNNEL INFECTIONS

Infections affecting the skin where the PD catheter exits from the peritoneal cavity *(exit-site infections)* are frequently observed. Redness or tenderness of the exit site may be the only signs of an infection. In more advanced cases, purulent drainage or crusts may form around the exit site. However, early treatment with oral antibiotics and vigorous local cleaning and local application of antiseptic agents usually leads to a cure. If left untreated, an exit-site infection can lead to the spread of infection into the subcutaneous tunnel through which the catheter burrows into the peritoneal cavity *(tunnel infection)* and subsequently to peritonitis. Tunnel infection is characterized by tenderness along the subcutaneous path of the dialysis catheter. In these cases, removal of the catheter and reinsertion at a different site, in addition to the antibiotic therapy, is often required for adequate treatment.

PERITONITIS

The leading complication of PD is peritonitis. At the time of introduction of CAPD, a high risk of infection constituted a limiting factor in its acceptability. However, as a result of improvements in the technique and equipment for dialysis, the risk of peritonitis has steadily declined over the last 10 years. Although the incidence of peritonitis varies from center to center, data from major pediatric dialysis centers show that the incidence of peritonitis is 1 episode every 12 to 13 patient treatment months.[58,59] In general, the incidence of peritonitis in CAPD and CCPD is similar.[60,61]

The symptoms of peritonitis include nausea, fever, and abdominal pain, and the returning dialysate becomes cloudy. Often only one or two symptoms are present early in the course of the disease; physical findings of abdominal tenderness, guarding and rebound tenderness appear later. These symptoms can evolve within a short period of time. Poor patient motivation is a major risk factor for dialysis-associated peritonitis. Most episodes of dialysis-associated peritonitis result from failure to maintain asepsis, such as not wearing a mask during an exchange, not wearing sterile gloves, not cleaning the connector well prior to connecting the dialysis bag, or accidentally contaminating the connecting tube spike prior to putting it into the dialysate bag.[60] Gram-positive organisms *(S. epidermidis, S. aureus)* cause infection in almost half of the cases of PD-associated peritonitis, gram-negative bacteria account for 30 to 40 percent of cases, and culture-negative peritonitis has been reported in 10 to 20 percent of cases.[61,62] Fungal peritonitis may occur rarely, especially in immunosupressed patients.

The incidence of culture-negative peritonitis varies from center to center and may depend on the diligence with which cultures of the peritoneal fluid are obtained. Culture negativity of peritonitis may result from (1) improper collection technique of the PD fluid (2) prior antibiotic treatment, and (3) fungal or tubercular peritonitis.

TREATMENT OF PERITONITIS

Most patients with dialysis-associated peritonitis can be treated at home; however, hospitalization must be considered if the patient develops vomiting, fluid and electrolyte imbalance or systemic toxicity or if the infection has failed to resolve with appropriate antibiotic therapy. After collecting the dialysate for cell count, Gram's stain, and culture, three rapid dialysis exchanges are performed in order to remove debris from the peritoneal cavity. Subsequent dialysis is conducted with antibiotics and heparin (500 units per liter bag) added to the dialysate. Patients on CAPD can be started on their regular dialysis schedule after the initial exchanges, while those on CCPD may be managed by a long dwell-time (4 h) exchange on the machine for the first 48 h, following which a regular CCPD schedule may be instituted if the patient shows clinical improvement.

Gram-staining of the dialysate is helpful in deciding the initial antibiotic therapy required for the patient. Intraperitoneal instillation of antibiotics is sufficient to treat most episodes of dialysis-associated peritonitis. Cephalosporin antibiotics provide sufficient coverage against most of the gram-positive organisms that cause peritonitis; however, initial therapy should also include coverage against gram-negative organisms. This is done by adding gentamicin or other aminoglycosides into the dialysate. In patients suspected of having sepsis, systemic antibiotic therapy must be instituted. The antibiotic coverage must be reevaluated once culture results are available. In dialysis centers where methicillin-resistant staphylococci are prevalent, vancomycin should replace cephalosporin as the drug of choice for coverage of gram-positive organisms. Dosages of various antibiotics used in the treatment of dialysis-associated peritonitis are given in Table 18–6.

If the dialysis effluent fails to demonstrate clearing and reduction in cell count after 48 h, the dialysate should be recultured and the sensitivity of the organism reevaluated. Failure to eradicate peritoneal infection may suggest a tunnel infection or bacterial colonization of the catheter. Bacterial colonization of PD catheters may be facilitated by bacterial exopolysaccharide (also known as biofilm or slime). Removal of the infected catheter and insertion of a new one at another anatomic location may be necessary to treat both tunnel infection and bacterial colonization of the catheter; additionally, systemic antibiotics are required to treat tunnel infection.[63] Some workers have suggested that intraperitoneally instilled streptokinase may be helpful in disrupting biofilm and bacterial colonization on the PD catheter.[64] Antibiotic treatment for dialysis-associated peritonitis should be continued for at least 10 days in case of gram-positive infection and 14 days for gram-negative infection.[65] Treatment of fungal peritonitis is often difficult and requires systemic antifungal therapy and removal of the PD catheter.[66]

PREVENTION OF PERITONITIS

The best method of assuring the success of PD therapy is the prevention of peritonitis. In one study, preventable causes were reliably documented as an etiology of peritonitis in 45 percent of the cases; these included not wearing a mask during the dialysis exchange, not washing hands prior to bag exchange, and touching the tubing spike prior to insertion into the bag.[60] Therefore, the careful teaching of sterile techniques for dialysis becomes critically important in preventing peritonitis. An instructional manual detailing the need and the methods of maintaining sterile dialysis techniques should be supplied to the patients. Patients who have had an episode of peritonitis should be reeducated in the procedure. It is also important for patients to report exit-site infections promptly to their dialysis unit and be started on appropriate antibiotic treat-

TABLE 18–6. Intraperitoneal Antibiotic Dosage for Treatment of Peritonitis in Patients Undergoing PD[a]

	Dose			
	Initial		Maintenance	
	mg/kg	mg/2-L Bag	mg/L	Mg, Each 2-L Bag
Aminoglycosides				
Amikacin	5.0–7.5	350–500	6–7.5	12–15
Gentamicin	1.5–1.7	120	4–6	8–12
Netilmicin	1.5–2.0	140	4–6	8–12
Tobramycin	1.6–1.7	120	4–6	9–12
Cephalosporins				
Cefamandole	—	1000	ND	ND
Cefazolin	—	500–1000	125–250	250–500
Cefoperazone	—	2000	500	1000
Cefotaxime	—	2000	250	500
Cefoxitin	—	1000	100	200
Ceftazidime	—	1000	125	250
Ceftizoxime	—	1000	125	250
Ceftriaxone	—	1000	ND	ND
Cefuroxime	—	1500	250	500
Cephalothin	—	2000	250	500
Moxalactam	—	1000	ND	ND
Cephradine	—	500	125–250	250–500
Pencillins				
Ampicillin	—	500	50	100
Aziocillin	—	500	250	500
Vancomycin and others				
Vancomycin	—	1000	15	30
Aztreonam	—	1000	250	500
Clindamycin	—		150	300
Erythromycin	—	300	75	150
Antifungal				
Amphotericin	—	0.5	0.5	1
Miconazole	—	100	50	100

[a]The pharmacokinetic data and dosing recommendations presented here are based on published literature reviewed through January 1987 and personal experience. Those dosage recommendations which differ from product labeling are based on more recent experience.

Note: There is no evidence that mixing different antibiotics in dialysis fluid (except for aminoglycosides and penicillins) is deleterious for the drugs or patients. Do not use the same syringe to mix the different antibiotics.

Source: Modified and reproduced by permission from Keane WF, Everett ED, Fine RN, et al: CAPD-related peritonitis management and antibiotic therapy recommendations. *Perit Dial Bull* 7:55, 1987.

ment. Several devices for reducing the chances of bacterial contamination of the dialysate have been developed; these include one-way bacterial filters, portable ultraviolet sterilization apparatus, and a Y-set connection filled with disinfecting solution for CAPD patients.

NONINFECTIOUS COMPLICATIONS

Other complications related to the access to the peritoneal cavity are (1) obstruction of the dialysate flow and (2) dislocation of the catheter. Obstruction of the dialysate flow is usually caused by fibrin clots or omentum wrapped around the drainage holes of the dialysis catheter. Fibrin clot in the catheter may cause difficulty in both the inflow and the outflow of the dialysate through the catheter. On the other hand, in the early stages of dialysis, omental wrap around the catheter usually manifests itself as outflow obstruction. Under both circumstances irrigation of the catheter with saline to expel the clot, fibrin, or omentum stuck in the catheter can be tried. Bergstein et al.[67] have suggested intracatheter instillation of streptokinase to dissolve fibrin clots in partially thrombosed PD catheters. However, if none of the above-mentioned maneuvers succeeds in achieving the patency of the catheter, the catheter must be replaced surgically if PD therapy is to be continued.

Various types of hernias have been described in PD; von Lilien et al.[68] reported that the incidence of hernias was 40 percent among children undergoing PD. The incidence of hernias was highest in the very young children, possibly because of their thin abdominal walls. The most common location of hernias is ventral, followed by inguinal, umbilical, and scrotal. Incisional or umbilical hernias may also occur in some patients. Management of hernias includes reduction of dialysate volume, discontinuation of daytime dwell in patients undergoing CCPD, or even conversion of CAPD patients to the CCPD mode of dialysis. Surgical repair of the hernia is required in 75 percent of cases and should be undertaken as an elective procedure.[68]

Leakage of the dialysate along the catheter path usually occurs if the catheter is used prior to adequate healing of the surgical wound, especially if a large volume of dialysate is used. Reduction of the volume of the dialysate is often helpful in stopping the leak. A bloody effluent may infrequently be observed, especially in young, menstruating adolescents. Often, however, no obvious reason for the bleeding can be found. To prevent formation of blood clots and blockage of the dialysis catheter, heparin should be added to the dialysate.

RENAL TRANSPLANTATION IN PD PATIENTS

The optimal treatment modality for patients with ESRD is a successful renal transplantation. Concerns about an increased risk of infectious complications after transplantation in patients undergoing PD have been expressed in the past.[69] However, published data indicate that the incidence of serious infectious complications in children is not higher than those observed in other renal transplant recipients.[70,71] Graft and patient survival rates are comparable to patients who received HD or no dialysis at all. The PD catheter does not pose a significant problem after transplantation and can be left in place. The timing for removal of the PD catheter can coincide with the return of adequate renal function following transplantation. If the allograft function does not improve soon after transplantation, the PD catheter may be used to perform dialysis.

SUMMARY

Both CAPD and CCPD are accepted forms of renal replacement therapy in children. Enormous technologic developments over the past 15 years have made it possible to provide chronic dialysis therapy for children of all ages, including neonates. New technologies have also led to the production of recombinant erythropoietin and recombinant growth hormone and are expected to have a favorable effect on the management of these patients. Since symptomatic treatment and dialysis therapy can only improve the clinical manifestations of uremia and not correct them entirely, renal transplantation continues to be the ultimate goal.

APPENDIX: RECIRCULATION OF BLOOD IN A VASCULAR ACCESS

Despite all attempts, significant recirculation of blood may occur within the vascular accesses used for HD. Recirculation is a common problem if dialysis is performed using a single-lumen catheter and a uniclamp device. Recirculation decreases the efficiency of dialysis, and recirculation exceeding 10 percent should be considered unacceptable for chronic HD access. The percentage of blood recirculating through a vascular access can be calculated by using the following formula:

$$R = \frac{(\text{SUN} - \text{IUN})}{(\text{SUN} - \text{OUN})} \times 100$$

where R = recirculation in percentage, SUN = systemic BUN concentration obtained in the opposite limb, IUN = BUN concentration of the blood entering into the dialyzer, OUN = BUN concentration of the blood leaving the dialyzer.

Management of End-Stage Renal Disease in the 1990s: A Commentary

Richard N. Fine

The potential to avoid the devastating consequences of renal osteodystrophy, improve the growth retardation and avoid the clinical consequences of anemia, as well as the side effects of blood transfusions, has markedly changed the approach to the child with chronic renal disease (CRD). Prior to the availability of 1, 25-dihydroxyvitamin D_3, renal osteodystrophy was a common clinical consequence of renal failure in pediatric patients. Not only did the resulting deformities impair growth, but they also inhibited adequate ambulation. Despite corrective surgery, the cosmetic results were frequently suboptimal. With the assiduous attention to limiting dietary phosphorus intake and controlling the serum phosphorus level with appropriate phosphate binders, secondary hyperparathyroidism can be adequately controlled with the use of 1, 25-dihydroxyvitamin D_3. It is important in the pediatric patient to eliminate any excessive aluminum intake; the phosphate binder should not contain any aluminum. Calcium carbonate- or calcium acetate-containing phosphate binders are effective. It, therefore, can be anticipated in the decade of the 1990s that the child with end-stage renal disease (ESRD) will not develop the osseous deformities associated with renal osteodystrophy and secondary hyperparathyroidism and that this clinical consequence of uremia will not dictate the need to precipitously initiate ESRD therapy.

Even if renal osteodystrophy is eliminated and specific attention is paid to correct acidosis and encourage adequate caloric intake, growth retardation is a frequent concomitant of CRD in children. Until recently, no specific therapeutic intervention was uniformly successful in correcting the growth retardation associated with CRD in children. The recent demonstration that supraphysiologic doses of recombinant human growth hormone (rhGH) can produce an acceleration in growth velocity in children with CRD has had a dramatic impact on this devastating clinical consequence. Although the numbers of children who have been treated for a protracted period of time are limited, it does appear from the available data that it is possible to correct the growth retardation to the extent that the patients achieve the fiftieth percentile for their mid-parental height. This can occur despite declining renal function and the need to initiate dialysis. In the past, persistent growth retardation has precipitated the need for preemptive dialysis and/or transplantation. It can be anticipated that during the decade of the 1990s such preemptive therapeutic interventions would be obviated with the availability of rhGH. Hopefully, such therapeutic intervention will assure that children with CRD will achieve their genetic adult height.

Anemia was a frequent consequence of chronic renal failure and usually has its onset when the glomerular filtration rate (GFR) approaches 30 mL/min/1.73 m^2. Until the recent availability of recombinant human erythropoietin (rHuEpo), the only treatment for symptomatic anemia in the pediatric patient with chronic renal failure was repetitive blood transfusions. The use of rHuEpo in such children has a remarkable effect on the symptomatology that in the past had been ascribed to uremia. Lethargy, anorexia, and lassitude have been replaced with a sense of well-being following the correction of anemia with the use of rHuEpo. This has facilitated participation in normal routine daily activities with appropriate functioning at school despite declining renal function. It would be anticipated in the 1990s that anemia would be totally avoided in a child with chronic renal disease and that rHuEpo would be initiated before any of the symptoms attributable to anemia would develop.

The utilization of 1, 25-dihydroxyvitamin D_3, rhGH, and rHuEpo to avoid renal osteodystrophy, growth retardation, and anemia will undoubtedly impact on the criteria utilized in the 1990s for initiating ESRD care. It can be anticipated that a child with the onset of renal insufficiency during the first year of life could go through puberty prior to the need for ESRD care and avoid the occurrence of bone disease, attain a normal stature, and have an adequate sense of well-being without concomitant anemia. If the above becomes a reality, the care of children with ESRD in the 1990s will change markedly.

REFERENCES

1. Potter DE, Holliday MA, Piel CF, et al: Treatment of end-stage renal disease in children: A 15 year experience. *Kidney Int* 18:103, 1980
2. Egger PW: Personal communication, 1990.
3. Rizzoni G, Ehrich JHH, Brunner FP, et al: Combined report on regular dialysis and transplantation in Europe. *Nephrol Dial Transplant* 4(suppl 4):31, 1989.
4. U.S Renal Data Systems: *USRDS 1990 Annual Data report.* Bethesda, Maryland, National Institute of Diabetes, Digestive and Kidney Diseases, August 1990, p A-1.
5. Avner ED, Harmon WE, Grupe WE, et al: Mortality of chronic hemodialysis and renal transplantation in pediatric end-stage renal disease. *Pediatrics* 67:412, 1981.
6. Foreman JW, Chan JMC: 10-year survey of referrals to a pediatric nephrology program. *Child Nephrol Urol* 10:8, 1990.
7. Rotundo A, Nevins TE, Lipton M, et al: Progressive encephalopathy in children with chronic renal insufficiency in infancy. *Kidney Int* 21:486, 1982.
8. Raskin HN, Fishman RA. Neurologic disorders in renal failure. *N Engl J Med* 294:143, 1976.
9. So SKS, Chang PN, Najarian JS, et al: Growth and development in infants after transplantation. *J Pediatr* 110:343, 1987.
10. Davis ID, Chang PN, Nevins TE: Successful renal transplantation accelerates development in young children. *Pediatrics* 86:594, 1990.
11. Reimold EW: Chronic progressive renal failure: Rate of progression monitored by change in serum creatinine concentration. *Am J Dis Child* 135:1039, 1981.
12. Fine RN: The therapeutic approach to the infant, child, and adolescent with end-stage renal disease. *Pediatr Clin North Am* 34:789, 1987.
13. Leichter HE, Salusky IB, Alliapoulos JC, et al: CAPD and CCPD: An experience of 3-1/2 years. *Dial Transpl* 13:382, 1983.
14. Balfe JW, Vigneaux A, Williamsen J, et al: The use of CAPD in the treatment of children with end-stage renal disease. *Perit Dial Bull* 1:35, 1981.
15. Warady BA, Hellerstein S, Alon U: Letter to the editors. *Pediatr Nephrol* 4:96, 1990.
16. Penn I, Renal transplantation for Wilms tumor: Report of 20 cases. *J Urol* 12:793, 1979.
17. Hutchings RH, Hickman R, Scribner BH: Chronic hemodialysis in a preadolescent. *Pediatrics* 37:68, 1966.
18. Pillion G, Maisin A, Macher MA, et al: Hickman catheter for hemodialysis in paediatric patients. *Pediatr Nephrol* 2:318, 1988.
19. Mahn JD Jr., Mauer SM, Nevins TE: The Hickman catheter: A new access device for infants and small children. *Kidney Int* 24:694, 1983.
20. Cheesbrough JS, Finch RG, Burden RP: A prospective study of infection associated with hemodialysis catheters. *J Infect Dis* 154:579, 1986.
21. Almirall J, Gonzalez J, Rello J, et al: Infection of hemodialysis catheters: Incidence and mechanisms. *Am J. Nephrol* 9:454, 1989.

22. Uldall PR, Merchant N, Woods F, et al: Changing subclavian hemodialysis cannulas to reduce infections. Lancet 1981; 1:1373.
23. Quinton W, Dillard O, Scribner BH: Cannulation of blood vessels for prolonged hemodialysis. *Trans Am Soc Artif Intern Organs* 6:68, 1960.
24. Franzone AJ, Tucker BL, Brennan LP, et al: Hemodialysis in children. *Arch Surg* 102:529, 1971.
25. Idriss FS, Nikaidoh H, King LR, et al: Arteriovenous shunts for hemodialysis in infants and children. *J Pediatr Surg* 6:639, 1971.
26. Brescia MJ, Cimino JE, Appel K, et al: Chronic hemodialysis using venipuncture and a surgically created arteriovenous fistula. *N Engl J Med* 275:1089, 1966.
27. Gagnadoux MF, Pascal B, Bronstein M, et al: Arteriovenous fistula in small children. *Dial Transplant* 9:318, 1980.
28. Sicard GA, Merrell RC, Etheredge EE, et al: Subcutaneous arteriovenous dialysis fistulas in pediatric patients. *Trans Am Soc Artif Intern Organs* 24:695, 1978.
29. Latimer RG, Gebhart WF, Freidell HV, et al: Comparison of chronic hemodialysis angioaccess procedures. *Dial Transplant* 9:499, 1980.
30. O'Regan S, Villemant D. Ducharme G, et al: Effects of Brescia-Cimino fistulae on myocardial function in pediatric patients. *Dial Transplant* 10:202, 1981.
31. Lazarus JM: Complications in hemodialysis: An overview. *Kidney Int* 18:783, 1980.
32. Graefe V, Milutinovich J, Follette WC, et al: Less dialysis-induced mortality and vascular instability with bicarbonate in dialysate. *Ann Intern Med* 88: 332, 1978.
33. Kjellstrand CM: Techniques of paediatric haemodialysis. *Gambro Symposium on Pediatric Hemodialysis, Lund, Sweden,* 1972, pp 18–34.
34. Leanza H, Ryan C, Rivarola G, et al: Very low-dose heparin hemodialysis in high-risk patients. *Dial Transplant,* 18:556, 1989.
35. Campese VM: Cardiovascular instability during hemodialysis. *Kidney Int* 33(suppl 24):S-186, 1988.
36. Sherman RA, Rubin MP, Cody RP, et al: Amelioration of hemodialysis-associated hypotension by the use of cold dialysate. *Am J Kidney Dis* 5:124, 1986.
37. Henderson LW, Koch KM, Dinarello CA, et al: Hemodialysis hypotension: The interleukin hypothesis. *Blood Purification* 1:3, 1983.
38. Mahida BH, Dumler F, Zasuwa G, et al: Effect of cooled dialysate on serum catecholamines and blood pressure stability. *Trans Am Soc Artif Intern Organs* 29:384, 1983.
39. Sherman RA, Goodling KA, Eisinger RP: Acute therapy of hemodialysis-related muscle cramps. *Am J Kidney Dis* 2:287, 1982.
40. Neal CR, Resnikoff E, Unje AM: Treatment of dialysis related muscle cramps with hypertonic dextrose. *Arch Intern Med* 141:171, 1981.
41. Raskin NH, Fishman RA: Neurologic disorders in renal failure. *N Engl J Med* 294:204, 1976.
42. Arieff AI, Massry SG, Barriendos A, et al: Brain water and electrolyte metabolism in uremia: Effects of slow and rapid hemodialysis. *Kidney Int* 4:177, 1973.
43. Arieff AI, Guisado R, Massry SA, et al: Central nervous system pH in uremia and the effects of hemodialysis. *J Clin Invest* 58:306, 1976.
44. Polinsky MS: Neurologic complications of ESRD, dialysis and transplantation, in: Fine RN, Gruskin AB (eds): *End Stage Renal Disease in Children.* Philadelphia, Saunders, 1984, 307–339.
45. Swartz RD: Hemorrhage during high-risk hemodialysis using controlled heparinization. *Nephrology* 28:65, 1981.

46. Gotch FA, Keen ML: Precise control of minimal heparinization for high bleeding risk hemodialysis. *Trans Am Soc Artif Intern Organs* 23:168, 1977.
47. Mannucci PM, Remuzzi G, Pusineri F, et al: Deamino-8-d-arginine vasopressin shortens the bleeding time in uremia. *N Engl J Med* 308:8, 1983.
48. Ganter G: Uber die Beseitigung giftiger Stoffe aus dem Blute durch Dialyse. *Münch Med Wochenschr* 70:1478, 1923.
49. Popovich RP, Moncrief JW, Decherd JB, et al: The definition of a novel portable/wearable equilibrium peritoneal dialysis technique. *Trans Am Soc Artif Intern Org* (Abstract) 5:64, 1976.
50. Esperanca MJ, Collins DL: Peritoneal dialysis efficiency in relation to body weight. *J Pediatr Surg* 1:162, 1966.
51. Gosselin RE, Berndt WO: Diffusional transport or solute through mesentery and peritoneum. *J Theor Biol* 3:487, 1962.
52. Rubin J, Nolph KD, Krfnia D, et al: Protein loss in continuous ambulatory peritoneal dialysis. *Nephron* 28:218, 1981.
53. Popovich RE, Moncrief JW, Nolph KD, et al: Continuous ambulatory peritoneal dialysis. *Ann Intern Med* 88:449, 1978.
54. Kohaut EC: The effect of dialysate volume on ultrafiltration in young patients treated with CAPD. *Int J Pediatr Nephrol* 7:13, 1985.
55. Tenckhoff H, Schecter H: A bacteriologically safe peritoneal access device. *Trans Am Soc Artif Intern Organs* 14:181, 1968.
56. Alliapoulos JC, Salusky IB, Hall T, et al: Comparison of continuous cycling peritoneal dialysis with continuous ambulatory peritoneal dialysis in children. *J Pediatr* 111:513, 1987.
57. Leichter HE, Salusky IB, von Lilien T, et al: Peritoneal clearances with different dialysis regimens in children undergoing continuous cycling peritoneal dialysis. *Nephrol Dial Transplant* 4:893, 1989.
58. Balfe JW, Vigneaux A, Williamsen J, et al: The use of CAPD in the treatment of children with endstage renal disease. *Perit Dial Bull* 1:35, 1981.
59. Fine RN, Salusky IB, Hall T, et al: Peritonitis in children undergoing continuous ambulatory peritoneal dialysis. *Pediatrics* 71:806, 1983.
60. Warady BA, Campoy SF, Gross SP, et al: Peritonitis with continuous ambulatory peritoneal dialysis and continuous cycling peritoneal dialysis. *J Pediatr* 105:726, 1984.
61. Southwest Pediatric Nephrology Study Group: Continuous ambulatory and continuous cycling peritoneal dialysis in children: A report of the southwest Pediatric Nephrology Group. *Kidney Int* 27:558, 1985.
62. Salusky IB, Koppel JD, Fine RN: Continuous ambulatory peritoneal dialysis in pediatric patients. *Kidney Int* 24(suppl 15):S101, 1983.
63. Paterson AD, Bishop MC, Morgan AG, et al: Removal and replacement of Tenckhoff catheter at a single operation: Successful treatment of resistant peritonitis in continuous ambulatory peritoneal dialysis. *Lancet* 2:1245, 1986.
64. Norris KC, Shinaberger JH, Reyes GD, et al: The use of intracatheter instillation of streptokinase in the treatment of recurrent bacterial peritonitis in continuous ambulatory peritoneal dialysis. *Am J Kid Dis* 10:62, 1987.
65. Keane WF, Everett ED, Fine RN: CAPD related peritonitis management and antibiotic therapy recommendations. *Perit Dial Bull* 7:55, 1987.
66. Rault R. Candida peritonitis complicating chronic peritoneal dialysis: A report of five cases and review of the literature. *Am J Kidney Dis* 5:544, 1983.

67. Bergstein, JM, Andreoli SP, West KW, et al: Streptokinase therapy for occluded Tenckhoff catheters in children on CAPD. *Perit Dial Bull* 8:137, 1988.
68. von Lilien T, Salusky IB, Yap HK, et al: Hernias: a frequent complication of children treated with continuous peritoneal dialysis. *Am J Kid Dis* 10:356, 1987.
69. Cardella CJ: Renal transplantation in patients on peritoneal dialysis. *Perit Dial Bull* 1:12, 1980.
70. Leichter HE, Salusky IB, Ettenger RD, et al: Experience with renal transplantation in children undergoing peritoneal dialysis. *Am J Kid Dis* 8:181, 1986.
71. Malgon M, Hogg RJ: Renal transplantation after prolonged dwell peritoneal dialysis in children. *Kidney Int* 31:981, 1987.

19

RENAL TRANSPLANTATION

Kanwal K. Kher
Philip C. Guzzetta
Lamya Alarif

Chronic renal failure poses a considerable risk of growth retardation, bone disease, and neurodevelopmental delay in children, particularly infants. Despite the provision of appropriate medical therapy, attention to nutrition, treatment of anemia, and institution of dialysis, the problems of children advancing to end-stage renal disease (ESRD) remain unremitting. Because of these concerns, renal transplantation is regarded as the ideal option for the treatment of such children. It is generally recommended that all children with ESRD be considered for renal transplantation as soon as such a therapy becomes necessary. In the United States, a large percentage of such children receive dialysis therapy prior to renal transplantation, but some undergo transplantation preemptively, without going through an interval of dialysis. The care of children with ESRD is ideally provided by a team made up of a nephrologist, transplant surgeon, dialysis nurse, nutritionist, and social service worker, all of whom are involved in pre- and posttransplant management. The ESRD team ensures appropriate perioperative and continued long-term care of children requiring renal transplantation.

HISTORICAL PERSPECTIVES

Although solid organ transplantation has been contemplated since antiquity, serious scientific studies have been performed only during the twentieth century. The development of vascular suturing techniques by Alexis Carrel, for which he was given the Nobel Prize in 1912, established the methods by which solid organs could be transplanted. In the early 1900s, attempts at transplanting renal xenografts from animals to the arms of uremic humans, met with almost immediate failure despite the technical success of the vascular anastomoses,[1] suggesting an unknown barrier to transplantation between species.

These early failures convinced many physicians that solid organ transplantation was not possible, and little further clinical experimentation was done until after 1950. In 1953, Michon[2] reported a renal transplant from a mother to her son, who had suffered the loss of his solitary kidney in an accident. The kidney allograft functioned for 22 days; then it failed acutely and the recipient died. The first successful renal transplant between identical twins was performed in 1954 by Murray[3] in Boston. For his pioneering work in the field of transplantation, Murray received the Nobel Prize in Medicine in 1990.

Although transplantation was now feasible technically, it was clear that the prevention of allograft rejection by the host constituted an essential key to the adoption of renal transplantation as a viable form of therapy. Attempts at total body irradiation as a method of immunosuppression led to the lethal consequences of radiation illness and infection.[4] The development of immunosuppression protocols using 6-mercaptopurine, its derivative azathioprine, and prednisone in the early 1960s made genetically disparate living related donor (LRD) and cadaver renal transplants a viable alternative to dialysis.[5,6] Interestingly, it was not until 1964 that genetically determined tissue typing of the donor and the recipient was utilized to select recipients for kidney allografts.[7] The next major advance in immunosuppression occurred with the development of polyclonal antibodies to human lymphocytes.[8] The use of cyclosporine, which became available in 1984, dramatically improved the success rate of kidney allografts, marking another important milestone in the history of transplantation.[9] The development of OKT3, a murine monoclonal antibody to human T-cell surface antigen, has significantly improved the outcome of patients with steroid-resistant acute rejection.[10] More potent and specific immunosuppressive agents are being developed, and the infusion of bone marrow from the kidney donor, in an attempt to induce a form of tolerance, is undergoing clinical trials.[11]

IMMUNOLOGY OF TRANSPLANTATION

In 1966, Van Rood[12] demonstrated that ABO blood group and HLA system antigens were both important to the survival of transplanted grafts. He found that the survival of skin transplants between twins who were HLA- and ABO-identical was significantly better than that of transplants between siblings who were identical for only one of these systems. Consequently, the genetically determined ABO blood group as well as the HLA system antigens were recognized as the primary immunologic barriers to transplantation. Antigens of the ABO system are present on the red blood cells, while those belonging to the HLA system are present on the surface of all nucleated cells.

ABO SYSTEM

ABO incompatibility between donor and recipient is considered to be an absolute contraindication to transplantation; the same rules that govern matching for ABO compatibility in blood transfusion apply for solid organ transplants. Accordingly, blood group O donors are considered "universal donors" and those with the blood group AB are the "universal recipients." Patients with blood group O can, obviously, receive allografts only from blood group O kidney donors. Renal transplantation between an ABO-incompatible donor and host results in hyperacute rejection of the allograft, but rare instances of ABO-incompatible renal transplantation have been recorded.[13] The Lewis blood group has also been considered to be important in transplantation by some,[14] but its significance has not been fully determined.

HLA SYSTEM AND TRANSPLANTATION

The HLA antigen system represents the major histocompatibility (MHC) antigens in man. The term *HLA* is derived from the fact that these antigens were discovered initially on the lymphocytes and were called the *human lymphocyte system A.*[15] Because of its convenience, usage of this term has continued. The HLA system is the most complex and highly polymorphic genetic system known in humans. Products of the HLA gene complex (antigens) are inherited in a Mendelian codominant fashion. Offspring will inherit one haplotype from each parent, and there is random segregation of the haplotypes; only 25 percent will be HLA-identical, 50 percent will be haplo-identical, and 25 percent will be nonidentical. Although full matching for all six HLA antigens routinely determined prior to transplantation in unrelated cadaver donor-recipient selection has been shown to improve long-term graft survival,[16] the extreme polymorphism* of this system makes the selection of HLA identity in the random population a rare event. The chance of being able to obtain an HLA-identical cadaveric donor varies from 1 in 100 to 1 in 10,000, depending on the gene frequency of the alleles in different ethnic and racial groups.

Clarification of the structure and function of the MHC (which is known as HLA in man) has taken place over the past 40 years. These efforts started with the description of HLA antisera in the early 1950s and culminated in the characterization of the three-dimensional structure of the HLA-A2 molecule by x-ray crystallography.[17] The HLA genetic unit is located on the short arm of chromosome 6 in humans and has three distinct genetic regions known as the HLA class I region, HLA class III region, and HLA class II region (also known as the HLA-D region).[18] These gene-bearing regions are not contiguous; class I and II regions are located toward the ends of the chromosome, while class III is interposed between them (Fig. 19–1). Genes in the HLA class I region code for HLA-A, B, and C antigens, which consist of a 45 kDa heavy-chain and a light-chain β_2-microglobulin. Genes in the class II region code for HLA-DR, DQ, and DP antigens. In addition, the class II region contains other genes whose genetic functions remain an enigma. Class II antigens consist of an α chain and a β chain. The Class III region contains at least 21 transcribed genes, some of which code for serum complement components C2 and C4 and properdin factor B. The class III region also contains the gene which codes for the enzymes 21 hydroxylase and tumor necrosis factors TNFα and TNFβ. Table 19–1 shows a recent listing of recognized HLA specificities.

*Polymorphism denotes the occurrence of two or more genetically determined forms of the gene.

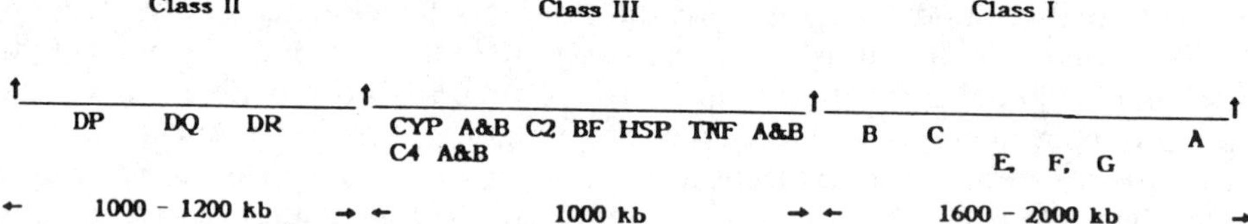

FIG. 19–1. Human HLA complex on the short arm of chromosome six. [From Dupont B: The HLA system: An introduction, in John Lee (ed): *The HLA System: A New Approach*. New York, Springer-Verlag, 1990, p 1. Reproduced by permission.]

TECHNIQUES OF HLA TYPING

Different techniques have been developed to detect HLA antigens (alleles) in humans; all those in current use utilize lymphocytes as the marker cells. Tissue typing and identification of class I alleles (antigens) is done by the serologic technique of complement-dependent microcytotoxicity test, which was first described by Terasaki and McClelland[19] in 1964 (Fig. 19–2). Class II alleles (DR, DQ, DP, Dw52, Dw53) may also be identified using serologic techniques of enriched B-cell preparation or two-color fluorescence.[20] Other D-region specificities are identified using cellular assays such as mixed leukocyte culture reaction (MLC), homozygous typing cells (HTC), and the primed lymphocyte test (PLT).[21] The originally described serologic techniques for identification of HLA alleles are being supplemented by molecular genetics technology such as gene amplification and sequence-specific oligonucleotide probe hybridization.[22] Further refinements of these techniques are expected in the future.

HLA MATCHING AND GRAFT SURVIVAL

Despite early enthusiasm, the value of HLA matching in renal transplantation is uncertain, and a clear understanding and consensus regarding the role of HLA matching in renal transplantation is controversial. Based on the currently available information, the following comments in relation to the role of HLA matching in renal transplantation can be made:

1. HLA matching cannot be considered the sole determinant of the outcome and survival of renal transplants.
2. Perfect or six-antigen HLA-match renal transplantation carries a better long-term survival rate than do grafts with a lesser degree of HLA matching.[16]
3. Renal transplantation with zero HLA match (or six-antigen mismatch) can be performed. Unlike ABO, such an incompatibility does not necessarily lead to hyperacute rejection of the allograft.[23,24]

PANEL REACTIVE ANTIBODY TESTING

Patients who require renal transplantation may develop anti-HLA antibodies, leading to hyperacute rejection of the allograft. Such HLA sensitization results

TABLE 19–1. HLA Specificities in Humans

A	B	C	D	DR	DQ	DP
A1	B5	Cw1	Dw1	DR1	DQw1	DPw1
A2	B7	Cw2	Dw2	DR2	DQw2	DPw2
A3	B8	Cw3	Dw3	DR3	DQw3	DPw3
A9	B1	Cw4	Dw4	DR4	DQw4	DPw4
A10	B1	Cw5	Dw5	DR5	DQw5(w1)	DPw5
A11	B14	Cw6	Dw6	DRw6	DQw6(w1)	DPw6
Aw19	B15	Cw7	Dw7	DR7	DQw7(w3)	
A23(9)	B16	Cw8	Dw8	DRw8	DQw8(w3)	
A24(9)	B17	Cw9(w3)	Dw9	DR9	DQw9(w3)	
A25(10)	B18	Cw10(w3)	Dw10	DRw10		
A26(10)	B21	Cw11	Dw11(w7)	DRw11(5)		
A28	Bw22		Dw12	DRw12(5)		
A29(w19)	B27		Dw13	DRw13(w6)		
A30(w19)	B35		Dw14	DRw14(w6)		
A31(w19)	B37		Dw15	DRw15(2)		
A32(w19)	B38(16)		Dw16	DRw16(2)		
Aw33(w19)	B39(16)		Dw17(w7)	DRw17(3)		
Aw34(10)	B40		Dw18(w6)	DRw18(3)		
Aw36	Bw41		Dw19(w6)			
Aw43	Bw42		Dw20	DRw52		
Aw66(10)	B44(12)		Dw21	DRw53		
Aw68(28)	B45(12)		Dw22			
Aw69(28)	Bw46		Dw23			
Aw74(w19)	Bw47		Dw24			
	Bw48		Dw25			
	B49(21)		Dw26			
	Bw50(21)					
	B51(5)					
	Bw52(5)					
	Bw53					
	Bw54(w22)					
	Bw55(w22)					
	Bw56(w22)					
	Bw57(17)					
	Bw58(17)					
	Bw59					
	Bw60(40)					
	Bw61(40)					
	Bw62(15)					
	Bw63(15)					
	Bw64(14)					
	Bw65(14)					
	Bw67					
	Bw70					
	Bw71(w70)					
	Bw72(w70)					
	Bw73					
	Bw75(15)					
	Bw76(15)					
	Bw77(15)					

Source: Dupont B: The HLA system: an introduction, in John Lee (ed): *The HLA System: A New Approach*. New York, Springer-Verlag, 1990, p 17. Reproduced by permission.

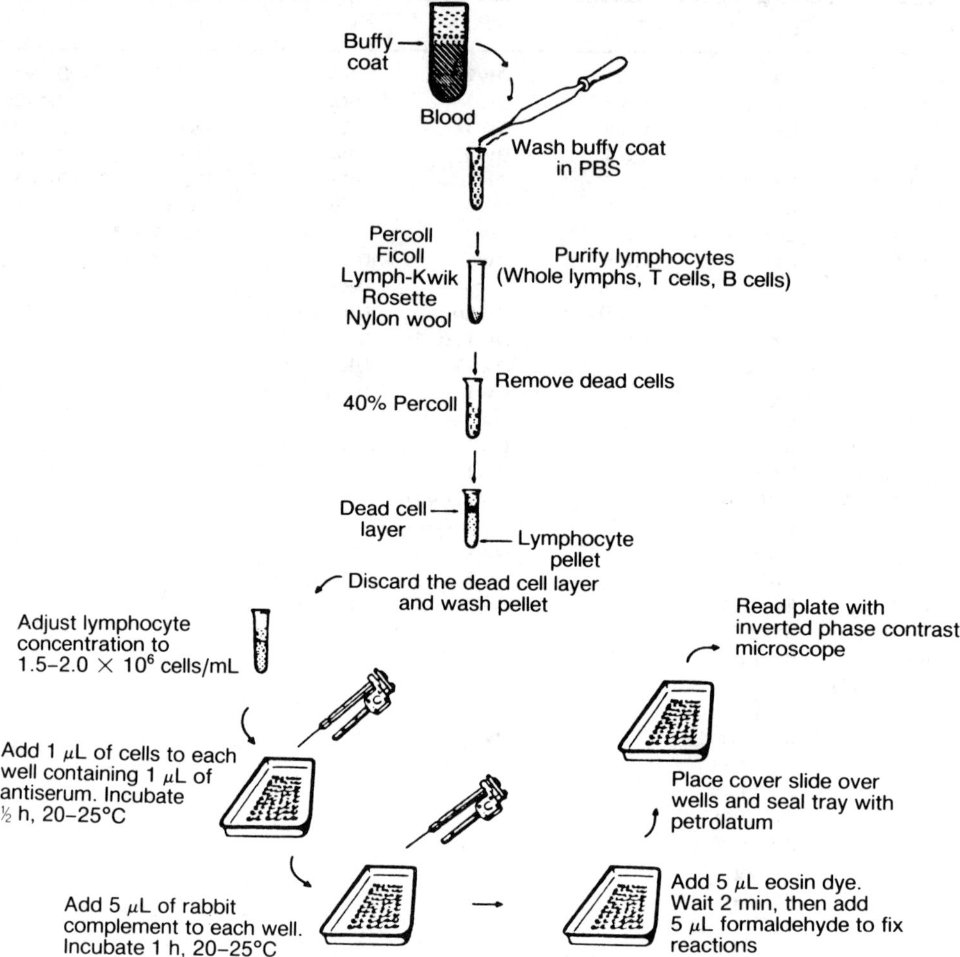

FIG. 19–2. The microdroplet cytotoxicity test procedure used for tissue typing. [From Cecka JM, Terasaki PI: Tissue typing and histocompatibility. In Toledo-Pereyra LH (ed): *Kidney Transplantation*. Philadelphia, F. A. Davis Company, 1988. Reproduced by permission.]

from three sources: pregnancy (HLA antigens from the father present on fetus's white cells), blood transfusions, and previous organ grafts. The serum of patients awaiting cadaver renal transplants is tested periodically (usually monthly) for such antibodies against a panel of lymphocytes (minimum of 60 cells) obtained from a randomly selected population. Such testing indicates the likelihood of finding preformed anti-HLA antibodies in the recipient that would result in a positive crossmatch if an organ were available for transplantation to the patient. This is commonly known as the *panel reactive antibody (PRA) test.* A potential transplant recipient is defined as being highly sensitized if his or her PRA $\geq$ 80 percent. These patients invariably come up positive on the final crossmatch. The accuracy and value of PRA testing depends on the choice of the test panel, the frequency of each HLA antigen tested, and data analysis to determine the exact sensitizing antigen, acceptable mismatches, and nonacceptable mismatches for each patient.

CROSSMATCHING

Crossmatching is the final critical test performed prior to renal transplantation. The patient's undiluted and diluted serum (up to 1:32) is reacted against the donor's lymphocytes in an effort to detect any preformed cytotoxic lymphocytotoxic antibodies in the recipient that are directed against that specific donor's T and B cells. These antibodies have been shown to cause hyperacute rejection.[25] Because of refinements in immunology techniques, the significance of a positive conventional lymphocytotoxic crossmatch has undergone some rethinking over the years. One of the recent findings is that autoantibodies of the IgM class can give rise to a false-positive crossmatch as well as high PRAs in patients awaiting renal transplantation[26]—a discovery that has led to modifications of the conventional crossmatch techniques. One of these modifications involves pretreatment of the recipients's serum with either dithiothreitol (DTT) or dithioerythritol (DTE). Both of these reducing agents degrade the S-S bonds of the IgM autoantibodies so that a true crossmatch with IgG antibodies can be evaluated. A negative crossmatch with DTE/DTT pretreated serum in face of a positive conventional lymphocytotoxic crossmatch may be interpreted to mean that renal transplantation could be undertaken without the danger of hyperacute rejection.[26] Another sensitive technique for performing lymphocytotoxic crossmatches, using flowcytometer technology, was developed in the 1980s. This test provides a quantitative and sensitive method (100 times more sensitive than the serologic method) of detecting T- and B-cell-bound class-specific antibody.[27]

CADAVER RENAL TRANSPLANTATION AND ORGAN SHARING

Because of a shortage of available organs for transplantation in the United States, Congress passed the National Transplantation Act in 1984 (Public Law 98-507). As a consequence, the Department of Health and Human Services established a Task Force on Organ Transplantation which recommended establishing an Organ Procurement and Transplantation Network (OPTN). The OPTN is currently operated under contract by a nonprofit organization known as the United Network for Organ Sharing (UNOS). The purpose of UNOS is to ensure a fair and an equitable distribution of available organs to all the patients in need of them. The UNOS runs a 24-h computerized network which allocates cadaveric kidneys that become available for transplantation throughout the United States. Those ESRD patients who opt for renal transplantation are registered with UNOS at their request through their respective transplant centers.

When a cadaver kidney becomes available for transplantation, the UNOS computer determines ranking and priority for each of the enrolled patients and formulates a list of potential recipients. The UNOS ranking list is based on a point system determined by the patient's age, length of time spent on dialysis, blood group, and PRA status. Children below 10 years of age, patients who have been on dialysis longer, and those with high PRAs are given extra points. Currently, there are over 17,000 patients awaiting cadaveric kidneys (UNOS update, September/October 1990). Children often do not effectively compete for the available organs because most have relatively low PRA titers. Although efforts are being made by UNOS to enhance a child's likelihood of receiving an organ, the organs offered to our patients continue to be from young pediatric donors. These, unfortunately, have a relatively low 1-year survival rate. With the 100-percent function rate of LRD transplants at our institution in the last 5 years and the distressing shortage of cadaveric kidneys from donors older than 5 years, we prefer LRD transplantation whenever possible.

PROCUREMENT AND ALLOCATION OF CADAVERIC KIDNEYS

Once a cadaveric kidney becomes available, the donor hospital contacts the organ procurement organization (OPO) operating in the region, which then enters donor data into the UNOS computer. The computer generates a list of potential recipients by rank. In general, UNOS policies advocate allocating available solid organs in the following order of preference: (1) locally, (2) within the UNOS region, and then (3) nationally. The next step requires the UNOS transplant coordinator to contact the transplant coordinators of all the OPOs on the computer-generated list, informing them of the availability of a kidney. The OPO transplant coordinator, in turn, contacts the transplant center physician of the listed patient(s) in the area. The contact physician for the patient decides whether the available kidney is suitable for the patient and if the patient is medically fit to undergo the procedure at that time. On the basis of the response of the transplant centers contacted, a revised rank-order list is developed. The organ is then air-shipped or surface-transported to the center where the patient ranking first on the UNOS list is located—provided, of course, that this patient is considered fit to undergo transplantation at that time. A crossmatch between the recipient's serum and the donor's lymph node or splenic tissue lymphocytes is then undertaken. If the crossmatch is negative, the transplant surgery proceeds. In case of a positive crossmatch, the kidney is sent to the transplant center that has the next eligible patient on the UNOS list.

HARVESTING AND RENAL PRESERVATION

Once the criteria for brain death[28] are met and the consent for organ donation is completed, the donor is taken to the operating room. Before surgery and during the harvesting procedure, efforts are made to maintain blood pressure, hydration, and urine output as close to normal as possible. Pressor agents other than dopamine in low dose should be avoided. Using standard sterile surgical techniques, each kidney with its respective blood vessels and an appropriate

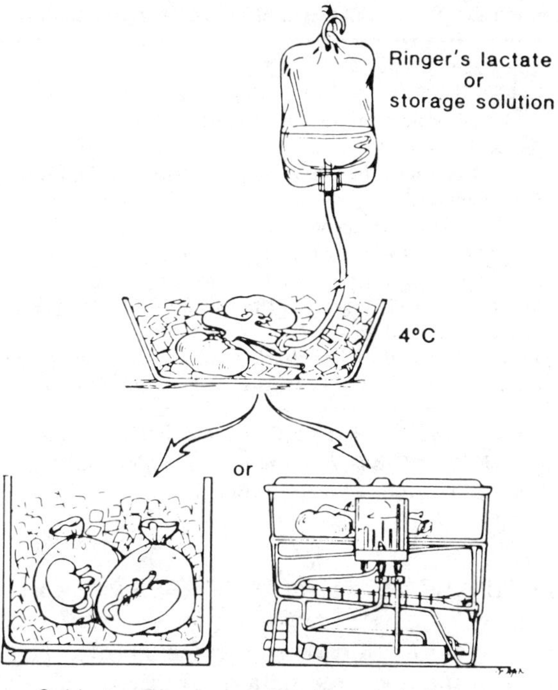

FIG. 19–3. Technique of flushing the kidney after removal from a cadaver donor and methods of transportation of the donated organ. [From Whitten JI, Toledo-Pereyra LH: Surgical techniques, Toledo-Pereyra LH (ed): *Kidney Transplantation*. Philadelphia, F. A. Davis Company, 1988, p 81. Reproduced by permission.]

length of ureter is removed. It is our practice to remove small kidneys from young donors (less than 5 years of age) en bloc; larger kidneys are removed and separated with a cuff of aorta and vena cava. The harvested organ is quickly cooled by placing it in sterile cold saline slush and rinsing it with a cold rinse electrolyte solution (University of Wisconsin solution, Collins'-type solutions, or other comparable rinse solutions) until the fluid returning from the renal vein is clear. The time taken to cool the kidney from the moment the renal artery is clamped (warm ischemia time) should be minimized as much as possible, preferably to less than 20 min.[29] Experimental evidence in dogs shows that warm ischemia time exceeding 30 min is associated with a significant increase in the incidence of allograft nonfunction.[30]

For the purpose of transportation, the harvested kidney either is preserved in a cold electrolyte solution or is perfused with cooled perfusion fluid by a mechanical pumping device (Fig. 19–3). The former method is convenient and is used more widely than the latter. Cold preservation involves placing the organ in a sterile plastic bag containing cold electrolyte solution, wrapping the package in a second plastic bag ("double bagging"), and packing the organ in a Styrofoam container filled with ice (not dry ice). The container is appropriately labeled and transported to the transplant center where the transplant is to be performed. Kidneys preserved in this manner can survive up to 48 h (cold ischemia time). The pulsatile pump preservation method involves continuous perfusion of the kidney with electrolyte solution via the renal artery. Organ preservation time can be extended beyond 48 h by this technique.[30]

TABLE 19–2. Screening Criteria for Cadaver Kidney Donors

Donor age < 65 years
No history of:
  Underlying hypertension requiring therapy
  Diabetes mellitus
  Malignancy other than localized intracranial tumor or treated skin cancer
No evidence of:
  Underlying primary renal disease
  Systemic viral or bacterial infection
Normal urine output (> 1 mL/kg/h)
Normal urinalysis (except for minor abnormalities associated with acute preterminal illness)
Normal BUN and creatinine
Warm ischemia time less than 60 min, preferably <30 min
Negative serology for hepatitis B and human immunodeficiency virus (HIV)

Source: Modified from Cosimi AB: The donor and donor nephrectomy, in Morris PJ (ed): *Kidney Transplantation—Principles and Practice.* Philadelphia, W. B. Saunders, 1988, p 93. Reproduced by permission.

RECIPIENT TRANSPLANT PREPARATION

When information about the availability of a cadaveric kidney is transmitted to the transplant center, data regarding the donor's clinical status prior to and during organ harvesting, blood group, HLA tissue type, and CMV status are usually available. The physician involved decides whether to accept the kidney that is being offered. This decision is based on the recipient's current medical status and the donor selection criteria listed in Table 19–2. If the kidney appears to be acceptable, the potential recipient is asked to report to the transplant center where blood is obtained for a final crossmatch. Since it takes 3 to 4 h for the crossmatch to be performed after the donor's tissue sample is received by the tissue typing laboratory, the patient may either stay in the hospital (without being admitted) or be advised to return to his or her home. The transplant surgery is undertaken if the final crossmatch proves negative.

DONOR EVALUATION FOR LIVING-RELATED RENAL TRANSPLANT

The first step in the selection of a living-related donor (LRD) is to establish the individual's willingness to donate the organ. This can be done formally or informally, using easily understood language. An interpreter may be necessary in situations where the donor does not understand English. Initial laboratory workup should consist of obtaining the donor's blood group, doing HLA typing, establishing a lymphocytotoxic crossmatch between the donor's peripheral blood lymphocytes and the recipient's serum, and obtaining cytomegalovirus (CMV) and human immunodeficiency virus (HIV) viral studies. All these studies can be performed in a phased manner. If the crossmatch is negative, the donor should undergo a thorough examination by a physician. The purpose of such medical evaluation is to determine whether there is any underlying renal or

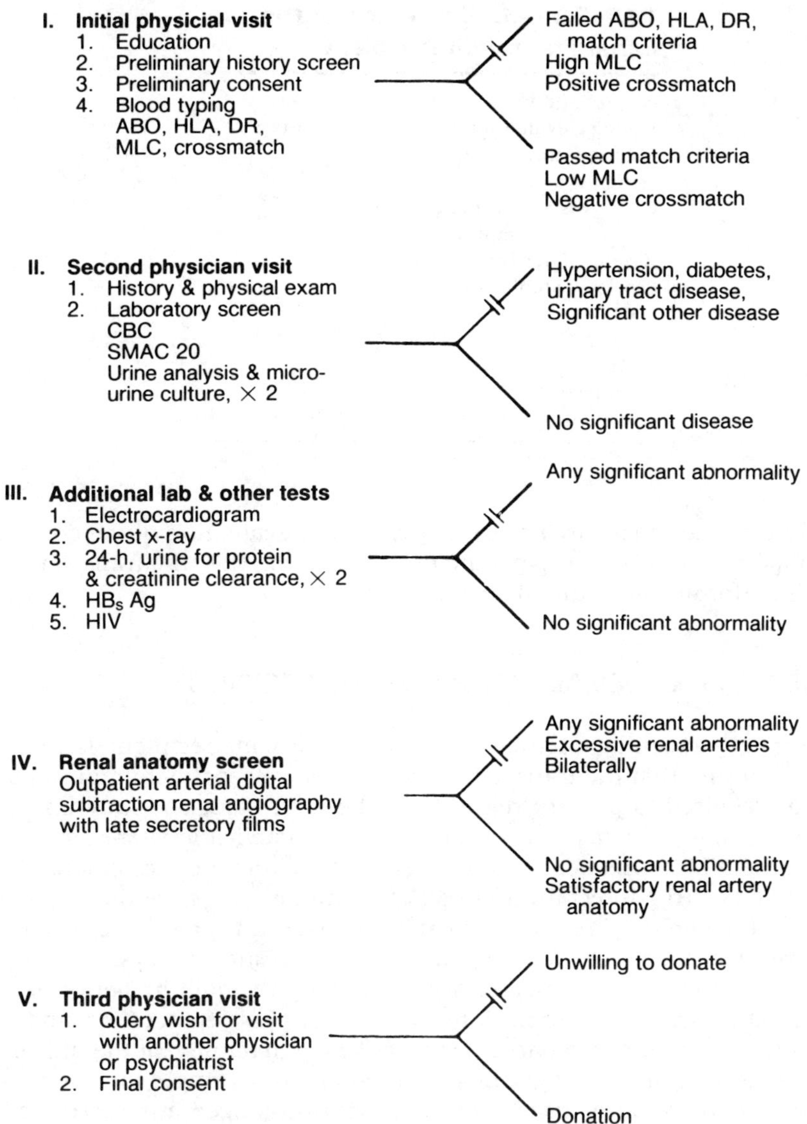

FIG. 19–4. A decision tree used in evaluating living related donors. A potential donor must pass each investigative step prior to initiating the next step. Failure (*broken lines*) results in disqualification of the individual as a renal transplant donor. (From Ogden DA: Living related transplantation, in Toledo-Pereyra LH (ed): *Kidney Transplantation*. Philadelphia, F. A. Davis Company, 1988, p 357. Reproducted by permission.)

systemic disease that may render the donor unsuitable for surgery and to ascertain if removal of one kidney would risk compromising his or her renal function in the future. Risks associated with donor surgery are assessed and discussed with the individual. A suggested outline for investigations of LRDs is given in Fig. 19–4. If the donor is deemed fit, a renal angiogram is performed

TABLE 19–3. Evaluation of the Renal Transplant Recipient

History and physical examination
Urologic evaluation, including a voiding cystourethrogram
Dental evaluation
Cardiovascular function and echocardiographic evaluation
Baseline liver function tests
Serologic studies for
CMV
Hepatitis B
HIV
Varicella
Chest radiograph and Tine (or PPD) test

to delineate the renal vasculature. A psychiatric evaluation of the donor is usually undertaken prior to organ donation. Following this, the transplant surgery can be performed at a suitable date.

PRETRANSPLANT EVALUATION OF THE RECIPIENT

A thorough screening of the prospective transplant recipient is required in order to ensure that the transplant surgery—as well as the immunosuppressive therapy required to prevent rejection of the graft—not pose any unusual risk for the patient. Patients at a serious risk for complications are advised about these potential consequences and offered other therapeutic options. In some cases, such as HIV infection, the risk of immunosuppressive therapy may outweigh the benefits of renal transplantation. Surgical procedures such as urologic reconstruction or nephrectomy (for polycystic kidneys, severe uncontrolled hypertension, or infected scarred kidneys) should be performed ahead of the actual transplant procedure. Some transplant centers are undertaking these elective procedures, particularly native nephrectomy, at the time of transplant surgery itself. Although the patient undergoes a single surgical procedure in the second scenario, risks associated with prolonged anesthesia and other complications must be evaluated on a case-by-case basis. Immunization against childhood diseases should also be completed prior to transplantation. Table 19–3 outlines the suggested pretransplant evaluation of children.

THE RECIPIENT'S TRANSPLANT ELIGIBILITY

MALIGNANCY

The transplant recipient should be free of malignancy at the time of transplantation. It is unclear how long the patient should be in remission before renal transplantation can be attempted. In children with Wilms tumor who have undergone a bilateral nephrectomy, it is customary to wait a year before transplantation. Earlier transplantation has been reported to be associated with a high recurrence rate of the tumor.[31,32]

OXALOSIS

Primary oxalosis is associated with the development of ESRD early in life and has been considered to have an unfavorable prognosis despite renal transplantation. Broyer et al.[33] recently reported a follow-up of 98 patients who received renal transplants for ESRD due to primary oxalosis. Three-year graft survival in these patients was 17 percent and 23 percent, respectively, for kidneys from cadaveric donors and LRDs. The authors of the study point out that in view of the metabolic nature of this disease, combined liver and renal transplantation may be a better solution and may be given consideration in the future.

CYSTINOSIS

Renal transplantation has been recommended for children with ESRD due to cystinosis. Although graft survival here appears to be comparable to that for control populations, the progression of systemic disease and involvement of other organs cannot be prevented by renal transplantation.[34]

CONGENITAL NEPHROTIC SYNDROME

Early planned transplantation has recently been recommended as the therapy of choice in infants with congenital nephrotic syndrome.[35] Such therapy involves elective bilateral nephrectomy followed by institution of peritoneal dialysis and subsequent renal transplantation. Improvement in growth and well-being has been reported with such an approach,[35] but long-term survival has yet to be reported.

SICKLE CELL DISEASE

Experience of renal transplantation of children with sickle cell disease (SCD) is limited. In a national study, Chatterjee[36] identified a total of 45 SCD patients (mostly adults) who had undergone renal transplantation. Of this group, 12 had SCD and the remainder had sickle cell trait. In the group as a whole, graft survival was comparable to that for patients without sickle cell disorders. One of the recommendations regarding the handling of the transplanted organ that emerged from this study was that in order to prevent sickling within the transplanted allograft, the donor kidney should be warmed to 37°C just prior to revascularization.

HIV INFECTION

Because of the danger of accentuating the state of immunodeficiency with immunosuppressive therapy, renal transplantation has not received active consideration in patients with HIV infection. This concern has been supported by a recent French report on 22 HIV-positive patients who had received renal transplants.[37] Five-year survival among these patients was reported to be 30 percent, and the outcome was worse in patients treated with triple immunosuppressive therapy (prednisone, azathioprine, cyclosporine) than in those who received only prednisone and azathioprine. Deaths were mostly due to AIDS-related infectious complications. The authors of the study concluded that in the absence of an effective anti-HIV drug therapy, chronic dialysis remains the most appropriate way of treating HIV patients with ESRD.

SURGICAL MANAGEMENT

TECHNICAL CONSIDERATIONS

The kidney is generally transplanted into the retroperitoneal space of the recipient's pelvic region. To avoid crossing of the donor renal vessels over those of the recipient, the right donor kidney is usually transplanted into the recipient's left side and vice versa. The incidence of renal artery stenosis is generally higher in pediatric transplant recipients than in adults,[38] and we believe that avoiding end-to-end anastomosis of the renal artery to the internal iliac artery minimizes that problem. Accordingly, our preferred method is end-to-end anastomosis of the renal vein to the external iliac vein and end-to-end anastomosis of the renal artery to the external iliac artery.

In small children (<20 kg) receiving adult kidneys, the renal artery and vein must be anastomosed to the side of the recipient's aorta and inferior vena cava, respectively, with the kidney placed in the retroperitoneum. It is surprisingly easy to place a large kidney into a small child,[39] particularly if the child has been on peritoneal dialysis; generally, there is no difficulty with renal transplant perfusion or hypotension due to diversion of the arterial flow away from the aorta and into the renal transplant.

INTRAOPERATIVE MONITORING

A Foley catheter is placed in the urinary bladder, which is filled with an antibacterial irrigant, and the drainage tube remains clamped until the neoureterocystostomy is completed. A single large-bore peripheral intravenous line is placed for the administration of medications, fluids, and blood. A percutaneous central venous catheter is placed for monitoring of central venous pressure (CVP) and postoperative administration of intravenous fluids and drugs, including antilymphoblast globulin (ALG) in patients receiving a cadaver kidney. We routinely administer mannitol (from 1 g/kg to 50 g, maximum) just prior to completion of the vascular anastomosis. The amount of intravenous fluid to be infused during the surgery is dictated by the CVP and the turgor of the kidney after the vascular clamps have been released. Ideally, the CVP should be maintained between 12 and 15 cmH_2O and the kidney should remain firm on pal-

TABLE 19–4. Immunosuppressive Protocol for Children Undergoing Living Related Renal Transplantation at the Children's National Medical Center, Washington, D.C.

Day − 1 (presurgery)	Cyclosporine 10 mg/kg po at midnight
Day 0	Azathioprine 2 mg/kg IV in OR
	Methylprednisolone 5 mg/kg IV in OR
	Cyclosporine 1 mg/kg IV q 8 h
Day 1	Azathioprine 2 mg/kg po qd
	Prednisone 2 mg/kg po bid
	Cyclosporine 5 mg/kg po bid[a]
	(check cyclosporine level qd)
Day 2	Azathioprine 2 mg/kg po qd
	Prednisone 1.5/kg po bid
	Cyclosporine 5 mg/kg po bid
Day 3	Azathioprine 2 mg/kg po qd
	Prednisone 1 mg/kg po bid
	Cyclosporine 5 mg/kg po bid
If the cyclosporine level is in the therapeutic range, continue prednisone taper.	
Days 4–6	Azathiorpine 2 mg/kg po qd
	Prednisone 0.75 mg/kg po bid
	Cyclosporine dose given po bid is based on blood level
Days 7–9	Azathioprine 2 mg/kg po qd
	Prednisone 0.50 mg/kg po bid
	Cyclosporine dose given po bid is based on blood level
Days 10–12	Azathioprine 2 mg/kg po qd
	Prednisone 0.50 mg/kg po qd
	Cyclosporine dose given po bid is based on blood level
Beyond day 12, same meds as for day 12	

[a]Intravenous cyclosporine may be continued if patient cannot tolerate oral feeds.

pation. Any transfused blood products must be washed and should also be CMV-negative in the CMV-negative recipient.

All our patients receive prophylactic antibiotics in the perioperative period. We use cefazolin in a dose ranging from 25 mg/kg to a maximum of 1 g/kg. Azathioprine and methylprednisolone are administered intravenously in the operating room as per our immunosuppressive protocols (Tables 19–4 and 19–5).

IMMEDIATE POSTTRANSPLANT MANAGEMENT

GENERAL

We prefer to place patients in the intensive care unit for the first 24 h following transplantation. Stringent isolation precautions for the moderately immunosuppressed patient are usually unnecessary.[40] A good hand-washing routine and the restriction of contact with people who have respiratory or skin infections

TABLE 19–5. Immunosuppressive Protocol for Children Undergoing Cadaveric Renal Transplantation at the Children's National Medical Center, Washington, D.C.

Day 0	Azathioprine 2 mg/kg IV in OR
	Methylprednisolone 5 mg/kg IV in OR
	Minnesota antilymphoblast globulin (ALG) 15 mg/kg IV via CVP line over 6 h (given immediately after surgery)
Day 1	Azathioprine 2 mg/kg po qd
	Prednisone 2 mg/kg po bid
	ALG 15 mg/kg IV via CVP line
Day 2	Azathioprine 2 mg/kg po qd
	Prednisone 1.5 mg/kg po bid
	ALG 15 mg/kg IV via CVP line
Day 3	Azathioprine 2 mg/kg po qd
	Prednisone 1.0 mg/kg po bid
	ALG 15 mg/kg IV via CVP line

After 14 days of ALG, the patient is transitioned to cyclosporine in the following manner:

Day 14	Azathioprine 2 mg/kg po qd
	Prednisone 1.0 mg/kg po bid
	ALG 15 mg/kg IV via CVP line
	Cyclosporine 5 mg/kg po bid
Day 15	Azathioprine 2 mg/kg po qd
	Prednisone 1.0 mg/kg po bid
	Cyclosporine 5 mg/kg po bid

Once the cyclosporine level is therapeutic for three consecutive days, the prednisone is tapered in the following manner, while maintaining the same azathioprine and cyclosporine doses:

Prednisone 0.75 mg/kg po bid × 3 days
Prednisone 0.50 mg/kg po bid × 3 days
Prednisone 0.50 mg/kg po qd thereafter

should, however, be enforced for all posttransplant patients. The child who has been severely immunosuppressed is confined to a single-bed private room for a week. Thereafter he or she is allowed gradual access to the rest of the hospital. Posttransplant patients are at a high risk of developing viral infections, such as CMV, especially if they have received antirejection therapy with steroid boluses, ALG, or OKT3.

FIRST POSTOPERATIVE DAY

Monitoring during the first day following renal transplantation focuses primarily on urine output, serum creatinine, blood pressure, and CVP. Some patients undergoing renal transplantation may still retain their native kidneys, which may contribute to their urine output; this must be kept in mind in assessing the function of their allografts. Large urine output (at least 2 mL/kg/h) is expected in well-functioning allografts, particularly in LRD transplant recipients.

The transplanted kidney is very sensitive to hypotension; therefore it is important to maintain normal blood pressure so as to prevent delayed graft function due to acute tubular necrosis. Many transplant recipients will, however, have problems because of hypertension resulting either from an underlying hypertensive disorder or from fluid overload in the perioperative period. The goals of fluid replacement following renal transplantation are to keep the kidney well perfused without causing fluid overload and its complications. Fluid replacement should consist of hourly urine output along with insensible and excessive losses such as from nasogastric drainage. The type of replacement intravenous fluid used usually consists of D_5W ½ normal saline with 10 meq of $NaHCO_3$/L. If the urine output is less than 4 mL/kg/h, all of it is replaced (milliliter for milliliter); but if the urine output is greater than 4 mL/kg/h, only 75 percent of the urine output is replaced in the following hour.

Serum creatinine serves as an excellent, practical marker for the assessment of posttransplant renal functions. It must be measured immediately after surgery and every 6 h thereafter for the first day. If the allograft begins to function promptly, it is not unusual to see the serum creatinine fall below 1.0 mg/dL within 24 h. If the creatinine is decreasing steadily, it is measured daily. Serum potassium and phosphorus may also demonstrate a prompt decline following transplantation and must be monitored closely. In the recipient of a cadaver kidney, we utilize Minnesota ALG until the kidney is functioning well (Table 19–5).

As soon as the patient has been stabilized following surgery, a radionuclide renal scan is obtained. The scan serves as a baseline parameter for renal blood flow and excretory function and is especially helpful as a point of comparison should renal dysfunction develop later on. The scan is also helpful in evaluating residual renal function in the patient's native kidneys. Within 24 h of surgery, renal transplant ultrasound and Doppler flow studies are obtained. The ultrasound study is useful in evaluating renal anatomy as well as ureteric and pelvic size and in localizing any fluid collection around the allograft (lymphocele). It also provides important baseline information on renal arterial blood flow (using Doppler ultrasound).

DAY TWO AND BEYOND

Daily monitoring of weight, intake-output charting, serum chemistry analysis of electrolytes, BUN and creatinine, blood cell counts, and cyclosporine blood level are essential in making decisions regarding the patient's clinical condition after transplantation. Additional laboratory studies may be performed as required by the patient's clinical status. In the absence of complications, patients with well-functioning renal transplants should be ready to leave the hospital in 2 weeks. Outpatient clinic visits are initially scheduled twice weekly; this interval is gradually lengthened if renal function remains stable. Outpatient clinic follow-up focuses on the evaluation of renal function, blood pressure, side effects of immunosuppressive therapy, and growth and development. Patients with significant bony deformities due to renal osteodystrophy will require orthopedic surgical correction when transplant function is stable and the dose of corticosteroids has been significantly reduced.

PHARMACOLOGY OF IMMUNOSUPPRESSIVE THERAPY

Immunosuppressive therapy is essential for preventing rejection of the renal allograft following transplantation. Over the last 30 years, several types of immunosuppressive agents—ranging from total lymphoid irradiation of the transplant recipient to the administration of specific monoclonal antibodies—have been developed. Some of these therapies have proved their usefulness in clinical transplantation and are widely used, while others have been abandoned because of their limited usefulness or high risk of side effects and toxicity. At present, the core group of immunosuppressive drugs used in clinical practice comprises azathioprine, glucocorticosteroids, and cylosporin A (CyA). Antilymphocyte globulin (ALG) is used as an adjunct immunosuppressive agent by some transplant centers, while monoclonal antibody OKT3 is generally recommended for the treatment of steroid-resistant acute allograft rejection. The sites of action of the commonly used immunosuppressive drugs in renal transplant recipients are shown in Fig. 19–5.

AZATHIOPRINE

Azathioprine, a purine analogue, was one of the first immunosuppressive agents used successfully in clinical renal transplantation.[6] Azathioprine is metabolized in the liver to its active compounds 6-mercaptopurine and 6-thioinosinic acid, which are eventually inactivated by the enzyme xanthine oxidase to 6-thiouric acid. Due to its primary hepatic elimination, the dose of the azathioprine need not be adjusted in renal failure.

Azathioprine is a nonspecific immunosuppressive agent whose precise mode of action is poorly understood. The active metabolites of azathioprine are incorporated into the DNA of rapidly dividing cells and thus interfere in the cellular proliferation, including that of activated cytotoxic lymphocytes.[41] The side effects of azathoprine are primarily related to hemopoietic suppression, increased risk of infections, and hepatic dysfunction. Azathioprine is available for oral use as tablets (50 mg) as well as a solution for intravenous administration. The usual immunosuppressive dose for the maintenance immunosuppression is 2 mg/kg/day.

GLUCOCORTICOSTEROIDS

Glucocorticosteroids were introduced as immunosuppressive agents in renal transplantation at almost the same time as azathoprine.[42,43] Despite their clinical use for some 25 years, the precise mechanism by which glucocorticosteroids abrogate rejection in renal transplantation is not fully clear. It is well known

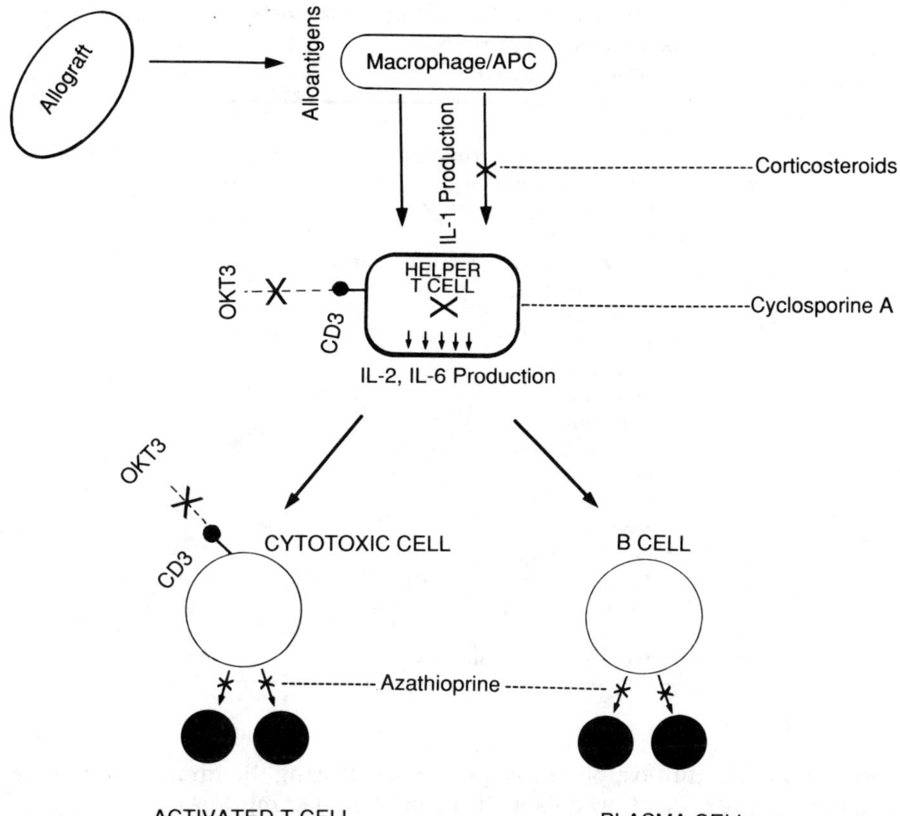

FIG. 19–5. Sites of action in the immune system of common immunosuppressive agents. [Modified from Handschumacher RE: Drugs used for immunosuppression, in Gilman AG et al (eds): *Goodman and Gilman's The Pharmacological Basis of Therapeutics,* 8th ed. New York, Pergamon Press, 1990, p 1265. Reproduced by permission of McGraw-Hill, Inc.]

that glucocorticosteroids act at several levels within the immune system.[41,44] Available experimental evidence suggests that they are able to prevent allograft rejection by suppressing the production of monocyte-derived interleukin 1 (IL-1), and by inhibiting the release of IL-1-dependent interleukin 2 (IL-2) from activated T cells.[45,45a,46] As a consequence of lack of these two trophic factors, proliferation of T cells in response to antigenic stimulation is prevented.[45] Administration of glucocorticosteroids is well known to cause lympholysis in experimental animals, but this phenomenon has not been confirmed in human beings.[47] The antiinflamatory property of glucocorticosteroids has been implicated as another possible mechanism by which they promote reversal of symptoms associated with acute allograft rejection.[48]

The two glucocorticosteroids currently used for immunosuppression in renal transplantation are prednisone and methylprednisolone. The choice of the agent is largely center-dependent and both drugs, in appropriate doses, are equi-

TABLE 19–6. Toxicities Observed with Long-Term Use of Corticosteroids

Metabolic
Abnormal fat distribution
Growth retardation
Sodium retention
Hypokalemia
Decreased carbohydrate tolerance
Gastrointestinal
Gastric ulceration
Esophagitis
Pancreatitis
Musculoskeletal
Myopathy
Avascular necrosis of bones
Osteoporosis
Cardiovascular
Hypertension
Neuropsychiatric
Mood changes, psychosis
Increased intracranial pressure
Eye
Posterior polar cataracts

potent in their immunosuppressive properties. During the immediate posttransplant period, the dose of prednisone is usually high (2 mg/kg/day), but a gradual reduction to 0.25 to 0.3 mg/kg/day is achieved by the end of first 3 to 6 months.[49] The manner in which this reduction is accomplished varies from center to center. Treatment of acute allograft rejection by glucocorticosteroids involves administration of a bolus dose (10 to 20 mg/kg/dose) of methylprednisolone (Solumedrol) on 3 consecutive days. The side effects associated with long-term glucocorticosteroid therapy are listed in Table 19–6.

CYCLOSPORIN A*

Cyclosporin A (CyA) is a unique immunosuppressive that was developed from the extract of a fungus *(Tolypocladium inflatum)* which was grown from soil samples obtained in Wisconsin and Hardanger Vidda, in Norway.[50] Most of the initial work in delineating the immunosuppressive properties of CyA was done in the laboratories of the Sandoz Pharmaceuticals, Basel, under the direction of J. F. Borel.

Cyclosporin A exhibits specific immunosuppressive properties and acts only on the activated T cells—not on all actively proliferating cells of the immune system, as do irradiation, azathioprine, and even glucocorticosteroids. Cyclo-

*Proposed international nonproprietary name for cyclosporin A is ciclosporin.

TABLE 19–7. Drugs That Affect the Blood Concentration and Toxicities of Cyclosporin A

Drugs that increase CyA level
Erythromycin
Ketoconazole
High-dose methylprednisolone
Verapamil
Danazol
Norethindrone
Drugs that lower CyA level
Phenobarbital
Phenytoin
Rifampin
Isoniazid
Intravenous trimethoprim
Drugs that may enhance CyA nephrotoxicity
Aminoglycoside antibiotics
Amphotericin B
Trimethoprim
Trimethoprim sulfamethoxazol
Melphalan

Source: Adapted from product information in *Sandimmune (cyclosporine). Clinical Management of the Transplant Patient.* East Hanover, New Jersey, Sandoz Pharmaceuticals, 1987.

sporin A inhibits IL-2 production by the activated helper T cells, preventing generation of the cytotoxic T cells involved in allograft rejection.[45,50,51]

Cyclosporin A is available for oral use in both liquid (in a lipid vehicle) and capsule forms as well as in an intravenously administered solution. Gastrointestinal absorption of CyA is poor (30 percent of the administered dose); this leads to significant variability in its peak and trough blood concentrations. The hepatic metabolism of CyA can be altered significantly by many drugs and may sometimes present therapeutic dilemmas. These drugs are listed in Table 19–7.

The blood concentration of CyA can demonstrate a variability from time to time in the same patient on a stable dose (intrapatient variability) as well as in the concentrations achieved in different patients on the same oral dose (interpatient variability).[52] Blood concentration of CyA is usually monitored as a 12-h trough. The therapeutic range of CyA depends on whether or not whole blood or plasma is used for assay and on the method of assay chosen. Traditionally, high-pressure liquid chromatography was used in assaying CyA. Not only is this method cumbersome but it measures the parent compound only, while the radioimmunoassay (RIA) method measures both CyA and its metabolites. A rapid method for assaying CyA (TDx method—Abbot Laboratories) has been developed recently. This technique, which also measures CyA and its metabo-

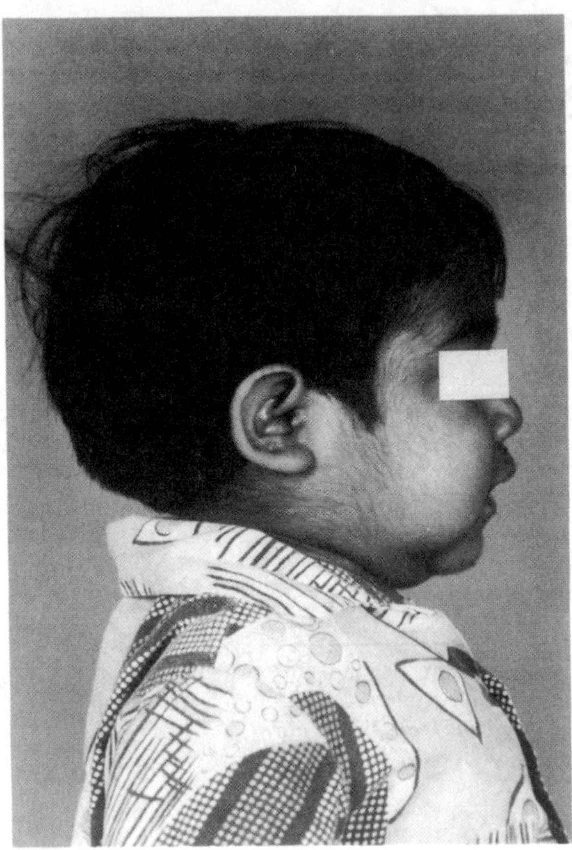

FIG. 19–6. Example of facial hair growth pattern in a transplant recipient receiving cyclosporin A.

lites, has been reported to correlate well with the RIA assay.[53] Several other specific and quick CyA assay methods are undergoing trials at this time.

Cyclosporin A is associated with several side effects including hepatotoxicity, excessive hair growth, gum hypertrophy, nephrotoxicity, hypertension, and seizures.[54] Excess hair growth usually occurs on the face, extremities, and back (Fig. 19–6). While hirsutism is not dose-dependent, the remaining side effects are generally due to toxic drug concentrations. The nephrotoxicity of CyA is of particular concern to transplant nephrologists, since it may affect long-term allograft function. Clinical suspicion of CyA nephrotoxicity is usually entertained in a patient who demonstrates a significant elevation of serum creatinine level without any concomitant features suggestive of acute allograft rejection. In cases of acute CyA toxicity, reduction of the CyA dose usually leads to a decrease in the serum creatinine concentration. The morphologic characteristics of CyA nephrotoxicity (Figs. 19–7 and 19–8) are listed in Table 19–8.

ANTILYMPHOCYTE GLOBULIN

Antilymphocyte globulin (ALG) was first used as an immunosuppressive agent in experimental transplantation in 1963[55] and was introduced into clinical renal

TABLE 19–8. Renal Morphologic Changes Associated with Use of Cyclosporin A

Site of Lesion	Morphologic Features
Tubulopathy	Vacuolization of tubular cells
	Tubular cell microcalcification
	Tubular cell inclusion bodies
	Giant mitochondira in tubular cells on electron microscopy
Interstitial lesions	Diffuse interstitial fibrosis
	Strip interstitial fibrosis consisting of areas of interstitial fibrosis and tubular atrophy
Arteriopathy	Lumpy proteinaceous deposits in the arterial wall
	Intimal thickening with narrowing of vascular lumen
	Deposits of IgM and/or C3 in the affected vessels
	Glomerular involvement is usually minimal

Source: Adapted from Pichlmayr R, Wonigeit K, Ringe B, et al: *Sandimmune (ciclosporin) in Renal Transplantation: A Diagnostic and Therapeutic Approach to Minimize Toxicity.* Basel, Switzerland, Sandoz Pharmaceuticals, 1985. Adapted and reproduced by permission.

transplantation by Starzl and colleagues[8] in 1967. ALG is a polyclonal antilymphocyte antibody that is obtained by immunizing rabbits or horses with human lymphoid cells (cultured lymphoblasts).[56] The plasma thus obtained is adsorbed with human red cells and platelets in order to reduce the content of antibodies

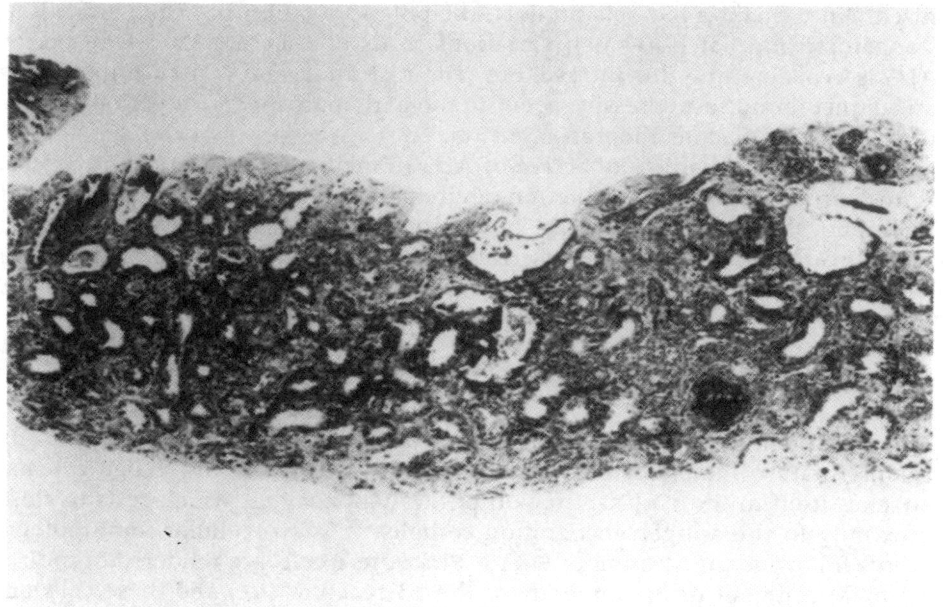

FIG. 19–7. Low-power view of a renal biopsy diffuse interstitial fibrosis associated with the use of cyclosporin A. (Photograph courtesy of Sandoz Pharmaceuticals, Hanover, New Jersey. Reproduced by permission.)

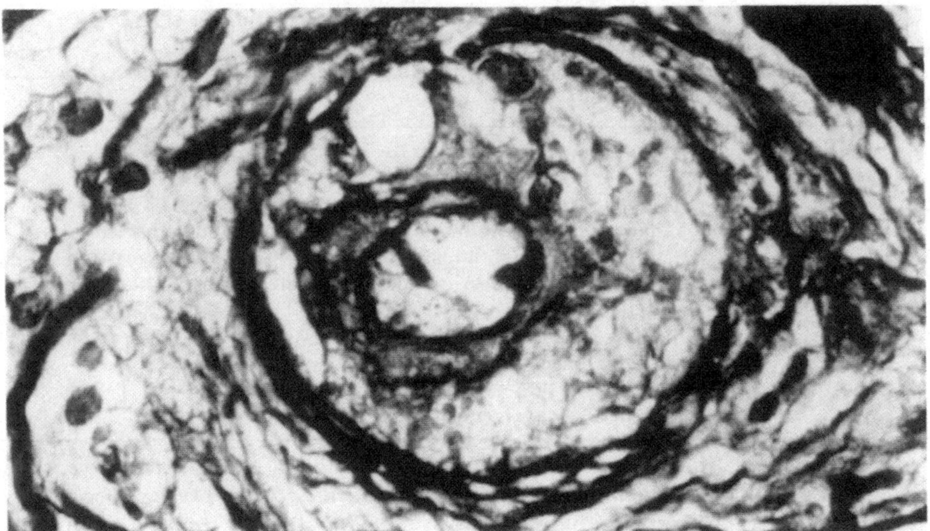

FIG. 19–8. Arteriopathy characterized by mucoid thickening and necrosis of smooth muscle cell associated with the use of cyclosporin A. (Photograph courtesy of Sandoz Pharmaceuticals, Hanover, New Jersey. Reproduced by permission.)

directed against these cellular hemopoietic components. The IgG fraction of the plasma, which contains the antilymphocyte antibodies, is separated and lyophilized. Since this is a biologic product, the potency of ALG has been difficult to standardize and batch-to-batch variations in its efficacy are known to occur. ALG is available only for intravenous administration and is used primarily as an adjunct immunosuppressive agent in the early posttransplant period and for the treatment of acute allograft rejection.

The precise mechanism of action of ALG in mediating its therapeutic effects is unclear, but a profound depletion of circulating lymphocytes, particularly of T lymphocytes, is seen following its administration.[41,56] Side effects associated with ALG therapy include hypersensitivity to the product, anaphylaxis, fever, chills, and increased susceptibility to infection.

MONOCLONAL ORTHOCLONE OKT3 ANTIBODY

The OKT3 antibody is a murine monoclonal antibody directed specifically against mature lymphocytes and thymocytes. This antibody recognizes and attaches itself to the T3 (CD3) region of the lymphocytes, which rests in close proximity to the antigen recognition complex.[57,58] Two cellular immunologic events follow administration of OKT3. First, the T cells are rendered opsonizable by attachment of the antibody to the T3 receptor site, and these cells are then cleared by the reticuloendothelial cells.[59] Second, the antibody attached to the CD3 receptor site damages it, with the result that the whole complex is shed from the T-cell surface.[57,60] Both these events essentially render the T cell non-

TABLE 19–9. Adverse Effects Associated with OKT3 Therapy

Adverse Reaction	Percent of Patients
Fever	73
Chills	57
Dyspnea	21
Chest pain	14
Vomiting	13
Nausea	11
Tremors	10
Less common side effects	
Headache	—
Meningismus	—
Development of antibodies against OKT3	80

Source: From Ortho Multicenter Transplant Study Group: A randomized clinical trial of OKT3 monoclonal antibody for acute rejection of cadaveric renal transplant. *N Engl J Med* 313:337, 1985. Reproduced by permission.

functional and incapable of developing killer cells. OKT3 exhibits its actions on the mature lymphocytes in circulation as well as on those within the allograft.[57]

OKT3 is administered intravenously as a rapid push without dilution of the drug. Significant side effects (Table 19–9) are encountered after the first dose, and these may extend into the second day of therapy.[10,61] These side effects are believed to result from mediators released from the lymphocytes that are damaged by the antibody.[10,62] Pretreatment with antipyretics, antihistamines, and particularly corticosteroids seems to mitigate the intensity of such "first-dose reactions."[61] It is also important to make sure that the patient is not overhydrated during OKT3 therapy, since pulmonary edema is particularly common in patients with fluid overload. Allergic reactions are uncommon with the first use of OKT3, but antimurine antibodies develop in 80 percent of patients during the second week of treatment.[10] The incidence of antimurine antibody formation can be decreased with concomitant use of azathioprine.

At present, OKT3 is used primarily for the treatment of acute allograft rejection, either as the first-choice drug or as a "rescue" agent when other antirejection therapy has failed.

COMPLICATIONS OF RENAL TRANSPLANTATION

PRIMARY NONFUNCTION OF THE KIDNEY TRANSPLANT

The term *primary nonfunction* refers to renal transplants that fail to function after blood flow through the allograft is established. According to the 1989 North American Pediatric Renal Transplant Cooperative Study (NAPRTCS), this prob-

TABLE 19–10. Common Causes of Early Renal Allograft Failure

Hyperacute allograft rejection
Acute renal arterial thrombosis
Acute tubular necrosis due to
  Prolonged warm ischemia time
  Use of vasoconstrictor drugs in the donor
  Recipient hypotension
Urinary obstruction due to
  Blood clots
  Urinary leak
  Obstructed Foley catheter

lem occurs in about 4 percent of children.[62] Possible causes of primary allograft nonfunction are given in Table 19–10.

Management of a primarily nonfunctioning allograft should be prompt. After ensuring that there is no urinary obstruction, a DTPA renal scan and an ultrasound study must be obtained. If renal perfusion is found to be poor, arterial thrombosis may be suspected. Under these circumstances, Doppler ultrasound may provide additional diagnostic information. Renal transplant arteriography may also be necessary in selected cases. Renal arterial thrombosis can also be a manifestation of hyperacute rejection. If renal perfusion is found to be satisfactory with the DTPA scan but the excretory function lags behind, it can be assumed that the patient has acute tubular necrosis. If hyperacute rejection is suspected or the viability of the allograft is in question, renal biopsy can provide valuable information. Exploratory surgery may be required in patients with primary nonfunction in whom the etiology is mechanical or technical. If the patient is suspected to have acute tubular necrosis (ATN), conservative management, including dialysis therapy, is instituted. Management of immunosuppressive medications becomes a challenge under these circumstances. Our approach to the patient with prolonged delay in allograft function has been to defer the use of CyA for at least 2 weeks so as to allow for the recovery of renal function.

The decision to perform a transplant nephrectomy for primary nonfunction is based on the viability of the allograft as determined by renal biopsy and the patient's general status. If the patient has developed infectious complications from the immunosuppressive therapy in addition to poor viability of the transplant, nephrectomy may have to be considered urgently. Otherwise, it is reasonable to wait for 6 to 8 weeks before removing the kidney.

ALLOGRAFT REJECTION

Rejection denotes destruction of the transplanted kidney tissues by the recipient's immune response. Three distinct clinicopathologic variants of renal allograft rejection are (1) hyperacute, (2) acute, and (3) chronic rejection.

HYPERACUTE REJECTION

Hyperacute rejection occurs within the first few minutes to an hour of perfusing the allograft with the recipient's blood. Often the kidney becomes hemorrhagic and cyanotic appearing while the patient is still in the operating room. Hyperacute rejection is caused by preformed circulating antibodies in the recipient that may be directed against the donor kidney's ABO or HLA antigens.[24] With the advent of routine crossmatching of the recipient's serum and the donor's lymphocytes prior to transplantation, hyperacute rejection has become rare. The pathologic hallmark of hyperacute rejection is the presence of fibrin and platelet thrombi in the glomerular capillaries and arterioles. Endothelial damage and detachment is commonly seen in the arterioles, while the interstitium is infiltrated with acute inflammatory cells such as neutrophils and mononuclear cells. Immunoglobulin (IgG and IgM), fibrin, and complement deposition occurs in the glomerular capillaries and the blood vessels.[63]

Hyperacute rejection is resistant to conventional antirejection therapy. Allograft nephrectomy is necessary after the diagnosis is confirmed on a frozen section of the renal biopsy specimen.

ACUTE REJECTION

Acute rejection can occur anytime following transplantation but is more common in the first 3 months of the posttransplant period. In the report of the 1989 NAPRTCS,[62] 24 percent of the LRD recipients and 28 percent of the cadaveric kidney recipients have had an episode of rejection by the fifteenth postoperative day. In the precyclosporine era, acute rejection was commonly seen between 7 to 10 days following transplantation. Rejection within the first week after transplantation is sometimes referred to as accelerated acute rejection and is usually associated with a poor outcome.[63]

Clinical features of acute rejection are fever, malaise, decreased urine output, hypertension, allograft tenderness, and rising BUN and serum creatinine. Fever is the most common sign of rejection in our patients, and careful assessment of the patient is mandatory to rule out an infective etiology. In children transplanted with adult kidneys who are treated with cyclosporine, signs of rejection can be quite subtle because of the large renal parenchymal reserve. DTPA renal scan is a sensitive investigative tool for detecting decreased function due to rejection, but it is not uncommon to find a lag time of 12 to 24 h before a renal scan would demonstrate unequivocal signs of acute rejection. Doppler ultrasound has also been suggested to serve as an adjunct to the diagnosis of acute rejection.[64] In patients with uncertain diagnoses, renal biopsy remains the confirmatory test. The biopsy is done under local anesthesia with sonographic guidance. The technique of renal transplant biopsy is discussed in Chap. 4.

The measurement of T-cell subsets may be useful in evaluating the renal posttransplant patient with a rising serum creatinine. When the CD4+/CD8+ (helper/suppressor) ratio is close to the control ratio (2:1), the patient is inadequately immunosuppressed and the risk of rejection is increased. Also, the percentage of IL-2 receptor positive cells and percentage of activated T cells can help differentiate rejection from viral infection.[65]

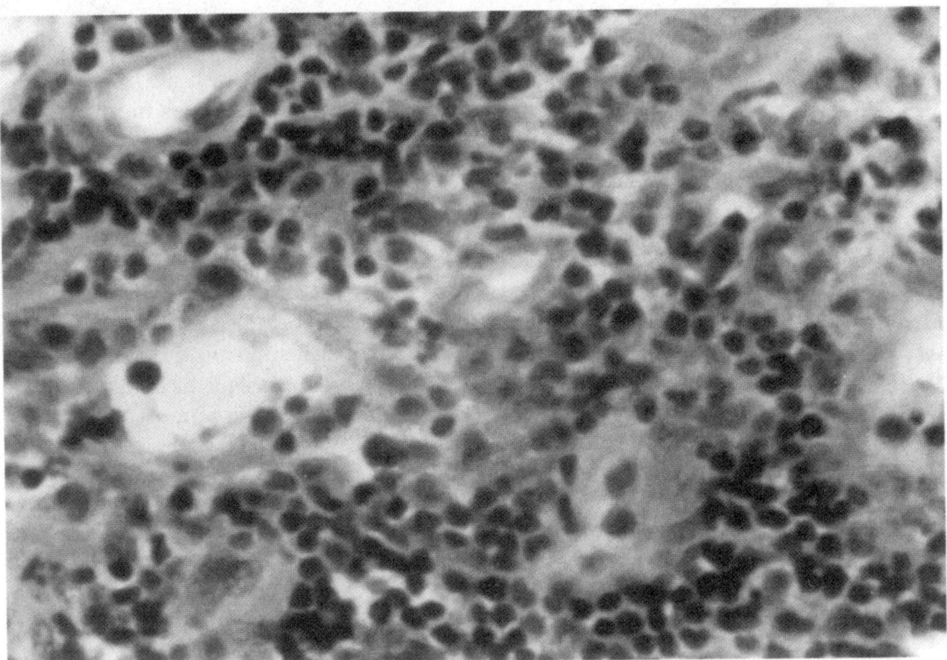

FIG. 19–9. Morphologic changes seen in acute allograft rejection. Mononuclear interstitial infiltrate is prominent. (Photograph courtesy of Sudesh Kapur, Children's National Medical Center, Washington, D.C.)

The characteristic morphologic feature of acute allograft rejection is the presence of interstitial mononuclear infiltrate, the glomeruli being relatively less affected (Fig. 19–9).[63] The interstitial cellular infiltrate consists of lymphocytes, plasma cells, and monocytes. Lymphocytes are seen invading the tubular cells and some may also be present within the tubular lumina, this phenomenon being referred to as *tubulitis* by some. In the more severe form of acute rejection (also known as vascular rejection), the vascular endothelium demonstrates damage characterized by endothelial cell swelling, detachment of the endothelium from internal elastic lamina, and infiltration of the mononuclear cells into the vessel wall (Fig. 19–10). Fibrin thrombi may also be present in the lumen of damaged blood vessels. Perivascular infiltration of mononuclear cells is common. Similar changes are usually exhibited by the glomerular capillaries. Acute inflammatory cells (polymorphonuclear cells and mononuclear cells) are seen in the mesangial areas, glomerular capillaries demonstrate endothelial damage, and fibrin thrombi may obstruct capillary lumens. As a result of poor glomerular perfusion, secondary changes may be seen in the tubules. Vascular and glomerular localization of IgM and complement (C1q, C3) are common features of acute vascular rejection.

Acute allograft rejection is a cell-mediated phenomenon elicited in response to the foreign antigens present in the allograft. Circulating antibody plays no role in acute rejection. A variety of cells infiltrate the interstitium of the allo-

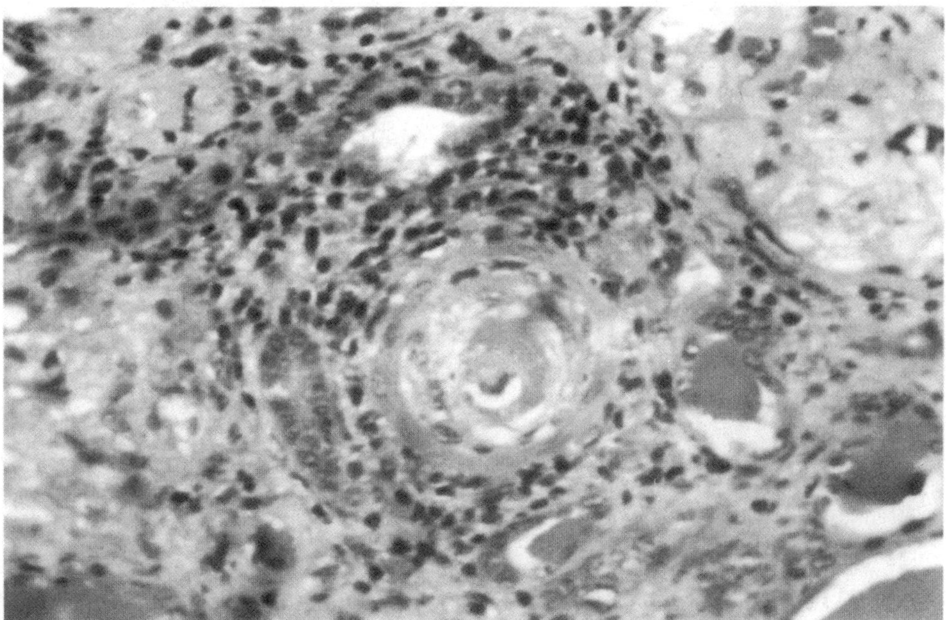

FIG. 19–10. Renal biopsy showing acute vascular rejection. The vessel wall is infiltrated with mononuclear cells. (Photograph courtesy of Sudesh Kapur, Children's National Medical Center, Washington, D.C.)

graft, commonly being T cells, B cells, monocytes, and HLA-DR-expressing mononuclear cells. Both T helper/inducer (T4) and suppressor/cytotoxic (T8) cells can be identified in the allograft by immunopathologic methods. The proportion of each of these cells within the allograft during acute rejection can vary, but T8 lymphocytes usually predominate.[66] The mechanisms involved in inducing organ damage in acute allograft rejection are depicted in Fig. 19–11.

Management of acute allograft rejection is given in Table 19–11. Acute rejection is reversible in more than half of the patients treated with steroid boluses. In steroid-resistant rejection, the rejection can be reversed in 85 percent of patients with OKT3. As mentioned earlier, special attention to the patient's fluid balance is mandatory prior to initiating OKT3 therapy. The side effects of the first dose of OKT3 can sometimes be severe; they include temperature elevation to over 40°C, shaking chills, and a flulike syndrome. Pretreatment with acetaminophen, steroids, and diphenhydramine may lessen these side effects, but in our experience fever and chills are common despite pretreatment. Fortunately, these side effects are much milder after the first dose of OKT3.

Recently, monoclonal antibodies directed against interleukin-2 receptor, which is important for T-cell growth, has also been shown to reverse acute renal allograft rejection.[67] Administration of prostaglandin E_1 analogue (misoprostol) has also been found to be of value in preventing acute allograft rejection.[68] Clinical application of both of these therapeutic modalities needs further evaluation.

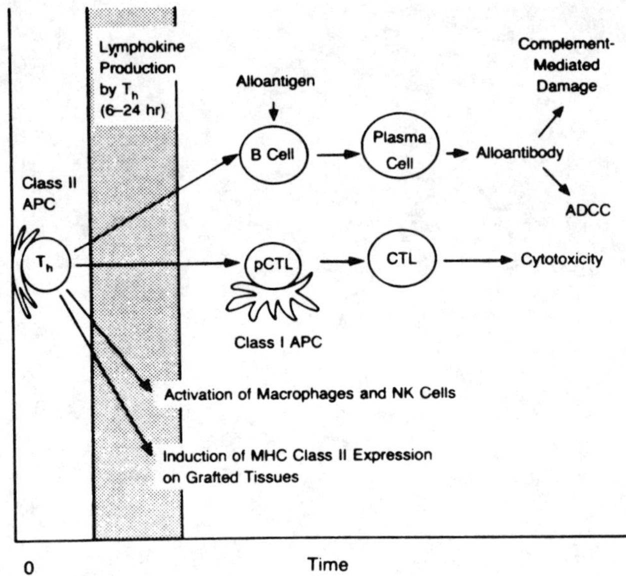

FIG. 19–11. Cellular interactions in transplant rejection. The diagram outlines activation of a T helper cell (T_h) by an antigen-presenting cell (APC) expressing MHC class II to produce lymphokines. These lymphokines promote the activation, proliferation, and differentiation of numerous effector mechanisms thought to contribute to transplant rejection. NK = natural killer, CTL = cytotoxic T-lymphocyte, pCTL = precursor CTL, and ADCC = antibody-dependent cell-mediated cytotoxicity. (From Krensky AM, Weiss A, Crabtree G, et al: T-lymphocyte-antigen interaction in transplant rejection. *N Engl J Med* 322:510, 1990. Reproduced by permission.)

CHRONIC ALLOGRAFT REJECTION

Chronic allograft rejection denotes a slow, progressive destruction of the renal transplant which leads to a gradual decline of renal function over months or years. The mechanisms leading to chronic rejection are poorly understood. Renal biopsy shows tubulointerstitial fibrosis, glomerular fibrosis, and evidence of arteriolar sclerosis. There is a striking lack of cellular infiltrates within the renal biopsy specimen (Fig. 19–12).[63] Most patients develop chronic rejection with little history of acute rejection, but a history of repeated episodes of acute rejection may be elicited in others. There is no effective treatment for chronic allograft rejection. These patients can be considered for repeat kidney transplantation once they reach ESRD.[69]

INFECTION

Patients undergoing renal transplantation are at a considerable risk for developing infectious complications. Although bacterial infections are common, many opportunistic infections by viruses, protozoa, and fungi can also occur. Susceptibility of transplanted patients results from nonspecific immunosup-

TABLE 19–11. Protocol for the Treatment of Early Allograft Rejection

Bolus Steroid Therapy

Days 1, 2, and 3: Solumedrol (methylprednisolone) 20 mg/kg (up to 1 g) IV qd

If the patient continues to show evidence of rejection or has a second rejection episode within several days of the first rejection and the cyclosporine level is therapeutic, OKT3 is begun.

OKT3 Therapy

Patient preparation

1. The patient must be euvolemic (less than 3% over dry weight) to prevent pulmonary edema. Obtain a chest x-ray.
2. OKT3 may be given through a good peripheral IV
3. Medications to prevent severe symptoms from OKT3 damage to the T cells with massive lymphokine release:
   a. Acetaminophen 10 mg/kg po or pr
   b. Diphenhydramine 1 mg/kg (up to 50 mg) IV or po
   c. Solumedrol 10 mg/kg IV over 20 min (first two doses of OKT3 only)
   d. Solu-Cortef (hydrocortisone sodium succinate) 2 mg/kg IV 30 min after OKT3 started (first dose of OKT3 only)

OKT3 Administration

1. 5 mg IV push qd for patients >30 kg
2. 2.5 mg IV push qd for patients <30 kg
3. 0.1 mg/kg IV push qd for small infants
4. Usual length of therapy is 10 days

Monitoring

1. Most severe symptoms occur with the first dose; a physician should be available to treat anaphylaxis or pulmonary edema. Temperature elevation to 41°C may occur, so appropriate equipment to treat fever must be available. Vital signs, including temperature, should be measured q 15 min for 2 h for the first two doses.
2. Blood for T-lymphocyte subset panel should be drawn before starting therapy, the next day, and twice weekly thereafter.
3. Draw blood for anti-OKT3 antibodies before starting therapy, at the end of therapy, and 6 weeks later.

Immunosupressive and other treatments

1. Prednisone 0.50 mg/kg po qd (withheld when IV steroids are given).
2. Azathioprine 2 mg/kg po qd unless WBC count is low.
3. Cyclosporine continued at doses necessary to keep at a low therapeutic blood level.
4. Acyclovir 100–200 mg po tid (after OKT3 is discontinued, it is given for 3 months)
5. The next-to-last day of OKT3 treatment, the prednisone and cyclosporine doses should return to prerejection doses.

pressive therapy used for prevention of allograft rejection. Unfortunately, as immunosuppressive drugs have become more effective in altering T-cell functions, the incidence of infectious complications has also risen. A list of common infections seen in renal transplant patients is given in Table 19–12.

CYTOMEGALOVIRUS INFECTION

Cytomegalovirus (CMV) infection is common in immunocompromised patients. About 70 percent of renal transplant recipients have been reported to acquire this infection.[70,71,72] CMV infection remains asymptomatic in a large number of patients, and symptomatic infection occurs in about 30 to 50 percent of those who are infected.[72] However, mortality is high (20 percent) in patients with

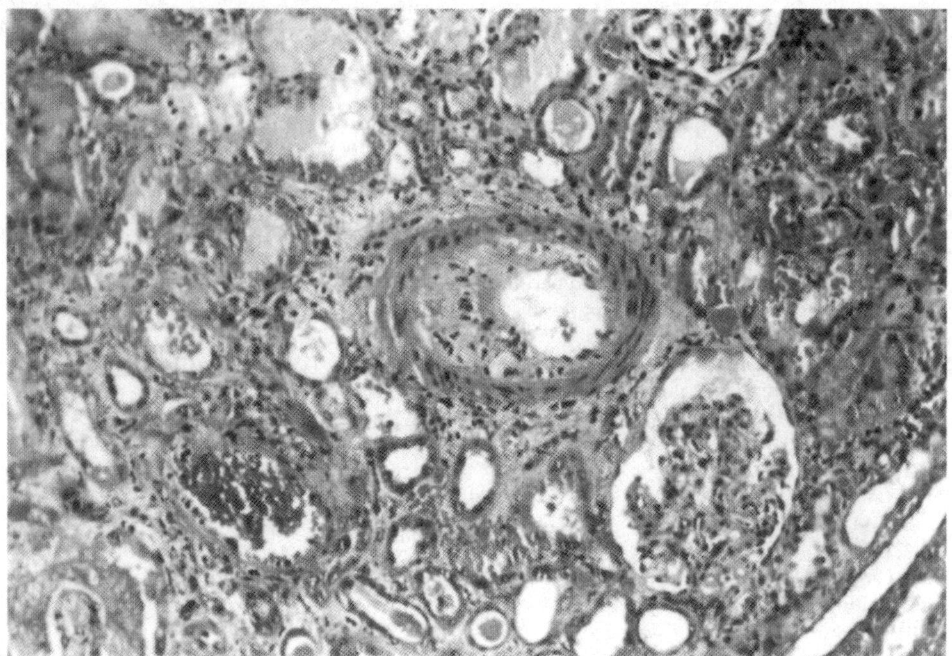

FIG. 19–12. Chronic allograft rejection, showing absence of interstitial inflammatory infiltration. Blood vessels demonstrate intimal hypertrophy and thickening. (Photograph courtesy of Sudesh Kapur, Children's National Medical Center, Washington, D.C.)

symptomatic disease.[73] Morbidity and mortality due to CMV infection is particularly high in patients undergoing immunosuppression with lymphocyte-depleting agents such as antithymocyte globulin or OKT3.[74]

CMV may be acquired in three distinct clinical settings.[75] First, in seronegative patients, primary CMV can result following transplantation of a CMV-positive allograft or by transfusion of blood products. Second, in a previously CMV-positive recipient, the latent virus can be reactivated by the immunosuppression required after transplantation. The third type of CMV transmission, known as superinfection, occurs in seropositive patients via an infected donor allograft; but, in contrast to reactivated disease, the donor virus strain proliferates and results in infection in the recipient. Patient-to-patient transmission of CMV appears to be unlikely.[76]

The clinical manifestations of CMV infection are varied and can result in a multisystemic disease.[77] Usually CMV infection becomes symptomatic during the first 3 to 4 weeks after transplantation; fever associated with leukopenia and thrombocytopenia may be the only initial manifestation. Subsequently, pneumonia, hepatitis, colitis, esophagitis, and chorioretinitis may evolve. CMV infection is known to produce endogenous immunosuppression.[78] A decrease in the $CD4^+$ T lymphocytes with an increase in $CD8^+$ lymphocytes is commonly noted and leads to a decrease in cell-mediated immunity.[75,79,80] Richardson et al[81] have described a peculiar glomerulopathy in association with CMV in renal transplant patients, but others have expressed doubts about the existence of

TABLE 19–12. Common Infectious Complications Associated with Renal Transplantation

One month
- Bacterial pneumonia
- Urinary tract infection
- Infection of vascular access lines
- Wound infection
- Peritonitis in patients who were receiving peritoneal dialysis therapy prior to transplantation
- Hepatitis B

One to three months
- Urinary tract infection
- Herpes simplex virus
- Cytomegalovirus
- Epstein-Barr virus
- *Pneumocystis carinii*
- *Aspergillus fumigatus* and other fungal infections

Beyond three months
- All infections listed in the above category
- Community-acquired viral infections, including influenza virus infection
- Community-acquired pneumonia
- Tuberculosis
- *Cryptococcus*

Source: Adapted from Rubin RH, Wolfson JS, Cosimi AB, et al: Infection in the renal transplant recipient. *Am J Med* 70:405, 1981. Reproduced by permission.

such a glomerular lesion.[82] A tubulointerstitial disease has also been reported in renal transplant patients suffering from CMV infection.[83]

Diagnosis of CMV rests on clinical manifestations, detection of CMV antibody by the complement fixation technique, enzyme-linked immunosorbent assay (ELISA) detection of CMV antibody (IgM and IgG), viral culture (throat, blood, and urine), and detection of the virus within pathologic specimens using hybridization and DNA amplification techniques.[84] A high degree of suspicion is required for the early diagnosis and treatment these patients.

Treatment of established cases of CMV infection is difficult and not always effective. Ganciclovir, a nucleoside with antiviral properties, has been found to be of therapeutic benefit in treating symptomatic disease in immunosuppressed patients.[85,86] Another new drug being considered for clinical use is foscarnet (trisodium phosphonoformate).[85] Clinical trials with this drug have yet to be completed and it remains experimental at this time.

Prophylactic use of CMV immune globulin in patients at risk to develop CMV (all patients receiving a CMV-positive kidney) has been shown to reduce the incidence of virologically confirmed CMV disease.[74] Acyclovir, an antiviral compound, has also been found to be effective as an agent for prophylaxis against CMV infection. Acyclovir, which has been suggested to be of particular benefit in preventing primary CMV infection, must be started at the time of transplantation and continued for 12 weeks.[85]

Pneumocystis carinii

Pneumocystis carinii is a protozoal infection that leads to pneumonia in immunocompromised patients. The incidence of *Pneumocystis carinii* pneumonia (PCP) in renal transplant patients is considerably lower than that of CMV infection. This type of pneumonia presents as an acute illness characterized by significant respiratory embarrassment and minimal clinical signs. Patients are usually hypoxic and the chest radiograph shows interstitial infiltrates. Diagnosis can be confirmed by bronchoalveolar lavage or lung biopsy, which shows intracellular organisms by silver stains. Treatment of PCP consists of intravenous administration of trimethoprim/sulfamethoxzole (20 mg/kg/day trimethoprim). Once acute symptoms have subsided, the same drug can be given orally for a total of 10 to 14 days.[87,88] Pentamidine has also been effectively used to treat PCP.[88] All infected patients are advised to take trimethoprim/sulfamethoxazole three times weekly (2 mg/kg/day trimethoprim) for chronic prophylaxis to prevent secondary recurrences of the disease.[89]

HYPERTENSION

Hypertension is a common clinical problem in renal transplant recipients. Broyer and colleagues[90] report that 85 percent of 334 children who received a functional cadaveric renal transplant developed hypertension during the posttransplant course. Others have reported similar results.[91] Hypertension in the immediate posttransplant period is often due to fluid overload, presence of native kidney, acute allograft rejection, and use of high-dose corticosteroid therapy. Chronic hypertension after the first month of transplantation may be due to renal artery stenosis, acute and chronic allograft rejection, or recurrent glomerulonephritis in the transplanted kidney. Cyclosporine and steroid therapy also contribute to the development of hypertension in the transplant patient. Table 19–13 lists the etiology of chronic hypertension in 209 transplant patients reported from Necker Hospital.

Renal artery stenosis is more common in pediatric patients than in adults.[12] The diagnosis of renal artery stenosis may be suggested by Doppler ultrasound or DTPA renal scan, particularly if the patient is pretreated with captopril.[92] The definitive diagnostic test for renal artery stenosis remains selective renal angiography. Transplant renal arterial stenosis may be treated by percutaneous transluminal angioplasty (PTA) a month after transplantation or by surgical correction. The success rate with PTA appears to be lower in children[93] than in adults.[94] Surgical repair of transplant renal artery stenosis in adults has an excellent success rate.[95]

MALIGNANCY IN TRANSPLANT RECIPIENTS

An increased incidence of cancer, particularly B-cell lymphoma, has been reported in renal and other transplant recipients.[96,97] Use of cyclosporine has

TABLE 19–13. Etiology of Posttransplant Hypertension in 209 Children Seen at Hôpital des Enfants Malades, Paris

Etiology	Number	Percentage
Chronic rejection	123	59.0
Renal artery stenosis	43	20.5
Native kidney	10	4.5
Recurrence of primary renal disease	9	4.5
Nonviable kidney	3	1.5
No obvious cause	21	10.0
Total	209	100

Source: From Broyer M, Guest G, Gagnadoux M-F, Beurton D: Hypertension following renal transplantation in children. *Pediatr Nephrol* 1:16, 1987.

been blamed for the increased frequency of these malignancies.[97] However, in a recently reported study in children, the incidence of malignancies was not reported to be high.[98] Of the 362 transplant patients, 3.6 percent of patients on conventional immunosuppressive therapy (azathioprine plus steroids) developed malignancies, while none taking cyclosporine developed them. The types of malignancies noted in this study were lymphomas and skin cancer. Despite the somewhat lower reported incidence of malignancies in children, all transplant patients must be monitored for the development of subsequent malignancies.

GLOMERULONEPHRITIS

RECURRENT GLOMERULONEPHRITIS IN THE ALLOGRAFTS

The recurrence of glomerulonephritis in the transplanted allograft is well known. However, the risk for such recurrent disease varies considerably, being highest in type II membranoproliferative glomerulonephritis (almost 100 percent) and focal and segmental glomerulosclerosis (up to 50 percent).[99–107] The diseases that are associated with recurrent glomerulonephritis in the allograft, ranked by their risk of recurrence, are given in Table 19–14.

DE NOVO GLOMERULONEPHRITIS IN THE ALLOGRAFTS

Glomerulonephritis in the allografts of patients who do not have any underlying glomerulonephritis is designated as de novo glomerulonephritis of the transplant. De novo membranous glomerulonephritis of renal transplants has been reported in children.[108,109] Habib et al.[109] reported that this was the commonest de novo glomerular disease in the renal transplants. Other types of glomerulonephritides seen by these workers were focal and segmental glo-

TABLE 19–14. Risk of Recurrent Transplant Glomerulonephritis in Patients with Underlying Glomerulonephritides

Category	Symptomatic Disease in Transplant	References
Diseases with High Risk for Recurrence		
Type II membranoproliferative glomerulonephritis	Common	99, 100
Focal and segmental glomerulonephritis	Common	100, 101
Hemolytic uremic syndrome	Common	102
Antiglomerular basement membrane disease	Common	103
Diseases with Moderate Risk for Recurrence		
IgA glomerulonephritis	Less common	100
Type I membranoproliferative glomerulonephritis	Uncommon	100
Henoch-Schönlein purpura	Uncommon	100
Diseases with Low Risk for Recurrence		
Alport syndrome	—	104
Congenital nephrotic syndrome	—	105
Membranous glomerulonephritis	—	100, 106
Lupus nephritis	—	104, 107

merulonephritis and antiglomerular basement membrane disease glomerulonephritis.

GROWTH FOLLOWING RENAL TRANSPLANTATION

Children suffering from ESRD are generally growth-retarded, which has been previously discussed in Chap. 16. The rate of growth may be enhanced in some of these children following renal transplantation, but it remains unpredictable. Most such children are, however, unable to attain normal adult height.[110,111] The etiology of growth retardation following transplantation has not been clearly evaluated but is believed to be related to the daily intake of corticosteroids used to prevent allograft rejection. Use of alternate-day corticosteroid in these children is associated with a better rate of linear growth.[112] The steriod-sparing effect of cyclosporine has also been credited with an improved prospect for growth.[113] Recently, recombinant human growth hormone has been advocated for the treatment of growth failure in children with chronic renal failure as well as for those who have undergone renal transplantation.[114] Initial results from these studies appear to be promising, but long-term follow-up of patients has not yet been reported.

DIALYSIS IN TRANSPLANT RECIPIENTS

Posttransplant dialysis is necessary in less than 20 percent of our cadaveric kidney recipients and has not been necessary in LRD kidney recipients in the last

10 years in our hospital. In those patients who require it, it is preferable to delay dialysis until the second postoperative day. Hemodialysis immediately after surgery predisposes the patient to bleeding in the retroperitoneum adjacent to the transplanted kidney. Careful fluid and electrolyte management should obviate the need for dialysis on the first postoperative day even if there is no renal function. It is best to avoid peritoneal dialysis (PD) immediately after surgery so as to prevent pain at the surgical site, although PD is less hazardous than hemodialysis.

OUTCOME

Since the introduction of cyclosporine in 1984, there has been a significant improvement in kidney allograft survival. Nevertheless, several nonimmunologic factors determine the survival of the patient and the kidney transplant. Recipient age appears to have an important bearing on the transplant survival. Although some centers have had excellent results with renal transplants in children less than 6 years of age,[115] the overall success rate continues to be lower than for older children, with a 66 percent 1-year function rate for children of age 6 or less compared to a 73 percent rate for older children receiving cadaveric kidneys.[62] Donor age in cadaveric renal transplants also affects outcome of the transplanted kidney. When the donor of a cadaveric kidney is less than 5 years of age, the 1-year survival of the grafts is less than (55 percent) when the donor is older (79 percent for $>$ 10 yr), regardless of the age of the recipient.[62,116,117,118]

Patient survival rate at 1 year, in most series, is greater than 90 percent for both LRD and cadaveric kidney recipients.[62,119,120] In the 1989 report of NAPRTCS, the patient survival at 1 year was 96 percent for LRD and 92 percent for cadaveric transplants.[62] The 1-year kidney allograft function rate for all children receiving LRD kidneys is excellent.[115,119,120] In the 1989 NAPRTCS report, the function rate for this group was 88 percent at 1 year.[62] The 1-year graft function rate for LRD at the Children's National Medical Center (CNMC) has been 100 percent for the last 5 years. Despite the use of cyclosporine, the overall function rate for cadaveric kidneys remains substantially lower than that for LRD. The 1-year function rate for cadaveric kidneys in the 1989 NAPRTCS report was 71 percent.[62] The 1-year function rate for cadaveric kidneys at the CHNMC has been 60 percent for the last 5 years—a reflection of the large number of kidneys from donors less than 5 years of age.

SUMMARY

Renal transplantation in children is a most rewarding endeavor because it can transform a chronically ill child into a robust one, free from the restrictions of dialysis in a matter of weeks. Attention to technical detail and meticulous management of immunosuppressive medications are mandatory because of the small safety margin in these patients. Despite early doubts about the advisability of recommending transplantation to the pediatric patient with ESRD, it is now clear that renal transplantation is the treatment of choice. Target-specific immunosupression may become a reality in the near furture with reduction in the risk of infectious complications commonly seen in transplant recipients. It is also likely that growth hormone may become an adjunt in the treatment of growth failure in children with chronic renal failure who undergo renal transplantation.

REFERENCES

1. Jaboulay M: Greffe de reins au pli du coude par soudures arterielles et veineuses. *Lyon Med* 107:575, 1906.
2. Michon L, Hamburger J, Oeconomos N, et al: Une tentative de transplantation renale chez l'homme: Aspects medicaux et biologiques. *Presse Med* 61:1419, 1953.
3. Murray JE, Merrill JP, Harrison JH: Renal homotransplanation in identical twins. *Surg Forum* 6:432, 1955.
4. Murray JE, Merrill JP, Dammin GJ, et al: Study on transplantation immunity after total body irradiation: Clinical and experimental investigation. *Surgery* 48:272, 1960.
5. Calne RY; The rejection of renal homografts: Inhibition in dogs by 6-mercaptopurine. *Lancet* 1:417, 1960.
6. Murray JE, Merrill JP, Dammin GJ, et al: Kidney transplantation in modified recipients. *Ann Surg* 156:337, 1962.
7. Terasaki PI, Vredevoe DL, Mickey MR, et al: Serotyping for homotransplantation: VI. Selection of kidney donors for thirty-two recipients. *Ann NY Acad Sci* 129:500, 1966.
8. Starzl TE, Marchioro TL, Porter KA, et al: The use of heterologous antilymphoid agents in canine renal and liver transplantation and in human renal homotransplantation. *Surg Gynecol Obstet* 124:301, 1967.
9. Canadian Multicentre Transplant Study Group: A randomized clinical trial of cyclosporine in cadaveric renal transplantation: Analysis at three years. *N Engl J Med* 314:1219, 1986.
10. Ortho Multicenter Transplant Study Group: A randomized clinical trial of OKT3 monoclonal antibody for acute rejection of cadaveric renal transplants. *N Engl J Med* 313:337, 1985.
11. Barber WH, Diethelm AG, Laskow DA, et al: Use of cryopreserved donor bone marrow in cadaver kidney allograft recipients. *Transplantation* 47:66, 1989.
12. Van Rood JJ, Van Leeuwen A, Schippers H, et al: Leucocyte groups and their relation to homotransplantation. *Ann NY Acad Sci* 129:467, 1966.
13. Slapak M, Digard N, Ahmed M, et al: Renal transplantation across the ABO barrier: A 9-year experience. *Transplant Proc* 22:1371, 1990.
14. Terasaki PI, Chia D, Mickey MR. The second histocompatibility locus in humans. *Transplant Proc* 1:21, 1988.
15. Dausset J. Iso-leuco-anticorps. *Acta Haematol (Basel)* 20:156, 1958.
16. Gjertson DW, Terasaki PI, Takemoto S, et al: National allocation of cadeveric kid-

ney by HLA matching: Projected effect on outcome and costs. *N Engl J Med* 324:1032, 1991.

17. Bjorkman PJ, Saper MA, Samraoui B, et al: Structure of the human class I histocompatibility antigen HLA-A2. *Nature* 329:506, 1987.
18. Dupont B. The HLA system, in Lee J (ed): *The HLA System: A New Approach.* New York, Springer-Verlag, 1990, p 15.
19. Terasaki PI, McClelland JD: Microdroplet assay of human serum cytotoxins. *Nature* 204:998, 1964.
20. Van Rood JJ, Van Leeuwen A, Ploem JS: Simultaneous detection of two cell populations by two colour fluorescence and application to the recognition of B-cell determinants. *Nature* 262:795, 1976.
21. Bach FH, Valentine EA, Alter BJ, et al: Typing for HLA-D: Primed LD typing and homozygous typing cells. *Tissue Antigens* 8:151, 1976.
22. Tiercy JM, Goumaz C, Mach B, et al: Application of HLA-DR oligotyping to 110 kidney transplant patients with doubtful serologic typing. *Transplatation* 51:1110, 1991.
23. Najarian JS, Migliori RJ, Simmons RI, et al: Effects of HLA matching in cadaver renal transplants. *Transplant Proc* 20(suppl 3):249, 1988.
24. Greenstein SM, Schechner RS, Louis P, et al: Evidence that zero antigen-matched cyclosporine-treated renal transplant recipients have graft survival equal to that of matched recipients. *Transplantation* 49:332, 1990.
25. Kissmeyer-Nielsen F, Olsen S, Patersen VP, et al: Hyperacute rejection of kidney allograft associated with pre-existing humoral antibodies against donor cells. *Lancet* 1:662, 1966.
26. Alarif LI et al. Transplantation of highly sensitized patients based on crossmatches using DTT-treated sera. *Transplant Proc* 21:742, 1989.
27. Garovoy MR, Rheinschmidt MA, Bigos M, et al: Flow cytometry analysis: A high technology crossmatch technique facilitating transplantation. *Transplant Proc* 15:1939, 1983.
28. President's Commission for the Study of Ethical Problems in Medicine: *Defining Death: A Report on the Medical, Legal, and Ethical Issues in the Determination of Death* (1982-371-059/8192). U.S. Government Printing Office, Washington, DC, 1982.
29. Toledo-Pereyra LH: Kidney harvesting and preservation, In Toledo-Pereyra LH (ed), *Kidney Transplantation.* Philadelphia, Davis, 1988, p 27.
30. Florack G, Sutherland DER, Ascherl R, et al: Definition of normothermic ischemia limits of kidney and pancreas grafts. *J Surg Res* 40:550, 1986.
31. DeMaria JE, Hardy BE, Brezinski A, et al: Renal transplantation in patients with bilateral Wilms tumor. *J Pediatr Surg* 14:557, 1979.
32. Penn I: Renal transplantation for Wilms tumour: Report of 20 cases. *J Urol* 122:793, 1979.
33. Broyer M, Brunner FP, Brynger H, et al: Kidney transplantation in primary oxalosis: Data from the EDTA Registry. *Nephrol Dial Transplant* 5:332, 1990.
34. Almond PS, Morel Ph, Troppmann C, et al: Progression of infantile cystinosis after renal transplantation. *Transplant Proc* 23:1386, 1991.
35. Holberg C, Jalanko H, Koskimies O, et al: Renal transplantation in small children with congenital nephrotic syndrome of Finnish type. *Transplant Proc* 23:1378, 1991.
36. Chatterjee SN: National study in natural history of renal allografts in sickle cell disease or trait: A second report. *Transplant Proc* 19(suppl 2):33, 1987.

37. Lang Ph, Niadaut P, and the Groupe Coopertif de Transplantation de L'Ile de France: Update and outcome of renal transplant patients with human immunodeficiency virus. *Transplant Proc* 23:1352, 1991.
38. Henning PH, Bewick M, Reidy JF, et al: Increased incidence of renal transplant arterial stenosis in children. *Nephrol Dial Transplant* 4:575, 1989.
39. Najarian JS, Frey DJ, Matas AJ, et al: Renal transplantation in infants. *Ann Surg* 212:353, 1990.
40. Nausef WM, Maki DG: A study of the value of simple protective isolation in patients with granulocytopenia. *N Engl J Med* 304:448, 1981.
41. Handschumacher RE: Drugs used for immunosupression. In Goodman AG et al (eds): *The Pharmacological Basis of Therapeutics,* Elmsford, NY, Pergamon Press, 1990, p 1264.
42. Murrey JE et al: Prolonged survival of human-kidney homografts by immunosuppressive drug therapy. *N Engl J Med* 268:1315, 1963.
43. Starzl TE, Marchioro TL, Waddell WR: The reversal of rejection in human homografts with subsequent development of tolerance. *Surg Gynecol Obstet* 117:385, 1963.
44. Bach J-F: Recent advances in steroid therapy. *Adv Nephrol* 5:173, 1975.
45. Strom TB: Immunosuppressive agents in renal transplantation. *Kidney Int* 26:353, 1984.
45a. Gillis S, Crabtree GR, Smith KA: Glucocorticoid-induced inhibition of T cell growth factor production: II. The effect on the *in vitro* generation of cytotoxic T cells. *J Immunol* 123:1632, 1979.
46. Snyder DS, Unanue ER: Corticosteroids inhibit murine macrophage Ia expression and interleukin-1. *J Immunol* 129:1803, 1982.
47. Dupont E, Berkenboom G, Leempoel M, et al: Failure of dexamethasone to induce *in vitro* lysis of human mononuclear cells. *Transplantation* 30:387, 1980.
48. Walker RG, d'Apice AJF: Azathioprine and steroids, in Morris PJ (ed): *Kidney Transplantation—Principles and Practices.* Philadelphia, Saunders, 1988, p 319.
49. Ettenger RB, Rosenthal JT, Marik J, et al: Successful cadaveric renal transplantation in infants and young children. *Transplant Proc* 21:1707, 1989.
50. Borel JF, Kis ZL: The discovery and development of cyclosporine (Sandimmune). *Transplant Proc* 23:1868, 1991.
51. Hess AD, Tutschka PJ, Santos GW: Effect of cyclosporine A on human lymphocyte response in vitro: III. CyA inhibits production of T lymphocyte growth factors in secondary mixed lymphocyte responses but does not inhibit the response of primed lymphocytes to TCGF. *J Immunol* 128:355, 1982.
52. Kahan BD, Reid M, Newburger J: Pharmacokinetics of cyclosporine in human renal transplantation. *Transplant Proc* 15:446, 1983.
53. Schroeder TJ, Brunson ME, Pesce AJ, et al: A comparison of the clinical utility of the radioimmunoassay, high-performance liquid chromatography, and TDx cyclosporine assay in outpatient renal transplant recipients. *Transplantation* 47:262, 1989.
54. Kahan BD, Flechner SM, Lorber MI, et al: Complications of cyclosporine-prednisone immunosuppression in 402 renal allograft recipients exclusively followed at a single center for from one year to five years. *Transplantation* 43:197, 1987.
55. Woodruff MFA, Aderson NF: Effect of lymphocyte depletion by thoracic duct fistula and administration of antilymphocyte serum on survival of skin homografts in rats. *Nature* 200:702, 1963.
56. Cosimi B: Antilymphocyte globulin, in Morris PJ (ed): *Kidney Transplantation—Principles and Practices.* Philadelphia, Saunders, 1988, p 343.

57. Goldstein G: Monoclonal antibody specificity: Orthoclone OKT3 T-cell blocker. *Nephron* 46(suppl 1):5, 1987.
58. Meuer SC, Acuto O, Hussey RE, et al: Evidence for the T3 associated 90 kd heterodimer as the T-cell antigen receptor. *Nature* 303:800, 1983.
59. Miller RA, Maloney DG, McKillop J, et al: In vivo effects of murine hybridoma monoclonal antibody in a patient with T-cell leukemia. *Blood* 58:78, 1981.
60. Chetenoud L, Baudrihaye MF, Kreis H, et al: Human in vivo antigenic modulation inducсd by the anti-T cell OKT3 monoclonal antibody. *Eur J Immunol* 12:979, 1982.
61. Chatenoud L, Legendre C, Ferran C, et al: Corticosteroid inhibition of the OKT3-induced cytokine related syndrome—dosage and kinetics prerequisites. *Transplantation* 51:334, 1991.
62. Alexander SR, Arbus GS, Butt KHM, et al: The 1989 report of the North American Pediatric Renal Transplant Cooperative Study. *Pediatr Nephrol* 4:542, 1990.
63. Croker BP, Salomon DR: Pathology of the renal allograft, in Tisher CC, Brenner BM (eds): *Renal Pathology with Clinical and Functional Correlation.* Philadelphia, Lippincott, 1989, p 1518.
64. Drake DG, Day DL, Letourneau JG, et al: Doppler evaluation of renal transplants in children: A prospective analysis with histopathologic correlation. *AJR* 154:785, 1990.
65. Siegel DL, Fox I, Dafol DC, et al: Discriminating rejection from CMV infection in renal allograft recipients using flow cytometry. *Clin Immunol Immunopathol* 51:157, 1989.
66. Bishop GA, Hall BM, Duggin GG, et al: Immunopathology of renal allograft rejection analysed with monoclonal antibodies to mononuclear cell markers. *Kidney Int* 29:708, 1986.
67. Soulillou P-J, Cantarovich D, Mauff BL, et al: Randomized controlled trial of a monoclonal antibody against the interleukin-2 receptor (33B3.1) as compared with rabbit antithymocyte globulin for prophylaxis against rejection of renal allografts. *N Engl J Med* 322:1175, 1990.
68. Moran M, Mozes MF, Maddux MS, et al: Prevention of acute graft rejection by the prostaglandin E_1 analogue Misoprostol in renal-transplant recipients treated with cyclosporine and prednisone. *N Engl J Med* 322:1183, 1990.
69. Kaiser BA, Polinsky MS, Palmer J, et al: Successful kidney retransplantation of children with stable but chronically rejecting allografts prior to dialysis. *Transplantation* 49:1009, 1990.
70. Pollak R, Barber PL, Prusak BF, et al: Cytomegalovirus as a risk factor in living-related renal transplantation: A prospective study. *Ann Surg* 205:302, 1987.
71. Ho M: Cytomegalovirus infection and indirect sequelae in the immunocompromised transplant patient. *Transplant Proc* 23(suppl 1):2, 1991.
72. Balfour HH Jr, Fletcher CV, Dunn D: Prevention of cytomegalovirus disease with oral acyclovir. *Transplant Proc* 23(suppl 1):19, 1991.
73. Rubin RH, Tolkoff-Rubin NE, Oliver D, et al: Multicenter seroepidemiologic study of the impact of cytomegalovirus infection on renal transplantation. *Transplantation* 40:243, 1985.
74. Snydman DR: Prevention of cytomegalovirus disease with intravenous immune globulin. *Transplant Proc* 23(suppl 1):20, 1991.
75. Rubin RH: Impact of cytomegalovirus infection on organ transplantation. *Rev Infect Dis* 12(suppl 7):754, 1990.
76. Tolkoff-Rubin NE, Rubin RH, Keeler EW, et al: Cytomegalovirus infection in dialysis patients and personnel. *Ann Intern Med* 89:625, 1978.

77. Hibberd PL, Rubin RH: Prevention of cytomegalovirus infection in the pediatric renal transplant recipients. *Pediatr Nephrol* 5:112, 1991.
78. Carney WP, Hirsch MS: Mechanism of immunosupression in cytomegalovirus mononucleosis. II. Virus-monocyte interaction. *J Infect Dis* 144:47, 1981.
79. Carney WP, Rubin RH, Hoffman RA, et al: Analysis of T-lymphocyte subsets in cytomegalovirus mononucleosis. *J Immunol* 126:2114, 1981.
80. Schooley RT, Hirsch MS, Colvin RB, et al: Association of herpes virus infection with T-lymphocyte subset alterations, glomerulopathy and opportunistic infections following renal transplantation. *N Engl J Med* 308:307, 1983.
81. Richardson WP, Colvin RB, Cheesman SH, et al: Glomerulopathy associated with cytomegalovirus viremia in renal allograft. *N Engl J Med* 305:57, 1981.
82. Herrera GA, Alexander RW, Cooley CF, et al: Cytomegalovirus glomerulopathy: A controversial lesion. *Kidney Int* 29:725, 1986.
83. Cameron J, Rigby RJ, Deth AG, et al: Severe tubulointerstitial disease in a renal allo-graft due to cytomegalovirus infection. *Clin Nephrol* 18:321, 1982.
84. Chou S: Newer methods for diagnosis of cytomegalovirus infection. *Rev Infect Dis* 12(suppl 7):727, 1990.
85. Balfour HH: Management of cytomegalovirus disease with antiviral drugs. *Rev Infect Dis* 12(suppl 7):849, 1990.
86. Reed EC: Treatment of cytomegalovirus pneumonia in transplant patients. *Transplant Proc* 23(suppl 1):8, 1991.
87. Medina I, Mills J, Leoung G, et al: Oral therapy for *Pneumocystis carinii* pneumonia in the acquired immunodeficiency syndrome. *N Engl J Med* 323:776, 1990.
88. Sattler FR, Cowan R, Nielson DM, et al: Trimethoprim-sulfamethoxazole compared with pentamidine for treatment of *Pneumocystis carinii* pneumonia in acquired immunodeficiency syndrome. *Ann Intern Med* 109:280, 1988.
89. Guidelines for prophylaxis against *Pneumocystis carinii* pneumonia for persons with human immunodeficiency virus. *MMWR* 38(suppl 5):1, 1989.
90. Broyer M, Guest G, Gagnadoux M-F, et al: Hypertension following renal transplant. *Pediatr Nephrol* 1:16, 1987.
91. Gordjani N, Offner G, Hoyer PF, et al: Hypertension after renal transplantation in patients treated with cyclosporine and azathioprine. *Arch Dis Child* 65:275, 1990.
92. Miach PJ, Ernest D, McKay J, et al: Renography with captopril in renal transplant recipients. *Transplant Proc* 21:1953, 1989.
93. Aliabadi H, McLorie GA, Churchill BM, et al: Percutaneous transluminal angioplasty for transplant renal artery stenosis in children. *J Urol* 143:569, 1990.
94. Lohr JW, MacDongall ML, Chonko AM, et al: Percutaneous transluminal angioplasty in transplant renal artery stenosis: Experience and review of the literature. *Am J Kid Dis* 7:363, 1986.
95. Dickerman RM, Peters PC, Hull AR, et al: Surgical correction of posttransplant renovascular hypertension. *Ann Surg* 192:639, 1980.
96. Penn I, Brunson ME: Cancers after cyclosporine therapy. *Transplant Proc* 20:885, 1988.
97. Wilkinson AH, Smith JL, Hunsicker LG, et al: Increased frequency of posttransplant lymphomas treated with cyclosporine, azathioprine, and prednisone. *Transplantation* 47:293, 1989.
98. Gruber SA, Chavers B, Skjei KL, et al: De novo cancer after pediatric kidney transplant. *Transplant Proc* 23:1373, 1991.
99. Eddy A, Sibley R, Mauer SM, et al: Renal allograft failure due to recurrent dense deposit disease. *Clin Nephrol* 21:305, 1984.

100. Habib R, Antignac C, Hinglias N, et al: Glomerulonephritis in the transplanted kidney in children. *Am J Kid Dis* 10:198, 1987.
101. Striegel JE, Sibley RK, Fryd DS, et al: Recurrence of focal segmental sclerosis in children following renal transplantation. *Kidney Int* 30:S110, 1986.
102. Hebert D, Kim E-M, Sibley RK, et al: Post-transplant outcome of patients with hemolytic-uremic syndrome: Update. *Pediatr Nephrol* 5:162, 1991.
103. Wilson CB, Dixon FB: Antiglomerular basement membrane antibody-induced glomerulonephritis. *Kidney Int* 3:381, 1973.
104. Advisory Committee to Renal Transplant Registry: Renal transplantation in congenital and metabolic diseases: A report from the ASC/NIH Renal Transplant Registry. *JAMA* 232:148, 1975.
105. Mahn JD et al: Congenital nephrotic syndrome: Evolution of medical management and results of renal transplantation. *J Pediatr* 105:549, 1984.
106. Virani R, Dan M: Membranous glomerulonephritis in renal transplant: A case report and review of literature. *Am J Nephrol* 2:316, 1982.
107. Fernandez JA et al: Recurrence of lupus nephritis in a renal allograft with histologic transformation of the lesion. *Transplantation* 50:1058, 1990.
108. Kher KK, Sheth KJ, Garancis JC: De novo membranous glomerulonephritis of renal transplant. *Int J Pediatr Nephrol* 2:139, 1981.
109. Habib R, Antignac C, Hinglias N, et al: Glomerulonephritis in the transplanted kidney in children. *Am J Kid Dis* 10:198, 1987.
110. Aschendorff C, Offner G, Winkler L, et al: Adult height achieved in children after kidney transplantation. *Am J Dis Child* 144:1138, 1990.
111. van Diemen-Steenvoorde R, Donkerwolcke RA, et al: Growth and sexual maturation in children after kidney transplantation. *J Pediatr* 110:351, 1987.
112. Kaiser B, Polinsky M, Stover J, et al: Growth after pediatric renal transplantation: Importance of alternate day steroids. *Kidney Int* 31:303, 1987.
113. Guest G, Broyer M: Growth after renal transplantation: Correlation with immunosuppressive therapy. *Pediatr Nephrol* 5:143, 1991.
114. Fine RN, Yadin O, Nelson PA, et al: Recombinant human growth hormone treatment of children following renal transplantation. *Pediatr Nephrol* 5:147, 1991.
115. Najarian JS, Frey DJ, Matas AJ, et al: Renal transplantation in infants. *Ann Surg* 212:353, 1990.
116. Ilstadt ST, Tollerud DJ, Noseworthy J, et al: The influence of donor age on graft survival in renal transplantation. *J Pediatr Surg* 25:134, 1990.
117. Rao KV, Kasiske BL, Odlund MD, et al: Influence of cadaver donor age on posttransplant renal function and graft outcome. *Transplantation* 49:91, 1990.
118. Arbus GG, Rochon J, Thompson D: Survival of cadaveric renal transplant grafts from young donors and young recipients. *Pediatr Nephrol* 5:152, 1991.
119. Potter D, Feduska N, Melzer J, et al: Twenty years of renal transplantation in children. *Pediatrics* 77:465, 1986.
120. Najarian JS, So SKS, Simmons RL, et al: The outcome of 304 primary renal transplants in children (1968–1985). *Ann Surg* 204:246, 1986.

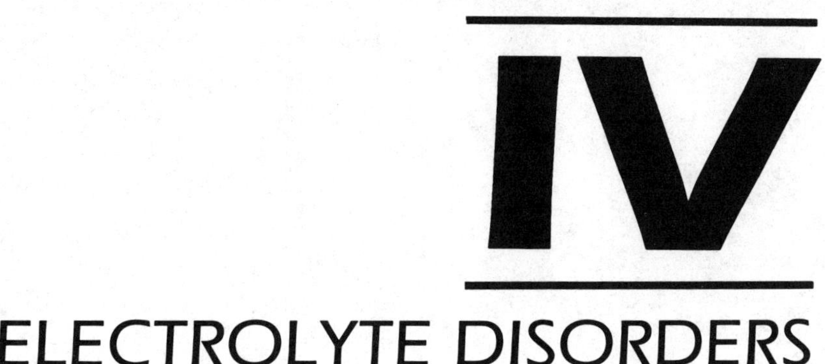

IV
ELECTROLYTE DISORDERS

20

METABOLIC ACID-BASE DISTURBANCES

Cynthia G. Pan

Metabolic derangements in acid-base equilibrium are commonly found in disease states and may be the first sign of an underlying primary metabolic disorder. They may also be serious indications of failing compensatory mechanisms, and if left untreated can lead to serious complications or death.

The diagnosis and treatment of metabolic acidosis and metabolic alkalosis rely on the understanding of normal acid-base physiology and the regulatory controls that govern blood pH. The purpose of this chapter is to summarize these systems and to review the clinical evaluation, diagnosis, and treatment of metabolic acidosis and alkalosis in pediatric diseases.

ACID-BASE EQUILIBRIUM

SOURCES OF HYDROGEN IONS

Hydrogen ions are produced in many metabolic reactions, the largest source being the oxidation of substrates to carbon dioxide. These substrates consist of neutral dietary precursors, such as glucose, and breakdown products of tissues. Carbon dioxide reacts with water within red blood cells to form carbonic acid. Carbonic acid quickly dissociates to hydrogen ion and bicarbonate. The reaction is facilitated by carbonic anhydrase (CA):

$$\underset{\text{(Hydration)}}{CO_2 + H_2O} \underset{CA}{\leftrightarrows} H_2CO_3 \leftrightarrows \underset{\text{(Dissociation)}}{H^+ + HCO_3^-}$$

In the lung, this reaction proceeds to the left and carbon dioxide is excreted efficiently through respirations. Acids excreted by the pulmonary system are termed *volatile acids. Nonvolatile acids* include sources of hydrogen ions produced daily during the catabolism of sulfur and phosphorus-containing proteins, mineralization of bones, and production of organic acids such as ketones or uric acid. These hydrogen ions are excreted via the kidney.[1] Under normal metabolic circumstances the body is faced with a potential positive hydrogen ion balance. The excretion of hydrogen ions by the kidney allows maintenance of a zero hydrogen balance.

MECHANISMS IN ACID-BASE EQUILIBRIUM

The physiologic maintenance of acid-base equilibrium is the result of the interaction of several mechanisms. Regulatory controls that maintain body pH between 7.35 and 7.45 require physiologic responses to be sensitive to changes in acid-base status. They must also be efficient, so that during fluctuations in metabolism or on exposure to exogenous sources of acid or alkali, pH is maintained constant.

The primary mechanism in maintenance of acid-base equilibrium is the body's set of buffers. These can be divided into bicarbonate and nonbicarbonate buffers. Buffers provide a rapid response to changes in acid-base equilibrium. Secondary physiologic mechanisms important in the regulation of the buffer system include the respiratory and renal responses. These systems are relatively slower in their response to regulate blood pH.[2]

BUFFERS

Buffers are defined as mixtures of weak acids and conjugate bases based on their ability to dissociate and associate with hydrogen ions.

Under normal conditions, estimates of 50 to 100 meq or 1 meq/kg of hydrogen ion is produced each day. Body buffers prevent wide fluctuations in body pH by removing free H^+ ions from solution instantly. Approximately half of buffering capacity is provided by the extracellular bicarbonate system. The other half is provided by nonbicarbonate intracellular buffers that include hemoglobin, plasma proteins, and phosphates. Together these buffer systems remain in equilibrium with each other. Therefore, changes occurring in hydrogen ion concentration cause changes in all buffers (isohydric principle). Maintenance of normal H^+ concentration requires generation of new bicarbonate, which in effect restores all buffer systems to their original state.[1]

Briefly, again, the relationship of species in the bicarbonate system is described as follows:

$$CO_2 + H_2O \leftrightarrows \underset{\text{Weak acid}}{H_2CO_3} \leftrightarrows \underset{\text{Conjugate base}}{H^+ + HCO_3^-}$$

The law of mass action states:

$$K = \frac{[H^+]\,[HCO_3^-]}{[CO_2 + H_2CO_3]}$$

$$[H^+] = \frac{K\,[CO_2 + H_2CO_3]}{[HCO_3^-]}$$

where K is constant.

A logarithmic transformation leads to the Henderson–Hasselbalch equation:

$$pH = pK + \log \frac{[HCO_3^-]}{[CO_2 + H_2CO_3]}$$

Dissolved CO_2 and carbonic acid in solution are in equilibrium to gaseous CO_2 which correlates to alveolar gas in the lung.[2] The Henderson–Hasselbalch equation can be rewritten to state

$$pH = pK + \log \frac{[HCO_3^-]}{S \times P_{CO_2}}$$

where P_{CO_2} is the partial pressure of carbon dioxide and S is its solubility factor.

SECONDARY PHYSIOLOGIC MECHANISMS

As seen by the above Henderson–Hasselbalch equation, the ratio of P_{CO_2} to bicarbonate concentration is directly proportional to $[H^+]$.

Clinical disturbances in acid-base equilibrium stem from changes in either of these two measurements. Classification of acid-base disorders is according to which variable is primarily disturbed (i.e., pH changes secondary to P_{CO_2} are respiratory disorders and those secondary to bicarbonate concentration are metabolic disorders). Primary disturbances of either variable result in a physiologic response by the other system, providing a compensatory mechanism to maintain hydrogen ion homeostasis.

Respiratory Regulation. Control of respirations or alveolar ventilation by the respiratory center is under the influence of several stimuli. Details of respiratory regulation are discussed by Cunningham et al.[3] In the context of this chapter, the reader should be aware that both blood pH and P_{CO_2} are strong stimuli for regulation of alveolar ventilation.

Renal Regulation. The kidney acts to regulate acid-base equilibrium by adjusting acid or alkali excretion. The overall result is maintenance of the bicarbonate buffer system. On a daily basis the kidney conserves existing bicarbonate stores and replenishes bicarbonate that is consumed in the process of buffering endogenous acids. When the body is presented with additional acid or alkali load, the normal kidney is able to adjust acid excretion quantitatively.

Reabsorption of bicarbonate. Bicarbonate concentration in glomerular filtrate is the same as that found in plasma. Approximately 80 to 90 percent of the freely filtered bicarbonate is reabsorbed in the proximal tubule, allowing almost complete conservation of bicarbonate prior to exiting the proximal tubule (Fig. 20–1). The presence of the enzyme carbonic anhydrase in the luminal proximal tubule's epithelium plays a key role in reabsorbing bicarbonate ion. This enzyme facilitates the intracellular hydration of CO_2 to carbonic acid. Carbonic acid proceeds to dissociation as hydrogen ion and bicarbonate ion. Details of renal tubular bicarbonate reabsorption are discussed by Gennari et al.[4] Other mechanisms such as direct bicarbonate or carbonic acid reabsorption may be involved, but their contribution is of little significance in normal conditions.

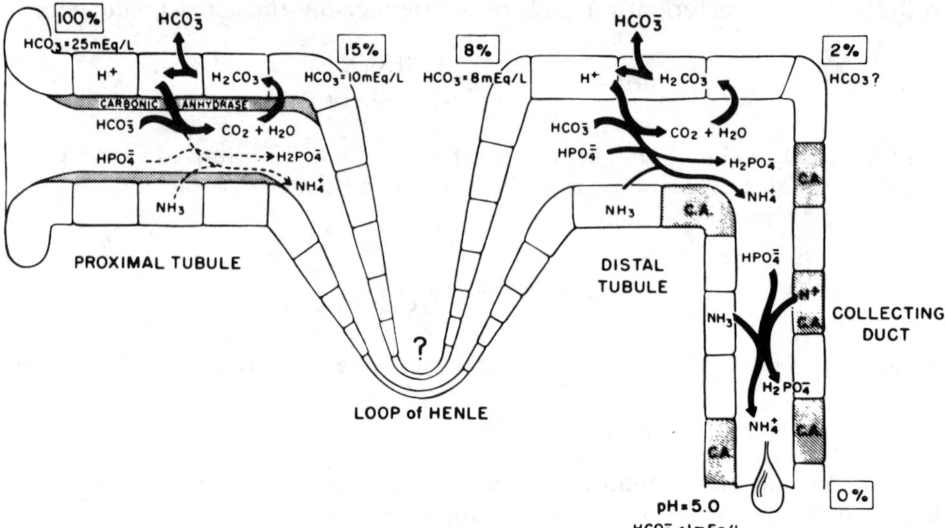

FIG. 20–1. The hydrogen ion secretory process in various segments of the nephron. The percentages shown in the boxes indicate fraction of filtered bicarbonate remaining in tubular urine; figures below the boxes indicate approximate bicarbonate concentration. (Reprinted with permission from Gennari FJ, Cohen JJ, Kassirer JP: Determinants of plasma bicarbonate concentration and hydrogen ion valence, in Cohen JJ, Kassirer JP (eds): *Acid Base,* 1st ed. Boston, Little, Brown and Company, 1982 p 64.)

Hydrogen ion excretion. The kidney excretes 50 to 100 meq per day (approximately 1 meq/kg/day) of hydrogen ions, but not as free hydrogen ions. Urinary buffer handles these hydrogen ions in the distal tubule such that the urine is rarely below pH 6.0 (Fig. 20–1). Filtered phosphate is the major urinary buffer and is termed the *titrable acid.* Hydrogen ions are also excreted by the conversion of urinary ammonia to ammonium. Ammonia, most of which is produced during glutamine metabolism, diffuses into the lumen from renal tubular epithelial cells. When combined with hydrogen ions, ammonia becomes ionized and thus trapped in the lumen and then excreted.

In the term newborn infant with a metabolic acidosis, the kidney is able to acidify the urine. The renal threshold for bicarbonate is slightly lower than that in adult kidneys (approximately 20 meq/L). In premature infants, net acid excretion during acidosis secondary to ammonium chloride loading is lower in the first 3 weeks of life than it is in the term infant.[5] When the rates of acid excretion in infants are compared to those of older children before and after an ammonium chloride load, the increase in acid excretion is less in infants.[6] This indicates less functional reserve in infants that may be required during physiologic stress.

METABOLIC ACIDOSIS

Metabolic acidosis is a disturbance in acid-base balance resulting from the lowering of bicarbonate concentration. The hydrogen ion concentration, or pH,

TABLE 20–1. Etiologies of Metabolic Acidosis

Loss of Bicarbonate
Gastrointestinal losses
Diarrhea
Ileus
Pancreatic drainage or fistula
Small bowel drainage or fistula
Biliary drainage
Ureterosigmoidostomies
Renal losses
Proximal tubular acidosis
Carbonic anhydrase inhibitors
Increased Hydrogen Ion Load
Exogenous administration
NH_4Cl, HCl
Toxins (aspirin, methanol, ibuprofen, ethylene glycol, etc.)
Endogenous production
Lactic acid
Diabetic ketoacidosis (acetoacetic acid, β-hydroxybutyric acid)
Inborn errors of metabolism (organic acids, amino acids)
Decreased Hydrogen Ion Excretion
Renal failure
Distal renal tubular acidoses

may not necessarily reflect this disturbance, as compensatory respiratory mechanisms may be working to preserve the normal state.

PATHOPHYSIOLOGY

Metabolic acidosis may occur through several mechanisms (Table 20–1). Loss of bicarbonate through the gastrointestinal tract or kidney can be of such magnitude as to result in the lowering of bicarbonate concentration. Second, the addition of acids to the body results in a hydrogen ion load that consumes bicarbonate, depleting the buffer system. Finally, failure to excrete hydrogen ions can result in depletion of bicarbonate stores. This typically occurs in renal failure, in which excretion of acid is impaired.

LOSS OF BICARBONATE

Gastrointestinal. In the pediatric patient, diarrhea is one of the leading causes of metabolic acidosis. Intestinal secretions distal to the pylorus are high in bicarbonate concentration, containing as much as 80 meq/L. Loss of small amounts of intestinal fluid via drainage, fistula, or diarrhea can lead to significant bicarbonate losses. With heavy losses of fluid, extracellular volume decreases as well, creating a smaller space for chloride. The end result is a hyperchloremic metabolic acidosis.

Surgical manipulations of the intestinal tract may create a source of fluid and electrolyte losses. In infants, ileostomies for necrotizing enterocolitis or meconium ileus may produce as much as 12 to 58 mL/kg/day of intestinal fluid. The development of hyperchloremic metabolic acidosis and hyponatremia has been shown to contribute to poor weight gain. With supplementation to correct for losses, weight gain may be more easily established.[7]

High rectourinary fistulas in imperforate anus may also lead to the development of a metabolic acidosis in infants. Reabsorption of urinary chloride and excretion of bicarbonate by the colon results in hyperchloremic metabolic acidosis.[8]

Renal. Clinical disorders characterized by renal bicarbonate wasting occur rarely. The proximal tubule is the major site for bicarbonate reabsorption. When it is injured or dysfunctional, the result is bicarbonate wasting and acidosis. Details regarding the etiologies of renal tubular acidosis and their diagnoses and treatments are provided in Chap. 21.

INCREASED HYDROGEN ION LOAD

There are many sources for exogenous or endogenous acids. Those that may be encountered more frequently or that are unique to the pediatric age group will be discussed.

Diabetic Ketoacidosis. Physicians caring for diabetic children are often faced with the medical emergency of diabetic ketoacidosis. Characterized by hyperglycemia, ketonemia, and acidosis, the events leading to diabetic ketoacidosis stem from insulin deficiency and the increase in counterregulatory hormones such as glucagon, cortisol, growth hormone, and epinephrine. Plasma bicarbonate falls in the process of buffering acetoacetic and β-hydroxybutyric acid. These acids are produced in excess by the liver as a consequence of the insulin deficiency which promotes lipolysis. Other catabolic hormones also increase lipolytic activity. The excess free fatty acids produced result in hepatic synthesis to ketoacids. Peripheral utilization and renal excretion of these acids may be able to keep up with this increased endogenous acid production in mild cases. In severe cases, however, the catabolic state overwhelms compensatory mechanisms and metabolic acidosis ensues (Fig. 20–2). Other contributing factors to metabolic acidosis are lactic acid production from hypoperfusion in severe dehydration and the hyperchloremic metabolic acidosis incurred during intravenous saline therapy.[9]

The symptoms of diabetic ketoacidosis will vary with the severity and length of the episode as well as the underlying illness that may have precipitated the metabolic disturbance. In severe diabetic ketoacidosis, hyperventilation is a prominent compensatory mechanism for the metabolic acidosis. Dehydration is often severe; as much as 10 percent of total body weight may be lost as a result of osmotic diuresis and complicating problems of vomiting and poor intake. Altered level of consciousness or coma may be present as well.

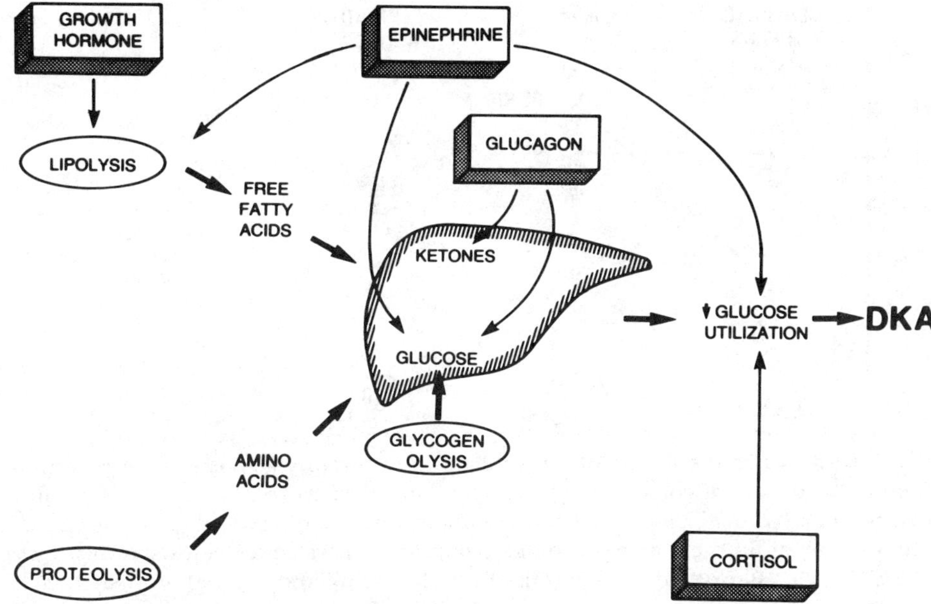

FIG. 20–2. The major sites of action of the counterregulatory hormones in diabetic ketoacidosis. (Reprinted with permission from Krane EJ: Diabetic ketoacidosis biochemistry, physiology, treatment, and prevention. *Pediatr Clin North Am* 34:938, 1987.)

Treatment of diabetic ketoacidosis is aimed at correcting the metabolic derangement with insulin therapy and repletion of the fluid and electrolyte losses. Correction of the metabolic acidosis usually occurs with this therapy. Ketogenesis is interrupted, ketones are metabolized peripherally, and bicarbonate stores are replenished. Treatment of severe acidosis with exogenous bicarbonate remains controversial.[10]

Because of the paradoxical fall in the pH of the cerebrospinal fluid (CSF) noted when systemic pH is corrected by intravenous bicarbonate therapy, aggressive bicarbonate replacement for treatment of diabetic ketoacidosis is not currently recommended. Lowering of the CSF pH may worsen the patient's state of consciousness in spite of an improvement in systemic pH and bicarbonate concentration. This phenomenon results from the differential permeability of the blood-brain barrier to CO_2 and bicarbonate, with CO_2 passing through this barrier relatively more easily than bicarbonate (Fig. 20–3). During correction of systemic acidosis, systemic P_{CO_2} rises as the stimulus for hyperventilation is resolved. The CSF P_{CO_2} rises without an accompanying rise in bicarbonate, resulting in a decrease in CSF pH.

Other reasons for withholding bicarbonate are based on changes in the hemoglobin-O_2 dissociation curve during acidosis. The "shift" of the curve to the right allows enhanced release of O_2 delivery to tissues during a state of decreased perfusion. Correction of pH may remove this mechanism from the patient who is dehydrated and poorly perfused.

Advocates of systemic bicarbonate therapy point to the detrimental effect of low pH (less than 7.1) on respiratory minute volume, the depressant effects of

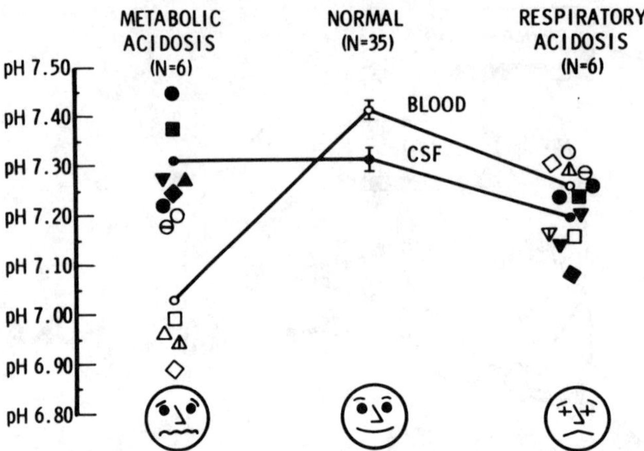

FIG. 20–3. Differing effects of metabolic and respiratory acidosis on cerebrospinal fluid pH and state of consciousness. Circles connected by solid lines represent mean values; open symbols, blood; and solid symbols, cerebrospinal fluid. (From Posner JB, Plum F: Spinal fluid pH and neurologic symptoms in systemic acidosis. *N Engl J Med* 277:611, 1967. Reprinted with permission of New England Journal of Medicine.)

acidosis on myocardial contractility, and the possible role of acidosis in insulin resistance. As a general guide, bicarbonate therapy is therefore reserved by many for use in diabetic ketoacidosis when the systemic pH is less than 7.1.[11]

Inborn Errors of Metabolism. The finding of metabolic acidosis in the newborn period should alert the physician to the possibility of an underlying inborn error of metabolism. Left unrecognized, many of these disorders can lead to significant mental retardation or death. Early recognition of several of these diseases and institution of specific therapy may prevent a devastating outcome.

Reviews of the clinical features of metabolic errors in newborns reveal that the signs and symptoms are nonspecific (Table 20–2). Most commonly found, however, are the symptoms of poor feeding and failure to thrive, followed by lethargy, vomiting, tachypnea, and seizures.[12,13] In most cases, these symptoms are manifested in the first week of life, often within the first 24 to 48 h.

Detailed descriptions of each metabolic error leading to acidosis can be found in several sources.[12,13] The disorders can be grouped into four major categories

TABLE 20–2. Clinical Manifestations of Inborn Errors of Metabolism

Failure to thrive
Lethargy
Vomiting
Seizures
Tachypnea
Jaundice
Hypotonia
Hepatomegaly

TABLE 20–3. Inborn Errors of Metabolism Associated with Metabolic Acidosis in the Neonatal Period

Disorders of Carbohydrate Metabolism
Hereditary fructose intolerance
Fructose-1,6-diphosphatase deficiency
Glycogen storage disease, type I (von Gierke's disease, glucose-6-phosphatase deficiency)
Glycogen storage disease, type III
Urea Cycle Defects
Carbamoylphosphate synthetase deficiency
Disorders of Amino Acid Metabolism
Pyroglutamic acidemia
Disorders of Organic Acid Metabolism
Methylmalonic acidemia
Propionic acidemia
Isovaleric acidemia
Butyric and hexanoic acidemia

Source: Adapted from Burton BK, Nadler HL: Clinical diagnosis of the inborn errors of metabolism in the neonatal period. *Pediatrics* 61:399, 1978. Reproduced by permission of American Academy of Pediatrics, ©1978.

and include those involving carbohydrate metabolism, the urea cycle, amino acid metabolism, and organic acid metabolism (Table 20–3). Initial laboratory workup for metabolic errors also shows overlap in the various disorders but may provide data that will aid in diagnosis. In disorders of carbohydrate metabolism, non-glucose-reducing substances in the urine along with direct hyperbilirubinemia may be the first laboratory indications of galactosemia. In urea cycle disorders, hyperammonemia is the predominant laboratory finding. Hyperammonemia may also be found in organic acid disorders, such as propionic acidemia, illustrating the need for definitive diagnostic tests to distinguish these disorders.[14]

Lactic Acidosis. Lactic acidosis has been defined as a blood lactate level greater than 2 meq/L (18 mg/100 mL). Lactic acid is the end product of anaerobic glucose catabolism. The ratio of lactate to pyruvate is determined by the relative oxidative state of tissue. Tissue hypoxia promotes an increase in the lactate-to-pyruvate ratio and has been observed in circulatory shock states, hypoxemia, and severe muscular exercise. In several of the inborn errors of metabolism, including glycogen storage disease type I, fructose diphosphatase deficiency, propionic acidemia, and methylmalonic acidemia, varying increases in lactate levels have been demonstrated. In such cases, if adequate tissue oxygenation is present, proportional increases in pyruvate are observed, the ratio remaining stable. Chronic idiopathic lactic acidosis in childhood is a rare disease and probably represents many different types of metabolic errors.[15]

Ingestions. The ingestion of several drugs and chemicals can lead to metabolic acidosis and pose health problems to the pediatric population.

Acetylsalicylic acid (aspirin). Toxic ingestion of acetylsalicylic acid is not uncommon, both in accidental and intentional overdose. Disturbances of acid-base equilibrium occur during acute salicylate poisoning through several mechanisms.

Increased alveolar ventilation is a well-recognized consequence of the ingestion of salicylates and is a result of their direct effect on the respiratory center, causing enhanced sensitivity to CO_2. This mechanism promotes hypocapnia and a primary respiratory alkalosis. Also contributing to the acid-base disturbance is an increase in O_2 consumption and CO_2 production secondary to salicylate's effect on the uncoupling of oxidative phosphorylation. This increase in CO_2 production becomes clinically significant with development of hypercapnia in patients with underlying pulmonary disease or central nervous system (CNS) depression in which the primary hyperventilation is impaired. In children, the most severe effect on acid-base equilibrium is the metabolic acidosis induced, the development of which largely depends on increased endogenous acid production. Salicylate metabolites may make a small contribution to the acidosis. Susceptibility to the development of this acidosis appears to be age-dependent. Children, particularly infants and those under the age of 4 years, are at a greater risk than are older children and adults.[16] Metabolic acidosis is a predominant feature in the infant, as opposed to the adult, in whom a primary hyperventilation and respiratory alkalosis are more often observed.

Clinical features of patients with salicylate intoxication include coma, altered mental status, convulsions, and hyperventilation. Fever may be seen in infants. The diagnosis is suspected by the history of ingestion, clinical symptoms, and the laboratory findings of acid-base disturbance and a positive urinary ferric chloride test. The definitive diagnosis is confirmed by an elevated salicylate level. The severity of the intoxication is best correlated with the salicylate level at the time of ingestion rather than that at the time of diagnosis. This can be estimated based on the pharmacokinetics of salicylate.[17]

Excretion of salicylate is primarily achieved through the kidney and is highly dependent on urinary pH. Reabsorption of nonionized salicylate is favored in an acidic urine. As urine pH becomes alkaline, salicylate clearance is enhanced. Treatment of salicylate intoxication is aimed at the correction of the metabolic acidosis and the enhancement of renal excretion through alkaline diuresis. Other methods of removal include peritoneal dialysis, hemodialysis, and hemoperfusion.[18]

Nonsteroidal anti-inflammatory drugs. Over-the-counter availability has brought attention to the potential hazards of these drugs. Ibuprofen overdosage has been reported to cause mainly gastrointestinal or neurologic symptoms, in addition to a metabolic acidosis.[19]

Ethylene glycol and methanol. Ethylene glycol is a solvent that is commonly used as an antifreeze agent in gasoline engines; it is extremely toxic when ingested. Its metabolites, glycolic acid and oxalic acid, produce a metabolic acidosis, and the latter compound may produce crystals that ultimately are responsible for the development of acute renal failure. The metabolic acidosis induced is often severe, with plasma bicarbonate levels below 5 meq/L.

Methanol, like ethylene glycol, produces severe toxicity in amounts as small as 30 mL. In addition to the metabolic acidosis, retinitis is a devastating complication. Metabolites include formic acid, a major anion contributing to the acidosis. Therapy for both methanol and ethylene glycol ingestion is aimed at correcting the acidosis with bicarbonate and removing the agent. Hemodialysis is indicated for removal of both ethylene glycol and methanol. Ethanol infusions slow the production of metabolites, as ethanol competes with alcohol dehydrogenase, an enzyme involved in the breakdown of both substances. The diagnosis of these poisonings must be made quickly. In the patient with severe metabolic acidosis who is suspected of an ingestion, the osmolal gap should be calculated. This measurement is the difference between the measured and calculated serum osmolality.

$$\text{Calculated osmolality} = 1.86\,[\text{Na}^+] + [\text{glucose}]/18 + [\text{urea nitrogen}]/2.8 + [\text{ethanol}]/4.6$$

The concentrations of each component of glucose, urea nitrogen, and ethanol are milligrams per 100 mL. If the osmolal gap is greater than 15 to 20 mOsm/kg, the diagnosis of methanol or ethylene glycol poisoning should be considered.[20]

DECREASED HYDROGEN ION EXCRETION

Renal Failure. The acidosis that develops with the onset of renal failure is a result of the inability to excrete acid. Regeneration of bicarbonate is consequently impaired and the daily production of endogenous acids soon begins to consume bicarbonate stores. In acute renal failure, if endogenous acid production is normal and there are no excessive pathologic states influencing acid-base balance, one can expect the serum bicarbonate level to decline by approximately 2 meq/L/day. Clinical situations in which endogenous acid production is increased (e.g., fever, surgery, diabetic ketoacidosis, infections) may induce a more severe acidosis.

In chronic renal failure, acidosis from the accumulation of anions is universal; its severity depends on the degree of renal impairment. Reductions in the glomerular filtration rate (GFR) to less than 25 percent of normal result in acidosis. However, in moderate renal insufficiency, a mild acid-base disturbance has also been observed.[21]

With prolonged untreated renal failure, serum bicarbonate levels rarely fall below 10 to 12 meq/L, in spite of the ongoing daily production of an acid load. This has been attributed to the buffering capacity of bone[22] and probably plays a role in the development of osteodystrophy, particularly in childhood disease.

Treatment of acidosis in both acute and chronic renal failure is aimed at normalization of plasma bicarbonate by administration of exogenous bicarbonate or by removal of organic acids by dialysis.

EVALUATION OF THE PATIENT WITH METABOLIC ACIDOSIS

Establishing the Diagnosis of Metabolic Acidosis. To make the diagnosis of an acid-base disorder, one must evaluate the clinical history. Often the primary diagnosis will be dependent on this data, as laboratory findings are not always definitive. Clues—such as the age of the patient, underlying medical diseases, or possible exposures to exogenous toxins—will aid in the diagnosis of metabolic acidosis.

Second, the establishment of the presence of a metabolic acidosis depends on appropriate laboratory tests. In a simple metabolic acidosis, a low serum bicarbonate and an accompanying lowered arterial P_{CO_2} establishes the diagnosis. Measurement of the serum pH is not always necessary unless the presence of acidemia is questioned or if there is a possibility that a mixed acid-base disturbance is present. Though this chapter will not address the details of diagnosing mixed acid-base disturbances, a few rules of thumb will help distinguish a pure metabolic acidosis from a complicated or mixed disorder.

Reduction in P_{CO_2} reflects respiratory compensation to a metabolic acidosis, the goal of which is to normalize serum pH. The expected serum P_{CO_2} in a simple, uncomplicated metabolic acidosis can be estimated from the serum bicarbonate level. This relationship is based on observations of the respiratory response to acidosis. A simplified, clinically usable equation in mild to moderately severe acidosis is

$$\Delta P_{CO_2} = 1.2 \times \Delta HCO_3^- \pm 2.0$$

where ΔP_{CO_2} represents the expected change in P_{CO_2} for the observed change in serum bicarbonate level. In severe acidosis (pH less than 7.1), bicarbonate levels may be less sensitive indicators of acidosis than pH. As a rule, if the pH is less than 7.1, the P_{CO_2} should be less than 18 mmHg; if the pH is less than 7.0, P_{CO_2} should be less than 15 mmHg.[23]

In cases where the P_{CO_2} is inappropriately high, an underlying pulmonary insufficiency causing a respiratory acidosis should be investigated. If the P_{CO_2} is lower than expected for the observed bicarbonate level, a primary respiratory alkalosis may be complicating the metabolic acidosis. In either of these situations, the inappropriate level of P_{CO_2} may also reflect a delay in compensation and may not necessarily represent a mixed disorder.

Anion Gap in the Diagnosis of Metabolic Acidosis. The anion gap can be calculated from routinely obtained laboratory measurements and is a useful tool in differentiating the causes of a metabolic acidosis. Normal physiology dictates that the sum of the total cations is equal to the sum of the total anions. The anion gap is derived from the following:

$$\begin{aligned}
\text{Total cations} &= NA^{+} + \text{unmeasured cations (UC)} \\
\text{Total anions} &= Cl^{-} + HCO_3^{-} + \text{unmeasured anions (UA)} \\
Na^{+} - (Cl^{-} + HCO_3^{-}) &= UA - UC \\
UA - UC &= \text{anion gap}
\end{aligned}$$

Unmeasured anions consist of proteins, sulfate, phosphate, and organic acids. Unmeasured cations consist of K^{+}, Ca^{2+}, and Mg^{2+} ions. K^{+} is often not included in the calculation of the anion gap because of its frequent fluctuations. The normal anion gap is 12 meq/L ± 2 meq/L.

Once the diagnosis of metabolic acidosis is made, the anion gap can be used to help differentiate the underlying etiology by identifying whether there is an elevated or normal anion gap (Table 20–4). In cases of an elevated anion gap, an unmeasured anion is the cause for the acidosis. Bicarbonate is consumed by the addition of an acid, and the anion formed from this acid is retained. The gap becomes increased as serum bicarbonate is lowered and the anion replacing it remains unmeasured. Examples of organic anions that can elevate the anion gap include ketoacids in diabetic ketoacidosis, lactate in lactic acidosis, and formic acid in methanol poisoning. The increase in anion gap may also be a result of changes in potassium, Ca^{2+}, phosphorus, or proteins.[24]

Metabolic acidosis with a normal anion gap usually occurs with bicarbonate losses, as in diarrheal illnesses or renal tubular acidoses. In these cases, there is a rise in serum chloride concentration equal to the lowering in bicarbonate concentration, thus keeping the anion gap unchanged.

Effects of Acute Acidosis. The physician should be knowledgeable about the acute effects of acidosis on the patient. Most devastating are the effects on the cardiovascular system. Acute severe acidosis (pH less than 7.1) may depress cardiac contractility and arteriolar tone leading to a state of shock. An increased venous tone secondary to acidosis may further complicate poor cardiac function and result in pulmonary edema. In a milder acidosis, an increase in heart rate and contractility is seen because of an increase in catecholamine production.[25]

TABLE 20–4. Use of the Anion Gap in Metabolic Acidosis

Normal Anion Gap Acidosis	Increased Anion Gap Acidosis
Gastrointestinal bicarbonate loss	Increased production of acid
Diarrhea	Diabetic ketoacidosis
Small bowel or pancreatic drainage	Inborn errors of metabolism
Ureterosigmoidostomies	Lactic acidosis
Renal bicarbonate loss	Starvation ketosis
Renal tubular acidosis	Ingestion of toxins
Carbonic anhydrase inhibitors	Salicylate
Hyperparathyroidism	Methanol
Hypoaldosteronism	Ethylene glycol
Other	Ibuprofen
Addition of HCl	Failure of excretion of acid
Dilutional acidosis	Renal failure

METABOLIC ALKALOSIS

Metabolic alkalosis is defined as the disturbance in acid-base equilibrium characterized by an elevated serum bicarbonate level, resulting in alkalemia. In a simple metabolic alkalosis, compensatory respiratory mechanisms raise P_{CO_2}, resulting in less change in serum pH.

PATHOPHYSIOLOGY

Hyperbicarbonatemia occurs when there is an addition or generation of new bicarbonate. Maintenance of alkalosis is promoted if compensatory mechanisms of renal bicarbonate excretion are absent or negated. Thus, the pathophysiology of metabolic alkalosis is often viewed in terms of *generation* and *maintenance* of hyperbicarbonatemia.

Generation of Alkalosis. Loss of body fluid low in bicarbonate concentration and high in chloride will cause the remaining bicarbonate to be distributed in a lesser fluid volume, leading to an elevated serum bicarbonate. Alkalosis produced under these circumstances is termed *contraction alkalosis* and can result from excessive fluid losses from the GI tract, kidney, or skin.

An increase in bicarbonate in the extracellular fluid (ECF) may also occur by addition of alkali from an exogenous source (iatrogenic) or by excess endogenous bicarbonate production. Exogenous sources of alkali include $NaHCO_3$, and salts of acids (e.g., lactate, acetate).

Alkalosis can also occur as a result of upper gastrointestinal loss of H^+, as with protracted vomiting or gastric drainage. Gastric parietal cells are responsible for the production of HCl in the gastric secretions. In this process, H^+ is secreted into the gastric lumen while HCO_3^- is returned to the systemic circulatory pool. Neutralization of the H^+ (in HCl) occurs downstream in the small intestines, where it combines with the HCO_3^- generated and secreted by the pancreatic cells. In the clinical situations where gastric H^+ is lost continuously, an equivalent systemic HCO_3^- accumulation ensues, leading to alkalosis.

The kidney also participates in endogenous alkali production. As discussed earlier in this chapter, the secretion of H^+ protons allows the reabsorption of a filtered bicarbonate in the proximal tubule and the generation of bicarbonate in the distal tubule (Fig. 20–1). The latter serves to restore bicarbonate that is consumed by the daily production of endogenous acid. When net acid excretion exceeds endogenous acid production, excess bicarbonate is generated and serum bicarbonate is increased. Factors that influence H^+ ion secretion, and thus bicarbonate generation, are listed in Table 20–5. Sodium is reabsorbed in exchange for each H^+ ion. Conditions favoring distal sodium reabsorption will increase H^+ ion secretion. These conditions include states of volume contraction and increased mineralocorticoids. Diuretic therapy leading to increased delivery of solute to the distal tubule, volume depletion, and stimulation of aldosterone is a classic example in which alkalosis is created. Aldosterone, secreted primarily or secondarily, will have a direct effect on Na^+-H^+ activity in the distal tubule.

TABLE 20–5. Factors that Influence Renal Hydrogen Ion Secretion

Potassium depletion
Mineralocorticoid excess
Diuretic therapy (increased sodium to the distal tubule, increased aldosterone)
Increased distal delivery of poorly reabsorbable anion

Other factors enhancing distal H^+ ion secretion include potassium depletion. Also, the increased delivery of a poorly reabsorbable anion to the distal tubule—such as sulfate, phosphate, or nitrate—will increase luminal negativity, thus favoring H^+ ion secretion. Chloride anions are the major anion of tubular fluid and easily reabsorbed. Therefore, in cases of severe chloride deficiency, poorly reabsorbable anions dominate, again favoring H^+ ion secretion.[26]

MAINTENANCE OF ALKALOSIS

Normally, increased renal excretion of bicarbonate is able to correct alkalosis. However, when the GFR is diminished (decreasing bicarbonate excretion) or circumstances for increased tubular reabsorption of bicarbonate exist, renal compensatory mechanisms are offset and alkalosis is maintained. Available evidence points to the fact that alkalosis itself promotes reduction of the GFR. The mechanisms involved in this process are not clearly understood but appear to be linked to tubuloglomerular feedback and volume contraction.[27,28] Factors enhancing tubular reabsorption of bicarbonate are decreased effective circulating volume, hypochloremia, hypokalemia, hyperaldosteronism, low circulating parathyroid hormone, hypercalcemia, and hyperphosphatemia.

CLINICAL STATES WITH METABOLIC ALKALOSIS

Vomiting. A classic example of moderately severe vomiting inducing a metabolic alkalosis in childhood is pyloric stenosis. Varying degrees of obstruction produce a wide range of clinical presentations, but typically the patient presents in the first month of life, at approximately 3 weeks of age, with protracted vomiting. As the obstruction worsens, the vomiting can be quite forceful, bringing the child to medical attention. As discussed earlier, with continued loss of gastric hydrochloric acid, there is a net gain of bicarbonate, leading to alkalosis. Maintenance of this increased extracellular bicarbonate is provided by other mechanisms, including volume contraction (from gastrointestinal fluid loss), hypochloremia, and potassium deficiency (Fig. 20–4). The degree of electrolyte and acid-base imbalance will vary depending on the severity of the patient's symptoms and the time at which the abnormality is diagnosed. Surgical correction of the lesion is the treatment of choice. Correction of severe electrolyte imbalance and alkalosis is advised preoperatively and can usually be done

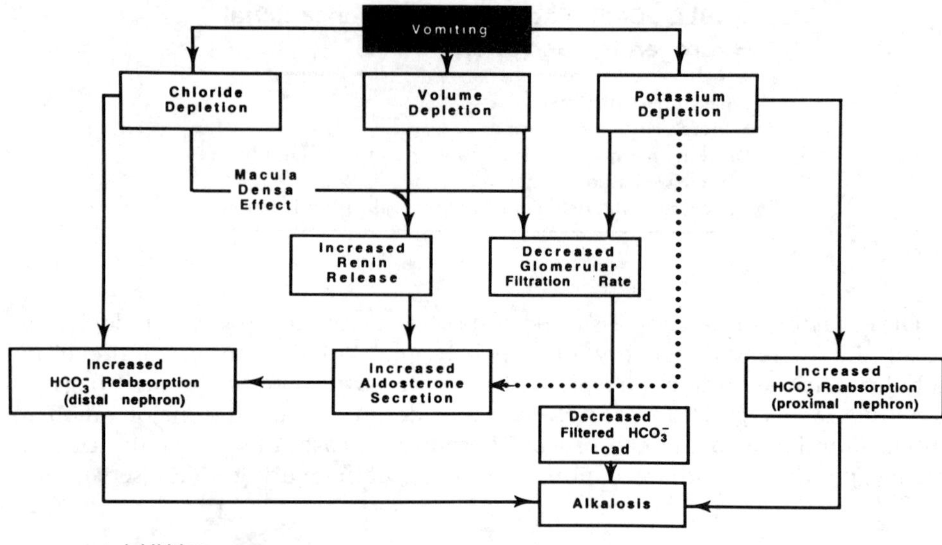

FIG. 20–4. Maintenance of alkalosis during vomiting. (Adapted and reproduced with permission from Galla JH: Pathophysiology of metabolic alkalosis. *Hosp Pract* 22(10):123, 1987. Illustration by Albert Miller.)

within the first 24 to 48 h. Fluid is administered to replete volume and correct potassium and sodium chloride deficits.

Other examples in which alkalosis has resulted from heavy gastric losses include gastric suction or drainage. A more difficult diagnosis is the patient with metabolic alkalosis secondary to self-induced surreptitious vomiting. A high level of suspicion may be needed to diagnose this potential etiology and to avoid unnecessary workup or invasive procedures.[29]

Diuretics. Prescribed for the treatment of hypertension, edema-forming states, and management of fluid overload, these agents may complicate the patient's state by inducing a metabolic alkalosis. In the pediatric age group, this is commonly seen in the neonatal intensive care unit. In one study,[30] approximately 25 percent of premature newborns admitted to one center received diuretics, primarily for respiratory distress syndrome as well as for fluid overload, congestive heart failure, and bronchopulmonary dysplasia. Electrolyte and acid-base abnormalities occurred in 23 percent of treated children. The major abnormalities were hypochloremia and metabolic alkalosis.[30] A contraction alkalosis, especially in severely edematous patients who lose substantial weight with diuretics, results from fluid losses high in sodium and chloride but relatively lower in bicarbonate. Several diuretics—including ethacrynic acid, furosemide, and metolazone—increase renal acid secretion, thus helping maintain a metabolic alkalosis. Hypokalemia and hypochloremia in chronic diuretic therapy ensue, the latter maintaining the alkalosis.[31]

Chloride-Deficient Diets. Metabolic alkalosis and hypochloremia secondary to an alkali load and insufficient chloride intake has been reported in infants receiving formulas with increased poorly reabsorbable unmeasured anions and low chloride content. The resulting failure to thrive also led to probable volume depletion and a contraction alkalosis. These abnormalities were all corrected with increasing dietary chloride.[32,33]

Congenital Chloride-Losing Diarrhea. Metabolic alkalosis has also been reported in other chloride-deficient states, such as congenital chloride-losing diarrhea. In this rare disease, a defect in chloride-bicarbonate transport results in high stool losses of chloride and protons, leading to a hypochloremic metabolic alkalosis.[34]

Cystic Fibrosis. Salt depletion in older children with cystic fibrosis is well recognized. Hyponatremia, hypochloremia, and metabolic alkalosis have also been reported in infants. This unusual presentation in infants is presumed to be a result of electrolyte losses via the skin in combination with losses due to a vomiting or diarrheal illness. In several cases, infants manifested their cystic fibrosis as hypoelectrolytemia and alkalosis on initial presentation. This warrants the consideration of this inherited disease when a disturbance in electrolyte or acid-base status in this age group cannot be explained.[35,36]

Mineralocorticoid Excess. Conditions associated with excess mineralocorticoids include primary aldosteronism and Cushing's syndrome, both rare diseases of childhood. The exact mechanism of the observed metabolic alkalosis is not completely understood. Increased delivery and reabsorption of sodium in the distal tubule and increased secretion of hydrogen ions as a consequence of aldosterone is one proposed mechanism. As opposed to patients with other forms of alkalosis, those with increased adrenocortical function are volume expanded.

Bartter's Syndrome. Characterized by normal blood pressure, hypokalemia, metabolic alkalosis, prostaglandinuria, hyperreninemia, and hyperaldosteronism, Bartter's syndrome comes to the attention of the pediatrician for the early failure to thrive observed in childhood. A primary defect in tubular function has been proposed, consisting of decreased distal chloride reabsorption accompanied by primary potassium wasting. Hyperreninemia and hyperaldosteronism are a consequence of the potassium deficiency, the latter exacerbating this deficiency. The increased production of renal prostaglandins is also stimulated and is felt to promote renin release as well. Therapy for Bartter's syndrome is aimed at potassium repletion and inhibition of renal prostaglandin synthesis using a prostaglandin synthetase inhibitor.[37]

Excess Alkali. In the presence of normal renal function, large amounts of alkali—such as sodium bicarbonate—administered continuously are needed to induce a metabolic alkalosis. A report of an alkalosis secondary to alkali exposure through use of baking soda for diaper rash has been reported.[38] Alkalosis secondary to excessive alkali is otherwise uncommon in the pediatric age group.

CLINICAL EVALUATION OF METABOLIC ALKALOSIS

The physiologic effect of metabolic alkalosis on ventilation is most dramatic in patients with an underlying chronic lung disease. In these patients, diuretic therapy may contribute to hypochloremia, hypokalemia, and alkalosis. Acidemia is a stimulus for ventilatory drive, and subtle changes in pH caused by a metabolic alkalosis may be substantial enough to depress ventilation.

Diagnosis of Metabolic Alkalosis. The presence of an elevated serum bicarbonate and an alkaline blood pH (greater than 7.45) indicates a metabolic alkalosis. Hypoventilation, allowing an increase in P_{CO_2}, is the proper respiratory response. The change in P_{CO_2} is predicted by the equation:

$$\Delta P_{CO_2} = 0.7 \times \Delta HCO_3^- \pm 5$$

where ΔP_{CO_2} is in mmHg and ΔH_{CO_3} is expressed in meq/L.

The approach to a patient with a metabolic alkalosis includes taking a detailed history of drug therapy, vomiting, nasogastric suctioning, and underlying illnesses. In cases suspected of surreptitious vomiting or diuretic abuse, the patient's own body image should be investigated. The physical exam should note the patient's growth and blood pressure in order to identify endocrine problems or Bartter's syndrome. Volume status should be assessed, but in many cases a decrease in extracellular volume sufficient to maintain an alkalosis may not be detectable by exam.

If renal function is normal, it is helpful to obtain the urinary chloride concentration. In metabolic alkaloses associated with volume depletion or hypochloremia, the urinary chloride is usually low—less than 10 meq/L or negligible. In cases of chronic diuretic therapy, the urinary chloride may be greater than 10 meq/L if a diuretic has recently been administered. Often termed *saline responsive,* or *chloride-responsive,* this group generally experiences improvement with the administration of NaCl or KCl.

The *chloride-resistant* group, in contrast, generally does not respond to a trial of NaCl or KCl. This group tends to have urinary chloride >10 meq/L. They may be volume-expanded and hypertensive (with the exception of Bartter's syndrome). In patients with hypertension, plasma renin and aldosterone levels will aid in separating cases of Cushing's syndrome and primary aldosteronism (Table 20–6).

THERAPY OF METABOLIC ALKALOSIS

Efforts to diagnose the etiology of a metabolic alkalosis will usually result in choosing a specific therapy. The most common causes—vomiting, diuretic ther-

TABLE 20–6. Diagnosis of Metabolic Alkalosis

Urinary Chloride <10 meq/L
Gastric losses (vomiting, nasogastric suctioning)
Low chloride intake
GI losses (congenital chloride-losing diarrhea)
Diuretic therapy
Urinary Chloride >10 meq/L
With normal blood pressure
Bartter's syndrome
Diuretic therapy (recently ingested)
With hypertension
Cushing's syndrome
Primary aldosteronism
Exogenous mineralocorticoids

apy, or nasogastric suctioning—are in the *chloride-sensitive* group and are corrected by appropriate replacement with sodium, chloride, potassium, and volume. In severe cases (pH > 7.55 and HCO_3^- >40 meq/L) or where metabolic alkalosis contributes to CNS or cardiotoxicity, intravenous HCl, 0.1 to 0.2 *M* solution, can be used to correct alkalosis. Intravenous HCl is given in a central line and the amount infused must be carefully titrated so as not to lead to overcorrection. Also, such therapy must be administered in a controlled setting for careful monitoring of acid-base status, volume status, and presence of infiltration of HCl from intravenous sites.[39] Knutsen[40] has advocated use of a 0.15 *M* HCl infusion by a peripheral intravenous line using a solution containing amino acids and fat. Arginine hydrochloride can be used in place of HCl and can be given by a peripheral intravenous route. The amount of HCl necessary to correct alkalosis is calculated by the following formula:

$$\text{HCl required (meq)} = 0.5 \times \text{weight (kg)} \times \text{desired decrement of plasma } HCO_3^-$$

Only half correction of the estimated HCl requirement should be undertaken initially; the rate of infusion (via a central line) should not exceed 0.2 meq /kg/h.[39] Carbonic anhydrase inhibitors such as acetazolamide induce a brisk bicarbonaturia, but treatment with them is usually reserved for severe alkalosis in edema-forming states and can result in hypokalemia. Finally, dialysis, either peritoneal or hemodialysis, can be adjusted such that dialysate fluids contain less bicarbonate or acetate or have other anions such as chloride substituted.

The *chloride-resistant* group may be more difficult to treat. Potassium repletion in hypokalemic patients may be helpful; in most cases, however, therapy is aimed at eliminating the source of excess mineralocorticoids.

SUMMARY

The pediatric patient may manifest a mild metabolic alkalosis or acidosis during the course of a common illness. When acid-base derangements become more severe, immediate attention is required. Because of this wide spectrum of severity, the physician must understand the physiology, etiologies, diagnosis, and treatment of these metabolic disorders.

REFERENCES

1. Johnston DG, Alberti KGMM: Acid-base balance in metabolic acidoses. *Clin Endocrinol Metab* 12:267, 1983.
2. Dell RB. Normal acid-base regulation, in *The Body Fluids in Pediatrics,* 1st ed. Boston, Little, Brown, 1973, pp 23–47.
3. Cunningham DJC, Robbins PA, Wolff CB: Integration of respiratory responses to changes in alveolar pressures of CO_2 and O_2 in arterial pH, in Cheniack NS, Widdicombe JG (eds): *Handbook of Physiology, Respiratory System—Control of Breathing.* Bethesda, Maryland, Am. Physiological Society, 1986, pp 475–528.
4. Gennari FJ, Cohen JJ, Kassirer JP: Determinants of plasma bicarbonate concentration and hydrogen ion balance, in *Acid-Base,* 1st ed. Boston, Little, Brown, 1982, pp 55–88.
5. Svenningsen NW: Renal acid-base titration studies in infants with and without metabolic acidosis in the postnatal period. *Pediatr Res* 8:659, 1974.
6. Edelmann CM JR: Physiologic adaptations required of newborn's kidney. *Contrib Nephrol* 15:1, 1979.
7. Bower TR, Pringle KC, Soper RT: Sodium deficit causing decreased weight gain and metabolic acidosis in infants with ileostomy. *J Pediatr Surg* 23:567, 1988.
8. Caldenone AA, Emmens RW, Rabinowitz R: Hyperchloremic acidosis and imperforate anus. *J Urol* 122:817, 1979.
9. Androgue HJ, Wilson H, Boyd AE, et al: Plasma patterns in acid-base diabetic ketoacidosis. *N Engl J Med* 307:1603, 1982.
10. Kaye R: Diabetic ketoacidosis—the bicarbonate controversy. *J Pediatr* 87:156, 1975.
11. Sperling MA: Diabetic ketoacidosis. *Pediatr Clin North Am* 31:591, 1984.
12. Barela TD, Johnson JD, Hayek A: Metabolic acidosis in the newborn period. *Clin Endocrinol Metab* 12:429, 1983.
13. Burton BK, Nadler HL: Clinical diagnosis of the inborn errors of metabolism in the neonatal period. *Pediatrics* 61:398, 1978.
14. Wolf BW, Hsia YW, Tanaka K, et al: Correlation between serum propionate and blood ammonia concentrations in propionic acidemia. *J Pediatr* 93:471, 1978.
15. Israels S, Haworth JC, Dunn HG, et al: Lactic acidosis in childhood. *Adv Pediatr* 22:267, 1976.
16. Winters RW, White JS, Hughes MC, et al: Disturbances of acid-base equilibrium in salicylate intoxication. *Pediatrics* 23:260, 1959.
17. Done AK: Salicylate intoxication: Significance of measurement in blood in cases of acute ingestion. *Pediatrics* 26:800, 1960.
18. James JA, Kimbell L, Read WT: Experimental salicylate intoxication: I. Comparison of exchange transfusion, intermittent peritoneal lavage, and hemodialysis as means for removing salicylate. *Pediatrics* 29:442, 1962.

19. Linden CH, Townsend PL: Metabolic acidosis after acute ibuprofen overdosage. *J Pediatr* 111:922, 1987.
20. Kaehny WD, Gabow PA: Pathogenesis and management of metabolic acidosis and alkalosis, in *Renal and Electrolyte Disorders,* 3rd ed. Boston, Little, Brown, 1986, p 165.
21. Widmer B, Gerhardt RE, Harrington JT, et al: Serum electrolyte and acid-base composition: The influence of graded degrees of chronic renal failure. *Arch Intern Med* 139:1099, 1979.
22. Lemann J, Jr, Litzow JR, Lennon EJ: The effects of chronic acid loads in normal man: Further evidence of the participation of bone mineral in the defense against chronic metabolic acidosis. *J Clin Invest* 45:1608, 1966.
23. Oh MS, Delmonte ML, Carroll HJ: Respiratory compensation in severe metabolic acidosis. *Kidney Int* 10:506, 1976.
24. Gabow PA, Kaehny WD, Fennessey DV, et al: Diagnostic importance of an increased serum anion gap. *N Engl J Med* 303:854, 1980.
25. Caroll HJ, Oh MS, eds: Disturbances in acid-base balance, in *Water, Electrolyte, and Acid-Base Metabolism,* 2nd ed. Philadelphia, Lippincott, 1989, p 236.
26. Narins RG, Jones ER, Townsend R, et al: Metabolic acid-base disorders: Pathophysiology, classification and treatment, in *Fluid, Electrolyte, and Acid-Base Disorders,* vol. 1. New York, Churchill-Livingstone, 1985, pp 269–384.
27. Berger BE, Cogan MG, Sebastian A: Reduced glomerular filtration and enhanced bicarbonate reabsorption maintain metabolic alkalosis in humans. *Kidney Int* 26:205, 1984.
28. Harrington JT: Metabolic alkalosis. *Kidney Int* 26:88, 1989.
29. Wallace M, Richards P, Chesser E, et al: Persistent alkalosis and hypokalemia caused by surreptitious vomiting. *Q J Med* 37:579, 1968.
30. Laudigon N, Campi A, Coupal L, et al: Furosemide and ethacrynic acid: Risk factors for the occurrence of serum electrolyte abnormalities and metabolic alkalosis in newborns and infants. *Acta Pediatr Scand* 78:133, 1989.
31. Schwartz WB, Van Ypersele de Strihou C, Kassirer JP: Role of anions in metabolic alkalosis and potassium deficiency. *N Engl J Med* 279:630, 1968.
32. Grossman H, Duggan E, McCamman S, et al: The dietary chloride syndrome. *Pediatrics* 66:366, 1980.
33. Roy S, III, Arant BS Jr: Hypokalemic metabolic alkalosis in normotensive infants with elevated plasma renin activity and hyperaldosteronism: Role of dietary chloride deficiency. *Pediatrics* 67:423, 1981.
34. Evanson JM, Stanbury SW: Congenital chloridorrhea or so-called congenital alkalosis with diarrhea. *Gut* 6:29, 1965.
35. Gottlieb R: Metabolic alkalosis in cystic fibrosis. *J Pediatr* 70:930, 1971.
36. Nussbaum E, Boat TF, Wood RE, et al: Cystic fibrosis with acute hypoelectrolytemia and metabolic alkalosis in infancy. *Am J Dis Child* 133:965, 1979.
37. Bartter FC, Rodriquez JA: Bartter's syndrome, in Frick P, Von Hornack GA, Koschsick K, et al: *Advances in Internal Medicine and Pediatrics.* Heidelberg, Springer-Verlag, 1982, pp 79–103.
38. Gonzalez J, Hogg RJ: Metabolic alkalosis secondary to baking soda treatment of a diaper rash. *Pediatrics* 67:820, 1981.
39. Galla JH, Luke RG: Pathophysiology of metabolic alkalosis. *Hosp Pract* Oct 15:123, 1987.
40. Knutsen DH: New method for administration of hydrochloric acid in metabolic alkalosis. *Lancet* 2:953, 1983.

21

RENAL TUBULAR ACIDOSIS

James D. Hanna
Fernando Santos
James C. M. Chan

INTRODUCTION

Metabolic acidosis caused by a defect in the excretion of hydrogen ions by the renal tubules is known as renal tubular acidosis (RTA). Depending on the tubular segment involved, the consequence of such a defect is either failure of the tubules to reabsorb filtered bicarbonate (type II RTA) or an inability to excrete the daily endogenous metabolic acid load (type I RTA); both circumstances lead to the development of metabolic acidosis.[1,2] RTA is characterized by failure to thrive as well as recurrent episodes of vomiting, dehydration, and constipation.[3,4] Nephrocalcinosis and nephrolithiasis are noteworthy complications of type I RTA, which results from hypercalciuria and hypocitraturia.[2,5–11] Most cases of RTA are sporadic, but familial cases with autosomal dominant transmission have been described. Renal tubular acidosis associated with genetically transmitted systemic diseases such as nerve deafness[12,13] or osteopetrosis[14,15] has also been reported. This chapter attempts to outline renal tubular handling of hydrogen ion and bicarbonate reabsorption, discuss clinical and laboratory features of various types of RTA, and recommend treatment for such patients.

RENAL HANDLING OF BICARBONATE

Bicarbonate reabsorption in the kidney takes place in both the proximal and distal nephrons. The majority of bicarbonate reabsorption, approximately 85 percent, occurs in the proximal tubule via the sodium hydrogen exchanger. This is a form of active transport, the energy for which is provided by the transcellular gradient for sodium. Once secreted, the hydrogen ion in the lumen combines with bicarbonate to form carbonic acid, which is rapidly broken down to carbon dioxide and water by the luminal-bound carbonic anhydrase. The carbon dioxide so formed rapidly equilibrates across the luminal membrane with intracellular carbon dioxide. Once inside the cell, carbon dioxide is hydrated with water via intracellular carbonic anhydrase and once again forms carbonic acid. Intracellular dissociation yields hydrogen ion and bicarbonate, which replaces the secreted hydrogen ion across the luminal membrane and yields a net movement of bicarbonate from the lumen into the cell, accompanied by sodium. Finally, the intracellular bicarbonate is transported from the cell to the peritubular capillary by an electrogenic sodium bicarbonate symporter, which is driven by the electrochemical gradient for bicarbonate from the cell into the peritubular space. Bicarbonate is then returned to the systemic circulation via the renal vein.

The reclamation of the remaining 15 percent of filtered bicarbonate is accomplished by the distal nephron through a sodium-independent electrogenic hydrogen (proton) translocating ATPase. Luminal secretion of hydrogen ion is balanced by the addition of bicarbonate across the basolateral membrane through the action of the chloride-bicarbonate exchanger. This process yields a secreted proton into the lumen and the return of bicarbonate to the systemic circulation.

RENAL HANDLING OF HYDROGEN ION

The Brönsted-Lowry concept defines an acid as a hydrogen ion donor and a base as a hydrogen ion acceptor.[16] A strong acid readily dissociates nearly completely into the hydrogen ion and the conjugate base. A weak acid dissociates only partially. There are two categories of acid: (1) metabolic acids and (2) nonmetabolic acids.[10] The *metabolic* acids are metabolized at the level of the liver and lungs into H_2O and CO_2, with the CO_2 exhaled by the lungs into the external environment (Fig. 21–1*A*). The *nonmetabolic* acids are excreted via the kidneys. The renal excretion of acid involves two mechanisms: the formation of titratable acid and ammonium. As shown in Fig. 21–1*B*, carbonic acid (H_2CO_3) dissociates into bicarbonate and hydrogen ion.[3,16] The bicarbonate is reabsorbed, and the secreted hydrogen ion is principally buffered by filtered phosphate into

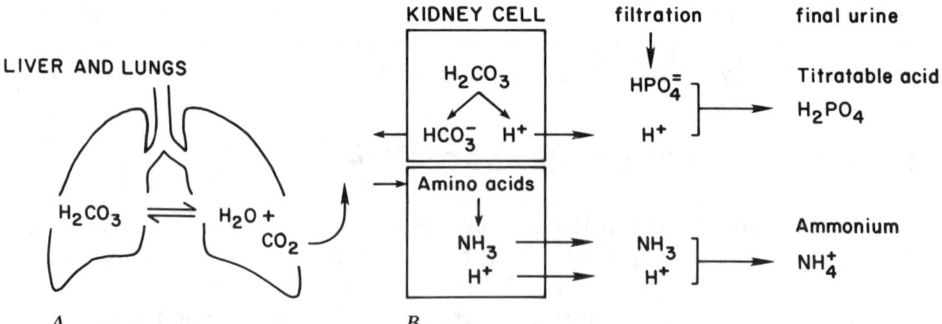

FIG. 21–1. Metabolic (*A*) and nonmetabolic (*B*) acids. H_2CO_3 = carbonic acid; H_2O = water; CO_2 = carbon dioxide; HCO_3^- = bicarbonate anion; H^+ = hydrogen ion; NH_3 = ammonia; NH_4^+ = ammonium; $HPO_4^=$ = monohydrogen phosphate; $H_2PO_4^-$ = dihydrogen phosphate.

titratable acid.[5,10] The other urinary buffers are citrate, creatinine, and uric acid. The pK of inorganic phosphate is 6.8. At the glomerular filtrate's pH of 7.25, 70 percent of the filtered phosphate exists as the conjugate base (HPO_4).[16] As the urinary pH drops to 6.8, 50 percent of the filtered phosphate is in the conjugate base form. A further drop in urine pH to 5.8 leaves only 10 percent of the phosphate in the conjugate form, virtually exhausting the buffering capacity of phosphate. At this point, the other urinary buffers begin to exert their effects, with the pKs of the creatinine and uric acid at 4.9 and 5.6, respectively.[16] These urinary buffers continue to be utilized until the pH declines to 4.4. In a physiological organism, the urinary pH does not drop much below 4.4.

In the past, the formation of ammonium (NH_4^+) ions was perceived as the result of ammonia (NH_3) formation by the action of glutaminase on glutamine (Fig. 21–2). The buffering of the luminal hydrogen ion (H^+) by ammonia gives rise to the formation of ammonium ion. The pK of ammonia, however, is 9.3, which means that almost all ammonia is already present as ammonium at the luminal pH of 7.3. Thus, renal ammoniagenesis is now viewed as the result of

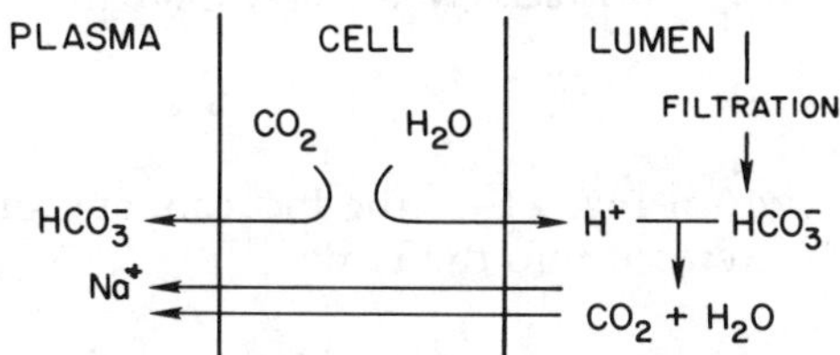

Bicarbonate Reabsorption

Formation of titratable acid

Formation of ammonium ions

FIG. 21–2. Bicarbonate reabsorption, formation of titratable acid and ammonium ions. Na^+ = sodium; H_2O = water; CO_2 = carbon dioxide; HCO_3^- = bicarbonate; H^+ = hydrogen ion; NH_3 = ammonia; NH_4^+ = ammonium; $HPO_4^=$ = monohydrogen phosphate. (Modified from Kildeberg P: *Clinical Acid-Base Physiology*. Baltimore, Williams & Wilkins, 1968, by permission.)

TITRATABLE ACID

$$pH - pK = \log \frac{HPO_4^{=}}{H_2PO_4^{-}}$$

AMMONIUM

$$\text{Glutamine} \rightleftharpoons 3\ CO_2 + 2\ NH_4^+ + 2\ HCO_3^-$$

$$\text{Glutamine} \rightleftharpoons \tfrac{1}{2}\ \text{glucose} + 2\ NH_4^+ + 2\ HCO_3^-$$

FIG. 21–3. Titratable acid and ammonium metabolism. CO_2 = carbon dioxide; HCO_3^- = bicarbonate, NH_4^+ = ammonium, HPO_4^- = monohydrogen phosphate; $H_2PO_4^-$ = dihydrogen phosphate. [Modified from Klahr S, et al.: in Chan JCM, Gill JR, Jr. (eds): *Kidney Electrolyte Disorders*. New York, Churchill Livingstone, 1990, by permission.]

the two pathways shown in Fig. 21–3; the bicarbonate returns to the plasma and the ammonium is excreted into the lumen.[17]

CLASSIFICATION

Primary RTA is a disorder resulting from a defect in proximal bicarbonate reabsorption and/or distal hydrogen ion secretion.[1–4] The most common biochemical characteristics are hyperchloremic metabolic acidosis and a normal or moderately reduced glomerular filtration rate. Characteristically, the anion gap is normal (Table 21–1).

TABLE 21–1. Metabolic Acidosis with Normal Anion Gap

- Renal tubular acidosis
- Early uremic acidosis
- Dilutional acidosis
- Acid loads
- Bicarbonate losses
  - Diarrhea
  - Ureterosigmoidostomy
  - Intestinal fistulas
  - Drugs
    - Calcium chloride
    - Magnesium sulfate
    - Cholestyramine

Three primary types of RTA are described. Type I RTA results from inadequate elimination of hydrogen ions in the distal nephron.[1,2,18] Type II RTA is characterized by massive bicarbonaturia secondary to defective proximal bicarbonate reabsorption.[3,4] Both type I and type II RTA are associated with hypokalemia.[1-4] In contrast, type IV RTA is characterized by *hyperkalemia* and is associated with a defect in ammonium excretion resulting from aldosterone deficiency or tubular resistance to actions of aldosterone.[19] Type I RTA associated with severe bicarbonate wasting was previously described as type III RTA. It is a hybrid form of RTA combining the distal acidification derangement with a defect in proximal bicarbonate reabsorption. Rather than being a distinct entity in itself, type III RTA is currently considered to be a variant of type I RTA, that is exclusively found in infants and children.

CLINICAL AND BIOCHEMICAL FEATURES

DISTAL RTA

Primary distal RTA presents clinically in infancy or early childhood.[3] Most commonly, these children present with a failure to thrive and are growth-retarded, their height and weight remaining at less than or equal to 2.5 standard deviations below the mean for age- and sex-matched controls.[20] Historically they are often reported as being listless,[20] irritable with stimulation,[4] having a poor appetite,[20] and—in extreme instances—as anorexic.[20] They have multiple episodes of emesis[20] and may have accompanying diarrhea,[4,21] but they may also have a history of constipation.[20] Despite their poor appetite and episodes of vomiting, their history will reveal polydypsia[3] and polyuria,[3] with an easy tendency to dehydration.[3] The polyuria has been found to occur as a result of a primary concentrating defect in the kidney.[2] Some patients present with nephrocalcinosis,[22-24] nephrolithiasis,[22] and/or pyelonephritis;[22] others develop these complications as the untreated disease progresses. Earlier reports made claim to an association of rickets, osteomalacia, and bone pain with distal RTA; however, an extensive study by Brenner et al.[25] did not support this contention. The prevailing view is that the aforementioned bone abnormalities are not seen with primary distal RTA in the absence of azotemia.

Physical examination of these children may reveal stunted growth,[3,4] gray pallor,[20] superficial venous spasm after phlebotomy,[20] proximal muscle wasting,[20] muscular weakness,[20] and hypotonia.[4] A developmental history may reveal a developmental delay.[4] As a rule the deficiency in hydrogen ion excretion is permanent, although temporary cases with reversal of the acidification defect have been reported.[4,26]

The majority of cases of isolated distal RTA occur sporadically,[22] but there are approximately 30 families in which familial occurrence has been reported.[22] These have shown mostly an autosomal dominant inheritance pattern,[20,22] but X-linked[22] as well as autosomal recessive[15,27] cases have been reported.

Renal tubular acidosis is hallmarked by hyperchloremic metabolic acidosis secondary to a defect in renal acidification, as manifest by an inappropriately high urine pH (reduction in net acid excretion), bicarbonaturia, or a dysfunc-

TABLE 21–2. Etiologic Spectrum of Type I RTA

Isolated primary defect	Genetically transmitted systemic diseases (Continued)
Secondary defects	Carbonic anhydrase deficiency
Tubulointerstitial renal disorders	Hereditary fructose intolerance
Obstructive uropathy	Fabry's disease
Medullary sponge kidney	Autoimmune disease
Renal transplantation	Sjögren syndrome
Nephrocalcinosis induced by metabolic and endocrine disorders:	Hypergammaglobulinemic disorders
Vitamin D intoxication	Systemic lupus erythematosus
Hyperparathyroidism	Chronic active hepatitis
Idiopathic hypercalciuria	Thyroiditis
Wilson's disease	Toxin or drug-induced
Hyperthyroidism	Amphotericin B
Genetically transmitted systemic diseases	Lithium
Ehlers–Danlos syndrome	Analgesics
Marfan syndrome	Cyclamate
Osteopetrosis with associated nerve deafness	Toluene
Sickle cell anemia	Hyponatriuric states
Elliptocytosis	Nephrotic syndrome
	Hepatic cirrhosis

tion of the distal nephron and its response to aldosterone (Tables 21–2 and 21–3). The hyperchloremic metabolic acidosis is associated with a normal serum anion gap of less than or equal to 12 meq/L[3] (Table 21–1). Another characteristic of these patients with type I RTA is a urine pH greater than 5.5 in the face of spontaneous or induced systemic acidosis[22] (CO_2 less than 17 mmol/L in infants, less than 20 mmol/L in an older child).[28] Net acid excretion in the face of systemic acidosis is less than 70 μeq/min/1.73 m^2, corresponding to a tubular lumen: plasma hydrogen ion gradient of 80:1 versus the normal tenfold greater increase of 800:1 seen in control subjects.[3] The hydrogen ion imbalance in distal RTA is related to a reduced net acid excretion; however, these patients also have increased endogenous acid production.[29] Patients with distal RTA who are given an oral alkali load, such as sodium bicarbonate, to increase their urine pH to greater than 7.8 reveal a subnormal increase in their urine minus blood P_{CO_2} difference. Their pressure gradient is less than 5 mmHg, as opposed to the greater than or equal to 30 mmHg increase found in healthy subjects (Table 21–4).[3] A mild degree of bicarbonaturia is present at all times in patients with classic distal RTA,[20] and a more severe degree of bicarbonaturia is present in those with type I RTA with bicarbonate wasting (old type III).[30] In the former, the magnitude and persistence of the bicarbonaturia is approximately 3 meq/kg/24 h,[20] which corresponds to a fractional excretion of less than 5 percent.[3] In the latter, the fractional excretion of bicarbonate ranges from 6 to 14 percent, and the bicarbonaturia is consequently higher (Table 21–4).[30]

Electrolytes can accompany the poorly reabsorbable bicarbonate anion in the distal nephron and collecting duct, and an associated wasting of sodium and especially potassium can be seen.[3] If wasting is present, fractional excretion of

TABLE 21–3. Etiologic Spectrum of Type II RTA

Isolated RTA	Vitamin D deficiency, dependence, or resistance
Primary (sporadic or familial)	Interstitial renal disease
Carbonic anhydrase inhibition	Sjögren syndrome
Acetazolamide	Medullary cystic disease
Mafenide (sulfamylon)	Renal transplantation rejection (early)
Carbonic anhydrase deficiency	Balkan nephropathy
Osteopetrosis with carbonic anhydrase II deficiency	Chronic renal vein thrombosis
Generalized	Toxins
Primary (sporadic or familial)	Outdated tetracyclines
Inborn error of metabolism	Lead
Cystinosis	Mercury
Lowe syndrome	Gentamicin
Hereditary fructose intolerance	Cadmium
Tyrosinemia	Maleic acid
Galactosemia	Coumarin
Wilson's disease	Streptozocin
Pyruvate carboxylase deficiency	Miscellaneous
Metachromatic leukodystrophy	Nephrotic syndrome
Glycogen storage disease	Paroxysmal nocturnal hemoglobinuria
Dysproteinemic states	Malignancy
Multiple myeloma	Congenital heart disease
Light chain disease	
Monoclonal gammopathy	
Amyloidosis	

sodium will be 2 to 3 percent;[22] potassium excretion can be greater than or equal to 40 meq/L, with a corresponding serum level of less than or equal to 3.8 meq/L.[3] The mechanism believed to be responsible for the perpetration of electrolyte loss is hyperaldosteronism resulting from extracellular fluid volume contraction; recent studies, however, have shown that hypokalemia is often absent in pediatric patients,[2,30] and the serum potassium levels are not uniform, showing variance from low to high.[4,31]

Urinary calcium excretion is increased to the level of 10 to 20 mg/kg/day, versus the normal value of less than 4 mg/kg/day.[3] Accompanying this hypercalciuria is hyperphosphaturia, as metabolic acidosis increases the renal clearance of both phosphate and calcium.[32,33] Additionally, hypocitraturia is induced by the metabolic acidosis through increased citrate oxidation in the proximal tubular mitochondria,[8,11] resulting in excretion of less than or equal to 23 mg citrate/g creatinine in the male (normal, greater than or equal to 128 mg citrate/g creatinine) and less than or equal to 71 mg citrate/g creatinine in the female (normal, greater than or equal to 300 mg citrate/g creatinine).[8] The resulting hypercalciuria, hyperphosphaturia, and hypocitraturia, combined with an alkaline urine, lead to precipitation of calcium phosphate as well as calcium oxalate and the subsequent development of nephrocalcinosis.[22] Urinary sulfate excretion has similarly been found to be increased (1.4 $\pm$ 0.5 meq/kg/day versus normal 0.7 $\pm$ 0.2 meq/kg/day)[34] and is believed to result in a pos-

TABLE 21–4. Clinical, Laboratory, and Treatment Characteristics of RTA in Children

	Type I (Classic, Distal)	Type II (Proximal)	Type III (Hybrid)	Type IV (Distal Nephron)
Growth failure	+++	++	+++	+++
Hypokalemic muscle weakness	++	+	+	Hyperkalemia
Nephrocalcinosis	Frequent	Rare	±	Rare
Renal insufficiency, obstructive uropathy, hypoaldosteronism, pseudohypoaldosteronism	Uncommon	Uncommon	Uncommon	Common
Low citrate excretion	+++	±	±	±
Plasma K^+	Low	Low	Low	High
Fractional excretion of filtered HCO_3 at normal serum bicarbonate levels, percent	<5	>15	5–15	<15
Urine anion gap	Postive	Normal	Variable	Positive
Glycosuria and aminoaciduria (Fanconi syndrome)	Absent	Present	±	±
Urine pH with acidosis	>5.5	<5.5	>5.5	Variable
Urine-blood P_{CO_2}	Low	Normal	Low	Low
Daily alkali treatment, meq/kg body weight	2 to 4	2 to 14	2 to 14	2 to 3
Daily potassium requirement	Decreases with correction	Increases with correction	±	±
Reponse to therapy	Good	Fair	Improves with time	Fair

Key: +, present; ++, +++, very common; −, not present; ±, variable.
Source: Modified from Chan JCM: *J Pediatr* 102:327, 1983. Reproduced by permission.

sible subclinical sulfate deficiency, impairing chondroitin sulfate incorporation into bone and potentially contributing to growth failure.[34]

Collagen metabolism, as well, is affected by metabolic acidosis, showing a marked elevation in the activity of a key biosynthetic enzyme during acidosis and returning to baseline within 24 h of correction of the imbalance.[35] Normal serum levels of vitamin D metabolites, calcium, phosphorus, and alkaline phosphatase[4] have been reported[4,36] in patients with this disorder. In fact, children, in contrast to adults, exhibit a positive calcium balance in metabolic acidosis.[37] In the initial stages of distal RTA, patients may have impairment of net acid excretion in the absence of detectable renal disease or a reduction in glomerular filtration rate (GFR). The degree of metabolic acidosis is, therefore, characteristically out of proportion to the reduction in GFR. Early in the disease process then, little to no impairment in GFR is evident;[3] however, as the disease progresses and its complications become manifest (i.e., calcium deposition/ nephrocalcinosis), mild to moderate reductions in the GFR may be seen. Often it is at this stage that referral and definitive diagnosis are confirmed. Rodriguez-Soriano et al.[2] have found that in type I distal RTA with bicarbonate wasting, there is an inverse linear correlation between the calciuria and plasma bicarbonate concentration, with the calciuria worsening as the serum bicarbonate level decreases. It is noteworthy that the bicarbonate wasting is of a transient nature, with the fractional bicarbonate excretion decreasing to the level of typical classic distal RTA during early childhood.[2] When quantitatively measured, the levels of fractional excretion tend to range from 6.8 to 15.1 percent during the first year of life and to decrease to 1.6 to 5.8 percent by age 4.[2] A special therapeutic note worthy of emphasis is that bicarbonate wasting may often increase after alkali therapy is begun, when rapid increases in growth velocity are seen.[38] Thus, type I RTA with bicarbonate wasting reveals a transient age-related proximal defect and a persistent distal tubular reabsorption defect that is permanent, resulting in sustained mild bicarbonate wasting typical of classic type I distal RTA.

PROXIMAL RTA

Proximal RTA presents with a feature common to all forms of RTA in that these children fail to thrive and exhibit a height and weight often below the 3rd percentile.[23] Almost invariably there is a history of excessive emesis, but otherwise these children are relatively free of symptoms if their defect is an isolated one and not part of the Fanconi syndrome (Table 21–3).[23] As opposed to distal RTA, a primary defect in the kidney's ability to concentrate is not present,[23] and these patients rarely, if ever, develop nephrocalcinosis.[3] In the absence of the Fanconi syndrome, which is associated with a generalized proximal tubular dysfunction, these patients do not experience osteomalacia, rickets, or bone pain.[3,25]

The biochemical features of proximal RTA are distinct from those of distal RTA because the distal tubule is not impaired; therefore, the untreated patient can acidify his urine to a pH of less than 5.5 when plasma bicarbonate concentration drops below the renal threshold for bicarbonate (Fig. 21–4).[20] As the plasma bicarbonate concentration is increased toward normal, bicarbonate reabsorption in the distal tubule is overwhelmed by the proximal wasting, and bicarbonaturia becomes evident (Fig. 21–4).[3,20] Maintenance of normal systemic bicarbonate levels is difficult secondary to the massive bicarbonaturia that occurs as the systemic bicarbonate levels are increased.[20] The accompanying urinary electrolyte loss (sodium and potassium) results in the contraction of extracellular fluid volume and secondary hyperaldosteronism.[20] The metabolic acidosis tends to be milder than in type I RTA[3] and, despite treatment, renal potassium wasting and hyperaldosteronism may persist in both types I and II RTA for reasons that are unknown.[3,39] Measurement of the fractional excretion of bicarbonate typically reveals a fractional excretion greater than 15 percent (Table 21–4).[3,20] Absence of associated hypercalciuria or hyperphosphaturia and presence of hypercitraturia leads to a virtual absence of nephrocalcinosis.[22] The

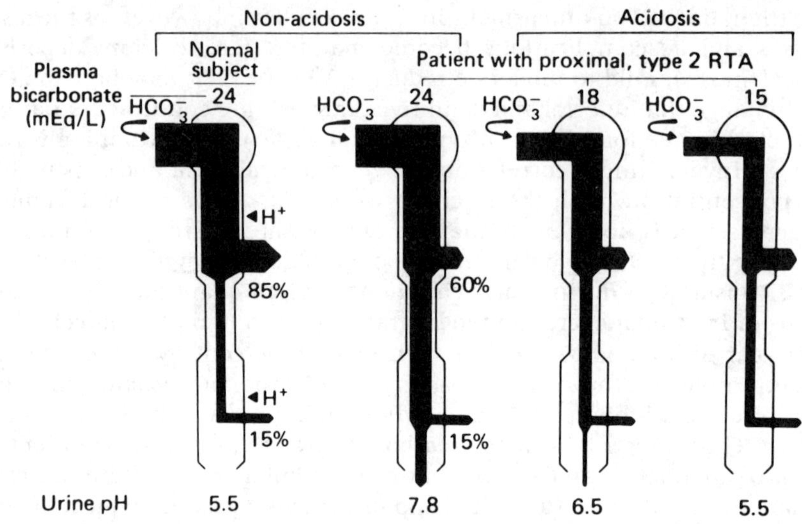

FIG. 21–4. Schematic representation of bicarbonate reabsorption and loss in patients with nonazotemic type II RTA. In a normal individual, the distal nephron reabsorbs 15 to 17 percent of filtered bicarbonate and excretes a normally acidified urine. In an individual with proximal RTA, the inability of the proximal tubule to adequately reabsorb bicarbonate delivers an increased load distally, which overwhelms the nephron's reabsorptive capacity. The result is a lowered systemic pH from renal bicarbonate loss and an increased urinary pH, also from bicarbonate loss. As the systemic bicarbonate level decreases below normal, the filtered load of bicarbonate is commensurately reduced and the distal nephron is no longer overwhelmed. Thus, normal terminal bicarbonate reabsorption occurs and an acidified urine is excreted. As the systemic pH is increased through bicarbonate supplementation, a reverse process occurs. HCO_3^- = bicarbonate, H^+ = hydrogen. (From McSherry E: Renal tubular acidosis in childhood. *Kidney Int* 20:800, 1981.)

GFR tends to be normal to slightly decreased in the untreated state.[3] After an ammonium chloride load, the urine pH decreases to less than 5.0 and the titratable acid and ammonium production from the distal nephron and collecting duct are normal.[23]

HYPERKALEMIC RTA (TYPE IV)

A recently recognized form of RTA is that associated with hyperkalemia or type IV renal tubular acidosis. This has become the most common form encountered in clinical medicine.[40] These infants, as in other types of RTA, present with growth failure.[3] Additionally, they have hyperkalemia, a fractional excretion of bicarbonate less than 15 percent,[3] variable hypercitraturia,[20] and variable generalized proximal tubular dysfunction.[3] They rarely exhibit nephrocalcinosis (Table 21–4).[3] Five subtypes of type IV RTA have been described (Table 21–5).

TABLE 21–5. Pathophysiologic Subtypes of Type IV RTA

Subtype		Clinical Finding						
Number	Mechanism and Designation	Plasma Renin Activity	Urinary Aldosterone	Blood/ Plasma	BP Volume	K	Salt Wasting	Response to Mineralocorticoid
1	Aldosterone deficiency without intrinsic renal disease Primary mineralocorticoid deficiency (Addison's disease; congenital adrenal hyperplasia; isolated hypoaldosteronism)	↑	↓	↓ →	↓ →	↑	+	Yes
2	Aldosterone deficiency with chronic hyporeninemia Primary hyporeninemia secondary hypoaldosteronism of azotemic adults (diabetes, gout, pyelonephritis, interstitial nephritis, nephrosclerosis)	↓	↓	↑ →	↑ →	↑	−	Yes
3	Adolescent hyperkalemic syndrome (chloride shunt)	↓	↓	↑	↑	↑	−	No
4	Reduced tubular responsiveness to aldosterone Pseudohypoaldosteronism (classic)	↑↑	↑↑	↓	↓	↑	+	No
5	"Early childhood" type IV RTA	Not ↓	Not ↓	Nml	Low Nml	↑	−	No

Key: ↑ = increased; ↓ = decreased; → = unchanged; + = present; − = absent; Nml = normal.
Source: Adapted from McSherry E: *Kidney Int* 20:799, 1981, and Chan JCM: *J Pediatr* 102:327, 1983. Reproduced by permission.

Subtype V is notable for its association with vomiting in addition to the shortness and stunted growth.[20]

Biochemically, hyperchloremic metabolic acidosis is accompanied by a normal anion gap, but, as opposed to classic hypokalemic distal RTA, hyperkalemia is present.[16] The ability to acidify the urine with accompanying acidosis, either systemic or induced, is intact.[20] As expected, both the metabolic acidosis and hyperkalemia are out of proportion to the reduction in GFR.[41,42] The proximal bicarbonate reabsorption is mildly impaired, and the fractional excretion of bicarbonate ranges from 3 to 10 percent (Table 21–4).[41,42]

Pathophysiologically, three general categories exist, which, in turn, have been further divided into subtypes. Type IV RTA can broadly be classified as a primary defect in the adrenal gland from either general dysfunction or deficiencies in mineralocorticoid synthesis, depressed stimulation of aldosterone release secondary to suppressed or inadequate renin/angiotensin production, or resistance of the collecting tubule to the action of mineralocorticoid (Table 21–5).

Subtype I is characterized by diminished urinary aldosterone, increased plasma renin, and salt wasting. The decrease in circulating aldosterone results in acidosis, hyperkalemia, and sodium chloride wasting.[20]

Subtype II, or, alternatively, hyporeninemic hypoaldosteronism, shows impaired renal renin production resulting from chronic interstitial damage, yielding reduced GFR, low aldosterone levels, hyperkalemia, and—as opposed to subtype I—lack of sodium chloride wasting.[20] Both subtypes I and II are characterized by hypercalciuria if sustained metabolic acidosis is present.[41,42]

Subtype III is called the *adolescent hyperkalemic syndrome* or *renal chloride shunt* and is accompanied by hypertension, hypervolemia, and hypoaldosteronism. This subtype is believed to be secondary to an increased reabsorption of chloride in the distal convoluted tubule.[20]

Subtype IV, or pseudohypoaldosteronism, is evidenced by increased urinary aldosterone, hyperkalemia, and sodium chloride wasting. It is believed to result from distal tubular unresponsiveness to circulating aldosterone.[20] There are two types of pseudohypoaldosteronism that are clinically distinguishable. Type I, or classic pseudohypoaldosteronism of infancy, can be familial and often shows salt wasting with a tendency toward hypotension.[22] It has also been associated with obstructive uropathy and concomitant bacterial infection of the urinary tract with *Escherichia coli.*[43] Classic pseudohypoaldosteronism tends to be a transient condition that abates after age 2 years.[20] Type II pseudohypoaldosteronism is seen in older children and adults and is characterized clinically by hypertension, volume expansion, and, as opposed to the classic form described above, by normal to low aldosterone levels.[22]

Subtype V or early childhood type IV RTA manifests itself as a hyperchloremic metabolic acidosis with accompanying hyperkalemia and aciduria. It would appear that the distal tubule is resistant to two of the three aldosterone-mediated functions normally accomplished at that site. Consequently, diminished potassium and hydrogen ion secretion with normal reabsorption of sodium is present. Sodium chloride wasting, azotemia, and hypertension are notably absent.[20] Renal bicarbonate wasting can be seen with high-dose alkali therapy, but—in contrast to type II proximal renal tubular acidosis—there is no associated kaliuria.[20] As in the case of the classic pseudohypoaldosteronism discussed above, patients with this form of type IV RTA outgrow their clinical manifestations by about age 5.[20] In contrast to subtypes I and II, this subtype has no hypercalciuria but rather a relative hyperreabsorption of calcium and a high urinary citrate excretion. Thus, nephrocalcinosis is absent.[20]

The hyperkalemia inherent in type IV RTA is itself partially responsible for the metabolic acidosis, as an elevated serum potassium level has been shown independently to inhibit renal ammoniagenesis, leading to decreased net acid excretion.[41]

DIAGNOSTIC STUDIES

There are three general abnormalities that result in acidification defects in the distal nephron and serve as the basis for a workup (Table 21–6). First, there can be an abnormal leaky pathway resulting in back diffusion of the bicarbonate, hydrogen ion, or both. Second, defective secretion of hydrogen ions may result from a voltage-dependent defect (luminal positive difference), inability to overcome an unfavorable chemical gradient (tubular pH less than systemic pH), or

TABLE 21–6. Possible Pathophysiologic Mechanisms Causing Distal RTA and Associated Response to Diagnostic Tests

Hypothetical Mechanism	Alkaline Urine (U-B P_{CO_2})	Phosphate Administration (U-B P_{CO_2})	Sulfate Infusion		Furosemide Test, U_{pH}	Clinical and/or Experimental Example
			U_{pH}	U_K		
Impaired H^+ secretion						
Proton pump failure	Low	Low	>5.5	Normal or high	>5.5	Primary nerve deafness
Inability to overcome an adverse gradient						
Electrical (voltage defect)						
Severe blockade of distal Na reabsorption	Low	Low	>5.5	Low	>5.5	Obstructive uropathy, amiloride
Reversible impairment of Na reabsorption	Low	Normal	<5.5	Normal	<5.5	Sickle cell anemia, lithium
Lack of Na available to be exchanged with H^+	Normal	Normal	<5.5	Normal	<5.5	Nephrotic syndrome
Back diffusion of acid						
Hydrogen ion	Normal	Normal	<5.5	Normal	<5.5	Amphotericin B

lack of sodium in the distal tubular fluid for exchange. Third, there can be an intrinsic pump defect with a reduced rate of transepithelial proton secretion.

AMMONIUM CHLORIDE TEST

When a normal individual is challenged by induction of metabolic acidosis, his or her urine pH decreases to less than 5 and his or her net acid excretion increases to more than 70 to 100 μeq/min/1.73 m^2.[3] In a patient suspected of having RTA, this response can be tested by several methods (Tables 21–4 and 21–6).

If a patient has a spontaneous metabolic acidosis of a moderate degree (infant, bicarbonate less than 17 mmol/L; child, bicarbonate less than 20 mmol/L),[28] a standard timed urine for net acid excretion can be collected. If the patient is not acidotic at the time of evaluation, metabolic acidosis can be induced with ammonium chloride (75 to 100 meq/m^2) administered orally over 1 h.[28,44,45] Total CO_2 concentration in the serum should be expected to decrease by 3 to 5 meq, and urine pH should be decreased to less than 5.5.[22] Alternatively, ammonium chloride can be given at a dose of 100 mg/kg/day over 3 to 5 days with maximal induction of ammoniagenesis after day three creating a three- to fivefold increase in hydrogen ion secretion.[46] An alternative agent which can be used to induce metabolic acidosis is calcium chloride at a dose of 2 mg/kg.[47] This may be especially important in a patient with liver disease. Last, arginine hydrochloride at a dose of 100 to 150 meq/m^2 IV[48] can be used, but this method is discouraged as it may induce proximal bicarbonate wasting.[22]

FRACTIONAL EXCRETION OF BICARBONATE

The calculation of fractional excretion of bicarbonate after an intravenous or oral load of bicarbonate or when plasma bicarbonate is in the normal concentration range yields useful information for distinguishing proximal RTA from other forms. The fractional excretion of bicarbonate is easily calculated by obtaining simultaneous serum and urine samples for bicarbonate and creatinine when the plasma bicarbonate is in the normal range of 22 to 24 meq/L. The bicarbonate samples, both serum and urine, can be run on a standard blood gas machine, and the clearance of bicarbonate is divided by the clearance of creatinine, obviating the need for a volume measurement. The fractional excretion of bicarbonate (urine/plasma bicarbonate divided by urine/plasma creatinine $\times$ 100 percent) is persistently elevated at greater than 15 percent in patients with proximal RTA when they have a concurrent normal plasma bicarbonate concentration level (Table 21–4). By contrast, classic distal renal tubular acidosis shows incomplete bicarbonate reabsorption at low levels of plasma bicarbonate but increasing bicarbonate resorption as the plasma bicarbonate level increases. Classic distal RTA usually shows a fractional excretion of bicarbonate of less than or equal to 5 percent,[3] while the hyperkalemic form, type IV, reveals values of 5 to 10 percent.[22] Distal RTA with bicarbonate wasting lies in the intermediate range of 5 to 15 percent (Table 21–4).[3,30]

Formal bicarbonate titration testing is seldom, if ever, done. This procedure would be applicable if the need to quantify bicarbonate loss were to arise, as in the differentiation of type II RTA from type I with bicarbonate wasting.

URINE-BLOOD P_{CO_2} TEST

The pressure gradient created between urine P_{CO_2} and blood P_{CO_2} after bicarbonate administration is also helpful in assessing the terminal nephron's response to acidosis. The increment in urinary P_{CO_2} during bicarbonate infusion or after an oral load, which results in excretion of a highly alkaline urine, creates a favorable chemical gradient for hydrogen ion secretion (urine pH greater than blood pH) and is a sensitive and reliable indicator of the terminal nephron's ability to secrete protons.[49] After sodium bicarbonate loading, urine P_{CO_2} should increase to greater than or equal to 70 mmHg, and this value should be at least 25 mmHg higher than systemic CO_2 levels.[50] Patients with distal renal tubular acidosis exhibit a less than or equal to 10 to 15 mmHg rise when the urine pH is greater than or equal to 7.5 (Table 21–4).[46] The basis for this test lies in the peculiar physiological and anatomic aspects of the distal tubular lumen, where secreted hydrogen ions enter the tubular lumen, combine with bicarbonate anions, and form carbonic acid, which is slow to dehydrate to water and CO_2.[21] Additionally, in the medullary collecting duct and lower urinary tract, CO_2 is trapped and diffuses slowly from the urine secondary to the unfavorable surface-to-volume relationship present at that site.[21] This test may be accomplished by infusing sodium bicarbonate (500 meq/L) at 3 mL/min and collecting timed urines 15 to 30 min apart. Urines can be considered ready for P_{CO_2} testing when three consecutive pH's exceed 7.5.[22]

An alternative method for measuring a urinary P_{CO_2} gradient is obtained by giving a neutral sodium phosphate load. Under normal conditions, administration of neutral sodium phosphate at 0.6 mmol/kg body weight diluted in 180 mL of normal saline infused at 1 mL/min for 3 h results in a two- to threefold increase in serum phosphorus concentration and an increased urinary phosphate concentration above 20 mmol/L.[21,22] Under conditions where the urine pH equals the pK of the phosphate buffer system (6.8), the phosphate acts as a nonreabsorbable anion enhancing distal sodium delivery and subsequently sodium-hydrogen ion exchange. The hydrogen secreted into the tubular lumen combines with phosphate to form acid phosphate, which reacts with a bicarbonate anion to form carbonic acid, which dehydrates to CO_2 and H_2O in the distal-most segments of the nephron and lower urinary tract.[21] Thus, urinary P_{CO_2} is increased greater than or equal to 25 mmHg above the systemic value for P_{CO_2}.[52,53] Patients with distal RTA will, as expected, show an impairment in their urinary P_{CO_2} to systemic P_{CO_2} gradient (Table 21–6).

A variant of the above test is to assess urinary pH following sodium sulfate infusion. In a normal individual in whom a state of sodium avidity has been induced, either by oral mineralocorticoid administration or a low-salt diet, infusion of sodium sulfate will result in a fall of urine pH to less than 5.5 and a kaliuric response.[52,54] Proton secretion is induced by sulfate, which, much like phosphate, acts as a poorly reabsorbable anion that increases distal nephron sodium delivery and promotes sodium-hydrogen ion exchange. The electronegative potential in the lumen created by the sulfate anion prevents back diffusion of the hydrogen ion. This test is accomplished by infusing sodium sulfate, 500 mL of a 4 percent sodium sulfate solution, over a period of 45 to 60 min.[52] In normal subjects given 1 mg of oral 9-alpha-fluorocortisone in the 12 h preceding the infusion of sodium sulfate, a fall in urine pH associated with increased excretion of sodium, potassium, and net acid is seen.[52] Similar results were obtained when normal children were given 0.1 mg fludrocortisone 12 to 14 h prior to 0.2 mmol sodium sulfate infusion. The infusion at onset was 5 mL/kg body weight $\times$ 0.3, followed by a continuous rate of 0.74 mL/min/1.73 m^2 for a 90-min period.[55]

Inadequate distal sodium delivery can result from the contraction of extracellular fluid volume, as seen in the child with protracted diarrhea. The response to acidifying agents (ammonium chloride, sodium sulfate, sodium phosphate) is in part dependent on sodium avidity and sodium delivery to the distal nephron and collecting duct for exchange with hydrogen ions.[56,57] Thus, when faced with the need to evaluate urinary acidification with the agents listed above, it is important also to assess distal sodium delivery.

FUROSEMIDE CHALLENGE TEST

In an effort to lessen the cumbersome task of sodium sulfate infusion, the administration of oral furosemide has been advocated to assist in assessing distal nephron acidification. Once again, a state of sodium avidity should be induced prior to furosemide administration. Encouragingly, the same results have been obtained when the two tests have been concomitantly compared.[58] One to two mg/kg body weight of furosemide (Lasix) given orally results in a marked reduction in urinary pH secondary to enhanced delivery of sodium chloride to the distal tubule by the furosemide. Once again, proton secretion is stimulated in exchange for the sodium as well as by the favorable electronegative lumen potential which is induced by the chloride anion (Table 21–6).[44,58]

URINARY ANION GAP

Recently, the urinary anion gap has been advocated as a rapid, immediate means of assessing ammonium excretion because this test may be accomplished on a spot urine. The test is based on the assumption that hyperchloremic metabolic acidosis secondary to bicarbonate loss outside the kidney (for example, diarrhea) should be accompanied by a high urinary ammonium concentration. In contrast, hyperchloremic metabolic acidosis secondary to a renal acidification defect would be expected to be associated with a low urinary ammonium concentration.[59,60] Urinary ammonium levels can be estimated indirectly by the urinary anion gap: urinary anion gap $= U_{Na} + U_K - U_{Cl}$.[59]

During systemic acidosis, the urinary anion (chloride) exceeds the sum of the urinary cations (sodium plus potassium), so that the anion gap is negative. This represents an appropriate increase in the urinary ammonium excretion and is opposite to the values seen with disorders of hydrogen ion excretion, such as type I renal tubular acidosis, where the urinary anion gap would be positive. One caveat in this test is that urinary pH should be less than 6.5, as at a pH of 6.5 the concentration of bicarbonate in the urine is less than 1 mmol/L and can be considered negligible. If urine pH exceeds 6.5, the concentration of bicarbonate must be considered in the urinary anion gap equation (Table 21–4).[60]

SUMMARY

Patients with hyperchloremic metabolic acidosis which cannot be ascribed to an extrarenal bicarbonate loss should be suspected of having a defect in urinary acidification (Fig. 21–5). Serum potassium may provide a clue to the type of defect, because classic distal RTA and proximal RTA patients usually have hypokalemia, while patients with type IV RTA are characteristically hyperkalemic. Additionally, if the urine pH in the presence of metabolic acidosis is less than 5.0, a defect may either reside in the proximal tubule or result from a generalized dysfunction of the distal nephron, with hyperkalemia reducing ammoniagenesis. In proximal RTA, urinary ammonium excretion would be expected to be intact and elevated, and the urinary anion gap would be negative to normal at 10 to 12 meq/L provided the urine pH were less than 6.5. In type IV, the urinary anion gap would be positive. A urine pH above 5.5 generally denotes a defect in distal nephron hydrogen ion secretion and can be confirmed by evaluating a urine-blood (U-B) P_{CO_2} gradient following a bicarbonate load. Typically, the U-B P_{CO_2} following a bicarbonate load is low in types I and IV RTA. However, the hyperkalemia present with the latter suggests simultaneous defects in hydrogen ion secretion and potassium secretion. The U-B P_{CO_2} gradient in proximal RTA will be normal.

TREATMENT OF RTA

Treatment of distal RTA, both classic and that associated with bicarbonate wasting, aims to achieve four goals: to (1) accelerate the growth rate, (2) reduce the risk and/or halt the progression of nephrocalcinosis, (3) preserve a normal GFR/prevent subsequent reduction in GFR, and (4) ameliorate the serum electrolyte abnormalities.[21] Correction of the metabolic acidosis is accomplished through the use of daily alkali supplementation. The dose is dependent on endogenous acid production and the magnitude of the bicarbonaturia. In adults, endogenous acid production is 1 meq/kg/day; in children, 2 meq/kg/day.[3] As noted above, the degree of bicarbonaturia is less than 5 percent in classic distal renal tubular acidosis[3] and can be as high as 6 to 14 percent in the type I with bicarbonate wasting form.[30] This increased requirement tends to decrease with age, such that by age 4 to 6 years, the dose of alkali supplement declines to an amount equal to that required by patients with classic RTA.[2] The goal is to achieve and maintain a normal plasma bicarbonate concentration of 22 to 24 meq/L. Caution should be exercised in dosing alkali therapy, and plasma bicarbonate levels should be followed closely, because lower doses of alkali therapy

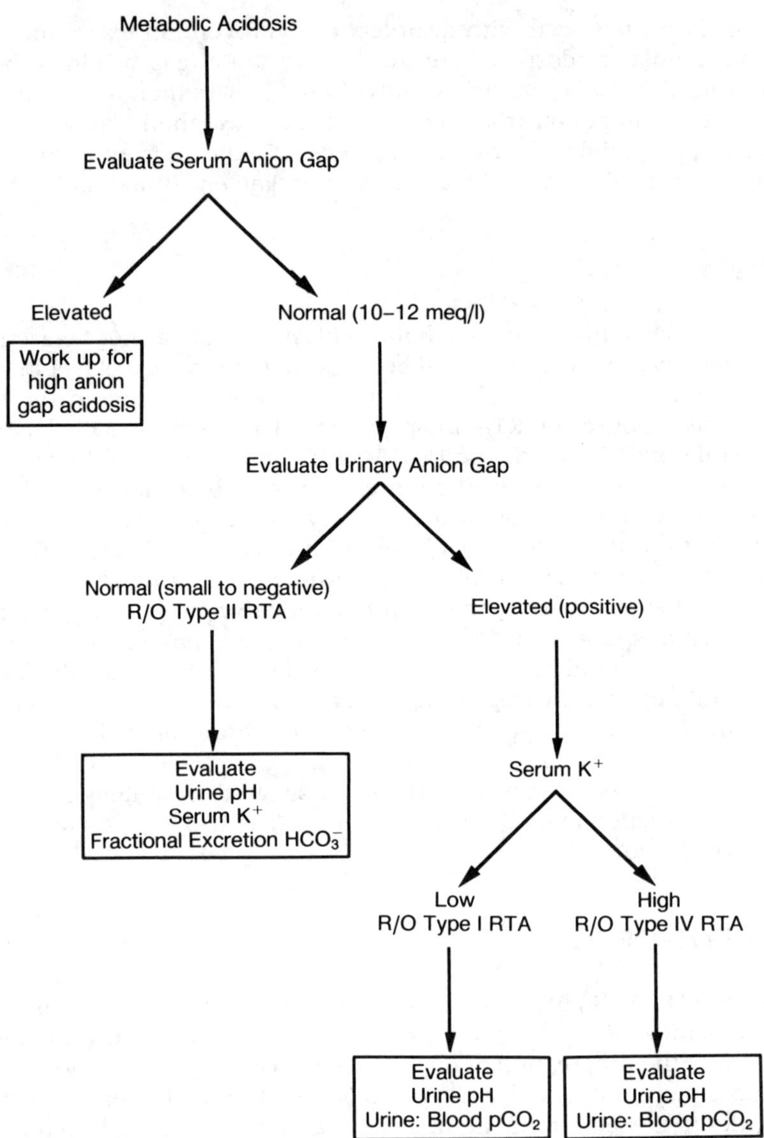

FIG. 21–5. Algorithm for diagnostic work-up of a patient with suspected renal tubular acidosis. K^+ = potassium; urine: blood P_{CO_2} = urine-blood P_{CO_2}, mmHg.

will not result in the desired therapeutic outcome and excessive doses may produce expansion of the extracellular fluid volume with a resultant exacerbation of urinary bicarbonate wasting.[21] Various preparations of alkali therapy are commercially available (Table 21–7). Two of the most frequently used oral preparations are sodium bicarbonate and Shohl's solution. Sodium bicarbonate may cause abdominal bloating and belching resulting from intragastric CO_2 production. Shohl's solution consists of a combination of sodium citrate and citric

TABLE 21–7. Commerical Preparations for Alkali Supplementation

Drug	How Supplied	Dosage Equivalent
Bicitra	Solution: 5 mL = 500 mg sodium citrate 300 mg citric acid	1 mL = 1 meq base
Calcium carbonate	Tablet: 420 mg, 650 mg	1 g = 22.3 meq base
	Powder: 1000 mg per ½ teaspoon	
Polycitra	Solution: 5 mL = 550 mg potassium citrate 500 mg sodium citrate 334 mg citric acid	1 mL = 2 meq base
Polycitra-K	Solution: 5 mL = 1100 mg potassium citrate 334 mg citric acid	1 mL = 2 meq base
Sodium bicarbonate	Tablet: 325 mg, 650 mg	325 mg = 4 meq base
	Solution: 1 mL = 1 meq	1 mL = 1 meq base
Shohl's solution	Solution: 1000 mL = 140 g citric acid 90 g hydrated crystalline sodium citrate	1 mL = 1 meq base

acid (98 g/L sodium citrate, 140 g/L citric acid). The citric acid is converted to CO_2 and water, the citrate to bicarbonate. Shohl's preparation can be rather unpalatable, and dilution with chilled ginger ale or fruit juice yields a more tolerable supplement.[21]

Sustained correction of metabolic acidosis promotes a significant improvement in growth rate, resulting in attainment of normal height provided the serum bicarbonate concentration is kept within the normal range.[38] Studies have shown that normal heights can be achieved within 6 months of starting therapy in infants and within 3 years of the initiation of therapy in stunted children.[38] The mechanism by which chronic metabolic acidosis produces impairment of growth currently remains unknown. It has been shown that the human growth hormone peak release after challenge with arginine or L-dopa is blunted in both acute and chronic acidosis.[20] Following correction of the acidosis, the peak release of growth hormone after stimulation returns to normal levels.[20] These data point to the plasma bicarbonate level as being a critical determinant of growth hormone release after a provocative stimulus. Collagen synthesis has similarly been shown to be affected by acidosis,[20] as reflected through measurement of the activity level of a critical enzyme, lysyl oxidase, in the biosynthetic pathway. The serum concentration of the enzyme was inversely correlated with the plasma bicarbonate level.[20] Moreover, sulfate excretion is elevated in type I RTA, which, through its effect on chondroitin sulfate incorporation into bone, may contribute to the growth failure seen in these patients.[34]

The hypercalciuria, hypocitraturia, increased renal phosphate clearance, and alkaline urine in a patient with distal renal tubular acidosis favor renal calcium deposition.[22] Correction of the acidosis with alkali treatment has been shown to normalize urinary citrate excretion.[8] The hypercalciuric effect of the metabolic acidosis appears to be mediated through decreased renal tubular calcium reabsorption. This is believed to be the result of impaired intracellular metabolism.[32,61] One study showed an inverse relationship between urinary calcium excretion and plasma bicarbonate concentration.[2] Other literature has not confirmed this observation.[21] Hypercalciuria is not an invariable finding in patients with untreated type I RTA.[4,36,37] An additional observation has been the role of sodium intake and its effect on the magnitude of urinary calcium excretion. A decreased sodium intake increases avidity for resorption of sodium and calcium in the nephron, resulting in decreased hypercalciuria.[61]

The potassium disturbances and hypokalemia normalize after sustained correction of metabolic acidosis. This is attributed to alleviation of the renal bicarbonate wasting secondary to alkali-induced reexpansion of the extracellular space, which results in removal of the stimulus for renin and aldosterone secretion. It is generally unnecessary, therefore, to continue long-term potassium supplementation in patients with distal renal tubular acidosis.[21]

The GFR does not appear to be affected early in the course of the disease. With time and the development of complications such as calcium deposition and nephrocalcinosis, variable reductions in glomerular filtration rate may be noted.[20,21] Therefore, it appears that the glomerular filtration rate does not usually deteriorate provided nephrocalcinosis and calcium deposition are prevented or arrested very early in the disease. If the disease is discovered in early infancy and alkali treatment is begun, nephrocalcinosis may not occur.[62] Interestingly, in a kindred from Philadelphia with members who had incomplete distal renal tubular acidosis, renal function remained stable and did not show deterioration to complete distal RTA until nephrocalcinosis was noted to have developed.[8]

PROXIMAL RTA

Isolated proximal RTA is also treated by supplementation of bicarbonate in amounts sufficient to replace the bicarbonaturia.[23] Since the underlying defect is in the proximal tubule and not the distal tubule, alkali replacement therapy reverses the metabolic derangement. However, the massive bicarbonaturia that occurs with proximal RTA may temporarily require potassium supplementation, and it may be difficult to fully correct the base deficit.

HYPERKALEMIC RTA

Therapy of type IV RTA centers on correction of the three metabolic abnormalities: (1) reduction in the serum potassium, (2) reversal of the acidosis, and (3) treatment of the primary hormonal deficiency/insufficiency.[22] Hyperkalemia is present, by definition, in all subtypes of type IV RTA and is treated by a reduction in dietary intake of potassium, the use of potassium-wasting diuretics such as furosemide or metolazone (Zaroxolyn), and, if necessary, the use of potassium-binding exchange resins such as sodium polystyrene sulfonate (Kayexalate).[3] The metabolic acidosis associated with this disorder is frequently ameliorated with a simple reduction in the serum potassium level, for reasons discussed above. If obstructive uropathy is present, a diuretic such as hydrochlorothiazide at a dose of 1 to 2 mg/kg/day alone or with alkali treatment is effective in reducing the hyperkalemia as well as reversing the metabolic acidosis.[3] The rationale of this treatment is that thiazides inhibit sodium chloride resorption in the loop of Henle, which, in turn, results in an increased delivery of sodium to the distal tubule, where it can be exchanged for potassium and hydrogen ion.

The dose of alkali therapy is determined in the same manner as it was for type I RTA, based on endogenous acid production and the magnitude of the associated bicarbonaturia.

If a primary hormonal deficiency is present, as in subtypes I and II, the use of a mineralocorticoid—such as 9-alpha-fludrocortisone at a dose of 0.05 to 0.2 mg/day[3]—in conjunction with measures for reducing serum potassium and maintaining a normal serum bicarbonate concentration, may prove useful. Care must be exercised when using mineralocorticoids in this condition as they may aggravate preexisting volume expansion, necessitating the simultaneous use of a loop diuretic such as furosemide. In states of tubular unresponsiveness to aldosterone, mineralocorticoids are often of no avail.[22] These patients should receive sodium chloride supplementation as well as alkali therapy in the form of sodium bicarbonate. This has been shown to reverse the hyponatremia and hyperkalemia, improve symptoms, and enhance growth.[46] In the subtype III with a chloride shunt, thiazide diuretics as well as dietary restriction of sodium chloride are useful in correcting the hyperkalemia and hyperchloremic metabolic acidosis.[20]

CONTROVERSIES

HYPERCALCIURIA IN RTA

Although distal RTA appears to be a reasonably straightforward diagnosis clinically, numerous controversies surround this disease. One of the most intriguing is the role of hypercalciuria and nephrocalcinosis in the impairment of acidification and in the progression from incomplete distal RTA to complete distal RTA. In the late 1950s, Wrong and Davis[44] noted some patients who had a demonstrable acidification defect in the absence of frank metabolic acidosis, a so-called incomplete distal RTA. It was notable, however, that some of these patients already had nephrocalcinosis coexistent with the acidification defect. A similar phenomenon was observed in a large Atlanta kindred spanning four generations with 64 members, in whom hypercalciuria was the presenting manifestation.[63] Buckalew et al.[63] subsequently proposed that hypercalciuria with progression of nephrocalcinosis and renal damage were the necessary predecessors to the development of a renal acidification defect. Further, nephrocalcinosis existing independent of a defect in acidification could not be demonstrated after an oral acid challenge in other kindred members. Norman and colleagues[8] studied a kindred from Philadelphia that had one member initially with incomplete distal RTA who progressed to complete distal RTA only after the appearance of nephrocalcinosis. This patient was not treated with an alkali preparation. Severe hypocitraturia was present in two members with complete distal RTA and in two members with incomplete distal RTA who were first detected by the abnormal citrate excretion. After high-dose alkali therapy, the rate of citrate excretion increased to normal.[8] The two cases of incomplete distal RTA were placed on an alkali preparation; whether they will develop or be spared nephrocalcinosis and progression to complete RTA is an open question. Coe and Parks[64] found that alkali therapy had little effect on reduced citrate excretion, but the supplement did eliminate hypercalciuria and reduce the frequency of nephrolithiasis. Finally, Hammett and coworkers,[65] following a kindred of four generations from Oklahoma, found hypercalciuria to be the most frequent renal abnormality to precede both the development of RTA and nephrocalcinosis. The questions of whether the combination of hypocitraturia and hypercalciuria are critical in the pathogenesis of nephrocalcinosis and progression of incomplete distal RTA to complete distal RTA or if sustained hypercalciuria in itself could damage the renal tubule with subsequent impairment of acidification and further progression to nephrocalcinosis remain unanswered. At present, it is unknown if hypercalciuria per se causes deterioration of renal function.

The origin of the hypercalciuria associated with type I RTA is itself a controversy. Earlier, it was believed that increased calcium mobilization and excretion through the kidney was secondary to the dissolution of bone matrix acting as a buffer for the acidotic state. However, radiologically visible bone lesions are absent in patients with type I RTA,[25] and subsequent studies revealed that chronic metabolic acidosis gives rise to hypercalciuria by decreasing renal tubular calcium resorption through a direct action on intracellular metabolism.[61,66] Recent reports have also shown that elevated calcium excretion is not invariably present in acidotic patients with type I RTA[36,37] and that hypercalciuria can persist even after correction of acidosis in some patients.[4] Thus, it has been suggested that hypercalciuria may result from a primary independent disorder of calcium metabolism.[67]

PREVENTING NEPHROCALCINOSIS

A logical question following from the preceding discussion is whether the complications discussed above can be prevented or whether retardation and/or regression of nephrocalcinosis in both the patient with existing RTA and the patient at risk for the development of RTA can be accomplished. As mentioned previously, alkali supplementation prior to the demonstration of nephrocalcinosis appears protective. In patients with existing disease, it is unknown if alkali therapy serves to retard further calcium deposition and progressive nephrocalcinosis. Recent work with rats placed into stable chronic renal insufficiency via subtotal nephrectomy has shown a protective effect of chronic verapamil administration with regard to calcium deposition, progressive nephrocalcinosis, and further renal deterioration.[68,69] Whether the administration of verapamil to a patient with demonstrable nephrocalcinosis will retard further progression or if administration to a high-risk patient prior to evidence of calcium deposition may prevent future development of nephrocalcinosis is open to speculation and will perhaps be explored in future human trials. Unfortunately, we have no medical means at present to initiate a regressive process on existing calcium deposits in the patient with nephrocalcinosis coexistent with RTA.

BICARBONATE REGENERATION IN DISTAL NEPHRON

A newly reopened area of controversy is the amount of bicarbonate regeneration that takes place in the distal nephron. It was previously believed that the distal nephron regenerated bicarbonate. Recently, this was reviewed and addressed by Halperin,[70] who estimates that, theoretically, new bicarbonate could be regenerated in the distal nephron provided there was a luminal hydrogen ion acceptor other than bicarbonate present. Currently, this is not believed to be the case, since only small amounts of monohydrogen phosphate are delivered to this segment of the nephron (10 mmol $HPO_4^=$) in conjunction with ammonium, which already contains an accepted proton. Rather, the author suggests that the distal nephron participates in acid-base homeostasis by secretion of hydrogen ion, and that new bicarbonate regeneration takes place more proximally in the thick ascending limb of the loop of Henle, where transfer of a proton from luminal ammonium, synthesized in the proximal convoluted tubule, helps to reclaim or recycle filtered bicarbonate that was not reabsorbed in the earlier nephron segments (Fig. 21–6).[70] Under such a theory, medullary

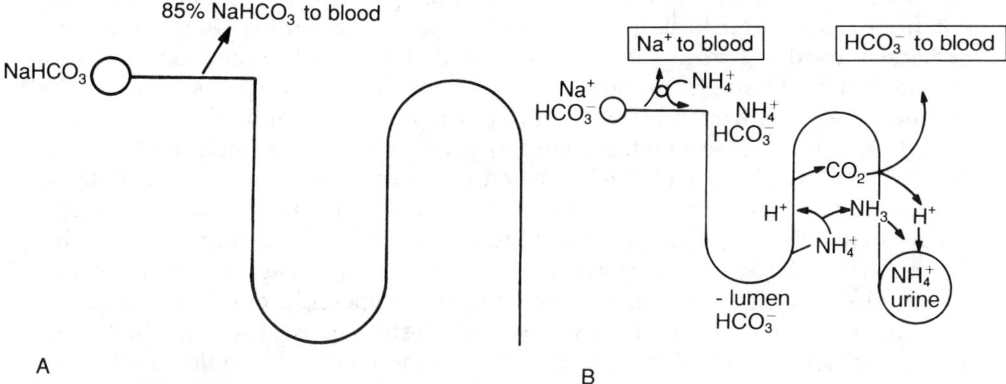

FIG. 21–6. Schematic representation of distal nephron bicarbonate regeneration. Most of the filtered bicarbonate is reclaimed by proximal nephron events. Much of that which escapes proximal reabsorption receives a proton from luminal ammonium, also generated from the proximal tubule, thus removing most of the luminal bicarbonate. The carbonic acid generated dissociates into carbon dioxide and ammonia to traverse to the collecting duct, where H^+ ATPase promotes hydrogen ion secretion, creating bicarbonate and ammonium. The bicarbonate is reabsorbed into the blood, the ammonium excreted in the urine. Na^+ = sodium; NH_3 = ammonia; NH_4^+ = ammonium; CO_2 = carbon dioxide; HCO_3^- = bicarbonate. (From Halperin ML: How much new bicarbonate is formed in the distal nephron in the process of net acid excretion? *Kidney Int* 35:1280, 1989.)

collecting duct hydrogen ion secretion would yield a tendency toward accumulation of medullary interstitial bicarbonate, tending to alkalinize the vicinity of the medulla and creating a high pH that ultimately may prove favorable for calcium deposition and development of nephrocalcinosis.

GROWTH FAILURE IN RTA

A cause of great concern for physicians treating this disease is the etiology underlying the growth failure common to all forms of RTA. The critical role of acidosis is revealed by the observation that those who receive high doses of alkali therapy resulting in sustained correction of the acidosis grow at a normal rate, while those receiving lower doses of alkali remain stunted in their growth.[23,38] Prior to the early 1980s, bone disease and growth retardation were believed to be a prominent feature of type I RTA. By extension, calcium and the vitamin D axis were thought to be involved through aberrant regulation. In 1982, Brenner et al.[25] clarified the issue of bone disease as a principal component of type I RTA. Subsequently, Chesney and coworkers[36] found normal serum calcitriol levels and a normal increase in 1,25-dihydroxyvitamin D following stimulation from hypophosphatemia in patients with distal RTA. In adults the negative calcium balance seen in RTA results from decreased intestinal calcium absorption and increased renal calcium excretion. In contrast, children with distal RTA have been found to have a positive calcium balance during acidosis.[37] Apparent from the above is that the vitamin D axis appears intact, and the role of calcium in growth failure remains unexplained. Another potential factor contributing to growth failure, suggested by Chan,[34] is sulfate deficiency resulting from significantly elevated urinary sulfate excretion producing impaired bone formation. Chondroitin sulfate, through its effect on the binding of sulfate, has an essential role in the formation of bone.

Additionally, collagen metabolism has been shown to be impaired by acidosis. Although the major part of collagen synthesis takes place intracellularly, the final enzymatic step to ensure normal strength and structural integrity occurs extracellularly through cross-linkage of the collagen molecule.[20] This process is mediated by the enzyme lysyl oxidase. The plasma activity of this enzyme has been elevated up to tenfold during hyperchloremic metabolic acidosis and returned to normal with correction of the acidosis through alkali therapy.[35] The significance of this observation is that acidosis has a direct effect on collagen metabolism, and it is tempting to speculate that the acidosis blocks/inhibits/steals an intermediary in the biosynthetic pathway leading to accumulation of the precursor enzyme.

The effect of acidosis on the secretion and peripheral action of growth hormone is a subject of ongoing research. McSherry et al.[71] have shown a blunted release of growth hormone provoked by arginine and L-dopa in both chronic acidotic states (children with distal RTA) and acutely induced acidotic states. Conversely, the release was normal following chronic or acute correction of the acidosis.[71] The role of insulinlike growth factors and growth hormone at the cellular level under acidotic conditions is currently being investigated.

NEWER INSIGHTS INTO THE MOLECULAR BASIS OF RTA

The recent recognition of RTA associated with osteopetrosis and cerebral calcification, the so-called carbonic anhydrase II deficiency syndrome, has shed new light on enzymatic insufficiencies/deficiencies present in this form of RTA.[72] Such deficiencies may help explain the pathophysiologic difference of type I RTA from type II RTA. In the carbonic anhydrase II deficiency syndrome, the RTA is usually of the mixed type; it is explained by Sly[72] through a model in which the functions of carbonic anhydrase II in the proximal and distal tubules are physiologically and biochemically distinct. In this model (Fig. 21–7), the major reclamation of bicarbonate in the proximal tubule is assigned to carbonic anhydrase IV rather than carbonic anhydrase II. The proximal tubule contains carbonic anhydrase IV on the luminal surface, which catalyzes the reaction of $H_2CO_3 \rightleftharpoons CO_2 + H_2O$. The CO_2 generated diffuses freely into the proximal tubular cell, where intracellular carbonic anhydrase II allows regeneration of carbonic acid, and by spontaneous dehydration bicarbonate is formed, which is transported to the peritubular capillary. The hydrogen ion left from spontaneous dehydration is once again secreted into the lumen, where the cycle recurs. In the distal tubule (Fig. 21–7), a hydrogen ion is secreted into the lumen by a magnesium ATPase pump, leaving an hydroxide ion in the distal tubular cell. Carbon dioxide diffuses freely into the cell and condenses with the hydroxide anion to form bicarbonate in a carbonic anhydrase II catalyzed reaction. The bicarbonate so generated is then transported across the basement membrane into the peritubular capillary.[72] In patients with carbonic anhydrase II deficiency, there is an inability to titrate the hydroxide anion by-product of the magnesium ATPase pump; this also reduces the ability to secrete hydrogen ion and acidify the urine appropriately. Theoretically, hydration of CO_2 to produce hydrogen ion and bicarbonate in the proximal tubule and the condensation of a hydroxide anion with CO_2 to produce bicarbonate in the distal tubule could be separately affected by different mutations in the carbonic anhydrase II gene. The characteristic differences of types I and II RTA then may be explained by different mutations affecting the rate of carbonic anhydrase II enzyme turnover in the proximal and distal tubular cells.

The ability to diagnose accurately a suspected patient with RTA through the use of a rapid screening method like the urinary anion gap or a more involved timed urine collection for citrate excretion opens yet another area of controversy. The screen would need to prove as accurate, reliable, and reproducible as the standard timed collection for net acid excretion. The answer to this question awaits further clinical analysis of these two methods and their comparison to the standard timed net acid excretion.

Case History 21–1. N.H., a black girl, was 4 years and 6 months old when she was admitted with end-stage renal disease. Seven days prior to her admission, she complained of dysuria and received symptomatic treatment at home. Five days prior to being admitted, she presented to the emergency room and was diagnosed as having a urinary tract infection. She was subsequently discharged on sulfisoxazole (Gantrisin). A urine cul-

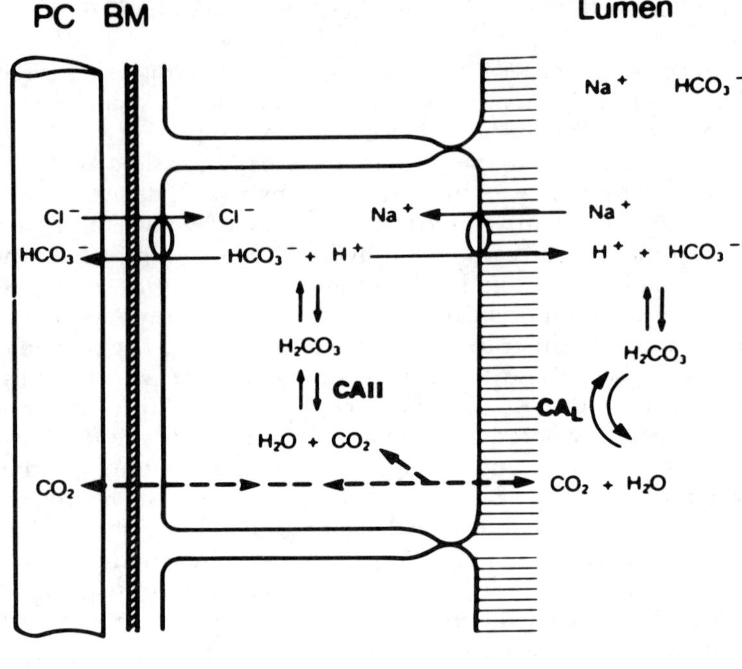

A

FIG. 21–7. *A* and *B*. Schematic representation of the proposed mechanism by which mutation of the carbonic anhydrase II gene could give rise to two distinct pathophysiologic entities such as type I and type II renal tubular acidosis. In the proximal cell, carbonic anhydrase IV allows generation of carbonic acid, which spontaneously dehydrates to CO_2 and H_2O. The CO_2 so generated diffuses into the cell, where carbonic anhydrase II enzyme allows carbonic acid to reform. Through dehydration, bicarbonate and hydrogen ion are generated. The bicarbonate is reabsorbed into the peritubular capillary and hydrogen ion is secreted into the tubular lumen, where the process recycles. In the distal tubule, a magnesium-dependent ATPase acts as a proton-translocating enzyme and gives rise to a hydroxide anion intracellularly and the hydrogen ion in the lumen. The hydroxide anion, under the influence of carbonic anhydrase II, combines with carbon dioxide and gives rise to bicarbonate, which is reabsorbed into the peritubular capillary. Inability to titrate condensation of the hydroxide anion with CO_2 because of carbonic anhydrase II deficiency would thus limit the ability to secrete hydrogen ions into the lumen and would produce an inability to acidify the urine appropriately. Na^+ = sodium; Cl^- = chloride; ADP = adenosine diphosphate; P_i = phosphate; H^+ = hydrogen; HCO_3^- = bicarbonate; CO_2 = carbon dioxide; H_2CO_3 = carbonic acid; CA II = carbonic anhydrase II; CAL = carbonic anhydrase IV; Mg^{++} ATPase = magnesium-dependent ATPase proton translocator. [From Sly WS: Carbonic anhydrase II deficiency syndrome: Osteopetrosis with renal tubular acidosis and cerebral calcification, in Scriver CR, Beaudet AL, Sly WS, et al (eds): *The Metabolic Basis of Inherited Disease,* New York, McGraw-Hill Information Services Company, 1989, p 2862. Reproduced by permission.]

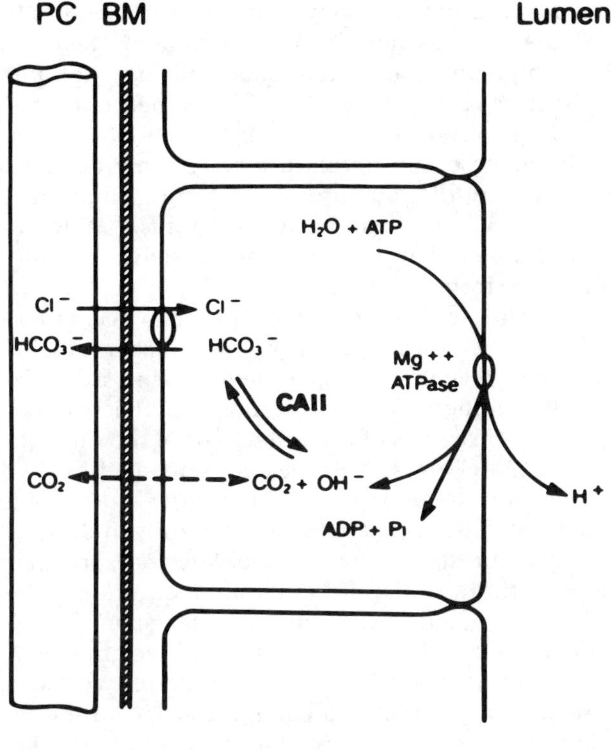

B

FIG. 21–7 (*Continued*).

ture grew 3500 colonies/mL of *Escherichia coli.* The following day, she was noted to be tachypneic, to be very weak and unable to stand, and to have constant tremors. Her temperature was 99° to 100°F orally, and she was noted to be more sleepy than usual and to have emesis after meals. For the next 2 days she ran a low-grade temperature, remained anorexic, and was constantly thirsty. The day prior to admission, she became delusional and febrile. On the day of admission, she had a nosebleed. She was taken to the ear, nose, and throat clinic, where her nose was cauterized. She was subsequently referred to the pediatric emergency room because she appeared pale. In the emergency room she had a low-grade temperature of approximately 100° orally. Her respirations were 40/min and regular. Her blood pressure was 100/60 mmHg. Her weight at age 4 ½ years was 15.88 kg (25th percentile) and height 97.8 cm (less than 5th percentile). The remainder of her physical examination revealed that she was pale but there were no neurocutaneous stigmata. Fundi were normal in appearance; however, the conjuctiva were pale. The lungs were clear, there was no murmur. Abdominal exam was soft and benign without organomegaly. Rectal exam was negative for blood. Her neurologic exam was recorded as having no deficits. Her emergency room laboratory studies revealed a white blood cell count of 13,400 cells/mm^2, her hemoglobin 4.8 mg/dL. A serum haptoglobin was normal, and so were coagulation studies (PT, PTT); however, a bleeding time was not obtained. Urinalysis revealed microscopic hematuria with greater then 5 red blood cells per high power field (HPF). Laboratory studies revealed a sodium of 136 meq/L; potassium, 5.4 meq/L; chloride, 102 meq/L; bicarbonate 23 meq/L; BUN 192 mg/dL; creatinine, 16.5 mg/dL; glucose, 92 mg/dL; urate, 11.2 mg/dL; calcium, 4.1 mg/dL; phosphorus, 4.0 mg/dL; total protein, 7.2 g/dL; albumin, 4.0 g/dL; alkaline phosphatase, 203 units/L; and LDH, 636 units/L. N.H. was subsequently admitted and underwent acute peritoneal dialysis. While on dialysis, her BUN dropped from 192 mg/dL to 43 mg/dL. Her creatinine declined from 16.5 mg/dL to 7 mg/dL. Her anion gap decreased from 31 meq/L to 14 meq/L. Further workup consisting of an abdominal x-ray and intravenous pyelogram revealed marked nephocalcinosis with normal renal size (Fig. 21–8). Radiographs of her hands and knees revealed irregularity at the metaphyseal regions of the distal ends of the radii, ulnae, and femurs, along with osteosclerosis. This was accompanied by evidence of subperiosteal reabsorption in the fingers and the inner aspects of the tibias consistent with renal osteodystrophy. N.H. subsequently underwent a renal biopsy, which revealed end-stage renal disease. She was subsequently discharged to home on peritoneal dialysis and oral medications.

N.H.'s past history revealed that she was a normal, spontaneous vaginal delivery after an uncomplicated pregnancy. Her birthweight was 7 lb 11 oz (50th to 60th percentile). Her developmental milestones were recorded as normal. She was seen by her pediatrician at age 2 years, 4 months for dysuria. Her weight at that time was 13.3 kg (75th percentile). Her height was 85 cm (30th percentile). The urinalysis at that time revealed a specific gravity of 1.007, red blood cells too numerous to count, protein 1+. Her next recorded visit to the pediatrician was at age 4 years 4 months, for upper respiratory tract infection with pharyngitis. Her weight at that time, 15.4 kg, had decreased to the 25th percentile. Her height, 97 to 98 cm, had decreased to the 10th percentile. A urinalysis at that time revealed specific gravity of 1.010 and red blood cells 1 to 3 per HPF, with the normal for the laboratory 0 to 1 per HPF. Protein reaction was 2+. Her next visit was her presentation to the emergency room for the admission described above, which revealed her weight to be 15.8 kg (25th percentile) and her height 97 to 98 cm (slightly less than the 5th percentile). Further past history revealed a greater than 1- to 1 ½-year history of polyuria, polydypsia, and enuresis, with daytime frequency such that the mother described a pattern of urinating up to 16 times a day.

Family history was noncontributory for renal disease on the mother's side. Father's family history was unknown. There was no history of sickle cell disease or tuberculosis.

Comment. There are three features in this case which lead to a suspicion of renal tubular acidosis. The first is growth failure. As noted at age 2 years 4 months, the patient's weight and height were at the 75th and 30th percentiles, respectively. By age 4 years 6 months, her weight was at the 25th percentile and height at less than the 5th percentile. Second, the microscopic hematuria from the age of 2 years, 4 months was evidenced

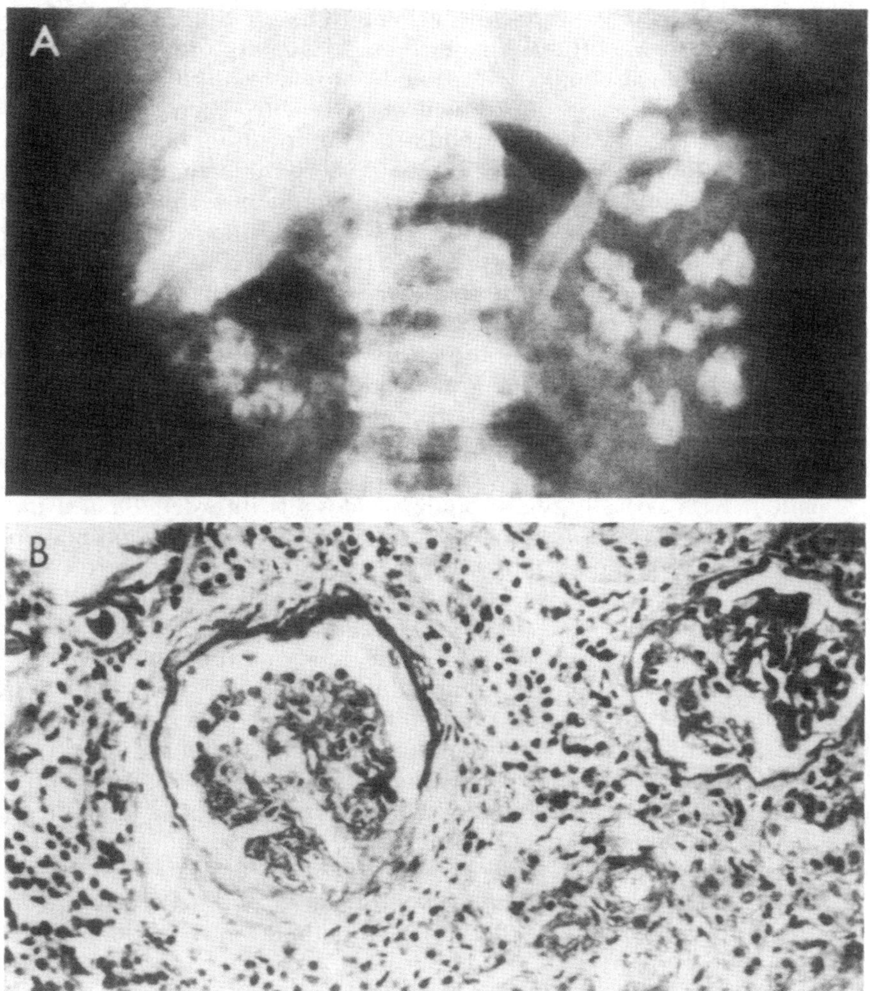

FIG. 21–8. *A* and *B*. Abdominal radiography and renal biopsy of N.H. at the time of her presentation with end-stage renal disease, demonstrating intrarenal calcification by x-ray and marked glomerular and tubular abnormalities by light microscopy. (Reprinted by permission from Chan JCM: Acid-base, calcium, potassium and aldosterone metabolism in renotubular acidosis. *Nephron* 23:152–158, 1979.)

by a urinalysis with too many red blood cells to count; at age 4 years, 4 months, the urinalysis still showed 3 red blood cells per HPF, which was abnormal for the reference laboratory. Third, she had at least a 1- to 1½-year history of polyuria, polydypsia, enuresis, and daytime frequency. At the age of 4 years, 6 months, improved bladder control consisting of daytime continence and near nighttime continence would be expected. N.H. exhibited a pattern contrary to this.

Our workup of this patient would begin by separating proximal from distal renal tubular acidosis. We would start by looking at a first morning urine for pH and concentrating ability, as this specimen would be expected to be more acidic and more concentrated than any other specimen during the day. If the urine pH was greater than or equal to 7 with a simultaneous normal serum bicarbonate, we would be suspicious of bicarbonaturia and possible proximal renal tubular acidosis. We would then proceed with the fractional excretion of the bicarbonate. If, on the other hand, the urine pH was greater than 5.5 with a simultaneous serum bicarbonate less than 21 meq/L, we would evaluate the distal hydrogen secretory mechanism through a sodium bicarbonate load and a urine minus blood P_{CO_2}. If this difference was less than 25 to 30 mmHg, we could consider a disorder compatible with inability to excrete endogenously produced hydrogen ions, such as type I or type IV renal tubular acidosis. To differentiate type I from type IV, we would next check the serum potassium. In type I renal tubular acidosis, the serum potassium would be expected to be low. In type IV, it would be expected to be high, consistent with aldosterone deficiency/insufficiency or resistance of the distal tubule to the actions of aldosterone.

A special note regarding the interpretation of urine pH in the workup of a patient with possible renal tubular acidosis is in order. First, urine pH should always be measured by the glass electrode method and not simply by the dipstick method, as the latter has a greater margin of error. Second, a random urine pH can be ambiguous with respect to urine ammonium excretion, especially with pH values close to 6. This is true because renal ammonium production in states of acute versus chronic acidemia is different. In acute acidosis, urine ammonium concentrations may be low from consumption of ammonia through buffering of hydrogen ions. When this occurs, urine pH rises to a value near 6. On the other hand, in chronic acidotic states, ammonia production is stimulated, allowing more buffering of the hydrogen ion and yielding increased concentrations of ammonia to buffer hydrogen ions in the urine. As the concentration of ammonia increases, the urine pH will be in the range of 6 or higher. Thus, a random urine pH without knowledge of the chronicity of the acidemic state or the status of other stimulators of renal ammoniagenesis yields ambiguous information.

ACKNOWLEDGMENTS

The authors thank Ms. M. Reilly for secretarial assistance. Supported by NIH grants T32 DK 07526 and DK 31370.

REFERENCES

1. Sebastian A, McSherry E, Morris RC Jr: Impaired renal conservation of sodium and chloride during sustained correction of systemic acidosis in patients with type I, classic renal tubular acidosis. *J Clin Invest* 58:454, 1976.
2. Rodriguez-Soriano J, Vallo A, Castillo G, et al: Natural history of primary distal renal tubular acidosis treated since infancy. *J Pediatr 101:669, 1982.*
3. Chan JCM: Renal tubular acidosis: Medical progress. *J Pediatr* 102:327, 1983.

4. Santos F, Chan JCM: Renal tubular acidosis in children: Diagnosis, treatment and prognosis. *Am J Nephrol* 6:289, 1986,
5. Chan JCM: Acid-base disorders and the kidney. *Adv Pediatr* 30:401, 1983.
6. Roth KS, Buckalew VM Jr, Chan JCM: Renal tubular disorders, in Gonick HC (ed): *Current Nephrology*. Chicago, Year Book Medical Publishers, 1985, pp 87–137.
7. Kainer G, Chan JCM: Renal tubular acidosis: Diagnostic work-up, treatment and mechanism of growth retardation. *Indian J Pediatr* 55:552, 1988.
8. Norman ME, Feldman NI, Cohen RM, et al: Urinary citrate in the diagnosis of distal renal tubular acidosis. *J Pediatr* 92:394, 1978.
9. Tsuru N, Chan JCM: Growth failure in children with metabolic alkalosis and metabolic acidosis. *Nephron* 45:182, 1987.
10. Chan JCM: Nutrition and acid-base metabolism. *Fed Proc* 40:2423, 1981.
11. Simpson DP: Citrate excretion: A window on renal metabolism. *Am J Physiol* 244:F233, 1983.
12. Dunger DB, Brenton DP, Cain AR: Renal tubular acidosis and nerve deafness. *Arch Dis Child* 55:221, 1980.
13. Donckerwolcke RA, Van Biervliet JP, Koorvaar G, et al: The syndrome of renal tubular acidosis with nerve deafness. *Acta Paediatr Scand* 65:100, 1976.
14. Whyte MP, Murphy WA, Fallon MD, et al: Osteopetrosis, renal tubular acidosis and basal ganglia calcification in three sisters. *Am J Med* 69: 64, 1980.
15. Sly WS, Hewett-Emmett D, Whyte MP, et al: Carbonic anhydrase II deficiency identified as the primary defect in the autosomal recessive syndrome of osteopetrosis with renal tubular acidosis and cerebral calcification. *Proc Nat Acad Sci USA* 80:2752, 1983.
16. Klahr S, Weiner ID: Disorders of acid-base metabolism, in Chan JCM, Gill JR Jr (eds): *Kidney Electrolyte Disorders.* New York, Churchill Livingstone, 1990, pp 1–58.
17. Schoolwerth AC, LaNova KF: Control of ammoniagenesis by X-keto glutamate in rat kidney mitochondria. *Am J Physiol* 244:F399, 1983.
18. Goodyear PR, Kalonstran VMD: Hereditary tubular transport abnormalities, in Spitzer A, Avner E (eds): *Inheritance of Kidney and Urinary Tract Diseases.* Boston, Kluwer Academic Press, 1990, pp 141–165.
19. Chan JCM, Duffee J, Kodroff MB: Dehydration, renal vein thrombosis and hyperkalemic renal tubular acidosis in a newborn. *Am J Nephrol* 3:329, 1983.
20. McSherry E: Renal tubular acidosis in childhood. *Kidney Int* 20:799, 1981.
21. Santos F, Kainer G, Chan JCM: Renal tubular acidosis, in Massry SG, Suki WN (eds): *Therapy of Renal Diseases and Related Disorders.* Boston, Martinus Nijhoff Publishing, 1991, pp 207–221.
22. DuBose TD Jr, Alpern RJ: Renal tubular acidosis, in Scriver CR, Beaudet AL, Sly WS, et al (eds): *The Metabolic Basis of Inherited Disease.* New York, McGraw-Hill Information Services, 1989, pp 2539–2568.
23. Nash MA, Torrado AD, Greifer I, et al: Renal tubular acidosis in infants and children: Clinical course, response to treatment, and prognosis. *J Pediatr* 80:738, 1972.
24. Convey WR, Pfister RC: The radiologic findings in renal tubular acidosis: Analysis of 21 cases. *Radiology* 105:497, 1982.
25. Brenner RJ, Spring DB, Sebastian A, et al: Incidence of radiographically evident bone disease, nephrocalcinosis and nephrolithiasis in various types of renal tubular acidosis. *N Engl J Med* 307:217, 1982.
26. Leumann EP, Skinmann B: Persistent and transient distal renal tubular acidosis with bicarbonate wasting. *Pediatr Res* 9:767, 1975.
27. Sly WS, Whyte MP, Sundaram V, et al: Carbonic anhydrase II deficiency in 12 fam-

ilies with the autosomal recessive syndrome of osteopetrosis with renal tubular acidosis and cerebral calcification. *N Engl J Med* 313:139, 1985.

28. Edelmann CM, Boichis H, Rodriguez-Soriano J, et al: The renal response of children to acute ammonium chloride acidosis. *Pediatr Res* 1:452, 1967.
29. Chan JCM: Acid-base, calcium, potassium, and aldosterone metabolism in renal tubular acidosis. *Nephron* 23:152, 1979.
30. McSherry E, Sebastian A, Morris RC Jr: Renal tubular acidosis in infants: The several kinds including bicarbonate wasting, classic renal tubular acidosis. *J Clin Invest* 51:499, 1972.
31. Narins RG, Goldberg M: Renal tubular acidosis: Pathophysiology, diagnosis and treatment. *Disease a Month* 23:1, 1977.
32. Lemann J Jr, Litzow JR, Lennon EJ: The effects of chronic acid loads in normal man: Further evidence for participation of bone mineral in the defense against chronic metabolic acidosis. *J Clin Invest* 45:1608, 1966.
33. Edelmann CM, Rodriguez-Soriano J, Boichis H, et al: Renal bicarbonate reabsorption and hydrogen ion excretion in normal infants. *J Clin Invest* 46:1318, 1967.
34. Chan JCM: Urinary sulfate excretion in children with classic renal tubular acidosis. *Nutr Metab* 22:257, 1978.
35. McSherry E, Morris RC Jr, Griger C, et al: Evidence that acidosis affects collagen metabolism in children with RTA. *Clin Res* 27:373A, 1979.
36. Chesney RW, Kaplan BS, Phelps M, et al: Renal tubular acidosis does not alter circulating values of calcitriol. *J Pediatr* 104:51, 1984.
37. Chan JCM: Calcium and hydrogen ion metabolism in children with classic (type I/ distal) renal tubular acidosis. *Ann Nutr Metab* 25:65, 1981.
38. McSherry E, Morris RC, Jr: Attainment and maintenance of normal stature with alkali therapy in infants and children with classic renal tubular acidosis. *J Clin Invest* 61:509, 1978.
39. Donckerwolcke RA, Van Stekelanburg GJ, Tiddens HA: A case of bicarbonate losing renal tubular acidosis with defective carbonic anhydrase activity. *Arch Dis Child* 45:769, 1970.
40. Morris RC, Jr: Renal tubular acidosis. *N Engl J Med* 304:418, 1981.
41. Schambelan M, Sebastian A, Hulter HN: Mineralocorticoid excess and deficiency syndromes, in Brenner BM, Stein JH (eds): *Contemporary Issues in Nephrology: Acid-Base and Potassium Homeostasis,* vol 2, New York, Churchill Livingstone, 1978, pp 232–268.
42. Perez GO, Oster JR, Vaamonde CA: Renal acidosis and renal potassium handling in selective hyperaldosteronism. *Am J Med* 57:809, 1974.
43. Rodriguez-Soriano J, Vallo A, Oliveros R, et al: Transient pseudohypoaldosteronism secondary to obstructive uropathy in infancy. *J Pediatr* 103:375, 1983.
44. Wrong O, Davis HEF: The excretion of acid in renal diseases. *Q J Med* 28:259, 1959.
45. Chan JCM, Alon U: Tubular disorders of acid base and phosphate metabolism. *Nephron* 40:257, 1985.
46. Batlle DC, Kurtzman NA: The defect in distal (type I) renal tubular acidosis, in Gonick HC, Buckalew VM Jr (eds): *Renal Tubular Disorders: Pathophysiology, Diagnosis and Management.* New York, Marcel Dekker, 1985, p 281.
47. Oster JR, Hotchkiss JL, Carbon M, et al: A short duration renal acidification test using calcium chloride. *Nephron* 14:281, 1975.
48. Loney LC, Norling LL, Robson AM: The use of arginine hydrochloride infusion to assess urinary acidification. *J Pediatr* 100:95, 1982.

49. DuBose TD Jr: Hydrogen ion secretion by the collecting duct as a determinant of the urine to blood pCO_2 gradient in alkaline urine. *J Clin Invest* 69:145, 1982.
50. Halperin ML, Goldstein MB, Richardson RMA, et al: Distal renal tubular acidosis syndromes: A pathophysiological approach. *Am J Nephrol* 5:1, 1985.
51. Halperin ML, Goldstein MB, Haig A, et al: Studies on the pathogenesis of type I (distal) renal tubular acidosis as revealed by the urinary P_{CO_2} tension. *J Clin Invest* 53:669, 1974.
52. Batlle DC, Sehy JT, Roseman MK, et al: Clinical and pathophysiologic spectrum of acquired distal renal tubular acidosis. *Kidney Int* 20:389, 1981.
53. Batlle DC, Kurtzman NA: Renal regulation of acid-base homeostasis: Integrated response, in Seldin DW, Giebish G (eds): *The Kidney: Physiology and Pathophysiology.* New York, Raven Press, 1985, p 1539.
54. Seldin DW, Coleman AJ, Carter N, et al: The effect of Na_2SO_4 on urinary acidification in chronic renal disease. *J Lab Clin Med* 69:893, 1967.
55. Rodriguez-Sorinao J, Vallo A, Castillo G, et al: Pathophysiology of primary distal renal tubular acidosis. *Int J Pediatr Nephrol* 6:71, 1985.
56. Schwartz WB, Jenson RL, Relman AS: Acidification of the urine and increased ammonia excretion without change in acid-base equilibrium: Sodium reabsorption as a stimulus to the acidifying process. *J Clin Invest* 34:673, 1955.
57. Batlle DC, Riotee A, Schlueter W: Urinary sodium in the evaluation of hyperchloremic metabolic acidosis. *N Engl J Med* 316:140, 1987.
58. Batlle DC: Segmental characterization of defects in collecting tubule acidification. *Kidney Int* 30:546, 1986.
59. Goldstein MB, Bear R, Richardson RMA, et al: The urine anion gap: A chemically useful index of ammonium excretion. *Am J Med Sci* 292:198, 1986.
60. Batlle DC, Hizon M, Cohen E, et al: The use of the urinary anion gap in the diagnosis of hyperchloremic metabolic acidosis. *N Engl J Med* 318:594, 1988.
61. Coe FL, Firpo JJ, Hollandsworth DL, et al: Effect of acute and chronic metabolic acidosis on serum immunoreactive parathyroid hormone in man. *Kidney Int* 8:262, 1975.
62. McSherry EM, Pokroy MV: The absence of nephrocalcinosis in children with type I RTA on high-dose alkali therapy since infancy. *Clin Res* 26:470A, 1978.
63. Buckalew VM Jr, Purvis ML, Shulman MG, et al: Report of a 64 member kindred with variable clinical expression including idiopathic hypercalcemia. *Medicine* 53:229, 1974.
64. Coe FL, Parks JH: Stone disease in hereditary distal renal tubular acidosis. *Ann Intern Med* 93:60, 1980.
65. Hammett IA, Czerwinski AW, Coats B, et al: Familial absorptive hypercalciuria and renal tubular acidosis. *Am J Med* 67:385, 1979.
66. Lemann J Jr, Litzow JR, Lennon EJ, et al: Studies of the mechanism by which chronic metabolic acidosis augments urinary calcium excretion in man. *J Clin Invest* 46:1318, 1967.
67. Nephrocalcinosis and renal tubular acidosis, editorial. *Lancet* 2:934, 1974.
68. Goligorsky MS, Chaimovitz C, Rapoport J, et al: Calcium metabolism in uremic nephrocalcinosis: Preventive effective of verapamil. *Kidney Int* 27:774, 1985.
69. Harris DCH, Hammond WS, Burke TJ, et al: Verapamil protects against progression of experimental chronic renal failure. *Kidney Int* 31:41, 1987.
70. Halperin ML: How much "new" bicarbonate is formed in the distal nephron in the process of net acid excretion? *Kidney Int* 35:1277, 1989.

71. McSherry E, Weberman J, Grumbach M, et al: The effect of acidosis on human growth hormone (HGHO) release in children with nonazotemic RTA. *Clin Res* 28:535A, 1980.
72. Sly WS: The carbonic anhydrase II deficiency syndrome: Osteopetrosis with renal tubular acidosis and cerebral calcification, in Scriver CR, Beaudet AL, Sly WS, et al (eds): *The Metabolic Basis of Inherited Disease.* New York, McGraw-Hill Information Services Company, 1989, pp 2857–2866.

22

URINARY STONE DISEASE

Kanwal K. Kher

Urolithiasis, or urinary stone disease, has been known to afflict humanity since ancient times. Urinary stones have been found in Egyptian mummies,[1] and the disorder was well known to Hippocrates.[2] Urolithiasis is not a common disorder in children; it has been estimated that about 1 percent of all cases occur in childhood.[3] In the industrialized Western countries, urinary stones most commonly affect the kidneys and the ureters. In contrast, bladder stones are more often seen in children from the less developed regions. Bladder stones are particularly prevalent in the so-called stone-belt countries of Turkey, Iran, the Indian subcontinent, Thailand, and Indonesia;[4,5] however, they appear to be uncommon in Africa.[6] In the United States, urolithiasis in children is more prevalent in the south eastern region (1 case per 1300 admissions)[7] and southern California (1 case per 1000 admissions)[8] as compared to the northern states (1 case per 7600 admissions).[9] Also, urolithiasis is reported to be less common among black or Hispanic individuals.[9] The last 10 years have seen a resurgence of interest among pediatric nephrologists and urologists in pediatric urolithiasis because of the demonstration of several underlying metabolic abnormalities in urinary calcium excretion in stone-forming children.[10,11]

This chapter focuses on the etiology, pathogenesis, clinical features, diagnostic investigation, and management of urinary stones commonly encountered in children.

ETIOLOGY

Urolithiasis affecting the upper urinary tract is commonly encountered under three circumstances: (1) urinary tract obstruction and structural malformations, (2) urinary tract infection, and (3) metabolic disturbance. Urinary tract infection as an underlying etiology of urolithiasis has been reported to be somewhat more common in European children,[12,13] while metabolic disturbances, especially hypercalciuria, predominate in the studies reported from the United States.[10,12] The incidence of urinary tract malformation as an etiology for urolithiasis varies in published studies but generally appears to be similar on both

TABLE 22–1. Etiology of Urolithiasis in Children from Europe and the United States

Etiology	North America n (%)	Europe n (%)
Developmental anomalies	160 (32.5%)	145 (30.1%)
Infection (no other underlying factor)	21 (4.3%)	209 (43.5%)
Metabolic disorders	162 (32.9%)	59 (12.3%)
Idiopathic hypercalciuria	39	36
Immobilization	39	4
Uric acid stones	22	2
Cystinuria	15	9
Hyperoxaluria	12	5
Renal tubular acidosis	10	2
Primary hyperparathyroidism	9	0
Hypercortisolism	6	1
Milk-alkali syndrome	4	0
Unexplained hypercalcemia	4	0
Idiopathic hypercalcemia of infancy	1	0
Calcinosis universalis	1	0
Endemic urate stones	10 (2.0%)	0
Others	139 (28.3%)	68 (14.1%)
Total	492	481

Source: Modified and reproduced with permission from Polinsky MS, Kaiser BA, Bluarte HJ: Urolithiasis in childhood. *Pediatr Clin North Am* 34:683, 1987.

sides of the Atlantic.[12,14,15] The reason for a higher incidence of metabolic disease as the etiology of urinary stones in U.S. children is unclear. Table 22–1 lists and compares the underlying causes of urolithiasis in children from Europe and the United States.

MECHANISM OF URINARY STONE FORMATION

Urinary stones are made up of aggregates of crystals that develop in an environment that favors their precipitation and growth. Calcium is a common component of urinary stones; other ions that may be encountered in such stones are oxalates, phosphates, urates, and cystine. The crystalline composition of common urinary stones is given in Table 22–2, and the frequency with which various types of renal stones are seen in children is given in Table 22–3. The mechanism by which various crystals precipitate and lead to stone formation within the urinary tract is not entirely understood. In general, three interactive processes which can be considered essential to the development of urinary stones are (1) urinary supersaturation, (2) factors promoting crystal growth, and (3) inhibitors of crystal growth.

Urolithiasis results from precipitation of various salts that are excreted in urine, often in abnormally high concentration. Precipitation of stone constituents such as calcium and oxalate and initiation of urolithiasis require the concentration of these ions to reach a critical level or supersaturation.[16] Sponta-

TABLE 22–2. Common Names and Chemical Composition of Various Types of Urinary Stones

Common Name	Chemical Name	Clinical Conditions Associated	Radiopacity
Struvite	Magnesium-ammonium-phosphate-hexahydrate	Urinary infection	Moderately opaque
Calcium stones			
Brushite	Calcium hydrogen phosphate dihydrate	Hypercalciuria	Highly opaque
Whewellite	Calcium oxalate monohydrate	Hypercalciuria, hyperoxaluria, hyperuricosuria	Highly opaque
Weddelite	Calcium oxalate dihydrate	Hypercalciuria, hyperoxaluria, hyperuricosuria	Highly opaque
Whitlockite	Tricalcium phosphate	Hypercalciuria	Highly opaque
Hydroxyapatite	Basic calcium hydrogen phosphate	Hypercalciuria	Highly opaque
Cystine stones			
	l-cystine	Cystinuria	Nonopaque/ partially opaque
Uric acid stones			
	Uric acid Uric acid dihydrate Monosodium urate monohydrate	Hyperuricosuria	Nonopaque

neous development of crystals (also known as *nucleation*) is impossible if the solution is undersaturated. Urinary supersaturation is influenced not only by the concentration of various urinary salts but also by urinary volume and pH. The influence of fluid intake and urine volume on the state of urinary supersaturation is, however, not well settled. Some investigators have demonstrated a high incidence of urolithiasis in countries and regions with tropical climatic

TABLE 22–3. Incidence of Various Types of Urinary Stones in Children

Type of Stone	Percentage
Calcium oxalate	31
Struvite (magnesium ammonium phosphate)	18
Calcium phosphate	13
Uric acid	8
Cystine	2
Not analyzed	28

Source: Modified and reproduced with permission from Gearhart JP, Herzberg GZ, Jeffs RD: Childhood urolithiasis: Experiences and advances. *Pediatrics* 87:445, 1991. Copyright © 1991 by American Academy of Pediatrics.

conditions.[17,18] This has been interpreted as suggesting a role for low urinary volume (as a consequence of evaporative water loss in hot weather) in enhancing urinary supersaturation. Others have found a marginal role for fluid intake in the pathogenesis of urolithiasis.[19,20] Supersaturation of urine can potentially occur at night, when the fluid intake is low, and in the postprandial period, when stone-forming ions may be excreted in the urine in an increased concentration.[21,22]

Urinary supersaturation can be assessed in a urine sample by measuring the concentration of ions in question and determining the activity products of the ions involved as precipitating salts in the stones.[23] Activity product is mathematically derived from the following formula:

$$\text{Activity product} = (\text{ion A} \times f_2)(\text{ion B} \times f_2)$$

where f_2 is the activity coefficient for the ion. As an example, in relation to calcium oxalate stones, calcium would represent ion A, while ion B would be oxalate.

Several computerized programs, such as EQUIL-2, are available for clinical evaluation of urolithiasis patients. They provide information on the activity product, free urinary ion concentration, and urinary saturation for common urinary salts involved in urolithiasis.[24]

It is now well established that normal urine contains constituents that inhibit the formation of urinary stones (Table 22–4). These inhibitory substances either retard crystal growth by attaching to existing crystal surfaces or chemically complex with various ions to reduce the potential for urinary supersaturation.[25] Some inhibitors of stone growth may also act as complexing agents. A good example of this is citrate, which inhibits stone growth while also reducing the urinary supersaturation of calcium by complexing with excreted urinary calcium. Magnesium can also act as an inhibitor and a complexor by binding to urinary oxalate. Nephrocalcin, a potent inhibitor of the calcium oxalate crys-

TABLE 22–4. Inhibitors of Crystal Formation

Calcium phosphate crystal system
Magnesium
Citrate
Pyrophosphate
Calcium oxalate crystal system
Citrate
Pyrophosphate
Tamm-Horsfall mucoprotein
Chondroitin sulfate
RNA fragments
Nephrocalcin

Source: Modified and reproduced with permission from Smith LH: Pathogenesis of renal stones. *Miner Electrolyte Metab* 13:214, 1987.

TABLE 22–5. Stone-Promoting Factors and Possible Mechanisms That Enhance the Risk of Stone Disease

Stone Promoting Factors	Possible Mechanism
Low fluid intake	Increasing urinary supersaturation of stone-forming salts
Animal protein and dairy products	Hypercalciuria; increased uric acid excretion
Vegetarian diet	Increased oxalate intake and urinary excretion
Immobilization	Induces hypercalcemia and hypercalciuria
Hypocitriuria	Lack of complexing between calcium and citrate enhances calcium oxalate supersaturation
Hypomagnesiuria	Magnesium is believed to complex oxalate; lack of magnesium in urine increases availability of oxalate and increases supersaturation of calcium oxalate

tal system, has been described recently. Absence of this glycoprotein may be an important predisposing factor for the formation of calcium oxalate stones in some patients.[26,27]

Factors other than supersaturation, such as decreased fluid intake and excess protein consumption, can also enhance stone growth. The mechanisms by which these factors promote stone formation are variable and are listed in Table 22–5.

CLINICAL MANIFESTATIONS

Urolithiasis is well known to be more common in males. The male/female ratio ranges from 1.5:1 to 2.0:1 in some studies,[28,29] while others have shown the distribution to be equal in both sexes.[30,31] Black children in the United States are reported to be less likely to develop urolithiasis than are children of other racial backgrounds.[11,28–30]

Abdominal or flank pain is an important manifestation of urinary stones. Colicky abdominal pain has been reported in some studies to be present in up to 50 percent of affected children.[15,28,30,32] In infants and younger children, the nature of this pain is often vague, and it may cause irritability. Some children describe the pain as being sharp and "cutting." Nausea and vomiting may accompany the pain, and localized tenderness along the flank may be present. Some patients may even be suspected of having appendicitis. Hematuria is another common manifestation of urolithiasis and is usually microscopic in nature. Microscopic hematuria has been reported in one large study to be present in 100 percent of children with urolithiasis.[31] Gross hematuria is seen in about 30 to 50 percent of these.[28,30,32] Less commonly, urinary stones can result in acute urinary tract obstruction and anuria.[33,34] Some 30 to 40 percent of children with urolithiasis may pass urinary stones spontaneously during voiding.[28,30]

About a third of children with urolithiasis have an underlying malformation of the urinary tract.[12,15,28] These children may either be known to have such urinary tract abnormalities or may first present with urinary stones. The association of urinary tract infection and urinary stones is well known.[14,29] In some instances urinary stones develop because of chronic and recurrent urinary tract infection; clinical features of urinary tract infection may predominate in such patients. In others, urinary tract infection may be the consequence of urinary stones. In a recent study reported from the Johns Hopkins Hospital,[28] the evidence of associated urinary tract infection was present in 47 percent of children with stones. Most of these children also had an underlying urinary tract malformation.

CLINICAL STATES ASSOCIATED WITH UROLITHIASIS

HYPERCALCIURIA

Calcium (complexed as oxalate or phosphate) is the commonest element found in urinary stones, being present in about 40 to 60 percent of patients.[28,35] Hypercalciuria is the most common metabolic disorder associated with urolithiasis in children.[12] The mechanism by which calcium is involved in the pathogenesis of urinary stone disease has been a subject of considerable scientific investigations in recent years. The role of hypercalciuria in causing clinical syndromes other than urolithiasis in children has also attracted a significant interest in the past decade.[10,11]

Hypercalciuria can be a manifestation of a number of clinical disorders, which are listed in Table 22–6. For the purpose of classification, hypercalciuria can be seen with either normocalcemia or hypercalcemia. When it is associated with hypercalcemia, disorders such as vitamin D intoxication, hyperparathyroidism, sarcoidosis, and malignancy must be considered as diagnostic possibilities in evaluating such patients. Hypercalcemia is not consistently present in patients with hypercalciuria due to prolonged immobilization. In one study of 14 patients with immobilization-induced hypercalciuria, hypercalcemia was not noted in any;[36] in another study, only 1 of 8 patients demonstrated hypercalcemia.[37] In the latter study, however, an increase in serum calcium concentration from baseline admission values (but not in the hypercalcemic range) was noted in all patients. Hypercalciuria due to immobilization is believed to result from the resorption of calcium from bones.[36] Dietary restriction of calcium does not prevent excess urinary calcium excretion in such patients.[36]

Normocalcemic hypercalciuria can result from enhanced gastrointestinal absorption of calcium *(absorptive hypercalciuria)* and from defective renal tubular reabsorption of the filtered calcium *(renal hypercalciuria)*. The relative frequency of absorptive types of hypercalciuria versus renal types of hypercalciuria in children remains unsettled. While Santos et al.[38] found absorptive hypercalciuria to be more common in their population of children, a large study reported by the Southwest Pediatric Nephrology Study Group[39] found renal hypercalciuria to be more prevalent.

Absorptive hypercalciuria has been further classified by Pak and colleagues[40] into type I and type II disorders. Type I hypercalciuria is characterized by increased intestinal calcium absorption and normal fasting urinary calcium excretion. Increased urinary calcium excretion is observed with both a calcium-restricted diet and an oral calcium loading test.[40] Type II hypercalciuria is similar to type I hypercalciuria except that hypercalciuria is not seen following

TABLE 22–6. Classification of Hypercalciuria

Normocalcemic Hypercalciuria
Absorptive hypercalciuria
Type I
Type II
Renal hypercalciuria
Idiopathic
Secondary
Loop diuretics
Immobilization
Phosphate depletion
Acidosis, including distal renal tubular acidosis
Unknown mechanism
Juvenile rheumatoid arthritis
Diabetes mellitus
Cystic fibrosis
Medullary sponge kidney
Wilson disease
Hypercalcemic Hypercalciuria
Immobilization
Vitamin D intoxication
Endocrine disorders
Hyperparathyroidism
Hyperthyroidism
Hyperadrenal corticoidism
Sarcoidosis
Malignancy

ingestion of low-calcium diet but manifests itself only after an oral calcium loading test.[40] Serum parathyroid hormone and 1,25-$(OH)_2D_3$ concentrations are low or normal in patients with both types of absorptive hypercalciuria.

Laboratory features of renal hypercalciuria include excessive renal calcium excretion in the fasting state and the presence of secondary hyperparathyroidism. Oral calcium loading does not significantly increase urinary calcium excretion, but some elevation from baseline values may be observed.[40] Renal hypercalciuria is encountered as an idiopathic disorder in many instances, but a secondary etiology may be present in others. Long-term use of loop diuretics is a frequent etiology of renal hypercalciuria and nephrocalcinosis in neonates.[41–43] Table 22–7 lists the laboratory features that are helpful in distinguishing the absorptive and renal variants of hypercalciuria.

The defect responsible for renal hypercalciuria has not yet been identified. Some patients with renal[44] and alimentary hypercalciuria may have a dysregulated vitamin D metabolism associated with an elevated serum concentration of 1,25-$(OH)_2D_3$.[45–48] Whether elevated serum 1,25-$(OH)_2D_3$ concentration is a primary abnormality in these patients or a consequence of another metabolic defect remains controversial.[48] It has also been suggested that some patients with alimentary hypercalciuria may absorb excess calcium because of an exaggerated intestinal response to circulating 1,25-$(OH)_2D_3$.[47] Decreased excretion of

TABLE 22–7. Laboratory Features Distinguishing Absorptive and Renal Hypercalciuria

Laboratory Test	Absorptive Type I	Absorptive Type II	Renal
Serum calcium	Normal	Normal	Normal
Fasting hypercalciuria	No	No	Yes
Urine calcium with oral calcium load	Increased	Increased	No change to slight increase
Hypercalciuria on calcium restricted diet	Yes	No	Yes
Serum parathyroid hormone	Low or normal	Low or normal	Elevated

urinary citrate has been demonstrated in some adult patients with calcium oxalate stones,[49] but this has not been observed consistently.[50] Urinary citrate concentration in hypercalciuric children has been found to be normal.[51] Several disease states such as juvenile rheumatoid arthritis,[52] diabetes mellitus,[53] cystic fibrosis,[54] medullary sponge kidney,[55,56] and Wilson disease[57] are associated with normocalcemic hypercalciuria, but the mechanism of hypercalciuria in these conditions has not been fully established.

Apart from being a risk factor for urolithiasis and nephrocalcinosis, hypercalciuria has been recognized as an etiology of microscopic and gross hematuria in children.[39,58,59] Hematuria in such cases is not associated with any clinical or laboratory evidence of glomerulonephritis. Characteristically, the syndrome of hypercalciuria-associated hematuria is seen in white male children who have a family history of urolithiasis.[39] Coexisting glomerulopathy—such as IgA nephropathy, thin basement membrane disease, and proliferative glomerulonephritis—may be seen rarely in patients with hypercalciuria and must be considered if appropriate clinical and laboratory evidence is present.[39]

INFECTION STONES

Urinary stones that develop as a result of urinary tract infection are referred to as *infection stones.* They are made up primarily of struvite or magnesium ammonium phosphate, but calcium-containing apatite or hydroxyapatite may also be present in some.[60] The characteristic feature of these stones is that they are large and irregular (staghorn calculi), often occupying the entire renal pelvis. Although infection stones can occur as primary disorders, they are more often seen in patients with malformed or obstructed urinary tracts and in those requiring chronic urinary catheterization.[61]

Only those organisms that produce the enzyme urease are capable of forming struvite urinary stones; the leading group in this category is the protease species. Other organisms that may also be associated with infection stones are *Staphylococcus aureus, Klebsiella pneumoniae, Serratia marcescens, Pseudomonas aeruginosa, Ureaplasma urealyticum,* some strains of *Candida,* and *Cryptococcus.*[62,63] Since *Escherichia coli* does not produce urease, infection by this organism does not result in infection stones. Urease produced by the above-mentioned organisms splits urea into ammonia and carbon dioxide. The product of these reactions is the formation of ammonium and hydroxyl ion.

$$H_2N-\underset{\underset{O}{\|}}{C}-NH_2 + H_2O \rightarrow 2NH_3 + CO_2$$

$$NH_3 + HO_2 \rightarrow NH_4^+ + OH^-$$

Hydration of CO_2 generates bicarbonate and consequently increases urinary pH.

$$CO_2 + H_2O \rightarrow H_2CO_3 \rightarrow H^+ + HCO_3^-$$

In the presence of alkaline pH, the supersaturated urine precipitates magnesium, ammonium, calcium, and phosphate, leading to stone formation.

RENAL TUBULAR ACIDOSIS

Patients with distal renal tubular acidosis (type 1 RTA) often develop nephrocalcinosis and, less commonly, renal stones. In a study of 44 patients with distal RTA, nephrocalcinosis was present in 56 percent while nephrolithiasis was seen in only 7 percent.[64] Proximal renal tubular acidosis (type 2 RTA) and hyperkalemic distal renal tubular acidosis (type 4 RTA) are not associated with either nephrocalcinosis or urolithiasis.[64] The pathogenesis of nephrocalcinosis and urinary stones in type 1 RTA has been linked to hypercalciuria[65] and decreased urinary excretion of citrate,[66] which is an important inhibitor of crystal growth. Nephrocalcinosis and urolithiasis in type 1 RTA are discussed in detail in Chap. 21.

Oxalate is the end product of glyoxylate and ascorbic acid metabolism. Its increased production, or hyperoxaluria, can occur in a variety of inherited and acquired disorders (Table 22–8). The primary clinical manifestation of hyperoxaluria is nephrocalcinosis and urolithiasis (stones are made up of calcium oxalate). Genetically determined or primary hyperoxaluria can present in childhood and is of two subtypes, based on the type of enzymatic defect. Type I primary hyperoxaluria is an autosomal recessive peroxisomal disorder characterized by a deficiency of hepatic peroxisomal alanine:glyoxylate aminotransferase.[67] Pyridoxine (vitamin B_6) is an essential cofactor for the conversion of glyoxylate to glycine in the peroxisomes. Consequently, as a result of the enzyme deficiency, glyoxylate is converted to oxalate and glycolate. Excess oxalate is then deposited in various tissues, causing organ damage. Type II primary hyperoxaluria is caused by a deficiency of the cytosolic enzyme D-glycerate dehydrogenase.[68] Type II primary hyperoxaluria is an extremely rare disease; for all practical purposes type I hyperoxaluria is the only clinically relevant form.

TABLE 22–8. Clinical Conditions Associated with Hyperoxaluria

Primary hyperoxaluria
Type I
Type II
Secondary hyperoxaluria
Gastrointestinal disorders
Regional enteritis
Blind loop syndrome
Small bowel bypass surgery for obesity
Biliary and pancreatic disease
Excessive dietary oxalate intake
Excessive or toxic intake of oxalate precursors
Ethylene glycol
Ascorbic acid
Methoxyflurane anesthesia
Pyridoxine deficiency

Many patients with type I primary hyperoxaluria may remain asymptomatic during childhood. They develop renal stones and consequent sequelae in late childhood or even adulthood.[69] A distinctly severe variant of type I primary hyperoxaluria, the infantile form, manifests early in life. These patients generally have a more progressive clinical course characterized by dense nephrocalcinosis, which leads to chronic renal failure.[70–72] Once acute renal insufficiency sets in and oxalate cannot be eliminated, it is deposited in a wide variety of tissues, including the bone marrow and corneas. Nephrolithiasis is uncommon in patients with the infantile variety of type I primary hyperoxaluria.[71,72] Some workers have designated the infantile form of type I primary hyperoxaluria as a *metabolic malignancy.*[68]

Secondary hyperoxaluria is commonly seen in patients with fat malabsorption and gastrointestinal disorders (enteric hyperoxaluria) such as biliary disease, pancreatic disease, inflammatory bowel disease, ileal bypass surgery, and bowel resection.[73] Calcium oxalate urolithiasis as a result of hyperoxaluria is a well-known complication of these disorders. The pathogenesis of hyperoxaluria and urolithiasis in bowel diseases is now believed to be related to fat malabsorption in these patients.[74] Normally a considerable amount of dietary oxalate is excreted in the stools as cacium oxalate complex. In patients with fat malabsorption, free fatty acids present in the gastrointestinal tract complex with calcium in the diet to form insoluble soaps, thus diminishing the calcium available for complexing with dietary oxalate. Consequently, free oxalate available in the gut is absorbed in the colon.

Excessive dietary intake of oxalates may also lead to elevated urinary oxalate excretion and may be causally linked to oxalate urolithiasis. Vegetables are the predominant source of oxalate in the diet. Table 22–9 lists the foods that are high in oxalate content. Some investigators have recently suggested that calcium oxalate stones may also be the consequence of a primary disorder in oxalate metabolism.[75] In this regard, a defect in red cell oxalate transport has been identified in 79 percent of calcium oxalate stone formers.[76] The mechanism

TABLE 22–9. Foods High in Oxalate Content

Vegetable Sources	Drinks
Rhubarb	Chocolate
Spinach	Cocoa
Turnips	Ovaltine
Beets	Tea
Sweet potatoes	Grape juice
Parsley	Orange juice
Dill	
Nuts	
Unripe bananas	

Source: Modified and reproduced with permission from Smith LH: Enteric hyperoxaluria and other hyperoxaluric states. *Contemporary Issues in Nephrology* 5:136, 1980. © 1980 by Churchill Livingstone, New York.

responsible for this defect has not yet been identified, but this observation may serve as a marker of impaired oxalate metabolism in such patients. These preliminary observations need to be confirmed and explored further.

CYSTINURIA

Cystinuria is a metabolic disease characterized by a defect in cystine transport across the renal tubules and the gastrointestinal tract.[77] The disorder is inherited in an autosomal recessive manner. Normally almost all (99 percent) of the filtered amino acids are reabsorbed in the proximal renal tubules and less than 1 percent of the filtered load is excreted in urine. In patients with cystinuria, cystine and other dibasic aminoacids (ornithine, lysine, and arginine) are not reabsorbed from the glomerular filtrate. Since cystine is insoluble, especially in the acidic environment, these crystals precipitate within the urinary tract, leading to urolithiasis.

Cystinuria predominantly affects adults in the second or third decade of life.[77,78] Recurrent urolithiasis and associated complications—such as infection, hematuria, renal colic, and obstruction—are common. Cystine crystals are soluble in an alkaline urine and may not be visible in the urine sediment unless the urine is concentrated and acidified. Cystine stones are radiolucent but may be radiopaque because of their high sulfur content. In addition, many such stones contain secondary calcium deposits, which also make them visible on a plain radiograph of the abdomen. Ultrasonography or intravenous pyelography is the procedure of choice for localizing cystine stones within the urinary tract. Cystine can be chemically detected in urine by using either the sodium nitroprusside test or by urinary amino acid screening.

It is essential to make a distinction between cystinuria and cystinosis. Cystinosis is a systemic defect affecting cystine metabolism wherein cystine crystals accumulate intracellularly, leading to widespread organ dysfunctions, primary among which is renal failure. Cystinuria, on the other hand, is not a systemic defect and intracellular accumulation of cystine does not occur.

HYPERURICOSURIA

Uric acid, which is produced in humans as an end product of dietary or endogenous purine metabolism, is freely filtered by the glomeruli but undergoes complex transport within the renal tubules. The net urinary excretion of uric acid depends on the balance between proximal tubular reabsorption (normal: 90 percent of the filtered load) and tubular secretion. The urinary solubility of uric acid is determined by pH. At a urinary pH of 5.0, the solubility limit of uric acid is only 15 mg/dL; while at pH 7.0, the solubility limit increases to 200 mg/dL.[79] Therefore, low urine pH favors the formation of uric acid stones.

Myeloproliferative disorders, especially following aggressive chemotherapy, constitute an important cause of hyperuricemia and hyperuricosuria in childhood. Less commonly, increased urinary excretion of uric acid may occur in patients receiving uricosuric drugs, such as salicylic acid and probenecid, or foods high in purine, such as meat, poultry and fish. Uricosuria may also be associated with gastrointestinal diseases such as ulcerative colitis, regional enteritis, and ileostomy, which are characterized by excessive loss of fluid and bicarbonate via the gastrointestinal tract.[79,80] Uric acid stones are presumed to result from dehydration and acidic urine formed under these circumstances.

Hyperuricemia and hyperuricosuria can result in three distinct types of clinical renal disorders: (1) interstitial deposition of uric acid and its salts, leading to chronic urate nephropathy ("gouty nephropathy"); (2) precipitation of uric acid in the collecting ducts, leading to acute urate nephropathy and acute renal failure; and (3) formation of uric acid–calcium oxalate stones. Of these three disorders, gouty nephropathy and uric acid–calcium oxalate urolithiasis are seldom observed in children, while acute urate nephropathy and acute renal failure can complicate myeloproliferative disorders.

A distinct association between hyperuricosuria and calcium oxalate stones is well described in adults. It has been suggested that uric acid crystals in the urine of such patients may either serve as a nidus for calcium-oxalate deposition[81] or promote precipitation of calcium oxalate by decreasing the concentration of inhibitors of calcium-oxalate lithiasis in urine.[82]

MISCELLANEOUS STONES

Several types of drugs that are excreted in urine can result in urinary supersaturation of drug crystals, leading to urolithiasis. Among the drugs that commonly lead to urinary stone formation are triamterene, sulfonamide, and acetazolamide.[83] Rarely, parents of patients or the patients themselves may falsely claim to have passed renal stones for the purposes of secondary gain or as a part of the Munchausen syndrome. The diagnosis of factitious calculi may be suspected in patients with behavioral problems, where there is failure to document urolithiasis radiologically and in the absence of any metabolic etiology predisposing to urolithiasis despite extensive laboratory evaluation. Chemical analysis of these patients' stones reveals quartz.[84]

EVALUATION OF UROLITHIASIS IN CHILDREN

Urolithiasis in children is always secondary to an underlying systemic or renal disease, and attempts should always be made to determine the etiology. Evaluation of such children can be divided into two categories: (1) establishing the diagnosis of urinary stones and (2) determining the etiology of urolithiasis. Tests included under both categories can be conducted simultaneously.

ESTABLISHING THE DIAGNOSIS

The diagnosis of urolithiasis can be established by (1) a careful review of the history, (2) physical examination, and (3) radiologic investigations of the urinary tract. As pointed out earlier, symptoms of stone disease include abdominal pain which may take the form of a renal or ureteric colic or be vague in its localization.

RADIOLOGY

While a plain radiograph of the abdomen can identify radiopaque stones such as those composed of calcium oxalate and calcium phosphate, stones made up of uric acid, xanthine, cystine, and triamterene are radiolucent and are not generally visible. Mixed uric acid–calcium oxalate stones are radiopaque and cystine stones are also radiopaque if the sulfur content of the stones is high. Infection or struvite stones exhibit a variable degree of radiopacity. Renal ultrasonography is another noninvasive and potentially useful radiologic method for identifying urinary stones and also provides information related to the secondary effects, such as hydronephrosis; detects structural renal abnormalities; and aids in the diagnosis of nephrocalcinosis. However, intravenous pyelography may be necessary to identify radiolucent stones within the urinary tract in many patients. In addition to confirming the presence of urinary stones, an intravenous pyelogram will also identify any abnormalities in the anatomy of the urinary tract.

DETERMINING THE ETIOLOGY OF UROLITHIASIS

URINALYSIS

Urinalysis, especially the microscopic examination, may be helpful in identifying crystals such as calcium oxalate, magnesium ammonium phosphate (triple phosphate), cystine, and urate in patients with urolithiasis. Such clues constitute an initial step in establishing the etiology of the stone. For example, the presence of calcium-oxalate crystals in the urine would suggest further evaluation of the patient for hypercalciuria, while the presence of cystine crystals in the urinary sediment establishes the diagnosis of cystinuria. The identification of urinary crystals is discussed in Chap. 2.

URINE CULTURE

Recurrent urinary tract infection is the etiology of urolithiasis in 20 to 30 percent of children in the United States; its incidence is higher in the European centers. Evidence for urinary tract infection should be sought by history, examination of the medical record, and by obtaining a urine culture. It must also be emphasized that, in some patients, urinary tract infection may be the consequence of urolithiasis and not its etiology.

SERUM ELECTROLYTES

Serum electrolytes, including calcium and phosphorus, should be obtained to determine whether the patient has hypercalcemia. If hypercalcemia is documented, the patient must undergo evaluation for the causes listed in Table 22–6. The presence of normal-anion-gap hyperchloremic acidosis would suggest the diagnosis of type 1 RTA.

RENAL FUNCTION

Serum creatinine and blood urea nitrogen (BUN) should be obtained for baseline evaluation of renal function. Patients who have sustained renal parenchymal loss as a consequence of complications (urinary tract infection or obstruction) resulting from urolithiasis may show an abnormal BUN and serum creatinine. Patients with the infantile variant of oxaluria may have established renal failure when first seen; serum creatinine and BUN will also be abnormal in such patients.

METABOLIC EVALUATION

Metabolic evaluation is necessary in about 40 to 50 percent of children with urolithiasis. Hypercalciuria is the most common metabolic cause of urolithiasis in children, and it should be looked for first. Investigations of less common disorders such as cystinuria and defects in uric acid metabolism may be considered later. Laboratory tests necessary for the metabolic evaluation of children with urolithiasis are given in Table 22–10.

URINARY CALCIUM EXCRETION

The diagnosis of hyperalciuria can be established by quantifying calcium in a 24-h collection of urine. The urine should be collected by the usual methods in a container, with no preservatives. Upper limit of daily urinary calcium excretion in healthy children ingesting an unrestricted diet is 4 mg/kg. Accuracy of urine collection is essential in determining hypercalciuria and should be

TABLE 22–10. Laboratory Tests Used in the Evaluation of Metabolic Etiology of Urolithiasis

Serum electrolytes
Serum creatinine and BUN
Serum calcium
Serum uric acid
Spot urine for calcium/creatinine ratio
24 hour urine for calcium and creatinine
Calcium loading test in hypercalciuric patients
Parathyroid hormone assay
Nitroprusside test for cystine (when suspected)
Stone analysis
Stone-risk profile in 24-h urine collection

checked by obtaining a simultaneous creatinine concentration in the 24-h urine sample.*

Screening for hypercalciuria can also be done in a spot urine sample by determining the ratio between urinary calcium and creatinine. A urine calcium/creatinine ratio (each measured in milligrams per deciliter) of 0.2 is regarded as the upper limit of normal, and a higher ratio indicates hypercalciuria.[85,86] The calcium/creatinine ratio is not affected by the patient's age, sex, or race.[86] A good correlation between calcium/creatinine ratio and 24-h urinary calcium excretion has been demonstrated in adult patients with hypercalciuria and urolithiasis.[87] The calcium/creatinine ratio can be used as a helpful tool in the diagnosis of hypercalciuria in children in whom a 24-h urine collection cannot be obtained; the test can also be utilized in following these patients and judging the effectiveness of therapy.

CALCIUM LOADING TEST

A test to differentiate alimentary hypercalciuria and renal hypercalciuria was proposed by Pak et al. in 1975 (sometimes referred to as the *Pak test*).[88] It is conducted by placing the patient on a fixed low-calcium diet (400 mg of calcium in adults) for 7 days prior to the day of the test. Patients are fasted overnight except for a fixed water intake (250 mL at 9 P.M. and at midnight). The first morning urine sample is voided and 250 mL of water is taken by the patient. Blood is drawn for fasting serum calcium concentration as well as parathyroid hormone assay (if not obtained previously). A 2-h urine sample is collected to measure baseline calcium and creatinine (for calcium/creatinine ratio). The patient is then given calcium glubionate syrup in a dose of 1 g/1.73 m^2 of body surface area. Urine is collected for the following 4 h for the estimation of calcium and creatinine. A standard 300-calorie breakfast comprising 25 meq sodium, 100 mg calcium, and 100 mg phosphorus is given the patient during the test period. Intake of tap water may also be encouraged. Differentiation between absorptive and renal hypercalciuria is made by features discussed in Table 22–8. Briefly, absorptive hypercalciuria is characterized by normal fasting calcium excretion (calcium/creatinine ratio), which increases with the intake

*Normal = 15 to 20 mg/L in children 3 to 18 years of age. Details are discussed in Chap. 1.

of calcium load. Renal hypercalciuria, on the other hand, is associated with high fasting hypercalciuria, which is affected marginally by calcium loading.[86,88] Serum parathyriod hormone concentration is normal in absorptive hypercalciuria and elevated in renal hypercalciuria.

STONE ANALYSIS

If a urinary stone has been passed and is available, its chemical composition should be determined. This is the most direct way of establishing the etiology of urolithiasis.

STONE-RISK PROFILE

A stone-risk profile study is commercially available for evaluation of patients with urolithiasis.[88] The test measures urine volume, pH, concentration of calcium, oxalate, uric acid, sodium, and magnesium. Relative supersaturation of each combination of urinary ions is then calculated and plotted in a graphic display.

MANAGEMENT STRATEGIES IN UROLITHIASIS

Patients diagnosed as having urolithiasis may be completely asymptomatic, may have severe abdominal pain, or may manifest complications such as urinary obstruction and urinary tract infection. Each of these clinical aspects must be addressed based on the clinical circumstance. Pain due to renal colic is usually not relieved by acetaminophen or salicylates; often narcotic analgesics must be employed. Appropriate therapy for urinary tract infection is indicated in patients with this complication. Urinary tract obstruction arising as a result of a calculus may require surgical treatment, and consultation with a pediatric urologist should be obtained.

As a part of general management, patients should be encouraged to drink water, especially at night, in order to reduce the urinary saturation of various stone-forming constituents. Because calcium supplementation has recently become a "home remedy" for the prevention of osteoporosis in adult life, hypercalciuria and urolithiasis may be seen in some patients taking large calcium supplements.[90] Patients should be asked about their intake of such supplements and advised against it. Patients should also be instructed to look for the passage of stone after voiding as long as stones are visualized radiologically in the urinary tract, and preferably, the urine should be strained through a sieve. Recovered stones should be sent for chemical analysis. Ultrasonography should be utilized to assess the extent of stone formation or resolution and to investigate obstruction of the urinary tract periodically.

TREATMENT OF SPECIFIC CONDITIONS

RENAL HYPERCALCIURIA

Thiazide diuretics are well known to reduce urinary calcium excretion and are used to treat patients with renal hypercalciuria with or without stones.[91] Thiazides reduce urinary calcium excretion by enhancing reabsorption of calcium in the renal tubules. Hydrochlorothiazide (HydroDIURIL) is commonly employed in a dose of 2 to 3 mg/kg/day in a divided dose (q 12 h). Other thiazides are equally effective and can be used in equivalent doses. Common side effects of thiazides include hypokalemia, hypercalcemia, and hyperuricemia.

ABSORPTIVE HYPERCALCIURIA

Patients with absorptive hypercalciuria should be instructed to decrease their daily calcium intake by modifying their diet. Dairy products are especially high in calcium and their intake should be restricted; however, this may not always be easy in children. Children may develop hypercalciuria and neprolithiasis while receiving enteral hyperalimentation containing excessive amounts of calcium. This form of absorptive hypercalciuria is treatable by decreasing the calcium content in the hyperalimentation formula.

Cellulose phosphate, which binds to calcium in the gut and prevents its absorption, has been used to treat absorptive hypercalciuria. This drug must be given with meals; its potential side effect is a negative calcium balance in a growing child. Also, increased urinary oxalate excretion can occur with orthophosphate therapy, which may, in fact, negate the advantages gained by the reduction of urinary calcium excretion. The mechanism of hyperoxaluria with this treatment is believed to be lack of any calcium available in the gut to complex with oxalate, which is left free to be absorbed. The dose of cellulose phosphate in children with hypercalciuria is not established.

RENAL TUBULAR ACIDOSIS

Treatment of nephrocalcinosis and nephrolithiasis associated with type 1 RTA should be directed at the correction of acidosis. Such therapy has been shown to reduce the incidence of nephrolithiasis in the affected patients.[92] It has been suggested that potassium citrate may be better than sodium citrate for this purpose.[93]

OXALURIA

Treatment of nonrecurrent oxalate urolithiasis should involve general measures such as increasing fluid intake and decreasing dietary sources of oxalate. Recurrent urolithiasis may be treated with (1) potassium citrate,[94] (2) thiazide diuretics,[67] (3) orthophosphate,[67] or (4) magnesium oxide.[95] While treatment of calcium oxalate urolithiasis with potassium citrate, thiazides, and orthophosphate is well accepted, therapy with magnesium supplements requires further evaluation. Treatment of the infantile form of primary oxaluria, which should be considered on an urgent basis, consists of administering large doses of pyridoxine, and oral orthophosphate and maintaining good hydration. Hemodialysis should be undertaken in patients with renal insufficiency in order to diminish the total body oxalate burden. Combined liver and renal transplantation has been advocated for these patients.[68,96] Patients with enteric hyperoxaluria require treatment of their underlying gastrointestinal condition. Their dietary fat intake should be reduced, and some patients may benefit from the use of cholestyramine.

URIC ACID

Acute urate nephropathy as well as uric acid lithiasis can be treated by maintaining a high urinary volume and alkalinizing the urine. Allopurinol should also be administered to patients with myeloproliferative disorders in order to diminish uric acid synthesis.

EXTRACORPOREAL SHOCK-WAVE LITHOTRIPSY

Spontaneous passage of urinary stones is common (30 to 40 percent) in children.[28] Surgical removal of the stones may become necessary in patients in whom complications such as urinary obstruction develop. Extracorporeal shock-wave lithotripsy (ESWL) is now available as a nonsurgical method for the removal of urinary stones. Experience with the use of this modality in children is limited but growing. However, such treatment is available in only a few medical centers at this time.

BLADDER STONES

Bladder stones were once a common occurrence in the Western world,[97] but with industrialization they have almost disappeared. However, this disorder still persists in southeast Asia.[4,5] Even there, bladder stones are more common among the poor than the well-to-do, suggesting that nutrition may be involved as a possible etiologic factor. The disease is typically seen in children below age 10, with a strong male dominance. The stones are usually large, sometimes almost filling the entire bladder.[5] Symptoms of renal colic are uncommon, but dysuria caused by either the stone itself or the associated urinary infection may be seen. Recurrence following surgical removal of the stone is unusual.[98]

CONCLUSION

Urolithiasis in children results from malformation of the urinary tract, recurrent urinary tract infection, or metabolic abnormalities. Metabolic abnormalities—mostly hypercalciuria—remain the predominant cause of urolithiasis in some regions of the United States. In evaluating these children, initial investigations should focus on ruling out underlying recurrent urinary tract infection, which may be associated with malformation of the urinary tract. Radiologic investigations are essential in identifying the site of urinary stones as well as in determining the anatomy of the urinary tract. Metabolic investigations of urolithiasis are cumbersome but may be required in a patient with recurrent stone disease. At times, however, even extensive investigations may not provide conclusive information as to etiology. Treatment of a patient with urolithiasis should be directed toward correcting the underlying causative factors.

Hypercalciuria: A Commentary

F. Bruder Stapleton

Urinary calcium excretion—what is normal, how much is too much, and what harm can it do to children? These questions are confronting pediatric nephrologists and pediatricians with increasing frequency. In 1981, we drew attention to the frequent association of urolithiasis and hypercalciuria in children. At the same time, the observation of nephrocalcinosis and urolithiasis in premature infants receiving furosemide therapy was published. Since then, greater attention has been directed toward the potential pathologic consequences of urinary calcium excretion as well as the pathogenetic mechanisms responsible for hypercalciuria.

Normal urinary calcium excretion is generally accepted to be <4.0 mg (0.1 mol)/kg/day for school-age children ingesting a routine diet. Similar normative standards are applicable in adults. There does not appear to be a major difference in urinary calcium excretion between males and females. Black adults excrete less calcium than do white adults; it is unknown whether racial differences in calcium excretion exist in children. The diagnostic criteria for excessive urinary calcium excretion have not been established with certainty in neonates and infants. Urinary calcium excretion is markedly influenced by the calcium and phosphorus content of infant formulas. Unquestionably, urinary calcium excretion is significantly greater per kilogram of body weight in early infancy, therefore the criteria used in older children are not appropriate for the youngest patients.

The preferred criteria for determining the diagnosis of hypercalciuria in a child remains somewhat controversial. Many authors recommend the use of the ratio of urinary calcium to creatinine (mg/mg) concentrations to assess urinary calcium excretion. In a 24-h urine, a urinary calcium/creatinine ratio of <0.2 is considered normal. This is reasonable if one assumes that urinary calcium excretion should be <4 mg/kg/day and the average urinary creatinine excretion of 20 mg/kg/day. This ratio also applies following an overnight fast. Due to diet-induced calciuria, this ratio will change following a meal. On the other hand, 24-h urines are extremely difficult to obtain in small children, and a postprandial urinary calcium:creatinine ratio of <0.2 is a useful screening tool to exclude hypercalciuria in infants. The oral calcium loading test has been advocated as a useful way of differentiating specific pathogenetic types of hypercalciuria and formulating appropriate therapeutic plans for adults with urolithiasis. While initial applications of this diagnostic test in children with urolithiasis were promising, subsequent experience has found it to be inconsistent and markedly influenced by dietary sodium. We do not recommend the oral calcium loading test as a routine clinical study in children with hypercalciuria.

Clinical manifestations of hypercalciuria include urolithiasis, nephrocalcinosis, isolated hematuria, and the frequency-dysuria syndrome. Hypercalciuria is the most common etiology of urolithiasis in both children and adults. In some children, hematuria alone may be an early manifestation of hypercalciuria and represent a harbinger of overt urinary stone disease. The following case exemplifies the association of hematuria with idiopathic hypercalciuria in a complex patient.

A 3-year-old white girl was diagnosed as having systemic juvenile rheumatoid arthritis with hectic fevers, polyarthritis, and lymphadenopathy. Before therapy with salicylates, microscopic hematuria was noted. At 4½ years of age she developed episodes of urinary incontinence, severe dysuria, and gross hematuria concomitant with fever and increased joint symptoms. Evaluation of the urinary tract at the onset of urinary symptoms yielded negative urine cultures and normal findings on intravenous pyelogram and voiding cystourethrogram.

The serum antinuclear antibody and IgM rheumatoid factor tests yielded negative results. Cystoscopic evaluation at 4½ years and at 5 years of age failed to reveal the source of hematuria. She was then referred for nephrologic consultation because of increasing episodes of dysuria and hematuria. At the time of evaluation, the patient was receiving tolectin sodium 200 mg three times daily for joint pain. There was no family history of renal disease or urolithiasis. No evidence of inflammatory bowel disease was found with barium enema studies. Physical examination revealed fusiform swelling of the interphalangeal joints of the hand and contractures of both elbows and knees. The urinalysis revealed a large reaction to hemoglobin, red blood cells "too numerous to count," proteinuria (1+), and many calcium oxalate crystals. Metabolic evaluation found creatinine clearance to be 110 m/min/1.72 m^2, normal uric acid and oxalate excretion, and increased urinary calcium excretion of 4.6 mg/kg/day. The serum calcium concentration was 9.5 mg/dL. At 5½ years of age the child spontaneously passed a calcium oxalate urinary calculus during an episode of dysuria and hematuria.

This patient demonstrated many of the clinical manifestations associated with hypercalciuria. The finding of unexplained hematuria has been noted in children with idiopathic hypercalciuria and in children with juvenile rheumatoid arthritis. The association of frequency and dysuria without urinary tract infection also is seen in some children with idiopathic hypercalciuria. Finally, urolithiasis is the end result of hypercalciuria in this patient. Our studies in children with juvenile rheumatoid arthritis have found that hypercalciuria occurs in as many as one-third of arthritic children in an outpatient setting. Hematuria may be found in as many as 50 percent of such children with hypercalciuria. The nature of the hypercalciuria appears to be resorptive and is responsive to hydrochlorothiazide. Frequently the hematuria associated with hypercalciuria will abate during treatment with hydrochlorothiazide.

The appropriate therapy for children with hypercalciuria remains controversial. In some patients, excessive urinary calcium excretion is related to enhanced absorption of gastrointestinal calcium and/or to excessive dietary sodium intake. A mild reduction in dietary calcium intake may lessen the risk for complications of hypercalciuria in such patients; however, care must be given to assure adequate calcium intake to meet the demands of growth. Similarly, a reduction in dietary sodium intake appears to be warranted in most children with hypercalciuria. The long-term effects of this form of treatment have not been established. The most debatable issue is whether to administer the anticalciuric diuretic hydrochlorothiazide. This agent has a number of important potential adverse effects. My personal opinion is not to administer hydrochlorothiazide to patients with hematuria. Hydrochlorothiazide (starting at 1 mg/kg/day and increasing to 2 mg/kg/day if necessary) is prescribed for children who have urolithiasis associated with persistent hypercalciuria. The appropriate length of such therapy has not been determined.

REFERENCES

1. Sigerist HE: *A History of Medicine,* vol 1: *Primitive and Archaic Medicine.* New York, Oxford University Press, 1955, p 63.
2. Mettler CC: *History of Medicine.* Philadelphia, Blakiston, 1944, p 696.
3. Lonsdale K: Human stones. *Science* 159:1199, 1968.
4. Aurora AL, Taneja OP, Gupta DN: Bladder diseases of childhood: I. An epidemiologic study. *Acta Paediatr Scad* 59:177, 1970.
5. Ashworth M, Hill SM: Endemic bladder stones in Nepal. *Arch Dis Child* 63:1503, 1988.
6. Andersen DA: The nutritional significance of bladder stones. *Br J Urol* 34:160, 1962.
7. Noe NH, Stapleton FB, Jerkins GR, et al: Clinical experience with pediatric urolithiasis. *J Urol* 129:1166, 1983.
8. Walther PC, Lamm D, and Kaplan GW: Pediatric urolithiasis: A ten-year review. *Pediatrics* 65:1068, 1980.
9. Troup CW, Lawnicki CC, Bourne RB, et al: Renal calculus in children. *J Urol* 107:306, 1972.
10. Stapleton FB, Noe HN, Jerkins GR, et al: Hypercalciuria in children with urolithiasis. *Am J Dis Child* 136:675, 1982.
11. Stapleton FB, McKay CP, Noe HN: Urolithiasis in children: The role of hypercalciuria. *Pediatr Ann* 16:980, 1987.
12. Polinsky M, Kaiser BA, Baluarte HJ: Urolithiasis in childhood. *Pediatr Clin North Am* 34:683, 1987.
13. Ghazali S, Barratt TM, Williams DI: Childhood urolithiasis in Britain. *Arch Dis Child* 48:291, 1973.
14. Diamond DA, Menon M, Lee PH, et al: Etiologic factors in pediatric stone recurrence. *J Urol* 142:606, 1989.
15. Choi H, Snyder HM III, Duckett JW: Urolithiasis in childhood: Current management. *J Pediatr Surg* 22:158, 1987.
16. Smith LH: Pathogenesis of renal stones. *Mineral Electrolyte Metab* 13:214, 1987.
17. Prince CL, Scardino PL, Wolan CT: The effect of temperature, humidity and dehydration on the formation of renal calculi. *J Urol* 75:209, 1956.
18. Better OS: Impaired fluid and electrolyte balance in hot climates. *Kidney Int* 32(suppl 21):S-97, 1987.

19. Miller LA, Stapleton FB: Urinary volume in children with urolithiasis. *J Urol* 141:918, 1989.
20. Ljunghall S, Felström B, Johansson G: Prevention of renal stones by a high fluid intake. *Eur Urol* 14:381, 1988.
21. Jenkins AD: Calculus formation, in *Adult and Pediatric Urology*. Gillenwater JY, Grayhack JT, Howards SS, et al (eds). Mosby Year Book, St. Louis, Missouri, 1991, p 403.
22. Pak CYC, Sakhaee K, Crowther C, et al: Evidence justifying a high fluid intake in treatment of nephrolithiasis. *Ann Intern Med* 93:36, 1980.
23. Pak CYC, Chu S: A simple technique for determination of urinary state of saturation with respect to brushite. *Invest Urol* 11:211, 1973.
24. Werness PG, Brown CM, Smith LH, et al: EQUIL 2: A BASIC computer program for the calculation of urinary saturation. *J Urol* 134:1242, 1985.
25. Smith LH: The pathophysiology and medical treatment of urolithiasis. *Semin Nephrol* 10:31, 1990.
26. Nakagawa YM, Ahmed SL, Hall E, et al: Isolation from human calcium oxalate renal stones of nephrocalcin, a glycoprotein inhibitor of calcium oxalate crystal growth: evidence that nephrocalcin in patients with calcium oxalate nephrolithiasis is deficient in τ-carboxyglutamic acid. *J Clin Invest* 79:1782, 1987.
27. Worcester EM, Nakagawa Y, Wabner CL, et al: Crystal adsorption and growth slowing by nephrocalcin, albumin, and Tamm-Horsfall protein. *Am J Physiol* 255:F1197, 1988.
28. Gearhart JP, Herzberg GZ, Jeffs RD: Childhood urolithiasis: Experiences and advances. *Pediatrics* 87:445, 1991.
29. Bensman A, Roubach L, Allouch G, et al: Urolithiasis in children. Presenting signs, etiology, bacteriology and localization. *Acta Paediatr Scand* 72:879, 1983.
30. Rainer D, Leumann EP, Stauffer U: Childhood urolithiasis. *Helv Paediatr Acta* 35:301, 1980.
31. Noronha RFX, Gregory JG, Duke JJ: Urolithiasis in children. *J Urol* 121:478, 1979.
32. Sinno K, Boyce WH, Resnick MI: Childhood urolithiasis. *J Urol* 121:662, 1979.
33. Kheradpir MH, Bodaghi E: Calculus anuria in childhood. *Child Nephrol Urol* 9:295, 1988.
34. Nicholson R, Hewitt I, Kam A: Ureteric sludge syndrome. *Arch Dis Child* 66:344, 1991.
35. Laufer J, Boichis H: Urolithiasis in children: current medical management. *Pediatr Nephrol* 3:317, 1989.
36. Stewart AF, Adler M, Byers CM, et al: Calcium homeostasis in immobilization: An example of resorptive hypercalciuria. *N Engl J Med* 306:1136, 1982.
37. Andrews P, Rosenberg AR: Renal consequences of immobilization in children with fractured femurs. *Acta Paediatr Scand* 79:311, 1990.
38. Santos F, Suárez D, Málaga S, et al: Idiopathic hypercalciuria in children: Pathophysiologic considerations of renal and absorptive types. *J Pediatr* 110:238, 1987.
39. The Southwest Pediatric Nephrology Study Group: Idiopathic hypercalciuria: Association with isolated hematuria and risk for urolithiasis. *Kidney Int* 37:807, 1990.
40. Pak CYC, Britton F, Peterson R, et al: Ambulatory evaluation of nephrolithiasis. Classification, clinical presentation and diagnostic criteria. *Am J Med* 69:19, 1980.
41. Atkinson SA, Shah JK, McGee C, et al: Mineral excretion in premature infants receiving various diuretic therapy. *J Pediatr* 113:540, 1980.
42. Hufnagle KG, Khan SN, Penn D, et al: Renal calcifications: A longterm complication of furosemide therapy in preterm infants. *Pediatrics* 70:360, 1982.

43. Ezzedeen F, Adelman RD, Ahlfors CE: Renal calcifications in preterm infants: Pathophysiology and long-term sequelae. *J Pediatr* 113:532, 1988.
44. Stapleton FB, Langman CB, Bittle J, et al: Increased serum concentrations of 1,25-$(OH)_2$ vitamin D in children with fasting hypercalciuria. *J Pediatr* 110:234, 1987.
45. Hymes LC, Warshaw BL: Families of children with idiopathic hypercalciuria. Evidence for hormonal basis of familial hypercalciuria. *Am J Dis Child* 139:621, 1985.
46. Broadus AE, Isogna KL, Lang R, et al: Evidence for disordered control of 1,25-dihydroxyvitamin D production in absorptive hypercalciuria. *N Engl J Med* 311:73, 1984.
47. Kaplan RA, Haussler MR, Deftos LJ, et al: The role of 1α, 25-dihydroxy vitamin D in the mediation of intestinal hyperabsorption of calcium in primary hyperparathyroidism and absorptive hypercalciuria. *J Clin Invest* 59:756, 1977.
48. Lemann J, Gray RW: Idiopathic hypercalciuria. *J Urol* 141:715, 1989.
49. Conte A, Roca P, Gianotti M, et al: On the relation between citrate and calcium in normal and stone-former subjects. *Int J Urol Nephrol* 21:369, 1989.
50. Parks JH, Coe FL: Urine citrate and calcium in calcium nephrolithiasis. *Adv Exp Med Biol* 208:445, 1986.
51. Miller LA, Stapleton B: Urinary citrate excretion in children with hypercalciuria. *J Pediatr* 107:263, 1985.
52. Stapleton FB, Hanissian AS, Miller LA: Hypercalciuria in children with juvenile rheumatoid arthritis: Association with hematuria. *J Pediatr* 107:235, 1985.
53. Malone JI, Lowitt S, Duncan JA, et al: Hematuria and hypercalciuria in children with diabetes mellitus. *Pediatrics* 79:756, 1987.
54. Katz SM, Krueger LJ, Falkner B: Microscopic nephrocalcinosis in cystic fibrosis. *N Engl J Med* 319:263, 1988.
55. Parks JH, Coe FL, Strauss AL: Calcium nephrolithiasis and medullary sponge kidney in women. *N Engl J Med* 306:1088, 1982.
56. Higashihara E, Nutahara K, Niijina T: Renal hypercalciuria and metabolic acidosis associated with medullary sponge kidney: Effect of alkali therapy. *Urol Res* 16:95, 1988.
57. Azizi E, Eshel G, Aladjem M: Hypercalciuria and nephrolithiasis as a presenting sign in Wilson disease. *Eur J Pediatr* 148:548, 1989.
58. Kalia A, Travis LB, Brouhard BH: The association of idiopathic calciuria and asymptomatic gross hematuria in children. *J Pediatr* 99:716, 1981.
59. Stapleton FB, Roy S III, Noe M, et al: Hypercalciuria in children with hematuria. *N Engl J Med* 310:1345, 1984.
60. Kristensen C, Parks J, Lindheimer M, et al: Reduced glomerular filtration rate and hypercalciuria in primary struvite nephrolithiasis. *Kidney Int* 32:749, 1987.
61. Donnelly J, Hackler RH, Bunts RC: Present urologic status of the World War II paraplegic: 25-year followup, comparison with the status of the 20-year Korean War paraplegic and 5-year Vietnam paraplegic. *J Urol* 108:558, 1972.
62. Griffith DP, Bruce RR, Fishbein WN: Infection (urease)-induced stones, Coe FL (Ed) in *Contemporary Issues in Nephrology* 5:231, 1980.
63. Grenabo L, Claes G, Hedelin H, et al: Rapidly recurrent renal calculi caused by ureaplasma urealyticum: A case report. *J Urol* 135:995, 1986.
64. Brenner RJ, Spring DB, Sebastian A, et al: Incidence of radiographically evident bone disease, nephrocalcinosis, and nephrolithiasis in various types of renal tubular acidosis. *N Engl J Med* 307:217, 1982.
65. Chan JCM: Calcium and hydrogen ion metabolism in children with classic (type I/distal) renal tubular acidosis. *Ann Nutr Metab* 25:65, 1981.

66. Norman ME, Feldman NI, Cohen RM, et al: Urinary citrate excretion in the diagnosis of distal renal tubular acidosis. *J Pediatr* 92:394, 1978.
67. Danpure CJ, Jennings PR: Peroxisomal alanine: Glyoxylate aminotransferase deficiency in primary hyperoxaluria type I. FEBS J 201:20, 1986.
68. Scheinman JI: Primary hyperoxaluria: Therapeutic strategies for the 90's. *Kidney Int* 40:389, 1991.
69. Morgan SH, Watts RWE: Perspectives in the assessment and management of patients with primary hyperoxaluria type I. *Adv Nephrol* 18:95, 1989.
70. De Zegher FE, Wolff ED, van der Heijden AJ, et al: Oxalosis in infancy. *Clin Nephrol* 22:114, 1984.
71. Leumann EP, Niederwieser A, Fanconi A: New concepts of infantile oxalosis. *Pediatr Nephrol* 1:531, 1987.
72. Latta K, Brodehl J: Primary hyperoxalosis type I. *Eur J Pediatr* 149:518, 1990.
73. Smith LH, Fromm H, Hofmann AF: Acquired hyperoxaluria, nephrolithiasis and intestinal disease. Description of a syndrome. *N Engl J Med* 286:1371, 1972.
74. Hofmann AF, Laker MF, Dharmsathaporn K, et al: Complex pathogenesis of hyperoxaluria after jejunoileal bypass surgery. Oxalogenic substances in diet contribute to urinary oxalate. *Gastroentrology* 84:293, 1983.
75. Borsatti A: Calcium oxalate nephrolithiasis: Defective oxalate transport. *Kidney Int* 39:1283, 1991.
76. Baggio B, Gambaro G, Marchini F, et al: An inheritable anomaly of red-cell oxalate transport in "primary" calcium nephrolithiasis correctable with diuretics. *N Engl J Med* 314:599, 1986.
77. Halperin EC, Thier SO: Cystinuria. *Contemp Issues Nephrol,* 5:208, 1980.
78. Jaeger P: Cystinuria: Pathophysiology and treatment. *Adv Nephrol* 18:107, 1989.
79. Fuiano G, Federico S, Conte G, et al: Uric acid and kidney. *Adv Exp Med Biol* 252:107, 1989.
80. Holmes EW: Uric acid nephrolithiasis. *Contemp Issues Nephrol* 5:116, 1980.
81. Milman S et al: Pathogenesis and clinical course of mixed calcium oxalate and uric acid nephrolithiasis. *Kidney Int* 22:366, 1982.
82. Pak CYC, Holt K and Zerwekh JE: Attenuation by monosodium urate of the inhibitory effect of mucopolysaccharide on calcium oxalate nucleation. *Invest Urol* 17:138, 1979.
83. Ettinger B, Oldroyd NO and Sorgel F: Triamterene induced nephrolithiasis. *JAMA* 244:2443, 1980.
84. Gault MH, Campbell NRC and Aksu AE: Spurious stones. *Nephron* 48:274, 1988.
85. Ghazali S and Barratt TM: Urinary excretion of calcium and magnesium in children. *Arch Dis Child* 45:97, 1974.
86. Stapleton FB, Noe N, Jerkins G, et al: Urinary excretion of calcium following an oral calcium loading test in healthy children. *Pediatrics* 69:594, 1982.
87. Matsushita K, Tanikawa K: Significance of calcium to creatinine concentration of a single-voided urine specimen in patients with hypercalciuric urolithiasis. *Tokai J Exp Clin Med* 12:167, 1987.
88. Pak CYC, Kaplan R, Bone H, et al: A simple test for the diagnosis of absorptive, resorptive and renal hypercalciurias. *N Engl J Med* 292:497, 1975.
89. Pak CYC, Skurla C, Harvey JA: Graphic display of urinary risk factors for renal stone formation. *J Urol* 134:867, 1985.
90. Pak CYC, Sakhee K, Hwang TIS, Preminger GM, et al: Nephrolithiasis from calcium supplementation. *J Urol* 137:1212, 1987.

91. Yendt ER, Cohanim M: Prevention of calcium stones with thiazides. *Kidney Int* 13:397, 1978.
92. Coe FL, Parks JH: Stone disease in hereditary distal renal tubular acidosis. *Ann Intern Med* 93:60, 1980.
93. Preminger GM, Sakhee K, Pak CYC: Alkali action on the urinary crystallization of calcium salts: Contrasting responses to sodium citrate and potassium citrate. *J Urol* 139:240, 1988.
94. Pak CYC, Fuller C: Idiopathic hypocitriuric calcium-oxalate nephrolithiasis successfully treated with potassium citrate. *Ann Intern Med* 104:33, 1986.
95. Hindeberg J: Effect of magnesium citrate and magnesium oxide on the crystallization of calcium salts in urine: Changes produced by food-magnesium interaction. *J Urol* 149:248, 1990.
96. McDonald JC, Landreneau MD, Rohr MS, et al: Reversal by liver transplantation of the complications of primary hyperoxaluria as well as the metabolic defect. *N Engl J Med* 321:1100, 1989.
97. Coulson WJ: The cause of stone, in Coulson WJ (Ed): *The Diseases of the Bladder and Prostate Gland.* New York, William Wood, 1881, p 221.
98. Aurora AL, Taneja OP, Gupta DN: Bladder stone disease of childhood: II. A clinicopathologic study. *Acta Paediatr Scand* 59:385, 1970.

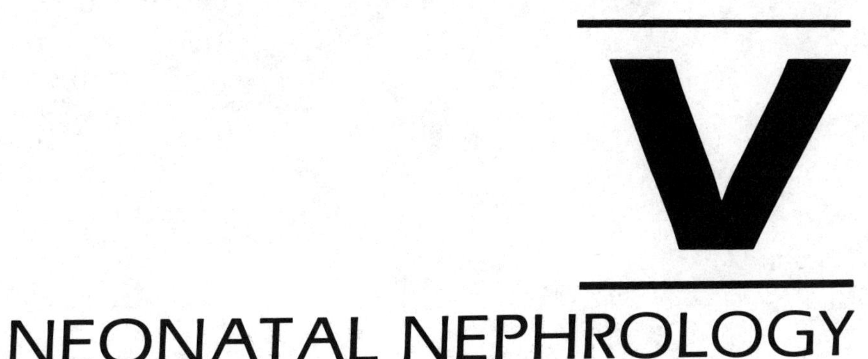

NEONATAL NEPHROLOGY

23

NEONATAL RENAL FUNCTION

Kanwal K. Kher

The placenta serves as the primary excretory organ for the developing fetus. The fetal kidneys begin producing urine during the latter part of the first trimester and are essential for maintaining the volume of the amniotic fluid. Renal maldevelopments that are associated with inadequate intrauterine urine output are characterized by oligohydramnios and its sequelae, such as pulmonary hypoplasia. Although renal function is not fully developed at birth, full-term neonates can effectively manage to maintain fluid, electrolyte, and acid-base balance. A premature neonate, on the other hand, may have difficulty in handling some of the metabolic tasks essential to extrauterine existence. This chapter discusses the various aspects of renal function that are unique to neonates.

INTRAUTERINE RENAL DEVELOPMENT

The urinary tract and kidneys develop from a mass of mesodermal cells, known as the *nephrogenic cord,* which is located along the dorsal aspect of the fetus. The intrauterine development of the kidney is characterized by the formation of three distinct but linked stages called the *pronephros,* the *mesonephros,* and the *metanephros.* The first two of these consist of primitive excretory organs that involute with advancing fetal development. The pronephros develops at about the third week of gestation and consists of nonfunctional excretory tubules that disappear by the fifth week. As the pronephros involutes, the mesonephros starts to form at its caudal end (Fig. 23–1). The development of these morphologically distinct structures overlaps considerably.[1] While the pronephric nephrons do not produce urine, the mesonephric nephrons have primitive glomeruli and are capable of performing excretory functions. The mesonephric nephrons produce urine by the ninth week of gestation and continue to do so until their involution, which occurs by the twelfth week.[2] Urine produced by the mesonephric nephrons is hypotonic in relation to plasma but is free of glucose, suggesting the development of significant tubular function.[3,4]

The metanephros or definitive kidney begins development at about 5 weeks

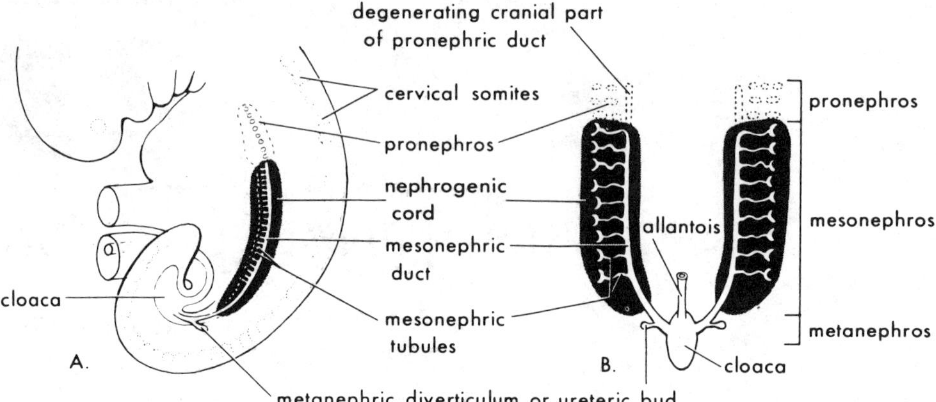

FIG. 23–1. Early development of the urogenital system showing differentiation of the nephrogenic cord into the pronephros, mesonephros, and metanephros (*A* and *B*). The pronephros is degenerating at this stage, while the mesonephros is well developed. The ureteric bud is in its early stage. (From KL Moore: *Before We Are Born—Basic Embryology and Birth Defects.* Philadelphia, Saunders, 1983. Reproduced by permission.)

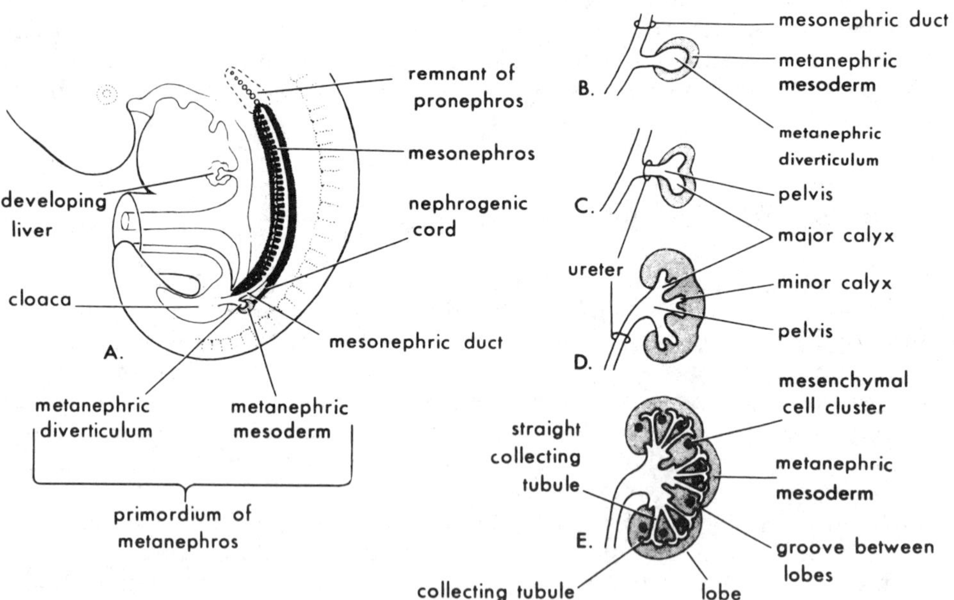

FIG. 23–2. Differentiation of the metanephric mesoderm into the nephrons and formation of the collecting system from the ureteric bud (*A* through *E*). (From KL Moore: *Before We Are Born—Basic Embryology and Birth Defects.* Philadelphia, Saunders, 1983. Reproduced by permission.)

of gestation with the formation of a tubular structure, called the *ureteric bud,* from the mesonephric duct. This bud grows and comes into contact with mesodermal cells of the nephrogenic cord (Fig. 23–2). Upon such contact, the cells of the ureteric bud divide and develop into structures that later form the collecting system. The proliferating cells of the nephrogenic cord give rise to tubular structures known as *metanephric tubules.* Blood vessels invaginate the proximal end of the metanephric tubules to form glomerular tufts, while the distal ends of the tubules connect with the elements of the proliferating ureteric bud, eventually forming a complete nephron. Nephrons in the fetal kidney develop centrifugally, younger nephrons being placed along the superficial cortex while the developmentally older nephrons are situated in the deeper cortex. Each kidney is endowed with approximately a million nephrons, and the embryogenesis of the nephrons is completed by the thirty-fifth week of gestation. Further nephronogenesis does not occur after this gestational age.[5]

CLINICAL ISSUES

Because of incomplete nephronogenesis in infants born prior to 35 weeks of gestation, their glomerular filtration rate (GFR) will be lower at birth than that of those born after the thirty-fifth week. Rapid improvement in most aspects of renal function, including GFR, occurs in all premature infants upon attainment of the conceptional age (gestational age plus postnatal age) of 35 weeks.[6,7] Some studies have also shown that extrauterine existence may, in itself, exert a positive influence on the maturation of renal function in premature infants.[6]

NEONATAL RENAL FUNCTION—DEVELOPMENTAL ASPECTS

Urine is an essential constituent of the amniotic fluid. Although metanephric nephrons begin to appear around the fifth week of gestation, sufficient urine production probably begins around the ninth week. By the twelfth week, the fetal kidneys are able to excrete radioisotope material administered to the mother.[8] Improvements in renal function occur throughout intrauterine life and continue outside the uterus. Renal function comparable to that of normal, healthy adults is attained by the second year of life.

FIRST VOID

About 20 to 25 percent of full-term and premature neonates void urine in the delivery room. Almost all normal healthy neonates (premature and full-term) void within 24 h of birth (Table 23–1).[9,10] The volume of the first voided urine is variable, ranging from a few milliliters to 20 mL. Fetal kidneys are unable to concentrate urine even by late gestation; therefore the first voided urine is hypotonic in relation to the serum (urine osmolality: 100 to 200 mosmol/kg).[11]

TABLE 23–1. Timing of First Urinary Voiding by Full-Term and Preterm Neonates following Birth[a]

	Full Term		Preterm	
	Kramer and Sherry,[9] Percent (n = 500)	Clark,[10] Percent (n = 395)	Kramer and Sherry,[9] Percent (n = 200)	Clark,[10] Percent (n = 80)
In delivery room	17.0	12.9	21.5	12.0
0–24 h	92.4	100.0	90.5	100.0
24–48 h	99.4	—	100.0	—
over 48 h	100.0	—	—	—

[a]Figures given represent percentages of total listed newborns.

Source: I Kramer, SN Sherry: The time of passage of the first stool and urine by the premature infant. *J Pediatr* 46:158, 1955. Also Clark DA: Times of first void and first stool in 500 newborns. *Pediatrics* 60:457, 1977. © 1977 *Pediatrics*. Data reproduced by permission.

CLINICAL ISSUES

A newborn infant that has not voided by the end of its first 24 h of life poses a serious management concern. Correction of hypovolemia and hypotension is an essential first step in anuric infants suspected of having prerenal azotemia. This therapeutic measure alone may improve renal perfusion and help establish urine flow. Failure to respond to volume replacement and normalization of blood pressure may indicate the onset of acute tubular necrosis (ATN). Evaluation of such infants should focus on ruling out, in addition to ATN, the diagnostic possibilities of obstructive uropathy and renal maldevelopment. Ultrasonographic examination of the kidneys and collecting system is immensely helpful initially in determining renal anatomy and evaluating obstructive lesions of the urinary tract. A radionuclide (DTPA) scan can be used to study renal perfusion and excretory functions. Intravenous pyelography is often not helpful in investigating a neonate's urinary tract, since the contrast material is poorly concentrated in its kidneys and the radiographic images obtained are often of poor interpretive quality. A voiding cystourethrogram may be necessary in a male infant in order to investigate the possibility of urinary tract obstruction due to posterior urethral valves.

RATE OF URINE FLOW

Direct measurement of urine flow rate is hazardous and difficult to justify in a normally growing fetus. The indirect technique of B-mode ultrasound studies, on the other hand, has been used to evaluate fetal urine production in normal pregnancies. Fetal urine output rises steadily between the thirtieth and fortieth weeks of gestation and keeps pace with the increase in fetal weight. A urine production rate of 9.6 ± 0.9 mL/h at 30 weeks of gestation increases linearly to reach 27.3 ± 2.3 mL/h at 40 weeks[12]. On the basis of fetal weight, it amounts to 6 to 10 mL/kg/h between 30 and 40 weeks of gestation. Retardation of fetal growth due to maternal causes such as hypertension, preeclampsia, and abnormal placental function adversely affects the fetus's hourly urine output. Following birth, the hourly urine output decreases dramatically in healthy full-term infants. After an initial period of postnatal adjustment, the urine flow rate diminishes and settles at about 2 to 3 mL/kg/h (range, 0.5 to 5.0 mL/kg/h).[11,13] Premature infants, however, void a larger volume of urine than normal full-term neonates. Sulyok et al.[14] have determined that premature infants (gestational age 28 to 35 weeks) void urine at a rate of 1.01 mL/min/1.73 m^2 by the end of the first week, which amounts to almost twice the rate (0.59 mL/min/ 1.73 m^2) observed in normal full-term infants at a comparable postnatal age. Urine output in premature infants continues to remain high during the initial 6 weeks following birth.[15]

CLINICAL ISSUES

A urinary flow rate of 2.0 to 3.0 mL/kg/h is considered normal in healthy full-term neonates. In the newborn infant, oliguria is defined as urine output below 1.0 mL/kg/h.[16,17] The adequacy of a newborn infant's renal function cannot be judged by the excretion of a "normal" urinary volume alone. In many infants with serious renal diseases such as dysplasia, renal cystic diseases, and nonoliguric ATN, urine volume may remain normal or even be "excessive" in the face of serious renal insufficiency. To depend on urinary output as the sole indicator of renal function under such circumstances in a newborn infant can be misleading. In neonates whose renal function is suspected to be compromised, renal function tests such as estimation of blood urea nitrogen (BUN) and serum creatinine should be obtained to settle the issue.

One study[18] has shown that painful stimuli (e.g., venipuncture) can decrease the rate of urine flow in premature neonates. A significant decrease in GFR was also noted in these infants during the application of painful stimuli. However, the relevance of these observations to clinical practice remains unknown and is probably insignificant.

GLOMERULAR FILTRATION RATE

The GFR is the most frequently employed test for the evaluation of renal function. Estimation of the GFR is commonly done by the method of creatinine clearance. The most reliable technique for measuring the GFR is, however, the inulin clearance test (Chap. 1). Despite some legitimate concerns about the significance of creatinine clearance in newborns, a good correlation between creatinine clearance and inulin clearance has been demonstrated.[19] During intrauterine development, the GFR increases slowly until the thirty-fifth week of gestation. This is followed by an accelerated phase of maturation.[6] Accordingly, the GFR in infants born prior to 35 weeks of gestation is considerably lower than that in those born at a later gestation (Fig. 23–3). Although a precise rea-

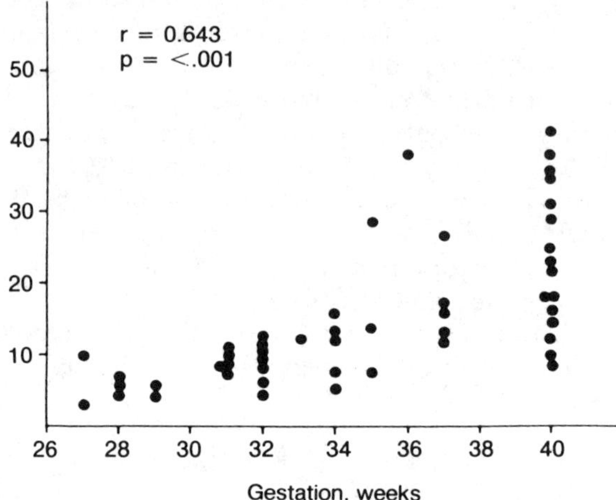

FIG. 23–3. Scattergram showing relationship of gestational age and GFR measured by creatinine clearance. Creatinine clearance was performed at 24 to 40 h after birth. (From SR Siegel, W Oh: Renal function as a marker of human fetal maturation. *Acta Paediatr Scand* 65:481, 1976. Reproduced by permission.)

son for the rapid maturation of the GFR after 35 weeks of gestation is not known, completion of nephronogenesis at this age has been suggested as a likely possibility.[6]

In full-term infants, the GFR is about one-fifth of the normal adult value (20 mL/min/1.73 m^2) at birth[19] It is even lower in premature infants (Table 23–2).

TABLE 23–2. Creatinine Clearance in Full-Term (39 to 40 Weeks), Preterm (32 to 34 Weeks), and Very Small Premature (28 to 32 Weeks) Infants during the First 5 Weeks of Extrauterine Life—Measured as mL/min/1.73m^2

Time	Very Small Preterm[a] (28–32 Weeks)	Preterm (32–34 Weeks)	Full Term (39–40 Weeks)
1–2 days	9.5 (6.9–12.7)	15.9 ± 1.9	20.8 ± 1.9
4–6 days	10.7 (9.4–15.3)	24.1 ± 1.7	46.6 ± 5.2
3–5 weeks	—	37.0 ± 3.7	60.1 ± 4.6

[a]Data represented as median values and ranges. Others (gestation 32 to 40 weeks) are represented as mean ± S.D.

Source: A Aperia, O Broberger, G Elinder, et al: Postnatal development of renal function in pre-term and full-term infants. *Acta Paediatr Scand* 70:183, 1981; also N Gordjani, R Burghard, JU Leititis, et al: Serum creatinine and creatinine clearance in healthy neonates and prematures during the first 10 days of life. *Eur J Pediatr* 148:143, 1988. Data reproduced by permission.

Postnatally, the GFR in full-term infants doubles during the first 7 to 14 days and triples by 3 to 5 weeks.[6,19] Although premature neonates also demonstrate a similar increase in GFR in the immediate postnatal period, their GFR—as compared to that of full-term infants—consistently remains lower during the first 4 to 6 weeks. The GFR in premature infants varies directly with the degree of prematurity and correlates well with conceptional age (gestational age plus postnatal age).[7] As an example, the GFR of a 7-week-old infant born at a gestational age of 28 weeks approximates the GFR of an infant of 35 weeks' gestation (28 weeks gestation plus 7 weeks postnatal age) at birth. Some studies[6,20] also suggest that postnatal existence enhances the pace of maturation of GFR in premature infants. For the sake of standardization, GFR has traditionally been represented in relation to body surface area (mL/min/m^2 or mL/min/1.73 m^2). Coulthard and Hey,[21] however, suggest that representing GFR in relation to body weight (mL/min/kg) may be not only convenient but also more accurate in neonates. This issue remains unsettled.

CLINICAL ISSUES

Because of the low GFR in newborn infants, the dose of drugs that are eliminated primarily via the kidneys requires adjustment. This is particularly true in premature infants, whose GFR can remain somewhat lower for up to 6 weeks following birth. In neonates with a history of perinatal asphyxia, especially those undergoing mechanical ventilation, the GFR is often lower than in non-asphyxiated neonates of similar gestation. The degree to which GFR is decreased in such instances correlates with the severity of hypoxia.[20,22,23] Polycythemic neonates also have a lower GFR than those with a normal hematocrit.[24] Following hemodilution, however, the GFR in these infants returns to normal.[24] Hyperbilirubinemia has also been reported to affect the GFR adversely during the neonatal period.[25] While providing increased fluid intake during the first week of life is ineffective in increasing GFR,[26–28] the rapid infusion of albumin (1 g/kg over 10 min) transiently increases systemic blood pressure as well as GFR in sick preterm neonates.[29]

SERUM CREATININE

In neonates, serum creatinine essentially reflects maternal serum creatinine concentration at birth.[30] During the first week of life, serum creatinine concentration decreases rapidly in most neonates, including those born prematurely.[30,31] Serum creatinine concentration is less than 1.0 mg/dL by the end of the first week of life (usually 0.5 mg/dL) in full-term infants. Wide variations in the rate of decline of serum creatinine concentration are, however, to be expected during this time, even among normal full-term infants.[32] Serum creatinine further declines during the remainder of the first month of life in full-term infants and settles at around 0.2 to 0.4 mg/dL.[19,30] Serum creatinine concentration in premature infants remains higher than in full-term infants of similar postnatal age throughout the first 4 to 6 weeks of life (Fig. 23–4 and Table

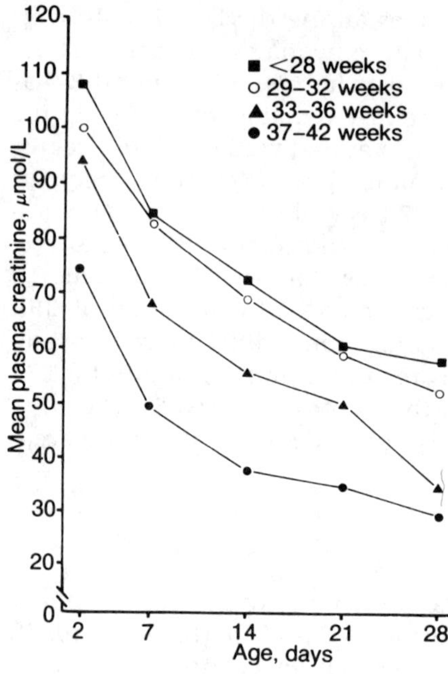

FIG. 23–4. Relationship between mean plasma creatinine concentration and postnatal age in different gestational groups. (From Rudd PT: Reference ranges for plasma creatinine during the first month of life. *Arch Dis Child* 58:212, 1983. Reproduced by permission.)

23–3).[30,31] It may take 6 to 8 weeks for very small premature neonates (26- to 28-week gestation) to achieve a stable creatinine concentration comparable to that observed in full-term infants at 4 weeks of postnatal age.

CLINICAL ISSUES

Serum creatinine concentration is an unreliable measure of renal function in neonates less than 1 week old. A downward trend in the serum creatinine concentration is to be expected in both full-term and premature infants during the first 4 weeks of life. Lack of the expected decline of serum creatinine or its actual rise during the early neonatal period is suggestive of renal insufficiency.

TABLE 23–3. Plasma Creatinine Concentration (mg/dL) in Infants of Various Gestational Ages during the First 4 Weeks of Life

Gestational	Postnatal Age (Days)				
Age, (Weeks)	2	7	14	21	28
28	1.3 ± .4	0.94 ± .3	0.81 ± .3	0.67 ± .3	0.6 ± .2
29–32	1.17 ± .4	0.93 ± .4	0.77 ± .3	0.66 ± .3	0.58 ± .3
33–36	1.05 ± .4	0.76 ± .4	0.62 ± .4	0.56 ± .4	0.39 ± .2
37–42	0.84 ± .4	0.56 ± .4	0.42 ± .2	0.39 ± .2	0.33 ± .2

Source: Adapted from PT Rudd, EA Hughes, MM Placzek, et al: Reference ranges for plasma creatinine during the first month of life. *Arch Dis Child* 58:212, 1983. Reproduced by permission.

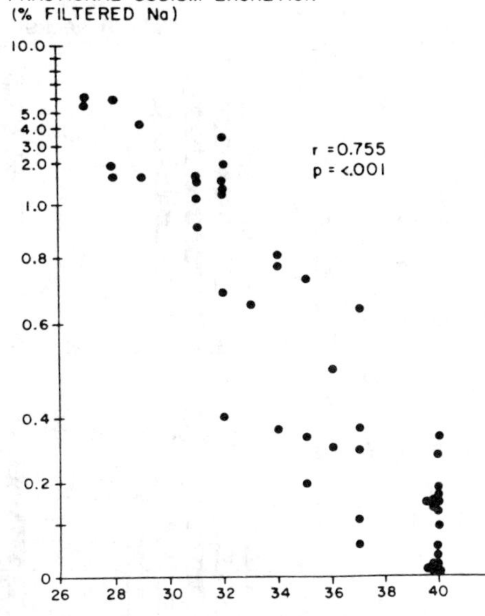

FIG. 23–5. Scattergram showing relationship between fractional sodium excretion and gestational age. (From SR Siegel, W Oh: Renal function as a marker of human fetal maturation. *Acta Paediatr Scand* 65:481, 1976. Reproduced by permission.)

SODIUM HOMEOSTASIS

Normal full-term neonates are generally in a positive sodium balance. On the other hand, normal premature infants demonstrate a high renal fractional excretion of sodium (FeNa)—that is, 2.0 to 2.5 percent compared to the 0.5 to 1 percent seen in full-term infants (Fig. 23–5).[3,33] Consequently, premature infants exhibit an obligatory renal salt-wasting tendency in early extrauterine life. While urinary sodium loss in a full-term infant rarely exceeds 0.5 meq/kg/day, this loss in premature infants may amount to as much as 2 to 3 meq/kg/day. Premature infants often develop a net negative sodium balance during the first 7 to 10 days of life when fed breast milk or unsupplemented formula (Fig. 23–6).[14,15,33,34] In them, FeNa declines to about 1 percent by the time they attain a conceptional age of 38 to 40 weeks.[35] Compared to stable premature infants of similar gestational age, sick premature infants excrete an even greater daily amount of urinary sodium.[36] Renal sodium loss in such infants may be as high as 4 to 5 meq/kg/day.

The underlying reason for renal sodium wasting in premature infants during early postnatal life is not well understood and is a matter of considerable debate. Some investigators believe that premature infants are born with a larger extracellular fluid volume than full-term infants. The sodium and water diuresis noted in them is, therefore, an expected physiologic response.[37] A similar response is noted in normal animals subjected to volume expansion.[38] Whether or not the atrial natriuretic factor participates in the natriuresis of premature newborns has not been well established. Early work suggests some role for this hormone in initiating diuresis in the postnatal period.[38a] An alternate view suggests that the renal salt wasting in premature infants results from immaturity

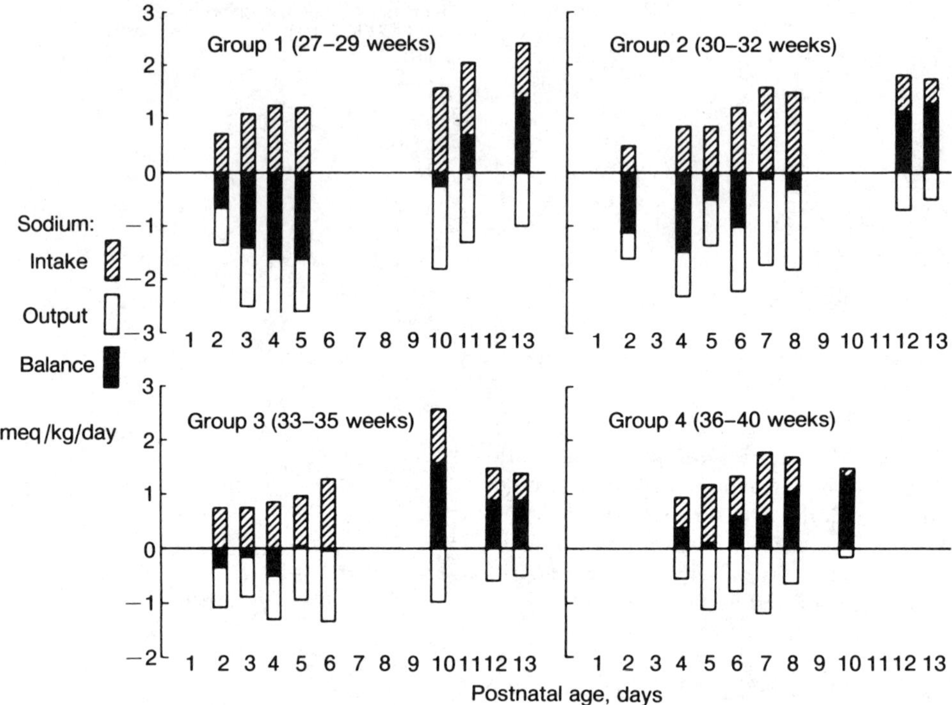

FIG. 23–6. Net sodium balance in newborn infants of various gestational ages during the first 2 weeks of life. Premature infants born at younger gestation have a greater net negative sodium balance. Most infants are in a positive sodium balance by the tenth to eleventh day of life. (From J Al-Dahhan, GB Haycock, C Chantler, et al: Sodium homeostasis in term and pre-term neonates. I: Renal aspects. *Arch Dis Child* 58:335. 1983. Reproduced by permission.)

of the renal tubules. Supporters of this hypothesis have proposed that there is a discordance between the rate at which the glomerular and tubular functions mature in the immediate postnatal period, with renal tubular maturation lagging behind while GFR increases rapidly. As a result, the renal tubules in premature neonates are unable to reabsorb the incoming sodium to the same degree as do those in full-term infants, resulting in renal salt wasting.[39,40] Aldosterone production (as judged by urinary excretion of aldosterone) has been reported to be normal or high in premature neonates; a deficiency of this sodium-conserving hormone is unlikely to be a factor involved in neonatal renal sodium wasting.[41] Renal tubular hyporesponsiveness to aldosterone may be present in premature infants and can conceivably contribute to their urinary salt wasting.

When challenged with an acute sodium load, both full-term and premature neonates demonstrate a limited capacity to eliminate it. Since premature neonates generally have a higher fractional excretion of sodium in the postnatal period, they exhibit a greater natriuretic response following sodium administration than do full-term neonates.[36,42] However, even in premature infants, the observed natriuretic response following sodium intake is five- to tenfold lower than that observed in older children.

CLINICAL ISSUES

Hyponatremia is a common clinical problem in sick premature neonates and is observed in two distinct postnatal phases. In some premature infants, hyponatremia is noted within the first few days of postnatal life *(early hyponatremia)*. Often these neonates are sick or require ventilator support.[43] Traditionally, early hyponatremia in such neonates has been attributed to excessive urinary sodium excretion.[34] However, the observation of Rees et al.[44] that urinary excretion of arginine vasopressin is elevated in such infants implicates the inappropriate secretion of the antidiuretic hormone (SIADH) as an etiology of early hyponatremia in some premature neonates.

Early hyponatremia in neonates may also result from the rapid administration of fluid to the mother. The bromide space, reflecting extracellular fluid volume, in infants born to mothers given rapid fluid infusions prior to delivery has been found to be significantly expanded.[45] The mechanism of excess water transfer from mother to fetus under such circumstances, however, remains conjectural. Obviously, hyponatremia in these infants is dilutional in nature, and fluid restriction rather than increased sodium administration is necessary to correct the hyponatremia.

Late hyponatremia is defined as hyponatremia occurring in premature infants during the second to the sixth weeks after birth.[43,46–48] The incidence of late hyponatremia in prematures varies from 30 to 50 percent and is more common in smaller infants.[33–35] Most premature infants with late hyponatremia appear healthy and are usually asymptomatic when the condition is first detected. Slowing of growth has, however, been reported in others.[43] The pathogenesis of late hyponatremia has been a matter of intense study and speculation. The primary mechanisms involved in the genesis of late hyponatremia are thought to be (1) excessive urinary sodium loss in premature infants compounded by (2) a low sodium intake as a result of unsupplemented breast milk or formula feeding. A role for aldosterone and arginine vasopressin in the pathogenesis of late hyponatremia has been suggested recently since urinary excretion of both aldosterone and vasopressin has been shown to be elevated in such neonates.[47,48] The postulated sequence of events involving these two hormones is that renal salt and water loss leads to a state of protracted intravascular volume depletion, which mediates an enhanced production of both aldosterone and arginine vasopressin. Despite an increased circulating aldosterone concentration, renal tubular sodium reabsorption does not increase because of the insensitivity of renal tubules to this hormone. In contrast, an increased circulating concentration of arginine vasopressin leads to enhanced water reabsorption in the renal tubules and the development of dilutional hyponatremia.[47,48] Prophylactic sodium supplementation in the diet of premature neonates often reduces the incidence of hyponatremia among them.[34] Such sodium supplementation should gradually be withdrawn after three or four weeks in order to reduce the risk of hypernatremia.

POTASSIUM BALANCE

Despite a lower GFR, both full-term and premature infants maintain a reasonable potassium balance. With increasing intake of potassium, renal potassium excretion is also enhanced.[33] A gradual increase in the serum potassium concentration during the first 3 weeks of life has been noted in premature infants, and serum concentrations up to 5.5 meq/L may be seen under normal circumstances.[49] Hyperkalemia has, however, been reported in the first 48 h in very small premature neonates, possibly due to inadequate renal function.[50] A negative potassium balance may be noted in some critically ill premature infants, especially with the use of diuretics.[51]

WATER BALANCE

The kidneys perform the important task of regulating fluid balance in children and adults. Premature as well as full-term infants respond to fluid deprivation by forming a concentrated urine and decreasing the urinary volume.[52–54] But neonates are unable to concentrate the urine to an osmolality higher than 400 to 600 mosmol/L (specific gravity: 1.015 to 1.020). This contrasts with a urinary osmolality of 900 to 1200 mosmol/L achieved with overnight fluid restriction in older children. Accordingly, newborn infants are unable to conserve water during states of fluid restriction as effectively as older children and adults and are at a greater risk of developing dehydration and hypernatremia.

The inability of neonatal kidneys to concentrate urine to the same degree as the kidneys of children and adults has been attributed to shorter tubules in the juxtamedullary nephrons and absence of the medullary hypertonic gradient required by the "countercurrent multiplier system." Increased protein feeding of neonates (9 g/kg/day) has been shown to enhance their concentrating ability significantly, possibly by providing urea necessary for the development of a medullary concentration gradient.[55] Excessive protein feeding is, however, not recommended in view of the increased solute load imposed on the kidneys by such a diet.

Full-term as well as premature neonates respond appropriately to sudden fluid intake by increasing their urinary volume and forming dilute urine.[18,26,27,56] Urinary osmolality as low as that observed in adults (40 to 45 mosmol/L) can be achieved by neonates during periods of excess fluid administration. It must be emphasized, however, that it takes neonates significantly longer to excrete a given fluid volume than it does older children and adults. McCance et al.[56] found that normal adult volunteers excreted 100 percent of the fluid challenge (approximately equaling 6 percent of body water) in 4 h while only 60 percent of an equivalent amount of fluid challenge was eliminated by normal full-term neonates during the same period of time.

CLINICAL ISSUES

Recommendations regarding fluid intake by neonates have undergone some remarkable changes in the last 25 years. While fluid restriction was in vogue in earlier times, liberalization of fluid intake to account for increased insensible losses associated with the use of radiant warmers and phototherapy in premature infants has been in practice for the last 15 years. However, with increasing fluid intake, a higher incidence of patent ductus arteriosus, congestive heart failure, respiratory distress syndrome, bronchopulmonary dysplasia, and necrotizing enterocolitis has been reported in premature infants.[57-60] Arant,[61] in a commentary on the subject, pointed out that the time may have arrived to consider a fluid intake below that traditionally recommended for premature infants. This may be physiologic as well as help reduce the incidence of the complications mentioned above.

ACID BASE BALANCE

The kidney performs crucial functions in regulating the acid base balance. Renal tubules reabsorb most of the bicarbonate that is filtered through the glomeruli and also eliminate hydrogen ions generated by dietary ingestion and endogenous metabolic activity (1 meq/kg/day). The process of tubular bicarbonate rebasorption and hydrogen ion excretion is discussed in detail in Chap. 21. Briefly, the proximal renal tubules reabsorb 85 percent or more of the bicarbonate present in the tubular fluid, the remainder being reabsorbed in distal segments of the nephron; none is excreted in urine. The process of bicarbonate reabsorption in the proximal tubule is not without limits. If plasma bicarbonate concentration is increased by exogenous intravenous infusion or oral intake of bicarbonate in normal adults, bicarbonate begins to appear in the urine when the serum bicarbonate concentration reaches 26 to 28 meq/L.[62] The serum concentration at which renal tubular bicarbonate reabsorption capacity is saturated and bicarbonate appears in urine is known as the *renal threshold for bicarbonate.* This threshold is considerably lower in neonates and remains so during the entire first year of life.[63,64] Svenningsen[64] reports that the renal threshold for bicarbonate in full-term and premature infants during the first 3 weeks of life is 21.1 and 21.8 meq/L respectively. A slight improvement in the renal threshold for bicarbonate was noted to occur during 4 to 6 postnatal weeks in both the premature and full-term infants. Edelmann et al.[63] found that the renal threshold for bicarbonate in normal infants 1 to 12 months of age continues to be lower than adults—21.5 to 22.5 meq/L. Renal bicarbonate loss consequent to a low renal threshold for bicarbonate is believed to be an important factor that renders newborn infants vulnerable to a lower plasma bicarbonate (total CO_2) concentration. Urinary acidification during the first 3 weeks of postnatal life has been reported to be significantly lower in premature infants than in normal full-term infants of like postnatal age.[63,65]

CLINICAL ISSUES

Metabolic acidosis is a common clinical problem in sick premature neonates and is usually due to perinatal events such as hypoxia, hypotension, and hypovolemia. A particular type of metabolic acidosis was noted by Kildeberg[66] in apparently healthy premature infants between 1 to 3 weeks of age and was

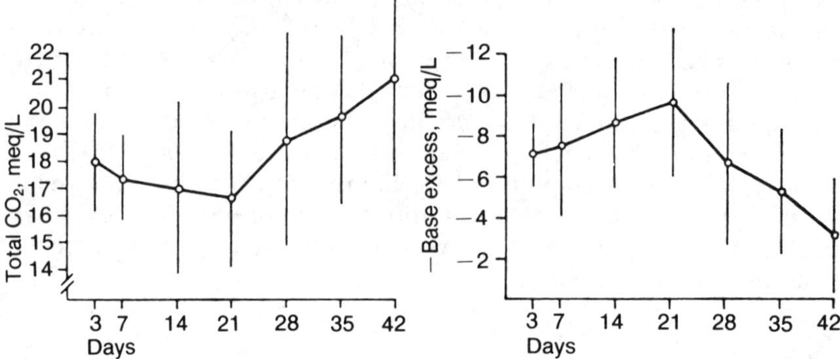

FIG. 23–7. Postnatal changes in plasma total CO_2 (tCO_2) and the base excess in clinically healthy premature infants. A decline in tCO_2 during the early neonatal course with a nadir around the third postnatal week is shown. Some have referred to this phenomenon as the late metabolic acidosis of prematurity. (From E Sulyok: The relationship between electrolyte and acid-base balance in the premature infant during early postnatal life. *Biol Neonate* 17:227, 1971. Reproduced by permission of S. Karger AG, Basel, Switzerland.)

termed the *late metabolic acidosis of prematurity.* Retardation of somatic growth has been described as a prominent feature in infants so affected. It was proposed that the late metabolic acidosis may be due to the high rate of endogenous acid production consequent to high-protein feeding (3 to 4 g/kg/day) and the kidneys' inability to excrete the excess hydrogen ions thus generated.[66] Others have disputed the existence of late metabolic acidosis of prematurity. These investigators suggest that the lower plasma bicarbonate concentration (up to 14.5 meq/L) noted in these premature infants is a normal finding, since such values fall within the two standard deviations of the mean value for the test at this age (Fig. 23–7).[67] In this view, late metabolic acidosis may be regarded as an extreme expression of the *physiologic acidosis* expected in premature infants at this age. Spontaneous improvement of the acidosis and normalization of plasma bicarbonate (total CO_2) occurs by 3 to 6 weeks after birth.[33,67] Treatment of this form of metabolic acidosis with sodium bicarbonate has not been found to enhance the rate of weight gain.[67]

SUMMARY

Although a full-term neonate has the same number of nephrons as a normal adult, their function is not completely developed. The preterm infant, on the other hand, is severely handicapped in that its nephrons lack not only full anatomic development but also complete functional maturation. In order to manage the metabolic problems of sick preterm and full-term infants, it is necessary to understand the developmental changes in renal function that occur during intrauterine and early extrauterine life. Other therapeutic interventions in the neonate, particularly the use of antibiotics, are also significantly guided by the level of renal function. This chapter has outlined the various aspects of neonatal renal function that are of clinical relevance and directly influence the care of these patients.

REFERENCES

1. Torrey TW: Early development of human nephros. *Contrib Embryol* 35:175, 1954.
2. Gersh I: The correlation of structure and function in the developing mesonephros and metanephros. *Contrib Embryol* 26:35, 1937.
3. Stanier MW: The function of mammalian mesonephros. *J Physiol (London)* 151:472, 1960.
4. Perry JS, Stanier MW: The rate of flow of urine of pigs. *J Physiol (London)* 161:344, 1962.
5. McCrory WW: *Embryologic Development of Kidney in Developmental Nephrology.* Cambridge, Massachusetts, Harvard University Press, 1972, pp 12–17.
6. Arant BS Jr: Developmental patterns of renal functional maturation compared in the human neonate. *J Pediatr* 92:705, 1978.
7. Leake RD, Trygstad CW, Oh W: Inulin clearance in the newborn infant: Relationship to gestation age and postnatal age. *Pediatr Res* 10:759, 1976.
8. Hutchinson DL, Gray MJ, Plentl AA, et al: The role of the fetus in the water exchange of the amniotic fluid of normal and hydramniotic patients. *J Clin Invest* 38:971, 1959.
9. Kramer I, Sherry SN: The time of passage of the first stool and urine by the premature infant. *J Pediatr* 46:158, 1955.
10. Clark DA: Times of first void and first stool in 500 newborns. *Pediatrics* 60:457, 1977.
11. Strauss J, Daniel SS, James LS: Postnatal adjustment in renal function. *Pediatrics* 68:802, 1981.
12. Waladimiroff JW, Campbell S: Fetal urine-production rates in normal and complicated pregnancy. *Lancet* 1:151, 1974.
13. Jones MD, Gresham EL, Battaglia FC: Urinary flow rates and urea excretion rates in newborn infants. *Biol Neonate* 21:321, 1972.
14. Sulyok E, Varga F, Gyory E, et al: On the mechanism of renal sodium handling in newborn infants. *Biol Neonate* 37:75, 1980.
15. Sulyok E, Varga F, Gyory E, et al: Postnatal development of renal sodium handling in premature infants. *J Pediatr* 95:787, 1979.
16. Mathew OP, Jones AS, James E, et al: Neonatal renal failure: Usefulness of diagnostic indices. *Pediatrics* 65:57, 1980.
17. Chevalier RL, Campbell F, Brenbridge ANAG: Prognostic factors in neonatal acute renal failure. *Pediatrics* 74:265, 1984.
18. Barnett HL, Vesterdal J, McNamara H, et al: Renal water excretion in premature infants. *J Clin Invest* 31:1069, 1952.
19. Aperia A, Broberger O, Elinder G, et al: Postnatal development of renal function in pre-term and full-term infants. *Acta Paediatr Scand* 70:183, 1981.
20. Svenningsen NW: Single injection polyfructosan clearance in normal and asphyxiated neonates. *Acta Paediatr Scand* 64:87, 1975.
21. Coulthard MG, Hey EN: Weight as the best standard for glomerular filtration in the newborn. *Arch Dis Child* 59:373, 1984.
22. Ross B, Cowett RM, Oh W: Renal function of low birth weight infants during the first two months of life. *Pediatr Res* 11:1162, 1977.

23. Guignard JP, Torrado A, Mazuni SM, et al: Renal function in respiratory distress syndrome. *J Pediatr* 88:845, 1976.
24. Aperia A, Bergquist G, Broberger O, et al: Renal function in newborn infants with high hematocrit values before and after isovolemic haemodilution. *Acta Paediatr Scand* 63:878, 1974.
25. Broberger U, Aperia A: Renal function in infants with hyperbilirubinemia. *Acta Paediatr Scand* 68:75, 1979.
26. Leake RD, Zakauddin S, Trygstad CW, et al: The effects of large volume intravenous fluid infusion on neonatal renal function. *J Pediatr* 89:968, 1976.
27. Aperia A, Herin P, Lundin S, et al: Regulation of renal water excretion in newborn full-term infants. *Acta Paediatr Scand* 73:717, 1984.
28. Coulthard MG, Hey EN: Effect of varying water intake on renal function in healthy preterm babies. *Arch Dis Child* 60:614, 1985.
29. Lay KS, Bancalari E, Malkus H, et al: Acute effects of albumin infusion on blood volume and renal function in premature infants with respiratory distress syndrome. *J Pediatr* 97:619, 1980.
30. Rudd PT, Hughes EA, Placzek MM, et al: Reference ranges for plasma creatinine during the first month of life. *Arch Dis Child* 58:212, 1983.
31. Stonestreet BS, Oh W: Plasma creatinine levels in low birth weight infants during the first three months of life. *Pediatrics* 61:788, 1978.
32. Sertel H, Scopes J: Rates of creatinine clearance in babies less than one week of age. *Arch Dis Child* 48:717, 1973.
33. Sulyok E: The relationship between electrolyte and acid-base balance in the premature infant during early postnatal life. *Biol Neonate* 17:227, 1971.
34. Al-Dahhan J, Haycock GB, Chantler C, et al: Sodium homeostasis in term and preterm neonates. I: Renal aspects. *Arch Dis Child* 58:335, 1983.
35. Engelke SC, Shah BL, Vasan U, et al: Sodium balance in very low-birth-weight infants. *J Pediatr* 93:837, 1978.
36. Aperia A, Broberger O, Thodenius K, et al: Developmental study of the renal response to an oral salt load in preterm infants. *Acta Paediatr Scand* 63:517, 1974.
37. Arant BS, Jr: Renal disorders of the newborn, in Brenner BM, Stein JH (eds): *Contemporary Issues in Nephrology,* vol 12. New York, Churchill Livingstone, 1984, p 111.
38. Kaloyanidesw GJ, Azer M: Evidence for a humoral mechanism in volume expansion natriuresis. *J Clin Invest* 50:1603, 1971.
38a. Rozycki HJ, Baumgart S: Atrial natriuretic factor and postnatal diuresis in respiratory distress syndrome. *Arch Dis Child* 66:43, 1991.
39. Rodriguez-Soriano J, Vallo A, Oliveros R, et al: Renal handling of sodium in premature and full-term neonates: A study using clearance methods during water diuresis. *Pediatr Res* 17:1013, 1983.
40. Aperia A, Broberger O, Broberger U, et al: Glomerulotubular balance in premature and fullterm infants. *Acta Paediatr Scand (Suppl)* 305:70, 1983.
41. Aperia A, Broberger O, Herin P, et al: Sodium excretion in relation to sodium intake and aldosterone excretion in newborn pre-term and full-term infants. *Acta Paediatr Scand* 68:813, 1979.
42. Aperia A, Broberger O, Thodenius K, et al: Renal response to an oral sodium load in newborn full-term infants. *Acta Paediatr Scand* 61:670, 1972.
43. Day GM, Radde IC, Balfe JW, et al: Electrolyte abnormalities in very low birth weight infants. *Pediatr Res* 10:522, 1976.
44. Rees L, Brooks CGD, Shaw JCL, et al: Hyponatremia in first week of life in pre-term infants. I: Arginine vasopressin secretion. *Arch Dis Child* 59:414, 1984.

45. Rojas J, Mohan P, Davidson KK: Increased extracellular water volume associated with hyponatremia at birth in premature infants. *J Pediatr* 105:158, 1984.
46. Roy RN, Chance GW, Radde IC, et al: Late hyponatremia in very low birth weight infants (<1.3 kilograms). *Pediatr Res* 10:526, 1976.
47. Sulyok E, Kovacs L, Lichardus B, et al: Late hyponatremia in premature infants: Role of aldosterone and arginine vasopressin. *J Pediatr* 106:990, 1985.
48. Kovacs L, Sulvyok E, Lichardus B, et al: Renal response to arginine vasopressin in premature infants with late hyponatremia. *Arch Dis Child* 61:1030, 1986.
49. Al-Dahhan J, Haycock GB, Nichol B, et al: Sodium homeostasis in term and preterm neonates. III: Effect of salt supplementation. *Arch Dis Child* 59:945, 1984.
50. Shortland D, Trounce JQ, Levene MI: Hyperkalemia, cardiac arrhythmias, and cerebral lesions in high risk neonates. *Arch Dis Child* 62:1139, 1987.
51. Engle W, Arant BS: Urinary potassium excretion in the critically ill neonate. *J Pediatr* 74:259, 1984.
52. Hansen JDL, Smith CA: Effect of withholding fluid in the immediate postnatal period. *Pediatrics* 12:99, 1953.
53. Auld PAM, Bhangananda P, Mehta S: The influence of an early caloric intake with IV glucose on catabolism of premature infants. *Pediatrics* 37:592, 1966.
54. Fisher DA, Pyle HR, Porter JC, et al: Control of water balance in the newborn. *Am J Dis Child* 106:51, 1963.
55. Edelmann CM Jr, Barnett HL, Troupkou V: Renal concentrating mechanism in newborn infants: Effect of dietary protein and water content, role of urea and responsiveness to antidiuretic hormone. *J Clin Invest* 39:1062, 1960.
56. McCance RA, Naylor NJB, Widdowson EM: The response of infants to a large dose of water. *Arch Dis Child* 29:104, 1954.
57. Bell EF, Warburton D, Stonestreet BS, et al: Effect of fluid administration on development of systemic patent ductus arteriosus and congestive heart failure in premature infants. *N Engl J Med* 302:598, 1980.
58. Bell EF, Oh W: Water requirement of premature newborn infants. *Acta Paediatr Scand*(Suppl) 305:21, 1983.
59. Bell EF, Warburton D, Stonestreet BS, et al: High fluid intake predisposes premature infants to necrotising enterocolitis. *Lancet* 2:90, 1979.
60. Lorenz JM, Kleinman LI, Kotagal UR, et al: Water balance in very low-birth-weight infants: Relationship to water and sodium intake and effect on outcome. *J Pediatr* 101:423, 1982.
61. Arant BS Jr: Fluid therapy in the neonate: Concepts in transition. *J Pediatr* 101:387, 1982.
62. Pitts RF: *Renal Regulation of Acid-Base Balance: Physiology of the Kidney and Body Fluids.* Chicago, Year Book Publishers, 1974, p 199.
63. Edelman CM Jr, Rodriguez-Soriano J, Boichis H, et al: Renal bicarbonate reabsorption and hydrogen ion excretion in normal infants. *J Clin Invest* 46:1309, 1967.
64. Svenningsen NW: Renal acid base titration studies in infants with and without metabolic acidosis in the postnatal period. *Pediatr Res* 8:659, 1974.
65. Svenningsen NW, Lindquist B: Postnatal development of renal hydrogen ion excretion capacity in relation to age and protein intake. *Acta Paediatr Scand* 63:721, 1984.
66. Kildeberg P: Disturbance of hydrogen ion balance occurring in premature infants. II: Late metabolic acidosis. *Acta Paediatr Scand* 53:517, 1964.
67. Schwartz GJ, Haycock GB, Edelmann CM Jr, et al: Late metabolic acidosis: A reassessment of the definition. *J Pediatr* 95:102, 1979.

24

NEONATAL DISORDERS

Kanwal K. Kher

Neonatal nephrology is a developing subject for the pediatric nephrologist as well as the neonatologist. Despite the enormous advances in this field in the last 15 years, more is yet to be understood about the functioning of the kidney in the very low birthweight premature infant. Unfortunately, many sick infants are susceptible to renal injury as a consequence of functional immaturity or exposure to invasive techniques and nephrotoxic drugs in the immediate neonatal period. The management of renal disorders in neonates presupposes the requisite of technical skills, a knowledge of neonatal renal physiology, and a capacity to innovate, since the physician must apply procedures that are essentially designed for adults and older children to the care of sick neonates. This chapter is devoted to a discussion of specific issues related to the etiology, diagnosis, and management of acute renal failure and hypertension in neonates. Developmental malformations commonly encountered in neonates and the increasingly recognized problem of nephrocalcinosis in premature infants are also briefly covered.

RENAL MALFORMATIONS

On the basis of autopsy studies, it has been estimated that asymptomatic undiagnosed malformations of the kidney and collecting system occur in 5 to 10 percent of the general population.[1,2] Recent data from the French Registry of Congenital Malformations have projected a lower incidence of congenital malformations of the urinary tract (3.5 per 1000 live births).[3] In another study, using ultrasound screening of healthy infants for urinary tract anomalies, Steinhart and colleagues[4] found the incidence of congenital urinary abnormalities to be 1.37 percent.

Congenital anomalies of the kidneys should alert the physician to the presence of associated anomalies affecting other organ systems. Developmental anomalies of the extraurinary system are present in 30 to 50 percent of individuals who demonstrate a congenital anomaly of the kidney or the urinary tract.[2,3] The organ systems most commonly affected by congenital anomalies in

TABLE 24–1. Incidence of Developmental Anomalies Affecting Nonrenal Organ Systems in Patients with Congenital Abnormalities of the Kidney and Urinary Tract

Organ System	Abnormalities, Percent
Cardiovascular system	25
Gastrointestinal system	18
Central nervous system	10
Skeletal system	9
Lungs	7
Face	7
Genito-reproductive system	4
Chromosomal aberrations	4
Others	8

Source: Barakat AJ, Drougas JG, Barakat R: Association of congenital abnormalities of the kidney and urinary tract with those of other organ systems in 13,775 autopsies. *Child Nephrol Urol* 9:268, 1988–89. Copyright © 1989 S. Karger AG, Basel, Switzerland. Reproduced by permission.

association with renal malformations are the cardiovascular system, the gastrointestinal tract, and the central nervous system (Table 24–1). Conversely, patients with spina bifida or with vertebral and anal anomalies have a higher incidence of malformations affecting the urinary tract.

RENAL AGENESIS

Renal agenesis is defined as the *congenital absence of any identifiable renal tissue;* it can affect one or both kidneys. Unilateral renal agenesis occurs in approximately 0.3 percent (or 3 per 1000) of the healthy general population screened for this abnormality.[5,6] Unilateral renal agenesis is compatible with a normal life span and normal renal function. Often unilateral renal agenesis is discovered by chance during an abdominal evaluation by ultrasound for an unrelated disorder.

Bilateral renal agenesis is a lethal disorder that manifests itself at birth with features of Potter syndrome, consisting of oligohydramnios, pulmonary hypoplasia, typical facies with low-set ears, parrot-beak nose, receding chin and redundant skin, and malformations of the limbs such as clubfoot, bowed legs, and dislocated hips. Rarely, patients with bilateral renal agenesis may be born without the characteristic features of Potter syndrome.[1] The incidence of bilateral renal agenesis has been reported to be 0.12 per 1000 births in studies done in Europe[7] as well as in North America.[8] A significantly higher incidence of unilateral renal agenesis (4.5 percent versus 0.3 percent in control) has been reported in first-degree relatives (parents and siblings) of infants born with bilateral renal agenesis.[5]

PROGRESSIVE NEPHRON DAMAGE IN UNILATERAL RENAL AGENESIS

Experimental investigations in rats have shown that reduced renal mass may render the residual nephrons vulnerable to progressive damage and lead to glomerular sclerosis.[9] This type of glomerular injury is believed to result from ongoing glomerular hypertension and hyperfiltration in the surviving nephrons.[10,11] Whether reduced nephron mass in human beings also leads to progressive glomerular injury remains unresolved. Several reports support the notion that diminished renal mass as a consequence of unilateral renal agenesis[12,13] as well as unilateral nephrectomy done during childhood[14] or later in life[15,16] for a variety of renal disorders can lead to focal glomerulosclerosis and proteinuria. This type of progressive renal damage is uncommon in healthy renal transplant donors,[17] but microalbuminuria and a higher incidence of systemic hypertension have been reported in them.[18] In a recent commentary on the issue, Fine[19] suggests that despite "normal" renal function tests, patients who have undergone uninephrectomy or who were born with unilateral renal agenesis must be followed for an extended period of time for evidence of progressive renal damage.

RENAL HYPOPLASIA

The term *renal hypoplasia* (or *simple hypoplasia*) is applied to kidneys that are normal in shape and architecture but are smaller than normal in size. The total number of nephrons in the kidney is reduced. Dysplastic elements such as cartilage, primitive renal tubules, fibrous tissue, or cysts are not present in kidneys affected by hypoplasia. Although it can occur unilaterally, renal hypoplasia generally affects both kidneys.[1] Ultrasonographic evaluation of such kidneys reveals normal contour and corticomedullary differentiation. Most patients maintain normal renal function, and chronic renal failure is uncommon. Developmental malformations of the cardiovascular and gastrointestinal systems may be seen in patients with renal hypoplasia.[1]

RENAL DYSPLASIA

Renal dysplasia is characterized by hypoplastic kidneys that also contain elements of primitive tubules, mesenchyme, immature glomeruli, and cartilage (Fig. 24–1). Cortical cysts may also be present in some cases. Multicystic renal dysplasia, a condition characterized by an enlarged nonfunctioning kidney with cysts, is discussed at length in Chap. 14. Renal dysplasia can occur unilaterally

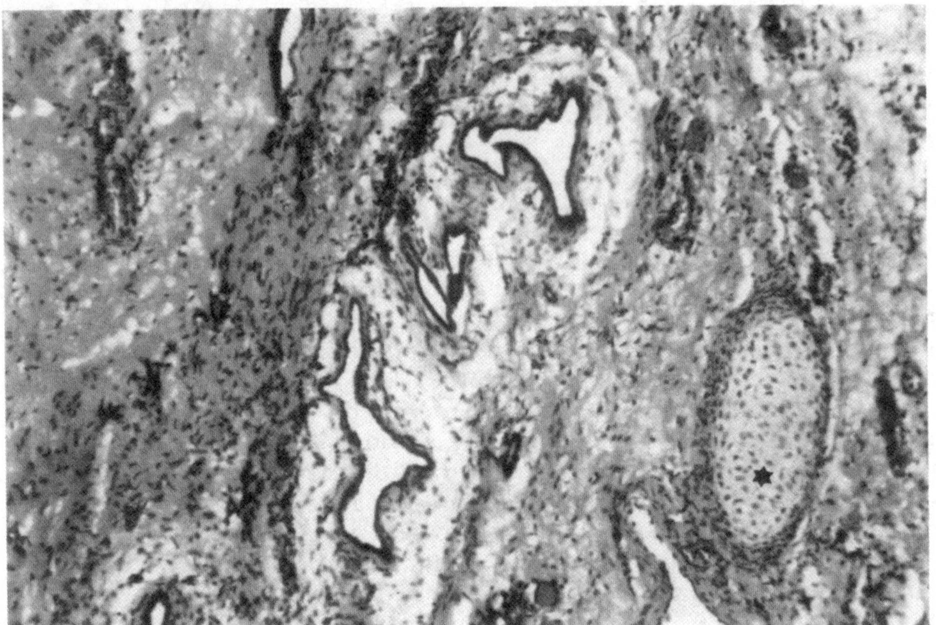

FIG. 24–1. Renal biopsy specimen showing an island of cartilage (*) in a patient with renal dysplasia. (Photograph courtesy of Kathleen Patterson, M.D., Children's Hospital National Medical Center, Washington, D.C.)

or in both kidneys and may be associated with obstruction or developmental anomalies of the urinary tract.[1]

Although renal dysplasia and urinary tract obstruction are frequently observed in the same patient, the role played by such an obstruction in the pathogenesis of renal dysplasia remains controversial. It has been shown that the timing of fetal urinary obstruction is a critical factor in determining whether the affected kidney will develop hydronephrosis or renal dysplasia. Evidence in the fetal lamb model suggests that ureteric obstruction induced early in the second trimester leads to renal dysplasia, while obstruction induced later in gestation results in hydronephrosis.[20] Also, early relief of fetal urinary tract obstruction has been shown to reverse the progression of renal dysplasia in the developing kidney,[21,22] lending support to the view that urinary obstruction may be causally related to renal dysplasia.

Clinical manifestations of renal dysplasia depend on its severity and whether or not both kidneys are involved. Unilateral dysplasia may remain silent, but an abdominal mass may be detected if multicystic dysplasia is present. These patients often develop hypertension early in life. Bilateral and severely dysplastic renal disease, particularly when associated with obstructive uropathy, may be associated with features of Potter syndrome, including pulmonary hypoplasia. Many such infants may not survive beyond the neonatal period because of severe pulmonary complications. With the now ubiquitous use of prenatal fetal ultrasound examination, renal dysplasia in infants is detected early. Diagnosis of renal dysplasia is established by ultrasound examination of the kidneys, which show small and dysmorphic renal architecture. Radionuclide scan diethylenetriaminepentaacetic acid (DTPA) usually shows both blood flow and function to be poor on the affected side. Multicystic renal dysplasia demonstrates characteristic large renal cysts in a dysmorphic organ on renal ultrasound and has poor blood flow and function on DTPA scan. Although confirmation of the diagnosis requires documenting the characteristic microscopic findings in renal tissue, this is usually not necessary.

Many patients with renal dysplasia manifest obligatory renal salt wasting and develop profound hyponatremia in the neonatal period. Supplementation of sodium should be provided in such patients. Hypertension in patients with renal dysplasia requires aggressive therapy. Angiotensin converting enzyme (ACE) inhibitor agents, such as captopril, are usually effective, but hyperkalemia resulting from such therapy must be monitored. Patients with bilateral renal dysplasia may develop end-stage renal failure at birth. This necessitates initiation of chronic dialysis in the neonatal period. Others with varying degrees of chronic renal failure can be managed by conservative treatment, as discussed in Chap. 17, until dialysis or transplantation becomes necessary.

Nephrogenic renal nodular blastema (nephroblastomatosis), a recognized precursor of Wilms' tumor,[23] may be seen histologically in multicystic dysplastic kidneys.[24] The incidence of such premalignant tissue in multicystic dysplastic kidneys is probably low. In two recent studies, 2 percent[25] and 6.5 percent[26] of surgically removed specimens of multicystic dysplastic kidney were shown, on careful microscopic examination, to contain blastematous tissue. Because of the potential risk of malignancy, surgical removal of multicystic dysplastic kidneys is considered the treatment of choice by some.

NEONATAL HYPERTENSION

Hypertension is an uncommon clinical problem in neonates, but the routine monitoring of blood pressure in sick neonates has increased awareness of this disorder. In the last 10 years, much has been learned about the etiology, diagnosis, treatment, and follow-up of neonates with hypertension. This condition in the neonate is always of secondary etiology; it is commonly due to renal or renovascular diseases. Significant morbidity such as intraventricular hemorrhage,[27] cerebral ischemia,[28] and myocardial dysfunction[29] can develop if hypertension in the neonate is left untreated. Diagnosis and treatment of hypertensive neonates requires joint efforts by the neonatologist and the nephrologist. The treatment of such patients has been made somewhat easier with the availability of ACE inhibitors and calcium channel blocking agents.

EPIDEMIOLOGY

Since blood pressure is not routinely monitored in healthy full-term neonates, the true incidence of neonatal hypertension is difficult to ascertain. Most case reports and studies dealing with hypertension in neonates have comprised sick

TABLE 24–2. Blood Pressure in Neonates[a]

	1 Day	2 Days	3 Days	4 Days	5 Days	6 Days
SP						
Awake	70.54 ± 9.13	71.65 ± 10.80	77.08 ± 12.34	78.85 ± 10.31	80.70 ± 10.72	75.75 ± 10.10
Asleep	70.41 ± 9.59	70.50 ± 8.96	74.47 ± 11.28	76.22 ± 10.26	77.13 ± 13.61	72.95 ± 11.18
DP						
Awake	42.73 ± 9.81	44.76 ± 11.15	49.33 ± 9.74	51.87 ± 12.03	51.12 ± 11.85	48.55 ± 11.02
Asleep	42.28 ± 11.97	43.69 ± 9.43	47.52 ± 10.29	46.45 ± 10.27	47.60 ± 11.22	45.45 ± 12.30
MAP						
Awake	55.32 ± 8.63	56.58 ± 10.28	63.44 ± 12.87	63.37 ± 11.11	64.54 ± 12.17	62.05 ± 11.82
Asleep	55.45 ± 11.35	55.69 ± 9.02	58.77 ± 9.25	58.45 ± 9.36	59.90 ± 11.79	57.50 ± 11.95

[a]Systolic (SP), diastolic (DP), and mean arterial blood pressure (MAP), represented as mean and standard deviations (mmHg) in full-term neonates during waking hours and sleep in the first 6 days of life.

Source: From Tan KL: Blood pressure in full-term healthy neonates. *Clin Pediatr* 26:21, 1987. Reproduced by permission.

full-term and premature infants almost exclusively. In one study, 2 percent of all neonates (gestational age, 25 to 41 weeks) admitted to the intensive care and the intermediate care nurseries in a tertiary care center were found to be hypertensive.[30]

NORMAL BLOOD PRESSURE IN NEONATES

Systolic blood pressure in full-term normal neonates approximates 70 mmHg systolic when measured indirectly either by Doppler ultrasound[31] or by the Dinamap apparatus (Table 24–2).[32] Diastolic blood pressure in the full-term healthy neonate, as measured by the Dinamap, is about 40 mmHg.[31] Similar readings have been reported by others using intraaortic blood pressure monitoring devices.[33] The systolic BP of full-term neonates shows an average daily increase of 1 to 2 mmHg during the first 2 weeks of life, followed by a slower rise for the next 4 weeks (Fig. 24–2).[31,34] By the end of week 6, the systolic BP in healthy neonates is generally slightly above 90 mmHg.[31] A similar trend in the postnatal development of blood pressure is also seen in low-birthweight infants.[35]

Apart from postnatal age, gestational age and birthweight also influence blood pressure in newborn infants.[33,36,37] There is no clear consensus about blood pressure norms in low-birthweight infants, partly because many such

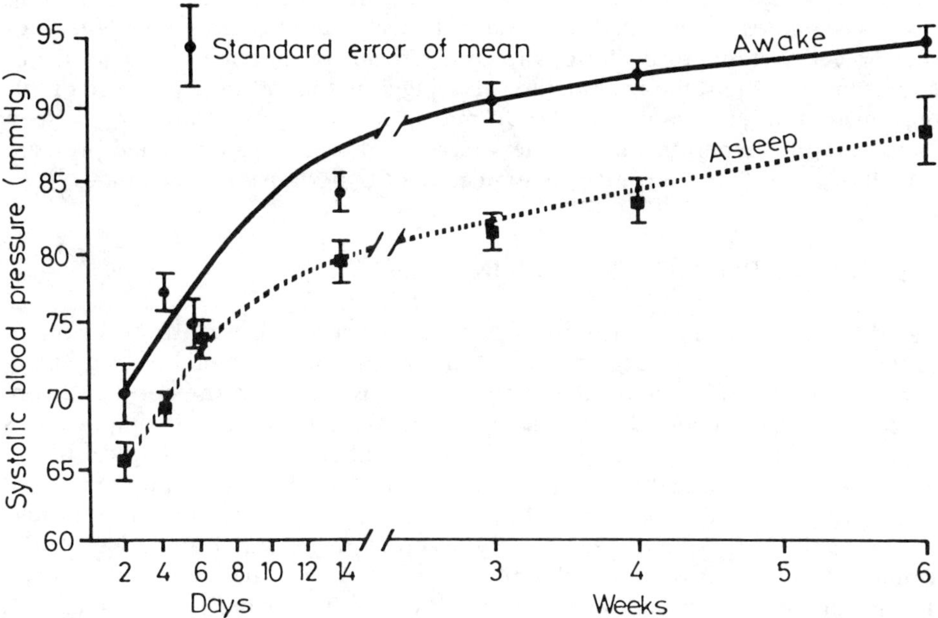

FIG. 24–2. Increase in systolic blood pressure in the first 6 weeks of life in full-term neonates in the waking and sleeping states. (From Earley A, Fayers P, Ng S, et al: Blood pressure in the first 6 weeks of life. *Arch Dis Child* 55:755, 1980. Reproduced by permission.)

TABLE 24–3. Mean Arterial Blood Pressure (MAP), Represented as Mean Pressure and Standard Deviation (mmHg), in Preterm Infants[a]

	<1.0 kg (n = 17)	1.0–1.5 kg (n = 41)	1.5–2.5 kg (n = 63)	>2.5 kg (n = 61)
At birth	32.9 ± 15.4	39.1 ± 18.2	42.4 ± 19.6	48.8 ± 19.4
At 7 days	41.4 ± 15.4	47.2 ± 18.2	50.4 ± 19.6	60.2 ± 19.4
At 14 days	44.6 ± 15.5	50.1 ± 18.2	53.2 ± 19.6	64.2 ± 19.4
At 28 days	47.6 ± 15.4	53.0 ± 18.2	56.1 ± 19.6	68.3 ± 19.4

[a]Blood pressure was recorded by an intraaortic blood pressure monitoring device or by Dinamap apparatus.

Source: From Stork EK, Carlo WA, Kliegman RM, et al: Hypertension redefined for critically ill neonates (abstract). *Pediatr Res* 18:321, 1984. Reproduced by permission.

infants are sick; they may have received intravenous fluids and been subjected to other resuscitative measures soon after birth. Some of the published normative data for mean blood pressure in premature infants of various birthweights are given in Table 24–3.

DEFINING HYPERTENSION

In view of a lack of agreement on normal standards, the definition of hypertension in neonates is unsettled. Adelman[38] has suggested that pressure readings that exceed 2 standard deviations from the mean for age may be regarded as hypertension. The same investigator also suggests that a blood pressure of 90/60 mmHg in a term infant and 80/50 mmHg in a premature one may be seen as pointing to hypertension.[38] Others have used mean arterial blood pressure (MAP) of more than 70 mmHg as indicative of hypertension in neonates.[30]

MEASURING BLOOD PRESSURE IN NEONATES

Blood pressure can be measured in neonates either by intraaortic instrumentation or indirectly in a large peripheral artery. Intraaortic blood pressure measurement utilizes an umbilical catheter, which is placed in the aorta and connected to a monitoring device through a pressure transducer. Complications associated with the insertion of an umbilical catheter (e.g., mechanical blockage of the catheter or failure of the transducer mechanism) limit prolonged monitoring of direct blood pressure via umbilical catheterization. Two noninvasive methods that have been widely accepted in neonatal nurseries are the Doppler technique (Arteriosonde) and the oscillometric technique (Dinamap). The advantage of the oscillometric method is that it provides systolic, diastolic, and mean arterial blood pressures, while the Doppler technique can measure only systolic pressure. The readings obtained by direct intraaortic monitoring correlate well with those determined by indirect methods, particularly the oscillometric method.[39,40]

The general principles of measuring blood pressure indirectly, using a cuff placed over a peripheral artery, are discussed in Chap. 10; they should also be adhered to in neonates. Specifically, the blood pressure cuff should cover at least 50 percent of the circumference of the arm[41]; also, the patient should be comfortably placed and not crying. When intraabdominal pressure is raised by external compression, an increased blood pressure reading may be obtained[42]; therefore this should be avoided during blood pressure monitoring.

It is unclear whether, in neonates, blood pressure is normally higher in the lower extremities, as it is in older children. While some have reported that the blood pressure in the upper limbs is identical to that in the lower limbs,[35,39] others have suggested that systolic blood pressure may actually be higher in the upper limbs in normal neonates even in the absence of coarctation of the aorta.[43] It has also been well established that blood pressure is higher during the waking state than during sleep.[31,34]

ETIOLOGY OF HYPERTENSION

Renovascular diseases such as renal arterial thrombosis, embolization, and developmental parenchymal renal disease are the leading but not the only causes of hypertension in neonates. Table 24–4 lists the etiologies that must be considered in the evaluation of a hypertensive neonate.

RENOVASCULAR HYPERTENSION

Renovascular disorders are the most common causes of hypertension in neonates. While congenital stenosis of the renal artery has been described,[44,45] acquired disorders are more frequently encountered as the etiology of neonatal hypertension. Of these, thrombosis of the renal artery following umbilical artery catheterization is a particularly common and well-described etiology.

Aortic and renal arterial thrombosis and renal infarction following insertion of an indwelling umbilical arterial catheter have been well described since the early 1970s.[45–49] The risk of thrombotic complication resulting from indwelling umbilical catheters is substantial; aortography of neonates with indwelling umbilical catheters in one study demonstrated aortic clots in 95 percent.[47] In another study, high-resolution ultrasound detected aortic clots in 26 percent of neonates with indwelling umbilical artery catheters.[50] The types of aortic clots that may be seen as a consequence of umbilical arterial catheterization are shown in Fig. 24–3.

Although mechanical blockage of the aortic lumen, especially in very small premature neonates, can cause aortic thrombosis, intimal damage induced by the catheter itself may be an important additional factor predisposing to such thrombotic events. In experimental studies conducted in rabbits, insertion of a polyvinyl chloride umbilical catheter, similar to that used in neonates, into the aorta results in endothelial disruption within 24 h, and thrombi are found on the damaged endothelial surface.[51] The severity of thrombosis in these instances

TABLE 24–4. Etiology of Hypertension in Neonates

Renovascular Disorders
- Renal artery thrombosis
- Aortic thrombosis
- Congenital renal artery stenosis
- Renal embolization from patent ductus arteriosus
- Intimal hyperplasia of aorta and renal arteries
- Renal vein thrombosis

Renal Parenchymal Disorders
- Multicystic renal dysplasia
- Other forms of renal dysplasia
- Polycystic kidney disease
  - Autosomal recessive polycystic kidney disease
  - Autosomal dominant polycystic kidney disease
- Urinary tract obstruction
- Ask-Upmark kidney
- Perinephric hematoma or urinoma

Cardiovascular Problems
- Coarctation of the aorta

Drugs
- Phenylephrine eye drops
- Corticosteroid administration
- Theophylline
- Neonatal cocaine exposure
- Withdrawal symptoms due to maternal use of heroin and methadone

Endocrine Disorders
- Hyperthyroidism
- Adrenogenital syndrome
- Hyperaldosteronism
- Neuroblastoma
- Pheochromocytoma

Miscellaneous Conditions
- Bronchopulmonary dysplasia
- Following pyeloplasty
- Closure of abdominal wall defects
- Acutely increased intracranial pressure

Unknown Etiology

was determined by the severity of endothelial damage and the length of time during which the catheter was left in place.[51]

Aortic clots resulting from umbilical arterial catheters cause hypertension by (1) occluding the ostia of the renal arteries, (2) extension of thrombosis into the renal arteries, or (3) microembolization of the kidney by fragments of the clot (Fig. 24–4). Hypertension usually appears within a few days of catheterization and is mediated by a high renin output from the affected kidney.[30,49]

RENAL ARTERIAL EMBOLISM

Renal embolism, presumably originating from patent ductus arteriosus, has been reported to cause severe hypertension in young infants.[52] This diagnosis

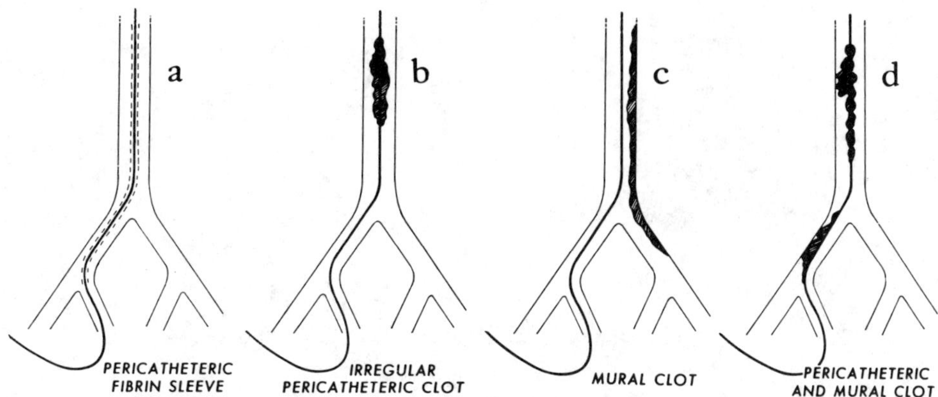

FIG. 24–3. The four common types of aortic clot configurations visualized by aortography in neonates with thrombosis related to umbilical arterial catheterization. (From Neal WA, Reynolds JW, Jarvis CW, et al: Umbilical artery catheterization: Demonstration of arterial thrombosis by aortography. *Pediatrics* 50:6, 1972, © 1972 by *Pediatrics*. Reproduced by permission.)

may be considered in patients who have not undergone umbilical arterial catheterization but have demonstrable evidence of renal embolism, either by a radionuclide renal scan or by an arteriogram. Obviously, a primary site for the development of arterial thrombi and emboli is a prerequisite for such a diagnosis. Plasma renin activity (PRA) is elevated in such patients.[52]

RENAL VEIN THROMBOSIS

Acute renal vein thrombosis is a less common cause of renovascular hypertension in neonates.[53] Severe hypotension, asphyxia, and dehydration are the common antecedents of renal vein thrombosis in neonates. In addition to hypertension, other manifestations of renal vein thrombosis include gross or microscopic hematuria and proteinuria, while renal function tests—blood urea nitrogen (BUN) and creatinine—can be normal. Kidneys are usually enlarged when visualized by ultrasonography but can be normal in some patients during the early course of thrombosis. Thrombus may also be visualized in the renal vein by ultrasonographic evaluation. Plasma renin activity is usually elevated in these patients.[53]

RENAL PARENCHYMAL DISORDERS

Hypertension is commonly seen in neonates with autosomal recessive and autosomal dominant polycystic kidney diseases. Multicystic dysplastic kidney also carries a high risk of hypertension in early infancy. Patients with hypoplasia do not usually develop hypertension, but those with hypoplastic dysplastic kidneys can do so.

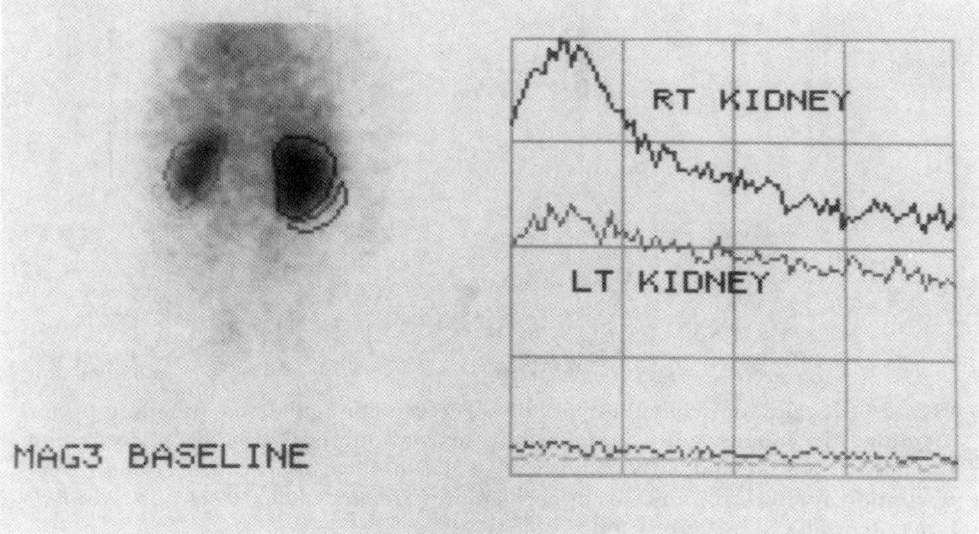

FIG. 24–4. Radionuclide scan (*A*) in a 9-day-old full-term male neonate with neonatal asphyxia who developed hypertension 2 days following insertion of an umbilical artery catheter. The scan shows poor uptake and excretion of the radionuclide by the left kidney. An ultrasound examination (*B*) demonstrated normal renal architecture and size, but a clot in the aorta that extended from the level of renal arteries to the bifurcation of the aorta was visualized. The clot resolved without therapy over the next 2 months, and blood pressure normalized as well.

COARCTATION OF THE AORTA

Coarctation of the aorta should be excluded in all patients with neonatal hypertension. The clinical tip-off suggesting this diagnosis is the demonstration of elevated blood pressure in the upper extremities only. Another common clinical feature of aortic coarctation is a delayed and weak femoral pulse, but this finding may not be present at birth and is usually detected between the third and the seventh days of life.[54] Upper-extremity hypertension may be absent in neonates with aortic coarctation who have coexistent cardiac failure. The diagnosis is established by echocardiography and angiography.

DRUGS

The exposure of neonates to pharmacologic agents can result in transient hypertension. Prolonged therapeutic use of a corticosteroid or theophylline in toxic concentration is often associated with hypertension. Fluid overload as well as the administration of vasoactive drugs are other common causes of transient hypertension. Hypertension due to the ophthalmic application of phenylephrine is well known.[55] Intentional or accidental exposure of the neonate to cocaine[56,57] and other illicit drugs can also result in hypertension and should be considered under the appropriate clinical circumstances.

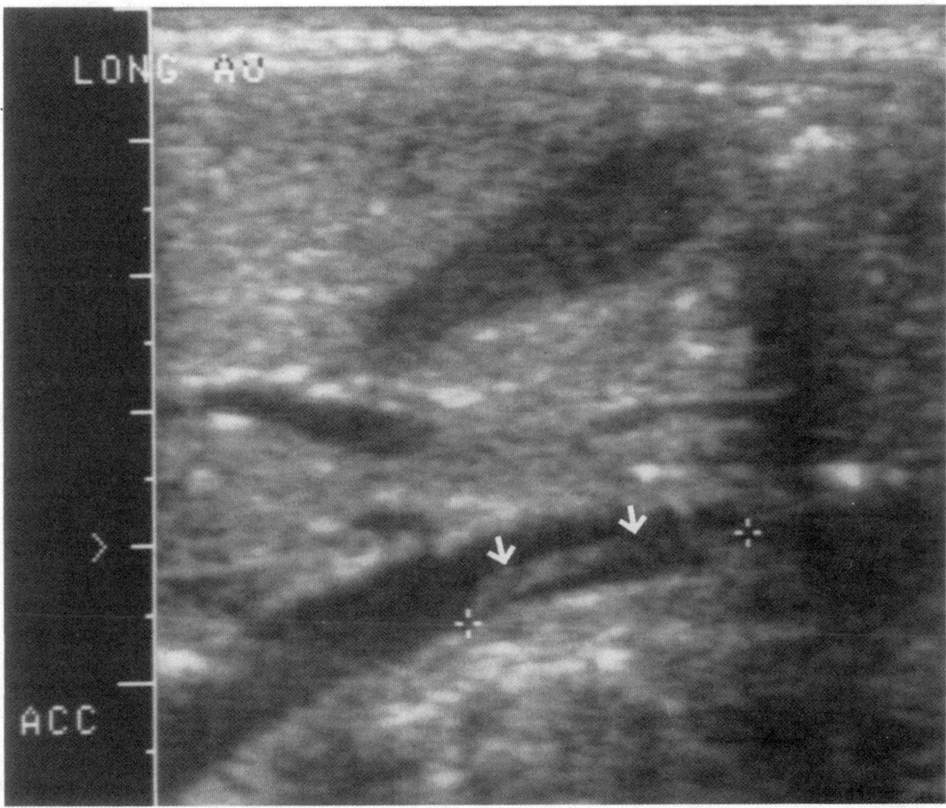

B
FIG. 24–4 (*Continued*).

ENDOCRINE DISORDERS

Endocrine disorders such as congenital adrenal hyperplasia[58] and hyperthyroidism[59] are rare but known causes of neonatal hypertension. Low-renin hypertension in infants has also been described.[60] *Pheochromocytoma* is an uncommon cause of hypertension in children[61] and is an even less common etiology of hypertension in the neonate. Because of their rarity, endocrine causes of hypertension should be considered only if clinical suspicion mandates it or when other causes of hypertension have been excluded.

MISCELLANEOUS CONDITIONS

There is a high incidence of hypertension among neonates with bronchopulmonary dysplasia.[62] The pathogenesis of hypertension in these neonates is unclear and may be multifactorial. The possible contributory factors include prolonged use of umbilical artery catheters as well as administration of a corticosteroid or theophylline. Other unusual circumstances reported to be associated with neonatal hypertension are hydronephrosis,[63] after earlier surgical repair of an obstructed ureteropelvic junction,[64] and following closure of defects in the abdominal wall.[65]

UNKNOWN ETIOLOGIES

Hypertension of undetermined etiology has been described in infants by Sheftel et al.[66] and in the extension of the same study by Friedman and Hustead.[67] Almost all the reported patients in these studies were born prematurely, and hypertension appeared in the period following discharge from the neonatal care unit. Response to antihypertensive drugs was often satisfactory, and the hypertension resolved by the age of 2 years. Even though no definable etiology of hypertension was demonstrated in the reported patients, they probably do not represent essential neonatal hypertension and should not be so categorized.

CLINICAL MANIFESTATIONS OF HYPERTENSION

As is the case in older children and adults, hypertension in neonates is largely an asymptomatic disorder. A high degree of suspicion and routine monitoring of blood pressure in high-risk neonates are the usual mode by which hypertension is detected in this age group. Surprisingly, most neonates tolerate hypertension well, and manifestations arising from associated or underlying disorders such as prematurity, meconium aspiration, respiratory distress syndrome, or sepsis predominate. Myocardial dysfunction in hypertensive neonates has been reported,[29] but congestive heart failure is uncommon unless other cardiac anomalies such as coarctation of the aorta or patent ductus arteriosus are also present. Significant left ventricular hypertrophy is commonly seen in neonates with sustained hypertension.[30]

Neonatal hypertension related to umbilical arterial catheterization manifests itself within a few days to a week following catheter placement. Other features of these patients are gross or microscopic hematuria and mild proteinuria. Similar findings may be observed in patients with renal vein thrombosis. A palpable renal mass is, however, rarely present in these patients. Excessive renal salt wasting and hyponatremia have been described in neonates with renovascular hypertension.[68] Although its precise mechanism remains unknown, it has been suggested that renal salt loss under these circumstances may be due to increased glomerular pressure (*pressure natriuresis*).

A unilateral renal mass may be present in patients with multicystic dysplastic kidney or hydronephrosis, while those with polycystic kidney disease may have bilaterally palpable renal masses. Patients with coarctation of the aorta characteristically develop weak femoral pulses, and elevated blood pressure is detected in the upper limbs only. Hypertensive retinopathy, in addition to left ventricular hypertrophy, may develop in neonates with sustained hypertension.[30,69]

CLINICAL COURSE

Published data relating to the long-term follow-up of patients who developed hypertension in the neonatal period are scant. Most patients with a renovascular etiology of hypertension respond to conventional antihypertensive treatment within 3 to 7 days. Slow resolution of the aortic and renal artery thrombus in a week to several months is seen in most cases even without any thrombolytic therapy.[70] The duration of antihypertensive treatment needed in patients with hypertension related to umbilical arterial catheterization varies from a few weeks to several months. The average duration of treatment reported in one long-term study was 4 months,[71] but longer treatment—up to 2 years—may be required in some cases.[72] Most children who survive the neonatal period remain normotensive after the antihypertensive therapy is discontinued, and most maintain normal renal function.[70–72] Renal atrophy or failure of renal parenchymal growth on the affected side may be evident during follow-up in patients with unilateral renal thromboembolic disease.

EVALUATION OF THE HYPERTENSIVE NEONATE

The extent to which hypertensive neonates are investigated is determined by institutional practices. Extensive investigations are not necessary in most patients in whom hypertension is suspected to be the result of umbilical arterial catheterization.[73] Coarctation of the aorta should be ruled out in all hypertensive neonates by clinical examination and an echocardiographic examination. The next task for the physician is to focus on renal and renovascular causes of hypertension. This requires obtaining routine laboratory tests such as urinalysis, complete blood count including platelet count, determination of BUN and serum creatinine, abdominal ultrasound examination, and DTPA renal scan. Doppler ultrasound study of the renal arteries and veins for blood flow provides further diagnostic information and may be undertaken if such studies are available. Intravenous pyelography and renal angiography are not required in most patients. It must be emphasized that many neonates with renal arterial thrombosis and embolization have only transient urinary abnormalities (hematuria) as well as normal renal function and do not manifest any abnormalities of renal size and architecture. The only positive diagnostic feature of these patients is the abnormality in renal blood flow seen by radionuclide scan. With time, however, the affected kidney becomes smaller in size, while the contralateral kidney often demonstrates compensatory hypertrophy.

Urologic and endocrine evaluation is not required for every hypertensive neonate; such evaluation should be dictated by leads obtained from clinical and initial laboratory studies. Neonates with sustained hypertension and those who require prolonged antihypertensive therapy should be followed periodically by echocardiographic examination in order to monitor left ventricular size (for hypertrophy) and function. Diagnostic tests used in the evaluation of hypertensive neonates are outlined in Table 24–5.

TREATMENT OF HYPERTENSION

The treatment of neonates with hypertension is determined by the underlying etiology. Those with renal arterial thrombosis or embolism can be managed by conventional antihypertensive agents in the dosages listed in Table 24–6.

TABLE 24–5. Diagnostic Tests Used for the Evaluation of Hypertensive Neonates

Test	Observation	Interpretation
Clinical		
Four-limb blood pressure	Upper-limb hypertension only	Coarctation of the aorta
Femoral pulses	Weak	Coarctation, aortic thrombosis
Abdominal palpation	Renal mass	Multicystic dysplastic kidney, hydronephrosis, polycystic kidneys
History of umbilical catheterization	Positive	Consider renal arterial thrombosis or renal embolization
Laboratory		
Urinalysis	Hematuria/proteinuria	Renal artery or venous thrombosis, embolism
Electrolytes, renal function tests	Abnormal renal function	Serious renal disease or renovascular accident. Renal function is usually normal in most cases of unilateral renal arterial thrombosis
Renal ultrasound	Normal size	Renal arterial embolism, early renal arterial and venous thrombosis
	Small size	Renal dysplasia, sequela of arterial renal arterial thrombosis
	Renal cysts	Multicystic dysplastic kidney, polycystic kidneys
	Hydronephrosis	Urinary obstruction
	Renal arterial or venous clot	Renal arterial or venous thrombosis
Renal scan	Poor renal blood flow and function, segmental filling defects	Renal arterial thrombosis
Plasma renin activity	Elevated	Renal or renovascular etiology

TABLE 24–6. Doses of Antihypertensive Drugs in Neonates

Drug	Usual Dose	Frequency of Administration
Hydralazine	1.0–4.0 mg/kg/day IV 1.0–10.0 mg/kg/day PO	q 4–6 h
Furosemide	1.0–2.0 mg/kg/day IV, PO	q 12–24 h
Propranolol	0.5–2.0 mg/kg/day PO	q 8 h
Captopril	0.05–0.5 mg/kg/day PO	q 8 h
Enalaprilat	5.0–25.0 μg/kg/day IV	q 12 h
Diazoxide	1.0–5.0 mg/kg/dose IV	q 4 h, sooner if necessary
Sodium nitroprusside	0.2–8.0 μg/kg/min IV	Continuous infusion

Hydralazine is often employed as the drug of first choice for the treatment of mild to moderately severe neonatal hypertension. One of the advantages of this drug is that it can be administered intravenously in a neonate whose gastrointestinal tract may not be functional. If necessary, diuretics or beta-blocking agents can be added as second-tier drugs. ACE inhibitors such as captopril should be used cautiously in neonates, especially in those who are born prematurely. Severe hypotension and acute renal failure have been reported with ACE inhibitor therapy in premature infants with renovascular lesions.[74] Another group of patients at high risk for acute renal failure as a consequence of ACE-inhibitor therapy are those with bilateral renal arterial lesions or those with a single kidney which involves a thrombotic lesion. Use of ACE inhibitors in neonates requires close monitoring of renal function and perfusion by radionuclide scans. Hypertensive emergencies can be treated by intravenous administration of either diazoxide or sodium nitroprusside.

Apart from appropriate medical therapy, surgical or other adjunctive therapy may be considered in some patients with neonatal hypertension. Thrombolytic drugs (streptokinase) and anticoagulant therapy (heparin) have been tried in some patients with large aortic thrombi. Results have varied,[57,75,76] and controlled trials using these modalities are lacking. Also, specific recommendations for the use of anticoagulant and thrombolytic therapy in aortic and renal artery thrombosis have not yet been established. However, some have advocated the use of these therapies in patients with symptomatic arterial obstruction such as decreased femoral pulse or cold lower extremities and in those with impending complete blockage of the lower extremities.[75] The risks associated with these therapeutic modalities—particularly intracranial bleeding and hemorrhage in other organs—must be considered carefully. Surgical removal of the aortic thrombus (thrombectomy) has been employed in some neonates, but these procedures should be reserved for severe cases and employed only in institutions where microvascular surgery can be performed. Nephrectomy may be necessary in a rare patient with hypertension due to unilateral renal arterial disease, which does respond well to antihypertensive therapy and cannot be dealt with surgically.[44]

ACUTE RENAL FAILURE

Acute deterioration of renal function and oliguria are common clinical problems for neonatologists and pediatric nephrologists. Often this results from correctable prerenal causes such as hypovolemia, hypotension, poor cardiac output, and diminished renal perfusion. Some of these patients, however, proceed to develop the syndrome of acute renal failure (ARF), which is characterized by the histologic features of acute tubular necrosis (ATN). Less commonly, ARF may result from developmental malformations and obstruction of the urinary tract. It has been estimated that 1 to 8 percent of neonates admitted to neonatal intensive care units suffer from ARF.[77–79] However, these figures probably represent an underestimation of the incidence of ARF, since many neonates (especially prematures) with nonoliguric ARF may go unrecognized and unreported.[79]

DEFINITION

Oliguric ARF is defined as a urine output below 1 mL/kg/h associated with a serum creatinine above 1.5 mg/dL at 2 to 5 days of age. Nonoliguric ARF, on the other hand, is associated with either a normal or excessive urine output while the serum creatinine remains elevated. It must be recalled that serum creatinine in the neonate reflects the maternal serum creatinine concentration (usually 1.0 mg/dL) and should decline during the first week of life. Lack of this expected decline or an actual increasing trend should alert the physician to deteriorating renal function and ARF. Acute deterioration of renal function resulting from reversible causes such as hypovolemia and hypotension should be considered under the category of prerenal azotemia.

ETIOLOGY

Hypoxic or hypovolemic renal injury resulting from perinatal events such as traumatic delivery, hypoxic episodes, hemorrhage, shock, respiratory distress syndrome, and sepsis are the commonest causes of ARF as well as prerenal azotemia in neonates.[77–83] Less commonly, neonatal ARF can result from congenital renal malformations, obstruction, and renal arterial or venous thrombosis. The use of nephrotoxic drugs for the treatment of sepsis or fungal infection should also be considered in the etiology of ARF in neonates. A multifactorial etiology of neonatal ARF is common; a frequent clinical scenario is perinatal hypoxia or hypovolemia, sepsis, poor cardiac output, and use of nephrotoxic agents for the treatment of presumed sepsis. Rarely, hemoglobinuria,[84] myoglobinuria,[85] hyperuricemia,[86] polycythemia,[87] and administration of radiologic contrast media and ACE inhibitors also play a role. Table 24–7 lists the causes of neonatal ARF.

DIAGNOSIS

The general principles of investigating patients with ARF discussed in Chap. 15 also apply to neonates. The overriding concern in a sick neonate is to exclude the possibility of a treatable cause of renal dysfunction such as prerenal azotemia. Consequently, careful attention should be paid to the neonate's intravascular volume status and blood pressure; a fluid challenge should be considered if any evidence for prerenal azotemia exists. Differentiation of prerenal azotemia from intrinsic ARF or acute tubular necrosis can be attempted using the urinary indices discussed in Chap. 15. However, several pitfalls of using these diagnostic tests to differentiate prerenal azotemia from established ARF in neonates must be pointed out (Table 24–8). Since urinary sodium excretion is normally high in premature infants, elevated urinary sodium excretion is not a dependable tool for differentiating prerenal azotemia from ARF. Although fractional excretion of sodium (FeNa) is considered a more reliable test in differentiating renal tubular damage associated with established ARF, its applicability to neonates with ARF is also conditional. Most studies suggest that FeNa

TABLE 24–7. Etiology of Acute Renal Failure in Neonates

Hypotension
Maternal antepartum hemorrhage
Twin-twin transfusion
Septic shock
Traumatic delivery
Neonatal hypoxia
Congestive heart failure

Intrinsic Renal Disorders
Bilateral renal dysplasia
Renal agenesis
Polycystic renal diseases
Severe and bilateral renal arterial and venous thrombosis
Intrarenal precipitation of
- Uric acid
- Myoglobin
- Hemoglobin

Nephrotoxic Drugs
Aminoglycosides
Indomethacin
ACE inhibitors
Contrast media

Urinary Tract Obstruction
Urethral obstruction
Ureteral obstruction in patients with a single kidney
Bilateral ureteral obstruction

exceeding 2.5 to 3.0 should be used as an index of established ARF in a neonate,[78,83] but the sharp demarcation between prerenal azotemia and established ARF is not always clear in this age group (i.e., the test has poor specificity).[88] Similarly, the extent to which BUN and serum creatinine are raised does not help to differentiate prerenal azotemia from established ARF.[78,88]

TABLE 24–8. Urinary Diagnostic Indices Helpful in the Differentiation of Prerenal Azotemia from Established Acute Renal Failure (ARF)

	Diagnostic Value		
Test	Prerenal	ARF	Comment
Urinary sodium	<20 meq/L[a]	>20 meq/L	Premature infants may normally have high urinary sodium. The test has poor specificity.
Urine-to-plasma osmolality ratio	>1.0	<1.0	
Fractional excretion of sodium	<2.5	>3.0	May be normally high in prematures. The test has poor specificity.

[a]Urinary sodium levels above 20 meq/L have been reported in neonates with well-documented prerenal azotemia.[83]

In recent years, attempts have been made to develop markers of renal tubular dysfunction that would help to predict renal tubular damage and aid in the diagnosis of ARF in neonates. These markers include β_2-microglobulin, myoglobin, retinol-binding protein, and N-acetyl-β-D-glucosaminidase (NAG).[89,90] Because these tests are not as yet readily available in most clinical laboratories, their use remains restricted to research investigations.

Urinary tract obstruction must be excluded in all patients with ARF and anuria. Apart from direct visualization of the external genitalia and catheterization of the urinary bladder, radiologic studies for evaluation of the anatomy of the urinary tract are indicated in neonates with ARF. Attention should be paid to renal size and shape and whether or not there are indications of bilateral urinary tract obstruction. Doppler ultrasound examination of the renal arterial tree and the renal vein is increasingly becoming a standard method of evaluating the patency of the renal vascular architecture. Radionuclide (DTPA) renal scan provides a reasonably accurate assessment of renal blood flow and function as well as renal anatomy. However, poor glomerular filtration may somewhat limit the usefulness of this investigation in neonates with advanced ARF. Intravenous pyelography should not be undertaken in a neonate with ARF because of the risk that the administration of a radiocontrast agent will compound renal parenchymal damage.

MANAGEMENT

It is essential that the etiology of oliguria in a sick neonate be determined as rapidly as possible. This usually requires providing a fluid challenge and obtaining the diagnostic urinary indices and necessary radiologic studies. If a patient is considered to be suffering from established ARF, the general principles related to the management of fluid and electrolyte balance, nutrition, and supportive care discussed in Chap. 15 must be followed.

Dialytic therapy should be considered if the regulation of fluids, acidosis, and hyperkalemia cannot be effectively managed by conservative therapy. Hemodialysis is technically difficult in neonates, mainly because of the difficulty of establishing adequate vascular access and the instability of the cardiovascular system and blood pressure encountered in such neonates. On the other hand, peritoneal dialysis provides an effective, technically easier dialysis therapy in neonates, especially in those with unstable blood pressure. Special modifications must be made in the peritoneal dialysis setup in order to deliver a small volume of dialysate accurately (Fig. 24–5). In patients in whom peritoneal dialysis is either not feasible or contraindicated—as in those with abdominal wall defects, necrotizing enterocolitis, or recent abdominal surgery—continuous arteriovenous or venovenous hemofiltration with dialysis may be an option.

As is the case in older children, nonoliguric ARF is considerably easier to manage than oliguric ARF. These patients require monitoring of fluid status, since dehydration and further compromise of renal function can result if close attention to such details is not provided. Hyponatremia, hypokalemia, and hypocalcemia are also common accompaniments in patients with nonoliguric ARF and must be corrected appropriately.

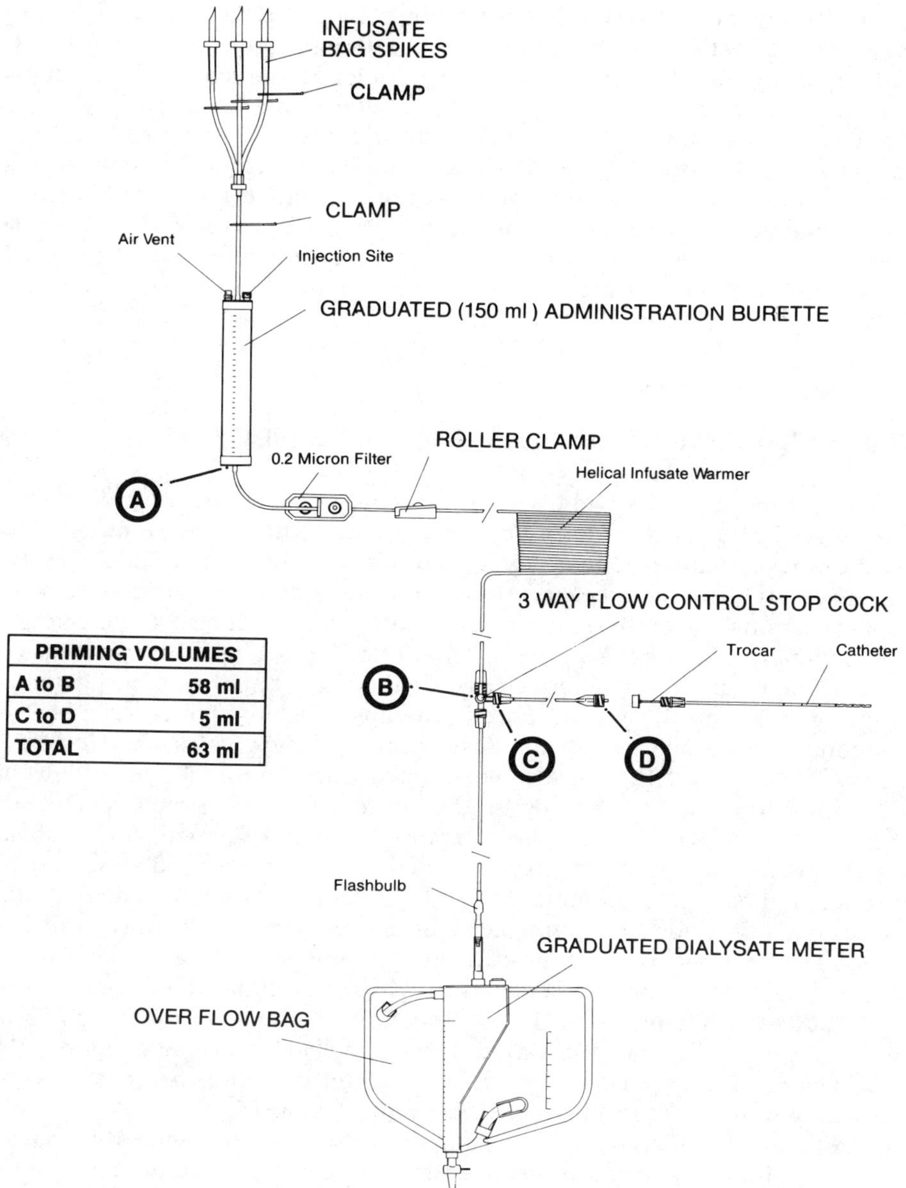

PRIMING VOLUMES	
A to B	58 ml
C to D	5 ml
TOTAL	63 ml

FIG. 24–5. A sketch diagram of Gesco Dialy-Nate, a commercially available peritoneal dialysis unit designed to be used in neonates. (Reproduced by courtesy of Gesco International Inc., San Antonio, Texas.)

OUTCOME

The outcome of ARF depends to a great extent on the underlying condition that precipitated the onset of renal dysfunction. Other factors contributing to acute patient mortality in ARF are fluid overload, congestive heart failure, and electrolyte derangements. Survival is determined by the type of ARF, prognosis being better in patients with nonoliguric ARF than in those with oliguria. The mortality from oliguric ARF reported by Chevalier and colleagues[77] was 50 percent, while all the patients with nonoliguric ARF in their study survived.

Residual abnormalities in glomerular filtration rate may persist in survivors of neonatal ARF,[77] especially in those with obstructive uropathy, renal arterial or venous thrombosis, and developmental renal anomalies. Defects in urinary concentrating capacity are also common following ARF in the neonatal period. Anand and colleagues[81] report defective concentrating ability in all their survivors, while such defects are reported in only 11.1 percent of patients by Zaramella et al.[91]

RENAL CALCIFICATION IN PREMATURE NEONATES

Nephrocalcinosis, or calcification within the renal parenchyma, as well as renal stones have been described in premature neonates. The incidence of renal calcification in premature neonates was reported to be 64.0[92] and 26.6[93] percent in 2 recent studies. Renal calcifications are usually detected during ultrasonographic examination of the abdomen of asymptomatic neonates. Hypercalciuria is the hallmark of neonates prone to renal calcification.[92–94] Other risk factors felt to be important in the pathogenesis of this disorder are hypophosphatemia, hypercalcemia, and the use of diuretic therapy.[93,94] Although furosemide has commonly been implicated in the development of hypercalciuria,[94] increased urinary calcium excretion has also been noted with the use of hydrochlorothiazide and spironolactone therapy in premature infants.[95] Oxygen dependency for more than 28 days has also been reported to be a risk factor for renal calcification. This probably reflects the severity of pulmonary disease, use of diuretics, and need for parenteral hyperalimentation in such patients.[93] Partial or complete resolution of nephrocalcinosis on follow-up has been reported.[94]

Therapy of patients with nephrocalcinosis should be aimed at removal of the precipitating events and the reduction of hypercalcemia and hypercalciuria when these are demonstrated. Discontinuation of diuretic therapy should be considered and fluid intake liberalized if the clinical circumstances permit. Use of thiazide diuretics to decrease urinary calcium excretion has been recommended by some,[94] but its efficacy remains undetermined.

Conditions other than prematurity and the use of diuretic agents that may be associated with renal calcifications in early life are distal renal tubular acidosis, primary hyperparathyroidism, oxaluria, and a variant of Bartter syndrome.[96]

SUMMARY

An understanding of the indicators of normal renal function in the neonate is essential to their appropriate interpretation and clinical usefulness. The care of sick and premature neonates has improved significantly in the last 15 years as a result of technologic advances. However, the survival of such neonates is not achieved without a "price." Iatrogenic disorders such as aortic and renal thrombosis leading to renovascular hypertension and acute renal failure are accepted as reasonable risks of treatment. Our understanding of developmental renal physiology has not kept pace with emerging clinical successes, particularly in the care of very low birthweight prematures. Sometimes we must depend on our experience with older neonates and those born at term to interpret the renal function of these very small prematures and to plan their treatment. Despite these shortcomings in our understanding, an attempt has been made in this chapter to unify investigative, therapeutic, and physiologic concepts for the effective management of neonates suffering from some of the more common renal disorders.

REFERENCES

1. Rubenstein M, Meyer R, Bernstein L: Congenital abnormalities of the urinary system: I. A postmortem survey of developmental anomalies and acquired congenital lesions in a children's hospital. *J Pediatr* 58:356, 1961.
2. Barakat AJ, Drougas JG, Barakat R: Association of congenital abnormalities of the kidney and urinary tract with those of other organ systems in 13,775 autopsies. *Child Nephrol Urol* 9:269, 1988–89.
3. Stoll C, Alembik Y, Roth MP, et al: Risk factors in internal urinary system malformations. *Pediatr Nephrol* 4:319, 1990.
4. Steinhart JM, Kuhn JP, Eisenberg B, et al: Ultrasound screening of healthy infants for urinary tract abnormalities. *Pediatrics* 82:609, 1988.
5. Roodhooft AM, Birnholtz JC, Holmes LB: Familial nature of congenital absence and severe dysgenesis of both kidneys. *N Engl J Med* 310:1341, 1984.
6. Longo VJ, Thompson GJ: Congenital solitary kidney. *J Urol* 68:63, 1952.
7. Carter CO, Evans K: Birth frequency of bilateral renal agenesis. *J Med Genet* 18:158, 1981.
8. Wilson RD, Baird PA: Renal agenesis in British Columbia. *Am J Med Genet* 21:153, 1985.
9. Schimamura T, Morrison AB: A progressive glomeruloscelerosis occurring in partial five-sixths nephrectomized rats. *Am J Physiol* 79:95, 1975.
10. Hostetter TH, Olson JL, Rennke HG, et al: Hyperfiltration in remnant nephrons: A potentially adverse response to renal ablation. *Am J Physiol* 241:F85, 1981.
11. Brenner BM: Nephron adaptation to renal injury or ablation. *Am J Physiol* 249:F324, 1985.
12. Thorner PS, Arbus GS, Celermajer DS, et al: Focal segmental glomerulosclerosis and progressive renal failure associated with a unilateral kidney. *Pediatrics* 73:806, 1984.
13. Kaneko K, Ohtomo Y, Fukuda Y, et al: Focal segmental glomerulosclerosis associated with a unilateral hypoplastic kidney. *Clin Nephrol* 33:52, 1990.
14. Welch TR, McAdam AJ: Focal glomerulosclerosis as a late sequela of Wilms tumor. *J Pediatr* 108:105, 1986.
15. Gutierrez-Millet V, Nieto J, Parga M, et al: Focal glomerulosclerosis and proteinuria in patients with solitary kidneys. *Arch Intern Med* 146:705, 1986.
16. Novick AC, Gephardt G, Guz B, et al: Long-term follow-up after removal of a solitary kidney. *N Engl J Med* 325:1058, 1991.

17. Vincentti F, Amend WJC Jr, Kaysen G, et al: Long-term renal function in kidney donors. *Transplantation* 36:626, 1983.
18. Watnick TJ, Jenkins RR, Rackoff P, et al: Microalbuminuria and hypertension in long-term renal donors. *Transplantation* 45:59, 1988.
19. Fine LG: How little kidney tissue is enough? *N Engl J Med* 325:1097, 1991.
20. Beck AD: The effect of intra-uterine urinary obstruction upon the development of the fetal kidney. *J Urol* 105:784, 1971.
21. Glick PL, Harrison MR, Noall RA, et al: Correction of congenital hydronephrosis in utero: III. Early mid-trimester ureteral obstruction produces renal dysplasia. *J Pediatr Surg* 18:681, 1983.
22. Glick PL, Harrison MR, Adzick NS, et al: Correction of congenital hydronephrosis in utero: IV. In utero decompression prevents renal dysplasia. *J Pediatr Surg* 19:649, 1984.
23. Machin GA: Persistent renal blastema (nephroblastomatosis) as a frequent precursor of Wilms' tumor: A pathological and clinical review. *Am J Pediatr Hematol Oncol* 2:353, 1980.
24. Cormie WJ, Engelstein MS, Duckett JW Jr: Nodular renal blastema, renal dysplasia, and duplicated collecting system. *J Urol* 123:100, 1980.
25. Noe HN, Marshall JH, Edwards OP: Nodular blastema in the multicystic kidney. *J Urol* 142:486, 1989.
26. Dimmick JE, Johnson HW, Coleman GU, et al: Wilms tumorlet, nodular renal blastema and multicystic renal dysplasia. *J Urol* 142:484, 1989.
27. Bada HS, Korones SB, Perry EH, et al: Mean arterial blood pressure in infants and those at risk for intraventricular hemorrhage. *J Pediatr* 117:607, 1990.
28. Watkins AMC, West CR, Cooke RWI: Blood pressure and cerebral hemorrhage and ischemia in very low birth weight infants. *Early Human Devel* 19:103, 1989.
29. McGonigle LF, Beaudry MA, Coe JY: Recovery from neonatal myocardial dysfunction after treatment of acute hypertension. *Arch Dis Child* 62:614, 1987.
30. Skalina MEL, Kliegman RM, Fanaroff AA: Epidemiology and management of severe symptomatic neonatal hypertension. *Am J Perinatol* 3:235, 1986.
31. Early A, Fayers S, Ng S, et al: Blood pressure in the first 6 weeks of life. *Arch Dis Child* 55:755, 1980.
32. Tan KL: Blood pressure in full-term healthy neonates. *Clin Pediatr* 26:21, 1987.
33. Kitterman JA, Phibbs RH, Tooley WH: Aortic blood pressure in normal newborn infants during the first 12 hours of life. *Pediatrics* 44:959, 1969.
34. De Swiet M, Fancourt R, Peto J: Systolic blood pressure variation during the first 6 days of life. *Clin Sci Mol Med* 49:557, 1975.
35. Tan KL: Blood pressure in very low birth weight infants in the first 70 days of life. *J Pediatr* 112:266, 1988.
36. Shortland DB, Evans DH, Levene MI: Blood pressure measurements in very low birth weight infants over the first week of life. *J Perinat Med* 16:93, 1988.
37. Weindling AM: Blood pressure monitoring in the newborn. *Arch Dis Child* 64:444, 1989.
38. Adelman RD: The hypertensive neonate. *Clin Perinatol* 15:567, 1988.
39. Baker MD, Maisel MJ, Marks KH: Indirect BP monitoring in the newborn: Evaluation of a new oscillometer and comparison of upper- and lower-limb measurements. *Am J Dis Child* 138:775, 1984.
40. Sonesson SE, Broberger U: Arterial blood pressure in the very low birth weight neonate: Evaluation of an automatic oscillometric technique. *Acta Paediatr Scand* 76:338, 1987.

41. Lum LG, Jones, MD: The effect of cuff width on systolic blood pressure measurement in neonates. *J Pediatr* 91:963, 1977.
42. Sinkin RA, Phillips BL, Adelman RD: Elevation in systemic blood pressure in the neonate during abdominal examination. *Pediatrics* 76:970, 1985.
43. Piazza SF, Chandra M, Harper RG, et al: Upper vs lower limb systolic blood pressure in full term normal newborn. *Am J Dis Child* 139:797, 1985.
44. Wilson DI, Appleton RE, Coulthard MG, et al: Fetal and infantile hypertension caused by unilateral renal arterial disease. *Arch Dis Child* 65:881, 1990.
45. Plumer LB, Kaplan GW, Mendoza SA: Hypertension in infants—A complication of arterial catheterization. *J Pediatr* 89:802, 1976.
46. Wigger HJ, Bransilver BR, Blanc WA: Thromboses due to catheterization in infants and children. *J Pediatr* 76:1, 1970.
47. Neal WA, Reynolds JW, Jarvis CW, et al: Umbilical artery catheterization: Demonstration of arterial thrombosis by aortography. *Pediatrics* 50:6, 1972.
48. Goetzman BW, Stadalnik RC, Borgren HG, et al: Thrombotic complications of umbilical artery catheters: A clinical and radiologic study. *Pediatrics* 56:374, 1975.
49. Bauer SB, Feldman SM, Gellis SS, et al: Neonatal hypertension: A complication of umbilical-artery catheterization. *N Engl J Med* 293:1032, 1975.
50. Seibert JJ, Taylor BJ, Williams BJ, et al: Sonographic detection of neonatal umbilical-artery thrombosis: Clinical correlation. *AJR* 148:965, 1987.
51. Chidi CC, King DR, Boles ET: An ultrastructural study of the intimal injury induced by an indwelling umbilical artery catheter. *J Pediatr Surg* 18:109, 1983.
52. Durante D, Jones D, Spitzer R: Neonatal renal arterial embolism syndrome. *J Pediatr* 89:978, 1976.
53. Evans DJ, Silverman M, Bowley NB: Congenital hypertension due to unilateral renal vein thrombosis. *Arch Dis Child* 56:306, 1981.
54. Ward KE, Pryor RW, Matson JR, et al: Delayed detection of coarctation in infancy: Implications for timing of newborn follow-up. *Pediatrics* 86:972, 1990.
55. Borromeo-McGrail V, Bordiuk JM, Keitel H: Systemic hypertension following administration of 10% phenylephrine in the neonate. *Pediatrics* 51:1032, 1973.
56. Chasnoff IJ, Bussey ME, Savich L: Cocaine intoxication in a breast-fed infant. *Pediatrics* 80:836, 1987.
57. Reznik VM, Anderson J, Griswold WR, et al: Successful fibrinolytic treatment of arterial thrombosis and hypertension in a cocaine-exposed neonate. *Pediatrics* 84:735, 1989.
58. Minouni M, Kaufman H, Roitman A, et al: Hypertension in a neonate with 11 beta hydroxylase deficiency. *Eur J Pediatr* 143:231, 1985.
59. Eason E, Costom B, Papagergiou AN: Hypertension in neonatal thyrotoxicosis. *J Pediatr* 100:766, 1982.
60. Feld ML, Roy S, Stapleton FB: Low-renin hypertension in young infants. *Am J Dis Child* 139:823, 1985.
61. Kaufman BH, Telander RL, von Herden JA, et al: Pheochromocytoma in the pediatric age group: Current status. *J Pediatr Surg* 18:879, 1983.
62. Abman SH, Warady BA, Lum GM, et al: Systemic hypertension in infants with bronchopulmonary dysplasia. *J Pediatr* 104:929, 1984.
63. Munoz AI, Pascual JF, Baralt Y, et al: Arterial hypertension in infants with hydronephrosis. *Am J Dis Child* 131:38, 1977.
64. Gilboa N, Urizar RE: Severe hypertension in a newborn after pyeloplasty of hydronephrotic kidney. *Urology* 22:179, 1983.

65. Adelman RA, Sherman MP: Hypertension in the neonate following closure of abdominal wall defects. *J Pediatr* 97:642, 1980.
66. Sheftel DN, Hustead V, Friedman A: Hypertension screening in the follow-up of premature infants. *Pediatrics* 71:763, 1983.
67. Friedman A, Hustead VA: Hypertension in babies following discharge from a neonatal intensive care unit. *Pediatr Nephrol* 1:30, 1987.
68. Blanc F, Bensman A, Baudon JJ: Renovascular hypertension: A rare cause of neonatal salt loss. *Pediatr Nephrol* 5:304, 1991.
69. Skalina MEL, Annable WL, Kliegman RM, et al: Hypertensive retinopathy in the newborn infant. *J Pediatr* 103:781, 1983.
70. Payne RM, Martin TC, Bower RJ, et al: Management and follow-up of arterial thrombosis in the neonatal period. *J Pediatr* 114:853, 1989.
71. Adelman RD: Long-term follow-up of neonatal renovascular hypertension. *Pediatr Nephrol* 1:35, 1987.
72. Caplan MS, Cohn RA, Langman CB, et al: Favorable outcome of neonatal aortic thrombosis and renovascular hypertension. *J Pediatr* 115:291, 1989.
73. Buchi KF, Siegler RL: Hypertension in the first month of life. *Hypertension* 4:525, 1986.
74. Tack ED, Perlman JM: Renal failure in sick hypertensive premature infants receiving captopril therapy. *J Pediatr* 112:805, 1988.
75. Vailas GN, Brouillette RT, Scott JP, et al: Neonatal aortic thrombosis: Recent experience. *J Pediatr* 109:101, 1986.
76. Corrigan JJ, Jeter M, Allen HD, et al: Aortic thrombosis in a neonate: Failure of urokinase thrombolytic therapy. *Am J Pediatr Hematol Oncol* 4:243, 1982.
77. Chevalier RL, Campbell F, Brenbridge ANAG: Prognostic factors in neonatal acute renal failure. *Pediatrics* 74:265, 1984.
78. Norman ME, Asadi FK: A prospective study of acute renal failure in the newborn infant. *Pediatrics* 63:475, 1979.
79. Stapleton FB, Jones DP, Green RS: Acute renal failure in neonates: Incidence, etiology and outcome. *Pediatr Nephrol* 1:314, 1987.
80. Dauber IM, Krauss AN, Symchych PS, et al: Renal failure following perinatal anoxia. *J Pediatr* 88:851, 1976.
81. Anand SK, Northway JD, Crussi FG: Acute renal failure in newborn infants. *J Pediatr* 92:985, 1978.
82. Jones AS, James E, Bland H, et al: Renal failure in the newborn. *Clin Pediatr* 18:286, 1979.
83. Mathew OP, Jones AS, James E, et al: Neonatal renal failure: Usefulness of diagnostic indices. Pediatrics 65:57, 1980.
84. Merlob P, Litwin A, Lazar L, et al: Neonatal ABO incompatibility complicated by hemoglobinuria and acute renal failure. *Clin Pediatr* 29:219, 1990.
85. Haftel AJ, Eichner J, Haling J, et al: Myoglobinuric renal failure in a newborn infant. *J Pediatr* 93:1015, 1978.
86. Gottlieb RP, Roeloffs S, Galler-Rimm G, et al: Transient renal insufficiency in the neonate related to hyperuricemia and hyperuricosuria. *Child Nephrol Urol* 11:111, 1991.
87. Herson VC, Ray JR, Rowe JC, et al: Acute renal failure associated with polycythemia in a neonate. *J Pediatr* 100:137, 1982.
88. Ellis EN, Watson WC: Use of urinary indexes in renal failure in the newborn. *Am J Dis Child* 136:615, 1982.

89. Tack ED, Perlman JM, Robson AM, et al: Renal injury in sick newborn infants: A prospective evaluation using urinary β_2-microglobulin concentration. *Pediatrics* 81:432, 1988.

90. Roberts DS, Haycock GB, Dalton RN, et al: Prediction of acute renal failure after birth asphyxia. *Arch Dis Child* 65:1021, 1990.

91. Zaramella P, Zorzi C, Pavanello L, et al: The prognostic significance of acute neonatal renal failure. *Child Nephrol Urol* 11:15, 1991.

92. Jacinto JS, Modanlou HD, Crade M, et al: Renal calcification incidence in very low birth weight infants. *Pediatrics* 81:31, 1988.

93. Short A, Cooke RWI: The incidence of renal calcification in preterm infants. *Arch Dis Child* 66:412, 1991.

94. Ezzedeen F, Adelman R, Ahlfors CE: Renal calcification in preterm infants: Pathophysiology and long-term sequelae. *J Pediatr* 113:532, 1988.

95. Atkinson SA, Shah JK, McGee C, et al: Mineral excretion in premature infants receiving various diuretic therapies. *J Pediatr* 113:540, 1988.

96. Welch TR, Resptrepo C, Hug G: Renal calcification. *Pediatrics* 82:287, 1988.

INDEX

Page numbers in *Italic* indicate figures; page numbers followed by t indicate tabular material.